Minimally Invasive Surgery and New Technology

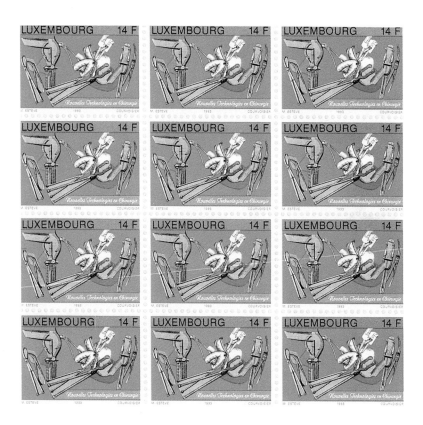

Minimally Invasive Surgery and New Technology

EDITED BY

Felicien M. Steichen, M.D.

Director, Institute for Minimally Invasive Surgery, St. Agnes Hospital, White Plains, New York;
F.M. Steichen Professor of Surgery, New York Medical College, Valhalla, New York

Roger Welter, M.D.

President, Association Européenne de Chirurgie Viscérale;
Chief of Surgery and Director Emeritus, Princess Marie-Astrid Hospital, Luxembourg

with 550 illustrations, including 150 in color

Quality Medical Publishing, Inc.

ST. LOUIS, MISSOURI
1994

Cover art:
Estève, Maurice (b. 1904, France).
Echafaudages (Scaffoldings).
Huile sur toile, 1944, 65 × 81 cm.

Frontispiece art:
Collage for a Stamp (1993) by Maurice Estève, issued by the
Luxembourg Post Office on May 10, 1993 to honor all surgeons
and scientists who have contributed to the Art and Science of
Surgery and to announce the next Congress on New Technology
and Advanced Surgical Techniques for 1995 in Luxembourg.

Printed in the United States of America.

PUBLISHER   Karen Berger

PROJECT EDITOR   Suzanne Seeley Wakefield

EDITING ASSISTANTS   Kathleen J. Jenkins, Suzanne Murat

PRODUCTION   Judy Bamert

BOOK DESIGN   Susan Trail

COVER DESIGN   Diane M. Beasley

Quality Medical Publishing, Inc.
11970 Borman Drive, Suite 222
St. Louis, Missouri 63146

LIBRARY OF CONGRESS CATALOGING-IN-PUBLICATION DATA

Minimally invasive surgery and new technology / edited by Felicien M.
   Steichen, Roger Welter.
         p.   cm.
      "Transactions of the Second Congress of Minimally Invasive Surgery
   and New Technology"—Pref.
      Includes bibliographical references and index.
      ISBN 0-942219-51-1
      1. Endoscopic surgery—Congresses.   2. Endoscopic surgery—
   Technological innovations—Congresses.   I. Steichen, Felicien M.
   II. Welter, Roger.   III. Congress of Minimally Invasive
   Surgery and New Technology (2nd : 1992 : Luxembourg, Luxembourg)
      [DNLM: 1. Surgery, Laparoscopic—congresses.   2. Suture
   Techniques—congresses.   3. Endoscopy—congresses.   WO 500 M6648
   1992]
   RD33.53.M57   1994
   617′.05—dc20
   DNLM/DLC
   for Library of Congress   93–38895
                                                              CIP

TH/WW/WW
5   4   3   2   1

Contributors

Murat Akyol, M.D.
Consultant Surgeon, Department of Surgery, University of Glasgow, Western Infirmary, Glasgow, Scotland

Jean-Luc Alain, M.D.
Professor, Department of Pediatric Surgery, CHU Dupuytren-Limoges, Limoges, France

David M. Albala, M.D.
Professor of Urology, Loyola University, Chicago, Illinois

Peter Alken, M.D.
Professor of Urology, and Director, Department of Urology, Klinikum Mannheim, University of Heidelberg, Mannheim, Germany

Ermanno Ancona, M.D.
Professor of Surgery, Department of General Surgery, University of Padua, Padua, Italy

John R. Anderson, B.Sc., M.B., Ch.B.
Senior Lecturer in Surgery, University Department of Surgery, Royal Infirmary, Glasgow, Scotland

Giuseppe Angiluetta, M.D.
Resident, Department of Gastrointestinal Surgery, Second University of Naples, Naples, Italy

Paolo Annessi, M.D.
Assistant Professor, I Clinica Chirurgica Policlinico Umberto I, University of Rome "La Sapienza," Rome, Italy

Francesco Ardissone, M.D.
Division of Thoracic Surgery, Ospedale San Luigi Gonzaga (University Hospital), Turin, Italy

Carlos J. Arenas-Linares, M.D.
Thoracic Surgeon, Department of Thoracic and General Surgery, University Hospital of Seville, Seville, Spain

Aly el Arini, M.D.
Tanta Cancer Institute, Cairo University, Tanta, Egypt

Bruno G. Audino, M.D.
Division of Thoracic Surgery, Ospedale San Luigi Gonzaga (University Hospital), Turin, Italy

Paolo Aurello, M.D.
Resident, I Clinica Chirurgica Policlinico Umberto I, University of Rome "La Sapienza," Rome, Italy

Orla M. Austin, M.B., B.Ch., Ba.O.
Department of Surgery, Beaumont Hospital, Dublin, Ireland

Francisco J. Ayarra, M.D.
Associate Professor of Surgery, Thoracic Surgeon, Department of Thoracic and General Surgery, University Hospital of Seville, Seville, Spain

Juan Santiago Azagra, M.D.
Chief, Department of Abdominal Surgery, CHU André Vesale, Montigny-le-Tilleul, Belgium

D. Azoulay, M.D.
Professor, Department of Hepato-Biliary Surgery, Liver Transplant Research Center, Paul Brousse Hospital, Villejuif, France

John V. Bagnato, M.D.
Chief of Surgery, Department of Surgery, Surgical Clinic Hattiesburg, Hattiesburg, Mississippi

M. Barban, M.D.
I Divisione Chirurgica, Presidio Ospedaliero Multizonale, Treviso, Italy

Romeo Bardini, M.D.
Associate Professor of Surgery, Department of General Surgery, University of Padua, Padua, Italy

Michael Barthel, M.D.
Department of General Surgery, University of Göttingen, Göttingen, Germany

Horst Dieter Becker, M.D.
Professor and Director, Department of General Surgery, Eberhard-Karls-University Hospital, Tübingen, Germany

Jacques Belghiti, M.D.
Professor, Department of Digestive Surgery, University of Paris VII, Xavier Bichat, Clichy, France

Graham Bell, M.B., Ch.B., Ch.M.
Consultant Surgeon, Department of Surgery, Inverclyde Royal Hospital, Greenock, Scotland

Siegfried Beller, M.D.
Department of Surgery, Landeskrankenhaus Bregenz, Bregenz, Austria

Claudio Belluco, M.D.
Assistant, Department of General Surgery, University of Padua, Padua, Italy

Philippe Bérard, M.D.
Professor, Department of Surgery, Hôtel Dieu, Lyon, France

George Berci, M.D.
Clinical Professor of Surgery Emeritus, School of Medicine, University of California–Los Angeles, Los Angeles, California

Jean-Paul Binet, M.D.
Professor and Director Emeritus, Department of Surgery, Hôpital Marie-Lannelongue, le Plessis Robinson, France

H. Bismuth, M.D.
Professor, Department of Hepato-Biliary Surgery, Liver Transplant Research Center, Paul Brousse Hospital, Villejuif, France

P. Blanc, M.D.
Department of Hepatology, Montpellier University School of Medicine, Montpellier, France

Oskar Boeckl, M.D.
Professor, First Surgical Department, Landes Krankenanstalten Salzburg, Salzburg, Austria

Stefano Bona, M.D.
Assistant Professor of Surgery, Department of General and Oncologic Surgery, University of Milan, Milan, Italy

Luigi Bonavina, M.D.
Assistant Professor of Surgery, Department of General and Oncologic Surgery, University of Milan, Milan, Italy

Piero Borasio, M.D.
Chief, Department of Thoracic Surgery and Professor, Department of Cardiovascular and Thoracic Surgery, University of Turin, Turin, Italy

J. Borelly, M.D.
CHU Central, Service de Chirurgie E, University of Nancy, Nancy, France

Marina Bortul, M.D.
Ricercatore Istituto, Clinica Chirurgica Generale e Terapia Chirurgica, University of Trieste, Trieste, Italy

David Bouchier-Hayes, F.A.L.S.
Professor, Department of Surgery, Beaumont Hospital, Dublin, Ireland

Jean Nicolas Boullenois, M.D.
Surgeon, Department of Digestive and General Surgery, Surgical Pavilion B, Les Hôpitaux Universitaires de Strasbourg, Strasbourg, France

Jacques-Henri Boverie, M.D.
Assistant Professor of Radiology, Department of Medical Imaging, Centre Hospitalier, University of Liège, Liège, Belgium

Laura Broglia, M.D.
Resident in Radiology, Department of Radiology III Cattedra, University of Rome "La Sapienza," Rome, Italy

Gerhard Buess, M.D.
Professor, Department of General Surgery, Eberhard-Karls-University Hospital, Tübingen, Germany

Paul E. Burke, M.B., B.Ch.
Senior Lecturer, Department of Surgery, Beaumont Hospital, Dublin, Ireland

Luca Busetto, M.D.
Istituto di Medicina Interna, Universita' Degli Studi di Padova, Padua, Italy

Dominique S. Byrne, M.B., Ch.B.
Registrar in Surgery, Department of Surgery, Stobhill General Hospital, Glasgow, Scotland

William John Byrne, M.D.
Department of Surgery, Ysbyty Gwynedd, Bangor, Gwynedd, Wales

C. Caldato, M.D.
I Divisione Chirurgica, Presidio Ospedaliero Multizonale, Treviso, Italy

Jerome Canady, M.D.
Chief Surgical Resident, Department of Surgery, McKeesport Hospital, McKeesport, Pennsylvania

Isaac Capela Fernandez, M.D.
Staff Surgeon and Clinical Chief, Department of General and Gastrointestinal Surgery, Hospital Ramon y Cajal, Universidad Alcala de Henares, Madrid, Spain

Pedro Carda-Abella, M.D.
Associate Professor, Staff Surgeon, and Clinical Chief, Department of General and Gastrointestinal Surgery, Hospital Ramon y Cajal, Universidad Alcala de Henares, Madrid, Spain

P. Declan Carey, M.D.
Academic Surgical Unit, St. Mary's Hospital Medical School, London, England

D. Castaing, M.D.
Department of Hepato-Biliary Surgery, Liver Transplant Research Center, Paul Brousse Hospital, Villejuif, France

M. Celerier, M.D.
Professor, Department of Surgery, Hôpital Saint-Louis, Paris, France

Michel Ceuterick, M.D.
Department of Abdominal Surgery, CHU André Vesale, Montigny-le-Tilleul, Belgium

Giorgio Chiampo, M.D.
Division of Thoracic Surgery, Ospedale San Luigi Gonzaga (University Hospital), Turin, Italy

G. Chiara, M.D.
I Divisione Chirurgica, Presidio Ospedaliero Multizonale, Treviso, Italy

Jean-Marie Collard, M.D.
Chef de Clinique Associé, Maître de Conference, Départment de Chirurgie Digestive, Cliniques Universitaires St.-Luc, Université Catholique de Louvain, Brussels, Belgium

Jordi Colomer Mascaro, Ph.D.
Servicio de Cirugia General, Hospital de Viladecans, Barcelona, Spain

W. Coosemans, M.D.
Department of Thoracic Surgery, University of Leuven, Leuven, Belgium

John D. Corbitt, Jr., M.D.
Chief of Surgery, Department of General Surgery, John F. Kennedy Medical Center, West Palm Beach, Atlantis, Florida

Vincenzo Costantino, M.D.
Surgical Researcher, Department of General and Pediatric Surgery, Semeiotica Chirurgica, University of Padua, Padua, Italy

Hugh A. Crispin, M.B., Ch.B., B.Sc.(Hons.), Edin.
Vascular Surgeon, University Department of Surgery, Stuivenberg University Hospital of Antwerp, Antwerp, Belgium

Jose M. Cuaresma-Ferrete, M.D.
Department of Thoracic and General Surgery, University Hospital of Seville, Seville, Spain

Luciano Curella, M.D.
Resident, I Clinica Chirurgica Policlinico Umberto I, University of Rome "La Sapienza," Rome, Italy

Jean-François Cuttat, M.D.
Attending Surgeon, Department of Surgery, Centre Hospitalier Universitaire Vaudois, Lausanne, Switzerland

Francesco D'Angelo, M.D.
Assistant Professor, I Clinica Chirurgica Policlinico Umberto I, University of Rome "La Sapienza," Rome, Italy

Thomas M. Daniel, M.D.
Professor of Surgery, Division of Thoracic and Cardiovascular Surgery, University of Virginia Health Sciences Center, Charlottesville, Virginia

Ara Darzi, M.D.
Academic Surgical Unit, St. Mary's Hospital Medical School, London, England

Renato De Angelis, M.D.
Assistant Professor, I Clinica Chirurgica Policlinico Umberto I, University of Rome "La Sapienza," Rome, Italy

Maurizio De Giuli, M.D.
Assistant, Department of Surgery, University of Turin School of Medicine, Turin, Italy

Olivier Delahaut, M.D.
Resident, Department of Surgery, CHU André Vesale, Montigny-le-Tilleul, Belgium

Alberto Del Genio, M.D.
Professor of Gastrointestinal Surgery, Department of Esophageal Surgery, Second University of Naples, Naples, Italy

Louis R.M. Del Guercio, M.D.
Professor and Chairman, Department of Surgery, New York Medical College, Valhalla, New York

Tom R. DeMeester, M.D.
Professor and Chairman, Department of Surgery, University of Southern California School of Medicine, Los Angeles, California

A. Dennison, M.D.
Department of Hepato-Biliary Surgery, Liver Transplant Research Center, Paul Brousse Hospital, Villejuif, France

Manuela DeVos, M.D.
Department of Surgery, Katharinen Hospital, Stuttgart, Germany

Hendrik Dienemann, M.D.
Department of Surgery, Ludwig-Maximilians-Universität, Munich, Germany

Raymond A. Dieter, Jr., M.D.
Chairman, Department of Surgery, Glen Ellyn Clinic, Glen Ellyn, Illinois

Natale Di Martino, M.D.
Associate Professor, Department of Gastrointestinal Surgery, Second University of Naples, Naples, Italy

James G. Docherty, M.B., Ch.B.
Research Fellow, Department of Surgery, University of Glasgow, Western Infirmary, Glasgow, Scotland

Josep Domingo Fontanet, Ph.D.
Servicio de Cirugia General, Hospital de Viladecans, Barcelona, Spain

Robert F. Dondelinger, M.D.
Radiologist-in-Chief and Professor, University Hospital Sart Tilman, Liège, Belgium

Ippolito Donini, M.D.
Director, Istituto di Clinica Chirurgica Generale, Universita' Degli Studi di Ferrara, Ferrara, Italy

Jean D. Doublet, M.D.
Department of Urology, Hôpital Tenon, Paris, France

F. Dubois, M.D.
Professor, Department of Surgery, Clinique de la Porte de Choisy, Paris, France

Michael Sean Dudeney, M.B., B.Ch., B.A.D. (NUI)
Department of Surgery, Beaumont Hospital, Dublin, Ireland

Ronald-Joachim Elfeldt, M.D.
Oberarzt, Department of General and Thoracic Surgery, University of Kiel, Kiel, Germany

Rainer Engemann, M.D.
Assistant Director, Chirurgische Universitätsklinik Würzburg, Würzburg, Germany

Giuliano Enzi, M.D.
Istituto di Medicina Interna, Universita' Degli Studi di Padova, Padua, Italy

Kurt Erhart, M.D.
Interne Medizinische Abteilung, Landeskrankenhaus Bregenz University, Bregenz, Austria

Harry J. Espiner, M.D.
Consultant Surgeon, University Department of Surgery, Royal Infirmary, Bristol, England

Serge Evrard, M.D.
Clinique Chirurgie A, Les Hôpitaux Universitaires, Strasbourg, France

F. Favretti, M.D.
Chairman, Department of Surgery, City Hospital, Belluno, Italy

Gianfranco Fegiz, M.D.
Professor and Chairman, I Clinica Chirurgica Policlinico Umberto I, University of Rome "La Sapienza," Rome, Italy

François Fekete, M.D.
Professor of Surgery, Chief, Department of Digestive Surgery, University of Paris VII; Hôpital Beaujon, Clichy, France

Jose Fernandez-Cebrian, M.D.
Staff Surgeon, Department of General and Gastrointestinal Surgery, Hospital Ramon y Cajal, Universidad Alcala de Henares, Madrid, Spain

Claudio Ferraro, M.D.
Division of Thoracic Surgery, Ospedale San Luigi Gonzaga (University Hospital), Turin, Italy

Valentino Festa, M.D.
Assistant, Department of Surgery, University of Turin School of Medicine, Turin, Italy

Frank L. Fontana, M.D.
Chairman, Department of Surgery, McKeesport Hospital, McKeesport, Pennsylvania

Morris E. Franklin, Jr., M.D.
Professor of Surgery, Department of Surgery, University of Texas Medical School, San Antonio, Texas

Virgilio Fresneda Moreno, M.D.
Chief of Surgery, Department of General and Digestive Surgery, Hospital Ramon y Cajal, Universidad Alcala de Henares, Madrid, Spain

Stephan M. Freys, M.D.
Department of Surgery, University of Würzburg, Würzburg, Germany

Karl-Hermann Fuchs, M.D.
Assistant Director, Department of Surgery, University of Würzburg, Würzburg, Germany

Uberto Fumagalli, M.D.
Assistant Professor of Surgery, Department of General and Oncologic Surgery, University of Milan, Milan, Italy

Michel Gagner, M.D.
Assistant Professor of Surgery, Department of Surgery, University of Montreal, Hôtel-Dieu de Montreal, Montreal, Quebec, Canada

David J. Galloway, M.D., M.B., Ch.B.
Consultant Surgeon, Department of Surgical Gastroenterology, Gart Navel General Hospital, Glasgow, Scotland

Manuel Garcia-Caballero, M.D.
Assistant Professor of Surgery, Department of Surgery, University of Malaga, Malaga, Spain

Fernando Jose Garcia-Diaz, M.D.
Associate Professor of Surgery, Department of Thoracic and General Surgery, University Hospital of Seville, Seville, Spain

Corrado Garrone, M.D.
Assistant, Department of Surgery, University of Turin School of Medicine, Turin, Italy

Bernard Gattegno, M.D.
Professor, Department of Urology, Hôpital Tenon, Paris, France

Dominique Geiger, M.D.
Anesthesiologist, Department of Digestive and General Surgery, Surgical Pavilion B, Les Hôpitaux Universitaires de Strasbourg, Strasbourg, France

Roberto Giardino, M.D.
Division of Thoracic Surgery, Ospedale San Luigi Gonzaga (University Hospital), Turin, Italy

Friedrich Gill, M.D.
Department of Obstetrics and Gynecology, K.A. Rudolfstiftung, Vienna, Austria

Serge Ginter, M.D.
Department of Gynecology and Obstetrics, Klinikum der Christian-Albrechts-Universität, Kiel, Germany

Juan Carlos Giron-Arjona, M.D.
Resident, Department of Thoracic and General Surgery, University Hospital of Seville, Seville, Spain

Heike Goebel, M.D.
Department of Digestive and General Surgery, Surgical Pavilion B, Les Hôpitaux Universitaires de Strasbourg, Strasbourg, France

Martine Goergen, M.D.
Resident, Department of Abdominal Surgery, CHU André Vesale, Montigny-le-Tilleul, Belgium

Fernando Gomez-Ferrer, M.D.
Professor and Chairman, Department of Surgery, University of Valencia, Valencia, Spain

Philip H. Gordon, M.D.
Professor of Surgery, McGill University; Director, Colon and Rectal Surgery, Sir Mortimer B. Davis Jewish General Hospital, Montreal, Quebec, Canada

Franck Gosset, M.D.
Resident, Department of Digestive and General Surgery, Surgical Pavilion B, Les Hôpitaux Universitaires de Strasbourg, Strasbourg, France

D. Gossot, M.D.
Attending Surgeon, Department of Surgery, Hôpital Saint-Louis, Paris, France

D.J. Gouma, M.D.
Department of Surgery, University Hospital, Maastricht, The Netherlands

Pierce A. Grace, M.B., B.Ch.
Consultant Surgeon, Department of Vascular Surgery, Hamersmith Hospital, London, England

Jacques F. Grenier, M.D.
Professor of Surgery, Head of the Surgical Department, Department of Digestive and General Surgery, Surgical Pavilion B, Les Hôpitaux Universitaires de Strasbourg, Strasbourg, France

F. Dean Griffen, M.D.
Clinical Professor of Surgery, Highland Clinic; Louisiana State University Medical Center, Shreveport, Louisiana

Fabrizio Grignani, M.D.
Department of General Surgery, University of Milan–S. Giuseppe Hospital, Milan, Italy

Wolfgang Grin, M.D.
Department of Obstetrics and Gynecology, K.A. Rudolfstiftung, Vienna, Austria

G. Grosdidier, M.D.
Professor, CHU Central, Service de Chirurgie E, University of Nancy, Nancy, France

Eberhard Gross, M.D.
Professor, First Surgical Department, Allgemeines Krankenhaus Barmbek–Hamburg, Hamburg, Germany

Dominique Grousseau, M.D.
Surgery Assistant, Department of Pediatric Surgery, CHU Dupuytren–Limoges, Limoges, France

Werner Grünberger, M.D.
Department of Obstetrics and Gynecology, K.A. Rudolfstiftung, Vienna, Austria

O. Gualandi, M.D.
I Divisione Chirurgica, Presidio Ospedaliero Multizonale, Treviso, Italy

Jörg Haberstroh, M.D.
Chirurgische Universtätsklinik Freiburg, Freiburg, Germany

Tapani Havia, M.D.
Assistant Professor, Department of Surgery, University of Turku, Turku, Finland

R.J. Heald, M.D.
Colorectal Research Unit, Basingstoke District Hospital, Basingstoke, England

Johannes Heimbucher, M.D.
Department of Surgery, University of Würzburg, Würzburg, Germany

M.P. Heinerman, M.D.
Department of Surgical Endoscopy, Landeskrankenaustalten Salzburg, Salzburg, Austria

Thomas O. Henkel, M.D.
Registrar, Department of Urology, Klinikum Mannheim, University of Heidelberg, Mannheim, Germany

Jonathan R. Hiatt, M.D.
Associate Professor, Department of Surgery, Cedars-Sinai Medical Center/UCLA School of Medicine, Los Angeles, California

A.D.K. Hill, M.D.
Surgical Registrar, Department of Surgery, St. Mary's Hospital, London, England

Hans Hoffmann, M.D.
Department of Surgery, Ludwig-Maximilians-Universität, Munich, Germany

Gérard Holbach, M.D.
Department of Surgery, Krankenhaus Gerresheim, Düsseldorf, Germany

Jörg Holste, Dr. Med. Vet.
Research Department, Ethicon GmbH u Cokg, Norderstedt, Germany

Alex Hubens, M.D., Ph.D.
Professor of Surgery, Stuivenberg University Hospital of Antwerp, Antwerp, Belgium

Peter Huber, M.D.
Department of General Surgery, Eberhard-Karls-University Hospital, Tübingen, Germany

Martin Hürtgen, M.D.
Department of General and Thoracic Surgery, Justus-Liebig-University, Giessen, Germany

Andreas Imdahl, M.D.
Chirurgische Universitätsklinik Freiburg, Freiburg, Germany

Marileda Indinnimeo, M.D.
Assistant Professor, I Clinica Chirurgica Policlinico Umberto I, University of Rome "La Sapienza," Rome, Italy

Calin Ionescu, M.D.
Resident, Department of Digestive and General Surgery, Surgical Pavilion B, Les Hôpitaux Universitaires de Strasbourg, Strasbourg, France

Joseph C. Iraci, M.D.
Attending Surgeon, Department of Surgery, Lenox Hill Hospital, New York, New York

Daniel Jacobs, M.D.
Adjunct Professor in Anesthesiology, Department of Anesthesiology, CHU André Vesale, Montigny-le-Tilleul, Belgium

Carol C. Jagdeo, M.D.
Clinical Instructor of Medicine, Georgetown University Hospital, Washington, D.C.

†David G. Jagelman, M.D.

J.J. Jakimowicz, M.D., Ph.D.
Professor, Department of Surgery, Catharina Hospital, Eindhoven, The Netherlands

Anton Jansen, M.D., Ph.D.
Department of General and Vascular Surgery, St. Antonius Ziekenhuis, Nieuwegen, The Netherlands

I.M.C. Janssen, M.D.
Department of Surgery, Community Hospital, Arnhem, The Netherlands

Rafael Jimenez-Merchan, M.D.
Resident, Department of Thoracic and General Surgery, University Hospital of Seville, Seville, Spain

Klaus-Peter Jünemann, M.D.
Associate Professor, Department of Urology, Klinikum Mannheim, University of Heidelberg, Mannheim, Germany
†Deceased.

P.J. Kestens, M.D.
Professor, Cliniques Universitaires St.-Luc, Université Catholique de Louvain, Brussels, Belgium

Karl Kipfmüller, M.D.
Attending Surgeon, Katharinen Hospital, Stuttgart, Germany

†P. Klementschitsch, M.D.

Charles D. Knight, Jr., M.D.
Clinical Associate Professor of Surgery, Department of Surgery, Highland Clinic; Louisiana State University Medical Center, Shreveport, Louisiana

Charles D. Knight, Sr., M.D.
Clinical Professor of Surgery, Department of Surgery, Highland Clinic; Louisiana State University Medical Center, Shreveport, Louisiana

M.O. Köppen, M.D.
First Surgical Department, Allgemeines Krankenhaus Barmbek–Hamburg, Hamburg, Germany

John G. Kral, M.D., Ph.D.
Professor, Department of Surgery, State University of New York Health Science Center at Brooklyn, Brooklyn, New York

Vincenzo Landolfi, M.D.
Assistant, Department of Gastrointestinal Surgery, Second University of Naples, Naples, Italy

Volker Lange, M.D., Ph.D.
Department of Surgery, Munich University, Munich, Germany

D. Larrey, M.D., Ph.D.
Professor, Department of Hepatology, Montpellier University School of Medicine, Montpellier, France

Aristotel Lazar, M.D.
Department of Surgery and Vascular Surgery, Heinz Kalk-Hospital, Bad Kissingen, Germany

Austin Leahy, M.B., B.Ch.
Consultant Surgeon, Department of Surgery, Beaumont Hospital, Dublin, Ireland

Aldo Leggeri, M.D.
Director and Professor, Department of General Surgery, Trieste University, Trieste, Italy

†Deceased.

G. Lepsien, M.D.
Department of Surgery, Städtisches Krankenhaus Lüneburg, Lüneburg, Germany

T. Lerut, M.D.
Professor, Department of Thoracic Surgery, University of Leuven, Leuven, Belgium

Marco Maria Lirici, M.D.
Assistant Professor of Surgery, Fourth Department of General Surgery, University of Rome "La Sapienza," Rome, Italy

Mario Lise, M.D.
Professor of Surgery, Second Department of Surgery, University of Padua, Padua, Italy

Eduardo Lobo Martinez, M.D.
Staff Surgeon, Department of General and Gastrointestinal Surgery, Hospital Ramon y Cajal, Universidad Alcala de Henares, Madrid, Spain

Patrice H. Lointier, M.D., Ph.D.
Professor of Digestive Surgery, Clinique La Chataigneraie, Beaumont, France

Pedro Lopez Hervas , M.D.
Staff Surgeon, Department of General and Gastrointestinal Surgery, Hospital Ramon y Cajal, Universidad Alcala de Henares, Madrid, Spain

Jesús Loscertales, M.D.
Professor of Surgery, Department of Thoracic and General Surgery, University Hospital of Seville, Seville, Spain

Udo Losert, M.D.
Center for Biomedical Research, University of Vienna, Vienna, Austria

Gerhard W. Lotz, M.D.
Allgemeinchirurgische Abtailung, St. Vincenz und Elisabeth Hospital, Mainz, Germany

Jean-Michel Loubeau, M.D.
Attending Surgeon, Department of Surgery, Lenox Hill Hospital, New York, New York

Christian J. Lukosch, M.D.
Surgeon, Department of General and Thoracic Surgery, Justus-Liebig-University, Giessen, Germany

Bernd Lünstedt, M.D.
Chirurgische Universitäts Klinik und Poliklinik Würzburg, Würzburg, Germany

Francesca Maccioni, M.D.
Radiologist, Assistant Professor, Department of Radiology II Cattedra, University of Rome "La Sapienza," Rome, Italy

Marco Maciocco, M.D.
Department of General Surgery, University of Milan–S. Giuseppe Hospital, Milan, Italy

T. Madhusudan, M.S.
Registrar, Department of Surgery, King George Hospital, London, England

Elena Manzone, M.D.
Division of Thoracic Surgery, Ospedale San Luigi Gonzaga (University Hospital), Turin, Italy

Jacques Marescaux, M.D.
Professor, Chirurgie A, Les Hôpitaux Universitaires de Strasbourg, Strasbourg, France

Claudio Mariani, M.D.
Department of General Surgery, University of Milan–S. Giuseppe Hospital, Milan, Italy

Philippe Marre, M.D.
Aneien Chef de Clinique Universitaire, Faculté de Médecine Paris St. Antoine, Department of Visceral Surgery, Saint-Germain-En-Laye, France

Andreina Martella, M.D.
Clinical Fellow, Department of Gastrointestinal Surgery, Second University of Naples, Naples, Italy

F. Martin, M.D.
CHU Central, Service de Chirurgie E, University of Nancy, Nancy, France

Enrique Martinez Molina, M.D.
Staff Surgeon, Department of General and Gastrointestinal Surgery, Hospital Ramon y Cajal, Universidad Alcala de Henares, Madrid, Spain

W. Martino, M.D.
Department of Hepato-Biliary Surgery, Liver Transplant Research Center, Paul Brousse Hospital, Villejuif, France

J. Marzelle, M.D.
Department of Surgery, Hôpital Marie-Lannelongue, le Plessis Robinson, France

Francescopaolo Mattioli, M.D.
Professor of General Surgery, Director of General Surgery Institute, First Clinica Chirurgica Generale e Terapia Chirurgica, Universita' Degli Studi, Genoa, Italy

Enda W.N. McDermott, M.D.
St. Vincent's Hospital, University College Dublin, Dublin, Ireland

John R. McGregor, M.D., M.B., Ch.B.
Lecturer in Surgery, Department of Surgery, University of Glasgow, Western Infirmary, Glasgow, Scotland

J. Barry McKernan, M.D., Ph.D.
Clinical Professor of Surgery, Department of Surgery, Medical College of Georgia, Augusta, Georgia

Herbert Mecke, M.D.
August-Viktoria Krankenhaus, University of Berlin, Berlin, Germany

Andreas Melzer, M.D.
Department of General Surgery, Eberhard-Karls-University, Tübingen, Germany

N. Menzies-Gow, M.D.
Academic Surgical Unit, St. Mary's Hospital Medical School, London, England

Peter Merkle, M.D.
Department of Surgery, Katharinen Hospital, Stuttgart, Germany

Roberto Merlino, M.D.
Resident in Radiology, Department of Radiology III Cattedra, University of Rome "La Sapienza," Rome, Italy

Guenther Meyer, M.D.
Department of Surgery, Klinikum Grosshadern, Ludwig-Maximilians-University, Munich, Germany

Hans-Joachim Meyer, M.D.
Chefarzt, Chirurgische Klinik, St. Martinus-Hospital Olpe, Olpe, Germany

H. Michel, M.D.
Professor, Department of Hepatology, Montpellier University School of Medicine, Montpellier, France

Claudio Miglietta, M.D.
Assistant, Department of Surgery, University of Turin School of Medicine, Turin, Italy

Stanley Scott Miller, Ch.M.
Consultant Surgeon in General and Pediatric Surgery, Department of Surgery, Aberdeen Royal Infirmary, Aberdeen, Scotland

John R.T. Monson, M.D.
Professor of Surgery and Head, Department of Academic Surgical Unit, The University of Hull, Castle Hill Hospital, Cottingham, North Humberside, England

T. Montariol, M.D.
Department of Visceral Surgery, Centre Hospitalier Général, Saint-Germain-En-Laye, France

Marco Montorsi, M.D.
Associate Professor of Surgery, Department of General and Oncologic Surgery, University of Milan, Milan, Italy

Vicente Morales Castiñeiras, M.D.
Associate Professor and Staff Surgeon, Department of General and Gastrointestinal Surgery, Hospital Ramon y Cajal, Universidad Alcala de Henares, Madrid, Spain

Jean Moreaux, M.D.
Professor, Department of Surgery, Clinique de la Porte de Choisy, Paris, France

Mario Morino, M.D.
Associate Professor of Surgery, Department of Surgery, University of Turin School of Medicine, Turin, Italy

Thorsten F. Morlang, M.D.
Department of Surgery, Städtische Kliniken Frankfurt-Höchst, Frankfurt, Germany

Claudio Mossetti, M.D.
Division of Thoracic Surgery, Ospedale San Luigi Gonzaga (University Hospital), Turin, Italy

Philippe Mouret, M.D.
Consultant and Attending Surgeon, Lyon, France

Christian Mueller, M.D.
Department of Surgery, Klinikum Grosshadern, Ludwig-Maximilians-University, Munich, Germany

James J. Murphy, M.D.
St. Vincent's Hospital, University College Dublin, Dublin, Ireland

Didier Mutter, M.D.
Chirurgie A, Les Hôpitaux Universitaires de Strasbourg, Strasbourg, France

Ulf Nahrstedt, M.D.
Department of General Surgery, AK Ochsenzoll, Hamburg, Germany

Gianluigi Natali, M.D.
Resident, Department of Radiology III Cattedra, University of Rome "La Sapienza," Rome, Italy

Giuseppe Navarra, M.D.
Researcher, Istituto di Clinica Chirurgica Generale, Universita' Degli Studi di Ferrara, Ferrara, Italy

Salvador Navarro Soto, Ph.D.
Servicio de Cirugia General, Hospital de Viladecans, Barcelona, Spain

Benoît Navez, M.D.
Department of Surgery, Hôpital St. Joseph, Charleroi (Gilly), Belgium

T. Neufang, M.D.
Department of Surgery, Städtisches Krankenhaus Lüneburg, Lüneburg, Germany

A.T. Nicholson, M.Sc., M.B., Ch.B.
Consultant Radiologist, Department of Radiology, Royal Hull Hospital Trust, Hull, Humberside, England

Enrico Nicolo, M.D.
Associate Chairman, Department of Surgery, McKeesport Hospital, McKeesport, Pennsylvania

Henning Niebuhr, M.D.
Department of General Surgery, General Hospital, Hamburg, Germany

Juan J. Nogueras, M.D.
Staff Surgeon, Department of Colorectal Surgery, Cleveland Clinic Florida, Fort Lauderdale, Florida

Douglas R. Norman, M.D.
Assistant Professor of Surgery, Department of Thoracic Surgery, Rush North Shore Medical Center, Rush Medical School, Chicago, Illinois

Corrado Novello, M.D.
Division of Thoracic Surgery, Ospedale San Luigi Gonzaga (University Hospital), Turin, Italy

Antonio Nuzzo, M.D.
Clinical Fellow, Department of Gastrointestinal Surgery, Second University of Naples, Naples, Italy

Jean-Baptiste Nyarwaya, M.D.
Fellow in Anesthesiology, Anesthésie et Réanimation Chirurgicale, CHU Bicêtre, Le Kremlin Bicêtre, Paris, France

H. Obertop, M.D.
Department of Surgery, University Hospital, Maastricht, The Netherlands

Savino Occhionorelli, M.D.
Fellow in Training, Istituto di Clinica Chirurgica Generale, Universita' Degli Studi di Ferrara, Ferrara, Italy

Patrick J. O'Dwyer, M.D.
Department of Surgery, University of Glasgow, Western Infirmary, Glasgow, Scotland

Niall J. O'Higgins, M.D.
Professor, St. Vincent's Hospital, University College Dublin, Dublin, Ireland

Douglas O. Olsen, M.D.
Assistant Clinical Professor of Surgery, Vanderbilt University; Department of Surgery, Baptist Hospital, Nashville, Tennessee

Franco Orsi, M.D.
Resident in Radiology, Department of Radiology III Cattedra, University of Rome "La Sapienza," Rome, Italy

Carles Ortiz Rodriguez, M.D.
Servicio de Cirugia General, Hospital de Viladecans, Barcelona, Spain

J.B. Otte, M.D.
Cliniques Universitaires St.-Luc, Université Catholique de Louvain, Brussels, Belgium

G.P. Pageaux, M.D.
Department of Hepatology, Montpellier University School of Medicine, Montpellier, France

†J. Papillon, M.D.

Karl-Joseph Paquet, M.D.
Department of Surgery and Vascular Surgery, Heinz Kalk-Hospital, Bad Kissingen, Germany

Christian Partensky, M.D.
Professor, Department of Surgery, Hôpital Edouard Herriot, Lyon, France

Margaret Paz-Partlow, M.A., M.F.A.
Clinical Project Associate, Department of Surgery, Cedars-Sinai Medical Center, Los Angeles, California

Vittorio Pedicino, M.D.
Medical Student, Department of Radiology III Cattedra, University of Rome "La Sapienza," Rome, Italy

Sergio Pedrazzoli, M.D., Ph.D.
Semeiotica Chirurgica, University of Padua, Padua, Italy

Marco A. Pelosi, M.D.
Associate Clinical Professor, University of Medicine and Dentistry of New Jersey, New Jersey Medical School, Newark, New Jersey; Director, Pelosi Women's Medical Center, Bayonne; Director, Department of Obstetrics and Gynecology, Bayonne Hospital, Bayonne, New Jersey

Marco A. Pelosi III, M.D.
Department of Obstetrics and Gynecology, New York Downtown Hospital, New York, New York

Alberto Peracchia, M.D.
Professor of Surgery, Department of General and Oncologic Surgery, University of Milan, Milan, Italy

Joaquin Perez de Oteyza , M.D.
Associate Professor and Staff Surgeon, Department of General and Gastrointestinal Surgery, Hospital Ramon y Cajal, Universidad Alcala de Henares, Madrid, Spain

Giuseppe Pezzuoli, M.D.
Professor of Surgery, Department of General and Oncologic Surgery, University of Milan, Milan, Italy

F. Pi, M.D.
Servicio de Cirugia General, Hospital de Viladecans, Barcelona, Spain

Dirk M. Potempa, M.D.
Registrar, Department of Urology, Klinikum Mannheim, University of Heidelberg, Mannheim, Germany

Giuseppe Pozzi, M.D.
Resident, I Clinica Chirurgica Policlinico Umberto I, University of Rome "La Sapienza," Rome, Italy

Giovanni Ramacciato, M.D.
Assistant Professor, I Clinica Chirurgica Policlinico Umberto I, University of Rome "La Sapienza," Rome, Italy

Raul Ramos, M.D.
Clinical Professor of Surgery, Department of Surgery, University of Texas Health Science Center at San Antonio, San Antonio, Texas

Jens J. Rassweiler, M.D.
Associate Professor, Department of Urology, Klinikum Mannheim, University of Heidelberg, Mannheim, Germany

Biagio Ravo, M.D.
Department of Surgery, Rome American Hospital, Rome, Italy

†Deceased.

Carlo Rebuffat, M.D.
Assistant Professor, Department of General Surgery, University of Milan–S. Giuseppe Hospital, Milan, Italy

H. Paul Redmond, M.B., B.Ch.
Department of Surgery, Beaumont Hospital, Dublin, Ireland

Katrin Reichenmiller, Cand. med.
Universitätsklinik Freiburg, Freiburg, Germany

Alain Remont, M.D.
Resident in Visceral Radiology, Department of Medical Imaging, Centre Hospitalier, University of Liège, Liège, Belgium

Antonio Rico-Alvarez, M.D.
Thoracic Surgeon, Department of Thoracic and General Surgery, University Hospital of Seville, Seville, Spain

Paul Damien Ridley, M.D.
Senior Registrar, Department of Thoracic Surgery, Frenchay Hospital, Bristol, England

Riccardo Rosati, M.D.
Assistant Professor of Surgery, Department of General and Oncologic Surgery, University of Milan, Milan, Italy

Mauro Roseano, M.D.
Ricercatore Universitario, Clinica Chirurgica Generale, University of Trieste, Trieste, Italy

Daniel Rosenthal, M.D.
Clinical Professor of Surgery, Department of Surgery, University of Texas Health Science Center at San Antonio, San Antonio, Texas

Plinio Rossi, M.D.
Chairman of Diagnostic Radiology, Department of Radiology III Cattedra, University of Rome "La Sapienza," Rome, Italy

T. Routiot, M.D.
CHU Central, Service de Chirurgie E, University of Nancy, Nancy, France

Giancarlo Roviaro, M.D.
Head, Department of General Surgery, University of Milan–S. Giuseppe Hospital, Milan, Italy

C.M.S. Royston, M.S.
Consultant Surgeon, Department of General Surgery, Royal Hull Hospitals, Hull, Humberside, England

Klaus Rückert, M.D.
Department of General Surgery, General Hospital, Hamburg, Germany

Alberto Ruol, M.D.
Assistant Professor of Surgery, Department of General Surgery, University of Padua, Padua, Italy

R. Christopher G. Russell, M.S.
Consultant Surgeon, Department of Surgery, Middlesex Hospital, London, England

Jonathan M. Sackier, M.D.
Associate Professor of Surgery, Department of Surgery, University of California at San Diego, San Diego, California

Samir Said, M.D.
Department of Surgery, University of Cologne, Cologne, Germany

Monserrat Salvi, M.D.
Assistant Professor of Surgery, Department of Surgery, University of Malaga, Malaga, Spain

Kamran Samii, M.D.
Professor, Department of Anesthesiology, CHU Bicêtre, Le Kremlin Bicêtre, Paris, France

Mirco Santini, M.D.
Fellow in Training, Istituto di Clinica Chirurgica Generale, Universita' Degli Studi di Ferrara, Ferrara, Italy

Paul Sauvage, M.D.
Professor, Chef de Service, Department of Pediatric Surgery, CHU Hautepierre, Strasbourg, France

Alain Sauvanet, M.D.
Department of Digestive Surgery, University of Paris VII, Xavier Bichat, Clichy, France

Silvio Marco Scalambra, M.D.
Department of General Surgery, University of Milan–S. Giuseppe Hospital, Milan, Italy

Andreas Schäfer, M.D.
Department of General and Thoracic Surgery, Justus-Liebig-University, Giessen, Germany

Anton Schafmayer, M.D.
Department of Surgery, Städtisches Krankenhaus Lüneburg, Lüneburg, Germany

Hans-Martin Schardey, M.D.
Department of Surgery, Klinikum Grosshadern, Ludwig-Maximilians-University, Munich, Germany

Friedrich-Wilhelm Schildberg, M.D.
Professor and Director, Department of Surgery, Klinikum Grosshadern, Ludwig-Maximilians-University, Munich, Germany

Jürgen Schleef, M.D.
Department of Surgery, Städtisches Krankenhaus Lüneburg, Lüneburg, Germany

Hans-Wilhelm Schreiber, M.D.
Professor and Director Emeritus, Department of Surgery, University of Hamburg, Hamburg, Germany

Detlev-Wilhelm Schröder, M.D.
Department of General Surgery, University of Kiel, Kiel, Germany

William W. Schuessler, M.D.
Privat Dozent, Department of Surgery, University of Texas Health Science Center at San Antonio, San Antonio, Texas

Konrad Schwemmle, M.D.
Department of General and Thoracic Surgery, Justus-Liebig-University, Giessen, Germany

Andrea Segalin, M.D.
Fellow in General Surgery, Department of General and Oncologic Surgery, University of Milan, Milan, Italy

Gianni Segato, M.D.
Assistant, Second Department of Surgery, University of Padua, Padua, Italy

J.C. Séguier, P.H.
Anesthesiologist, Department of Anesthesiology, Centre Hospitalier General, Saint-Germain-En-Laye, France

Kurt Semm, M.D.
Professor, Department of Gynecology and Obstetrics, Klinikum der Christian-Albrechts-Universität, Kiel, Germany

Helga Siegl, M.D.
Center for Biomedical Research, Allgemeines Krankenhaus, University of Vienna, Vienna, Austria

Enrique Sierra Gil, Ph.D.
Servicio de Cirugia General, Hospital de Viladecans, Barcelona, Spain

P. Sinda, P.H.
Anesthesiologist, Department of Anesthesiology, Centre Hospitalier General, Saint-Germain-En-Laye, France

Steven J. Snooks, M.D.
Consultant Surgeon, Department of General Surgery, King George Hospital, London, England

César Solis, M.D.
Resident, Department of Digestive and General Surgery, Surgical Pavilion B, Les Hôpitaux Universitaires de Strasbourg, Strasbourg, France

Andrea Sortini, M.D.
Associate Professor, Istituto di Clinica Chirurgica Generale, Universita' Degli Studi di Ferrara, Ferrara, Italy

Felicien M. Steichen, M.D.
Director, Institute for Minimally Invasive Surgery, St. Agnes Hospital, White Plains, New York; F.M. Steichen Professor of Surgery, New York Medical College, Valhalla, New York

Wolf J. Stelter, M.D.
Professor, Department of Surgery, Städtische Kliniken Frankfurt-Höchst, Frankfurt, Germany

Paul Sungler, M.D.
First Surgical Department, Landeskrankenaustalten Salzburg, Salzburg, Austria

Gerhard Szinicz, M.D.
Department of Surgery, Landeskrankenhaus Bregenz University, Bregenz, Austria

Paola Tabbi, M.D.
Resident, I Clinica Chirurgica Policlinico Umberto I, University of Rome "La Sapienza," Rome, Italy

Andrew Damian Taylor, M.D.
Consultant Radiologist, Department of Radiology, Hull Royal Infirmary, Hull, Humberside, England

Pierre Testas, M.D.
Professor of Gastrointestinal Surgery, Department of Surgery, Centre Hospitalier Kremlin-Bicêtre, Paris, France

Philippe Thibault, M.D.
Professor and Chairman, Department of Urology, Hôpital Tenon, Paris, France

Arnulf Thiede, M.D.
Professor, Direktor der Klinik, Chirurgische Universitäts-klinik und Poliklinik–Würzburg, Würzburg, Germany

T. Tommaseo, M.D.
Chairman, I Divisione Chirurgica, Presidio Ospedaliero Multizonale, Treviso, Italy

Reinhold Tschada, M.D.
Associate Professor, Department of Urology, Klinikum Mannheim, University of Heidelberg, Mannheim, Germany

Bernward Ulrich, M.D.
Professor and Director of Surgery, Department of Surgery, Krankenhaus Gerresheim, Düsseldorf, Germany

Stefano Valabrega, M.D.
Assistant Professor, I Clinica Chirurgica Policlinico Umberto I, University of Rome "La Sapienza," Rome, Italy

Jean-Stephane Valla, M.D.
Professor of Pediatric Surgery, Hôpital Lenval, Nice, France

Van L. Vallina, M.D.
Assistant Professor of Surgery, Rush North Shore Medical Center, Rush Medical School, Chicago, Illinois

Jaume Vall-Llovera Gambus, M.D.
Servicio de Cirugia General, Hospital de Viladecans, Barcelona, Spain

M.N. van der Heyde, M.D.
Community Hospital, Arnhem, The Netherlands

D. Van Raemdonck, M.D.
Department of Thoracic Surgery, University of Leuven, Leuven, Belgium

Carlos Vara-Thorbeck, M.D.
Professor of Surgery, Department of Surgery, University of Malaga, Malaga, Spain

J.S. Varma, M.D.
Senior Lecturer in Surgery, Department of Surgery, University of Newcastle Upon Tyne School of Medicine, Newcastle Upon Tyne, England

Federico Varoli, M.D.
Assistant Professor of Surgery, Department of General Surgery, University of Milan–S. Giuseppe Hospital, Milan, Italy

Frédéric Vaxman, M.D.
Surgeon, Department of Digestive and General Surgery, Surgical Pavilion B, Les Hôpitaux Universitaires de Strasbourg, Strasbourg, France

Philippe Vaysse, M.D.
Professor, Department of Pediatric Urology, University of Toulouse, Toulouse, France

Jose M. Velasco, M.D.
Associate Professor of Surgery, Department of Surgery, Rush North Shore Medical Center, Rush Medical School, Chicago, Illinois

Contardo Vergani, M.D.
Department of General Surgery, University of Milan–S. Giuseppe Hospital, Milan, Italy

Albert Verhulst, M.D., B. Eng.
Consultant in Vascular Surgery, Department of Surgery, Stuivenberg University Hospital of Antwerp, Antwerp, Belgium

Siegbert Vogel, M.D.
Surgeon, Universitätsklinik und Poliklinik–Würzburg, Würzburg, Germany

Pierre-Philippe Volkmar, M.D.
Surgeon, Department of Digestive and General Surgery, Surgical Pavilion B, Les Hôpitaux Universitaires de Strasbourg, Strasbourg, France

J. Waninger, M.D.
Chefarzt, Chirurgische Abteilung, Städtisches Krankenhaus Lörrach, Lörrach, Germany

György Weber, M.D., Ph.D.
First Assistant, Department of Surgery, Pécs University Hospital, Pécs, Hungary

Kevin Roy Wedgwood, M.D., B.Sc.
Consultant Surgeon, Department of General Surgery, Castle Hill Hospital, Cottingham Hull, England

Roger Welter, M.D.
President, Association Européenne de Chirurgie Viscérale; Director Emeritus, Department of Surgery, Princess Marie-Astrid Hospital, Luxembourg

Steven D. Wexner, M.D.
Residency Program Director and Director, Anorectal Physiology Laboratory, Department of Colorectal Surgery, Cleveland Clinic Florida, Fort Lauderdale, Florida

Franz Wierrani, M.D.
Department of Obstetrics and Gynecology, K.A. Rudolfstiftung, Vienna, Austria

Robert Graeme Wilson, M.D.
Senior Registrar in Surgery, Wards 9/10, Royal Infirmary of Edinburgh, Edinburgh, Scotland

Ursula Windberger, D.V.M.
Center for Biomedical Research, University of Vienna, Vienna, Austria

†R. Wittmoser, M.D.

†Deceased.

Preface

Primum non nocere has been guiding surgeons in the treatment of the sick and injured since before Hippocrates formulated the concept as a principle for all medical science and practice. This prescription rules the daily activities of the surgical craftsman in his or her use of therapeutic techniques: control of bleeding, prevention or treatment of infection, gentle handling and expert repair of tissues, avoidance of pain, and early return to optimal form and function. Our rich heritage is filled with names and deeds of surgeons who, throughout history, have contributed advances—some momentous, other more modest—to the scientific base and artful craft of surgery.

Cutting and sewing is an important part of the skills required in operative surgery. In patiently trained and dexterous hands, the ability to perform both functions well contributes significantly to a technically satisfactory operative result. In a long succession of improvements in sewing materials and machines over the last two centuries, mechanical sutures have reached a state of the art that has provided surgeons with optimal methods and results.

Minimally invasive surgery, with a reduced incision for gaining access to the chest or abdomen, is another advance in the never-ending search for improved surgical treatment modalities. Conceptually and in practice, stapling and laparoscopy or thoracoscopy are natural partners in this continual quest for improvements in patient care. Whereas the 1988 Européenne Congress of the Association Européenne de Chirurgie Viscérale was entirely devoted to the fields of application of surgical stapling, the 1992 Luxembourg Congress featured both stapling and minimally invasive surgery, with a predominant portion devoted to minimal access operations.

We hope that this book, which contains the important transactions of this Second European Congress in Luxembourg (September 10-12, 1992) on Minimally Invasive Surgery and New Technology will reflect the excitement and hope conveyed by these new and meaningful technological advances and operative techniques in surgery.

Roger Welter

Coming Home to Luxembourg

An Essay on the Venue of the Congress of Minimally Invasive Surgery and New Technology

This essay was originally written as a message of welcome to all the participants in the September 1992 Congress in Luxembourg and appeared in the program. It represented sentimental memories and feelings of pride for the country of birth of both senior editors. The message is reproduced in this book, which contains the transactions of the Congress, as an expression of gratitude by all the participants to the country and its people who made the Congress such an impressive event.

If "small is beautiful," Luxembourg possesses both attributes—a proud and peaceful claim that is in part the result of history but is also a gift of nature. To a large extent this claim is also founded on the fierce determination of the Luxembourg people to be free and live in peace and harmony with the world that surrounds them. Over more than a thousand—often tumultuous, sometimes painful—years of existence, the citizens of Luxembourg have created the political, cultural, and economic basis to support these aims. They have protected a pleasant human and natural environment that favors visits by neighbors and friends the world over.

Luxembourg, now known as a modern financial center, owed its earlier prominence to the fortress built on the natural ramparts of the capital city by Count Sigefroi in 963 and during the years that followed before the end of the tenth century. Because of the tactics of warfare prevailing throughout the Middle Ages, up to and including the French Revolution, the Napoleonic Wars, and two world wars, some of the visits were not always in the spirit of neighborly love and warm fellowship. Nevertheless, these are feelings that the people of Luxembourg enjoy for themselves and give freely—while maintaining an appearance of crusty individualism—to their friends, neighbors, and visitors.

Throughout history Luxembourg changed rulers frequently, often through the vagaries of fate, such as princely marriages, royal alliances, and state treaties. The country was governed at various times by Burgundy, Spain, France, Austria, and Holland from the mid-fifteenth century to 1839, the official date of independence, finally guaranteed by the great European powers in 1867 at the treaty of London.

However, Luxembourg has not always passively tolerated such changes in governance: during the fourteenth century Luxembourg experienced its first European calling under John I, "the Blind," Count of Luxembourg and King of Bohemia. He died at the battle of Crécy in 1346 (during the Hundred Years' War), fighting for Phillip VI, King of France. His daughter, Bonne of Luxembourg, was married to John II, "le Bon," son of Phillip VI and his successor as King of France. John I of Luxembourg was the son of Emperor Henry VII and the father of Emperor Charles IV—both of the Holy Roman Empire of German origin. His uncle Baudouin was archbishop and prince-elector of Trier, and another Luxembourger, Pierre d'Aspelt, held the position of archbishop and prince-elector of Mainz. Throughout the centuries that followed, the Luxembourg territory was progressively reduced in size, while the fortress continued to be coveted by various powerful neighbors.

The treaty of the Pyrénées in 1659 gave a large southwestern portion of the country, with the cities of Thionville and Montmédy to France. At the treaty of Vienna in 1815, Luxembourg ceded all its lands to the east of the rivers Moselle, Sûre, and Our to Prussia and was rewarded by becoming an independent Grand Duchy. Finally, in 1839, at the conclusion of the Belgian revolt against Holland, the entire "Quartier Wallon" was separated from Luxembourg as the "Province du Luxembourg Belge." At the time the great powers were probably self-conscious of the ridicule they would be exposed to by elevating 999 square miles to a kingdom, and they gracefully refrained from this step.

Since 1851 William I of the House of Orange had been King of Holland and Grand Duke of Luxembourg, while the two countries were established as constitutionally independent entities. This political arrangement was reaffirmed by the treaty of 1839, in which Belgium separated from Holland. After the death of William III, Grand Duke of Luxembourg and King of Holland (1890), the Royal House of Orange was without a male heir. The constitution of Luxembourg did not accept a female line of succession at the time. Therefore a cousin of William III, Duke Adolphe of Nassau, who had relinquished his country to the reorganization of the German Empire under Prussian hegemony, became Grand Duke of Luxembourg. His son, Guillaume IV, Grand Duchess Marie-Adélaide, her sister the beloved Grand Duchess Charlotte, and at present the very popular Grand Duke Jean and Grand Duchess Joséphine-Charlotte have given Luxembourg for well over 100 years a strong identity and the stability of a constitutional monarchy. The legislative, executive, and judiciary branches are separated as in all democracies, with an elected parliament and executive government based on political majorities of the popular vote. Needless to say, with the accession of Grand Duchess Marie-Adélaide, Luxembourg amended part of its constitution.

During this period of extraordinary political and economic stability, only temporarily derailed by two world wars, Luxembourg changed from an agrarian economy to a prosperous industrial base, mostly in steel production, to which has been added more recently a thriving service economy in consumer goods, banking, international finance, and worldwide audiovisual communications. And throughout this period, Luxembourg has known a second European and international calling that radiates far beyond its narrow borders. Realizing that for a small country true peace of mind and body can be achieved only by harmonious coexistence with all mankind, Luxembourg statesmen and leaders of industry and finance have been active often as prime movers to a degree that belies the territorial importance of the country they represent.

The peace conference in The Hague before World War I (Paul Eyschen), activities at the League of Nations (Joseph Bech), and the founding of the German-French Committee for Mutual Understanding as well as the International Steel Confederation between the world wars (Emile Mayrisch), the creation of the Werner Plan for Monetary European Union (Pierre Werner), and the Presidency of the United Nations General Assembly and of the European Community Commission (Gaston Thorn) are but a few examples of these efforts. Robert Schuman, the French statesman who can rightfully claim to be the founder of the new Europe together with Adenauer and De Gasperi, was born of French parents in Luxembourg. He learned the French and Luxembourg languages as a child; German was added as he entered the public school system. Later he would often refer to his years of elementary and high school as the basis of his understanding of problems that faced Europe and of the ways to remedy these problems.

The Charlemagne Medal, conferred by the city of Aachen to individuals who have made outstanding contributions to European unity and understanding, was bestowed in 1958 on Robert Schuman and in 1961 on Joseph Bech—longstanding Luxembourg Minister of Foreign Affairs. In 1986 this distinction was granted to the entire nation "in grateful recognition for its exemplary, principled support of unity amongst Europeans."

A visit to Luxembourg will not reveal grandiose monuments made by human hand, nor spectacular natural vistas; yet within its narrow borders the countryside can vary from gentle fields to rolling hills covered by forests, with unforgettable effects of light and color, depending on the season and the time of the day. Rivers meander through valleys that deepen as the visitor moves from south to north. In the east the wide valley of the Moselle River has been a fertile ground for vineyards and wine making since Roman times.

In the northern part of the country, called Oesling or Ardennes, the valleys are deep and the hills rise more sharply and steeply. The natural contours of the land favored the construction of fortified castles in medieval times. Many of these are in ruins now; others are beautifully reconstructed. Among them are Vianden and Bourscheid, with towns nestled in the surrounding valleys and houses clinging precariously to the hillside. Victor Hugo, the French poet and author of *Les Misérables*, found refuge in Vianden during his early days of voluntary exile from the France of Napoleon III. Sleepy villages, their inhabitants gone to work in the fields at early dawn, and bustling towns and small cities offer the visitor a beautiful panorama of charmingly decorated farmhouses and artfully preserved urban centers adapted to life in the twentieth century. Villages and towns often resemble a public garden or park: abundant flowers alternate with green lawns and wooded areas that are permeated by light and dappled shade, leading one's mind to that enjoyable state between dream and reality.

Nowhere is this impression more vivid than on a visit to the city of Luxembourg. Goethe, the German poet, anatomist, and statesman, said of the still-existing fortress at the end of the eighteenth century that it was "the most wondrous place, unique perhaps on the face of the earth." Were he to revisit the capital city today and approach it as he did then through the original suburbs of Grund, Clausen, and Pfaffenthal, to ascend the castle road and cross the permanent bridge that has replaced Sigefroi's drawbridge, he would be pleased to see how the fortress, dismantled in 1867, and the dwellings in and around it have aged. His eyes, taking in the panoramic view before him from the rocky promontory called "Bock" on which the original castle was built, would light with the joy of old found treasures: the original suburbs, with all their colorful diversity, and across from where he stands, the majestic elevation called "Plateau du Rham" with its hospice (now a retirement home) and remnants of the ring of fortified walls built in the fourteenth century. His gaze would almost certainly carry him to his left and bring back the delightful memory of the "Three Acorns," an elegant link in what was once an impregnable, fortified city.

But his enjoyment of the aesthetic marriage of old and new would suffer a sudden jolt at the view of a high-rise structure to the left surrounded by a confusion of buildings distinguished by a function-oriented, bureaucratic style. Penetrating into the city, he would be elated to find the Spanish governor's—now the Grand Duke's—Palace and House of Representatives, the Jesuit Church, now enlarged to a cathedral, the elegant and daring bridges, and so much of what has distinguished the city since his last visit. Coming from an age when most transactions were in cash, he would be surprised by the proliferation of banks and the steel and glass cubicles housing their headquarters in places where proud patrician villas once stood. In the spirit of tolerance that he quietly favored, Goethe would accept the proposition that in its desire to welcome the political and economic institutions of a unifying Europe, Luxembourg was moved more by what is practical than by what is beautiful. He would encourage his fellow visitors to concentrate their attention on what is beautiful, with the knowledge that what man's hand has spoiled, man's mind and hand can restore. He would be delighted to know that efforts of merging old and new aesthetically and symbolically are at work once again, exactly where his gaze caressed the silhouette of rocks, woods, and the fort of the Three Acorns, hopefully soon to become a modern museum—a monument to peace in the ruins of war. Goethe the landscape painter, were he to catch a glimpse of architect I.M. Pei moving with great purpose from old to new, would smile in recognition and encouragement across the ramparts and 200

years of history. And if Goethe the tourist or his modern successors felt a need for intellectual and religious contemplation, in search of a soul among this collection of old stones and new glass and concrete, they would be attracted to Echternach, the venerable city that owes its reputation to a small monastery established in the seventh century by 12 missionary Benedictine monks. It was expanded by Willibrord from Northumberland into an Abbey in 698. Willbrord was the Apostle of Friesen and Archbishop of Utrecht, and together with his companions he brought the Christian faith to the Low Lands and Northern Germany, as well as great knowledge and education. The scriptorium in Echternach was a center from which all available science and knowledge was transmitted far and wide. A romanesque basilica dating from the eleventh century, with gothic features harmoniously incorporated, was faithfully reconstructed after World War II; it gives repose to the ashes of St. Willibrord in its original crypt. The old town hall nearby served also in the dispensation of justice during the Middle Ages.

The days of St. Willibrord are gone, and Luxembourg has no claim of being the sole repository from which all knowledge and truth emanate. But in the spirit of St. Willibrord, his companions, and their modern successors, the Luxembourg statesmen with a European vision and international vocation, President Roger Welter welcomes surgeons to Luxembourg in 1995 for another meeting of the minds, an exchange of ideas, and a pledge of good fellowship by, from, and for surgeons the world over.

Acknowledgments

We are very grateful to H.R.H. Grand Duchess Joséphine-Charlotte for her gracious participation and continued interest in the program of this Second Luxembourg Congress on Minimally Invasive Surgery and New Technology. Their Excellencies Prime Minister Jacques Santer and Minister of Health Johny Lahure, the Honorable Lydie Wurth-Polfer, Mayor, and Anne Brasseur, first Alderman of the City of Luxembourg, Dr. D. Hansen-Koenig, Director of Public Health, and their associates gave the support of state and city governments. We thank them for this and their personal commitment to the cause of public health.

A special tribute should go to the many scientific associations that participated in the organization and smooth execution of the various proceedings and parallel programs. *Primum inter pares* in this glittering array of prestigious national and international surgical societies is the Association Européenne de Chirurgie Viscérale, its President, Roger Welter, and his devoted, hard-working staff, whose proficiency and organizational skills were so evident throughout the meeting, down to the most exquisite details of simultaneous translation into five languages, high-quality audiovisual equipment, timely choice of subject matter, and great hospitality.

An effort of this magnitude depends entirely on the expertise of the faculty and the enthusiasm of the participants. Success in these areas represents the ultimate recompense for all the trials and tribulations of the organizers. In this they were richly rewarded by the faculty of leading surgeons, physicians, and scientists from all over the world who gave clear and exhaustive presentations of the state of the art in their various specialties and spheres of scientific interest. Similarly, some 1700 participants from 34 countries followed the presentations with good-spirited perseverance and participated in the discussions with intelligent vigor.

Turi Josefson, her staff from Autosuture Europe, and the many other exhibitors deserve a special citation of merit for their exemplary support within the framework of ethical standards, guiding the cooperation between medical academia and industry.

Last but not least, we would like to recognize the limitless energy and devotion to perfection of our publishers at Quality Medical Publishing: Karen Berger, David Miller, Beth Campbell, and especially Suzanne Wakefield, for whom the word impossible is not part of the editorial vocabulary. Judy Bamert's superb page layouts present the technically complex contents in an elegant fashion. We also thank our secretaries, Ruth Haynes and Marlene Callaro, who have labored mightily to keep us and our manuscripts on track.

Felicien M. Steichen

Contents

Common Bile Duct

Complications of Operations on the Biliary Tract

X *Videoendoscopic Hernia Repairs*

XI *Videoendoscopic Small and Large Bowel Surgery*

XVI *Videoendoscopic Gastroduodenal Surgery*

XVII *Reconstructive and Corrective Procedures in the Upper Gastrointestinal Tract*

Minimally Invasive Surgery
and New Technology

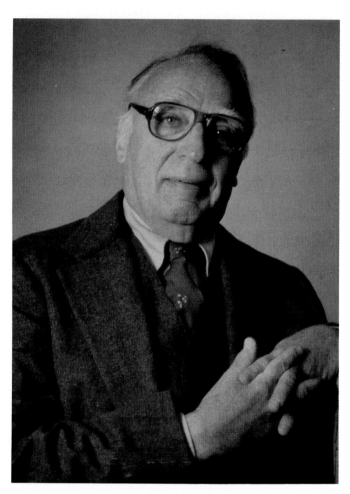

Mark M. Ravitch
1910–1989

The Library of Mark M. Ravitch

Enrico Nicolo

It was in Luxembourg, at the last conference he attended, the Second International Symposium and First European Congress on Stapling in Surgery in June 1988, that Mark M. Ravitch enjoyed to the fullest his undisputed status as a cosmopolitan teacher and surgical leader. During his entire life, and since his death on March 1, 1989, Mark Ravitch has been widely acclaimed as an inspiring teacher, a prolific clinical investigator, scholar, and an exemplary figure in surgery. His life and work made an enduring impression.

Mark Ravitch was the traditional "*Homo chirurgicum*," an eminently practical man, and at the same time a sentimentalist. A practical man: by the range of his intellectual inquiries, by the freshness of his clear skepticism, and by the sharpness of his observations, he gave impetus to the surgical world of the twentieth century. A sentimentalist: a lover of the poetry of surgical history, he found inspiration from noble and courageous sentiments and acts of the past through his passionate interest and scholarly study and interpretation of the history of medicine and mankind.

Mark Ravitch dedicated himself to the cause of collecting books, and he added his name to the long and glorious list of such medical bibliophiles as Hunter, Osler, and Cushing, whose main objective has been to "keep alive an interest in the great men of the past, and not alone in their works that they cherish, but in their lives, which they emulate . . . and who have combined intellectual preeminence with nobility of character."

Deeply interested in old surgical books, Mark Ravitch, with admirable patience, strong determination, and the fine taste of a connoisseur, never lost any opportunity to search for and acquire them. He collected more than 350 rare books. From the oldest, *Observationes Chirurgicae* by Giralamo Fabrizzi (1598), the collection covers many of the significant achievements in the development of surgery during the past four centuries and contains the names of some of the illustri-ous pioneers who occupy a pedestal in the history of surgery by virtue of their achievements in the art and science: John Hunter, Percival Pott, Astley Paston Cooper, Antonio Scarpa, William Halsted, Edoardo Bassini, August Gottlieb Richter, Benjamin Travers, and Wenzel Treitz.

Mark Ravitch developed a strong predilection for writings about hernia. "I have long been a student of the development of the operation for inguinal hernia. I have long made a specialty of the important books on hernia," he wrote in a letter in 1978. In fact, he collected more than 190 rare books on hernia. Beginning with Cellarius Fridericus' *Disputatio Medical de Hernia* (1656), the collection includes the brightest stars in the luminous firmament of the history and development of hernia surgery: Pieter Camper, *Incones Herniarum* (1801); Antonio Scarpa, *Sulle Ernie* (1809); Astley Paston Cooper, *The Anatomy and Surgical Treatment of Inguinal Hernia* (1804); Antonio DeGimbernat; Franz Kaspar Hesselbach; Jules Cloquet; Pott; Richter; Joseph-François Malgaigne; Lucas Championaire; Henry O. Marcy; John Ferguson; Wiliam S. Halsted; Wood; Treitz; and finally, as Ravitch wrote, "the Great Surgeon, Edoardo Bassini of Padua, essentially the creator of the modern operation for inguinal hernia." Including more than 20 oversized volumes, rare monographs, foreign doctoral theses, and unique pamphlets, the hernia materials represent one of the most comprehensive collections in this specialty.

Since April 9, 1992, the Mark M. Ravitch History of Surgery Collection has been permanently housed in the Mark M. Ravitch History of Medicine Room in the Falk Library of the Health Sciences at the University of Pittsburgh.

We can conclude with this statement: as he turned back to find his companions in the great past, we too may turn back to find in Mark Ravitch a companion and a friend.

I

Methods of Learning and Teaching New Surgical Techniques

1   *The Dynamics of Progress in the Art and Science of Surgery*

Felicien M. Steichen

Ambroise Paré (1510-1592) (Fig. 1), the great and humane military surgeon, clinical scientist, and therapeutic innovator, counselor to four kings of France (Henri II, Francois II, Charles IX, Henri III) and modest companion to soldiers and field commanders, once made the famous statement, "Je le pansay, et Dieu le guarit" ("I dressed his wounds, and God restored his health").[1] Thus he defined the then-existing state of the art—or craft—and science in surgery. The craft, in which he was a gifted and compassionate master and reached universal recognition, undiminished by the passage of time. He had less fascination with the science of understanding and influencing the pathophysiological processes of disease because of his commitment as a clinician to relieving individual suffering.[6,13,31] As a professional healer he was deeply committed to the spiritual values of religious tolerance—he was a Huguenot—and to

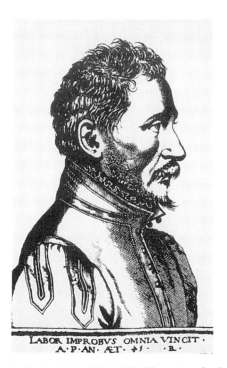

Fig. 1. Ambroise Paré, 1510-1590. (Engraving by Jean Le Royer, 1561.)

social justice and respect for moral principles. He attributed the physiological function of wound repair and healing to acts of God, because his rational understanding of the level of scientific knowledge as it existed during his lifetime left no place for a different concept. His statement was perhaps also a reference to the powers of the unknown concealed in each human being. It is an image still used by men and women of the healing arts the world over, although today scientific methods explain God's participation, as Paré perceived it.

The contributions of Paré and of surgeons since then represent a classic model for the definition of qualities that lead to progress in surgery:

- The timely recognition and possible prevention of health problems.
- An open, searching, and at times lucky human mind to develop ideas and solutions and submit them to the rigors of experimental methods.
- Verifiable scientific methods that withstand critical examination and the ultimate trial of clinical application.
- Clinical acceptance that is governed by an absolute code of ethics and that should be cautiously progressive, of real benefit, and available to all.
- The necessary technology that can be satisfied by existing materials and methods or new ones specifically developed for a given purpose. Without the essential human and financial resources, progress is laborious at best.
- Finally, all improvements are illusory and temporary if knowledge, experience, and skills cannot be or are not transmitted to future generations of practitioners of the art and science of surgery.

RECOGNITION AND PREVENTION OR TREATMENT OF A HEALTH PROBLEM

As surgeons we are called upon to treat the pain and suffering of individual patients and to mend broken bodies rather than to prevent the disease or accident that led to the condition in the first place. Surgeons have had no real experience through clinical practice and research with the prevention of disease and injury. This often requires that they undertake the strange venture of a sociopolitical crusade. An outstanding exception to this was the successful campaign waged by Alton Ochsner, Richard Overholt, and Dwight Harken against smoking, which has been statistically proven to increase the risk of lung cancer and heart disease. They faced well-organized and -financed opposition but succeeded in North America. It is to be hoped that their message will soon have the same effect in Europe and other parts of the world. As chest surgeons, they placed the common goal before personal interest, a good lesson in everyday medical ethics.

In contrast to the surgeon's concern with restoring form and function, pediatricians, gynecologists, and specialists in communicable and infectious diseases divide their clinical activities between curative and preventive methods. The interest of public health officials is oriented almost entirely toward prevention of an epidemic, its containment in case of an outbreak, and protection by medication, immunization, or both.

A nice example in modern times is the conquest of the poliomyelitis virus that had produced disease of endemic proportions in North America. It is hoped that the HIV virus will follow a similar fate, after political posturing and pressure-group antics have been eliminated. In the case of poliomyelitis it took the mobilization of a whole continent, orchestrated by the March of Dimes and inspired by President Roosevelt, who had had poliomyelitis himself. The virus was isolated from the feces of patients by Landsteiner and Poppen in 1903. It was later cultivated and found to multiply in tissue cultures of non-nervous origin by Enders, Weller, and Robbins. This work was a stepping stone in the research of Jonas Salk who developed an effective vaccine in 1954 and Albert Sabin who introduced the oral preparation of the vaccine.[25] Similar efforts in the past have led to the elimination or control of the various pestilences of the Middle Ages, the ravages of tropical diseases, and the burdens of communicable conditions.

Modern society has created a series of endemic, even epidemic, conditions that are not recognized as such because they are not transmitted by a microbe or virus. Their names are man's inhumanity to man, substance abuse, highway slaughter, industrial accidents, and sports follies. Surgeons must work to eliminate some of these conditions that keep them professionally occupied at present, just as Drs. Ochsner, Overholt, and Harken did in the case of cigarette smoking. They are joining with laypeople in the American Trauma Society, the Handgun Control Association, the Occupational Safety and Health Administration (OSHA), and the Highway Safety Office, to name but a few organizations interested in controlling modern, mechanical epidemics. The ultimate purpose of any social or health care agency or group of professionals should be to eliminate the reason for which they were created—and then self-destruct, or change course and direct their energies and resources to a new need, such as the March of Dimes did in the case of birth defects, after poliomyelitis had been vanquished.

DISCOVERY AND THE ROLE OF THE SCIENTIFIC HUMAN MIND

In his presidential address on "The Nature of Discovery" to the American Surgical Association in 1956, Alfred Blalock, surgical scientist, pioneer cardiac surgeon, and educator (Fig. 2), defined the methods by which discoveries are made and distinguished four categories: (1) chance or accident, (2) intention or design,

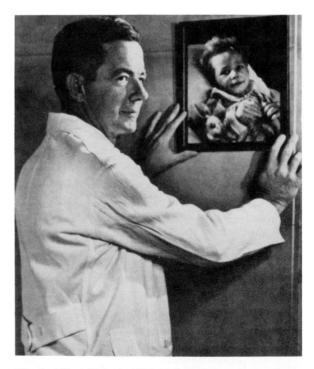

Fig. 2. Alfred Blalock, 1899-1964. (Photograph by Karsh, 1950.)

THE SCIENTIFIC HUMAN MIND

Discovery is an idea tested by the experimental method.

CLAUDE BERNARD

Discoveries are made:
  By the prepared mind through chance or accident
  By the searching mind through design or intention
  By the serendipitous mind through intuition or
    inspiration

ALFRED BLALOCK

---

(3) intuition or inspiration, and (4) a combination of some or all (see the box).[7]

Discoveries are made by humans who find and develop an idea and submit it to the scrutiny of the experimental method, according to Claude Bernard (1813-1878), the author of *An Introduction to the Study of Experimental Medicine*.[5]

Discovery by Chance or Accident

Discoveries made by chance are the result of an unexpected observation that becomes a discovery only if the observer recognizes its importance. Louis Pasteur (1822-1895) expressed this relationship clearly and succinctly: "In the field of observation, chance favors only the *prepared mind*."[4,7]

Examples of such events abound throughout the history of the biological sciences. The study of what seems like so many anecdotes not only lightens the tedium of more serious reading, but also gives deep insights into achievements made possible by an open, curious, motivated human mind.

A well-documented discovery by chance concerns Ambroise Paré and the treatment of wounds. During his first campaign as surgeon to Maréchal de Montéjan, the French army pursued Charles V into Italy and laid siege to Turin (1536). Paré found himself treating many soldiers wounded by firearms, and he ran out of the oil of elder mixed with a little theriaca that was used, scalding hot, to cauterize the wounds. He was constrained to apply in its place a digestive made of egg yolks, oil of roses, and turpentine. Early the next day "I found those on whom I had put the digestive medicament feeling little pain and their wounds without inflammation or swelling. The others to whom I had applied the said boiling oil, I found feverish with great pain and swelling about their wounds. Then I resolved with myself never more to burn thus cruelly poor men wounded with gunshot."[4,31]

Edward Jenner (1749-1823) observed that dairymaids who had "the pockmarks" of cowpox did not contract smallpox. After a discussion with John Hunter, his friend and teacher (Fig. 3), he tried the critical test, which resulted in planned vaccinations in 1798 and the elimination of smallpox. This event also represents one of the earliest recorded incidents of a human immune reaction with successful result.[4]

The prepared mind of Louis Pasteur (Fig. 4) led him to the surprise observation that when in one of his experiments he inoculated fowls with an old bacterial culture, they became sick but did not die. He postulated and then proved that the injection of progressively more virulent bacteria builds up the immune response to infection. This rediscovery of immunization found lifesaving applications against rabies in man, still a public health problem at the time, and against anthrax in sheep.[4,13]

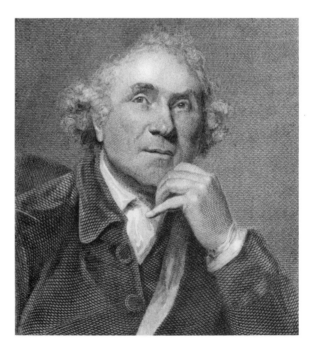

Fig. 3. John Hunter, 1728-1793. (Engraving by W. Sharp, 1788.)

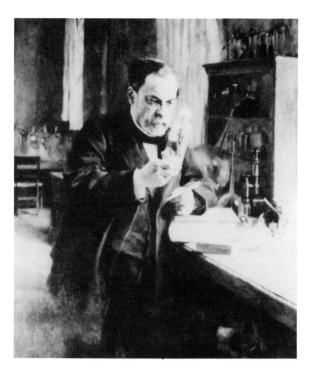

Fig. 4. Louis Pasteur, 1822-1895. (Photograph by Albert-Gustaf Edelfelt.)

Wilhelm Konrad Röntgen (1845-1923), professor of physics and rector of the University of Würzburg, was working on November 8, 1895 with a Hittorf-Crookes' tube he had covered with black cardboard. To test the opacity of the cover he darkened the room and noticed that a screen covered with barium platinocyanide would fluoresce as it became exposed to the rays of the tube. Named *X* (meaning unknown) *rays* by Röntgen, these invisible rays would penetrate flesh to show bones and expose photographic plates that were protected from visible light. A new, revolutionary mode of diagnosis had been discovered.[4]

In 1916 Dr. George Papanicolaou (1883-1962), working as a researcher at New York Hospital, was studying oocytes and the menstrual cycle in guinea pigs. He used a nasal speculum to inspect the guinea pig's vagina and found changes of the menstrual cycle in the scraped cells, which in turn allowed him to predict ovarian activity. Recognizing the potential of his findings by 1920, Dr. "Pap" began to study cell scrapings of the vagina and cervix in women and soon discovered carcinoma of the cervix uteri. His results were first presented in 1928 and were received with great skepticism. The validity of the Pap smear in the detection of carcinoma of the cervix uteri was finally established in 1941, and by 1960 the worldwide mortality rate from cancer of the cervix had decreased dramatically, thanks to this "simple" screening test.[3]

The discovery of penicillin has benefited mankind, not only because of its direct impact on bacterial disease, but also because of the continued development of various antibiotics. Pasteur and Joubert observed in 1877 that contamination of cultures by airborne molds prevented further growth of bacteria. They predicted that this phenomenon could become the basis for treating infections.

In 1929 Alexander Fleming (1881-1955) noticed that the accidental contamination of a staphylococcal culture by a mold created a clear area around the mold. He realized that the mold produced a substance that killed bacteria, and he tried to isolate the active principle.[4] This was ultimately achieved by Howard Florey and Ernest Chain in 1940 at Oxford University and represents a brilliant example of discovery by design or intention, the next category in our descriptions.[11]

A more contemporary chance observation led to the brilliant discovery of external cardiac compression in modern cardiopulmonary resuscitation, a method that has saved thousands of lives the world over in the last 32 years.

Under a grant from the Consolidated Edison Electric Company of New York City, concerned by electric shock accidents and deaths, Professor W.B. Kouwenhoven of the Department of Engineering at Johns Hopkins University had been studying the effects of electric shock on physiological parameters and of ventricular fibrillation since 1928.

In the 1950s, Professor Kouwenhoven, Dean and then Dean Emeritus of the School of Engineering, had expanded his activities to work in the Surgical Research Laboratory at the Johns Hopkins Hospital on an alternating-current external defibrillator. His research team included G. Guy Knickerbocker, Postgraduate Fellow in Engineering, and James R. Jude, Assistant Resident and Research Fellow in Surgery at Johns Hopkins Hospital (Fig. 5).

In the spring of 1958, while applying the heavy electrodes of the defibrillator to the highly angled and elastic chest of a dog, Kouwenhoven and Knickerbocker observed a blip of vascular pressure on the strain gauge amplifier recording the blood pressure from the cannulated femoral artery. They discussed

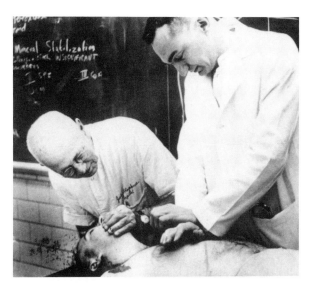

Fig. 5. James Jude demonstrating cardiopulmonary resuscitation on G. Guy Knickerbocker, while W.B. Kouwenhoven performs mouth-to-mouth resuscitation.

this observation with James Jude, who was by then Senior Assistant Resident in Surgery. Together the three researchers developed techniques and projects by which the defibrillator paddles were replaced by their hands for rhythmic compression. The efficiency of the method and rate of success were studied in animals with prolonged fibrillation, for whom external manual compression and defibrillation were employed. In addition, they explored the effects of administering epinephrine, calcium chloride, sodium bicarbonate, and other medications to victims of cardiac arrest.[14–16,21]

In 1958 the technique became sufficiently established for Henry Bahnson, then guiding the Cardiovascular Surgical Division at Hopkins, to apply external cardiac compression to a 2-year-old child whose heart was in ventricular fibrillation; the baby was successfully resuscitated.[42] Shortly thereafter, James Jude applied external cardiac compression to an obese woman whose respirations and pulse ceased while she was receiving halothane—a new anesthetic at the time—in preparation for urgent removal of an acutely inflamed gallbladder. Jude applied rhythmic 60-per-minute compressions over the lower sternum, the patient recovered a normal heartbeat, and the operation was successfully concluded. By applying his experimental expertise to the clinical setting, Jude proved

that the chest wall did not have to be pliable as in dogs or in babies, but above all he demonstrated the pathway of an idea submitted to the scrutiny of scientific method and then transposed to its ethical, clinical application. Knickerbocker and Kouwenhoven rediscovered an observation made by Boehm in Germany, who had studied the effects of chloroform on cardiac action in cats 80 years earlier and had noted that by squeezing the cats' chests, asystole could be reversed. The prepared minds of these investigators gave them the necessary genius to take this one step or many steps further through the teamwork with Jude, first experimentally and then clinically.[15,21,42]

Discovery by Intention or Design

The results obtained by design or intention are due to a planned, systematic investigation of a problem. The majority of discoveries were and are made this way in the era of modern medicine. During the contemporary period of medical research, both basic and clinical, prospective, randomized, double-blind studies have become the standard for discoveries by design to satisfy statistical analysis and validity.

The second contribution by Paré, individual ligature of major vessels, happened by design. Until 1552 he had still recommended cautery for hemostasis, but he had given considerable thought to using ligatures for major vessels. Paré discussed this with several colleagues, and at the siege of Danvilliers during the Lorraine campaign, an officer of Viscount de Rohan, the army commander, was shot in the leg. Paré tied off the vessels in the amputated stump and spared the officer the hot iron. Although known to Hippocrates, ligature of vessels had been practically abandoned since antiquity, and it is Paré's merit to have returned it to permanent importance as a basic surgical technique.

While we mentioned earlier that Pasteur rediscovered immunization by chance and that he had made the statement that "chance favors the prepared mind," the prodigious scientific contributions by the genius of his prepared mind were mostly the result of planned, systematic, diligent investigation.[4,13,25] Besides the ability to discover new facts, he was able to adapt his scientific findings to practical applications in medicine and industry and to teach and inspire others. Although he started his career as a chemist and became a self-taught microbiologist and immunologist, his life could well serve as the model for a career in surgical research: proof that microbes are reproduced from parent organisms, not through spontaneous generation, and that germs cause disease; creation of vaccines for virulent disease; and as a "sideline occupation" he found solutions to many industrial biochemical problems. His experiments to demonstrate the efficacy of the anthrax vaccine were conducted by using 50 sheep, 25 of which were vaccinated and 25 used for control. All were inoculated with anthrax 1 month after vaccination, and 2 days later all 25 control animals were dead, but all vaccinated sheep survived. Even today Pasteur's methods could withstand the scrutiny of statistical analysis. However, such an experiment might well not take place today because of protests by animal rights advocates.

The development of antisepsis by Joseph Lister (1827-1912) (Fig. 6) of Glasgow also belongs in the category of discoveries by design. A year after Pasteur's demonstration of the "germ theory" in 1864, Lister used carbolic acid to disinfect the wound of James Greenlee's compound fracture at the Glasgow Infirmary. Starting on August 12, 1865, Lister treated the wound with carbolic acid for 6 weeks, and it healed without infection.[4,25,26]

Since living organisms cause suppuration, a method had to be found to eliminate germs by a reliable substance. Lister chose carbolic acid because it had been effective when sprayed on sewage. From this first success, Lister expanded his principle to the treatment of ordinary wounds and abscesses with equal success (1867). He then applied his concepts to the preparation of antiseptic silk and catgut and developed the idea of creating an antiseptic environment (1871) by using a solution of 1:100 carbolic acid for scrubbing hands, soaking instruments, preparing the patient's skin, and spraying the operating room air. Lister eliminated postoperative suppuration, tetanus from use of catgut, erysipelas, puerperal fever, and hospital gangrene. Although he had an enthusiastic following among his students, Lister had a difficult time convincing his fellow surgeons. This is a sad commentary on the ability of surgeons (or any professionals) to recognize progress when it takes place and abandon time-honored but experimentally discredited beliefs and biases.[44]

During the 1880s the antiseptic method was developed into aseptic techniques in Germany and France. This had been heralded by Pasteur, who stated in 1874, "If I had the honor of being a surgeon I would never introduce into the human body an instrument without having passed it through boiling water or better still, through a flame and rapidly cooled right before operation."

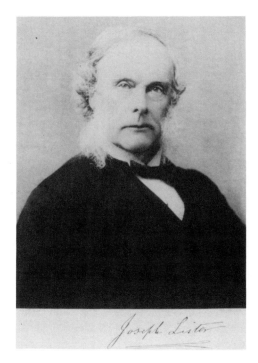

Fig. 6. Joseph Lister, 1827-1912.

Another example of the systematic, tenacious pursuit of a solution to a problem, in this case spirochetal infection, was the search by Paul Ehrlich (1854-1915) for a "magic bullet to strike at parasites and at parasites only and to learn how to do this with chemical substances."[4,13] The six hundred and sixth compound tested by his co-worker, Dr. Sahachiro Hata, proved to be effective experimentally and improved patients dramatically (1910), although these therapeutic effects of Salvarsan and later Neo Salvarsan No. 914 would be surpassed by penicillin. Dr. Ehrlich's success was the first example of treatment with a chemical substance—chemotherapy.[4,25]

The second component of modern cardiopulmonary resuscitation is a patent airway and adequate ventilation. As a student in the emergency department of the Billroth clinic during the Battle of Vienna in 1945, Peter Safar had become particularly interested in the need for better early resuscitation efforts in trauma victims, in the field and during transportation.[40] During his years of training in anesthesiology he continued to search for a simple method of ventilation and learned at the Anesthesiology Congress of October 1956 that J.O. Elam's work and results on mouth-to-mask exhaled air ventilation for army nerve gas casualties was neither widely known nor recognized as a useful method for civilian application. The Red Cross was still teaching manual chest pressure–arm lift (Silvester) artificial ventilation, which Safar and many of his colleagues knew to be unsatisfactory, judging from their clinical experience of intubating patients and doing mouth-to-tracheal tube inflation to check the placement of the tube. Indeed, the Silvester method did not provide the backward head-tilt and forward jaw-thrust to ensure a patent airway, nor sufficient force of ventilation to maintain satisfactory oxygenation.[38]

Following conversations with Dr. Elam that triggered curiosity and stimulated a well-entrenched enthusiasm for hard work and physiological research, Peter Safar set out to compare manual chest pressure–arm lift artificial ventilation with mouth-to-mouth and mouth-to-airway ventilation for practical, general use. From this point on it was step-by-step, systematic effort in the research laboratory, on volunteers (I was one of them), and finally on patients in need of resuscitation that led to the development of the cardiopulmonary-cerebral resuscitation system of basic (in conjunction with the previously described cardiac compression), advanced, and prolonged life support for use in ambulances, emergency situations, and intensive care units. A whole new world of patients "rising from the dead" was developed and continues to evolve.[37,40] While communicable diseases may dampen some of the enthusiasm for techniques of direct contact with a patient outside the hospital environment, the basic steps of the pulmonary and cardiac resuscitation remain valid. Gadgets and methods will be found to eliminate any concern for direct airway-to-airway transmission of disease.

Many other examples of discovery by design could be described here. Two momentous ones will be reviewed in greater detail later: the development of closed and open heart surgery in the treatment of congenital and acquired heart disease and the application of immunology to the practical solutions of clinical transplantation of organs.*

Discovery by Intuition or Inspiration

Sometimes discoveries occur when a solution to a problem one is intensely interested in suddenly enters conscious thought. Typically it happens during the study of the problem; at other times it will occur serendipi-

*References 8, 23, 29, 34, 35, 44.

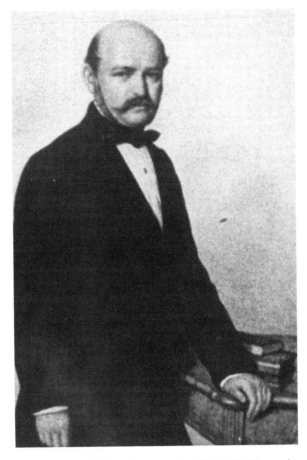

Fig. 7. Ignaz Philipp Semmelweis, 1818-1865. (From the Ignaz Semmelweis Museum, Budapest, Hungary; painted 1857.)

tously when work on the problem has been laid aside temporarily. The "inspiration" comes to a scholarly mind and represents an advance in thinking that goes well beyond simple observation and average interpretation. Sir Isaac Newton is said to have stated that no great discovery was ever made without a bold guess.[7]

A discovery that fits this category is the prevention of puerperal fever by Hungarian physician Ignaz Philipp Semmelweis (1818-1865) (Fig. 7). While an assistant at the first obstetrical clinic of Vienna's Allgemeines Krankenhaus, he concerned himself intently with the fact that in his clinic, 11.4% women died of the dreaded condition, whereas in the second clinic, all staffed by midwives, mortality was only 2.7%. Women delivered at home also had a lower death rate. Semmelweis found no answer to this problem, until his friend Kolletschka died of fulminating systemic blood poisoning from a small scalpel wound, suffered during a postmortem examination. Necropsy of Kolletschka's body revealed the same pathological changes as those observed in women who had died of puerperal fever. The inspiration or revelation then came to Semmelweis that he and his students were examining women's wounded genitalia with hands that came directly from examining patients in autopsy and that just as Kolletschka had suffered, these women would die of poisons entering the body through the wounds. Midwives did not attend autopsies, and hence the rate of puerperal fever was much less in the second clinic. He therefore instituted a routine that all students and physicians who wanted to examine a patient had to scrub their hands in a chlorinated lime solution with clean sand until all odors from the autopsy room were removed. While in April 1847, 18% of all women died, the number fell to 2.38% in June 1847 and to 1.2% in July after the introduction of the hand scrubbing procedure. Semmelweis also insisted on hand scrubbing between each patient examination and on isolation of patients with open wounds to protect the others from airborne infections. However, his strict routine was resented and he was ridiculed; in 1851 he returned to Budapest, where his theories were only marginally more accepted.[4,13,25] He became increasingly despondent and died in a mental institution on August 13, 1865—ironically, of blood poisoning, a day after Lister had for the first time used carbolic acid in the treatment of a compound fracture, guided by the work of Pasteur on germs and airborne infection. As we have seen already, Lister initially suffered the same fate of rejection and ridicule but ultimately was given the recognition he deserved, and he became the first British surgeon elevated to peerage. In his writings he always gave full credit to Semmelweis, who had blindly applied principles of antisepsis to obstetrical and gynecological procedures some 18 years earlier.

Of special interest is the discovery of insulin, in part because of the role Frederick Grant Banting, a 29-year-old orthopedic surgeon, played in it.[4] While preparing for a lecture on the pancreas for students on October 30, 1920, he read an article in *Surgery, Gynecology and Obstetrics* by Dr. Moses Barrow of the University of Minnesota in which the author commented on the work of Minkowski and von Mering and suggested that if they had persevered in their efforts, a substance secreted by the pancreas that could alleviate diabetes mellitus might have been discovered. Barrow also pointed out the similarity in degenerative changes of the acinar cells of the pancreas with experimental ligation of the pancreatic duct and blockage by a gallstone. Banting had a hunch and wrote a note to himself that night: "Ligate the pancreatic duct of dogs. Wait 6 to 8 weeks for degeneration. Remove the residue and extract." He hoped to obtain an extract of the islet cells, free from the destroying influence of trypsin of the acinar cells that had slowly degenerated as a result of the ductal blockage.

Banting took his idea to professor John James Rickard MacLeod, head of the Department of Physiology at the University of Toronto, and met with a lot of resistance initially. In the spring of 1921, Banting repeated his request for laboratory space and animals and was granted both, together with a volunteer, Charles Best, who was about to graduate in the class of physiology and biochemistry. This was a fortunate choice. The two men became lifelong friends and made a superb team. On April 14, 1921, Banting and Best started their work to prove Banting's hunch or intuition. They tied the pancreatic ducts of a number of dogs, experienced many reverses, such as dissolution of the catgut ligature used initially, as well as infection and death of test animals. But at the end of July 1921 they were able to extract their precious substance from the shriveled pancreas with atrophied acinar cells and healthy islets of Langerhans. On the night of July 30, 1921, Banting and Best injected 5 ml of the extracted solution into a diabetic dog and found that blood sugar levels had been halved and the urine was free of any sugar.[4,13,25]

Alain Carpentier, the successor to the great tradition in cardiac surgery of Francois Gaudart d'Allaines and Charles Dubost of the Broussais Hospital in Paris, became intently concerned with valvuloplasty by plicating sutures in the early 1970s. A young child had died because the sutures used to narrow the mitral valve (then the accepted technique) had cut through the valvular annulus. Three months after this event, while crossing the entrance of the hospital on his way home, Carpentier suddenly had the answer: prosthetic rings of appropriate shape and size could remodel the valvular annulus and distribute the stress of the reconstruction to the multiple sutures used to maintain the ring in position. The prosthetic ring annuloplasty for the mitral and tricuspid valves was thus conceived and then realized after much experimental work.[9]

The impetus to expand pelvic celioscopy and diagnostic peritoneoscopy to therapeutic laparoscopy came from Philippe Mouret, who had trained as a general and gynecological surgeon and was practicing both specialties in Lyon with a heavy emphasis on pelvic endoscopic procedures. Since the earlier days of Professor Palmer in Paris there had been a great tradition of gynecological pelvic endoscopy in France, and Hubert Manhés from Vichy had performed the first cure of an ectopic pregnancy by celioscopic procedure in 1972.[28]

One day Philippe Mouret, while doing a pelvic endoscopy, had the inspiration to turn the celioscope "upward" (*vers le haut*) after having inspected the pelvis, and he was amazed at the potential for therapeutic laparoscopic procedures that literally lay before his eyes and suddenly entered the stage of conscious planning and experimental exploration.[27] The solutions in this case were based on an extensive experience in pelvic procedures and the intense interest of the surgeon to rise above a line connecting both anterior and superior iliac spines. After a suitable experimental and clinical preparation, Mouret performed a laparoscopic lysis of adhesions in 1972, a laparoscopic appendectomy in 1983, and the first laparoscopic cholecystectomy in 1987. As Edward Jenner, believing in his discovery, had inoculated his wife and children against smallpox early on, Mouret performed a laparoscopic appendectomy on his son very early in his experience with the procedure. His conviction was strong that this was the right way and that his family should not be deprived of this approach.[28]

The first laparoscopic appendectomy had been performed in 1980 and its report published in 1982 by Kurt Semm of Kiel, Germany, who at the time was severely criticized by some of his peers. He had based his approach as a gynecologist on a vast experience with pelviscopy (20,000 procedures performed between 1970 and 1992) and had created in a planned, systematic manner the instruments that would allow him to perform appendectomy. He then accomplished the first appendectomy after careful transition from designing and constructing instruments to using them clinically. Semm's approach was more by design than intuition.[41] At the time Mouret performed his first appendectomy, he was not aware of Semm's earlier achievement.

Discovery by a Combination of Some or All Modes

The conquest of pain is as important to the practice of surgery as are the treatment of wounds, the restoration of form and function, the control of bleeding, and the prevention or treatment of infection (see the box). However, it is difficult to assign a clear mode of discovery to one of the three original anesthetic agents or give pri-

---

THE SURGEON'S GOALS AND MEANS

To repair and heal wounds
To restore form and function
To control loss of blood and body fluids
To eliminate or reduce pain
To prevent or treat infection

---

ority for its clinical application to one of the four men who each claimed that honor individually. These men entered into an acrimonious debate rather than share a glory that would have given fame, respect, and honor to each one of them.[4,25,33]

In Britain, Humphrey Davy, studying the effects of nitrous oxide in 1800, Michael Faraday those of ether in 1818, and Henry Hill Hickman those of carbon dioxide in 1824, all came to the conclusion that these substances could abolish pain. No physician of their day recognized the importance of their findings. Samuel Guthrie, a physician-chemist of upper New York state, was distilling a "sweet whiskey" from chloride of lime and alcohol in 1831 at about the same time Soubeiran in France and Liebig in Germany independently developed the heavy, sweet, volatile "chloric ether," which was given the name chloroform in 1834 by Dumas, a French chemist. Even though Guthrie's 8-year-old daughter fell asleep while playing about a vat, chloroform's great promise escaped the country doctor's attention—an example of an unprepared mind.

Laughing gas parties and ether frolics, commonly held in the 1840s, were the demonstrations, albeit of popular science, that emboldened Long, Wells, and Morton to attempt anesthesia for patients undergoing surgical procedures by inhalation of these little-known gaseous compounds. As such, the mode of discovery by these three men could be a combination of design and intuition.

It is not my purpose to enter into arguments of priority, at the time muddled by patent claims and royalties—a situation not unlike the present state with HIV testing. Plus ça change, plus c'est la même chose.

Historically, physician Crawford Williamson Long (1815-1878) first used ether as an anesthetic in his practice in Jefferson, Georgia on March 30, 1842. Horace Wells (1815-1848), dentist, used nitrous oxide in his dental practice in Hartford, Connecticut as early as December 1844. William Thomas Green

Morton (1819-1868), a dentist and previous associate of Wells's, first demonstrated the use of ether at the Massachusetts General Hospital (October 16, 1846) on patient Gilbert Abbott, who was undergoing removal of a tumor of the jaw by Dr. John C. Warren. Later, Charles Thomas Jackson challenged Morton's contribution, suggesting that he had led Morton to experiment with highly purified ether, a fact that Morton had never disputed. But historically the credit of a discovery goes to the person who recognized a new concept and made it work. In this case the merit is clearly Morton's.[33]

The events described in this chapter stress the importance of the human mind and spirit, the willingness to work hard, and the ability to be curious, imaginative, and patient. The character traits of humility for dealing with success and accepting criticism, honesty in research, scientific discipline to admit contrary results, and scholarship and generosity to colleagues and patients are also important. No single human being possesses all of these ideal qualities; none of the scientists described in the previous pages held all of them. But many did enjoy a combination of the most essential traits and were willing to compensate throughout their careers for early cumbersome inadequacies. The scientist as a brilliant intellectual, somewhat detached from reality, is a popular conception that is quite unfounded.[29]

All of these scientists were well educated and solidly informed, although not on every detail of their ultimate discovery, especially if it happened by chance or intuition. Banting was not ignorant of his subject, but had he known every detail of previous work done he might well not have tried at all. Exacting criticism of one's own work, failure to record observations, excessive credence given to fixed ideas of senior investigators, and blind acceptance of "authoritative" observations can lead to total unproductivity. On the other hand, too much enthusiasm, ignorance of previous work, and intellectual arrogance may lead to costly duplication and inaccuracy.

Alfred Blalock summed it all up by saying, "Fortunate are those who have the proper combination of enthusiasm, critical judgment, and open mind."[7]

VERIFIABLE SCIENTIFIC METHODS AND RESULTS

We have seen how scientists and surgeons have contributed to progress in surgery, sometimes working in isolation from one another, more often as a cooperative group by exchange of information and skills or as a coherent, purpose-oriented, functional research team. In today's world, where high technology is often involved, a well-balanced team of surgeons, with scientists from other disciplines, is essential. Since the results of such a research group should ideally benefit patients, the clinicians who are part of the team should also be scientists, such as the surgeon-scientist that Dr. Joseph E. Murray described in his I.S. Ravdin Lecture at the Clinical Congress of the American College of Surgery on October 23, 1991.[29] Many role models for this title, past and present, join the list. With apologies to all possible candidates, two surgeon-scientists come to mind whose contributions have left a special memory of excitement with me and have given all of us the joy and pride to be surgeons. These are Alfred Blalock, who performed the first operation for treatment of an intracardiac defect and opened the way for the phenomenal developments in heart surgery since 1945,[23,34,44] and Joseph E. Murray, Nobel Prize recipient in medicine in 1990 for his basic science and clinical contributions to the first successful renal transplantation,[29] which since 1954 has given impetus to the present state of the art in kidney, liver, heart, lung, and pancreas transplantation (Fig. 8).

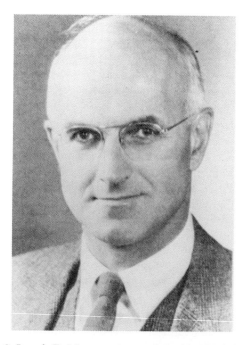

Fig. 8. Joseph E. Murray, winner of the 1990 Nobel Prize in Medicine.

Alfred Blalock (1899-1965) had earned his membership in the ranks of surgical scientists with his research and definitive contribution to the understanding and treatment of surgical shock during the "Vanderbilt years" (1925-1940) of his illustrious career. In a series of simple, even somewhat crude experiments by today's standards of sophisticated laboratory instrumentation, Blalock proved that surgical shock is caused by a decrease in circulating blood volume, not by the elaboration of toxins nor by reflex neurological mechanisms, theories that were proposed at that time.[44]

When he was presented in 1943 by Dr. Helen B. Taussig with the problem of cyanotic congenital heart disease, Blalock realized that his subclavian-to-pulmonary artery anastomosis—which he had done experimentally to study pulmonary hypertension long before it was recognized as a problem—might be the answer. He then showed in the laboratory that this operation would increase blood flow to the lungs and relieve cyanosis under experimental conditions. It took great courage, determination, and skill to make the first "blue baby operation" on November 29, 1944, a success, using the most primitive vascular instruments and very basic anesthetic support. This seminal step in the history of cardiac surgery has saved thousands of lives by leading to the development of techniques for mechanically redirecting blood to compensate for anatomical and physiological problems within the heart.[8,23,34,44]

The impetus that led to the first successful kidney transplantation also came from an internist, George W. Thorne at Peter Bent Brigham Hospital, who felt in the 1940s that hypertension in patients with Bright's disease could be cured if the diseased kidneys could be removed. Under the leadership of Francis D. Moore, Chief of Surgery, a broad experimental program was started and extended to human transplantation. David Hume performed a series of cadaveric renal transplants into the thighs of unmodified recipients; these transplants functioned for months during these early years of the program, and this gave the team at the Brigham some optimism about the clinical potential of transplantation.

The first successful kidney transplantation was the happy result of complete immunocompatibility between identical twins. In Dr. Murray's own words: "Dr. James B. Brown at Barnes Hospital in St. Louis, Missouri, stimulated by observations of skin allografts in burned patients, cross skin–grafted a pair of monozygotic twins and achieved permanent survival. By the 1950s I had developed in the dog a model renal transplantation operation that could maintain prolonged normal function. Thus the stage at the Brigham Hospital was set when identical twins, one healthy and the other in terminal uremia, were referred to Dr. John Merrill, our nephrologist.

"After extensive discussions with the patients and their families, and critical soul-searching by the team, a decision was made to remove a normal kidney from a healthy person, not for his own benefit but for someone else's. The immediate success of the transplanted kidney in December 1954 had a worldwide impact and demonstrated conclusively that organ transplantation under favorable circumstances could be lifesaving. The patient lived a normal life for 8 years until he succumbed to recurrence of the nephritis in the transplanted kidney. He married the recovery room nurse who had cared for him. Just last week we had a nostalgic luncheon with her, their two daughters, and the donor and his wife. All of them expressed gratitude and satisfaction for the whole experience. Incidentally, the donor, now 59 years old, has led a perfectly normal, healthy life with his one remaining kidney."[29]

Since this pioneering event, immunosuppressive drug therapy has made possible allografts of almost any human organ, to the extent that a major problem is not so much the surgical technique and creation of immunological tolerance, but the procurement of transplantable organs.

Besides their tremendous accomplishments, however, Drs. Blalock and Murray, like all other surgeonscientists, demonstrated a change in the approach to problem solving that is a major component of all progress in surgery: the experimental and scientific exploration of a health problem, followed by careful application to human patients—a reversal of the hippocratic sequence of the art and science of surgery to the science and craft or art of surgery of the modern era.[35,36]

Since their original laboratory work in which Blalock and Murray tested an idea by the experimental method, comparing results obtained by their approach to those found in controls, the research methodology has changed. For reasons of statistical validity, research, especially in the clinical areas, has to be accomplished through prospective, randomized, double-blind studies. Barring such sophisticated niceties, these two surgeonscientists demonstrated the principles of basic and clinical research—the scientific proof that sustains and drives the clinical art or craft. This proof is obtained through a scholarly approach, rigorous testing, and honesty in analyzing and interpreting the results. Above all, the end product has to be beneficial to the patient and should lead to new research projects.

ETHICAL AND CLINICAL ACCEPTANCE

The transfer of new knowledge to practical clinical implementation has to respect all ethical considerations and fulfill a clear goal of diagnosis or treatment or both. Throughout the history of surgery and medicine, an idea and its realization—as brilliant as they may be—have survived only if they were ethically acceptable and generally useful.

The trigger is at times a single patient or disease for which no other treatment is available, yet failure to treat would make matters worse. Such was the case for Paré's wound treatment, Blalock's blue baby operation, Murray's transplantation of a kidney from a healthy identical twin to his twin brother in renal failure, and a host of other achievements.

At other times a group of patients is involved, and the solution becomes a public health measure, often preventive in nature. Such were the vaccinations of Jenner and Pasteur, Lister's antisepsis, Semmelweis's serendipitous use of asepsis, Banting's and Best's discovery of insulin, and so many others. We have seen the need for surgeons to become more involved with solutions to public health problems of modern times: vehicular, industrial, and sports accidents and their prevention through safety measures; and violent crime and substance abuse and their prevention by eliminating the instruments of crime and abuse, along with providing the necessary education.

New diagnostic means almost invariably benefit large groups of patients, such as cytological studies of the uterine cervix and the application of the principles thus derived to other organs. The x-rays of Röntgen deserve their discoverer's original definition of "unknown" rays, since with time they revealed themselves to be beneficial in diagnosis and treatment if dosages were controlled, and deleterious if the exposure to them was unprotected. They are an early illustration of the modern dilemma with more and more invasive techniques for diagnosis, where the risk-to-benefit ratio has to be carefully evaluated, since a possible serious procedural complication could not be balanced against a potential therapeutic gain.

The transition from research to clinical trial in each institution is supervised by committees that follow strict, detailed federal guidelines of ethics, patients' rights, and actual benefit of the proposed diagnostic and/or therapeutic methods. Because of the continued uncontrolled

rise in health care costs in all industrialized countries, the concept of actual or real benefit will not only clearly estimate the advantages and harms, but will also incorporate the costs of our decisions into practice guidelines. For the qualitative idea of potential benefit will be substituted the quantative notion of actual or real benefit.[10] Such a transition presents a challenge for the future, not without some nostalgia for what seemed like a gentler past.

But the desire to protect the ethics and the actual benefit to patients may spin out of the profession's control and fall into the domain of bureaucratic and legalistic decision makers who have no real insights or competence in the doctor-patient relationship. A case in point is the explosively developing field of laparoscopic and thoracoscopic surgery, for which established surgeons have to do some reeducation and some retooling, with the understanding that the new technique does not entail changes in the actual anatomical performance of a given, established surgical operation, but only in the surgeon's approach through the abdominal and chest walls. Under the influence of sensational, poorly documented articles in the lay press, based on a total disregard of comparative statistics, some state regulatory agencies have introduced the notion of special credentialing.[1,2] This vitiates the smoothly functioning medical educational system by which surgeons learn from each other and help each other until a technique is mastered during their years of training and those of continued learning in practice, lasting a lifetime. That is not to say that the rodeo-like atmosphere, with surgical and legal bounty hunters, was not disquieting in the developing stages of these techniques and still is of some concern.

However, in today's world one could wonder who would or should have credentialed a Blalock, a Murray, or the many surgeons they taught worldwide, after these visitors returned home from their trips to Baltimore and Boston? In fact, it could be stated that Norman Shumway lost the well-deserved satisfaction of doing the first heart transplant, a technique on which he had worked with Lower in the laboratory since 1960, because the public environment was not ready in the United States when the first human cardiac transplant was performed by Christiaan Barnard in 1967 in Cape Town, South Africa.[45]

The recent controversy over the use of intravascular ultrasonography and the demand by insurers and government agencies for proof of performance and cost efficiency, without participating in the start-up expenses, is a good example of how progress can be slowed in the name of a good but poorly formulated and inappropriately applied cause. Will the hidden desire or misplaced zeal for saving on high-tech costs ultimately *increase* health care costs?[20]

The ethics of the transfer of new knowledge to human use and medical practice are well defined by Judeo-Christian moral traditions and, in fact, by the moral principles of all major religions throughout the world. For the practitioners of the science and art of healing they are reinforced by the hippocratic oath, freely consented to by all physicians. The discourse on ethics establishes principles of action for the scientist and physician. Since the time of the Babylonian ruler Hammurabi, who promulgated the code of regulatory laws named after him around 2000 BC, and throughout history, but especially in modern times, ethical precepts have been supported and enforced by the legal concept of human rights and responsibilities, individual or collective.[4,22]

Because of this we have to establish both the ethical and legal grounds in decisions of life and death and respect the wishes of the individual, with the exception of never giving a deadly drug or creating harm knowingly.[17] The twin principles of ethical and legal behavior will help society in solving present dilemmas, without violating the human aspect by a given decision, or the individual's rights, but understanding also that personal responsibility can have no substitutes.[22] Health care of the highest possible quality should be available to all, and the cost should be borne by a common effort of financial solidarity of all potential beneficiaries.

MATERIALS AND RESOURCES

The importance of the human factor—mind over matter—was given preference in the preceding pages. But it is quite certain that many of the discoveries would not have been possible without the availability of the necessary materials, the required financial resources, and the fiscal discipline by the public and political leadership to accept the cost of research and ensure equal distribution of health care. In fact, without a parallel evolution of the minds, the methods, and the means, no progress can occur in medical-surgical science and practice, just as in any of the other noble human endeavors.

The essential concurrence of ideas and materials in the development of surgical technology at any time period is easily demonstrated by historical comparisons. Trephining of the skull can be traced to prehistoric man. The Peruvian surgeons of the Paracas tribe developed great mastery and success during the first century, using knives of glasslike obsidian, stone, and bronze to trephine the skull in the treatment of skull fractures and relief of headaches and mental disease.[4] Yet despite good evidence that patients survived such practices, nobody would dispute the fact that mind and matter were harmoniously combined by Harvey Cushing (1869-1939) in developing techniques and the many fine stainless steel instruments to open and close the skull safely in the early 1900s—almost two millennia after the earlier crude attempts.[4,36]

Of the two topics that are the theme of this Congress, surgical stapling was developed in 1908 by Hültl of Hungary, because fine metal wires could be used and formed into B-shaped staples. The instrument maker Fischer was also able to create a device that would place rows of B-shaped staples through various mechanical transfers activated by the surgeon's hands. All of this would have been unthinkable when Benjamin Travers in 1812 and Antoine Lembert in 1826 described manual bowel sutures and John B. Murphy published his experience with a mechanical compression anastomotic button in 1892. Hültl's and Fischer's contributions were the result of methodical investigation and development to satisfy Hültl's desire to avoid peritoneal contamination by closing the bowel before transection. Later improvements—to satisfy increasing technical sophistication and aims—by various authors in the 1920s and the 1930s, the Moscow Institute for Surgical Instrumentation in the 1940s, and the first American manufacturer in the 1960s were all the result of systematic planning and development. While the clinical applications of Russian and American instruments by Ravitch and Steichen were all based on methodical research and transfer to human operations in carefully planned steps, the initial impetus for the functional end-to-end anastomosis—the anchor technique of early stapling methods—was a chance discovery based on comparison with the two-stage Mikulicz resection of colon cancer.[43]

Endoscopy of hollow viscera and various body cavities, known and practiced since the late 1800s, gained its present prominence because of significant simultaneous advances in light sources, optical systems, light conduction through fiberoptic bundles, and transmission of enhanced visual fields to television monitors, all advances that were quite unthinkable in the days of Hermann L.F. von Helmholtz (1821-1894), physicist and physician, inventor of the ophthalmoscope in 1850.[4] We have seen how the inspiration of Philippe Mouret to turn the celioscope upward rather than use it only in pelvic operations in 1968 led to the first laparoscopic lysis of adhesions for intestinal obstruction in 1972, appendectomy in 1983, and cholecystectomy in 1987. Kurt Semm's earlier appendectomy in 1980 evolved after careful planning and development of the necessary technology from a base of gynecological celioscopy.[12,27,28,30,41]

However, even the most brilliant mind, using sophisticated methods and state-of-the-art materials, cannot be productive without the *financial means* to sustain all of its aspirations for progress. Advances in any civilization are closely related to economic well-being. Once the Mediterranean shores and sea were home to Western civilization, after it moved along the trading and migration routes in Asia Minor and brought economic well-being to land routes and sea lane terminals. Medical care, often associated with religion and philosophy, was well-developed in ancient Egypt (3000-300 BC), Mesopotamia (2000 BC), and Greece (500 BC-500 AD), with the religious cult of Aesculapios, culminating in the work of Hippocrates, the "father of medicine," from the island of Cos (460 BC-366 BC) (Fig. 9). Galen (130-200 AD) (Fig. 10) traveled widely between Greece and Rome and left his imprint, for good and bad, on medicine for 1500 years. Much of the Greco-Roman medical knowledge was preserved and improved during the early Middle Ages by Arabic medicine—the

Persians Rhazes (865-925) and Avicenna (980-1037), and Syrians, Jews, and Christians writing in Arabic. This occurred at a time when Western Europe lay wasted from waves of barbaric invasions and epidemic plagues and the Moslem Arabs were in full military, political, and economic expansion across North Africa and into southern Spain and France.[4]

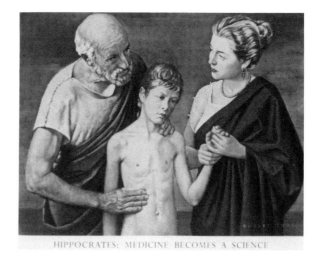

HIPPOCRATES: MEDICINE BECOMES A SCIENCE

Fig. 9. Hippocrates, the "father of medicine," 460-366 BC.

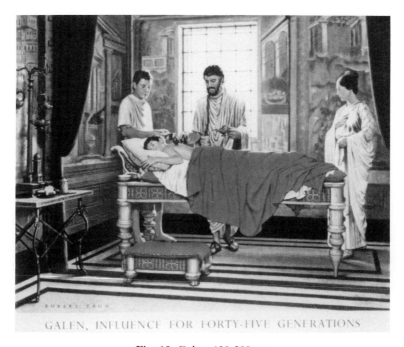

GALEN, INFLUENCE FOR FORTY-FIVE GENERATIONS

Fig. 10. Galen, 130-200 AD.

With the return to political stability (Charlemagne, 768-814; end of the Western caliphate, 1266; Venetian Republic, 820-1517), some of the great institutions of higher learning and medical schools were founded on the prosperous shores and lands of the Mediterranean sea: Bologna, 1158, Montpelier, 1180, Padua, 1222. It is therefore of more than passing interest that the three greatest medical texts ever written, laying the base of modern medicine, were authored by teachers and a student of Padua, part of the stable and prosperous Venetian Republic, during the Renaissance and its aftermath. The first was *De Humani Corporis Fabrica* (1543) by the Brussels-born innovator and master of anatomy Andreas Vesalius (1514-1564), professor of surgery and anatomy at the University of Padua (1537-1543) (Fig. 11).[13] *Exercitatio Anatomica de Motu Cordis et Sanguinis in Animalibus* (1628), a modestly printed book of 72 pages, was written by English physician and scientist William Harvey (1578-1657), a student at the University of Padua from 1597 to 1602; he graduated from Padua and Cambridge Universities in 1602. The discovery of the circulation of the blood established a new concept of the function of the human body and laid the groundwork of modern physiology.[13]

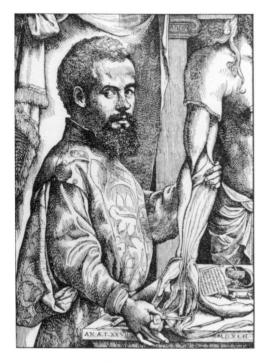

Fig. 11. Andreas Vesalius, 1514-1564, shown in this engraving at age 28 in 1543.

De Sedibus et Causis Morborum per Anatomen Indagatyis Libri Quinque (1761), a five-book, two-volume opus presenting 70 lectures and findings in 700 autopsies with commentaries, was assembled during some 50 years of teaching by Giovanni Battista Morgagni (1682-1771), professor of medicine and anatomy at the University of Padua (1711-1771). Morgagni is remembered as founder of a new branch in medical science—pathological anatomy.[13]

The three publications represent an orderly sequence of medical and scientific progress: from the anatomical form of the human body (Vesalius, 1543) to its physiological function (Harvey, 1628) and the results of malfunction of specific organs and tissues (Morgagni, 1761), there is a logical evolution.

With the discovery of America by Christopher Columbus in 1492 and later the development of the industrial revolution in the eighteenth century, economic and political preeminence moved west and north, from the shores of the Mediterranean to those of the Atlantic.[24]

The modern world has never remained without a medical mecca, often identified by the fact that it attracted "pilgrims" from all over the world, especially during the nineteenth century from the impatiently developing North American continent. During the first half of the nineteenth century this mecca was France, where clinicians had established the hospital as the center of medical teaching and research. The emphasis was on bedside observation and training and on astute clinical diagnosis and correlation with pathological findings; statistical techniques were introduced in clinical research.[24] Medical education was conducted in the tradition of such great clinical predecessors and contemporaries as Paré (1510-1590), Laënnec (1781-1826), Larrey (1766-1842), Dupuytren (1777-1835), Malgaigne (1806-1865), Broca (1824-1880), and Charcot (1825-1893).

However, the purely clinical approach to surgery and medicine—brilliant and original as it may have been then and still is now—has its limits, as all empiricisms have, unless it is enlarged by the input of basic biological sciences and experimental research. The reluctance of the French clinicians to include experimental investigation into their highly developed art or craft is the result of the separate evolution of hospital and university and is surprising, since the same academic environment had produced two of the greatest medical scientists of all times: Claude Bernard (1813-1878), physician, physiologist, and ironically, the author of *An Introduction to the Study of Experimental Medicine*, and Louis Pasteur (1822-1895).

This period in French medicine developed against a background of European political stability and the progressive economic well-being of the industrial revolution, only temporarily derailed by the revolution of 1848 and the Franco-Prussian war of 1870-1871, in retrospect a "regional" war although it laid some of the grounds for World War I.

After the middle of the nineteenth century, together with a growing economy, the momentum moved east, across the Rhine. The strength of this new approach was based on the use of experimental methods and the insight that basic science branches were indispensable to the understanding of disease. The homes for this movement were the universities, often with hospitals and laboratories side by side, in Germany, Austria-Hungary, and German-speaking Switzerland. Throughout the second half of the nineteenth century discoveries by German scientists, physicians, and surgeons attracted students from all over, especially the United States after the Civil War (1861-1865) but also England, Italy, Greece, Russia, Japan, and South America.[24] The list of discoveries and accomplishments includes the cell theory of Schleiden (1804-1881) and Schwann (1810-1882) and continued advances in physiology by Müller (1801-1858) and his pupils Helmholtz (1821-1894), du Bois-Reymond (1818-1890), of French extraction, and Carl Ludwig (1816-1895). The theory of cellular pathology was developed by Virchow (1821-1902), who besides a monumental contribution to pathology found the time to become a political opponent of Otto von Bismarck, the "iron" chancellor of Prussia. Julius Cohnheim (1839-1884) and Carl Weigert (1845-1904) advanced this work further through original contributions in experimental histology and pathology. Robert Koch (1843-1910) discovered the bacillus of tuberculosis in 1882 and proved that each infectious disease is caused by a specific microorganism.

In surgery, among the many outstanding clinics none was more famous than that of Billroth (1829-1894) in Vienna where the university remained a medical mecca until World War I.

Toward the end of the nineteenth century and especially after World War I, the tide turned west once more under the impetus of the returning American scientists, who accepted the experimental approach over simple observation and the effective role of the full-time teacher and investigator to accomplish the task. The modern American universities included medical education within their responsibilities around the turn of the century and provided a continuum of education and research in their basic laboratories and affiliated hospitals, sometimes by owning them outright.[24]

The flow of students changed at about the turn of the century with the emergence of the American university. What was a mere trickle before World War I became a steady stream between both wars and a torrent after World War II. Visitors from all over the world were coming to American medical schools and university hospitals to study and take home the new methods and progressive technology in neurosurgery, general thoracic surgery, cardiac surgery, radical cancer operations, and organ transplantation, as well as in the surgically related fields of anesthesia and resuscitation, a completely American creation of the mid-nineteenth century. I was a happy participant and grateful recipient of the educational bounty given so generously after World War II.

An example of this spectacular reversal is the professional life of Harvey W. Cushing (1869-1939), the Ohio-born, Yale- and Harvard-educated, Hopkins-trained pioneer of neurological surgery. Following his residency (1896-1900) under William S. Halsted (1852-1922), surgeon-scientist, innovator, and teacher par excellence, Cushing sailed in June 1900 to Europe, visiting Sir Victor Horsley (1857-1916) in London. Then at the University of Berne in Switzerland he became associated with Theodor Kocher (1841-1917), the Nobel Laureate, famous for his work on the thyroid, and worked in the laboratory of the physiologist Hugo Kronecker (1839-1914). His earlier interest in neurosurgery (nonexistent at the time as a specialty) then took a firm hold on Cushing after a conversation on the subject with Professor Kocher. By 1931, Cushing, now chief at the Peter Bent Brigham Hospital and Harvard University, had operated on 2000 patients with verified brain tumors and had established himself as an outstanding endocrinologist and surgeon of the pituitary and adrenal glands. By the time of his retirement in 1937 Dr. Cushing had literally educated and trained the neurosurgeons of the world, either directly or through his pupils and their pupils.[4]

In his book, *The Rise and Fall of the Great Powers*, Professor Paul Kennedy, historian at Yale University, suggests that there is a long-term relationship between economic development and productive capacity, and the position occupied by individual powers on the international scene.[19] He also makes the point that there is a clear correlation over a prolonged period between a great power's economic rise and fall and its growth and demise as an important political and military force. For a given power all of these relationships are relative, as compared with its neighbors. But their existence shows that it takes economic resources, the political responsibility on the part of the leaders to mobilize them, and in modern times, fiscal discipline on the part of the taxpayers to consent to their use, not only to support a military establishment, but also, preferably, a first-class education and health care system; scientific and artistic endeavors; healthy economic, military, and political statesmanship; and scholarship in philosophy and religion.

The flow of trade from the Mediterranean to the Atlantic and northwestern Europe from the sixteenth century onward and the relative shift of industrial productivity away from western Europe in the decades after 1890 are good examples of the changing balance of not only new military-political powers, but also thriving civilizations that have a high esteem for their scientists, artists, teachers, and doctors. A close correlation exists between a strong economy and flourishing activities in the healing arts and sciences, moving both in the same geographical direction as described previously. While a single event does not define a historical trend, one could wonder if the discovery and rapid expansion of videscopically guided surgical operations is one expression of new, unstifled scientific vigor in a Europe with a rising economic identity.[27]

It has been stated that while most great military power struggles have no intrinsic virtue, they do have some redeeming values in that they produce scientific advances and industrial improvements as fringe benefits. Inasmuch as war is an expression of vitality and drive, better results could be obtained by channeling these energies and resources into peaceful economic, scientific, and artistic competitions. Many mostly young, potentially productive lives would be saved. And while wars—cold or hot—produce no real winners and make both sides pay dearly,[18] the one nation that has to relent loses everything—to wit, the eclipse of the splendid German scientific establishment after World War I.

TRANSMISSION OF KNOWLEDGE

For a real scientific contribution to become progress it must not only resist critical laboratory investigation and be useful in clinical practice; it must also merit transmission to the next generations and demonstrate some staying power.

Norman Barrett's adage, "publish or perish," to characterize self-promotion in modern academia rather than the advancement of a worthwhile idea also has a literal

---

THE IMPORTANCE OF THE WRITTEN WORD

Publish or perish.
> N.R. BARRETT

VOX AUDITA PERIT, litera scripta manet.
> LATIN PROVERB

---

significance, inasmuch as verbal transmission usually perishes or becomes blurred (see the box).

The power of the written word was as important in Paré's contributions as were the contributions themselves. And since he was not able to do this in Latin, the accepted scientific language of his time, he wrote in simple, conversational French, comprehensible to all of his students, to guide them through apprenticeships and independent practice.

The example of John Hunter (1728–1793), called the founder of scientific surgery, is even more striking, since many of his biographies have stated that as a youth in Scotland he did not let a formal school regimen interfere with his education. His curiosity, intellectual drive, and powers of observation prepared John Hunter to become a self-taught scientist, acquiring some polish and discipline for his boundless energy during his early years through an association with his brother, William, a respected anatomist in London. John Hunter, ill at ease as a lecturer, attracted pupils such as Edward Jenner and Astley Paston Cooper more by the example of his life than by his spoken words. He introduced to the surgical world a system of thinking and observing based on scientific methods of gathering and judging the evidence. Besides his contributions to comparative anatomy, dentistry, and his great "Treatise on the Blood, Inflammation and Gunshot Wounds," Hunter left the world his monumental collection of 13,682 specimens of comparative anatomy, which was unfortunately reduced to some 1100 items by a direct bomb hit of the Royal College of Surgeons during the London blitz of 1940.[32]

From the earliest beginnings of transmission of empirical knowledge and then scientific proof, to the more formal teaching of students and training of apprentices, later residents in the hospital setting, teaching and training in modern times are most completely ensured by a balanced curriculum of basic and clinical sciences delivered in the laboratories and hospitals of a university. Here we find, ideally, men and women who are not only medical practitioners and scientists but also competent teachers and educators, with an optimal teacher-to-students ratio. The control of the teaching hospital by the university—ideally, its ownership by the academic institution—is essential, although unfortunately this has been threatened in recent times by practical financial considerations. While the full-time faculty concept was so successfully demonstrated at the Johns Hopkins University when it opened its doors in 1893 to highly qualified students who were interested in clinical excellence, research, and new ways of medical education, this model is endangered by today's fiscal and budgetary constraints in most places of higher learning.

To maintain excellence in teaching, training, and research, academic institutions must find ways to protect the time and activities of basic and clinical scientists alike from the intrusions of administrative overloads and unbalanced teaching and research responsibilities and find the necessary means to support all these activities, most often not or only minimally compensated by clinical activities. Fortunately these new stresses on the fabric of all institutions of higher learning are controlled through a patchwork of creative, at times innovative and unorthodox, funding. We can only hope that calmer seas will follow present waves of instability.

Finally, no idea or concept is valid unless it has been submitted to critical scientific evaluation and confirmation in the meetings and congresses of our professional societies, to frank and impartial discussion of qualities and deficiencies, and to the trial of practical application. The present Congress, beautifully organized, and encyclopedic on the subject of new technology in surgery, is a good example of this approach to the dissemination of knowledge.

PERSPECTIVE AND EXPECTATIONS

And now, let us imagine that Ambroise Paré has returned and is participating in this magnificent Congress. With his sixteenth century perspective, he would be immensely surprised but also inordinately proud of his successors. They give honor to his efforts for having elevated surgery from the hands of the barber-surgeons and the intrigues of the brothers of the College of St. Côme to the level of a masterful craft, inspired by his personal example and scholarly writings.

But after this initial astonishment Paré would soon realize that the basic goals of surgery, especially in wound care, have not changed. With the advent of manual and mechanical sutures the implementation of wound closure and intestinal anastomosis has become safer for the patient and technically easier for the surgeon. Paré would salute the developing endoscopic techniques as a fundamental contribution worthy of his own and those of Hunter, Lister, and Morton. Through these new techniques all the goals and means of the surgical act are addressed: minimal wounds, improved healing, reduced potential for infection, less postoperative pain, and earlier return to normal activities. Control of bleeding is secure and the loss of body fluids into large operative incisions is avoided.

But in an age when surgeons can repair and heal the wounds of man's inhumanity to man, repair or replace almost at will organs abused by disease, and restore to form and function children born with congenital malformations—all achievements that Paré would have attributed to God or the gods of pagan days—he would realize that the modern lifestyle has created a malaise that did not exist in his days because of lower expectations then. The God of today has surrendered the scientific secrets of earlier days but has kept control of what has always been a sacred prerogative: the right for each human being to live and die, protected by a divine code of ethics and morality. Paré would agree that doctors should give no deadly drugs, but he would also feel with his colleagues these dilemmas: when life does not yet exist, the early course of reproduction can be interrupted for valid reasons, and when life has become meaningless, it should not be prolonged by extraordinary means. In an age of seemingly limitless scientific and technological possibilities providing the sick and their families with high hopes, he would be concerned about the increasing disparity between available resources and rising demand: unequal levels of health care, futile efforts at resuscitation and misuse of high-tech procedures without actual benefit, and the discrepancy between the need for and availability of donor organs for transplantation.

Based on the past progress in surgery, Paré could confidently predict solutions to organ procurement through the use of animals that are genetically similar to humans and especially through the continued development of artificial organs. He could also conceive of advances in the treatment and cure of two major ills, cancer and atherosclerosis, not so much by surgical means alone, but rather by preventive measures and control of etiological agents and causes. He would strongly urge programs of early cancer detection and the effective use of proven traditional treatment modalities, while the

---

ADAPTED AND UPDATED FROM THE WRITINGS OF AMBROISE PARÉ

Je l'ai pansé, je l'ai guéri
   Que Dieu nous accompagne!
I dressed his wounds and restored his health
   May God be at our side!

EXPECTATION

Je l'ai pansé, je l'ai guéri
   Dieu est-il toujours notre compagnon?
I dressed his wounds and restored his health
   Is God still our partner?

PERSPECTIVE

"magical" chemical or immune "bullet" is being developed through basic and clinical research.

Being a real believer in and imbued by a sense of social justice, he would once more counsel his fellow surgeons to strive for and reach the highest moral and ethical grounds—symbolically God's conscience in each human being (see the box). And he would pray that this God be at our side on this extended journey into an uncertain future: "Que Dieu nous accompagne!"

Or would he be concerned that mankind has lost its soul to technology, abandoned its mind to the computer, sacrificed compassion to efficiency, and surrendered originality and courage to conformity? And would he therefore worry that humanity, created in the image of God, has abandoned its noble destiny? "Dieu est-il toujours notre compagnon?"

REFERENCES

1. Altman LK. Surgical injuries lead to new rule. New York Times [Metro], June 14, 1992.
2. Altman LK. When patient's life is price of learning new kind of surgery. New York Times [Medical Science], June 23, 1992.
3. Barter JF. The life and contributions of Doctor George Nicolas Papanicolaou. Surg Gyn Obstet 174:530-532, 1992.
4. Bender GA, Thom RA. Great moments in medicine, Parke Davis & Co and Detroit Northwood Institute Press, 1966.
5. Bernard C. Introduction à l'Etude de la Médecine Expérimentale. In Bourquin C, ed. Geneva: Editions du Cheval Ailé, 1945.
6. Binet JP. L'Acte Chirurgical. Editions Odile Jacob. Paris, 1990.
7. Blalock A. The nature of discovery. Ann Surg 144:289-301, 1956.
8. Blalock A. The expanding scope of cardiovascular surgery. Br J Surg 42:3, 1954.
9. Carpenter A. Biological tissues and surgical issues. Bull Am Col Surg 77:13-16, 1992.
10. Eddy DM. Medicine, money and mathematics. Bull Am Col Surg 77:36-49, 1992.
11. Ellis H. Cases from out of the past: Howard Florey—the first clinical use of penicillin. Contemp Surg 40:42-44, 1992.
12. Flowers JL, Zucker KA, Imbembo AL, Bailey RW. Laparoscopic cholecystectomy. Surg Rounds 4:271-282, 1991.
13. Garrison FH. An Introduction to the History of Medicine. Philadelphia: WB Saunders Co, 1929.
14. Jude JR, Kouwenhoven WB, Knickerbocker GG. A new approach to cardiac resuscitation. Ann Surg 154:311-319, 1961.
15. Jude JR. Rediscovery of external heart compression in Dr. William Kouwenhoven's laboratory. In Safar P, Elam J, eds. Advances in Cardiopulmonary Resuscitation: Historical Vignettes. New York: Springer-Verlag, 1975.
16. Jude JR. Personal communication, September 10, 1992.
17. Kass LR. "I will give no deadly drug." Bull Am Col Surg 77:6-17, 1992.
18. Kennan GF. The GOP won the Cold War? Ridiculous. New York Times, October 28, 1992, p LA21.
19. Kennedy P. The Rise and Fall of the Great Powers. New York: Random House/Vintage Books, 1987.
20. Kolata G. When doctors say yes and insurers no. New York Times [Business]. August 16, 1992.
21. Kouwenhoven WB, Jude Jr, Knickerbocker, GG. Closed-chest cardiac massage [Landmark Perspective]. JAMA 173:1064-1067.
22. Long M. L'Ethique Médicale, Le Corps Médical (Luxembourg) 19:666-676, 1991.
23. Longmire WP Jr. Alfred Blalock, His Life and Times. Private Printing, Author, 1991.
24. Ludmerer KM. Learning to Heal—the Development of American Medical Education. New York: Basic Books, 1985.
25. Lyons AS, Petrucell RJ. Medicine, An Illustrated History. New York: Harry N Abrams, 1978.
26. Mason ML. Joseph Lister—hospitalism and the antiseptic principle. Q Bull NW Univ Med Schl 33:2, 1959.
27. Mouret P. A look into the future of minimally invasive surgery and new technology. Congress on Minimally Invasive Techniques and New Technology, Luxembourg, September 12, 1992.
28. Mouret P. Personal communication, September 12, 1992.
29. Murray JE. The role of surgeon-scientists in medical progress. Bull Am Col Surg 77:22-28, 1992.
30. Nogueras JJ, Wexner SD. Laparoscopic colon resection. Perspect Col Rectal Surg 5:79-97, 1992.

31. Nuland SB. The Most Expert Chirurgeon, Ambrose Paré. Birmingham, Ala: Classics of Surgery Library, Gryphon Edition, 1984.
32. Nuland SB. Nature's High Priest—John Hunter. Birmingham, Ala: Classics of Surgery Library, Grypon Edition, 1985.
33. Nuland SB. The Origins of Anesthesia. Birmingham, Ala: Classics of Surgery Library, Gryphon Edition, 1988.
34. Ravitch MM. The contributions of Alfred Blalock to the science and practice of surgery. Johns Hopkins Med J 140:57-67, 1977.
35. Ravitch MM. The American Surgical Association, the peaks of excitement. Ann Surg 192:282-287, 1980.
36. Ravitch MM. Century of surgery, 1880-1980, Philadelphia: JB Lippincott, 1981.
37. Safar P. Initiation of closed-chest cardiopulmonary resuscitation: basic life support. A personal history. Resuscitation 18:7-20, 1989.
38. Safar P. From back pressure-arm lift to mouth-to-mouth control of airway and beyond. In Safar P, Elam J, eds. Advances in Cardiopulmonary Resuscitation: Historical Vignettes. New York, Springer-Verlag, 1975, pp 266-275.
39. Safar P. History of cardiopulmonary-cerebral resuscitation. In Kaye W, Bircher N, eds. Cardiopulmonary Resuscitation. New York: Churchill Livingstone, 1989, pp 1-53.
40. Safar P. Personal communication. September 11, 1992.
41. Semm K. Endoscopic appendectomy. Paper presented at Congress on Minimally Invasive Surgery and New Technology, September 1992, and personal communication, September 11, 1992.
42. Sladen A. Closed-chest massage: Kouwenhoven, Jude, Knickerbocker [Landmark Perspective]. JAMA 251:3137-3140, 1984.
43. Steichen FM, Ravitch MM. Stapling in Surgery. Chicago: Year Book Medical Publishers, 1984.
44. Thomas VT. Pioneering research in surgical shock and cardiovascular surgery. Philadelphia: University of Pennsylvania Press, 1985.
45. Naef AP. The Story of Thoracic Surgery. Toronto: Hogrefe & Huber Publishers, 1990, p 501.

2 Philosophy and Rationale in the Development of Surgical Techniques

Francescopaolo Mattioli

When I was a youngster, I attended a rock-climbing school. I had no fear while I was climbing, yet when I watched my fellow climbers I was terrified. I again had that uncomfortable sensation when I first saw a video tape on laparoscopic surgery. Today I perform this new surgical technique, but the long experience and proficiency acquired through daily practice have not relieved the anxiety and preoccupation associated with approaching something entirely new. I experience precisely the same feelings that I had when I performed my first operation, a hernia repair.

When I was asked to prepare this paper, my thoughts returned to the beginning of my surgical career; I felt that to reflect together on who we are as surgeons, on surgery, and on the consequences of surgery, from a philosophical as well as a pragmatic viewpoint, reviewing the newly developed techniques and the evolving technologies, could be of interest and benefit to us all.

Surgery has seen continuous technical progress over the last 100 years. However, the last few decades have witnessed the explosion of advances in technology more than in new techniques. In turn, advanced technology has led to the development of original operative procedures—some of them radical departures—that are replacing others that had previously been considered satisfactory. As is peculiar of the modern age, these changes are extremely rapid in "real time," as we say. Often they challenge our ability to absorb and apply them, leaving us with neither the time nor the patience to evaluate their importance or to forsee their positive or negative consequences. It is also hard to predict their effect on the surgical staff and their environment. To

24

better understand these problems, we should briefly analyze the elements of the trinomial: the surgeon, the art and science of surgery, and the new surgical techniques.

THE SURGEON

All of us are aware of who we are and what we do, so it may be pleonastic to reiterate the concept. However, in this case I must ask your indulgence; sometimes repeating what is obvious can assist ones reasoning process, making it possible to reach solutions and conclusions more quickly.

The Greek words *cheir* and *ergon* explain who the surgeon is: one who works with his hands. It does not mean that he impersonates the famous arm controlled by someone else's mind. Everyone knows that an individual's hands are an extension of his or her cerebral activity and that it is precisely the hand that differentiates humans from their close animal relatives. The hand of the pianist, of the painter, of the sculptor, the hand of the creator of the Sistine Chapel, the hand of the surgeon translate thought to deed. In this era of technicism, it may seem rhetorical to continue to compare surgical work with that of an artist. However, an intense mental activity is always present behind our manual efforts, even when surgery seems a matter of routine and practiced movements.

Creativity, imagination, and reasoning are always the basis, the essential premise of a good surgeon; manual ability and proficiency are equally fundamental. In 1888 Theodor Billroth wrote that a surgeon should combine both a Dionysian and an Apollonian nature. Surgeons, like any other artists, are in a "Dionysian" state of mind when they conceive an endeavor but must have a complete control over their manual technique to fulfill their intellectual concepts. These attributes may seem academic, philosophical, and distant from reality. But there are other attributes, other conditions that determine the surgeon's caliber and that today constitute perhaps what can be summarized by an obsolete and outmoded term: *vocation.*

We have all met surgeons who did not like to operate and for whom any excuse was good enough to stay out of the operating room. However, it is necessary to feel pleasure when operating, almost a physical pleasure, which has led psychiatrists to develop strange and questionable theories about what compels one to become a surgeon. Obviously, they entertain distorted and exaggerated views; however, there is undoubtedly such a thing as surgical sensuality: the physical contact with the object of one's theoretical studies, the object of one's

imagination. It is the pleasure of anatomical confirmation, the pleasure of weaving the cloth precisely as we designed it: the surgeon's senses.

Pleasure, then, and often ambition in the noblest sense of the word, are inherent—but none of this without courage. A surgeon must be someone who is able to worry, someone who understands fear. The surgeon's courage is to venture forth as far as possible, fully conscious of the human being facing him.

A surgeon is a physician who cures with his hands, but also with his mind and heart. The objective is the recovery of the patient through an act that must be at the same time necessary and beneficial, at the cost of being difficult.

The concept of courage is fundamentally a concept of surgical ethics. A surgeon is always a scientist, because he or she observes, classifies, and interprets. The surgeon must always be a teacher, so that others may learn and pass on this science in continuous progression.

ART AND SCIENCE OF SURGERY

Many bridges have been crossed since the days when surgery was a manual cure for external lesions and considered a poor alternative to the far more noble field of internal medicine. Besides an art, surgery has become a science, a very complex science that is rapidly progressing. It has become an integral and essential part of all medical science, and it is only right that in Italy the M.D. degree has kept its double denomination of "medicine and surgery," precisely to underscore that surgery is essential in medical training. Actually, surgery has become a multidisciplinary science, which is why it has recorded such spectacular progress and become an essential part of general medical studies.

The merging of the surgeon's charisma, imagination, creativity, intelligence and technique with knowledge, which is a continually expanding process, provided the spark that gave surgery its well-known characteristics and allows us to hypothesize unpredictable future developments.

Surgery has become an enormous field of study, a central subject that links many different branches. However, continual expansion and constant probing into the various sectors have created and are still creating an opposite effect: specialization. Specialization is unquestionably inevitable and can even be positive if the general sense of surgery is preserved. That is within a strategy that unites all surgical specialties, integrating the various fields and preventing dispersion. Inversely, it is easy to fragment the discipline, hence generating a negative event through the loss of the multidisciplinary vision distinctive to modern general surgery.

Considerable effort at various levels is required to safeguard this general goal. Many say that there are too many congresses being held. I claim, however, that these are needed because they may represent the only way to keep relationships open not only between the different branches of surgery but even within the framework of general surgery itself. The difficulty in keeping up to date and in remaining interested in the various fields compels one to favor some at the expense of others. Conventions often rekindle old interests and one's desire to emulate and therefore play the important role of bringing and keeping together a discipline that would otherwise fall prey to strong centrifugal tensions. It is precisely surgical charisma together with knowledge that leads to new techniques and technological developments in the surgical field that could in turn provide additional stimulus to superspecialization.

NEW SURGICAL TECHNIQUES

New techniques and new technologies are not one and the same. New techniques are created by surgeons—by their experience, by their resourcefulness, by their studies of physiopathology, by their experimenting. New technologies are generally a consequence of new techniques; however, new technologies often originate outside surgery and are applied therein by virtue of a variety of needs and demands for progress.

Surgeons are accustomed to innovation: every patient is different, every surgeon is different; operations always present something new and original. It is well established that repetition tires the surgeon and can lead to errors. Variety, innovation, and changes stimulate the surgeon's attention and therefore his or her operative excellence.

Surgeons constantly renew and update their technique as their experience grows, acquiring additional knowledge of pathogenesis and physiopathology and trying new materials and/or instruments. Applying new techniques always implies speculation, experimentation, and testing on the patient, which presents problems of ethics and informed consent that are not always easily solved. New techniques require confirmation of their validity through controlled trials and discussion during congresses.

Many techniques and surgical procedures have ap-

peared, but not all have been proved valid; today many procedures are only of historical and speculative value. Generally a new technique creates a new surgical treatment for a disease that had been treated differently until then. Sometimes a new technique generates better results than previous ones or provides an alternative. There are times when new techniques lead to the design of new instruments and equipment; other times it is the new equipment, perhaps designed in an experimental laboratory, that affects surgical technique by facilitating variants or even totally new procedures.

There are two definitions of technology in the dictionaries. The first is the noblest: "The science devoted to the practical rules of the various arts, sciences and professions and of their subsequent advancements." The second is less idealistic, but more closely related to modern reality: "The study of the procedures and equipment necessary for the transformation of a given matter into an industrial product." The first definition carries with it the concept of art and of the means capable of perfecting it, whereas the second stresses the concept of the practical use of raw material and subsequent profit. In other words, a surgical stitch can be perfected by technology to achieve an improved end-product and, at the same time, this same surgical stitch could represent the raw material capable of being transformed into an industrial product. This is the business of biomedical technology, an extremely important phenomenon from many viewpoints, both positive and negative. On the positive side: the motivation to experiment, the drive to improve available techniques, the inclusion of the surgeon in mostly international trials, the support—even financial—of a series of initiatives facilitating research: congresses, continuing education, residencies, surgical training. Among the negative aspects are the extreme consequence of the positive aspects I have just mentioned, the excessive incitement in particular. The infinitive "to press," besides other meanings, also carries the sense of "to instigate or to pressure continuously and insistently," and the adjective "pressing" also implies the concept of urgency, as in "pressing business." Technology can become pressing for surgeons, who can be pressured by their own instincts to attempt adventure, to apply innovation, to be modern and up to date. To exploit a surgeon's competitive spirit, to not be less than his or her competitors, to be faster than the others; to exploit the desire to improve a professional position. There are times when even the press is involved: an Italian daily newspaper boasting a large circulation recently published an article on videolaparoscopic cholecystectomy under the heading "Ol ed il calcolo se ne va" (Say hey and your stone will go away). Negative aspects; fortunately, amply compensated by the true expression of new technology: progress.

Still, there is one more aspect that deserves to be considered that can threaten anything new in the surgical environment, especially in the sphere of advanced technology, and that happens not solely in the surgical domain: politics. In a recent collection of articles by journalist Giovanni Ansaldo, a leading article from 1934 tells of the outbreak of cholera in Genoa, in 1854. At that time there were two schools of thought, the "contagionists" and the "anticontagionists." The first, Ansaldo reports, "Held true the old teaching that cholera was a disease of Asian origin, transmissible by contagion, meaning the direct contact of the ill with the healthy. . . . The route of infection, carriers, form of contamination were unknown, since Pasteur was still a student at this time." The others, the anticontagionists, disbelieved that cholera was spread through contact. They thought that cholera was an endemic disease occurring in certain people as a consequence of alimentary disorders and excesses, such as overdrinking and overeating.

The contagionists, being traditionalists in science, were reactionary, or to say the least, conservative in everything else. Their proclamation that to defend the country against cholera it would be necessary to seal off its borders was in keeping with the overall approach of the tyrannical government in power at that time. The aim was to keep nations separated by impeding the passage of people, books, and ideas. Not only did contagionists fear the spread of cholera, but other forms of contagion as well—especially those brought on by impassioned words and audacious purposes. Interestingly, in 1854 the most stringent quarantine enforcers were the Russian Empire and the Kingdom of Naples and the most committed contagionists were Czar Nicholas I and the Bourbon King.

Ansaldo relates that the anticontagionists all believed in free trade, supported the usefulness of speedy communications between countries, and devoted their efforts to making it possible for people, books, ideas, and formulas to cross borders as quickly as possible. The remedies they proposed to prevent the spread of cholera had a flavor of "illuminism" and "progressivism": gut out the old cities, tear down the old neighborhoods,

teach the people how to wash and how to take laxatives. They believed that all of these things could fight the spread of cholera, and those concepts combined very well with their tastes and progressivist and humanitarian ideals. As Ansaldo puts it, "A different concept of cholera, a different concept of life, a matter of words, a matter of politics."

Having dissected the elements of our trinomial—actually a polynomial, since besides surgeons, surgery, and new techniques we picked up new technology along the way—let us now try to put them back together again. Research, teaching, training are not the institutional duties of university surgeons only but of other surgeons as well, regardless of their affiliation. These are the duty of all physicians. There are surgeons who are excellent technicians, but their work is somewhat sterile with respect to "surgery," within quotation marks. I believe that this should be pointed out to the new generation, who often prefer the technical and applicative aspects of the surgical art. Surgery, new techniques, new technology: one could build an algorithm revealing the interactivity and interdependence of these three components: surgery creates new techniques, and it is not infrequent that new techniques create more new techniques, or perhaps modifying preexisting techniques for the sake of adaptation. For example, the Billroth II gastroenteroanastomosis using a linear stapler transforms an end-to-side gastrojejunal anastomosis into a side-to-side one. There are many similar examples.

Do new technologies also change the time honored and proven principles of surgical procedures? It would appear so, although we still have no idea whether this is an advantage. A current example: Endoscopic transduodenal approach to the choledocus has made it easy to perform a papillotomy and to remove biliary stones through this pathway. In many cases this has made preoperative radiomanometry and surgical treatment of common duct stones redundant. In laparoscopic cholecystectomy most surgeons choose to omit radiomanometry, which is optional, and to neglect the length of the cystic duct stump. It will probably be demonstrated that until now we have believed in dogmas that were either untrue or unimportant. However, given current conditions, it is a matter of concern to watch the sacrifice on the altar of technology of the principles on which we used to base viable surgical techniques.

As always, what is needed are practical implementation and decanting of data: Many uninspiring techniques have later become well-established procedures, and apparently solidly established procedures have failed the trial of time.

New techniques, new technology, advanced technology—so much for a surgeon to stay abreast of. Every day there is something new; a moment's distraction could mean missing the latest novelty. New suturing materials, artificial implants, mechanical staplers, ultrasound scalpels, laser scalpels, endoscopic surgery, videolaparoscopic surgery, radioimmunoguided surgery, transplant techniques, artificial organs, and on and on and on. Should a surgeon know how to do everything? The categorical reply is: the surgeon must know everything, must accept everything in advance, without refusing innovation, must separate everything that is useful from what is not or from what is even harmful.

Then, as always, there are those who prefer one type of surgery, others who prefer another. It is especially important not to use innovation as a "phosphorescent dye" at the service of one's self-regard. There is no surgeon who is first-class simply because he or she disposes of advanced techniques or technologies. A surgeon can be first-class even if he works with his hands, bare handed. When Ton That Tung proposed his classic hepatic digitoclasty, a number of Western surgeons refused to employ this technique because they felt it was primitive and manual. They were wrong: one should never forget that a surgeon's main instrument is his hands, even when he is holding sophisticated instruments.

The circle is thus closed: we started out with a man tempting the unknown, conquering his fear with the power of his hands and his mind, then everything—surgical science, technique, technology—returns and takes shape in the human surgeon. Human-surgeon, always alone facing another human, the patient, and confronted by conscience, forever ready to violate the boundaries between life and death, armed with his *virtude*, in the words of Dante. "Virtude" means courage, power, passion, love. The surgeon is sustained, at all times and in spite of everything, by his desire to discover his limits beyond those pillars of Hercules, which in the end are the ultimate threshold of life.

3   *Essential Concepts and Skills in Laparoscopic Surgery*

J. Barry McKernan

Since the time it was first performed in France in 1987[1,2] and in the United States in 1988,[3] laparoscopic cholecystectomy has been adopted by medical centers, general surgeons, and patients with astounding rapidity. Numerous articles involving series of several hundred to more than 1000 patients have appeared that detail favorable results with laparoscopic cholecystectomy.[4-9] The rate at which other traditional open procedures are being adapted to a laparoscopic approach is phenomenal. Laparoscopic inguinal hernia repair,[10,11] appendectomy,[12,13] highly selective vagotomy,[14,15] and antireflux procedures[16-18] have all been reported in the literature, and with the increasing availability of instruments specific for laparoscopic surgery, it appears as if the future holds no boundaries for this approach.

Despite the enthusiastic reception given to laparoscopic surgery, it is essential to remember that this area is one of evolving knowledge and skills. As the general surgical community struggles with issues raised by the rapid, widespread acceptance of operative laparoscopy, such as training and accreditation and demonstration of principles comparable with those of traditional techniques, we as practicing surgeons must keep our primary focus on safeguarding the well-being of our patients. This can best be achieved by keen attention to the three basis tenets of surgery:

- Patience in the approach
- Finesse in the execution
- Respect for fundamental principles

These tenets refine our focus and remind us that we cannot afford to rush, but should instead be committed to a very deliberate, planned approach. This is particularly true in laparoscopic surgery, where it is essential that structures be systematically and cautiously delineated until the anatomy is absolutely clear. Furthermore, proficiency with the use of the videoscope and all accessory instruments is critical to prevent complications. This article will outline the fundamentals that are necessary to perform successful laparoscopy and will detail the training philosophy adopted at our center for teaching and training surgeons so they can perform laparoscopic surgical procedures.

FUNDAMENTAL PRINCIPLES OF LAPAROSCOPIC SURGERY

To be adept at performing intra-abdominal or thoracic surgery under endoscopic observation, projected onto video monitors, it is essential that surgeons be proficient in the following areas:

- Bimanual surgical operative skills
- Endoscopic knot-tying techniques
- Use of angled scopes

It bears repeating that successful completion of any procedure demands an intimate knowledge of the anatomy of the region. Because the operative field is restricted with laparoscopic surgery as compared with traditional open surgery, careful and methodical visual exploration and gentle dissection are of paramount importance to avoid unnecessary complications. In accordance with this philosophy, some surgeons advocate intraoperative cholangiography for every patient undergoing laparoscopic cholecystectomy to delineate the common duct and to avoid operative injury to the bile ducts.[19,20] We rely on an intraoperative cholangiogram to detect stones in the common duct and to determine the length and course of the cystic duct only in those cases in which dissection of the cystic duct–common duct junction proves difficult.

Bimanual Surgical Skills

In performing our first laparoscopic cholecystectomy in June 1988, we employed a two-handed technique.[3] Although no surgical procedure is absolutely fail safe, having now used this technique in numerous laparoscopic procedures, I am convinced that bimanual surgery is the approach of choice, particularly for difficult cases. In addition to allowing the surgeon ultimate control, bimanual surgery affords a greater degree of safety and accuracy by providing excellent visualization and control of vital structures. We have also successfully applied the bimanual approach to a variety of operative laparoscopic procedures, including appendectomy, inguinal hernia repair, Nissen fundoplication, highly selective vagotomy, colectomy, and intestinal adhesioly-

sis. In particular, this technique facilitates dissection since one hand can be used to manipulate the tissue via grasping forceps, while the other hand can operate the scissors, electrocautery, or an irrigator-aspirator.

Endoscopic Knot-Tying Techniques

As more and more conventional procedures are being adapted to a laparoscopic approach, endoscopic suturing and ligating techniques—along with the necessary attendant instrumentation—for abdominal and thoracic surgery have been developed and refined. Adeptness with the following suturing and knot-tying techniques is necessary in performing laparoscopic surgery: ligature loop, endoligature with extracorporeal or intracorporeal knotting, sling suture, and continuous suture. An excellent review of these techniques has recently been published.[21]

Use of Angled Scopes

Angled scopes (e.g., 30-degree and 45-degree) maximize visualization of the operative field, and their use is particularly helpful in performing advanced gastric and intrathoracic videoscopically guided procedures. For example, in performing laparoscopic surgery for duodenal ulcer or gastroesophageal reflux disease, angled scopes facilitate activities on the posterior aspects of the stomach or esophagus. We also use a 45-degree scope when performing an inguinal hernial repair laparoscopically to dissect the peritoneum from the rectus muscle and to expose the internal ring and indirect sac, if present.

TRAINING IN SURGICAL LAPAROSCOPY

To perform operative laparoscopy safely and competently demands that surgeons develop considerable skills with a variety of nontraditional surgical instruments and operative techniques. As the first stage in educating surgeons who have no laparoscopic experience, our center mandates that they complete a basic course along with hands-on experience in diagnostic laparoscopy. Next they participate as camera operators, assistants, and surgeons under the guidance of a preceptor before performing operative laparoscopy procedures as the surgeon of record. This experience includes 25 to 50 diagnostic laparoscopies under direct supervision by a surgical preceptor. Following satisfactory completion of this initial orientation to laparoscopy, the surgeon is then trained to perform surgical laparoscopic procedures. This training consists of two phases. The first phase takes place in a simulation laboratory, where surgeons are given ample opportunity to practice the techniques used in laparoscopic surgery until they can execute them perfectly. The objective of this inanimate laboratory training is to provide an environment for the practice of endoscopic instruments used for grasping, tissue manipulation, and application of clips, ligatures, or staples, along with cutting and dissecting techniques. Repetition, coupled with a nonthreatening learning environment, promotes the development of dexterity with the exceptionally long instruments used in laparoscopy. Furthermore, it permits the surgeon to become comfortable with remote operations using video observation. Use of laparoscopic instruments with video observation requires a complete reorientation of both tactile and visual skills. The entry port into the abdomen acts as a fulcrum and causes movements to appear reversed; further disorientation of the field in the form of diminution or magnification may occur based on the distance of the telescope objective lens from the observed structure.

The second phase of training involves applying the skills used in the inanimate laboratory to surgery in live animals after adequate skills in the simulation laboratory have been demonstrated. The pig is the animal model of choice for laparoscopic cholecystectomy because of the similarity in choledochal anatomy to that of humans. Other institutions have also advocated that training in laparoscopic surgery include both didactic instruction and hands-on experience with live animals.[22,23]

Following laboratory and clinical training in both diagnostic and operative laparoscopic procedures, it is still necessary for the surgeon to gain experience in humans by assisting another surgical team in performing a procedure. Our center also requires surgeons to receive instructions during at least five operations on humans before being permitted to perform the specific laparoscopic procedure at our facility. We believe that this comprehensive training and accreditation process for laparoscopic surgery is absolutely necessary to ensure the safety of the patient.

CONCLUSION

The laparoscopic cholecystectomy procedure heralded an innovative era in general surgery. The remarkable advantages of laparoscopic surgery in terms of diminished postoperative pain and disability, shorter hospitalization, and quicker recovery have stimulated widespread and rapid dissemination of the technique and have defied attempts at controlled, randomized studies. It is imperative, however, that we not be blinded by the benefits of operative laparoscopy and lose sight of the fact that the patients' safety remains of paramount importance. We must adhere to the basic precepts of our general surgical training and insist that the outcome for all laparoscopic surgical procedures be, at a minimum, comparable with that of conventional open techniques.

REFERENCES

1. Mouret P. La chirurgie coelioscopique. Evolution ou revolution? Chirurgie 116:829, 1990.
2. Dubois F, Icard P, Bewrthelot G, et al. Coelioscopic cholecystectomy: Preliminary report of 36 cases. Ann Surg 211:60, 1990.
3. McKernan JB, Saye WB. Laparoscopic general surgery. J Med Assoc Ga 79:157, 1990.
4. Berci G, Sackier JM. The Los Angeles experience with laparoscopic cholecystectomy. Am J Surg 161:382, 1991.
5. Cuschieri A, Dubois F, Mouiel J, et al. The European experience with laparoscopic cholecystectomy. Am J Surg 161:385, 1991.
6. Reddick EJ, Olsen D, Spaw A, et al. Safe performance of difficult laparoscopic cholecystecotomies. Am J Surg 161:377, 1991.
7. Southern Surgical Group. A prospective analysis of 1518 laparoscopic cholecystectomies. N Engl J Med 324:1073, 1991.
8. Stoker ME, Vose J, O'Mara P, et al. Laparoscopic cholecystectomy: A clinical and financial analysis of 280 operations. Arch Surg 127:589, 1992.
9. Voyles CR, Petro AB, Meena AL, et al. A practical approach to laparoscopic cholecystectomy. Am J Surg 161:365, 1991.
10. McKernan JB, Laws HL. Laparoscopic preperitoneal prosthetic repair of inguinal hernias. Surgical Rounds. July, 1992, p 597.
11. Ger R. Laparosckopische hernienoperation. Chirurgie 62:266, 1991.
12. Valla JS, Limmone B, Valla V, et al. Laparoscopic appendectomy in children: Report of 465 cases. Surg Laparosc Endosc 1:166, 1991.
13. Peir A, Gotz F, Bacher C. Laparoscopic appendectomy in 625 cases: From innovation to routine. Surg Laparosc Endosc 1:8, 1991.
14. Katkhouda N, Mouiel J. A new technique of surgical treatment of chronic duodenal ulcer without laparotomy by videocoelioscopy. Am J Surg 161:361, 1991.
15. Laws HL, Naughton MJ, McKernan JB. Thorascoscopic vagectomy for recurrent peptic ulcer disease. Surg Endosc 1992. (In press.)

16. Dallemagne B, Weerts JM, Jehaes C, et al. Laparoscopic Nissen fundoplication: Preliminary report. Surg Laparosc Endosc 1:138, 1991.
17. Geagea T. Laparoscopic Nissen fundoplication: Preliminary report on ten cases. Surg Endosc 5:170, 1991.
18. Nathanson LK, Shimi S, Cuschieri A. Laparoscopic ligamentum teres (round ligament) cardioplexy. Br J Surg 78:947, 1991.
19. Rossi RL, Schimer WJ, Braasch JW, et al. Laparoscopic bile duct injuries: Risk factors, recognition and repair. Arch Surg 127:596, 1992.
20. Berci G, Sackier JM, Paz-Partlow M. Routine or selected intraoperative cholangiography during laparoscopic cholecystectomy? Am J Surg 161:355, 1991.
21. Ko ST, Airan MC. Therapeutic laparoscopic suturing techniques. Surg Endosc 6:41, 1992.
22. Dent TL. Training, credentialling, and granting of clinical privileges for laparoscopic general surgery. Am J Surg 161:399, 1991.
23. Society of American Gastrointestinal Endoscopic Surgeons. Granting of privileges for laparoscopic (peritoneoscopic) general surgery. Los Angeles: Society of American Gastrointestinal Endoscopic Surgeons, 1990.

4 *Extended Nonoperative or Minimally Invasive Operative Treatment*

H. Michel, D. Larrey, P. Blanc, and G.P. Pageaux

Since the first laparoscopic cholecystectomy performed by Mouret in 1987, numerous indications for laparoscopic operations on the digestive organs have been established.[1] It is not a new but a different approach to the comparable "open" operation, resulting in minimal anatomical access, less postoperative pain, a shorter hospital stay, a swift return to normal activities, and small scars—advantages already known within the gynecologist's experience. Because the hepatogastroenterologist lacks randomized controlled studies with numerous patients and long-term results, it is difficult to choose between this "minimally invasive" surgery and a nonoperative treatment of long duration.

We will discuss these alternative treatments for three conditions: cholecystolithiasis, chronic duodenal ulcer, and recurrent gastroesophageal reflux.

CHOLECYSTOLITHIASIS

Cholecystolithiasis occurs frequently; in the French population, 20% of adults 20 to 60 years of age have gallstones. Prevalence increases with age. Sixty percent of individuals older than 80 years have one or several gallstones.[2] The rate of asymptomatic gallstones, increasingly detected by ultrasonography, is 75%; that of symptomatic gallstones is 25%. Among them, 6% will be treated with biliary acids, either with or without lithotripsy, and 8% will undergo a cholecystectomy, resulting in 70,000 cholecystectomies performed annually. Considering the advantages of laparoscopic surgery, cholecystolithiasis has become the main indication for this procedure. It becomes necessary to know if prophylactic cholecystectomy is indicated for patients with paucisymptomatic or even asymptomatic gallstones. There are arguments for and against this hypothesis.

Arguments For Prophylactic Laparoscopic Cholecystectomy

Arguments for performing prophylactic laparoscopic cholecystectomy are as follows:

1. Removal of the gallbladder is responsible for any sequelae. The gallbladder plays only an accessory role during digestion, contrary to the belief that a special diet is needed after cholecystectomy. Bile stockage, contraction, and emptying of the gallbladder after meals are of little interest. Oddi's sphincter plays the main role in emptying bile in the duodenum and in promoting digestion.

2. There are numerous advantages for laparoscopic

cholecystectomy: minimal postoperative pain, no ileus or eventration, early feeding and walking, and scarcity of thromboembolic complications. Thus consequences are a shorter hospital stay (3.3 days after laparoscopic surgery versus 5.1 days after conventional open surgery), a shorter convalescence (17 versus 33 days), a swifter return to professional activities (18 versus 49.7 days), and consequently, a lower cost.[3,7,8] These advantages prompt physicians to propose an operation especially for symptomatic gallstones to avoid 6 to 18 months of treatment with biliary salts. This is particularly true for floating stones of less than 10 mm, which are always cholesterolic, and small stones resulting from extracorporeal shock wave lithotripsy, which require long-term oral dissolution therapy. In all cases laparoscopic cholecystectomy offers fast and definitive recovery, whereas oral dissolution therapy exposes patients to a recurrence rate of approximately 10% per year (i.e., 50% at 5 years).

3. This easy and safe procedure, confirmed by more than 5000 laparoscopic cholecystectomies prevents complications such as cholecystitis, acute obstructive cholangitis, pancreatitis, and for some authors, carcinoma of the gallbladder[3,7-11]; consequently, mortality is reduced. After conventional open cholecystectomy, the postoperative mortality rate is low: 0.1% to 0.2%. However, the mortality rate increases with age: 0.2% before 60 years, 3% after 60 years, and 5.8% after 70 years. Thus conventional cholecystectomy itself is responsible for 250 deaths of older patients among 70,000 operations.

4. The cost of this procedure is lower compared with that for medical therapy (dissolution and/or lithotripsy) and conventional open cholecystectomy. On the other hand, minilaparotomy would result in the same economic advantages.

Arguments Against Laparoscopic Cholecystectomy

Arguments against performing laparoscopic cholecystectomy are as follows:

1. Complications may occur after laparoscopic cholecystectomy. The classic complications of conventional cholecystectomy include propulsive diarrhea (rather unusual but uncomfortable); increased risk of colorectal cancer (debatable); and duodenogastric reflux, a factor in gastritis. In addition, complications of laparoscopic cholecystectomy occur more frequently and are directly related to the surgeon's training. French, American, and Belgian publications have noted mortality rates between 0.1% and 0.4% (0.1% in conventional cholecystectomy) and morbidity rates between 5% and 8% (i.e., cystic artery and bile duct injury). Morbidity can be lower with conversion of difficult laparoscopic cholecystectomy to conventional open cholecystectomy.[4]

2. The lack of short- or long-term prognostic factors: neither age, sex, gallbladder morphology, nor gallstone characteristics (i.e., number, size, transparency) allow assessment to determine whether asymptomatic cholecystolithiasis will become symptomatic. Indeed, most patients with cholecystolithiasis experience neither pain nor complications during life. Only a very low ratio (0.5% to 4%) will have cholecystolithiasis disease every year.

3. Performing prophylactic cholecystectomy for dyspepsia, headache, vomiting, fat intolerance, diarrhea, or constipation is useless and presents unnecessary risk. These signs are seen in patients without cholecystolithiasis and spontaneously disappear with time. The mortality risk in these patients is increased. Thus if we transpose the mortality rate of elective cholecystectomy to prophylactic cholecystectomy, we could imagine 875,000 operations in which 2500 deaths occur among younger patients. In fact, the only accepted indication for prophylactic cholecystectomy is to prevent severe infection in candidates for organ transplantation (in this case, the conventional procedure is preferred).

4. Efficacy of medical therapy (dissolution, lithotripsy) is not negligible.[14] Ursodeoxycholic acid (13 to 15 mg/kg/day), used for cholesterolic gallstones inside a functional gallbladder, allows total dissolution in 50% of patients when stone size is less than 15 mm and in 75% of patients when stone size is less than 5 mm. Approximately 15% of patients will have a less painful crisis, and 5% to 10% of patients will be definitively cured. This kind of therapy is used for patients with cardiorespiratory failure, ones older than 70 years, those who refuse an operation, or those with residual gallstones after endoscopic sphincterotomy. In this last case, 60% of gallstones disappear. Extracorporeal shock wave lithotripsy associated with ursodeoxycholic acid therapy eliminates approximately 10% of cholesterolic gallstones. These two therapies do not affect the gallbladder itself, which is a recurrence factor for gallstone formation.

In conclusion, there is consensus between European hepatologists not to extend the indications for cholecystectomy beyond symptomatic cholecystolithiasis, particularly when there are no complications.[2] Meanwhile, it is logical to think that, considering its advantages and greater acceptance among patients, indications for laparoscopic cholecystectomy are less restrictive for (1) cholecystolithiasis revealed by one or two painful crises and (2) some gallstones that, until then, had been thought cured with dissolution therapy or lithotripsy.

CHRONIC DUODENAL ULCER

Chronic duodenal ulcer affects 10% of the French population, with an incidence of 2%, or 100,000 new cases each year. The mortality rate is 1% to 2%, or 500 to 1000 ulcer patients each year in France.

In the past, drug therapy had little effect. Patients with recurrent ulcer underwent vagotomy, with or without antrectomy.[16] Currently drug therapy is very effective for both the acute phase and as long-term therapy to avoid recurrence. The number of consultations and hospitalizations for noncomplicated gastroduodenal ulcers has clearly decreased; therefore the number of surgical operations, both vagotomy and antrectomy, has declined. Thus, except for emergency situations, during the last 3 years we as surgeons have noted that one third of physicians have never entrusted patients to surgeons and two thirds have entrusted fewer than three patients.[17]

Long-term therapy is prescribed by 78% of physicians for 36% of patients who smoke, for 41% of stressed patients, and for 80% of patients with previous hemorrhage or who are taking nonsteroidal anti-inflammatory drugs.[18] The duration of long-term therapy varies from 1 year (36%) to 5 years (42%). This treatment accounts for biological and economic consequences.[19] The question is when to use this long-term therapy instead of laparoscopic vagotomy.

Arguments For Maintenance Medical Therapy

Arguments for maintenance medical therapy include the following:

1. Present medical treatment is effective. The number and duration of recurrences decrease: 60% to 80% of patients receiving long-term therapy do not have a recurrence versus 33% receiving a placebo who do.[20] Ulcer complications (hemorrhage, perforation, stenosis) are very unusual, even for patients with previous complications who are taking nonsteroidal anti-inflammatory drugs. Furthermore, the longer this treatment, the rarer, shorter, and less severe are the recurrences (15% with long-term therapy versus 87% at 5 years without it). Moreover, *Helicobacter pylori*, which is detected in 90% of duodenal ulcers, would promote recurrence, and it would seem that its eradication would make healing easier. At 1 year, the recurrence rate would be 72%

to 80% if *H. pylori* were present and 0% to 23% if it were absent.[21] *H. pylori* as a promoting factor of recurrence would be as important as smoking, stress, and overworking. Long-term therapy should be used in the following cases: patients who want it after receiving proper information, patients with contraindications to an operation, patients needing nonsteroidal anti-inflammatory drugs, patients with disabling diseases (e.g., cirrhosis, respiratory failure, cardiac failure), patients older than 65 years.[22]

2. This long-term therapy is not necessary throughout life. It is not certain that ulcer disease is an all-life disease; thus medical therapy must be definitive. The natural history of duodenal ulcer disease is characterized by painful crisis and recurrences with complications; nevertheless, this disease gradually turns asymptomatic in 70% of patients after 10 years of follow-up. Fry[16] ascertained that among 212 ulcer patients followed 10 years, only 5% were symptomatic.

3. This long-term therapy is well tolerated. It provides comfort to the patient. Side effects are of little importance (i.e., no alteration of gastric bacterial flora, mild hypergastrinemia).[20,22] In long-term achlorhydric patients, gastric cancer risk is always possible, but medical treatment never causes complete and definitive achlorhydria, contrary to surgical treatment. As for *H. pylori* infection, it remains a medical problem.

4. This therapy is economically reasonable, although the surgeon's and the physician's points of view differ.[31] Physicians believe that long-term medical treatment costs are 25% of the estimated total cost of ulcer disease in patients without this treatment.[18] There are savings in consultations, hospitalizations, fibroscopy and time lost from work. Cost of this therapy is lower than that of operative treatment.[24] More than 30 years of anti–*H. pylori* administration would cost no more than supraselective vagotomy! Surgeons have the opposite opinion.[25] Cost is evaluated as $1000 per patient per year during the first 2 years of treatment: 39% for consultations and studies, 23% for medicines, and 5% for time off from work.[26]

Arguments For Laparoscopic Operative Therapy

Arguments for performing laparoscopic operative therapy include the following:

1. Hyperselective vagotomy, or Taylor's procedure (anterior seromyotomy with posterior vagotomy), is effective and feasible with laparoscopic surgery. With conventional open surgery, this procedure cures 70% of patients with duodenal ulcers with a very low morbidity

rate (0% to 1%) and a functional complication rate (diarrhea, dumping syndrome) of approximately 10% to 12%. Nevertheless, recurrences increase with time (10% to 15% after 10 years of follow-up). The mortality rate is 0.1%.[27] As with H_2 blocker drugs, Taylor's procedure reduces acid secretion approximately 80% except that the operation is definitive; thus if atrophic gastritis occurs, gastric cancer risk increases.

2. This is the only therapy to propose for (1) patients with resistant ulcers after appropriate treatment for 2 years, (2) geographically and financially underprivileged patients with recurrent hemorrhage and, more rarely, stenosis, and (3) patients who are noncompliant with maintenance medical treatment. Adherence to this therapy depends on the information given and the patient's understanding of it; more than half of patients are unaware of smoking's toxicity in ulcer disease and the possibility of recurrence.

In conclusion, it is difficult to choose between maintenance medical therapy and laparoscopic surgery. Follow-up is only 2 years; 5 years are needed to appreciate results, yet first results are encouraging. Laparoscopic vagotomy is well tolerated, and work recovery is swift.[1] Mouiel et al.[28,29] have performed the laparoscopic procedure on 50 patients, 48 with Taylor's procedure and two with truncal vagotomy. All patients improved clinically. Legrand et al. and Weerts et al., in 1991, achieved good results on nine and 21 patients, respectively.

RECURRENT GASTROESOPHAGEAL REFLUX

Gastroesophageal reflux is frequent and perhaps even is a physiological state. In the United States 44% of the population has pyrosis once in a month and 7% every day.[3] Reasons for gastroesophageal reflux are multiple: (1) ineffective esophageal clearance, (2) mechanical lack of esophogastric junction, (3) gastric emptying delay, and (4) type of components that flow back (i.e., acid, pepsin, bile). Corpulence, hiatal hernia, and scleroderma are factors promoting pathological reflux.[3] Medical therapy, using assorted antacids, prokinetics, and antireflux measures, improves 95% of patients and avoids severe complications (hemorrhage, stenosis). With recent use of more potent acid secretion blockers (proton pump inhibitors) and more effective esophageal prokinetics (cisapride), persistent reflux is unusual. In our experience, one to two patients per year undergo operative treatment. Nevertheless, in 10% to 20% of patients recurrence of painful symptoms when treatment is stopped makes long-term therapy necessary.

Can laparoscopic therapy of reflux take the place of medical treatment? Two facts make the decision difficult: (1) gastroesophageal reflux causes functional symptoms, with different clinical manifestations according to patients; and (2) the severity of symptoms and the lesions caused by reflux lack correlation.

Arguments For Medical Therapy

The following arguments support the use of medical therapy:

1. Medical therapy is effective. Noncomplicated gastroesophageal reflux is improved by dietetic and postural measures. If the use of H_2 blockers is necessary, reflux usually is controlled. Furthermore, with omeprazole, failure of treatment is the exception and often is related to poor compliance. Long-term therapy is necessary for 10% of patients and protects them from recurrence and complications. In any case of complicated reflux (i.e., peptic ulcer, stenosis, esophagitis, Barrett's esophagus), medical treatment is indicated first; operative treatment is often necessary after manometric, pH metric, and scintigraphic evaluations.[32]

2. Gastroesophageal reflux is irregular. It is triggered or worsened (half of patients) by work activity, stress, and an inappropriate diet.[31,37] As in ulcer, it is not an all-life disease. With H_2-blockers or proton pump inhibitors, 58% and 83% of patients, respectively do not experience recurrence after 6 months of treatment.[34] Such an improvement spontaneously persisted through 9 years of follow-up in 75% of patients[35] and up to 10 years with mild treatment, even in cases of initial severe esophagitis.[36] It is likely that improvement in the causes—decrease of reflux severity and decrease of symptoms—is of some importance.

3. Only medical therapy is able to improve reflux related to esophageal[37] or gastric[38] emptying failure. Thus operative pyloroplasty could be responsible for worsening alkaline reflux. Using associated vagotomy as an antireflux procedure is not always of interest.[39] Gastric hyperacidity is not always significant in patients with reflux, so vagotomy is useless and impairs gastric emptying.

4. Conventional surgery for gastroesophageal reflux can eliminate failure or complications. So it probably does also with laparoscopic surgery. Failures (12% according to the investigation of French Surgery Association in 1989) are characterized by reflux recurrence early after intervention; thus approximately 60% of failures occur during the first 3 years, 33% between 3 and 10 years, and only 7% after 10 years. Nissen's procedure can cause complications such as postfundoplication

syndrome, inferior migration of fundoplication, and ulcer. Classic postfundoplication syndrome is characterized by dysphagia and inability to belch or vomit. This syndrome is explained by too effective an antireflux technique and occurs in 5% to 44% of patients, particularly those with preexisting esophageal propulsive disorders. Inferior migration of fundoplication on the upper zone of the stomach is also responsible for dysphagia and recurrent reflux. Fundoplication becomes uncomfortable during gastric emptying. Postfundoplication ulcers occur in 3% to 5% of patients, either inside or below the fundoplication.

Arguments For Surgical Therapy

The following arguments support the use of surgical therapy:

1. Nissen fundoplication is very effective. According to the French Surgery Association, with a follow-up period of 1 to 20 years, patients' rates without recurrence is 84% to 96% when using conventional surgery. In addition, pH monitoring is standardized, and lower esophageal sphincter pressure is multiplied fourfold. Still, fundoplication is more effective when there is associated hiatal hernia (92% of good results).

2. This operative therapy can be adapted to reflux pathophysiology. Monitoring of pH with esophageal manometry is needed before antireflux surgery to demonstrate the reality of acid reflux and to prevent operating for stasis esophagitis or propulsive disorders related to esophagitis. The Nissen procedure must be avoided in case of altered lower esophagus function.

3. Indications for surgery in patients with gastroesophageal reflux include typical clinical symptoms with severe resistant or recurrent esophagitis after 6 months of therapy and complications (stenosis, Barrett's esophagus, secondary asthma, laryngitis, recurrent pneumopathy). The aim of surgery is to avoid subsequent complications (hemorrhage, pneumopathy, hypothetical cancer evolution) or frequent endoscopic observation.

4. First results of the antireflux operation with the laparoscopic procedure are attractive.[40,41] Mouiel and Katkhouda[42] have performed this procedure on eight patients: seven were improved, and one had persistent reflux. Dallemagne[43] had no failure with 179 patients. Nevertheless, the follow-up time is too short to change physicians' treatment of reflux.

CONCLUSION

Laparoscopic surgery represents a technical revolution. This procedure provides unquestionable advantages, but we lack prospective controlled studies to determine whether to choose conventional surgery or laparoscopic surgery. Undoubtedly, laparoscopic cholecystectomy represents progress, which is not absolutely true for ulcer and gastroesophageal reflux surgery. Studies are still necessary. Maybe after improvement of materials and changes in the education of surgeons to achieve optimal clinical activity and results, this mini-invasive operative procedure (well accepted by patients) will allow an increase in operative indications.

REFERENCES

1. Testas P, Delaitre B. Chirurgie Digestive Par Voie Coelioscopique, vol 1. Paris: Maloine Edit, 1991.
2. La lithiase vésiculaire: Stratégie thérapeutique. Conférence européenne de consensus. Ann Gastroenterol Hepatol 28:157-162, 1992.
3. Mouiel J. Principles of safety in laparoscopic cholecystectomy. Presented at Second European Congress Viscero-Synthesis. Luxembourg, Sept. 10-12, 1992.
4. Morlang Th, Umscheid Th, Stelter WJ. Laparoscopic cholecystectomy on unselected patients. Minimally invasive surgery and new technology. Presented at Second European Congress of Viscero-Synthesis. Luxembourg, Sept. 10-12, 1992.
5. Etienne J. Laparoscopic cholecystectomy: The Belgian Registry. Minimally invasive surgery and new technology. Presented at Second European Congress of Viscero-Synthesis. Luxembourg, Sept. 10-12, 1992.
6. Wynne K. Laparoscopic cholecystectomy for the acutely inflamed gall bladder. Minimally invasive surgery and new technology. Presented at Second European Congress of Viscero-Synthesis. Luxembourg, Sept. 10-12, 1992.
7. Farello G, Cerofolini A, Bergamaschi G, et al. Laparoscopic cholecystectomy: Analysis of our experience in 519 patients. Minimally invasive surgery and new technology. Presented at Second European Congress of Viscero-Synthesis. Luxembourg, Sept. 10-12, 1992.
8. Ribet-Reinhart N, Amar L, De Watteville JC, et al. Comparison of postoperative pain for patients with laparoscopic cholecystectomy versus open surgery: Preliminary results. Minimally invasive surgery and new technology. Presented at Second European Congress of Viscero-Synthesis. Luxembourg, Sept. 10-12, 1992.
9. Fresneda V, Fernandez-Cebrian JM, Capela I, et al. Minimally invasive surgery and new technology. Presented at Second European Congress of Viscero-Synthesis. Luxembourg, Sept. 10-12, 1992.
10. Vazzana G, Champault G, Boutelier PH. Post-operative analysis of 200 laparoscopic cholecystectomies. Minimally invasive surgery and new technology. Presented at Second European Congress of Viscero-Synthesis. Luxembourg, Sept. 10-12, 1992.

11. Jiru P, Lederer K, Waneck R, et al. Laparoscopic chole-cystectomy as a routine procedure: Our experience of 700 operations. Minimally invasive surgery and new technology. Presented at Second European Congress of Viscero-Synthesis. Luxembourg, Sept. 10-12, 1992.

12. Go PM. A comparison of cost-effectiveness of conventional cholecystectomy and laparoscopic cholecystectomy. Minimally invasive surgery and new technology. Presented at Second European Congress of Viscero-Synthesis. Luxembourg, Sept. 10-12, 1992.

13. McGregor JR, O'Dwyer PJ, McDermott EWM, et al. Laparoscopic or mini-laparotomy cholecystectomy. Minimally invasive surgery and new technology. Presented at Second European Congress of Viscero-Synthesis. Luxembourg, Sept. 10-12, 1992.

14. Erlinger S. Le traitement médical de la lithiase vésiculaire est-il obsolète? Actualités digestives médico-chirurgicales. In Mouiel J, ed. Paris: Masson & Cie, 1992, pp 139-141.

15. Capron JP, Davion T, Dupas JL, et al. Les conséquences de la cholécystectomie (Première de deux parties). Gastroenterol Clin Biol 9:886-892, 1985.

16. Fry J. Peptic ulcer: A profile. Br Med J 2:809-821, 1964.

17. Boutelier PH, Chipponi J. Le traitement chirurgical du reflux gastro-oesophagien de l'adulte. Paris: Masson & Cie, 1989.

18. Mignon M. Prévention des rechutes et des complications ulcéreuses dans la maladie ulcéreuse duodénale. Traitement d'entretien. Gastroenterol Clin Biol 14:T1-T7, 1990.

19. Mignon M, Ruszniewski PH, Alberola B, et al. Groupe d'Etudes de la Maladie Ulcéreuse Duodénale (GEMUD). La gastrinémie basale est normale lors du traitement préventif à long terme des récidives d'ulcère duodénal par ranitidine 150 mg par jour. Gastroenterol Clin Biol 14: 407-408, 1990.

20. Ruszniewski PH, Mignon M, Slama A, et al. Two-year maintenance treatment of duodenal ulcer (DU) with ranitidine[R] 150 mg: A double-blind multicentric randomized study. Gastroenterology 100:A150, 1991.

21. Hentschel E, Nemec H, Schutze K. Duodenal ulcer recurrence and *Helicobacter pylori*. Lancet 338:569, 1991.

22. Susi D, Neri M. The natural history of duodenal ulcer disease is modified after discontinuing a five years maintenance therapy with ranitidine. Gastroenterology 100: A170, 1991.

23. Osterhaus J, You S, Hwang S, et al. Health and economic impact of ranitidine in a randomized controlled study for patients with a recent severe duodenal ulcer hemorrhage. Gastroenterology 98:A5, 1990.

24. Sonnenberg A. Costs of medical and surgical treatment of duodenal ulcer. Gastroenterology 96:1445-1452, 1989.

25. Champault G, Pautot V, Lauroy J. Ulcère duodénal chronique: Qu'attendre de la chirurgie en 1991? Actu-

alités digestives médico-chirurgicales. In Mouiel J, ed. Paris: Masson & Cie, 1992, pp 164-170.

26. Pym B, Sandstad J, Seville P, et al. Cost effectiveness of cimetidine maintenance therapy in chronic gastric and duodenal ulcer. Gastroenterology 99:27-35, 1990.

27. Taylor TV, Glunn AA, Mac Leod DAD, et al. Mortality and morbidity after anterior curve seromyotomy with posterior truncal vagotomy for duodenal ulcer. Br J Surg 72:950-951, 1985.

28. Mouiel J, Katkhouda J, Gugenheim J, et al. Traitement de l'ulcère duodénal par vagotomie tronculaire postérieure et séromyotomie fundique antérieure sous vidéo-laparoscopie. Chirurgie 116:546-551, 1990.

29. Mouiel J. Laparoscopic vagotomies. Minimally invasive surgery and new technology. Presented at Second European Congress of Viscero-Synthesis. Luxembourg: Sept. 10-12, 1992.

30. Bayerdorffer E, Mannes GA, Sommer A, et al. High dose omeprazole treatment combined with amoxicillin eradicates *Helicobacter pylori*. Eur J Gastroenterol Hepatol 4:697-702, 1992.

31. Demeester TR. Diagnosis and operative indications in gastro-esophageal reflux. Minimally invasive surgery and new technology. Presented at Second European Congress of Viscero-Synthesis. Luxembourg, Sept. 10-12, 1992.

32. Cargill G. Explorations fonctionnelles manométriques, pHmétriques et scintigraphiques. In Boutelier PH, Chipponi J, eds. Le Traitement Chirurgical du Reflux Gastro-Oesophagien de l'Adulte. Paris: Masson & Cie, 1989.

33. Spechler SJ, Department of Veterans Affaires Gastroesophageal Reflux Disease Study Group. Comparison of medical and surgical therapy for complicated gastroesophageal reflux disease in veterans. N Engl J Med 326:786-792, 1992.

34. Koelz HR, Birchler R, Bretholz A, et al. Healing and relapse of reflux esophagitis during treatment with ranitidine. Gastroenterology 91:1198-1205, 1986.

35. Palmer ED. The hiatus hernia-esophagitis-esophageal stricture complex: Twenty-year prospective study. Am J Med 44:566-579, 1968.

36. Behar J, Brand DL, Brown FC, et al. Cimetidine in the treatment of symptomatic gastroesophageal reflux: A double-blind controlled trial. Gastroenterology 74:441-448, 1978.

37. Dedieu P, Gaillard F, Lavignolle A, et al. Oesophagite par reflux: Aspects épidémiologiques, anatomopathologiques et évolutifs (123 cas). Gastroenterol Clin Biol 5:266-274, 1981.

38. Galmiche JP, Guillard JF, Denis P, et al. Etude du pH oesophagien en période post-prandiale chez le sujet normal et au cours du syndrome de reflux gastro-oesophagien. Intérêt diagnostique d'un score de reflux acide. Gastroenterol Clin Biol 4:531-539, 1980.

39. Rossetti M, Hell K. Fundoplication for the treatment of gastroesophageal reflux and hiatal hernia. World J Surg 1:439-444, 1977.

40. Cushieri A. Antireflux surgery: Laparoscopic cardiapexy. Minimally invasive surgery and new technology. Presented at Second European Congress of Viscero-Synthesis. Luxembourg, Sept. 10-12, 1992.

41. Gayet B. Laparoscopic hemifundoplication. Minimally invasive surgery and new technology. Presented at Sec-ond European Congress of Viscero-Synthesis. Luxembourg, Sept. 10-12, 1992.

42. Mouiel J, Katkhouda N. Reflux gastro-oesophagien. Expérience laparoscopique. Compte-rendu XVIe Journées Nicoises de Pathologie et Chirurgie Digestives et Vidéo-Laparoscopie. Nice: Feb. 14-15, 1992.

43. Dallemagne B. Laparoscopic Nissen fundoplication. Minimally invasive surgery and new technology. Presented at Second European Congress of Viscero-Synthesis. Luxembourg, Sept. 10-12, 1992.

5   *The Place of Laparoscopy in Modern Surgical Training*

Jonathan R. Hiatt, Jonathan M. Sackier, George Berci, and Margaret Paz-Partlow

New techniques in laparoscopic surgery provide a challenge for general surgery training programs. To ensure a complete surgical education for the residents and continuing education of the medical staff, didactic and technical instruction in these procedures must be offered and a healthy balance between laparoscopic and open operations must be preserved. We report a didactic, laboratory, and clinical strategy that has been designed to meet these goals.

MATERIALS AND METHODS

Cedars-Sinai Medical Center (CSMC) is an 1100-bed hospital with residency training programs in all major disciplines. The general surgery teaching program ensures the training of 25 residents who learn from and fully participate in the day-by-day decisions and operative procedures initiated by the attending and teaching staff. Both private and nonprivate patients are treated. A program in endoscopic surgery developed by one of the authors of this chapter (George Berci) offered experience in laparoscopic general surgical procedures, the number of which, especially that of laparoscopic cholecystectomy, began to increase in 1989 (Table 1). From the program's inception in 1989 to June 30, 1992, general surgeons performed 1755 laparoscopic procedures, most of which were part of the surgical teaching services. CSMC also has active programs in hepatobiliary surgery and in liver transplantation.

Surgical staff members were quick to recognize the importance of laparoscopic procedures and to integrate them into clinical practice. This enthusiasm and the eagerness of the advanced-level residents to learn the procedures during residency training stimulated the development of an educational system with the following elements.

Didactic program. A lecture series, *Principles of Endoscopic Surgery*, was incorporated into the Grand Rounds program. The course material encompasses basic elements and clinical applications of all commonly

Table 1. Biliary procedures performed at Cedars-Sinai Medical Center

Procedure	1988	Sept 1989–June 1992
Cholecystectomy		
Open surgery	271 (100%)	214 (12.5%)
Laparoscopic surgery	0	1503 (87.5%)
TOTAL	271	1717
Common Bile Duct Exploration		
Open surgery	35	72 (44%)
Laparoscopic	0	91 (56%)
TOTAL	35	163

used endoscopic techniques, such as gastrointestinal endoscopy, diagnostic and therapeutic laparoscopy, and laparoscopic procedures that include a reconstructive stage.

Laboratory program. This program has three components: a course in basic techniques, which is taken by all junior residents[3]; participation by senior and chief residents in advanced courses approved by the Society of American Gastrointestinal Endoscopic Surgeons (SAGES), and taught by members of the CSMC faculty[4]; and instruction in endoscopic procedures that is included in the curriculum of a weekly skills practicum for residents, taught in the vivarium. The porcine model is used in the laboratory courses because of its favorable correlation with human biliary anatomy.

Clinical program. Each resident receives a graded operative exposure to all laparoscopic procedures performed by members of the teaching faculty and thus gains experience as camera person, assistant, and finally as primary operating surgeon.

Research. Stimulated by the intensity of faculty interest in laparoscopy, residents have been participants in basic and clinical research. This participation was encouraged even before the introduction of laparoscopic cholecystectomy into clinical practice.

Education in open techniques. An educational strategy overseen by members of the liver transplant team was devised to provide training in hepatobiliary surgery. Surgical residents are involved with nontransplant hepatic resections and biliary reconstructions that are performed on the general surgery teaching service. The residents also learn open hepatobiliary anatomy and operative techniques by participation in liver transplant harvest and implantation into a recipient. Finally, laparoscopy used primarily to stage hepatobiliary malignancies has been integrated into the clinical activities of this service.

All data related to the residents' activities are collected on an ongoing basis in a computer-based registry.

RESULTS

From September 1, 1989 to June 30, 1992, surgical residents at CSMC participated in 752 laparoscopic procedures. In 430 of these procedures, residents served as primary operating surgeons; in 322, they were assistants (Table 2). All procedures were supervised by a senior member of the attending staff. The only major complication in a laparoscopic procedure performed by a resident was a lateral common bile duct injury during

Table 2. Resident participation in laparoscopic procedures, 1989-1992

Type of Procedure	No. of Procedures Performed
Cholecystectomy	497
Diagnostic	161
Appendectomy	70
Other	24
TOTAL	752

a cholecystectomy caused by the dissecting hook. This injury was recognized immediately and was repaired via laparotomy. The rate of conversion from laparoscopic to open procedures was 5%.

During the same period, the chief residents performed 72 major hepatobiliary procedures, including liver resections and biliary-enteric bypasses. The residents also participated in 130 orthotopic liver transplants.

As a consequence of the programs in clinical and basic research, the residents presented and/or published 15 manuscripts on topics related to laparoscopy and minimally invasive surgery.

DISCUSSION

The introduction of laparoscopic procedures in general surgery, which has occurred with unprecedented speed, has produced unique stresses that require retraining of a generation of surgeons. Although attention has been directed to credentialing and privileging for performance of these procedures,[5] less has been said about the effect on surgical training programs.[6,7]

Resident training must provide instruction and experience in procedures performed by general surgeons. Implicit in this expectation is a balance between laparoscopic and open operation. For biliary procedures, this may be difficult: patients or referring physicians often demand laparoscopy, and contraindications to the procedures decrease as experience in a technique increases. Acute cholecystitis, choledocholithiasis, previous abdominal operations, and other traditional obstacles can now be managed by the seasoned laparoscopist. From 1988 to 1991, the CSMC surgical staff performed twice the annual number of cholecystectomies; the number of open procedures decreased 16-fold.

The structured approach described in this chapter is compatible with primary educational goals in surgery, which include an understanding of basic science, an appreciation of clinical application, a graded exposure to operative technique, and a contribution to surgical research.

After having completed structured didactic and laboratory programs, residents achieve increasing operative responsibility in laparoscopic procedures. When laparoscopic cholecystectomy is performed, our teaching faculty members have exercised a liberal conversion policy: the laparoscopic approach has been aborted if unfamiliar anatomy, severe inflammation, technical difficulty, or inability to perform cholangiography is encountered.[8]

The educational goals of open procedures are similar to those of laparoscopic techniques, but the clinical number of open operations has declined. Programs in hepatobiliary surgery and liver transplantation characterized by similar didactic, clinical, and laboratory elements have contributed to a structured, educational approach to anatomy and operative techniques for surgical residents. Liver transplantation, which is a complement to the value of experience in liver resections and complex biliary reconstructions, offers many lessons for the general surgeon that may be learned by participation in the donor and recipient operations. These lessons include knowledge of the ligamentous attachments of the liver and methods of exposure and mobilization, upper abdominal vascular anatomy, anatomical variations in the biliary tract, and techniques for biliary reconstruction. Removal of a normal gallbladder from every grafted liver may constitute the only remaining large series of open cholecystectomies.

As a consequence of advancing technology, residency training carries—less than ever—a lifetime guarantee of maintaining up-to-date competence and knowledge of the progress in the craft as it influences the science of surgery, and vice versa. A program that is successful in preparing "surgical recruits" for making rational decisions should provide an education that furnishes young and mature surgeons with the intellectual skills that allow graduates and practitioners to make proper and responsible application of new techniques.

REFERENCES

1. Bailey RW, Imbembo AL, Zucker KA. Establishment of a laparoscopic cholecystectomy training program. Am Surg 57:231-236, 1991.
2. Berci G, Cuschieri A, eds. Practical Laparascopy. London: Ballière-Tindall, 1984.
3. Sackier JM. Training for laparoscopic biliary surgery. In: Cuschieri A, Berci G, eds. Laparoscopic Biliary Surgery. London: Blackwell, 1992.
4. Sackier JM. Training for minimal access surgery. Curr Prac Surg 1992 (in press).
5. Dent TL. Training, credentialling, and granting of clinical privileges for laparoscopic general surgery. Am J Surg 161:399-403, 1991.
6. Schirmer BD, Edge SB, Dis J, Miller AD. Incorporation of laparoscopy into a surgical endoscopy training program. Am J Surg 163:46-52, 1992.
7. Baird DR, Wilson JP, Mason EM, Duncan TD, Evans JS, Luke JP, Ruben DM, Lucas GW. An early review of 800 laparoscopic cholecystectomies at a University-affiliated community teaching hospital. Am Surg 58:206-210, 1992.
8. Sackier JM, Berci G, Phillips E, Carroll B, Shapiro S, Paz-Partlow M. The role of cholangiography in laparoscopic cholecystectomy. Arch Surg 126:1021-1026, 1991.

6   *The Place and Role of Minimally Invasive Surgery*

Philippe Mouret

The long-term future of minimally invasive surgery is impossible to determine. As astrophysicist Hubert Reeves notes in speaking of evolutionary phenomena, there are always limits to the "predictive horizons," particularly in the presence of a great many complex interacting factors. Surgery is so complex, so human, so social that the factors are incalculable, and our predictive horizon cannot go much farther than what we see today. Therefore let us analyze what we *can* ascertain about this new technology.

WHAT IS MINIMALLY INVASIVE SURGERY?

Minimally invasive surgery is not limited to a single technique or even a collection of techniques. We could define it as a *state of mind* or a focus that underlies the conduct of a surgical procedure, seeking to reduce the extent of the anatomical approach while maintaining its operational efficiency. We can readily see the difficulty in defining minimally invasive surgery in the number of names we have tried to give it: "minimal access surgery," "closed abdominal surgery," "Band-aid surgery" or "surgery without a scar" by the media, "patient-friendly surgery" by Hans Troidl, and so on. Each of these names captures a portion of the definition but focuses on only one aspect. None of these descriptive terms is quite on target. *Minimally invasive surgery* is the least limiting definition and therefore the most complete. Personally, I also like the term *minimally offensive surgery*, because it is even more general. More precisely, it is the operative technique in which the human body and tissues are exposed to a minimal surgical offense to achieve an optimal therapeutic result.

We will not find the perfect phrase, but we should notice that all of the definitions include the word *surgery*. Surgery is defined by its goals; therefore an innovative technique does not represent a revolution in surgery, but merely an advance to a hopefully higher level in the continuum of surgical progress. The goal of minimally invasive surgery is to reduce the area of access to a body cavity or organ lumen, to lessen the harm or damage to the area's tissues (minimal offense), and to focus on the selectivity of the surgical action. Thus the new techniques do not reflect a new surgical philosophy, but represent an elegant refinement of the hippocratic *Primum non nocere* and of William Halsted's concern for the precise and gentle handling of human tissues during an operation.

WHAT HAS BEEN THE IMPETUS IN THE EXPLOSIVE DEVELOPMENT OF MINIMALLY INVASIVE SURGERY?

I would analyze this by suggesting that the technical aspects in the fields of general and gastrointestinal surgery had been stagnant for some years; established procedures had become routine and no excitingly original ideas filled the surgical horizons. Suddenly, surgical celioscopy "parachuted" into our midst—and we were as surprised as if we were viewing an extraterrestrial event. "It is the Devil," said some. "It is the Messiah," said others. I would simply say this is the most recently born child of the surgical family. Of course, this little one was enthusiastically welcomed into the minimally invasive fraternity: claims to be the parent or even just the godparent suddenly defied all established biological laws. (Please excuse the metaphor I use in describing the birth of celiosurgery—but the reactions that it has brought throughout the surgical world can best be likened, it seems to me, to the arrival of a much desired infant.)

Techniques in gastrointestinal surgery appeared to be stagnant, or boring, by contrast with other specialties in which minimally invasive surgery was progressing: microsurgery, cardiovascular catheterization and manipulation stereotaxic procedures, and many more. In the gastrointestinal area, no such new techniques were being employed. And more than getting bored, gastrointestinal surgery was growing thin, eaten at the edges, leaving a large part of its substance to gastrointestinal endoscopy—to such a degree that some were predicting its eventual demise.

But as soon as this little lastborn cried with the joy, and some anxiety, of freedom from the confining but also protecting womb, it was hailed as a prodigy, capable of all achievements, even to the point of entirely overshadowing its mother.

MINIMALLY INVASIVE SURGERY: NEW DISCIPLINE OR NEW METHOD?

However, let us look beyond the emotional impact of this newcomer and examine some facts. Keeping in mind that minimally invasive surgery represents a larger concept than celiosurgery, I will nevertheless focus primarily on an analysis of celiosurgery because that is my area of expertise. I have given as an axiom that the art and science of surgery does not change in its essential mission and goals; change occurs only in methodology. I would like to try to demonstrate the following:

- It is a false premise to contrast two techniques: open and closed, traditional and modern.
- It is a false debate to argue for the creation of distinguishing boundaries between the two that divide rather than harmoniously integrate basic surgical concepts.
- It is far more important to respect the ground rules that govern strategy and technique of operative procedures, allowing the art or craft and science of surgery to progress, whatever the method.

The surgical procedure is the realization of a technical act using technological means. It starts from an *indication* for operation, which always proceeds from the comparative estimation of the procedure's benefits and risks to the patient. The method is determined by the surgeon—and it always represents a compromise between the various factors that compare the eye or mind and hand or instrument coordination. Some preliminary steps are required before the definitive surgical act: exposure and exploration of the pathological site, dissection and liberation of the specimen, presentation, and evaluation of the clinical alternatives. The first therapeutic action is often simple in its technical concept; to ligate, to amputate, to excise, to resect, to drain. This ablative or destructive stage is ideally and most often followed by reconstruction and restoration of lost form and function. In this effort the entire register of exquisite manual dexterity—science of surgery—is mobilized: sutured repair, anastomosis, temporary or permanent bypass or exclusion, organ substitution, reimplantation, transplantation. Ablation and restoration are the two essential and interdependent acts of a surgically therapeutic endeavor. They should always be surrounded and contained by the framework of the operative indication, established by the rational and scholarly intellect of the surgeon—thoughtful man of action.

All other factors are but utilities or, to make a comparison with the performing arts, accessories. Celioscopic surgery modified only the accessories without changing the principles of the intra-abdominal procedure. But the modification was so spectacular in its appearance and created a new surgical environment so that we thought everything had been altered.

There *has* been another, more profound technical evolution that concerns the realization of the surgical act itself. I am speaking of stapling. It has been accepted much more deliberately and as its merits were debated, the arguments were far less passionate than those used for or against celioscopy or laparoscopy. But there is a definite parallel between stapling and celiosurgery. The two have a very close conceptual relationship: each calls for technological resources to accomplish part of the surgical act. Each has a clearly defined objective of progress: to have fewer surprises and fewer mishaps due to the surgical activity. Each is clearly intended and capable to see its field of application extended. Stapling has become the technique of choice in celioscopic procedures that include a reconstructive phase. As instrument designers and manufacturers adapt to new demands the appropriate instruments will evolve. Nevertheless, there are some limits to the uses of stapling in unusual circumstances in which only a manual suture will suffice.

DREAM OR REAL PROMISE OF MINIMALLY INVASIVE SURGERY?

Celioscopic surgery is traveling along a path to acceptance similar to the one stapling accomplished before. It will establish a secure base as an adjuvant technical resource. Therefore it is also obvious that when the conditions of a normal and justifiable application are not met, celioscopy will have to give way to time tested, traditional techniques, capable of resolving the difficulties and complexities of unusual findings, beyond the technical potential of minimally invasive surgery.

Celiosurgery has modified some accessories so profoundly that in its wake the whole surgical atmosphere was changed. Even our symbol of the scalpel or bistoury has been replaced by the video monitor, which has now a central place in the operating room. For me, celiosurgery is defined uniquely by the substitution of the eye to hand coordination through a traditional surgical incision by an optically enhanced view that guides hands and their extensions—appropriate surgical instruments—through a minimal anatomical access. It is said to be a spectacle; indeed it becomes a show that can experience fearsome as well as beneficial consequences.

The surgical act has emerged from a narrow circle of primary participants through the phenomenon of television. Any viewer, competent or not, who watches a tennis match can judge at his leisure the merits or mistakes of the foremost players of the tennis world. Surgeons will not be exempt from the phenomenon of uninitiated appraisal. Obviously, vision enhanced by optical magnification and projection on a video screen is superior to that of the naked eye. Therefore this is *microsurgery* by virtue of the optics and by the definition of the televised picture. The view is *telescopic* in the way that it places the surgeon's eyes where he wishes them to be, and where he was never before able to place them, regardless of the site of incision or anatomic intrusion. Finally, and this is an important corollary, the entrance doors available to the eyes and hands are not limiting the intracavitary or intraluminal activity, thanks to the instrumental extensions of mind, eyes, and hands.

Personally, I wish we could stop at one criterion as to what constitutes a celiosurgical procedure and that we could eliminate any other modifiers of the definition. Everything would be simpler. In fact, let us decide that the definition of celiosurgery is: a procedure in which for all or part, the celioscope is used for visual exploration.

It may not be useless to recall that the celioscopy created by Palmer was an *exploratory* act. Why would we want to forget that function and move on to more complex applications? The benefits for gynecology are sufficiently obvious to demonstrate its advantages: disappearance of the exploratory laparotomy; complementary information or rectification of the diagnosis with possibilities far superior to those of laparotomy in the differential topographical diagnosis and the recognition of pathological associations. It also provides the possibility, as Maurice Antoine Bruhat underscores in gynecology, to extend the celiosurgical potential and accomplish the ultimate goals of a given therapeutic indication.

If the preliminary steps of exposure, dissection, and evaluation common to any operative procedure are given added comfort and security by celiosurgery, it is obvious that the procedure will expand along the concepts of minimally invasive surgery: *therapeutic celiosurgery*. The traditional intra-abdominal procedure will be simplified and the surgical openings adapted to the minimal requirements of the celiosurgical instruments and techniques.

EXPANDING CONCEPTS AND INTEGRATION INTO THE SURGICAL FAMILY

The attempt to place the boundary between celiosurgery and classic surgery at the level of integral realization of the operation by either method stems from a kind of *integrity*. If I use that term it is to emphasize that it proceeds from a certain rigidity, a certain intolerance, but surely not from an idea of evolution or progress.

If therefore we extend the concept of celiosurgery, some interesting consequences follow. The concept of *conversion* loses its connotation of failure, always badly felt, by the surgeon and by the patient. Besides, this misguided perception leads to curious consequences: while unavoidable, some authors came to consider that a normal rate of conversion was an indispensable criterion for judging the validity of a statistic. Brought back to what it is (e.g., a step of operative tactics), there is no longer a reason for conversion to be viewed as a shame or a glory.

In the teaching phase of celiosurgery, this strategy of progressive movement toward a wider use of the celioscopic approach represents a progression we must emphasize. This was the strategy of all those who were pioneers of celiosurgery. The progressive acquisition of mastery of the procedures seemed necessary to them. Why would it be impossible today to have the same pedagogical value? While the visualization with celioscopic surgery presents advantages, it is not natural and we have to recreate all the necessary cerebral reactions for its interpretation. This requires extensive practice.

The rising use of celioscopy in colon surgery often adopts the strategy of association. We speak of celiosurgical colectomy in "association with minilaparotomy." This connotes a casuistic subtlety, even though it is simpler to speak of colectomy assisted by celiosurgery. If we engage in other procedures even more complex, analogous strategies will have to be developed.

To imagine remains the attitude that we must keep. Our professional rules, as rigorous as they must stay, must not be sterilizing. The introduction of celioscopy in surgery is the result of a little bit of imagination. The sphere of imagination is far from being sterile on the surgeon's side or on the side of industry.

Today no one can guess the range in which celioscopic assistance will be useful nor the areas where total substitution by celioscopy will be possible; but it isn't necessary to guess. Each surgeon contributing to the body of celioscopic knowledge will play a large or small role in making celiosurgery an integrated process with traditional techniques.

Celioscopy brings advantages whenever it is useful, if it is utilized by the largest possible number of surgeons, for the maximum benefit of patients.

The attitude that the frontiers of celiosurgical procedures have all been charted and mastered could lead to focus on the technical aspects only to the detriment of the spirit of minimally invasive surgery and create an unjustified partition. Less partisan intolerance would lead the whole body of surgeons to accept the strategy and practice of minimally invasive surgery.

Thus all surgery in which celioscopy has its advantages could benefit from this approach. Indeed, it is in abdominal emergencies, gynecology, hernias, and others—that the minimally invasive concept can be most readily demonstrated to benefit the patients' well-being.

EVALUATION AND QUALITY CONTROL

It seems to me important that we do a *conceptual redefinition of celiosurgery* and that we place it back in the continuum of surgery as a major discipline of the healing arts.

Critical evaluation. All surgical procedures must be evaluated. Are we rigorous in our scrutiny of all procedures? I remember that for Pierre Testas, who wished to produce a statistical comparison between endoscopic cholecystectomy and classic cholecystectomy, it was easier to assemble a significant series of the celioscopic cholecystectomy than of a comparative open procedure. Of course, this does not diminish the fact that evaluation is a necessity, but it must not become an obsession. Not everything that is logically sound can be scientifically *validated.*

When B. Dallemagne presents the celioscopic technique of fundoplication and when he *shows* that it is in conception and realization the same as the open technique, there is no need to prove that the greater part of the evaluation is already done by the past experience; it is in evidence. It is the same for J. Mouiel and N. Katkouda with the Taylor technique, and many more examples could be given.

I would insist, on the other hand, on the technique for cure of a hernia, because in that particular case, the surgeon's technical choices to which celiosurgery led were not the standard transfers from the open technique. They focus on the principle of the *prosthetic hernioplasty* by Stoppa, to the exclusion of classic herniorrhaphy.

Was the hernioplasty, until now of limited usefulness, a minor technique? I do not think so, but it was more invasive in its realization. The celioscopic contribution reduces this invasion and provides other advantages in spite of the need for general anesthesia. This is enough to justify a clinical study to find statistical validity.

ACCREDITATION

The explosive and uncontrolled diffusion of this new technique gave us an infrastructure problem at the beginning. I hope this was only a temporary phenomenon, and from now on the teaching will be normalized and has regained the curriculum of the university. We have discovered on this occasion that there are complementary means to this traditional modality: on one side the guild and on the other side the participation of the industry. Each has natural processes that we were wrong to neglect. Concerning the industry, in all the professions having a technological part (surgery has a big one; celiosurgery has an even bigger one), the industry directly participates in the surgeon's taking a new instrument in hand and the initial use of its own products. Who would be surprised, indeed, to see a fighter pilot go to the manufacturer of his plane to acquire the first elements of his qualification? We must be careful to avoid possible conflict. To stay with the same metaphor, we must be assured that the flight instructors are not constituted into a fighter squadron or worse, into instigators of war. I do not think we are at that point!

In the teaching of celioscopy, the tendency to look for the spectacular, for the leading edge, and not basic surgery is very tempting. Nevertheless, it is obvious today that most of the accidents of celiosurgery, and gynecologists had proved this before, concern more basic than advanced procedures. It seems revolting to me that we want to discover or to learn the celioscopic colectomy when we do not master a difficult appendectomy, or when we keep a high rate of selection or conversion in cholecystectomy.

Applying a less invasive method cannot justify some "normal losses." In fact, and to sum up, it does not seem to me that celioscopic surgery brings enough innovations to the surgical principles to modify basic rules of surgical behavior. I do not believe that we can see an individual future for it, but we can consider or wish, as I do, that it may be an important, *incorporated* part of the future of all surgery.

Specific technical details do not justify the creation

of new rules. On the contrary, the thought and reality of an innovative phenomenon only emphasizes old rules, those of *ethics*.

CODE OF ETHICS AND CLINICAL REALIZATION

The *ethics rules* are the ones that must control the technical and technological factors that are part and parcel of the surgical art and science. Celioscopy is not exempted. The ethical rules must impose themselves as elements of control of the different actors in the surgical world, who, if we do not pay attention, constitute pressure groups, with everything that may imply power and the capacity for conflicts of interest.

Surgeons themselves are susceptible to setting up a lobby for and a lobby against. I think my arguments demonstrate the futility of such a partition. *The industry* is of course our ally. It brings us our instruments; from its performance will depend our results. It has its interests and therefore its strategies, which must nevertheless follow our rules of ethics.

Finally the patients themselves are of course the first interested in results of minimally invasive surgery and its future. Instinctively the patients can only be seduced by the spirit of minimally invasive surgery. The pressure they exercise can be powerful. This introduces the implicit demand of a *limitation of surgical choices and means.* Although they are the most directly concerned, the patients are rarely making decisions themselves, but they receive powerful information and advice:

Information—the media are generally the main purveyors, but often ethics has a hard time imposing itself on them.

The advice comes from the doctors and pharmacists, often advisers to their patients in France. So that their advice may be clarified, pharmacists and other do-gooders must themselves be well informed. They can only be so if we remember to associate them into our educational efforts, and to recognize that they have a real and natural arbitral power.

Finally, the economic criteria will be decisive in the years to come. Obviously as with all technological advances minimally invasive surgery represents an overcost in time, in tools, in personnel, in competence. This overcost cannot be accepted and will not be by the purse-string holder, except if we are able to bring proof by an argued and assessed evaluation that indeed this is a progress. In terms of linking quality and price, the result must be positive and the overcost of surgery must be balanced by a reduction of the follow-up period and the after-effects.

This economic study, which some have already started, comes up against a major problem, identical to the one which we evoked concerning the technical comparisons: the lack or the inadequacy of the evaluation of results with traditional surgery. Besides, the celioscopic practice makes it clear that we need to put the emphasis on the importance of the postsurgical lack of pain and functional disturbances. Its estimation will stay more qualitative than quantitative.

CONCLUSION

Such are the thoughts that I wanted to express on the future of minimally invasive surgery. If the observations I made today have only a positive view, I see the merit to have provoked active and global thought.

Who would have imagined only 4 years ago that we would witness a phenomenon of such extent? One of today's sessions' Presidents, Professor Puig LaCalle will remember certainly with amusement a video forum session over which he was presiding in May 1988 where my friend Hervé Marsaud and I, with the complicity of Jean Henri Alexandre, had the audacity to present a tape whose title was "Celioscopic approach to painful syndromes of the right iliac fossa." The reception from the audience had been reserved, to say the least, as he will recall.

Today I have the satisfaction of not having been completely wrong. We had been, at the time, I admit it, purposely provocative. But our conviction, progressively established in 20 years of experience, was already profound. It is the same today and to express it, I would like to give you this very personal thought: let us suppose that the power of some modern inquisition (maybe technocratic) imposed on me the retreat from the front-line of research. With a heavy heart, I believe I would bow and simulate retraction, adding a commentary, mezzo voce, "And even so, it was working." But if I were forced today to leave aside the celioscopy of exploration, the appendectomy, or the endoscopic cholecystectomy, the celioscopic gynecology, the staging of cancers, the cure of gastroesophageal reflux, the cure of hernias of the groin by laparoscopy, then I assure you that like Servatius and unlike Galileo, I would let myself be burned for my convictions . . . which means, to be less dramatic, that I would abandon the practice of surgery.

The Congress of Luxembourg demonstrates that

minimally invasive surgery has attained a healthy level of maturity. As often happens after a major meteorological disturbance or when a storm causes limited visibility, the horizon eventually becomes clear. The specialists talk about the "skyline." There is the ambiance of a "skyline" that we have seen in this Congress. There are still many obscure points, a lot of little clouds, but beyond them there are glimpses of sunlight and still farther beyond that, forecasts of a calm sky. This is my optimistic vision, which I invite you to share.

7 *The Present and Future Role of Conventional Invasive Surgery*

Jean Moreaux

THE CURRENT STATE OF CONVENTIONAL SURGERY

Traditional surgery of the digestive tract is on the decline for two reasons: (1) the recent rapid expansion of the field of celioscopic surgery and (2) the decrease in the amount of surgical literature that has been available over the last 5 years. The following additional factors have contributed to this decline:

- The large pharmaceutical companies have developed newer and more efficient drugs.
- Endoscopists are now able to remove polyps from the digestive canal, sclerose esophageal varices, extract stones from the biliary canal and Wirsung's canal, and provide palliative treatment for some forms of cancer.
- Radiologists can biopsy tumors, drain cystic cavities or suppurated collections, and sometimes even create portocaval anastomoses.
- Radiotherapy and chemotherapy can cure certain types of cancer.

All of these techniques can be associated with or used in place of surgery, which means a permanent modification of therapeutic measures. When dramatic results are achieved with medication, as in the case of gastroduodenal ulcers or peptic esophagitis, there is a tendency to postpone surgery, since no surgical technique can guarantee a 100% success rate in the long term. Thus entire facets of digestive surgery are in danger of disappearing.

A second reason, which appears to contradict the first, is that traditional surgery has made significant progress over the last 20 years and has achieved a degree of success and reliability. This progress includes improvements in surgical procedures, but even more important this success involves all aspects of these surgical procedures. The duration of surgery is no longer relevant, nor is the age of the patient. When surgery is indicated in elderly patients, there are no longer any restrictions.

Conventional surgery has become much less invasive. It is often elective, procedures are as short as possible, and incisions are usually transverse for better preservation of the abdominal wall. Hemorrhaging is minimal due to improved hemostasis techniques, and blood transfusions are no longer required in the majority of patients. Drainage of the abdominal cavity has become less traumatic, and the need for colostomy for ileostomy has decreased. Organ transplants have taken on a major role in digestive surgery, and liver transplantation has become a therapeutic modality in many hepatic diseases. There has been a decrease in both postoperative morbidity and mortality. The following examples are taken from some of our experiences over the past 20 years with conventional digestive surgery. The first concerns a prospective study of 5000 operations and reoperations for biliary lithiasis conducted between 1970 and 1990. There was only one accidental injury of the main biliary duct during cholecystectomy and six cases of brief external biliary fistula after cholecystectomy for acute cholecystitis. The hospital mortality rate was 0.09% in the absence of associated abdominal surgery. There were no postoperative deaths associated with elective surgery for gallbladder disease and lesions of the main biliary canal, and the mortality rate was 0.8% for emergency surgery. It was 0.6% for patients 75 years of age or older. During that same period, among 1027 operations for single colon cancer, there was evidence of anastomotic disunity without fecal peritonitis in only three patients, and there were eight postoperative deaths, only four of which occurred after curative surgery.

The success of conventional surgery is undeniable, but we must not allow ourselves to become complacent or think that treatment of a given disease has achieved such a degree of perfection that it cannot be improved. Only by constant evaluation can we progress.

THE FUTURE OF CONVENTIONAL SURGERY

The future of conventional surgery again depends on two factors: the future of celioscopic surgery and the future of digestive surgery in general, if one agrees that the major diseases of the twenty-first century will be the same ones that predominated in the twentieth century.

The bright future of celiosurgery has been outlined by Mouret. It is very difficult to predict the percentage of operations that will be performed celioscopically compared with those performed by conventional open techniques. Celioscopy could represent 80% of digestive surgery in some specialized centers if one separates gynecological surgery. Indeed, the place of celiosurgery will vary greatly from one center to another, and it will be possible to combine the two methods, leading to a new discipline.

What is more important is the future of digestive surgery: will celiosurgery allow us to regain ground already lost and to raise the banner of digestive surgery? Surgeons actually force themselves to adapt to celiosurgery those traditional operations that have proved their efficacy. Celiosurgery will have to be evaluated to determine whether it is as effective as traditional surgery. Finally, comparative economic studies will have to be carried out to show that a simple procedure requiring a shorter hospitalization and less time lost from work is less costly to the society than life-long drug therapy. Even if a surgical solution is the most advantageous economically and if health care systems are operating at a deficit, will authorities be able to stop reimbursement for medicine and force patients to undergo surgery for primarily economic reasons?

Might we not witness a progressive decline in all types of digestive surgery despite the resurgence brought about by celiosurgery? The future of this area of surgery is very difficult to predict. According to Bernard,[1] cancer surgery could disappear around the year 2030. Biliary lithiasis surgery might also disappear, but no one dares to mention a date. Under the direction of the Public Assistance Plan of Paris, a group was organized in 1986 and 1987 to conduct a prospective study concerning hospitals of the twenty-first century. This group predicted that the overall number of hospitalizations will decrease considerably and entire facets of surgery will disappear, for example, general surgery and digestive surgery, but not including transplantation and urology. At the same time health care costs will continue to increase. According to INSEE and OCDE, they will go from 13.9% of the family budget in 1985 to 20% at the beginning of the twenty-first century.

Similar studies have been conducted in other countries. From what we have read, predictions of a decline in general surgery are unanimous, but there is no consensus as to the significance of this decline. Some are very pessimistic and others are more reassuring. The total elimination of cancer surgery and of the complications of biliary lithiasis is unimaginable, as in nonsurgical treatment of appendicitis, peritonitis, digestive hemorrhage, intestinal occlusions, and all diseases of the abdominal wall. The Council on Long Range Planning and Development of the American Medical Association[3] believes in the survival of general surgery, especially because of the aging of the population, provided that methods are innovative and can be adapted to allow for continuing improvements in technology.

This uncertainty about the future of general and digestive surgery has led to a state of crisis. Interns are jumping ship. This disaffection could result in difficulties of installation and in living conditions estimated too painful and without compensation. General surgery, the main area common to all specialties, which had brought glory to surgery, is threatened to be relegated to the last position, behind specialties and even pseudospecialties. Scientific societies that want to stay general are no longer able to attract surgeons scattered into specialized societies.

The following steps must be taken to prepare for the future and maintain the present superior level of digestive tract surgery before its possible disappearance:

1. We must try to adjust the number of general and digestive surgeons to meet the needs of society. In 1986

there were 31,200 general surgeons in the United States. Many of them are young, and 65% will still be practicing by the year 2000. According to the predictions of the Council on Long Range Planning and Development, compared with the increases in surgical pseudo-specialties, the rate of increase in the number of general surgeons has been very low since 1980 but will reverse after the year 2000. In France, unfortunately, to our knowledge there are no such statistics.

2. We must accept the teaching of new techniques but also continue the teaching of traditional surgical procedures. This may be complex, and our current teaching and training programs are not satisfying this double goal. Today's interns adapt much more quickly than their elders to celiosurgery, but the problem remains to train them in traditional surgical procedures. Surgeons who have made a successful transition from traditional surgery to celiosurgery consider the conversion as essential, because they can see the advantages. But will future surgeons have sufficient knowledge of traditional surgical techniques to save their patients in cases of catastrophic occurrences, and will they be able to correct their own mistakes? It is possible that we will need to create a group of surgeons highly trained in conventional surgery to operate on difficult cases and treat pathological conditions for which celiosurgery is unsuitable, for example, some tumors of the liver or pancreas? They would be the "general general surgeons," a phrase coined by Longmire,[5] or the general supersurgeons.

3. Private surgical institutions and hospitals must also be able to adapt. Isolated and independent general surgeons are destined to disappear, along with the small facilities where they work. All centers, public or private, will revolve around a main core made up of a large technical staff, combined medicosurgical teams, numerous consultants, and a bed count far more limited than the current numbers. All deterrents to these objectives are destined to disappear. Doctors, surgeons, endoscopists, and radiologists will have to work in close collaboration and if possible in perfect harmony, which will permit each patient to choose the least aggressive and most appropriate therapy and in turn will provide the maximal chance of success.

4. We must improve the organization of organ transplantation, which will have a favored status within di-gestive surgery in the twenty-first century. These transplants would be performed in specially developed centers, where highly trained teams would concentrate on essential procedures and technology. These centers, with their complex organization and their use dependent on economic considerations, could be financed outside the limits of medical insurance.

All these reflections concern the future of surgery in wealthy countries, but we must not forget that all over the world the status of surgery is often catastrophic. With advances in technology, the gap between surgery in wealthy countries and poor countries will widen. Conventional surgery remains in all these less developed countries an unattainable goal because of a lack of financial resources and often an absence of the most basic hygiene. One must have visited hospitals in Africa or Asia to fully realize the extent of their needs. We must help all of these countries far more than we do now to ensure their survival and preserve our own. We can even imagine a future in which our interns travel to these places for initial training in traditional surgical techniques.

CONCLUSION

The future of traditional digestive tract surgery cannot be predicted. Current operative indications will decrease, but GI surgery will retain its overall status for many years to come. Surgical procedures may change, hospitals will change, but the concerns of patients do not. In the face of modern technology, we must not forget that our mission is to meet the needs of our patients, answer their questions, and to relieve their anxiety and suffering.

REFERENCES

1. Bernard J. The surgery of the year 2077. Nouv Presse Med 6:3123-3130, 1977.
2. Binet JP. The honor of surgery. Presse Med 14:2076-2079, 1985.
3. Council on Long Range Planning and Development. The future of general surgery. JAMA 262:3178-3183, 1989.
4. Jolly D. The hospital of the 21st century. Paris: Economica Edit, 1988.
5. Longmire WP. Am Coll Surg 69:2-6, 1984.
6. Organ CH. The future of general surgery. Arch Surg 125:145-146, 1990.

8   *Healing Hands or Healing Instruments: Enduring Surgical Principles for Minimally Invasive Operations*

Jean-Paul Binet

Modern surgery that heals the patient without undue risk is relatively new; it dates from the second quarter of the twentieth century, when all essential conditions for its safe practice were met. Historically, the discovery of such essential safety features as the "three *A*'s"—anesthesia, antisepsis, and asepsis—meant that the conditions ensuring lasting success, the "three *R*'s," had to be addressed: resuscitation, reeducation, and readaptation. The greater part of the nineteenth and twentieth centuries was spent in these endeavors. In the midst of the ongoing technological explosion, we must not forget what has been accomplished in past centuries and who accomplished these feats: among the many, Hippocrates, Vesalius, Ambroise Paré, Hunter, and Larrey. It would be unthinkable to forget Pasteur, who was not a surgeon, but who brought about changes that had such enormous impact on operative procedures by mastering, if not eradicating, the greatest of dangers—infection.

In the past 50 years—that is, during the lifetime of a mere generation or two of surgeons—we have seen 10 surgical specialties evolve from general surgery, as branches grow from the main trunk of a tree. In fact, general surgery in some ways has even been overshadowed by the specialties. Yet the ageless practice of the surgeon's mind that guides his hands and coordinates the use of instruments ensures the smooth transition and harmonious progress from the ancient craft of the barber-surgeon to today's practitioner of the art of minimally invasive surgery. More than ever before, mastery of operative surgery mandates technical skill. As Lord Joseph Lister stated: "To intrude an unskilled hand into such a piece of divine mechanism as the human body is indeed a fearful responsibility."

This responsibility is heightened by the ethical dictates and technical demands on the merits of a new procedure based on advanced technology. In the words of Alfred Blalock, surgeon-scientist and pioneer in cardiac surgery, "It usually requires a considerable time to determine with certainty the virtues of a new method of treatment—and usually still longer to ascertain the harmful effects." We must not, in our desire to achieve progress, implement a new surgical technique with some haste and disregard the cardinal principles on which the art and science of surgery is based. Despite technological sophistication, the surgeon's mind and hands are supreme and must move with the sure knowledge of the underlying anatomy, even when it is viewed on a television monitor.

Not much could be added to the artistic and practical significance that Paul Valery attached to the hand in 1937. We now know, thanks to ultrasonography, that in the fetus the hand is the first part of the body that moves; we have also learned that if a toe is implanted microsurgically to replace a congenitally missing finger before a child is 2 years of age, the toe as it grows will take the shape and function of the finger it replaces.

Thousands of tools are currently available to expand the capabilities of the surgeon's hands. Before World War II there were fewer than 100; now there are more than 300 kinds of artificial prostheses just for the bony joints. Mechanical sutures, particularly of the colon, are done readily with staples applied in one single motion, all automatically. By contrast, our older generation learned through painful failure and repetitious practice that the most important aspect of quality sutures was that they not be seen outside the bowel lumen. The tying of knots via videoscopic monitoring requires the ultimate coordination of the mind, the eyes, the hands, and their extension, the instruments of the operating surgeon.

When we felt entitled to believe that we had reached a certain perfection in the established, "classic" surgical procedure, with an operative mortality reduced to virtually nil (there are no longer any exploratory operations for ill-defined and life-threatening conditions), this new approach to the body cavities and visceral lumina was born and rapidly developed to an advanced, and (it is to be hoped) soon perfect level of technical accomplishment—an approach that uses the natural passages without opening the body or that finds access to body cavities through minimal incisions. Today many vascular, abdominal, thoracic, and gynecological operative procedures are done through small ports that accept placement of a telescope and camera—an extension of the surgeon's eyes (similar to a periscope on a submarine)—and of special instruments: elongations of the surgeon's fingers. The coordination of mind, eyes, and hands is guided by viewing the findings and operative action on a television monitor and adjusting the steps in technique according to visual and transmitted tactile perceptions.

It is apparent that the surgeon can no longer be the one individual capable of performing the essential steps of an operation; he or she now stands *at the center of a team*, and the interdependent role of the team members has replaced the obsolete role of "God's gift to surgery." Only a team of doctors and highly skilled technicians could have mastered cardiac surgery and organ transplantation, among the most sophisticated and complex applications of surgical therapy. And now every day brings news of yet another complex operation that is being undertaken through a minimally invasive approach—truly an ongoing revolution in operative surgery.

It would be neither just nor correct to relegate the art and science of surgery, as some have a tendency to do, to the ranks of a simple set of operative techniques. Surgery is a discipline within the body of the healing arts and sciences that demands a constant search and unfaltering effort in achieving a perfect match between intellect and dexterity, always at the highest level. This daily renewal in striving for the ideal result becomes even more challenging now, since surgical thought and action are often a multidisciplinary endeavor. This constant search and struggle for optimal outcome are unique and doubly fundamental: they reach structures and functions of what is a human life, and they are exercised on behalf of a patient—our brother or sister or neighbor—whose destiny is in our hands, without our having any right to error in creating the ideal therapeutic environment and accomplishment.

II

Diagnostic Techniques

9   *Ultrasonography in the Course of Laparoscopic Surgery*

J.J. Jakimowicz

A prospective study evaluating intraoperative ultrasonography and cholangiography during biliary tract surgery led my colleagues and me to the conclusion that ultrasonography is a reliable diagnostic tool, and when used as a screening procedure during biliary surgery, it offers certain advantages. Its application is not restricted to the biliary tract but can also be used in the course of the staging laparotomy. Ultrasonography is highly reliable in detecting and localizing pathological findings. It provides important information about the anatomy and has a potential for wide application. Use of intraoperative ultrasonography appears cost effective, and with proper training and equipment, it is easy to perform. From previous experience with ultrasonography, we have concluded that this method can become an effective substitute for cholangiography as a screening procedure for common bile duct pathology during cholecystectomy.[1-5]

The dynamic developments of laparoscopic techniques and the introduction of laparoscopic cholecystectomy turned our attention to the potential application of ultrasonography during laparoscopic surgery, both during laparoscopic cholecystectomy and in the course of diagnostic staging laparoscopy, particularly in patients with gastrointestinal malignancies. We focused on three applications of ultrasonography: (1) using ultrasonography to evaluate the final state of the biliary tract after completion of laparoscopic cholecystectomy, (2) evaluation for the presence or absence of biliary tract pathology before attempting laparoscopic cholecystectomy, and (3) in the course of diagnostic laparoscopy for screening of the liver, detection of lymph nodes, and localization and identification of anatomical structures.

MATERIALS

The Aloca 650 real-time mobile scanner is used. This system makes possible the use of a linear-array transducer, and if necessary, a mechanical sector transducer may also be used. The system has a Doppler option, which is particularly helpful in identifying vessels during diagnostic laparoscopy. In the preliminary stage

Table 1. Ultrasonography during laparoscopic surgery—transducer equipment

Transducer	Linear Array
UST 5522, 7.5 MHz (Aloca)	Length, 35 cm Diameter, 10 mm Screening surface, 38 mm Depth of view field, 6 cm Doppler capability

of our experience with intraoperative ultrasonography of the biliary tract, the endorectal transducer probe (UST 660, 7.5 MHz) was used. This transducer, which is 16 mm in diameter, could be applied only for assessment of the biliary tract after removal of the gallbladder because the umbilical wound must be dilated for introduction of this transducer's probe. This transducer has been superseded by a newly developed laparoscopic transducer probe specifically for use during laparoscopy. The technical data about this transducer are shown in Table 1.

METHODS AND RESULTS

In the early stage of our experience in assessing for the presence or absence of biliary tract pathology at the beginning of laparoscopic cholecystectomy, after the introduction of the first trocar, we faced a handicap because of the absence of a specific ultrasound transducer for this particular application. The available linear-array transducer usable for this purpose was the one for the endorectal application, which is 17 mm in diameter; thus it could not be passed through the trocar we used. So we were forced to restrict the evaluation in the early stage to an estimate of the final state of the common bile duct after removal of the gallbladder. Thus we used the ultrasound as an alternative for cholangiography to exclude common bile duct pathology.

Table 2. Results of ultrasonography during laparoscopic cholecystectomy

	Group 1	Group 2
Successful examination	76	53
Failure	3	1
Quality of visualization of CBD		
Good	69	50
Moderate	7	3
Diameter of CBD (mm)	0.3-12	0.3-0.8
Visualization of CBD (median)	0.4	0.4
Up to liver	74 (+) 2 (−)	50 (+) 2 (−)
Down to papilla	60 (+) 7 (−)	50 (+) 1 (−)
Maximal visible length of one section of CBD	2.0-5	3.7-5.1
Median	3.4	4.1
Time required for screening (min)	5-10	5-10
Pathology observed (no. of patients)	3	2
TOTAL	79	53

CBD = common bile duct.

The technique of examination is as follows. After final removal of the gallbladder, the ultrasound transducer is passed into the peritoneum through the umbilical incision. For visual control the laparoscope is placed through the midline trocar to see the hepatoduodenal ligament. The transducer is placed under direct vision on the anterior aspect of the common bile duct. The screening movements include a slight rotation of the transducer and forward and backward movement while the transducer is slowly pulled backward through the place of insertion. The common bile duct is seen and can be followed all the way to the papilla. Sometimes saline solution is introduced into the peritoneum via one of the trocars to submerge the common bile duct and create a better contact between the transducer probe and the duct. When a laparoscopic transducer is used, it is passed through one of the access ports, depending on the target of screening, and principles similar to those of contact screening are followed.

In the preliminary study we focused our attention on assessing the method's visibility when used as a perioperative screening procedure of the biliary tract. The preliminary results are summarized in Table 2. When a new technique is introduced, a learning curve is present, as reflected in the results achieved when using the endorectal transducer probe. The experience with laparoscopic transducer probes specifically for this purpose are shown in Table 2. By improving the examination technique and using improved equipment, we can achieve better results: in this case, a longer segment of the duct can be visualized in one section, and examination of the papilla is easier and more reliable. The rate of unsuccessful or incomplete screenings is reduced (see Table 2).

Intraoperative ultrasonography during diagnostic laparoscopy or when laparoscopic bowel resection was attempted was used in 14 patients. In all of these patients screening of the liver was performed. In two patients unexpected liver metastases were detected. Ultrasonography assisted laparoscopic colon resection in eight patients. It helped to localize a tumor in one patient, and enlarged lymph nodes along the ileocolic artery were detected in two patients. In patients with biliary and pancreatic tumors laparoscopic ultrasonography was important in final decision making. It was applied in three patients. In one patient unexpected liver metastases were detected (see Fig. 3). In a second case tumor infiltration of a gallbladder carcinoma into the liver was demonstrated. When applying ultrasonography in the course of pelvic lymphadenectomy in patients with prostatic carcinoma, lymph nodes could be demonstrated, and ultrasonography allowed easy localization of the surrounding vessels. The examples of different findings during the screening are shown in Figs. 1 through 3.

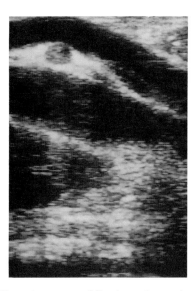

Fig. 1. Normal common bile duct, 4 mm in diameter, with the portal vein in the background in between cross section of hepatic artery.

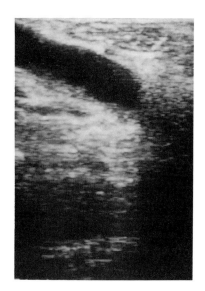

Fig. 2. Distal part of the common bile duct.

DISCUSSION

The use of ultrasonography in the course of laparoscopic surgery, particularly during laparoscopic cholecystectomy, was first reported by Jakimowicz and Ruers[1] in 1991. Already this preliminary experience has allowed the conclusion that ultrasonography can be applied successfully during laparoscopic surgery, but the development of specific equipment for this particular application is a must. The laparoscopic linear-array transducer UST 5522, 7.5 MHz (Aloca), became available in January 1992 for clinical evaluation. The reliability of this specific equipment allowed us to apply this method of examination not only to screening of the biliary tract but also to screening of the liver, examination of the pancreas, localization of bowel tumor, evaluation of the tumor and presence of metastases, and detection of lymph nodes; in addition, ultrasonography supported by Doppler could be used successfully to recognize the anatomical structures and allow safe dissection.

Our preliminary experience gained with this modality implies that with the further improvement of screening technique and equipment, intraoperative ultrasonography during laparoscopic surgery will provide certain benefits. When applied in the course of staging laparoscopy for a patient with a gastrointestinal malignancy or as a screening test of the biliary tract, it could limit the excessive preoperative diagnostic workup. It allows estimation of the extent of the patient's patho-

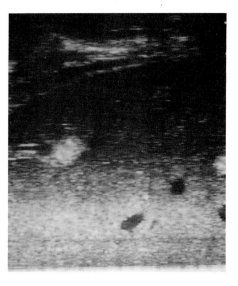

Fig. 3. Liver metastases detected by ultrasonography during staging laparoscopy.

logical condition and allows detection of unpredicted lesions.

CONCLUSION

When operating on patients with obscure anatomy and an inflammatory mass or tumor, intraoperative ultrasonography supported by Doppler can clarify the anatomy before dissection. Operative decision making can be supported by the outcome of the ultrasound examination and allow the choice of the optimal therapeutic option. When applied for screening of the biliary tract during laparoscopic cholecystectomy, ultrasonography provides valuable information on the status of the biliary tract. Measurement of the internal diameter of the common bile duct is possible and provides important diagnostic information. We know from previous experience not to expect any pathological findings in patients who have an internal diameter of the common bile duct of less than or equal to 5 mm.[2-4] If patients have a common bile duct with an internal diameter of 6 mm or more and if no pathology is found by ultrasonography, cholangiography should be considered. The preliminary experience implies that in the future intraoperative ultrasonography during laparoscopic surgery will be a simple and safe procedure, providing information for operative decision making.

REFERENCES

1. Jakimowicz JJ, Ruers TJM. Ultrasound-assisted laparoscopic cholecystectomy: Preliminary experience. Dig Surg 8:114-117, 1991.
2. Jakimowicz JJ. Intraoperative and postoperative biliary endoscopy; Intraoperative ultrasonography and sonography during laparoscopic cholecystectomy. Probl Gen Surg 8:442-457, 1991.
3. Jakimowicz JJ, Rutten H. Intraoperative ultrasonography of the biliary tract, an alternative to intraoperative cholangiography. In Ultra-shall in der Chirurgie (Simanowski/Mendel). New York: Springer-Verlag, 1991, pp 79-86.
4. Jakimowicz JJ, Rutten H, Sommeling C, et al. Intraoperative ultrasonography of the biliary tract, equipment, technique and results. In Brinkman EE, ed. Sonography in der Chirurgie. Hamelen: TM Verlag, 1990, pp 89-97.
5. Sigel B. Operative Ultrasonography. Philadelphia: Lea & Febiger, 1982.

10 The Value of Preoperative and Postoperative Ultrasonography in Minimally Invasive Surgery

Ulf Nahrstedt, Henning Niebuhr, and Klaus Rückert

In the context of minimally invasive procedures, the role of ultrasonography is increasing. Preoperatively, ultrasound enables the surgeon to view the organs to be treated in the upper or lower abdomen (e.g., gallbladder or inflamed appendix). In the case of the appendix, it can be used to demonstrate inflammation of the wall.[1,2] An inflamed appendix can be seen in approximately 90% of all cases.[2] A *target phenomenon* is often visible—that is, dark and light layers of gut wall and inflamed tissue around the appendix[1-3] (Fig. 1). Typical of this phenomenon is the nonexistence of peristasis in this area and the pressure pain that can be reproduced by the ultrasound applicator.[2] Particularly with a difficult diagnosis such as appendicitis in geriatric patients or in young women, this type of examination provides more reliable signs on which to base a diagnosis.[4] Also, certain differential diagnoses can be excluded on the basis of ultrasonography—for example, biliary colic, gallstones, symptomatic kidney stones, and early pregnancy.[5] Salpingitis as an important differential diagnosis, as opposed to appendicitis, cannot be demonstrated directly, but if the appendix is not inflamed, it is unlikely that the patient has appendicitis. With this method the rate of *negative laparotomies* can be reduced from 25% to 30% to 10% to 15% of all cases.[2,4,6]

For the appendix in particular, it is important to use modern equipment such as a 5 or 7.5 MHz scanner, to obtain a clear view, directly under the skin of the abdomen, in an area 40 by 80 mm. The level of experience of the examiner is also important, because often this procedure must be carried out quickly to obtain the correct view. This method should be learned under careful supervision and with hands-on experience.

In diseases of the gallbladder, a diagnosis of gallstones made by ultrasonography will be correct nearly 100% of the time. Many other pathological conditions can also be seen on sonogram, including polyps and vari-ous degrees of inflammation of the gallbladder wall[7,8] (Fig. 2). Thus there is much evidence to support the surgeon's decision to use a conservative or minimally invasive procedure. The width of the common bile duct as indirect evidence of common bile duct calculi can be measured by ultrasound.[9]

Other questionable findings (tumor of the gallblad-

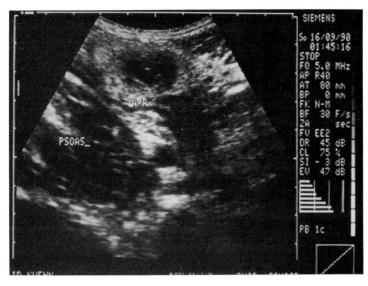

Fig. 1. Sonogram of patient with acute appendicitis.

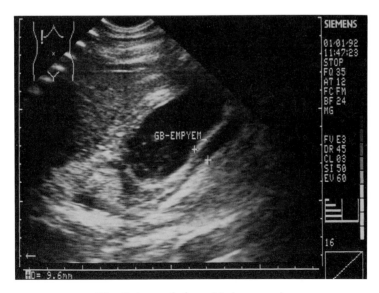

Fig. 2. Acute cholecystitis (empyema).

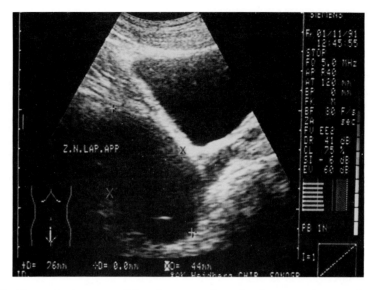

Fig. 3. Abscess in the space of Douglas; scan taken after laparoscopic appendectomy.

der or cecum or perityphlitis) are also revealed. Especially in the case of an uncertain diagnosis of appendicitis, this method helps to discriminate different diagnostic possibilities. Postoperatively, ultrasound makes complications more visible and easier to treat by percutaneous puncture or drainage (subhepatic fluid collection or abscess in the space of Douglas)[7,10,11] (Fig. 3).

PATIENTS

Preoperatively and postoperatively, 126 patients with symptomatic gallstones and 47 patients with acute appendicitis were examined with ultrasound (from January to June 1991). Solitary calculi were found in 45 patients and multiple stones in 79. An inflamed appendix could be seen in 43 of 47 patients with acute appendicitis. After laparoscopic cholecystectomy, subhepatic fluid collection was observed in 11 patients. Two of them were treated percutaneously under ultrasound guidance. After laparoscopic appendectomy, Douglas' abscess developed in two patients. One abscess was drained transvaginally and the other transrectally.

CONCLUSION

Ultrasound is an excellent diagnostic instrument in the surgeon's hands for better preoperative evaluation and decision making. Postoperatively, complications resulting from minimally invasive surgery can be handled percutaneously by the surgeon.[10,11] An inflamed appendix

can be seen preoperatively in nearly 90% of all cases by an examiner with some experience and modern equipment.[2] Postoperative complications such as Douglas' abscess are visible and can be treated by transcutaneous drainage guided by ultrasound.[11] In the same way, gallstones of all sizes can be seen with a high degree of reliability. An acutely inflamed gallbladder with a thick multilayered wall is visible in 90% of all cases and provides the surgeon with information pertaining to the decision to treat conventionally or with a minimally invasive procedure.

Ultrasonographic imaging of cancer of the gallbladder is not as reliable. In this case CT scans are preferable. Also, direct evidence of stones in the biliary duct is difficult to detect, and only 20% to 30% of these stones are visible. Indirect evidence is a common bile duct wider than 6 mm—thus all bile ducts wider than 6 mm should be examined with other diagnostic techniques such as preoperative or intraoperative contrast x-ray imaging or endoscopic retrograde cholangiography.

Postoperatively, ultrasonography should be used in all patients during follow-up, since it allows detection of fluid collection of more than 10 ml in the subhepatic space or the upper portion of the pouch of Douglas. Therefore drainage will not be necessary in all laparoscopic operations.[7] Patients with symptoms of subhepatic hematoma or a biloma can be treated with ultrasound-guided transcutaneous drainage, which is usually done under local anesthesia. Ultrasound examination before or after this type of operation is a noninvasive but extremely reliable measure. It is an ideal complement to the new minimally invasive surgical techniques in that it is nontraumatic with a high degree of safety.

REFERENCES

1. Schwerk WB, Wichtrup B, Rüschoff J, et al. Acute and perforated appendicitis: Current experience with ultrasound-aided diagnosis. World J Surg 14:271, 1990.

2. Zielke A, Malewski U. Sonographie bei Verdacht auf akute Appendicitis: Möglichkeit oder Notwendigkeit für den Chirurgen? Chirurg 62:743-749, 1991.

3. Borushok KF, Jeffrey RB, Laing FC, et al. Sonographic diagnosis of perforation in patients with acute appendicitis. AJR 154:275, 1990.

4. Puylaert JB, Rutgers P, Labisang, et al. A prospective study of ultrasonography in the diagnosis of appendicitis. N Engl J Med 317:666-669, 1987.

5. de Dombal FT. Diagnose und Operationsindikation bei der akuten Appendicitis: Wieviele Irrtümer sind vermeidbar? Chirurg 50:291, 1979.

6. Paterson-Brown S. Strategies for reducing inappropriate laparotomy rate in the acute abdomen. Br Med J 303:1115, 1991.

7. Hölscher AH. Ultraschalldiagnostik des akuten, nicht traumatisierten Abdomens. Chir Praxis 34:29, 1985.

8. Ralls PW, Colleti PM, Lapin SA. Real-time sonography in suspected acute cholecystitis. Radiology 155:767, 1985.

9. Lutz H. Ultraschalldiagnostik bei akutem Abdomen. Ultraschall Klin Prax 2:19, 1987.

10. Gronvall S, Gammelgaard J, Haubek A, et al. Drainage of abdominal abscesses guided by sonography. AJR Am J Roentgenol 138:527, 1982.

11. Hölscher AH. Sonographie im postoperativen Verlauf (Bauch und Thorax). Chirurg 63:606-611, 1992.

III

Anesthesia

11 *The Perioperative Conduct of Anesthesia for Endoscopic Surgery*

Jean-Baptiste Nyarwaya and Kamran Samii

Recent developments in endoscopic surgery techniques have provided a new opportunity for less invasive approaches to the management of intra-abdominal, intrathoracic, and extraperitoneal diseases, which previously required open surgery.

Although laparoscopy has been practiced for decades and proved safe by gynecologists, additional physiopathological changes may arise from these new intra-abdominal operative procedures. Therefore coexisting diseases, especially cardiorespiratory ones, should be carefully assessed and their risk/benefit ratio evaluated when intraoperative complications may outweigh postoperative comfort. The safety of the procedure probably depends more on the duration of the operation, close intraoperative monitoring, and the experience of both anesthesiologist and surgeon than on a particular anesthetic technique. Consequently, the technique demands a significant commitment from the anesthesiologist who must recognize occurring physiopathological changes and develop appropriate anesthetic planning and management.

PATHOPHYSIOLOGICAL CHANGES OF THE HEMODYNAMIC STATUS

Independent from the operative site, the concomitant pathophysiological alterations are proportionate to the compressive effect of the insufflated gas on the cardiorespiratory system, its absorption from the abdomen, and the positioning required during the laparoscopic procedure.

Animal experiments and clinical studies have demonstrated that changes in intra-abdominal pressure (IAP) vary the pressure and flow in the inferior vena cava (IVC). Guyton and Adkins[1] studied the gradient of pressure along the IVC in supine dogs. Although the IAP was normal (mean, $+0.7$ cm H_2O), the pressure in the IVC decreased progressively from its origin ($+1$ cm H_2O) to its end in the right atrium (RA) (-1 cm H_2O). An increase of the IAP up to 35 cm H_2O was followed by an increase of the pressure in the IVC. However, the pressure in the IVC remained always superior (2 to 3

cm H_2O) to that of the IAP except in the last intra-abdominal portion. Within this terminal part, a sudden decrease of the pressure was noted.[1] This high gradient is evident when the IAP is higher than 25 cm H_2O, and is a function that happens when stenosis in the suprahepatic part of the abdominal IVC is observed.[2,3] This phenomenon depends on neither the animal's position nor diaphragmatic level but expresses a hydraulically reproducible event that happens when a liquid runs through a flexible pipe from a high-pressure to a low-pressure cavity. Accordingly, many authors have noted a diphasic evolution of the cardiac output (CO) when the IAP is increased by insufflation of a gas. At the beginning and as long as the IAP is lower than 5 to 7 cm H_2O, the CO increases because of emptying of the collapsing intra-abdominal veins.[2,4-6] Thereafter when the pressure increases, the CO declines quickly and strictly parallels the decrease of the flow in the IVC. Ivankovitch et al.[4] observed a decrease in CO to 50% and to 65% when the IAPs were, respectively, 32 and 47 cm H_2O. This decrease is followed by an increase of the pressure measured in the RA. This increase results from transmission of the intrathoracic pressure through the elevated diaphragmatic domes. The transmural pressure in the RA (pressure in the RA minus intrathoracic pressure), representing the hemodynamically effective pressure, declines. However, during all these studies the heart rate was faster and the mean arterial pressure (MAP) increased because of increased diastolic pressure induced by the baroreflex mechanism and compression of the abdominal aorta.

Ivankovitch et al.[4] did not observe any difference when the abdominal cavity was insufflated with nitrous oxide (N_2O) or CO_2, although with the latter the arterial carbon dioxide pressure ($PaCO_2$) increased 8 mm Hg. Therefore the increase of the $PaCO_2$ has no effect on the changes noted. Nevertheless, the hemodynamic changes observed during laparoscopic procedures are confusing and show disagreements. Kelman et al.[7] noted an increase in CO ($+10\%$) as long as the IAP was less than 30 cm H_2O. Thereafter, when the IAP increased, the CO declined but remained higher than control values.

Motew et al.[8] did not observe any significant change in CO during gynecological laparoscopy with the patient in the Trendelenburg position, even when the IAPs were up to 30 cm H_2O. On the contrary, Marshall et al.[9] observed a 30% decrease with an IAP of 30 cm H_2O. The insufflated gas seems not to explain these differences. The sole variables likely to affect the findings of these studies in humans may be the mode of ventilation and the steepness of head-down tilt.

Recent hemodynamic studies performed during laparoscopic cholecystectomy with abdominal CO_2 insufflation of less than 15 mm Hg showed a modest decrease in stroke volume index (SVI) and cardiac index (CI) occurring in the first 5 minutes.[10,11] Later, the CI rose gradually as the heart rate and SVI increased, despite a significant decrease in end-diastolic volume index (EDVI).[11] When other hemodynamic parameters are considered, there is agreement between the results: the heart rate, MAP, right atrial pressure (RAP), systemic vascular resistance (SVR), and pulmonary artery pressure (PAP) increase. The transmural pressure, reflecting the mechanically effective pressure, follows that of the CO.

In conclusion, since low increases of IAP lead to increased venous return and higher increases in pressure (<30 to 35 cm H_2O) induce a fall of CO, it is not easy to determine the critical IAP at which the CO begins to decline. Experimental studies suggest that this pressure could be estimated as 7 to 10 cm H_2O in a horizontal or a moderate Trendelenburg position. However, this critical IAP may even be lower in patients with impaired cardiac function or because of the operative positioning. We propose this last assumption, according to the study of Matalon and Farhi,[12] who showed a decline of CO of 10% in conscious volunteers when they were placed in head-up tilt of 15 degrees. Although the Trendelenburg position increases the venous return, it does not completely improve the hemodynamic alterations induced by the pneumoperitoneum because the increased intrathoracic pressure impedes the filling of the RA.[7] During laparoscopic procedures, the hemodynamic status may also be modified by the dysrhythmias induced by increased $PaCO_2$[13] or vagal bradycardia[8] and is dramatically altered when a gaseous embolism happens.

Transthoracic endoscopic surgery may also induce hemodynamic changes. Therefore investigations to quantify the limit of tolerance are needed. Unequal pressures within the two thoracic cavities may cause mediastinal displacement with a serious hemodynamic effect. Furthermore, suction used to clear blood, smoke, and irrigation fluid from the surgical field may cause large negative intrathoracic pressures. N_2O diffusing into the closed cavity also can cause pressure changes.

Concerns remain about the effect of a pneumoperitoneum on the blood flow through the intra-abdominal organs, especially the liver and kidney. With regard to renal blood flow, Harman et al.[14] showed that compression of the IVC with a pressure of 20 mm Hg induces a marked decrease in glomerular flow resulting from dramatically increased renal vasoconstriction (up to 550%) and decreased glomerular filtration.

Respiratory Changes

Ventilatory gas exchange depends closely on the ventilatory and hemodynamic state expressed as ventilation to perfusion (V/Q) ratio. Impaired gas exchange frequently complicates general anesthesia,[15] particularly during abdominal surgery. During laparoscopic surgery, abdominal insufflation may contribute to the worsening of this impairment because of extra shifting of the diaphragm.[16] The underlying mechanisms include reduced functional residual capacity (FRC), airway closure, and dependent atelectasis in the dependent lung. An increased physiological shunt fraction (QS/QT) is observed in this zone of low V/Q.[17] However, this phenomenon may present a matter of little concern for anesthesiologists. Our unpublished data show that the calculated QS/QT did not significantly change during laparoscopic cholecystectomy in American Society of Anesthesiologists (ASA) class I and II patients. Important intrapulmonary shunting may be observed during a transthoracic procedure requiring one-lung ventilation with a collapsed upper lung in the lateral decubitus position. On the other hand, the V/Q ratio may increase as a result of decreased CO and an increased physiological dead space (VD_{phys}) in the upper pulmonary zone during abdominal endoscopic surgery in the dorsal decubitus position. During gynecological laparoscopy, Puri and Singh[18] noted a slightly increased VD_{phys} and dead space/tidal volume (VD/VT) in patients insufflated with IAP of 12 to 14 mm Hg while in 15 to 20 degrees of head-down tilt and with minute ventilation (VE) of 100 to 120 ml/kg^{-1}.

The contributive effect of operative positioning on alterations of V/Q ratio has not yet been evaluated clearly. Further upper diaphragmatic shifting may be assumed from head-down tilting with a more decreased V/Q ratio, whereas an important decrease in CO concomitant to head-up positioning may enlarge the zone of higher V/Q ratio. With regard to this last positioning, Matalon and Farhi[12] noted an increase in FRC ($+10\%$) and partial pressure of end tidal CO_2 ($PetCO_2$) ($+25\%$) in conscious volunteers as they passed from a horizontal position to a 15 degree tilt. However, Brown et al.[19] did not observe a significant impairment of gas exchange caused by the combined effect of the pneumoperitoneum (12 to 18 cm H_2O) and the Trendelenburg tilt (20 degrees) despite a significant decrease in V_T, vital capacity (VC), and V_E during laparoscopic procedures performed with the patient under local anesthesia. These patients minimized ventilatory work by increasing respiratory rate, with a resultant decrease in V_T.

Since CO_2 is used for abdominal insufflation, its homeostasis is a matter of concern. Seed, Shakespeare, and Muldoon[20] observed an increase of $PetCO_2$ and $PaCO_2$ during subumbilical laparoscopies that lasted 30 minutes. However, the rise of CO_2 (VCO_2) did not show a statistically significant increase. During a study comparing two groups, Magno et al.[21] noted a net increase of $PaCO_2$ in the group insufflated with CO_2, but in the group insufflated with N_2O, the CO_2 level did not change significantly. In a recent study Sagnard et al.[22] demonstrated that VCO_2 ($+25\%$) and $PetCO_2$ ($+26\%$) increased and reached a plateau without an increase in oxygen consumption after 20 minutes in a patient insufflated with CO_2 for laparoscopic cholecystectomy. These studies provide evidence that CO_2 is slowly absorbed from the peritoneal cavity.[22]

Effects on the Gastrointestinal Tract

During laparoscopic surgery, several factors, increase the IAP and may cause gastroesophageal regurgitation. They include abdominal insufflation, lithotomy position, and steep head-down tilt.[23] Furthermore, the functional integrity of the lower esophageal sphincter (LES) can be affected by many drugs used in anesthetic practice, especially any drug that is known to decrease the LES tone.[24]

This accepted clinical teaching in anesthesia is challenged by the low incidence of regurgitation demonstrated by patients in most studies performed during laparoscopic procedures.[25-27] Investigators who have examined the functional integrity of the LES observed that if the gastric pressure increases, there may be an increase in LES pressure, with no decrease in barrier pressure and consequently no increased tendency to regurgitation. Therefore the overall resistance to gastroesophageal reflux (GER) can be expressed by calculation of the barrier pressure, that is, the differential pressure between the LES and the stomach (bar-

rier pressure equals LES minus gastric pressure). Evidence of a normal adaptive response of the LES to increased IAP was provided first by Lind, Warrian, and Wankling.[28] Jones, Mitchell, and Hindocha[29] also demonstrated corresponding increases in LES pressure and gastric pressure in response to raised IAP during insufflation of the peritoneal cavity with CO_2 for laparoscopy. Illing, Duncan, and Yip[30] demonstrated by monitoring the pH in the lower esophagus that there was no correlation between the pH change with position and IAP. This finding provides more evidence that traditional descriptions of patients at risk may not be valid. However, their results suggest that acute physical effects that modify the gradient between the abdominal cavities (e.g., coughing or airway obstruction) may be commonly associated with GER.

The physiology of GER seems complex. The site of insertion of the upper leaf of the gastrophrenic ligament[31] and the length of the LES within the abdominal cavity[32] may play important roles in the competence of the gastroesophageal sphincter. Insufflation may flatten the intra-abdominal esophagus, adding to overall barrier pressure. In addition, the passive diaphragmatic movements of controlled ventilation produce smaller oscillations in LES pressure than during the intrinsic diaphragmatic contractions of spontaneous breathing.[33]

ANESTHETIC MANAGEMENT IN LAPAROSCOPY
Preoperative Evaluation

An important goal of preoperative assessment is to elicit the severity, progression, and functional limitations of coexisting disease. An accurate history requires a review of past and current medical records in addition to direct questioning of the patient. Specific areas to explore are taken from the patient's history, especially those presenting a potential interaction with pathophysiological changes induced by laparoscopic procedures. When severe cardiorespiratory impairments exist, the risk/benefit ratio must be considered, and appropriate monitoring must be available. Although the list of contraindications is narrowing with experience, acute glaucoma, intracranial hypertension, peritonitis, and poor cardiorespiratory risks remain absolute contraindications.

Premedication

Premedication is used to reduce apprehension and is based on the anesthetist's preference. Generally a sedative drug is prescribed the evening and the morning before the surgical procedure. The anesthesiologist should be aware that GER and aspiration may occur at any time perioperatively and postoperatively in patients at risk. In addition, laparoscopy is a risk factor for postoperative nausea and vomiting,[34,35] and residual quantities of anesthetic drugs may depress airway reflexes in spite of attempts to perform an awake intubation. Narchi, Edouard, Bourget[36] showed that a combination of a nonparticulate antacid and a histamine H_2 receptor antagonist (effervescent cimetidine) given immediately before anesthetic induction increases gastric pH in a significant and reliable manner. Although the threshold of residual gastric volume in humans is still controversial,[37] animal studies have shown that pH plays a predominant role in the occurrence of severe pulmonary morbidity due to acid aspiration,[38,39] with the worst risk an aspirate with a pH of 1 and a volume of $0.6\,\mathrm{ml/kg^{-1}}$.[38]

Anesthetic Induction and Positioning

When the patient's hands are positioned by his or her side and are inaccessible during the procedure, an extension to an intravenous cannula is attached to the tubing so that the injection site is situated conveniently. The monitoring equipment should include, in addition to routine sphygmomanometer cuff and cardioscope, a pulse oximeter and capnometer since their reliability has been demonstrated in stable patients, ASA classes I and II, during laparoscopic cholecystectomy.[40] In a retrospective analysis, Wittgen et al.[41] showed that invasive hemodynamic monitoring is required in a patient presenting with cardiovascular disease.

The most appropriate technique of providing anesthesia for laparoscopic surgery is no longer a matter for debate. The current operative laparoscopic requirements (duration, operative sites) leave little room for local or regional anesthesia. The sensitive epidural or spinal blockade needed must extend from the sacral area (S2 to S5) to the peritoneum (T4). According to Lefebvre et al.,[42] the sensitive blockade is excellent in only 20% and satisfactory in 70% of cases, despite obtaining adequate proximal sensitive blockade. However, when used, local anesthetic technique showed a lower incidence of postoperative sequelae.[43]

General anesthesia for digestive tract laparoscopic procedure should include tracheal intubation with controlled ventilation and good relaxation. With evidence of a low incidence of passive regurgitation,[25-27] tracheal intubation is still necessary for other reasons associated with adequacy of ventilation and better operating conditions. A cuffed orotracheal tube is used and its position

checked after abdominal insufflation and change of operative positioning. Heinonen, Takki, and Tammisto[44] have shown there is upward displacement of the hilus of the lung when an intubated patient is tipped headdown. Since the trachea is fixed in position, the result may be an inadvertent bronchial intubation. General anesthesia with double-lumen endobronchial tubes allowing one-lung ventilation[45] is needed in case a transthoracic endoscopic procedure is necessary. Contrary to widespread assumption, laparoscopy is not a minor event. Although the skin incision is small, the abdominal insufflation induces stressful stimulation requiring the adequate titration of short-acting narcotic analgesic and relaxant.[46] On the other hand, myorelaxation must be adequate, especially since abdominal distention must be sufficient with minimal insufflation (≤ 15 mm Hg). Furthermore, efficient relaxation allows the prevention of the acute physical effects of briskly increased intraperitoneal pressure on intrapulmonary pressures that are likely to worsen the pathophysiological changes described previously.

Anesthesia is maintained with N_2O/O_2 and a halogenated inhalational anesthetic. When a gas embolism is suspected, N_2O should be discontinued. Theoretically, the volume of an air cavity can increase to 200% to 400% of its original volume in the presence of 50% and 75% N_2O, respectively. When a venous gas embolism occurs in the presence of N_2O, the intravascular bubble will increase in size because N_2O diffuses into the bubble more rapidly than nitrogen diffuses out.[47] The rapid fall of PetCO$_2$ preceding cardiovascular collapse constitutes the most common early sign. However, a marked decrease in oxygen saturation[48] and a rapid but transient rise of PetCO$_2$ preceding its rapid fall[49] may constitute early warnings of a low-grade embolism. Ventilation is controlled by a volume-limited ventilator provided with respirometers and gas analyzer to monitor V_T, V_E, frequency (f), inspired and expired gases, and inspiration to expiration (I:E) ratio. Our recent study has demonstrated that a moderate hyperventilation ([$V_E = 1\,\mathrm{dl/kg^{-1}}$], with f = 12 min^{-1}, fraction of inspired oxygen [FIO_2] = 0.35 − 0.4, and I:E = 1:2) provided an adequate pulmonary exchange during laparoscopic cholecystectomy.[40] The gradient between arterial and end-tidal CO_2 remained within previously described limits in anesthetized humans.[50]

Providing anesthesia for complex endoscopic thoracic surgery poses ventilatory problems. Methods of improving arterial oxygen saturation (SaO$_2$) include careful patient positioning, adequate neuromuscular blockage to minimize intrathoracic pressure, optimization of CO to reduce venous admixture, adjustment of VT, and application of positive end-expiratory pressure (PEEP) to the ventilated lung.[51,52] The use of low-dose dobutamine infusion also has been reported as useful.[53] Application of continuous positive airway pressure (CPAP)[54] and insufflation of the collapsed lung with O_2 are also known to improve SaO_2. However, CPAP and, to a lesser extent, O_2 insufflation can cause partial expansion of the collapsed lung, hindering surgical access. Since the body temperature changes are similar to those happening with open surgery, equally comprehensive thermal monitoring and management using low-flow ventilation or warming of inspired gas are required.[55]

Intraoperative placement of a gastric tube allows decompression of gastric contents and may reduce the risk of visceral puncture at the time of creation of pneumoperitoneum. Also, gastroduodenal decompression can improve laparoscopic visualization and ease retraction of the upper quadrant structures. Tilt of the operative table and IAP should be carefully monitored. The positioning of the patient depends on the operative site. In subumbilical procedures the patient normally is placed in the Trendelenburg position to keep the small bowel and colon out of the pelvis. Head-up tilt improves the downward shifting of the abdominal contents. In our institution we observe the "rule of two 15s" with regard to abdominal insufflation and tilt of operative table: the use of an abdominal insufflator provided with a barostat allows maintenance of the IAP at >15 mm Hg; and after the abdominal insufflation has been completed, the operative table is tilted as required by the surgeon but without exceeding 15 degrees. Padded braces are positioned over the acromial processes and at the popliteal fossae. At the end of the procedure, the table is brought back to the horizontal position before the gas is vented.

During exsufflation of the pneumoperitoneum, some hemodynamic changes may happen. These alterations may be due to the redistribution of blood and to a sudden influx of a large quantity of acidic substances from blood pooling in the lower limbs. Therefore exsufflation should be performed in a progressive manner. The pharynx is inspected and any secretion sucked out before extubation. Residual myorelaxation is treated with a narcotic antagonist when necessary. However, because there are minimal skin incisions, the terminal stage of laparoscopic procedure is usually very short. This short time does not permit sufficient elimination of residual anesthetic drugs to allow performance of an awake extubation. Consequently, our patients frequently remain intubated when they go to the recovery ward. When intolerance to the endotracheal tube begins, as evidenced by bucking, it is preferable to perform the extubation. In fact, Illing, Duncan, and Yip[30] observed that gastroesophageal regurgitation and pharyngeal reflux commonly occur during emergence from anesthesia and during bucking while the endotracheal tube is still in place.

Complications of Endoscopic Surgery

Recent developments in endoscopic surgery for major procedures may result in new and important hazards. Gas embolism is potentially the most dangerous complication. In a review of 63,845 diagnostic laparoscopies, Bruhl[56] found only one case of gas embolism among 1594 serious complications. In a prospective study with a Doppler ultrasonic instrument, Wadhwa et al.[57] did not find a gas embolism in 100 patients undergoing tubal ligation. In 1976 Philips et al.[58] reported an incidence of 15 gas embolisms per 113.253 laparoscopic cases in a 1-year period. The incidence may be higher when laparoscopy is associated with hysteroscopy.[59] This low incidence and the relative safety of gynecological laparoscopic procedures shown by these results[56-58] may lead to complacency and a reluctance to use the expensive, but more sensitive (ultrasonic device) or invasive monitoring systems routinely. Therefore more surveys are needed to determine the current incidence of gas embolism with the new developments in endoscopic surgery. CO_2 embolisms associated with laparoscopic cholecystectomy have been reported recently.[60] Potential causes of gas embolism are perforation of a blood vessel, injection of gas into an abdominal viscus, and traumatic lysis of adhesions. Pneumothorax[61] and surgical emphysema extending from neck to groin[62] also have been reported as complications of laparoscopic cholecystectomy.

Although pneumothorax or pneumomediastinum can be caused by escape of gas through anomalies or from tears of the diaphragm, the common complications of a pneumoperitoneum are due to incorrect positioning of the Veress needle and trocar. Thus parietal or subcutaneous emphysema can be caused by failure of the Veress needle to penetrate the peritoneum. Visceral and vascular puncture and lacerations have been reported.[63] Once we observed a case of gastric perforation in our hospital during a hyperselective vagotomy, and the operation was continued through an open approach.

During a transthoracic endoscopic procedure, with the proximity of the heart to the surgical site, accidental physical irritation of the heart may be inevitable, especially because the video view is restricted. Ventricular ectopic beats may occur and precipitate malignant ventricular arrhythmias with hemodynamic problems. Inadvertent application of diathermy to the heart produces areas of myocardial damage that may become foci of arrhythmias. Diathermy to the epicardial blood vessels may provoke vasospasm and thrombosis, leading to myocardial ischemia.[64]

In view of the escalating enthusiasm for the laparoscopic technique among surgeons, the anesthesiologist will encounter these cases more often and should be aware of associated complications. Therefore years and many realistic reports are needed to reveal all the preventable complications and to improve intraoperative and postoperative monitoring.

POSTLAPAROSCOPIC PERIOD
Immediate Recovery Room Management

During the recovery time hypercarbia may be observed because of persistent absorption of CO_2 from the peritoneal cavity and the effect of residual curare. Venous CO_2 embolism, not evidenced in the operative room, has been reported and must be considered in the differential diagnosis of cardiovascular collapse or delayed awakening.[65] Therefore hemodynamic and ventilatory monitoring should continue until the complete recovery from anesthesia. Supplementary O_2 should be provided when desaturation is detected. Although saturation is monitored reliably by pulse oximetry, it is not easy to perform capnography on an extubated patient.

More serious complications related to gas diffusion, namely embolism,[65] pneumothorax, pneumomediastinum, and hemorrhage,[66] should be sought when any cardiorespiratory problem happens during the postoperative period. Recently we observed a case of severe hemorrhage occurring 48 hours after laparoscopic cholecystectomy. It was due to the detachment of a clip from the cystic artery.

Postoperative Sequelae and Complications

Certain aspects of the laparoscopy itself probably contribute to postoperative morbidity. They include the combination of required positioning, pneumoperitoneum, and the length of the procedure. Among cited postoperative sequelae, vomiting and nausea, pain, and respiratory alterations are frequently found.[67,68]

Factors associated with an increased risk of postoperative emesis include age, gender (menses), obesity, previous history of motion sickness, anxiety, gastroparesis, and type and duration of surgical procedure.[35] Laparoscopic surgery has been demonstrated as a risk factor for higher incidence of postoperative nausea and vomiting.[35,68] Anesthesiologists have little, if any, control over these surgical factors. However they can control other factors that influence postoperative emesis (e.g., preanesthetic medication, anesthetic drugs and technique of administration, and postoperative pain management). With regard to anesthetic choice, De Grood et al.[70] have demonstrated that the use of propofol, even associated with fentanyl and N_2O, ensures recovery with a low incidence of nausea and vomiting. Concerns about the ability of N_2O to cause emesis recently were discussed by Taylor et al.[71] who demonstrated that there was no difference in vomiting after anesthesia either with or without N_2O for laparoscopic cholecystectomy.

Although routine use of antiemetic prophylaxis clearly is not justified, patients at high risk for postoperative emesis should receive special consideration with respect to an antiemetic drug. Minimally effective doses of an antiemetic drug can be administered to reduce the incidence of sedation and other deleterious side effects. Gentle handling in the immediate postoperative period is also essential. If emesis does occur, aggressive intravenous hydration and pain management are important components of the therapeutic regimen, along with the antiemetic drugs. If one antiemetic does not appear effective, use of another drug with different site of action should be considered.[35] Patients should be warned of the side effects they are likely to feel, particularly neck and shoulder pain, which would be unexpected. Cigarini et al.[67] demonstrated while comparing pain scores between open and laparoscopic cholecystectomy, there was no significant difference, except on day 2 when pain was less severe after laparoscopy. However, overall analgesic requirements, especially opiates, were significantly reduced in the laparoscopic group. This claim is in accordance with the finding of Rose[68] who revealed a higher percentage (13% versus 2.6%) of excessive pain after open cholecystectomy. Postlaparoscopic pain may be attenuated or prevented by preoperative or perioperative administration of nonsteroidal anti-inflammatory drugs.[72-74] Potent nonopioid analgesics (e.g., Ketorolac) used to control pain allow avoidance of some of the opioid-related side effects, especially nausea and vomiting. In a study performed during laparoscopy,

Narchi, Benhamou, and Fernandez[75] showed that the application of a local anesthetic also reduced the postoperative need for analgesics.

Recent literature reveals that, similar to open upper abdominal surgery, upper abdominal laparoscopic surgery induces postoperative respiratory changes. Cigarini et al.[67] found the forced vital capacity (FVC) was reduced less after laparoscopic than after open cholecystectomy. This restrictive syndrome has been detected in the immediate postoperative period.[16,76] Sha, Ohmura, and Yamada[16] suggested that this may be due to diaphragmatic dysfunction, which had been observed previously in patients after upper open abdominal surgery.[77]

In the same study, Sha, Ohmura, and Yamada[16] showed by chest x-ray films that there was a marked cephalad shift of the inspiratory and expiratory position of the diaphragm, which induced basal atelectasis in 33% of patients. According to Toussignant et al.,[78] the recovery from the pulmonary alteration 24 hours after laparoscopic cholecystectomy was less complete in patients older than 50 years of age. Although desaturation is less frequent (8% versus 33.8%) as demonstrated by Rose,[68] these results suggest that any measures such as adequate analgesia, early ambulation, and exercises that reduce the extent of postoperative pulmonary complications must be emphasized, although laparoscopic cholecystectomy is considered less invasive.

Because of venous pooling in lower limbs induced by pneumoperitoneum and head-up tilt, the risk of thromboembolism may be increased, especially during a long-lasting laparoscopic procedure. Therefore this risk deserves investigation, and the use of preventive measures should be considered, such as intermittent and sequential compression devices for the lower extremities.

Despite these adverse complications, with some relevant to anesthetic management in the operating room and the recovery ward, advantages of laparoscopic surgery compared to open surgery are evident. Because the operation is performed through a few small puncture wounds in the abdominal wall rather than through a true surgical incision, patients suffer minimal pain immediately afterward.[67] This allows a quick return to normal activities and has obvious cosmetic benefits. In addition, because postoperative ileus is rare, patients can take oral feedings almost at once. As compared to open surgery, the hospital stay is shortened by 2 days after appendectomy[79] and 4 days after cholecystectomy.[80] Patients can resume normal activities after 7 days, whereas they must wait 3 to 7 weeks after open cholecystectomy.[80]

CONCLUSION

Although still a recent discovery, videoendoscopic abdominal and thoracic surgery are gaining worldwide acceptance, both because of its benefits and the method's potential to reduce the morbidity and costs associated with open surgery when performed by experienced surgeons. For anesthesiologists, the potential incidence of hemodynamic and respiratory embarassment in patients with a borderline cardiorespiratory function must be addressed in planning future anesthetic management. Further studies are needed to predict the criteria for good tolerance and to delineate clearly the contraindications.

We would like to thank Mrs. G. Rosine for her technical assistance.

REFERENCES

1. Guyton AC, Adkins LH. Quantitative aspects of collapse factor in relation to venous return. Am J Physiol 177:523, 1954.
2. Rubinson RM, Vasko JS, Doppman JL, et al. Inferior vena cava obstruction from increased intra-abdominal pressure. Arch Surg 94:766, 1967.
3. Doppman J, Rubinson RM, Rockoff D, et al. Mechanism of obstruction of the infradiaphragmatic portion of the inferior vena cava in the presence of increased intra-abdominal pressure. Invest Radiol 10:676, 1966.
4. Ivankovitch AD, Miletich DJ, Albrecht RF, et al. Cardiovascular effects of intraperitoneal insufflation with carbon dioxide and nitrous oxide in dog. Anesthesiology 42:281, 1989.
5. Richardson JD, Trinble JK. Hemodynamic and respiratory alterations with increased intra-abdominal pressure. J Surg Res 20:401, 1976.
6. Diamant M, Benumoff JL, Saidman LJ. Hemodynamics of increased intra-abdominal pressure. Interaction with hypovolemia and halothane anesthesia. Anesthesiology 18:23, 1978.
7. Kelman GR, Benzie RJ, Gordon LM, et al. Cardiovascular effects of peritoneal carbon dioxide insufflation for laparoscopy. Br J Anaesth 44:719, 1972.
8. Motew M, Ivankovitch AD, Bieniarz J, et al. Cardiovascular effects and acid-base and blood gas changes during laparoscopy. Am J Obstet Gynecol 115:1002, 1973.

9. Marshall RL, Jebson PJR, Davie IT, et al. Circulatory effects of peritoneal insufflation with nitrous oxide. Br J Anaesth 44:680, 1972.

10. Andel H, Grabner V, Zadrobilek E, et al. Cardiopulmonary effects of laparoscopic cholecystectomy. Anesth Analg S8, 1992.

11. Reid CW, Martineau RJ, Hull KA, et al. Haemodynamic consequences of abdominal insufflation with CO_2 during laparoscopic cholecystectomy. Can J Anaesth 39:S132, 1992.

12. Matalon SV, Farhi LE. Cardiopulmonary readjustments in passive tilt. J Appl Physiol 47:503, 1979.

13. Scott DB, Jullian DG. Observation on cardiac arrhythmias during laparoscopy. Br Med J 1:411, 1972.

14. Harman PK, Kron IL, MacLachlan AE, et al. Elevated intra-abdominal pressure and renal function. Ann Surg 196:594, 1982.

15. Froese AB, Bryan AC. Effects of anesthesia and paralysis on diaphragmatic mechanics in man. Anesthesiology 41:242, 1974.

16. Sha M, Ohmura A, Yamada M. Diaphragm function and pulmonary complications after laparoscopic cholecystectomy. Anesthesiology 75:A255, 1991.

17. Hedenstierna G, Tokics L, Stranberg A, et al. Correlations of gas exchange impairment to development of atelectasis during anaesthesia and muscle paralysis. Acta Anaesthesiol Scand 30:183, 1986.

18. Puri GD, Singh H. Ventilatory effects of laparoscopy under general anesthesia. Br J Anaesth 68:211, 1992.

19. Brown DR, Fishburne JI, Roberson VO, et al. Ventilatory and blood gas changes during laparoscopy with local anesthesia. Am J Obstet Gynecol 124:741, 1974.

20. Seed RF, Shakespeare TF, Muldoon MJ. Carbon dioxide homeostasis during anaesthesia for laparoscopy. Anaesthesia 25:223, 1970.

21. Magno R, Medegard A, Bengtsson R, et al. Acid-base balance during laparoscopy. Acta Obstet Gynecol Scand 44:81, 1979.

22. Sagnard P, Vlale JP, Annat G, et al. Diffusion du gaz carbonique dans l'organisme au cours de la cholecystectomie par voie coelioscopique. Ann Fr Anesth Reanim 10:R50, 1991.

23. Lamberty JM. Gynecological laparoscopy. Br J Anaesth 57:718, 1985.

24. Cotton BR, Smith G. The lower oesophageal sphincter and anaesthesia. Br J Anaesth 56:37-46, 1984.

25. Duffy BL. Regurgitation during pelvic laparoscopy. Br J Anaesth 51:1089, 1979.

26. Roberts CJ, Goodman NW. Gastroesophageal reflux during elective laparoscopy. Anaesthesia 45:1009, 1990.

27. Heijke SA, Smith G, Key A. Effect of the Trendelenburg position on lower oesophageal sphincter tone. Anaesthesia 46:185, 1991.

28. Lind JF, Warrian WG, Wankling WJ. Response of the gastroesophageal junctions zone to increases in abdominal pressure. Can J Surg 9:32, 1966.

29. Jones MJ, Mitchell RW, Hindocha N. Effects of increased intraabdominal pressure during laparoscopy on lower esophageal sphincter. Anesth Analg 68:63, 1989.

30. Illing L, Duncan PG, Yip R. Gastroesophageal reflux during anaesthesia. Can J Anaesth 39:466, 1992.

31. Bombeck CT, Dillard DH, Nyhus LM. Muscular anatomy of the gastroesophageal junctions and role of phrenoesophageal ligament. Autopsy study of sphincter mechanism. Ann Surg 164:643, 1966.

32. O'Sullivan GC, De Meester TR, Joelson BE, et al. Interaction of lower esophageal sphincter pressure and length of sphincter in the abdomen as determinants of gastroesophageal competence. Am J Surg 143:40, 1982.

33. Boyle JT, Altshuler SM, Nixon TE, et al. Role of diaphragm in the genesis of lower esophageal sphincter pressure in cat. Gastroenterology 88:723, 1985.

34. Forrest JB, Beattie WS, Goldstein CH. Risk factors for nausea and vomiting after general anaesthesia. Can J Anaesth 39:S90, 1992.

35. Watcha MF, White PF. Postoperative nausea and vomiting. Its etiology, treatment and prevention. Anesthesiology 77:162, 1992.

36. Narchi P, Edouard D, Bourget P. Oral effervescent cimetidine in daycase anesthesia: Effects on pH and volume. Anesthesiology 73:A6, 1990.

37. Hardy JF. Large volume gastroesophageal reflux: Rationale for risk reduction in the perioperative period. Can J Anaesth 35:162, 1988.

38. Raidoo DM, Brock-Utne JG, Roche DA, et al. The critical volume in acid aspiration. Anesthesiology 71:A879, 1989.

39. James FC, Modell JH, Gibbs CP, et al. Pulmonary aspiration: Effects of volume and pH in the rat. Anesth Analg 63:665, 1984.

40. Nyarwaya JB, Samii K, Mazoit JX, et al. Are pulse oximetric and capnographic monitoring reliable during laparoscopic surgery? Anesthesiology 75:A453, 1991.

41. Wittgen CM, Andrus CH, Fitzgerald SD, et al. Analysis of the hemodynamic and ventilatory effects of laparoscopic cholecystectomy. Arch Surg 126:997, 1991.

42. Lefebvre G, Vauthier-Bronzes D, Darbois Y, et al. La coelioscopie sous anesthésie péridurale: Technique, indications, résultats à propos de 220 cas. J Gynecol Obstet Biol Reprod 20:355, 1991.

43. Raeder JC, Bordahl P, Nordentoft J, et al. Local anaesthesia versus general anaesthesia for out-patient laparoscopic sterilization. Eur J Anaesth 9:A8, 1992.

44. Heinonen J, Takki S, Tammisto T. Effect of the Trendelenburg tilt and other procedures on the position of endotracheal tubes. Lancet 1:850, 1969.

45. Benumof JL, Alfrey DD. Anesthesia for thoracic surgery. In Miller RD, ed. Anesthesia, 3rd ed. New York: Churchill Livingstone, 1990, p 1517.
46. Cooper GM, Scoggins AM, Ward ID, et al. Laparoscopy—A stressful procedure. Anaesthesia 37:266, 1982.
47. Nunn JF. Controlled respiration in neurosurgical anesthesia. Anesthesia 14:413, 1959.
48. Michael S, Fraser RB, Reilly CS. Intra-operative embolism. Detection by pulse oximetry. Anaesthesia 45:225, 1990.
49. Shulman D, Aronson HB. Capnography in the early diagnosis of carbon dioxide embolism during laparoscopy. Can Anaesth Soc J 31:455, 1984.
50. Nunn JF, Hill DW. Respiratory deadspace and arterial to end-tidal CO_2 tension difference in anesthetized man. J Appl Physiol 15:383, 1960.
51. Cohen E, Thys DM, Eisenkraft JB, et al. PEEP during one-lung anesthesia improves oxygenation in patients with low arterial PaO_2. Anesth Analg 64:201, 1985.
52. Katz JA, Laverne RG, Fairley HB, et al. Pulmonary oxygen exchange during endobronchial anesthesia: Effect of tidal volume and PEEP. Anesthesiology 56:164, 1982.
53. Nomto Y, Kawamura M. Pulmonary gas exchange effects by nitroglycerin, dopamine and dobutamine during one-lung ventilation in man. Can J Anaesth 36:273, 1989.
54. Capan LM, Turndorf H, Patel C, et al. Optimization of arterial oxygenation during one-lung anesthesia. Anesth Analg 59:847, 1980.
55. Wallasvaara A, Paloheimo M. Ventilation and body temperature during laparoscopic vs open cholecystectomy [abstract]. Anesth Analg 74:S340, 1992.
56. Bruhl W. Complications of laparoscopy and liver biopsy under vision: The results of a survey. German Med Monthly 12:31, 1967.
57. Wadhwa RK, McKenzie R, Wadhwa SR, et al. Gas embolism during laparoscopy. Anesthesiology 48:75, 1974.
58. Philips J, Keith D, Hulka B, et al. Gynecologic laparoscopy in 1975. J Reprod Med 16:105, 1976.
59. Gomar C, Fernandez C, Villalonga A, et al. Carbon dioxide embolism during laparoscopy and hysteroscopy. Ann Fr Anesth Reanim 4:380, 1985.
60. Greville AC, Clements EAF, Erwin DC, et al. Pulmonary air embolism during laparoscopic laser cholecystectomy. Anaesthesia 46:113, 1991.
61. Gabbot DA, Dunkley AB, Roberts FL. Carbon dioxide pneumothorax occurring during laparoscopic cholecystectomy. Anesthesia 47:537, 1992.
62. Lew JKL, Gin T, Oh TE. Anaesthetic problems during laparoscopic cholecystectomy. Anaesth Intensive Care 20:91, 1992.
63. Calverley RK, Jenkins. The anaesthetic management of pelvic laparoscopy. Can Anaesth Soc J 20:679, 1973.
64. Chui PT, Gin T, Chung SCS. Anaesthesia for a patient undergoing transthoracic endoscopic vagotomy. Br J Anaesth 68:318, 1992.
65. Root B, Levy MN, Pollock S, et al. Gas embolism death after laparoscopy delayed by trapping in the portal circulation. Anesth Analg 57:232, 1978.
66. Chapin JW, Hurlbert BJ, Sheer K. Hemorrhage and cardiac arrest during laparoscopic tubal ligation. Anesthesiology 54:342, 1980.
67. Cigarini I, Joris J, Jacquet N, et al. Pain and pulmonary dysfunction after cholecystectomy under laparoscopy and laparotomy. Anesthesiology 75:A122, 1991.
68. Rose DK. Laparoscopic cholecystectomy. Is it better? Can J Anaesth 39:A110, 1992.
69. Palazzo MGA, Strunin L. Anaesthesia and emesis. I. Etiology. Can Anaesth Soc J 31:178, 1984.
70. De Grood PMRM, Harbers JBM, Van Egmond J, et al. Anesthesia for laparoscopy. Anaesthesia 42:815, 1987.
71. Taylor E, Feinstein R, White PE, et al. Anaesthesia for laparoscopic cholecystectomy. Is nitrous oxide contraindicated? Anesthesiology 76:541, 1992.
72. Gillberg LE, Harsten AS, Stahl LB. Effect of diclofenac sodium on postlaparoscopy pain. Anesthesiology 75:A21, 1991.
73. Rosenblum M, Weller RS, Conard PL, et al. Ibuprofen provides longer lasting analgesia than fentanyl after laparoscopic surgery. Anesth Analg 73:255, 1991.
74. De Lucia JA, White PF. Effect of intraoperative Ketorolac on recovery after outpatient laparoscopy. Anesthesiology 75:A14, 1991.
75. Narchi P, Benhamou D, Fernandez H. Intraperitoneal local anaesthetics for shoulder pain after day case laparoscopy. Lancet 338:1569, 1991.
76. Shear JM, Holtmann B, White PF. Pulmonary function following laparoscopic cholecystectomy. Anesth Analg 7:S286, 1992.
77. Simonneau G, Vivien A, Sartene R, et al. Diaphragm dysfunction induced by upper abdominal surgery: Role of postoperative pain. Am Resp Dis 128:899, 1983.
78. Toussignant G, Wiesel S, Laporta D, et al. The effect of age on the recovery of pulmonary function after laparoscopic cholecystectomy. Anesth Analg 74:S368, 1992.
79. McAnena OJ, Austin O, Hederman WF, et al. Laparoscopy versus open appendicectomy. Lancet 338:693, 1991.
80. Shirmer BD, Edge SB, Dix J, et al. Laparoscopic cholecystectomy. Treatment of choice for symptomatic cholelithiasis. Ann Surg 213:665, 1991.

12 *Should Acidosis Limit Anesthesia Time for Celiosurgery With Intraperitoneal CO₂?*

J.C. Séguier, P. Sinda, Philippe Marre, and T. Montariol

Anesthesia has been used for many years in celioscopy for gynecological indications. In the late 1980s additional indications for celioscopy appeared in surgery of the GI tract. The development of the capnometer allows the anesthetist to once again use rebreathing circuit ventilation with the safety of knowing the amount of exhaled and inhaled CO_2.

During laparoscopic surgery some anesthesiologists have observed an increase in end-tidal CO_2 pressure with no clinical manifestations. Most of the time this hypercapnia is moderate and usually appears after 60 minutes of insufflation of CO_2. Sometimes severe hypercapnia is observed in patients with subcutaneous emphysema unrelated to the duration of surgery. The aim of our study was to compare the changes in arterial CO_2 pressure ($PaCO_2$) determined by arterial blood gas sampling and end-tidal CO_2 pressure measured by capnography. At the same time we evaluated the changes in pH in arterial blood gases.

MATERIALS AND METHODS

Thirty-three patients were studied from December 1990 to September 1991. They were categorized as ASA class I or II and had no pulmonary disease. Their principal characteristics are presented in Table 1.

All patients undergoing laparoscopic cholecystectomy were examined by an anesthesiologist 1 week before the operation; explanations were given to all patients concerning the type of anesthetic and the laparoscopic cholecystectomy. Patients were premedicated with midazolam, given by mouth 30 minutes before induction of anesthesia.

General anesthesia was induced with midazolam (0.07 mg/kg), fentanyl (3 μg/kg), propofol (1.5 mg/kg), and atracurium (0.6 mg/kg). To maintain anesthesia we used propofol (3 to 10 mg/kg/h), fentanyl (2 μ/kg) in relation to inadequate analgesia because of surgical stimulation, and atracurium every 20 minutes. An antibiotic (cefotetan, 2 g) was administered prophylactically at the induction of anesthesia.

After endotracheal intubation and controlled ventilation were achieved with an ABT 4.3.0.0 ventilator (Roche Kontron) with a semi-rebreathing circuit, ventilation was monitored continuously with a capnograph (Datex Capnomac). No inhalation agent other than nitrous oxide was added. The inspiratory ratio of oxygen was 50%. At the beginning of anesthesia the respiratory parameters included a tidal volume of 8 ml/kg and a ventilation rate of 11/min. If the end-tidal CO_2 was above 38 mm Hg, the ventilation rate was increased to 15/min. If it was not sufficient after 15 minutes, the tidal volume was increased to 12 ml/kg. If it still was not sufficient after another 15 minutes, the ventilation rate was increased to 20/min.

Table 1. Evolution of mean values in relation to time: Semirebreathing circuit in celioscopic surgery

Time (min)	PaCO₂ (mm Hg)	PETCO₂ (mm Hg)	pH	Gradient	No. of Patients
T −5	37.74 ± 4.7	32.34 ± 4.3	7.42 ± 0.04	05.32 ± 4.1	33
T +15	42.16 ± 6.4	33.51 ± 5.7	7.38 ± 0.05	06.69 ± 4.8	33
T +60	44.26 ± 8.4	35.31 ± 6.4	7.36 ± 0.05	10.07 ± 7.9	33
T +120	46.23 ± 7.9	35.10 ± 7.2	7.34 ± 0.05	14.0 ± 11.7	21
T +180	47.66 ± 5.2	35.66 ± 4.08	7.30 ± 0.04	10.88 ± 2.1	7

Samples for determination of arterial blood gases were drawn through a 22-gauge arterial cannula. These samples were measured at the following intervals: 5 minutes before insufflation of CO_2, 15 minutes after the beginning of insufflation, and 60 minutes after the beginning and every hour thereafter. The usual parameters of expired and inspired gases were noted 5 minutes before insufflation, at the beginning of insufflation, 15 minutes after insufflation, and every 30 minutes thereafter. The following additional parameters were continuously monitored: arterial blood pressure, heart rate, pulsed oxymetry, and cardioscopic analysis.

Laparoscopic cholecystectomy was performed by two surgeons with a four-trocar technique. CO_2 was insufflated intraperitoneally during laparoscopy with an EID insufflator.

RESULTS

The mean duration of anesthesia was 187.8 minutes. No deaths or accidents occurred as a result of anesthesia. Three operations were discontinued. The first one was stopped 60 minutes after CO_2 insufflation because adhesions made it impossible to proceed. The second operation was stopped 60 minutes after insufflation because of hypercapnia (74 mm Hg) and a pH of 7.19, both of which proved impossible to lower. It was decided to perform open surgery. Thirty minutes later the $PaCO_2$ had returned to 45 mm Hg and the pH to 7.35 with the usual parameters of ventilation. The third operation was stopped at T + 150 minutes after cholecystectomy for removal of a splenic cyst. At the end of the laparoscopy $PaCO_2$ was 47 mm Hg, pH 7.34, and $PETCO_2$ 34 mm

Hg. Thirty minutes later at open surgery $PaCO_2$ was 32 mm Hg, pH 7.47, and $PETCO_2$ 25 mm Hg.

One patient developed subcutaneous emphysema at T + 150 minutes, a short time before the end of the procedure. $PaCO_2$ was 61 mm Hg and pH was 7.26; we did not stop the procedure but administered an inspiratory ratio of oxygen at 100% and increased the rate and tidal volume of respiratory parameters. The values improved (pH, 7.32 and $PaCO_2$, 52 mm Hg).

Table 1 shows the results for $PETCO_2$, $PaCO_2$, pH, and gradient. Taking into account the modifications of ventilation, $PETCO_2$ remained constant. Fig. 1 shows the evolution of pH in relation to time.

DISCUSSION

The evolution of $PaCO_2$ shows a progressive increase related to duration. The gradient is multiplied by two, which demonstrates that perioperative capnography often produces a false reading and shows that it might be necessary, after 1 hour of celioscopy, to check the value of the gradient. This will allow control of the acid-base equilibrium of the patient.

Indeed the evolution of pH as early as the first hour is an indication of respiratory acidosis that has not been corrected by adaptation of the ventilation parameters. This acidosis may lead to the interruption of celioscopy. We encountered no cardiovascular accidents in our experience, so we are uncertain as to the true significance of this acidosis, which is unrelated to the appearance of emphysema.

Parmentier et al.[1] reported similar results and noted that this acidosis may lead to the interruption of ce-

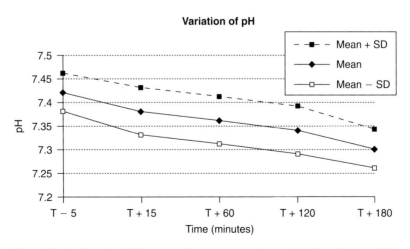

Fig. 1. Evolution of pH levels during operation (normal pH = 7.40 ± 0.02).

liosurgery. Sagnard et al.[2] obtained a permanent measurement of $PETCO_2$ by mass spectrometry without comparing their results with the blood gas values. These investigators found $PETCO_2$ to be stable after 20 minutes of insufflation, which demonstrates the balance between the introduction of CO_2 and its elimination by leakage and by the lungs. In contrast to conditions in our study, the CO_2 insufflation pressure in Sagnard's study was constantly maintained below 15 cm H_2O.

We are now repeating this same study with a new insufflator, which appears to have better control over intra-abdominal pressure. Initial results show less acidosis; in addition, the duration of surgery is shortened with improved experience.

CONCLUSION

We conclude that respiratory monitoring has its limits and underestimates the real $PaCO_2$; in addition, the respiratory acidosis that appears and increases with the duration of surgery is not controlled by modification of the ventilation. This suggests that there could exist safety limitations with regard to the duration of anesthesia for laparoscopic surgery with CO_2 insufflation.

REFERENCES

1. Parmentier G, Baudaux J, Dot K, et al. Anesthésie et chirurgie digestive sous coelioscopie: Incidents, précautions. J Chirurgie Colombes 1992.
2. Sagnard P, Viale JP, Annat G, et al. Diffusion du gaz carbonique dans l'organisme au cours de la cholécystectomie par voie coelioscopique. Ann Fr Anesth Réanim 10:R50, 1991.

13 *Hemodynamic Changes During Prolonged Laparoscopic Surgery*

Ursula Windberger, Helga Siegl, and Udo Losert

Laparoscopic operative techniques have quickly established themselves as an effective alternative to standard operative approaches in the treatment of different abdominal diseases. Several years ago hemodynamic changes during short-term diagnostic laparoscopy using CO_2 or N_2O as insufflation gas in human patients and in experimental animals were evaluated. An intra-abdominal pressure exceeding 15 mm Hg was found to be dangerous for the patient.[1-3] However, even at lower pressures, significant hemodynamic and pulmonary changes can be expected during laparoscopy.[4-6] With the development of prolonged operative techniques requiring longer insufflation times, other compensatory processes may develop.

In our experiments we used laparoscopic operative techniques for the resection of the sigmoid colon in swine.[7] The abdominal cavity was inflated with CO_2 to a pressure of 13 ± 2 mm Hg, and the pigs were positioned in modified Trendelenburg position (head down 20 to 25 degrees) for 2 hours. The purpose of this experiment was to evaluate hemodynamic changes during long-term laparoscopic surgery.

MATERIALS AND METHODS
Anesthesia

Seven healthy female Edelschwein pigs (35 ± 1 kg) were fed a standardized ration as desired and had free access to water. The animals received no food for 24 hours before surgery and were preanesthetized with 20 mg/kg ketamine hydrochloride and intubated after thiopentone (10 mg/kg) was given as a bolus. Anesthesia was maintained using a mixture of O_2 and N_2O by ventilator, intravenous Piritramid (15 mg) and pancuronium bromide (4 mg) by bolus and continuous infusion (100 µg/kg/min Piritramid and 6.6 µg/kg/min pancuronium bromide). Fraction of inspired oxygen (FIO_2) and positive end-expiratory pressure (PEEP) were maintained at 0.35 and 2 cm H_2O respectively, using a fixed inspirator volume. After physiological basal arterial partial pressure of carbon dioxide (PCO_2) was achieved, the inspiratory volume was not changed until the end of the experimental protocol to enable registration of changes in plasma PCO_2 during insufflation.

The animal experiments were carried out according to the principles of the Austrian law for animal experiments and the guidelines of the European Convention for the Protection of Vertebrate Animals Used for Experimental and Other Scientific Purposes (Strasbourg, 1986).

Hemodynamic Monitoring

Pressure catheters were placed into the brachiocephalic trunk, the femoral vein, the caudal caval vein, and the thoracic and abdominal cavity. A 5 Fr Swan-Ganz catheter was inserted, with the tip located in the main trunk of the pulmonary artery. A Millar tip catheter was placed into the left ventricle, and an electromagnetic flow probe was placed around the femoral artery. A pressure catheter was fixed to the endotracheal tube to record the inspiratory pressure, and another catheter was inserted into the abdominal cavity to measure the intra-abdominal pressure. The position of all catheters was validated at necropsy. All catheters were connected to Bell and Howell physiological pressure transducers for on-line monitoring (Hellige). Data were recorded digitally using a PC-based computerized system.[8]

Mean values were obtained for the arterial pulmonary (MAP) and central venous pressures (CVP) in the caudal caval vein, the peripheral venous pressure in the femoral vein (FVP), and the intra-abdominal pressure (IAP). From the left ventricular pressure, the systolic value (LVP) and the left ventricular end-diastolic pressure during inspiration ($LVEDP_{insp}$) and expiration ($LVEDP_{exp}$) were recorded. Heart rate (HR) was calculated from the electrocardiogram. Values during inspiration and expiration were taken from the pulmonary artery pressure (PAP), the right atrial pressure (RAP), and the intrathoracic pressure (ITP) (i.e., PAP_{insp}, PAP_{exp}, RAP_{insp}, RAP_{exp}, ITP_{insp}, and ITP_{exp}). The peak inspiratory (PIP_{peak}) and the plateau pressure ($PIP_{plateau}$) were estimated from the inspiratory pressure. Transmural pulmonary artery pressure (PAP_{trans}) during inspiration and the transmural right atrial pressure (RAP_{trans}) during inspiration were calculated as the difference between the inspiratory intraluminal pressures and the intrathoracic pressure during inspiration. Cardiac output (CO) was measured by thermodilution.

Blood Samples

Arterial, venous (CVP line), and pulmonary blood was collected for the estimation of blood gas values (Blood Gas Analyzer 995, AVL, Graz, Austria; OSM Hemoximeter, Radiometer, Copenhagen, Denmark), electrolyte determinations (Nova 6 Electrolyte Analyzer, Nova Biomedical, Massachusetts), and hematocrit values. For the estimation of noradrenalin, 10 ml of pulmonary blood was put into cold tubes containing EGTA plus trifuged 10 minutes at 2000 rpm. The plasma samples were then collected and stored at $-70°$ C for 2 months; at that time they were assayed by high-performance liquid chromatography (cation exchange, electrochemical detection).

Experimental Protocol

CO and blood samples were taken in fixed intervals before (-10 minutes) and after ($+10$, $+30$, $+60$, $+90$, $+120$ minutes) the start of the peritoneal insufflation. Pneumoperitoneum using CO_2 was maintained during the 2-hour operative procedure at a pressure of 10 to 15 mm Hg except for a brief interval (approximately 10 minutes) during which the resected specimen was removed from the abdominal cavity.

Statistics

All data, including the hemodynamic values chosen from the on-line data before (-10 minutes) and after ($+2$, $+5$, $+7$, $+10$, $+30$, $+60$, $+90$, $+120$ minutes) insufflation, were statistically evaluated with the analysis of variance for repeated measures using the Fisher PLSD test.

RESULTS
Hemodynamic Results (Figs. 1 to 7)

Table 1 shows the hemodynamic and pulmonary data throughout the study protocol. IAP increased in each experiment from 0 to 12 ± 3 mm Hg. MAP and LVP increased in parallel immediately ($+2$ minutes) after the onset of the insufflation and remained elevated until the end of the experimental protocol. CO increased after insufflation and remained at this increased level, whereas HR increased continuously (all $p < 0.05$). $LVEDP_{insp}$ and $LVEDP_{exp}$ did not change. Femoral blood flow (Q_{fem}) did not change uniformly. In two pigs Q_{fem} increased; but in four pigs Q_{fem} remained relatively stable, and in one pig Q_{fem} decreased. Figs. 1 through 4 show the course of MAP, LVP, CO, and HR during the experimental protocol.

Table 1. Hemodynamic and pulmonary changes during laparoscopic surgery (mean ± SD)

	−5	+2	+5	+7	+10	+30	+60	+90	+120 min
MAP (mm Hg)	133 ±11	148 ±16	146 ±19	148 ±17	143 ±14	144 ±15	142 ±14	145 ±21	146 ±13
LVP (mm Hg)	150 ±13	171 ±23	167 ±22	167 ±22	162 ±18	165 ±17	162 ±14	165 ±25	162 ±15
$LVEDP_{insp}$ (mm Hg)	17 ±5	22 ±7	29 ±15	27 ±14	22 ±5	24 ±9	23 ±13	28 ±15	26 ±13
$LVEDP_{exp}$ (mm Hg)	12 ±5	17 ±8	19 ±11	18 ±10	15 ±6	14 ±6	19 ±12	19 ±14	16 ±11
RAP_{insp} (mm Hg)	9 ±3	11 ±3	13 ±3	14 ±3	13 ±2	13 ±2	13 ±4	14 ±3	16 ±4
RAP_{exp} (mm Hg)	6 ±2	7 ±2	8 ±3	8 ±2	7 ±3	7 ±4	7 ±4	7 ±3	7 ±3
RAP_{trans} (mm Hg)	4 ±3	5 ±4	6 ±3	5 ±3	5 ±4	4 ±6	6 ±3	5 ±3	6 ±2
CO (L/min)	4.2 ±1	—	—	—	5 ±1.4	4.8 ±1.3	5.6 ±2.3	5.4 ±1.2	5.2 ±1.2
HR (BPM)	120 ±20	122 ±23	124 ±30	124 ±28	123 ±22	130 ±29	142 ±34	144 ±39	150 ±31
$LV_{dp/dt}$	1745 ±252	1800 ±275	1818 ±255	1804 ±207	1816 ±248	1822 ±194	1876 ±172	1870 ±191	1890 ±118
PAP_{insp} (mm Hg)	25 ±5	29 ±3	33 ±8	32 ±6	31 ±6	32 ±7	34 ±8	39 ±8	38 ±7
PAP_{exp} (mm Hg)	20 ±5	23 ±3	24 ±10	26 ±6	25 ±6	26 ±6	28 ±8	19 ±15	16 ±11
PAP_{trans} (mm Hg)	21 ±5	23 ±5	25 ±9	25 ±7	24 ±7	24 ±9	25 ±13	30 ±8	28 ±4
PIP_{peak} (mm Hg)	13 ±2	13 ±1	16 ±2	15 ±2	15 ±1	17 ±4	16 ±2	17 ±1	19 ±2
$PIP_{plateau}$ (mm Hg)	11 ±1	12 ±2	12 ±5	13 ±2	13 ±1	14 ±2	14 ±2	15 ±2	16 ±3
ITP_{insp} (mm Hg)	4 ±3	6 ±3	9 ±3	8 ±2	8 ±5	9 ±5	7 ±3	9 ±2	10 ±3
ITP_{exp} (mm Hg)	−0.5 ±1	0.4 ±1	0.4 ±1	0.7 ±2	1 ±2	1.3 ±4	0.1 ±1	0.8 ±2	0.1 ±1.3
CVP (mm Hg)	6 ±3	7 ±4	9 ±3	9 ±3	9 ±3	11 ±4	12 ±3	13 ±4	14 ±4
FVP (mm Hg)	11 ±4	14 ±3	17 ±3	18 ±4	17 ±2	18 ±3	19 ±5	22 ±8	23 ±5
Q_{fem} (ml/min)	89 ±25	96 ±34	89 ±35	93 ±37	81 ±40	81 ±30	85 ±22	95 ±44	91 ±36

FVP, CVP, and RAP_{insp} increased at +5 minutes and were elevated until the end of the study protocol. RAP_{trans} did not change. PAP_{insp} and PAP_{exp} increased at +5 minutes. PAP_{insp} remained increased, whereas PAP_{exp} decreased below baseline after +90 minutes. ITP_{insp} increased at +5 minutes and remained elevated. PAP_{trans} was increased from +60 minutes to the end of the study protocol. PIP_{peak} and $PIP_{plateau}$ increased at +5 minutes and remained at the increased level (all $p < 0.05$). Figs. 5 and 6 show the course of PAP_{insp} and PIP_{peak}, and Fig. 7 shows the nonparallel increase of RAP_{insp} and FVP.

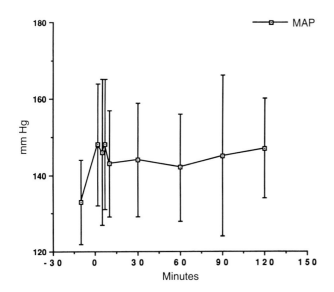

Fig. 1. Mean arterial pressure (MAP) during 120 minutes of laparoscopic surgery.

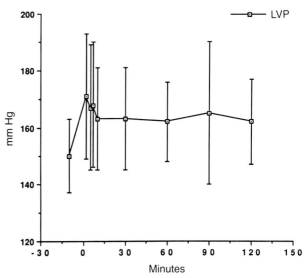

Fig. 2. Left ventricular pressure (LVP) during 120 minutes of laparoscopic surgery.

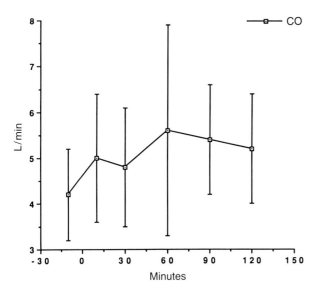

Fig. 3. Cardiac output (CO) during 120 minutes of laparoscopic surgery.

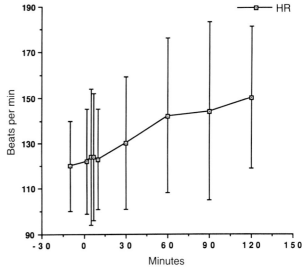

Fig. 4. Heart rate (HR) during 120 minutes of laparoscopic surgery.

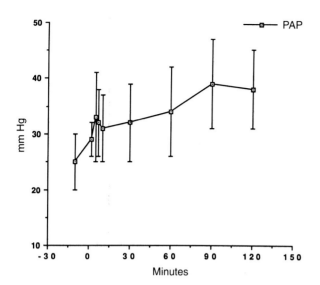

Fig. 5. Pulmonary artery pressure during inspiration (PAP$_{insp}$) during 120 minutes of laparoscopic surgery.

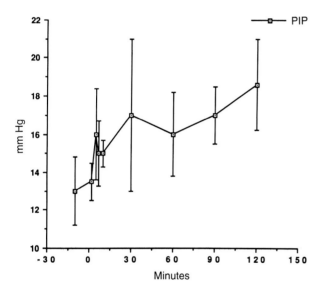

Fig. 6. Peak inspiratory pressure (PIP$_{peak}$) during 120 minutes of laparoscopic surgery.

Blood Samples

Table 2 shows the changes in norepinephrine, arterial, pulmonary, and caval partial pressure of oxygen (PO$_2$), O$_2$ saturation (SaO$_2$), PCO$_2$, and pH. Norepinephrine showed an increasing trend ($p = 0.08$). Pulmonary and caval PO$_2$ and SaO$_2$ increased continuously. Arterial SaO$_2$ (SaO$_{2\,art}$) decreased but remained in a physiological range

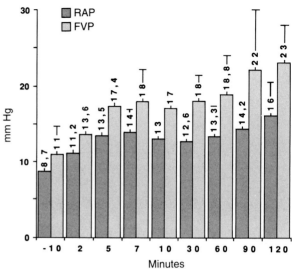

Fig. 7. Right atrial pressure during inspiration (RAP$_{insp}$) and femoral venous pressure (FVP) during 120 minutes of laparoscopic surgery.

PCO$_2$ increased, and pH decreased in each sample. Plasma sodium and potassium levels increased in each sample but remained within physiological concentrations (all $p < 0.05$). Plasma bicarbonate and hematocrit levels did not change.

Necropsy

Atelectasis and dystelectasis were present in the basal lung regions, whereas emphysematous tissue was found in the apical lung regions of every pig.

DISCUSSION

Laparoscopic technique offers important advantages for the patient, primarily the reduction of operative trauma. However, occasional anesthetic problems of unknown etiology have been observed.[5,6,9,10] Several years ago studies showed that the initial influence of increased intra-abdominal pressure on arterial pressure, CO, and blood gas values indicated the risks involving high intra-abdominal pressure and demonstrated the necessity for controlled ventilation[1,3,11,12] Prolonged pneumoperitoneum at 10 to 15 mm Hg, together with surgical manipulation in the modified Trendelenburg position, can influence hemodynamic homeostasis. The net effect on hemodynamics depends on the extent of intra-abdominal pressure, body position, and the adaptability of the patient.

In parallel with the increase in intra-abdominal pressure, the arterial, ventricular, pulmonary, intrathoracic,

Table 2. Norepinephrine and changes in PO_2, O_2 saturation, PCO_2, and pH during prolonged laparoscopic surgery (mean $\pm$SD)

	−5	+10	+30	+60	+90	+120 min
Norepinephrine (pg/ml)	637 ±235	1130 ±694	885 ±215	942 ±388	1271 ±737	1115 ±364
PO_2 art	145 ±15	142 ±27	140 ±25	133 ±18	130 ±14	134 ±22
PO_2 pulm	43 ±5	50 ±6	52 ±5	51 ±7	53 ±6	55 ±6
PO_2 cava	50 ±7	56 ±5	56 ±6	59 ±7	61 ±7	62 ±8
SaO_2 art	98.2 ±0.7	97.7 ±0.7	97.7 ±0.6	97.7 ±0.6	97.3 ±0.7	97.2 ±0.6
SaO_2 pulm	63 ±8	67 ±7	69 ±7	67 ±8	69 ±5	71 ±4
SaO_2 cava	74 ±8	77 ±5	74 ±6	77 ±7	79 ±5	77 ±7
PCO_2 art	37 ±4	44 ±2	46 ±3	48 ±4	49 ±5	53 ±6
PCO_2 pulm	41 ±4	50 ±1	55 ±3	56 ±4	58 ±5	61 ±5
PCO_2 cava	41 ±4	48 ±3	53 ±3	55 ±5	56 ±5	59 ±4
pH art	7.47 ±0.05	7.39 ±0.02	7.35 ±0.03	7.34 ±0.04	7.30 ±0.04	7.30 ±0.04
pH pulm	7.44 ±0.04	7.35 ±0.02	7.31 ±0.02	7.30 ±0.03	7.28 ±0.03	7.26 ±0.04
pH cava	7.44 ±0.05	7.37 ±0.03	7.33 ±0.03	7.31 ±0.04	7.30 ±0.03	7.27 ±0.03

and venous pressures were elevated and remained so as long as the intra-abdominal pressure was increased. CO paralleled this observation. The increase of MAP after short-term pneumoperitoneum is a known effect[11-13]; however, the elevated pressure over the 120-minute time frame was unexpected. Increase of central blood volume and the influence of neurological and humoral effects may have been responsible for the maintenance of this pressure elevation.[14-16] Increase in intra-abdominal pressure may decrease the splanchnic capacitance and therefore shift vascular volume toward the central compartment, thus increasing CO according to Starling's law. However, it is likely that more complex mechanisms function to effect cardiovascular changes in such instances. During pneumoperitoneum within the abdominal pressure limits used for gastrointestinal operative procedures, a close relationship exists between the increase of circulating blood volume effecting increased venous return and the reduction caused by compression of the caudal caval vein.[17] At low intra-abdominal pressures the CO increases as the blood volume increases, whereas at higher pressures the CO decreases, probably because of the further increase of resistance to venous return. This association can also be seen in a study in dogs.[1] At low abdominal pressure the vena caval flow and the arterial pressure were increased, whereas a dramatic decrease of caval flow, together with a decrease in CO, occurred at intra-abdominal pressures exceeding 15 mm Hg.

Under normal circumstances an increase of blood volume as shown after intravenous infusion is compensated initially by the increase of volume in the capacitance vessels, by stress relaxation of veins, by transcapillary fluid shift, and later by renal excretion.[18,19] During our study the CO did not decrease until the end of the operative procedure. The reason for this observation is unclear and can only be hypothesized. One explanation is that the great splanchnic reservoirs are unable to accept the excess volume because of extramural compression by sustained higher intra-abdominal pressures. Since the renal blood flow during laparoscopic procedures has not been described in the literature, the reduction in intravascular fluid volume as a result of urinary output remains an unknown factor. Transcapillary fluid shift could readily decrease the intravascular volume, especially in the case of increased peripheral venous pressure, although the unchanged hematocrit value in this experiment does not support this concept.

During the 60- to 120-minute interval, the HR increased, contributing to the increase in CO. Whether this increase is the result of stretch receptor stimulation or of sympathetic stimulation or if it is simply the effect of pancuronium bromide has not been investigated.

Acute arterial hypertension is rapidly and effectively regulated by the baroreceptors in the arterial and venous systems of a normal individual. It remains unclear why the increase of MAP remained for 120 minutes. The lack of arterial pressure decrease despite a decrease of CO at high intra-abdominal pressure[1] indicates that some other mechanisms are involved in the sustained arterial hypertension. Norepinephrine levels showed a trend toward higher values through the inflation period in our study. Stress,[20] acidosis,[21] or increased PCO_2[22] may influence the vasomotor center. However, we realize that the plasma concentration of catecholamines depends on reuptake and clearance, which cannot automatically be equated with increased sympathetic tone. Other humoral factors such as vasopressin[15,16] may play a significant role but were not investigated in this study.

Like the systemic arterial pressure, the PAP increased during the study protocol. PAP and to a lesser extent systemic arterial pressure increased during the inspiratory phase as mechanical ventilation effected an increase in intrathoracic pressure. The presumed main reason for this increase was inspiratory augmentation of intrathoracic pressure associated with diaphragmatic excursion. However, since the PAP_{trans} increased as well, other effects must also be involved. Increased pulmonary blood flow usually does not significantly change pulmonary pressures in normal individuals.[23,24] Therefore the increase in CO alone is rather unlikely to increase the PAP because of the autoregulatory potential of the lung vasculature. Sympathetic activation, however, could increase the pulmonary resistance by decreasing the compliance of the pulmonary arteries. Acidosis is also a known stimulus for pulmonary vasoconstriction. PIP was increased in our experiments, although it remained within a normal range. Under these circumstances, the pressure in the alveoli probably will be increased, thus affecting the PAP. The increased $PIP_{plateau}$, which may indicate decreased pulmonary compliance, is consistent with these findings. At necropsy, basal atelectases were present in each animal. However, these results did not significantly affect PO_2; thus it was not necessary to increase the FIO_2 or the PEEP during the experiment. Close monitoring of blood gas parameters is recommended,[4] not only because of the decrease in oxygenation, but more specifically because of the continuous increase of PCO_2 to beyond normal physiological values when tidal volumes were not adjusted.

This study supports the view that prolonged laparoscopic procedures with an inherent increase in intra-abdominal pressure should be undertaken with care and reservation in those patients with underlying pulmonary and cardiovascular disease or in patients receiving medication that affects their ability to compensate for pressure-induced compensatory processes.

REFERENCES

1. Ivankovich AD, Miletich DJ, Albrecht RF, et al. Cardiovascular effects of intraperitoneal insufflation with carbon dioxide and nitrous oxide in the dog. Anaesthesiology 42:281, 1975.

2. Motew M, Ivankovich AD, Bieniarz J. Cardiovascular effects and acid base and blood gas changes during laparoscopy. Am J Obstet Gynecol 115:1002, 1973.

3. Diamant M, Benumof JL, Saidman LJ. Hemodynamics of increased intra-abdominal pressure. Anaesthesiology 48:23, 1978.

4. Wittgen CM, Andrus ChH, Fitzgerald SD, et al. Analysis of the hemodynamic and ventilatory effects of laparoscopic cholecystectomy. Arch Surg 126:997, 1991.

5. Klaiber Ch, Metzger A. Komplikationen laparoskopischer Operationen aus anästhesiologischer Sicht. Toronto: Verlag Hans Huber, 1992, p 49.

6. Hasnain JU, Matjasko MJ. Practical anaesthesia for laparoscopic procedures. In Zucker KA, ed. Surgical Laparoscopy. St. Louis: Quality Medical Publishing, 1991, p 77.

7. Függer R, Herbst F, Gnant M, et al. Die experimentelle laparoskopische Sigmaresektion. Min Invasive Chir 1:167, 1992.

8. Stöhr HG, Faworka R, Losert U, et al. On-line Datenacquisition, Darstellung und Langzeitspeicherung von biologischen Meßgrößen mit einem freiprogrammierbaten PC-orientierten System. Biomed Tech 33:195, 1988.

9. Wieden TE, Wieden M, Foitzik H, et al. Emphysem und akute Hyperkapnie während der laparoskopischen Cholezystektomie. Min Invasive Chir 1:20, 1992.

10. Brantley JC, Riley PM. Cardiovascular collapse during laparoscopy: A report of two cases. Am J Obstet Gynecol 159:735, 1988.

11. Marshal RL, Jebson PJR, Davie IT, et al. Circulatory effects of carbon dioxide insufflation of the peritoneal cavity for laparoscopy. Br J Anaesth 44:680, 1972.

12. Kelman GR, Swapp GH, Smith I, et al. Cardiac output and arterial blood-gas tension during laparoscopy. Br J Anaesth 44:1155, 1972.

13. Johannsen G, Andersen M, Juhl B. The effect of general anaesthesia on the haemodynamic events during laparoscopy with CO_2-insufflation. Acta Anaesthesiol Scand 33:132, 1989.

14. Cooper GM, Scoggins AM, Ward ID, et al. Laparoscopy—A stressful procedure. Anaesthesia 37:266, 1982.

15. Solis Herruzo JA, Castellano G, Larrodera L, et al. Plasma arginine vasopressin concentration during laparoscopy. Hepatogastroenterology 36:499, 1989.

16. Melville RJ, Fricis HI, Forsling ML, et al. The stimulus for vasopressin release during laparoscopy. Surg Gynecol Obstet 161:253, 1985.

17. Kashtan J, Green JF, Parsons EQ, et al. Hemodynamic effects of increased abdominal pressure. J Surg Res 30:249, 1981.

18. Guyton AC. Textbook of Medical Physiology, 7th ed. Philadelphia: WB Saunders, 1986, p 272.

19. Rothe CF. Venous system: Physiology of the capacitance vessels. In Handbook of Physiology. The Cardiovascular System. Peripheral Circulation and Organ Blood Flow, vol 3. Bethesda, Md: American Physiology Society, 1983, p 397.

20. Fitzgerald RD, Dechtyar I, Pöschl G, et al. Euroanaesthesia 92 [abstract]. March 20-21, 1992, Mannheim.

21. Guyton AC. Textbook of Medical Physiology, 7th ed. Philadelphia: WB Saunders, 1986, p 244.

22. Price HL. Effects of carbon dioxide on the cardiovascular system. Anaesthesiology 21:652, 1960.

23. Guyton AC. Textbook of Medical Physiology, 7th ed. Philadelphia: WB Saunders, 1986, p 287.

24. Grover RF, Wagner WW, McMurphy IF, et al. Pulmonary circulation. In Handbook of Physiology. The Cardiovascular System. Peripheral Circulation and Organ Blood Flow, vol 3. Bethesda, Md: American Physiology Society, 1983, p 103.

IV

Endoscopic Dissection, Hemostasis, and Retrieval Devices

14 Lasers in Minimally Invasive Surgery

Serge Evrard, Didier Mutter, and Jacques Marescaux

The laser was first used in medicine 25 years ago. Although it is employed routinely in specialities such as ophthalmology, dermatology, and otolaryngology, the extent of its application in intra-abdominal surgery is unclear, except for laser use in gynecology. Lasers are less helpful to the general surgeon. Their cost and limited indications for use in visceral surgery restrict the use of this device.

However, the emergence of minimal access surgery may cause a new interest in laser technology. Laser light is easily conducted by flexible quartz optical fibers and is as readily adapted to the minimal access of trocars as it is to use with the flexible endoscope. Laser technology is progressing, especially in nonthermal applications, and new areas of use will be found in the near future.

In this chapter, the principles of laser technology are described and the current applications and the potential of laser use in minimal access surgery are discussed.

SCIENTIFIC BACKGROUND
Principles

The concept that led to the development of laser technology originated in the quantum theory published by Einstein[1] in 1917. *Laser* is the acronym for light amplification by stimulated emission of radiation[2] and was used to refer to the first device developed by Maiman in 1960. The principle of the laser is the stimulation of the emission of coherent monochromatic photons. *Monochromatic* means that photons are emitted at a single wavelength that corresponds to temporal coherence. *Spatial coherence* means that all wavefronts are in phase (Fig. 1).

The lasing medium, on which the specific wavelength of the laser depends is placed in a cavity with optical resonator properties. Schematically, this lasing cavity consists of two mirrors facing each other, one of which is 98% reflective. The small quantity of light passing through this mirror is the collimated beam. The lasing medium may be a gas (e.g., CO_2, helium-neon), a solid (e.g., ruby, titanium-sapphire), a liquid (e.g., Kiton red, rhodamine), or a metal vapor (e.g., of copper, gold). The lasing medium is stimulated (or pumped) by energy that can be a high-voltage supply or an intense light flash or that can originate in another laser (for example, a dye laser may be pumped by an argon laser). The excited molecules of the lasing medium are raised to higher metastable states for very short periods of time. They return to the ground state with emission of photons by three different mechanisms: spontaneous emission, absorption, and stimulated emission. Stimulated emission of radiation yields photons coherent in time and space: the laser beam (Fig. 2).

Wavelength. Wavelength is specific to the lasing medium. Wavelengths of medical lasers range from the ultraviolet to the near infrared (Fig. 3). Light of visible (400 to 700 nm) and near infrared part of the spectrum is easily transmitted along flexible quartz fibers. Far infrared light (the CO_2 laser) is transmitted by articulated mirrors, and the ultraviolet (the Excimer laser) by multifiber catheters.

Laser output. Laser output is expressed by its power, which is the time rate of energy flux in watts (w) and its energy, which is the power multiplied by the unit of time (w × seconds, joules [J]). Power and energy may be plotted to the surface of the light area delivery given the power density (in w/cm^{-2}) and the energy density (in J/cm^{-2}). Laser light can be used by the surgeon

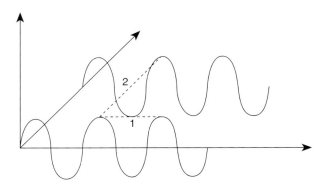

Fig. 1. Coherence of laser light **A,** Temporal coherence–inducing monochromatic light. **B,** Spatial coherence.

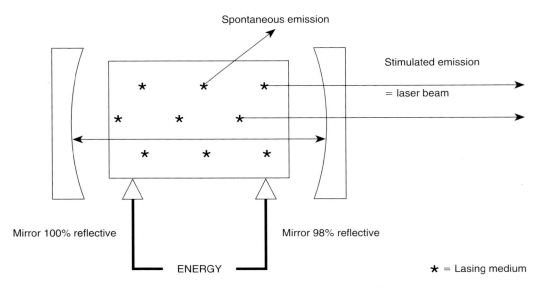

Fig. 2. Schematic representation of a laser.

Wavelength	Thermal lasers	Nonthermal lasers
193		
248	Excimer	
351		
488	Argon	
510	Copper vapor	
514	Argon	Dye lasers
578	Copper vapor	
628	Gold vapor	
633	Helium-neon	
1064	Nd-YAG	
10600	CO2	

Fig. 3. Wavelengths of medical lasers (nm).

at thermal or nonthermal intensities: At <50 J/cm^{-2}, there is no thermal effect; between 50 and 400 J/cm^{-2}, gradual tissue dehydration and coagulation occur; and at >400 J/cm^{-2}, tissues are vaporized.

Laser energy output can be produced by either a continuous wave or by energetic pulses.

Interaction of light with tissues. The interaction of light and tissues is complex.[3] Light incident upon tissue may be reflected, absorbed, scattered, or transmitted.[3] The biological chromophores on which absorption depends are hemoglobin and water. Tissular light behavior also depends on the laser wavelength.

Wavelength. For wavelengths of the visible spectrum and the near infrared, the longer the wavelength, the deeper the tissular distribution. In the far infrared range, light transmission into the tissues decreases considerably. Tissular penetration is about 1 mm for ultraviolet light, 2 to 4 mm for green light, 5 to 10 mm for red light, 10 to 30 mm for the near infrared, and only 0.05 to 0.1 mm for far infrared. Laser light with a low transmission and a high absorption rate dissipates its energy in a small volume; this induces vaporization. Laser light with a high transmission rate dissipates its energy in a larger volume with a lesser thermal effect.

Tissue. The heterogeneity of the tissue (vessels, fat, parenchyma, and so on), its blood flow rate, and the concentration of pigments or chromophores markedly affect the intratissular light behavior. Laser light that is absorbed by chromophores is converted into kinetic energy: heat for thermal power densities and photooxidation for nonthermal power densities.[4]

MEDICAL LASERS
Types of Lasers

Carbon dioxide laser. This laser uses a mixture of carbon dioxide (CO_2) and nitrogen gas. At a wavelength of 10,600 nm, the energy of a CO_2 laser is absorbed 100% by the tissue; none is absorbed by air. Because its output is invisible, it is coupled with a red helium-neon pilot laser for targeting. Water strongly absorbs CO_2 laser light; this results in the vaporization of a superficial layer of tissue. When the size of the spot is >600 μ, the CO_2 laser is ideal for cutting.[5] Peripheral coagulation is slight, but is sufficient to ensure sealing of vessels of 0.5 mm in diameter.[6]

However, there are disadvantages to the use of a laparoscopic CO_2 laser. CO_2 laser light transmission requires a series of mirrors and a cumbersome articulating arm, although flexible quartz fibers will probably soon be substituted for this arrangement. CO_2 pneumoperitoneum absorbs part of the CO_2 laser beam energy. Tissue vaporization induces considerable vapor; this necessitates ventilation of the pneumoperitoneum. Centering of the spot by means of the helium-neon laser guide is often difficult because of dazzling that results from the intense laparoscopic light source.

Argon laser. The argon laser produces two wavelengths: 488 nm and 514 nm. Heavily absorbed by hemoglobin, the depth of its tissular penetration is approximately 1 mm. Hemostasis of 1 mm diameter vessels is attained. Smoke production is slight. Light transmission by flexible quartz fibers is available.

However, cutting with an argon laser requires peripheral tissular coagulation, and the cost of the device is higher than that of the CO_2 laser.

Neodymium:yttrium-aluminum-garnet (Nd:YAG) laser. The Nd:YAG laser, which uses a crystal of yttrium-aluminum-garnet doped with a small quantity of ions of the rare earth metal neodymium, produces a 1060 nm invisible infrared light that is easily transmitted by optic fibers. This laser light is less specifically absorbed by hemoglobin and water than are CO_2 or argon lasers.[7] Tissue penetration is excellent, and vessels of 3 mm in diameter can be coagulated.[6] Visceral applications include surgical debulking and hepatic and spleen resections. The KTP laser is an Nd:YAG laser with a doubled frequency or a halved wavelength (532 nm). Its green light is useful for coagulation, and it has been used for laparoscopic cholecystectomy.[8] The

disadvantage of the KTP laser during laparoscopic use is an obliteration of the television image.

Excimer laser. Excimer (*EXCI*ted di*MER*) lasers are ultraviolet sources that produce very short energy pulses.[9] All excimer lasers use a gas mixture of approximately 0.1% halogen (xenon chloride or argon fluoride), 1% rare gas, and a buffer gas (either helium or neon or both). Excimer lasers can be used for the microsurgical welding of sutures. There is no indication for its use in minimal access surgery.

Diode laser. Semiconductor technology has produced a new laser concept: the diode laser. This small laser, which is the size of a matchbox, can be tuned. The wavelength can be varied, and the laser exhibits high electrical-to-optical efficiency.[10] With its relatively low cost and its performance in constant progress, the diode laser is the tool of the future in medical laser technology, especially in microsurgical welding and photodynamic therapy.

Copper-vapor and gold-vapor lasers. The lasing species of these pulsed lasers are neutral metal atoms. The copper-vapor laser has high efficiency and power with strong output lines at 510 and 578 nm. It is used in photodynamic therapy, either directly[11] or to pump a dye laser.[12] It has also been tested in vitro for use in the fragmentation of mixed and bilirubinate gallstones.[13] The gold-vapor laser emits, in the red at 628 nm, an absorption peak of hematoporphyrin derivatives, which are the photosensitizers most often used in photodynamic therapy.

Dye laser. In the dye laser, the lasing medium is a dye in the liquid state that is energized by different types of lasers, such as the argon laser, the metal-vapor laser, and the diode laser, or by light flashes. The dye laser can be tuned. In Table 1 the dyes available for photodynamic therapy and their lasing ranges are summarized.

Delivery systems. The delivery of laser energy for minimal access surgery by the flexible quartz fiber is

Table 1. Dye lasers available for photodynamic therapy

Dye	Lasing Range (nm)
Rhodamine 6G	570-650
Rhodamine B	601-675
DCM	615-745
Kiton red	580-630

optimal for both noncontact or contact applications. A quartz lens usually couples the laser beam with the fiber, which has a central core of high-quality glass coated with a thin layer of glass of a slightly lower refractive index. Light is transmitted along the fiber by total internal reflection. Fibers range from approximately 0.1 to 1 mm in diameter. Bare fibers can be used in a noncontact mode (coagulation), a near-contact mode (vaporization), or a contact mode (purely thermal).[8] The sides of bare fibers, which can accidentally deliver laser energy to adjacent organs, cannot be used.

Recently a variety of industrial sapphire and ceramic contact tips for hand-held or endoscopic use have been introduced. The sides of the fibers can be used for cutting and provide the surgeon with tactile feedback.[8] Contact fibers have the disadvantages of being slightly more expensive and of staying hot for 10 seconds after use, which can result in contact burns to adjacent organs.

Laser devices. Small laser devices are now available; they have a place in the operating theater with the preoperative ultrasonographic scanner or the ultrasonographic dissector (Fig. 4). Their prices, which vary with the type of lasing medium, range from approximately

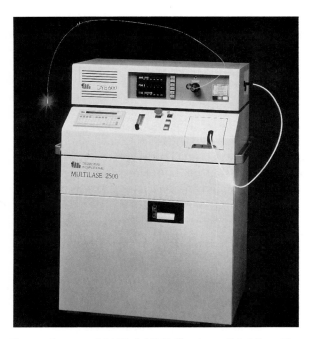

Fig. 4. Compact Nd:YAG/KTP/dye laser (Multilase Dye 600, Technomed International).

$20,000 to more than $200,000. Periodic maintenance of laser devices and fibers is necessary.

LASER APPLICATIONS IN MINIMALLY INVASIVE SURGERY
Thermal Applications

The laser can be used as a thermal scalpel to incise tissue and to achieve hemostasis simultaneously. The thermal applications of lasers have been used in minimal access surgery in the sites listed subsequently.

The liver. Experimental studies indicate that portions of the liver may be resected with CO_2 or Nd:YAG lasers or with the simultaneous use of both. Tranberg et al.[14] compared the Nd:YAG laser and the ultrasonographic dissector with the routine blunt dissection method of liver resection. They observed that the noncontact Nd:YAG laser resulted in a significant reduction of operating time when compared with that required by the other two methods and in a decreased perioperative blood loss but in more extensive tissue necrosis. Joffe et al.[15] demonstrated the superiority of the contact artificial sapphire technique as opposed to the noncontact approach in the rat model, as did Schroder et al.[16] in the canine model.

Recently Katkhouda et al.[17] reported the first case of laparoscopic laser resection of a liver hydatid cyst. The authors state that this technique, in which an Nd:YAG laser was used, may be indicated in small liver metastases or benign tumor resections. Palliative vaporization of scattered hepatic metastases, especially in tumors of endocrine origin, is also favored.[18]

The biliary tract. Laparoscopic laser cholecystomy has been proposed as an alternative to electrocautery.[8,19] No prospective data are available on this subject. Electrosurgical dissection may be faster and is less costly; laser dissection may be more precise.[8] Some authors deny the role of lasers in laparoscopic cholecystectomy.[20]

Stones in the common bile duct may be fragmented by the photoacoustic effect of a laser beam. In this contact technique, the laser light induces a plasma by means of heat, and the hot plasma produces a shock wave that fractures the stone.[21] The most appropriate type of laser for this procedure seems to be the pulsed dye laser, a high-energy pulsed device that reduces the size of the stone with minimal thermic effect. In this way common bile duct stones can be treated at the time of laparoscopic cholecystectomy in one procedure, thus obviating both conversion to an open common bile duct exploration and the need for a second procedure of endoscopic retrograde cholangiography, papillotomy, or stone extraction. A laparoscopic flexible choledocoscope driving the quartz fiber may be introduced either by the cystic duct or by choledocotomy. Irrigation by rapid saline flow then moves the stone fragments through the sphincter of Oddi into the duodenum.

The pancreas. Joffe et al.[22] have performed experimental and clinical pancreatic resections with the Nd:YAG laser. Total pancreatectomies have also been performed with the CO_2 laser in the dog model.[23] Significant reductions in operating time and blood loss were reported.

The spleen. Dixon et al.[24] have described an open technique for segmental or partial splenectomy that involves the ligature of selected hilar vessels and Nd:YAG vaporization of the splenic capsule, superficial sinusoidal tissue, and smaller peripheral vessels. Coagulated material was aspirated. As the hilum was approached, larger vessels were divided and clipped. Laparoscopic splenectomies have been performed, and lasers may be useful in partial resection.

The stomach. The contact Nd:YAG laser has been used for visceral incisions (especially in the stomach and intestine) during open procedures.[25,26] Laparoscopic surgery will profit from the use of this laser scalpel because no accurate cutting laparoscopic instrument exists. Hunter et al.[27] have reported a laser version of the Taylor procedure that was used in the dog model. Posterior vagotomy was performed conventionally, but an argon laser myotomy was performed along the anterior curvature. Serosa and muscularis were coagulated, but mucosa was not. Secretory studies were satisfactory.

Nonthermal Laser Applications

Photodynamic therapy. The principles of photodynamic therapy have been known for a century.[28] This anticancer technique is applied with increasing frequency in dermatology,[29] urology,[30] gastroenterology,[31] ophthalmology,[32] and neurosurgery.[33] It consists of a systemic injection of a photosensitizer that is preferentially taken up in tissues of strong mitotic activity and in pathological stroma.[34] Hematoporphyrin derivatives and dihematoporphyrin ether (Photofrin) are the most frequently used compounds, especially in clinical practice, but new photosensitizers with improved photophysical and biochemical properties, such as chlorines,[35] pheophorbide,[12] and phthalocyanines,[36] are being investigated.

Photosensitizers do not result in spontaneous toxicity; they must be excited by photons to produce cytotoxic free radicals such as singlet oxygen or superoxide radicals.[37] These transitory radicals are thought to damage blood vessel endothelium, which causes the destruction of tumor microcirculation.[38] Direct disruption of cell membranes[39] and subcellular organelles[40] has been described.

The efficiency and relative selectivity of photodynamic therapy and the body's tolerance suggest its use to complement curative surgical intra-abdominal procedures. The limiting factor of an extensive parenchymal resection is micrometastases in the areolar tissue and lymph nodes. In spite of large visceral resections, micrometastases frequently remain and may cause locoregional or metastatic recurrence.[41-43]

To our knowledge, there are only four reports[44-47] of intra-abdominal photodynamic therapy administration in humans. These papers reported phase I feasibility studies, of which were completed preoperatively and one of which was postoperative.[46] In the first two studies, which were conducted by Roswell Park Memorial Institute, photodynamic therapy was used as an adjuvant treatment after surgical debulking but only at second-look surgery for recurrences. The first report[44] addressed the treatment of pelvic recurrence of colorectal cancer, and the second[45] concerned the retroperitoneal recurrence of liposarcoma. The third study[47] was a case report of a common bile duct carcinoma treated by photodynamic therapy; a 4-year remission resulted. The final published report[46] from the National Cancer Institute was devoted to the treatment of peritoneal carcinomatosis.

The excitation of the photosensitizer by the incident photon produces the reemission of the fluorescent photon that can be used to localize the reaction. Detection of this fluorescence might be used to demonstrate small tumor deposits. Although the fluorescence detection signal is limited by tissue autofluorescence,[48] Herrera-Ornelas et al.[44] found a correlation between observed sites of fluorescence and tumor occurrence in biopsies of the same sites. Additional studies of sensitivity and specificity are necessary to determine the diagnostic importance of photodynamic therapy.

Photodynamic therapy is developing in conjunction with the concept of neoplastic cell targeting. Its technology is well adapted to minimal access surgery and is especially appropriate for iterative access to the intra-abdominal cavity. Laparoscopic photodynamic diagnosis and therapy may be useful in the management of digestive cancers, in which the diagnosis of recurrence and the destruction of peritoneal deposits or lymph node metastases would probably improve prognosis.

Miniaturized robotic guiding. Instrumentation of laparoscopic surgery is in its infancy, and considerable progress will soon be achieved. Three-dimensional imaging and microinstrumentation are especially desirable. Computer-assisted miniature robots that can cut with precision or perform endocorporeal knots are within the realm of possibility. Research is in progress. Lasers would be as useful in piloting these microdevices as they are in performing certain military functions.

CONCLUSION

There is no advantage to the use of lasers in open abdominal surgery, and very few gastrointestinal surgeons use lasers for that purpose. Minimal access surgery may change this attitude as it did in gynecological laparoscopic surgery. In a paper devoted to the future of laparoscopic surgery, Alfred Cuschieri said, "There are some disadvantages to the use of laser light energy with the existing generation of equipment.... On the other hand, there is no question that laser will be needed for the future development of minimal access surgery."[49]

REFERENCES

1. Einstein A. Zur Quantentheorie des Strahlung. Physikalische Zeitschrift 18:121, 1917.
2. Maiman TH. Stimulated optical radiation in ruby. Nature 187:493, 1960.
3. Svaasand LO, Doiron DR. Thermal distribution during photoradiation therapy. In Kessel D, Dougherty TJ, eds. Porphyrin Photosensitization. New York: Plenum Press, 1983, p 77.
4. Foote CS. Light, oxygen and toxicity. In Autor AP, ed. Pathology of Oxygen. New York: Academic Press, 1982, p 21.
5. Bruhat M, Mage G, Manhes M. Use of CO_2 laser via laparoscopy, laser surgery, vol 3. In Kaplan I, ed. Proceedings of the Third International Society for Laser Surgery. Tel Aviv, 1979, The Society.
6. Fuller T. Fundamentals of lasers in surgery and medicine. In Dixon JA, ed. Surgical Applications of Lasers. Chicago: Year Book, 1983, p 11.
7. Dixon JA, Berenson MM, McCloskey DW. Neodymium YAG laser treatment of experimental canine gastric bleeding. Gastroenterology 77:647, 1979.
8. Hunter JG. Laser or electrocautery for laparoscopic cholecystectomy. Am J Surg 161:345, 1991.
9. Linsker R, Srinivasan R, Wynne JJ, Alonso DR. Far-ultraviolet ablation of atherosclerotic lesions. Lasers Surg Med 4:167, 1984.
10. Thompson GBH. Physics of semiconductor laser devices. New York: John Wiley & Sons, 1980, p 28.
11. Allardice JT, Grahn MF, Rowland AC, Durcan JJ, Griffith A, Van der Walt JD, Williams NS. Safety studies for intraoperative photodynamic therapy. Laser Med Sci 7:133, 1992.
12. Evrard S, Jeannin E, Tsuji M, Damgé C, Marescaux J, Aprahamian M. Photodynamic therapy (PDT) of a pancreatic cancer in the rat. Br J Surg 79:575, 1992.
13. Dayton MT, Decker DL, McClane R, Dixon JA. Copper vapor laser fragmentation of gallstones: In vitro measurements of wall heat transmission. J Surg Res 45:90, 1988.
14. Tranberg KG, Ricotti P, Brackett KA. Liver resection—a comparison using the Nd:YAG laser, ultrasonic dissector or conventional blunt dissection. Am J Surg 151:368, 1986.
15. Stephen NJ, Brackett KA, Sankar MY, Daikuzono N. Resection of the liver with the Nd:YAG laser. Surg Gynecol Obstet 163:437, 1986.
16. Schroder T, Sankar MY, Brackett AKM. Major liver resection using contact ND:YAG laser. Lasers Surg Med 7:89, 1987.
17. Katkhouda N, Fabiani P, Benizri E, Mouiel J. Br J Surg 79:560, 1992.
18. Dixon JA. Current laser applications in general surgery. Ann Surg 207:355, 1988.
19. Reddick EJ, Olsen DO. Outpatient laparoscopic laser cholecystectomy. Am J Surg 160:485, 1990.
20. Voyles CR, Meena AL, Petro AB, Haick AJ, Koury AM. Electrocautery is superior to laser for laparoscopic cholecystectomy. Am J Surg 160:457, 1990.
21. Gitomer SJ, Jones RD. Modeling laser ablation and fragmentation of renal and biliary stones. In Conference on Lasers and Electro-Optics. Baltimore: Society of Lasers and Electro-Optics, 1987.
22. Joffe SN, Sankar MY, Salzer B. Preliminary clinical application of the contact surgical rod and endoscopic microprobes with the Nd:YAG laser. Lasers Surg Med 5:188, 1985.
23. Donna GD. Total pancreatectomy with the carbon dioxide laser. In Atsumi K, Nimsakul N, eds. Laser Tokyo '81. Tokyo: Inter-Group, 1981, p 43.
24. Dixon JA, Miller F, McCloskey D. Laser partial splenectomy. Surg Res 10:116, 1980.
25. Hira N, Moore KC. The use of the ND:YAG contact laser in abdominal surgery. Lasers Surg Med 7:86, 1987.
26. Skobelkin OK, Breckow EI, Smoljiniov MB. Resection of hollow abdominal organs with lasers. Lasers Surg Med 7:101, 1987.

27. Hunter JG, Becker JM, Dixon JA. Lesser curvature laser myotomy. Lasers Surg Med 8:362, 1984.
28. Raab O. Uber die wirkung fluoreszierender Stoffe auf Infusoria. Z Biol 39:524, 1900.
29. McCaughan JS, Guy JT, Hicks W, Laufman L, Nims TA, Walker J. Photodynamic therapy for cutaneous and subcutaneous malignant neoplasms. Arch Surg 124:211, 1989.
30. Schumacker BP, Hetzel FW. Clinical laser photodynamic therapy in the treatment of bladder carcinoma. Photochem Photobiol 46:899, 1987.
31. Patrice T, Foultier MT, Adam F, Audoin AF, Galmiche JP, Le Bodic L. Traitement palliatif par photochimiothérapie de 54 cancers digestifs. Essai clinique de phase 1. Ann Chir 43:433, 1989.
32. Murphree AL, Cote M, Gomer CJ. The evolution of photodynamic therapy techniques in the treatment of intraocular tumors. Photochem Photobiol 46:919, 1987.
33. Kostron H, Weiser G, Fritsch E, Grunert V. Photodynamic therapy of malignant brain tumors. Clinical and neuropathological results. Photochem Photobiol 46:937, 1987.
34. Bugelski PJ, Porter CW, Dougherty TJ. Autoradiographic distribution of hematoporphyrin derivative in normal and tumor tissue of the mouse. Cancer Res 41:4606, 1981.
35. Ris HB, Altermatt HJ, Inderbitzi R, Hess R, Nachbur B, Stewart JCM, Wang Q, Lim CK, Bonnett R, Berenbaum MC, Althaus U. Photodynamic therapy with chlorins for diffuse malignant mesothelioma: Initial clinical results. Br J Cancer 64:1116, 1991.
36. Barr H. Tralau CJ, MacRobert AJ, Krasner N, Boulos PB, Clark CG, Bown SG. Photodynamic therapy in the normal rat colon with phthalocyanine sensitisation. Br J Cancer 56:111-118, 1987.
37. Foote CS. Light, oxygen and toxicity. In Autor AP, ed. Pathology of Oxygen. New York: Academic Press, 1982, p 21.
38. Star WM, Marijnissen HPA, Van Den Berg Blok AE. Destruction of rat mammary tumor and normal tissue microcirculation by hematoporphyrin derivative photoradiation observed in vivo in sandwich obervation chambers. Cancer Res 46:2532, 1986.
39. Valenzeno DP. Photomodification of biological membranes with emphasis on singlet oxygen mechanisms. Photochem Photobiol 46:147, 1987.
40. Gibson S, Hilf R. Photosensitization of mitochondrial cytochrome C oxidase by hematoporphyrin derivative and related porphyrins in vitro and in vivo. Cancer Res 43:4191, 1983.
41. Warshaw AL, Swanson RS. Pancreatic cancer in 1988. Possibilities and probabilities. Ann Surg 208:541, 1988.
42. Quirke P, Durdey P, Dixon MF, Williams NS. Local recurrence of rectal adenocarcinoma due to inadequate surgical resection. Lancet :996, 1986.
43. Gunderson LL, Sosin H. Adenocarcinoma of the stomach: Areas of failure in a reoperation series (second or symptomatic look). Clinicopathologic correlation and implications for adjuvant therapy. Int J Radiat Oncol Biol Phys 8:1, 1982.
44. Herrera-Ornelas L, Petrelli NJ, Mittelman A, Dougherty TJ, Boyles DG. Photodynamic therapy in patients with colorectal cancer. Cancer 57:677, 1986.
45. Nambisan RN, Karakousis CP, Holyoke ED, Dougherty TJ. Intraoperative photodynamic therapy for retroperitoneal sarcomas. Cancer 61:1248, 1988.
46. Sindelar WF, DeLaney TF, Tochner Z, Thomas GF, Dachowski LJ, Smith PD, Friauf WS, Cole JW, Glatstein E. Technique of photodynamic therapy for disseminated intraperitoneal malignant neoplasms. Arch Surg 126:318, 1991.
47. McCaughan JS, Mertens BF, Cho C, Barabash RD, Payton HW. Photodynamic therapy to treat tumors of the extrahepatic biliary ducts. Arch Surg 126:111, 1991.
48. Baumgartner R, Fisslinger H, Jocham D, Lenz H, Ruprecht L, Stepp H, Unsöld E. A fluorescence imaging device for endoscopic detection of early stage cancer—Instrumental and experimental studies. Photochem Photobiol 46:759, 1987.
49. Cushieri A. Minimal access surgery and the future of interventional laparoscopy. Am J Surg 161:404, 1991.

15 *The Argon Beam Endoscopic Coagulator: A First Experimental and Clinical Report*

Jerome Canady, Carol C. Jagdeo, Enrico Nicolo, and Frank L. Fontana

MATERIALS AND METHODS

We will describe the first application of the Canady argon beam endoscopic polypectomy snare coagulator used in conjunction with flexible endoscopic instruments. The Canady argon beam coagulator consists of a reusable handle and disposable or reusable Silastic tubing (2.8 mm in diameter) delivering a 40 to 150 W radio frequency current traveling in a coaxial argon gas jet, delivered through a tungsten flexible wire with a snare at the end (1.0 mm in diameter). The flexible wire cable is enclosed in the Silastic tubing and connected to a handle (Fig. 1). The Silastic tubing, with its flexible wire, can be passed through the working channel of a flexible gastroscope, colonoscope, laparoscope, and other flexible endoscopic instruments. A single-pedal foot switch activates the unit, and a patient grounding plate is used for return of the radio frequency current to the generator. The inert, noncombustible argon gas provides the medium through which the current travels at room temperature. Conventional unipolar cautery is also incorporated into the catheter (Fig. 2). The argon beam coagulator (ABC) generator uses two cylinders that contain high-purity (99.9%) argon gas, which is stored in a portable generator with a variable gas flow rate of 1 to 12 L/min. When the tip of the catheter comes within 1 cm of the tissue, current is activated by depressing the foot pedal. The recommended flow rate for coagulation is 1 to 2 L/min with 40 to 80 W of power.

RESULTS

We have used the Canady argon beam endoscopic coagulator in six patients. The endoscopic procedures consisted of colonoscopic polypectomies, reduction of gastric varices via gastroscope, ablation of esophageal polyps, and coagulation of a liver biopsy site via flexible laparoscope (Fujinon):

  Colonic polyps
  Esophageal polyps
  Gastric varices
  Bleeding at liver biopsy sites

All patients responded well to the argon gas, and there was no mortality or morbidity.

The ABC delivers a depth of injury of 2 mm or less to tissue. Figs. 3 and 4 demonstrate a 4 cm sessile polyp of the transverse colon, which was removed by the Canady argon beam flexible polypectomy snare catheter.

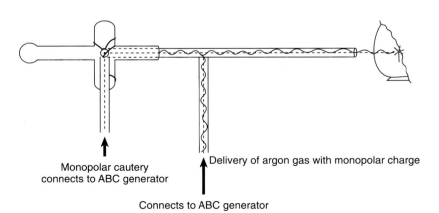

Monopolar cautery
connects to ABC generator

Delivery of argon gas with monopolar charge

Connects to ABC generator

Fig. 1. The flexible wire cable is enclosed in the Silastic tubing and connected to a handle.

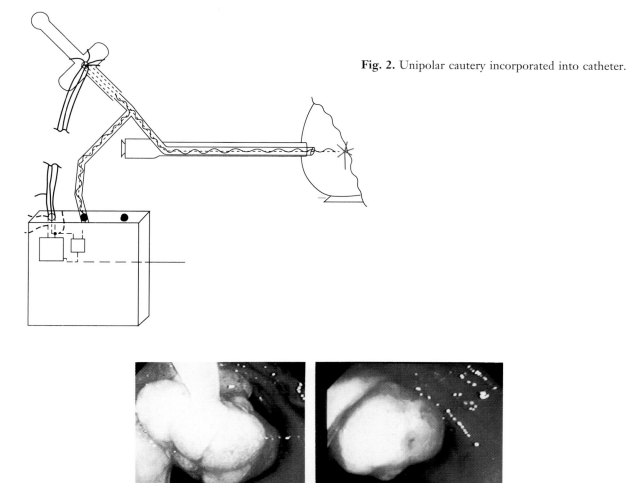

Fig. 2. Unipolar cautery incorporated into catheter.

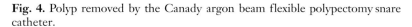

Fig. 3. A 4 cm sessile polyp of the transverse colon.

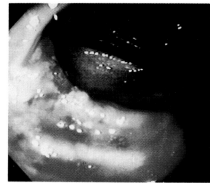

Fig. 4. Polyp removed by the Canady argon beam flexible polypectomy snare catheter.

DISCUSSION

We have described the use and development of the argon beam coagulator in flexible endoscopic instruments. Use of the argon beam coagulator in conjunction with flexible endoscopic instruments will be a quantum leap in the technological management of gastric and colonic bleeding, removal of polyps, and coagulation and dissection of tissue in the abdominal and thoracic cavities via flexible gastroscope, colonoscope, bronchoscope, thoracoscope, laparoscope, and cystoscope.

REFERENCES

1. Van Way CW, Ketch L, Stiegman A, et al. A comparison of ionized noble gas electrocoagulation with spray model electrocoagulation in canine liver and spleen. Scientific poster. Presented at the Seventy-Second Annual Clinical Congress, American College of Surgeons. New Orleans, 1986.
2. Henderson MR, Link WJ, Incropera FP, et al. Gas transport resulting from plasma-scalpel surgery. Med Biol Engl 12:208, 1974.
3. Ward PH, Castro D, Ward S. A significant new contribution to radical head and neck surgery. The argon beam coagulator as an effective means of limiting blood loss. Arch Otolaryngol Head Neck Surg 115:921-923, 1989.
4. System 6000 Argon Beam Coagulator tissue effects. Technical document. Bard Electro Medical Systems, Inc., Englewood, Colo, Jan. 1988.

---

16   *Laser Surgery Versus Electrosurgery: Point and Counterpoint*

Jean-François Cuttat

With the development of laparoscopic and thoracoscopic surgery, new instruments have been developed, in particular, instruments for the dissection of tissues. In addition to scissors for celioscopy, which are used the same way as in standard surgery, new instruments for laparoscopic applications, such as those using laser beam and electrical current, have been developed.

Since its description in 1928 by Harvey Cushing, electrosurgery has become a basic and standard procedure in surgery. Lasers were developed at the beginning of the 1950s and have been used routinely in certain surgical units for more than 20 years, especially in the United States.

Electrosurgery and lasers use thermal energy to obtain a surgical effect. Five points about these two techniques are discussed in parallel with respect to their application in minimally invasive surgery: production of energy, transport of energy from the generators to the tissues, action of the energy on the tissue, types of laser, and future technologies.

In this chapter only the use of thermal lasers is discussed. Other lasers are used in medical treatments but do not produce thermal reactions. They produce photochemical effects or shock waves or have highly specialized applications. Similarly, only high-frequency electrosurgical instruments are discussed.

WHAT IS A LASER IN SURGERY?

The word *laser* is the acronym for *l*ight *a*mplification by *s*timulated *e*mission of *r*adiation. However, for the surgeon a laser simply is an instrument that can *cut, coagulate*, and *vaporize* tissues. The key word is *instrument*, something with which to work. Electrosurgical instruments use electrons for cutting or coagulating tissues, whereas lasers use photons for cutting, coagulating, and vaporizing tissues. Laser or electrosurgical instruments cut by tissue suppression like a saw does, contrary to a surgical blade, which cuts like a knife.

Theoretically, lasers produce a *coherent* (waves of light are in phase), *monochromatic* (only one wavelength of light

94

or color) light in *collimation* (all photons directed in the same direction). However, theory becomes myth when the laser is used in surgery. All the lasers except the argon laser produce a light that is more or less monochromatic. That the laser light is more or less monochromatic is unimportant, even though the coagulation reactions of the tissue depend more on the color than on vaporization. All lasers produce a coherent light (i.e., the light waves are in phase), but the phase is not quite exact for lasers applied in surgery, because the distance between mirrors may vary as a function of changes in temperature or because of vibrations (e.g., when the apparatus is moved). This coherence is useless in surgical lasers because it has no effect on tissues, and even if lasers produce a coherent light, this coherence would be lost or is lost as the light travels through the optical fiber. Finally, all lasers produce a light that is very directed without being collimated because this would considerably reduce their efficacy. This aspect of the laser makes it possible to focus the light on a target quite small in diameter.

Creation of Energy

Three elements are essential for creation of laser light. The *active agent* is the gas within which the laser is created. The *source of energy* is electricity. The *oscillation cavity* consists of two or more mirrors that send each other the light in a way that only light beams directed in a certain direction are reflected. The creation of laser energy starts with activation of an energy source; thus surgical lasers need electrical current in the operating room. The electricity enters directly into the active medium, or it is used to spark a light, which produces photons that circulate in the active medium.

At the atomic level of the active medium, the electrons orbit around a central nucleus and normally are at rest. When an exterior energy is introduced, the electrons are temporarily deplaced at a higher orbit *(excitation)*, an orbit on which they rest for a brief moment before falling back to their regular orbit. Falling back, the originally absorbed energy becomes free in the form of a photon (spontaneous emission). The photon has a characteristic wavelength, which is a quality of the medium used. Once free, the photon can activate another atom. Returning to its equilibrium, the atom will liberate two identical photons *(stimulated emission)*. Because the process is evolving in a confined space with parallel mirrors at each extremity, the number of free photons will increase in the same direction *(amplification)*. One of the mirrors of the oscillation chamber is slight-

ly translucent, which permits a small quantity of light to escape. It is this portion of energy that is used to produce a surgical effect.

The thermic effect in electrosurgery is due to electrons produced from an electrical source. A radio frequency between 100 kHz and 4 MHz can be used, but the majority of systems on the market today produce a current between 500 and 750 kHz. At frequences below 100 kHz, muscles and nerves are stimulated by the current. At the other spectrum of frequencies, the capacity and inductance make it difficult to confine the current strictly to the direction defined by the electrical cable.

The equipment used in high-frequency surgery until approximately 1980 was composed of a vacuum tube and a discharger. The vacuum tube produced high-frequency tensions, which are not modulated and are used for cutting with a small hemostatic effect. The discharger produced high-frequency tensions with strong modulations of the amplitude for cuts with a strong hemostatic effect. The high-frequency energy produced by the two generators could be adjusted independently. New equipment based on semiconductors has been produced since the 1980s. The only difference in the properties of the cutting is the variation in depth of coagulation, resulting in modification of both amplitude and modification of the high-frequency current.

The generator of electrosurgery produces three types of current: (1) For *cutting*, the current is a regular sinusoidal wave, an alternating current that produces the highest local heat. (2) For *coagulation*, the current consists of thousands of short discharges of sinusoidal waves that are separated. A current with strong modulation of the amplitude, it is humidified temporarily to reduce the heating process and thus produce a hemostatic effect, which is more important. (3) A *mixed* current consists of discharges that alter high and low voltages, thus allowing presetting of the quality of cutting and the depth of coagulation.

In addition, there are different types of lasers that have characteristic effects. The effects of the lasers are due to length of the waves and depend primarily on the active medium. They are described in more detail below.

Transport of Energy From the Generator to the Tissue

To function, the electrical energy must be in a closed circuit. The generator of electrosurgery requires the connection of two cables to the patient. In general, a monopolar system is used for laparoscopic surgery (the body of the patient is one part of the circuit). With this type of system, the electrical energy is delivered through a unique electrical cable attached to the electrosurgical instrument, and the current returns through an electrical wire attached on the surface of the patient, generally located in the very low back or thigh.

Wire connections specific for electrosurgical instrumentation must be used to prevent the possible stimulation of the neuromuscular system.

When lasers are used, transport of light energy must be done with maximal security. There are two means to transport this light to the tissue level: through an assembly of articulated arms with mirrors or through optical fibers. The tubes with articulations and mirrors are quite unhandy and fragile, and their light transmission is rather complicated. At their extremity are lenses to concentrate the light beam. Optical fibers, on the other hand, allow great flexibility, do not require optical lenses to focus the light energy, and are easily adaptable in endoscopy and in surgical laparoscopy. Because of the absence of an optical lens at the outlet of the optical fiber, the light beam will diverge with an angle of approximately 15 degrees. Thus the diameter of the target will increase by 1 mm as the distance separating the outlet of the fiber from the target tissue increases by 4 mm. For CO_2 lasers, a hollow waveguide tube can be used (Excellit, manufactured by Coherent), which can be connected to the articulated arm. As with optical fibers, the absence of an optical lens at its outlet means the light will diverge. Even though rigid and fixed to the *bras articulé* (mobile, articulated extension), these instruments are easily used in surgical laparoscopy. If a convergent cone *(sapphire)* is added at the extremity of the fiber, the light energy is transformed into heat. This permits good section capacity but poor or mediocre coagulation capacity. The optical fibers are disposable, primarily because they are rapidly degraded and lose their transmission capacity after a number of sterilizations. Finally, they are fragile and break easily.

Effect of Energy on the Tissue

The effects of laser and electrical current are similar in some points. Cutting or coagulation is a function of the quantity of delivered and absorbed energy and of the surface of the tissue to which this energy is directed.

For a laser four effects result from conversion of the light energy to thermic energy: *reflection, absorption, dispersion,* and *transmission* (Fig. 1). Of all these effects, dispersion is the most important. The light current disperses or rebounds on the tissue until it is absorbed, in-

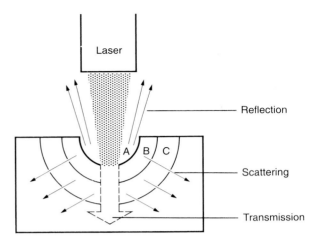

Fig. 1. Cells absorbing the laser beam directly will be vaporized by intracellular boiling. Nonabsorbed photons will be reflected, scattered, or transmitted, resulting in cellular necrosis or reversible cellular injury. A = zone of vaporization; B = zone of necrosis; C = zone of edema.

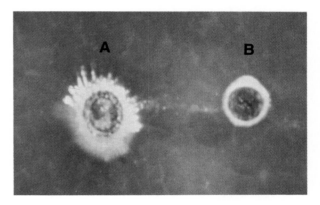

Fig. 2. Nd:YAG laser, A, and CO_2 laser, B, focused on the liver (power, 25 W). On the surface, lateral thermal damage of the Nd:YAG is important.

ducing a lateral damage that is responsible for coagulation. The surface of dispersion and the extent of lateral damage vary as a function of the length of the light wave. The CO_2 laser produces the least lateral damage with the least dispersion, whereas the Nd:YAG laser produces the most dispersion. The damage from the potassium, titanil, and phosphate (KTP) and the argon lasers falls between the other two. *If there is no dispersion, there is no lateral damage and thus no hemostatic effect* (Figs. 2 to 5).

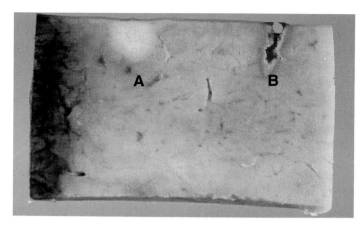

Fig. 3. Sagittal view of the liver: Nd:YAG laser, *A*, and CO_2 laser, *B* (power 25 W). CO_2 laser produces less scatter, and Nd:YAG, laser produces more.

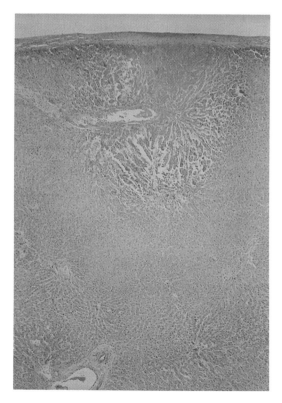

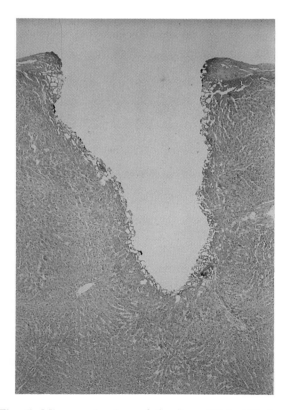

Fig. 4. Microscopic view of the liver. With Nd:YAG laser (power, 25 W), internal dispersion is high, and there is lateral thermal damage with a zone of thermal necrosis.

Fig. 5. Microscopic view of the liver. With CO_2 laser (power, 25 W), internal dispersion is low.

Absorption is variable, depending on the laser in use and on the tissue in question. The CO_2 laser beam, for example, is highly absorbed in water, whereas those from all other lasers are only slightly absorbed. In hemoglobin the Nd:YAG laser beam is only slightly absorbed, whereas all the other laser beams are highly absorbed. The best wavelength for coagulation is that of the Nd:YAG laser, the one least absorbed in hemoglobin. The coagulation capacity for wavelength depends on the absorption, and *as absorption increases, coagulation capacity decreases.*

In electrosurgery the electrical energy is converted into heat as a function of tissue resistance and of the level of energy used. In the case of a laser or an electrosurgical instrument used to evaporate tissue, a part of the heat necessary for vaporization is dispersed in the tissue, which leads to what is called *lateral damage*, thus an effect of coagulation.

Lasers that transmit easily through water but not through blood can be used for hemostatic purpose while the wound is constantly washed. This is an important advantage when compared to electrosurgery because water is an excellent conductor of electrical energy. The energy used in laser surgery is calculated as a function of the power of the beam, time of exposure, and surface exposed:

$$\text{Surgical dose} = \frac{\text{Power} \times \text{Time}}{\text{Tissue surface}}$$

Variation in surgical dose induces several phenomena: *denaturation, coagulation, necrosis,* and *vaporization* (Fig. 6). They are caused by the increase in tissue temperature. Up to 40° C there is no significant tissue damage. Between 40° and 50° C cellular damage and tissue damage are reversible as a function of exposure time. Between 50° and 70° C damage is irreversible, which corresponds to the phenomenon of denaturation. Above 70° C collagen is transformed into glucose, and coagulation is obtained. Above 100° C a transition phase occurs with evaporation of tissue water and extracellular water (i.e., vaporization). Tissues are quickly desiccated. Glucose becomes an adherent compound after such dehydration. Above approximately 200° C carbonization, which corresponds to fourth degree burning, occurs. Finally there is production of smoke as tissue temperature rises. This escalation in tissue effects is not quite linear, but the order of appearance remains constant. CO_2 lasers require the lowest surgical dose to obtain an effect. However, it is difficult to obtain a coagulation effect with this laser. The Nd:YAG laser requires a very high surgical dose to produce vaporization, but it has

a large area of application to obtain coagulation. The effects of KTP and argon lasers fall between the other two (Fig. 7).

During a laparoscopic procedure, power generally is not or is just slightly modified. The variables affecting the tissue surface can be adjusted by modification of

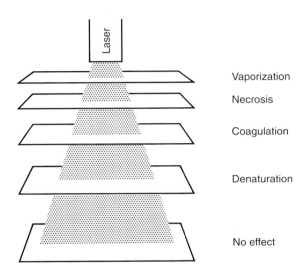

Fig. 6. Tissue effect is relative to the surgical dose applied.

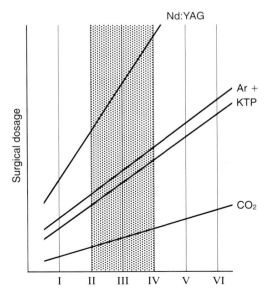

Fig. 7. Rate of work for various laser wavelengths. *I* = Denaturation; *II* = coagulation; *III* = necrosis; *IV* = vaporization; *V* = carbonization; and *VI* = incandescence.

the distance between the extremity of the fiber and the tissue and modification of exposure time. The longer the laser is applied to a particular surface, the greater the increase in heat flowing to adjacent tissue, leading to increasing damage of neighboring tissue. Currently, most laser products can produce a beam in a continued mode either pulsed or superpulsed to modulate the type of application.

In electrosurgery variation in surgical dose can also modify the ultimate effect on tissue. Treating big surfaces with high voltage and high power will produce coagulation, whereas treating small surfaces with low voltage and high power will produce dissection effects.

When an optic fiber is used in what is called *contact technique*, it produces a dissection. At a small distance it produces vaporization, and at a larger distance *(noncontact technique)* it produces a coagulation effect (Fig. 8). With the use of sapphires, only dissection can be obtained.

In electrosurgery biological tissues can be cut only if the tension between electrodes and tissue is sufficiently high to produce electrical sparking, which leads to a concentration of the electrical current at one specific point of the tissue. The temperature produced at this point where the electric sparks touch the tissue like microscopic lightning is so high that tissue immediately evaporates or burns. As the electrode dissects the tissue, the electrical sparks are continuously produced where the distance between the electrode and the tissue is sufficiently reduced. This way the cut is fabricated. In conclusion, the electrical current will rapidly increase tissue temperature, leading to vacuolization of cells. Because this phenomenon is happening extremely rapidly, heat does not have time to dissipate throughout the tissue; thus there is no hemostatic effect. Once an electrical arc is installed between the instrument and the tissue, the latter will heat as a function of its own resistance to electrical current, and the energy produced by the spark itself will also lead to tissue damage. These two types of heat cause the cell to explode and produce the dissection effect.

When a tissue is coagulated using the contact technique in electrosurgery, there is no electrical spark. The term *desiccation* is used for this effect. The term *fulguration* denotes tissue coagulation resulting from close contact with the electrical spark. Desiccated tissue has a soft, slightly brownish wound, whereas fulgurated tissue has a hard and blackish wound. To stop the reaction, the surgeon must withdraw his or her foot from the switch, or the water must be removed from the tissue so that it becomes a bad electrical conductor.

Laser Types

Carbon dioxide (CO_2) laser. CO_2 lasers (Coherent) emit a light 10,590 nm long (infrared part of the light spectrum). Because of its long wavelength, it cannot be delivered through an optical fiber and needs an articulated arm with mirrors at each articulation to direct the light of the laser into the needed direction. Because this light is invisible to the eye, it needs another light beam that is visible; in general, a helium neon laser is used. Approximately 90% of the laser energy is absorbed and transformed into heat within the first 0.2 mm of the exposed tissue. This leads to instant ebullition of the intracellular water and then to an explosion of the cell because of vaporization of the intracellular water. The

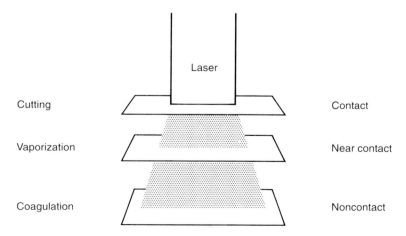

Cutting — Laser — Contact

Vaporization — Near contact

Coagulation — Noncontact

Fig. 8. Contact, near-contact, noncontact techniques.

CO_2 laser beam is absorbed in water; thus the water content of the exposed tissue determines its response to the laser beam. Because most tissues are composed of more than 80% water, the energy of the CO_2 laser can vaporize superficial tissue with minimal necrotic effect and thus with a small coagulation capacity. In contrast, in tissues with low concentration of water absorption becomes weak, which leads to more extended coagulation. These characteristics justify the use of CO_2 lasers in laparoscopy for cutting and coagulating adherences (low water content) while saving digestive structures, which constantly are moist. The beam must be focused on the side of treatment to produce its dissecting effect. Standard laparoscopes for CO_2 lasers are equipped with optical lenses that can focus between 300 and 3150 mm, with optimal focusing power approximately 2 cm below the distal end of the instrument, resulting in a diameter of the target of approximately 5 mm. To obtain coagulation or superficial vaporization, it is sufficient to defocus the light beam and thereby reduce the density of power and increase the treated surface.

The power density currently used is 2500 to 5000 W/cm^2 in continuous mode. It is necessary to use instruments with a rough surface while using CO_2 lasers to reduce the phenomenon of reflexion. Instruments that are only blackened cannot absorb the energy of the CO_2 lasers because black objects reflect infrared radiation and lead to the risk of tissue damage in neighboring tissue. Using instruments covered with titanium sand for "backstop" instruments is preferred.

Argon laser. The energy of the argon laser produces approximately 10 monochromatic colors at the same time. However, two colors (blue and blue-green) are most important at wavelengths of 488 and 514.5 nm, respectively. The energy can be delivered through optical fibers with a diameter of 0.3 to 0.6 mm. The beam can travel through water with minimal absorption. It reacts with red tissues and is absorbed by tissue pigments such as hemoglobin or melanin. Approximately 1 mm of tissue is penetrated, and the argon laser can be used for coagulation of small vessels and capillaries. Major disadvantages of this laser include the fact that a surgeon must wear protective eye wear and its relatively high cost.

For coagulation the fiber is placed 1 to 4 cm above the tissue zone exposed with a power of 2 to 5 W in continuous mode. Vaporization is obtained using a power of 5 to 10 W in continuous mode, and section is obtained in the same way, using a power of 10 to 15 W.

Nd:YAG laser. The active elements of the Nd:YAG laser are yttrium aluminum garnet (YAG) to which neodymium (Nd) is added. The wavelength of the produced light is 1060 nm, which is in the infrared range of the light spectrum. This light is invisible, and a lead beam of helium neon is added as for CO_2 lasers. As with argon lasers, the light of the Nd:YAG laser can be transmitted through optical fibers and delivered across flexible endoscopes. It can travel through water without difficulty and can be used in the urinary bladder or other cavities filled with liquid. The laser beam travels through tissues with a penetration up to 5 mm. It is absorbed by tissue protein and delivers a thermal effect, which is nonspecific and is an excellent coagulator even during active hemorrhage. These advantages have justified the use of this laser type in thoracopulmonary surgery, whether by thoracotomy or thoracoscopy. The major problem with Nd:YAG lasers is that the light is dispersed when it reaches the tissue; thus it loses much of its energy. With the development of sapphires, depth, penetration, and the problem of dispersion can more easily be controlled. This also allows its use in contact technique, which allows the surgeon to have tactile control. The major disadvantages of sapphires are their high cost and the fact that much attention is required not to touch neighboring organs with the sapphire because it remains very hot for several seconds after its use. The Nd:YAG laser remains one of the most reliable lasers at disposition.

KTP laser. Crystals of potassium (K), titanil (T), and phosphate (P) placed in the beams of certain lasers modify their wavelength. This phenomenon is called *doubling of frequence*. The KTP-532 laser (Laserscope) uses the YAG laser as an energy source. It emits a green light with a wavelength of 532 nm, which is twice the wavelength of the YAG laser. It allows the surgeon to cut or to coagulate. In contact technique it has a good capacity to section, whereas in noncontact technique the light beam is defocused and allows good coagulation.

KTP-YAG laser. Some lasers combine the principles of the two lasers separately to produce two types of effects, also separately but within the same instrument. For example, the KTP-YAG (Laserscope) associates the KTP-532 effects to those of the YAG laser and thus increases application possibilities.

FUTURE TECHNOLOGY

The importance of lasers in laparoscopic and thoracoscopic surgery is not yet clearly established. Their characteristics and advantages are not overwhelming as compared to electrosurgical means, particularly if attention is given to cost. As discussed previously, each laser has its own characteristics. Probably for surgeons the CO_2, YAG, and eventually KTP lasers are the most useful ones.

Two novelties in the domain of lasers must be discussed. As noted previously, the useful surgical dose of lasers is a function of the application time. There are three modes of applications: continuous, pulsed, and superpulsed. A new product on the market is a CO_2 laser called *Ultrapulse* (Coherent). It is, in fact, a high-energy pulsed laser, similar to the superpulsed laser, that delivers repetitive series of rapid pulsations with very short breaks in between but at very high energy (> 200 mJ for a pulsation of 600 μ), that is, five times the energy from other CO_2 lasers. The possible advantage of this type of laser is the ability to obtain vaporization with minimal thermal damage to neighboring tissue. This laser is called a *cold* laser. Another novelty is the appearance of new types of lasers, particularly the Two Point One Holmium:YAG laser (Coherent). With a wavelength of 2100 nm, the light of the Holmium laser is transmitted through optical fibers. It is highly absorbed by skin, and its depth of penetration is approximately 0.4 mm. It seems particularly efficient for surgery of the bone and the cartilage.

For electrosurgery, too, are new systems equipped with electronic monitors. They automatically monitor the high frequency to optimize the power permanently during a section or a coagulation. In addition, these generators interrupt automatically at the moment optimal coagulation is obtained, thus preventing carbonization (Erbe).

A new concept of coagulation in electrosurgery has also appeared, associating electrosurgery with argon laser beams. The field of coagulation is swept by a flux of argon laser light, which uses all the local oxygen and permits coagulation without risk of carbonization, maintenance of a low temperature at the coagulated surface with minimal necrosis, cleansing of the coagulation field, and eliminates smoke through the breeze of the argon jet (Erbe Beamer). This type of system should find numerous applications in laparoscopy and thoracoscopy. Finally, the first electrosurgery systems that allow bipolar section are now on the market. Since electrical energy needs a closed circuit, included are both monopolar and bipolar systems. In monopolar systems the electrical energy arrives through the instrument and

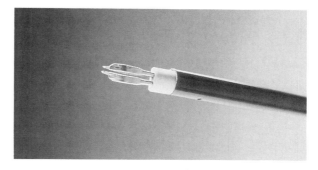

Fig. 9. Bipolar hook to allow dissection and coagulation in safety.

passes through the target tissue and then through the body. The body of the patient is an integral part of the electrical circuit. In bipolar electrosurgery (e.g., with tweezers) the current arrives through one part of the instrument, traverses the tissue, and leaves through the other part of the instrument. The body of the patient no longer is an integral part of the electrical field. These techniques are currently used in coagulation. With monopolar current, diffusion of the energy through the organism can induce lesions distant from the target tissue. This is a known risk during laparoscopy. For dissection in electrosurgery, only the possibility of a monopolar hook or of scissors with monopolar current is left. Thus during adhesiolysis, the risk of diffusing the energy through intestinal loops is important. To address this problem, many research activities to allow the development of a bipolar hook that allows dissection in safety without diffusion of electrical current are underway (Fig. 9). Because the body does not contribute to the diffusion of electrical energy, this type of section is possible even in a moist environment. It is an important new element in laparoscopic and thoracoscopic surgery.

CONCLUSION

New technical acquisitions both in laser and electrosurgical technology help to obtain a better effect with maximal security. The best laser is probably the laser of tomorrow. Perhaps one day will see lasers with cursors that allow modification of the wavelength at choice to produce a desired effect. In electrosurgery generators that control the effects of coagulation and instruments of bipolar dissection are probably important new helps to laparoscopic and thoracoscopic surgery.

17   *The Dangers of and Correct Procedures in Laparoscopic Electrosurgery*

Pierre Testas

Statistics of sequelae occurring from cholecystectomy indicate an increase in local complications (particularly in biliary tract trauma) as a result of laparoscopic cholecystectomy.[1,2] These complications may be caused by the surgeon's lack of experience or attention[3] or by the incorrect application of electrosurgical procedures.[4-7] In this chapter I will review safety procedures for the use of high-frequency currents required by laparoscopic surgery.

BASIC ELECTROSURGERY

High-frequency electrosurgical methods have been used for more than 50 years to produce coagulation or to dissect and liberate tissue samples. Its thermal effect is produced by an electric current that is passed through tissue, a procedure that does not lead to electrolytic or persistant side effects in nerves and muscles. Alternating currents at frequencies below 300 kHz are used during electrosurgery. Tissue transsection is obtained when the voltage between the surgical electrodes and the tissue to be cut is high enough to produce electric arcs. A sudden evaporation of water in the cells, which explode on contact with a small electrode, results from this high voltage. Hemostasis occurs at a lower average temperature (70° to 90° C); this results in colloidal coagulation. Thus high-frequency current leads to an increased tissue temperature (the joule effect), which is inversely correlated to the size of the active electrode surface and to a higher density of current at an equivalent electric force. To obtain a local temperature $\geq 100°$ C, formation of a high-energy arc (and sparks) is necessary. If the electrode is large, this energy discharge results in adhesion and clogging.

The two primary modes of high-frequency energy are monopolar and bipolar.

Monopolar mode. In monopolar mode, the active electrode affects the operating field at the level of the target tissue. As it leaves the organism, the current is collected by a neutral electrode with a large surface plate, which prevents an increase in temperature and subsequent burns.

Bipolar mode. In bipolar mode, active and neutral electrodes that are attached to the generators are connected to the jaws of forceps and are thus isolated. The tissue between the jaws is coagulated. In the monopolar mode, high-frequency currents (particularly square-wave currents) produce electromagnetic waves that can cause disturbances from diffusion at a distance. In the bipolar mode, the circuit is not affected by grounding; the electromagnetic disturbance is reduced or is nonexistent, and the electric field is concentrated. A recent circular from the French Ministry of Health described serious sequelae from the use of electric surgical knives on patients with pacemakers. If electrosurgery is necessary in these patients, then bipolar coagulation should be used.

In the monopolar mode, the apparatus is in direct and permanent contact with the patient by means of the electrode or plate, which is used to collect the current over a large area to prevent tissue burns. An alarm that indicates tissue burns, if the surface area of contact and tissue resistance is a potential cause for injury, can be incorporated in the plate. The plate position, which should be near the surgical site, is important. The plate should be applied by a cable to a large, regular cutaneous area. Modern plates have "floating" circuits, which are grounded.

In the monopolar mode, the circuit passes through the plate. However, some current leaks occur; they occur less often when a high-frequency (500 kHz) current is used, but even at a relatively low capacity, a high-frequency current with power surges can leak through some insulation. In a floating circuit, high-frequency current can be observed at the level of some contact and burn zones. Intra-abdominal or visceral burns can result from an increase in density that is required to obtain electrical arcs. Serious cutaneous burns can result when current leaks are formed or if the contact of current with wet clothes or a metal instrument should occur.[8]

In laparoscopic electrosurgery there is reduced control of the surgical field. Phenomena that occur beyond the field of vision during operation may not be treated immediately. Current may pass through a funicular structure that is coagulated in the monopolar mode. If this current contacts viscera, an electric arc that causes burns may result, especially if the high voltage required for fulguration is used.

The increase in the electrical resistance of tissue during coagulation may also result in injury. For example, in the coagulation of intestinal obstructions, if the first coagulation is directed toward the plate, the coagulated structure acquires greater electrical resistance. If a second coagulation is performed, the current is directed to return to the neutral electrode by an indirect route that offers less electrical resistance. The previous site of coagulation, which has a higher electrical resistance than do the viscera, can divert the current. This diversion is directed particularly toward the duodenum in biliary surgery but also toward the jejunum and ileum. Electric arcs are formed by a high-frequency current that can coagulate the intestines and can result in undetected tissue injury.

Another disadvantage of high-voltage coagulation is that the electrical arcs can heat the ends of the coagulating device, hook, or other coagulating instrument to temperatures $\geq 500°$. After the generator stops, several minutes pass before the device cools to room temperature; burns can occur when a heated instrument is removed while touching the intestines.

In the monopolar mode, prevention is the best method of avoiding the production of these electrical arcs and intestinal fulgurations. A low voltage must be used to whiten tissues; this requires time and patience from the surgeon. The controls must be set at low values to prevent sparks and thus avoid fulguration. When low electrical settings are used, desiccation and coagulation occur slowly, which increases the surgeon's control of the procedure. However, most of these problems can be avoided by use of the bipolar mode, in which two active electrodes of the same value are contained in a single instrument. The high-frequency current flows through tissue between these electrodes of the same value. The risk of the patient's incurring burns is negligible. In addition, the risk of electrical disturbance to the monitoring equipment attached to the patient, such as electrocardiogram, a cardiac pacemaker, or television

monitors, is low. Thus use of the bipolar technique is preferable in almost all cases that involve laparoscopic surgery.

DISCUSSION

Monopolar coagulation can result in the patient's being burned. During celioscopy, these burns may not be recognized because the entire area affected by the electric currents may not be visible. These undiscovered burns may also result in secondary fistulas of the principal biliary tract, gynecological problems, or postoperative duodenal, jejunoileal, or esophageal functional disorders, the causes of which may be difficult to determine.

One of the causes of laparoscopically induced biliary tract trauma is an increase in voltage in the electric surgical knife; this results in immediately visible coagulation that approaches fulguration. As a result of this high voltage, the peri-instrumental atmosphere heats and produces ischemia in adjacent tissue, sclerosis, and (later) biliary stenosis several months after operation.[9] Thus in surgical procedures that involve the use of high frequencies, low voltage and careful technique are essential. The bipolar mode is preferable to the monopolar mode. Although adequate electrosurgical instruments are available, careful selection and correct maintenance of the equipment are important. In laparoscopic electrosurgery, low voltage in the monopolar mode can be used with careful technique. The bipolar mode offers safer coagulation. Technical safety, proven methods, and good surgical training are the essential elements of successful laparoscopic surgery.

REFERENCES

1. Delaitre B, Testas P, Dubois F, Mouret P, Nouaille JM, Suc B, Collet D. Complications des cholécystectomies par voie coelioscopique. Chirurgie 1992 - 118 sous presse.
2. Moosa AR, Easter DN, Van Sonnonberg E, Casola G, d'Agostino H. Laparoscopic injuries to the bile duct. A cause for concern. Ann Surg 215:203-208, 1992.
3. Testas P. La formation à la chirurgie par coelioscopie et ses aspects médico-légaux in chirurgie digestive par voie coelioscopique. Paris: Maloine, 1991, pp 198-202.
4. Dubois F, Berthelot G, Levard H. Cholecystectomie par coelioscopie. Presse Med 18:980-982, 1989.
5. Perissat J, Collet D, Belliard R. Gallstones. Laparoscopic treatment intracorporeal lithotripsy followed by cholecystectomy or cholecystostomy. A personal technique. Endoscopy 21:373-374, 1989.

6. Davidoff AM, Pappas TH, Murray EA, Hillerm D, Johnson RD, Baker ME, Newman GE, Cottin PB, Meyers WC. Mechanisms of major biliary injury during laparoscopic cholecystectomy. Ann Surg 215:196-202, 1992.
7. Hunter JG. Avoidance of bile duct injury during laparoscopic cholecystectomy. Am J Surg 162:71-76, 1991.
8. Hunter JG. Laser or electrocautery for laparoscopic cholecystectomy? Ann J Surg 161:345-349, 1991.
9. Liguory CI. Complications biliaires de la cholécystectomie coelioscopique. Traitement endoscopique à propos de 22 cas. Illème Congrès Mondial de Chirurgie Endoscopique, Bordeaux, June 18-20, 1992.

18 Tissue Retrieval Devices and Techniques for Laparoscopic Surgery

Harry J. Espiner

The laparoscopic approach has found widespread acceptance because it replaces a painful incision with simple punctures for access. However, when the operation produces a bulky or friable specimen and the tissue is infected or cancerous, the problem of removal becomes significant.

In simple cholecystectomy, with a gallbladder that is not inflamed, removal through the umbilical or upper midline port is straightforward, using an instrument to widen the wound if necessary. However, when we adopted an "all comers" policy in our approach to symptomatic gallstone disease, we quickly encountered cases of severe inflammation and obstructive cholecystitis, together with empyema and gangrenous changes that presented problems. Frequently the pathological process had destroyed Hartmann's pouch and so the integrity of the gallbladder was compromised; under these circumstances it was very easy to lose stones into the peritoneal cavity, with the risk that complications would follow; these have already been reported. To overcome this problem we devised a retrieval system that allows safe and simple extraction in all circumstances without enlargement of the access puncture.

The following features were considered important in the design of the retrieval bag:

Strength of material: It should resist puncture with pointed instruments and withstand considerable force in traction.

Tear resistance: If the bag is punctured, tearing should not follow if further traction is applied; sac integrity must be preserved.

Thickness of material: The material must be lightweight so that a large-capacity bag can be fashioned for easy capture of the specimen.

Ease of deployment: The construction and shape of the bag should allow easy manipulation; a tether would prevent loss of the device from the field of view. This could also act as one point of fixation, leaving two hands free for tissue handling.

Ripstop nylon was the material selected; it is very strong but very light and resists tearing if punctured; the hole tends to close rather than enlarge. A single piece of material is used to construct the bag, which includes a long retaining tail. A single stitch line incorporates an external sleeve for use in deployment. The material is coated with polyurethane in a special formulation that renders the bag impermeable to biological fluids. The shape, which was computer designed, achieves a large capacity yet allows easy deployment (Figs. 1 and 2).

For gallbladder extraction the bag is deployed across the anterior surface of the liver from the upper midline port. It can easily be placed and opened in this position by passing 5 mm forceps down the sleeve on the side of the sac and placing the length of the sac in the 10 mm cannula. Withdrawing the forceps to the mouth and gripping the sac again in this position allows further deployment of the sac through the cannula and into the abdominal cavity. The bulk of the bag prevents loss of pneumoperitoneum initially, but a previously placed reducing sleeve on the 5 mm forceps can be slid into the cannula to retain the pneumoperitoneum as the bag enters the abdomen. The midclavicular line forceps are

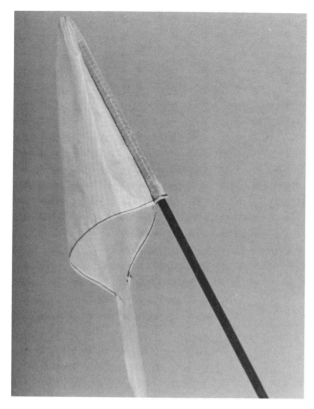

Fig. 1. A 5 mm grasping forceps is placed in the sleeve on the outer surface of the bag for easy introduction.

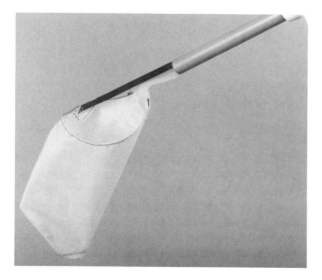

Fig. 2. The wide mouth opens automatically when the bag is deployed.

used to hold the lip of the bag open in direct view of the telescope and tension on the integral tail stabilizes the bag for easy placement of the gallbladder within it. Traction on the tail through the cannula while the trumpet or flap valve is open allows the bag to be drawn with a drawstring-like action into the mouth of the cannula and to be completely closed before withdrawing cannula and sac together through the abdominal wall.

Once through the wall, the cannula can be removed from the tail, the mouth of the bag can then be grasped and held externally, and access is freely available from the outside to the contents held within the sac, which is still inside the abdomen. The gallbladder neck is opened, the contents aspirated, the wall incised and removed, and the stones either aspirated or crushed as required to facilitate removal. With very large, hard stones, the use of a contact electrohydraulic lithotriptor facilitates removal without enlargement of the midline incision. In a consecutive series of over 400 cholecystectomies there has been no requirement for an enlargement of the puncture site for gallbladder or stone extraction using this technique.

In difficult cases it has been our policy to deploy the bag over the anterior surface of the liver, with the bag retained by its thin tail through the cannula; then we continue the removal, which frequently includes in situ destruction of the gallbladder to facilitate the procedure. As large stones enter the field they can be quickly placed within the bag and retained securely for final extraction when the remains of the gallbladder have been freed and placed within the bag.

With very thick-walled gallbladders containing large stones, we have found it useful to open the gallbladder deliberately after it is placed within the retrieval bag (still within the abdomen) to free the stones, cut the wall into pieces, and begin to morcellate the stones under direct vision. Once this procedure has been completed, extraction can follow and the fragments are more easily removed through the narrow 10 mm access puncture. This is only possible because the bag is impermeable and its large capacity allows extensive manipulation to be carried out without risk of puncture of the wall.

As our laparoscopic experience has increased we have developed smaller-sized bags for lymphadenectomy biopsy procedures and for appendectomies. We believe that it is wise to use such a device for retrieval in difficult cases of appendicitis, because disruption of the organ during removal could lead to loss of an unsuspected carcinoid tumor in the tip of the appendix or release mucus-secreting epithelium within the abdominal cavity. Deployment of the device during ovarian cystectomies has been valuable; with dermoid tumors there is always a risk of rupture, but holding the bag beneath the ovary collects any debris and irritant material likely to escape should the cyst be opened during dissection, and all the wall can be safely incorporated within the device for safe extraction.

We have extended our retrieval system to accommodate colonic specimens and have successfully completed right hemicolectomy for carcinoma. During this operation the bulky mass of tissue can be placed within a larger version of the bag, in fact, a sac, which can be carefully deployed over the anterior surface of the liver toward the diaphragm, occupying the right half of the abdominal cavity. Retrieval then can be through a minor extension of the umbilical access port before we internally reconstruct the bowel using endostapling instrumentation.

Current research is progressing to allow dissection and disintegration of a tumor within the sac so that any parietal incision is avoided. It is necessary, however, to have tissue sampling for a full histological workup; hence complete morcellation and disintegration of the specimen should be avoided.

We believe that this approach to laparoscopic surgery limits complications by protecting the access puncture sites from contact with potentially infected tissue; wound infection should be reduced and the absence of a parietal incision for extraction should also reduce the likelihood of incisional hernia and the risk of bowel strangulation. By eliminating contact of potentially cancerous tissue with the access tract, implantation should be avoided; already there have been case reports of secondary deposits from unsuspected carcinoma of the gallbladder occurring at the umbilicus as a direct result of extraction at this site. At present most colonic operations are laparoscopically assisted rather than performed through entirely laparoscopic methods. Small incisions are used for retrieval of the whole specimen and the smaller they are the greater the risk of implantation. A retrieval system as outlined here would avoid the risk and also allow the possibility of completing the whole operation within the abdomen so retaining the advantage of minimal access surgery.

V

Videoendoscopic Surgery of the Biliary Tract, Liver, and Pancreas

19 Preoperative Investigations for Laparoscopic Cholecystectomy

Kevin Roy Wedgwood, A.T. Nicholson, Andrew Damian Taylor, and C.M.S. Royston

With the advent of laparoscopic cholecystectomy there has been increasing controversy as to the need for intraoperative cholangiography. This ranges from the opinion that it should not be performed at all to the belief that since intraoperative cholangiography was performed in open cholecystectomy this practice should be continued with the laparoscopic technique.[1-3] However, there is no doubt that this procedure does add considerable time to the laparoscopic procedure and it is technically more difficult than intraoperative cholangiography performed during open cholecystectomy.

The following three potential courses of action can be tried to identify those patients who may be at risk of having common bile duct stones: (1) preoperative assessment of the biliary tract by endoscopic retrograde cholangiopancreatography (ERCP), (2) intraoperative assessment by intraoperative cholangiography, or (3) postoperative assessment of patients who have complications after laparoscopic cholecystectomy.

Among these options difficulties arise with the first one in that ERCP is both time consuming and costly to perform in all patients awaiting cholecystectomy, and there is significant morbidity associated with this investigation. Most surgeons now favor a selective approach to the examination of the biliary tract in patients undergoing cholecystectomy. Patients with either clinical, biochemical, or radiological evidence of common duct stones in the presence of known gallstones, who are considered suitable candidates for laparoscopic cholecystectomy, are assessed by preoperative ERCP. Common bile duct stones can be treated by sphincterotomy should any be found. Problems related to the second option have been discussed previously. Investigating patients postoperatively, after complications have arisen, increases morbidity. We therefore describe a modification of a radiological technique of intravenous cholangiography that we have used to identify patients who may have common bile duct stones.

MATERIALS AND METHODS

From October 1991 to July 1992, patients with ultrasound-proven gallstones awaiting laparoscopic cholecystectomy included those with a history of either pancreatitis or jaundice that resolved spontaneously, those with a raised liver enzyme profile, and those with a dilated common bile duct on ultrasound examination, who instead of undergoing routine ERCP had intravenous cholangiography. In addition, two patients who had undergone prior cholecystectomy and had symptoms after cholecystectomy had this procedure rather than ERCP. In total there were 61 patients (19 men and 42 women) with a mean age of 57 years (range, 30 to 82).

Technique

Patients are fasted for at least 6 hours before the investigation, although they are allowed free access to clear liquids, since it is important that they be well hydrated. From a 500 ml bag of saline solution, 100 ml are aspirated and discarded. This is replaced by 100 ml of Biliscopin (Schering) and the solution is mixed well. An intravenous cannula is inserted and the Biliscopin solution is then infused into a peripheral vein over a period of 3 to 3½ hours. The patient is then sent to the radiology department with the infusion continuing to run approximately 3 hours after it was begun. A plain x-ray film of the biliary tract is obtained followed by selective tomography, after which the patient is allowed to go home.

RESULTS

Results of this study are summarized in Fig. 1. In one patient the infusion of contrast medium was discontinued after approximately 5 minutes, because the patient complained of feeling faint and became hypotensive. It is of interest to note that this patient had an intense fear of needles and became faint when the intravenous cannula was inserted before beginning the in-

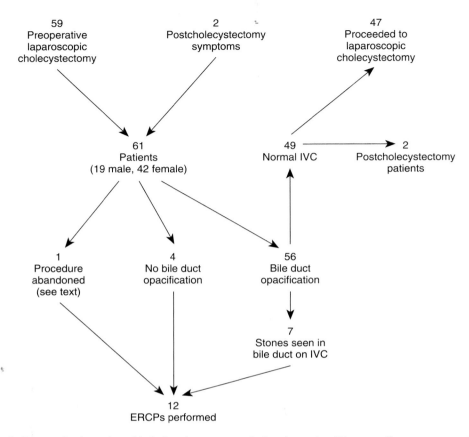

Fig. 1. Summarized results of infusion intravenous cholangiography. The overall success rate of the technique was 56/60 (93%); stones were found in 7 of 56 patients (12.5%). ERCP was performed in 12 of 61 patients (20%).

fusion. This patient underwent ERCP; the results were normal. Among the remaining 60 patients in whom this technique was performed, the outcome was successful in 56, in that the bile ducts were opacified and flow into the duodenum was observed. This represents a success rate of 93% for this technique (Fig. 2).

There were four failures in which bile duct opacification was not observed. In two of these cases failure was attributed to technical difficulties in that the time required for the infusion was in excess of 3 hours and the infusion had completely run out before the patients reached the radiology department. In a third patient the reason for failure could not be ascertained. All of these patients had undergone ERCP and the findings were normal in all three. The fourth patient was admitted with jaundice that resolved spontaneously, but gallstones were identified by ultrasonography. Following

unsuccessful intravenous cholangiography, this patient was further investigated by ERCP and found to have cholangiocarcinoma.

Of the 56 patients in whom the technique was successful, seven were shown to have stones within the common duct (Fig. 3). These seven underwent ERCP and stones were identified in six; those patients were managed with sphincterotomy. In one patient no stones were found in the duct at ERCP. This patient had a past history of jaundice that had resolved spontaneously, suggesting that the stone or stones may have been passed before ERCP was performed. In the remaining 49 patients the bile ducts were clearly visible, and there was no evidence of a filling defect. These patients proceeded directly to laparoscopic cholecystectomy with no need for further investigation. To date none has had symptoms attributable to retained stones.

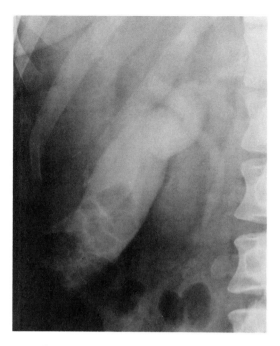

Fig. 2. Infusion intravenous cholangiogram showing normal duct anatomy with no common bile duct stones.

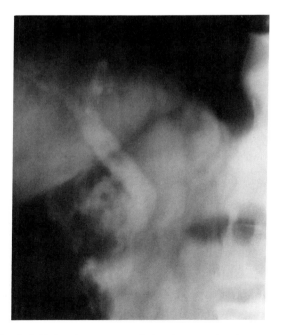

Fig. 3. Infusion intravenous cholangiogram showing stones within the common bile duct. This patient underwent ERCP and sphincterotomy prior to laparoscopic cholecystectomy.

DISCUSSION

The advent of laparoscopic cholecystectomy has revolutionized the management of cholelithiasis. However, concern has been expressed that with the arrival of this new technique surgical principles are being abandoned; for example, intraoperative investigation of the biliary tract is no longer being performed routinely. It should be stated, however, that many surgeons now believe that routine intraoperative cholangiography is unnecessary, and these surgeons have adopted a selective policy of intraoperative cholangiography. Although it is possible to perform intraoperative cholangiography in patients undergoing laparoscopic cholecystectomy, it is thought that this is more difficult than open intraoperative cholangiography, and it adds considerable time to the procedure, which at least in the surgeon's early learning curve is longer than that for open cholecystectomy; many surgeons have thus abandoned any type of biliary imaging with the laparoscopic technique. There remains, however, a small number of patients who present with cholelithiasis who have a history or clinical, biochemical, or radiological findings that would indicate investigation of the biliary tree is necessary. Ultrasound imaging is still utilized as the first line of investigation to confirm cholelithiasis and may be able to demonstrate stones in the common bile duct. Its role is clearly limited, however, since common bile duct stones can only be identified in approximately 1% of patients with normal-caliber ducts and in 60% of patients with dilated ducts.[4] This limitation thus renders ultrasonography less than ideal for investigation of the biliary tree. Intravenous cholangiography as practiced in the past has been abandoned because of poor image quality and was never fully accepted as a method by which the biliary tree could be successfully imaged to exclude common bile duct stones. We have therefore modified the technique of intravenous cholangiography by using an infusion technique, which in our initial series of 61 patients has had a success rate of 93% and has accurately demonstrated the presence of gallstones in the common bile in seven patients. We believe the reason for the success of this modified technique is the improvement in the quality of the image that is obtained; this has been achieved by an overall increase in the amount of contrast agent used. The contrast medium is infused intravenously and by an active transport mechanism is excreted into the bile duct. We believe that by ensuring a slow but constant delivery of the contrast medium intravenously, the active carrier transport mechanism is not overwhelmed, and therefore the total dose actually excreted via the liver is increased, thus enhancing the picture quality. In addition, we have taken particular care to ensure that all of the patients are well hydrated, since this also improves the carrier transport from the blood into the bile.

There were five failures in our study. Two resulted from technical difficulties in that the infusion had completely run out before the patient was transported to the radiology department; in both cases this occurred in the early part of the study. In the third patient, who had a history of jaundice that resolved spontaneously, ultrasound imaging showed the presence of gallstones in the gallbladder and grossly dilated intra- and extrahepatic bile ducts. Further investigation showed this patient to have cholangiocarcinoma. In one patient there was no satisfactory explanation as to why the infusion was unsuccessful. This patient also had a history of spontaneously resolving jaundice. This patient subsequently underwent ERCP, the results of which were entirely normal. In the last patient the procedure was abandoned shortly after intravenous infusion of contrast medium was begun, because the patient complained of feeling faint and became hypotensive. Whether this was a true reaction to the contrast medium is difficult to ascertain, since this patient was extremely anxious and became sweaty and faint when the intravenous cannula was inserted before commencing the infusion. The theoretical risk of anaphylaxis with the contrast material used is approximately 1 in 5000. This compares very favorably with the known risk of 1% to 3% for ERCP.

We believe that this technique has several advantages over the standard procedures used elsewhere; they are as follows: (1) This procedure unlike ERCP is inexpensive and is technically easy to perform. It does not require endoscopic expertise and requires only that the radiographer be capable of taking plain films and tomograms of the biliary tree. The cost of this procedure in our institution is approximately £45 to £50 per patient compared with approximately £400 to £450 for diagnostic day case ERCP. (2) This technique reduces the requirements for ERCP; that is, among the 61 patients in whom this technique was attempted, only 12 have required ERCP for evaluation (these being the seven patients with stones reported in the duct and the five failures). Therefore time and money are saved. In addition, in our institution the size of the common bile duct is sometimes overestimated by ultrasonography, which could potentially result in further unnecessary ERCPs; this technique would obviate that occurrence. (3) Inasmuch as this investigation is performed prior to laparoscopic cholecystectomy, information on the biliary tree is available and negates the need for intraoperative investigations. This reduces the operating time and also renders laparoscopic cholecystectomy a straightforward procedure without the need to cannulate the cystic duct. Furthermore, since it is performed prior to surgery, should any stones be found in the common duct by intravenous cholangiography, they can be managed by preoperative ERCP and sphincterotomy. (4) Finally, since this technique is performed preoperatively, concerns about postoperative complications arising as a result of retained stones are diminished. Although this technique may miss very small stones at the lower end of the common bile duct, we believe it is unlikely that these will cause untoward problems and may well be passed spontaneously. Since we have been using this method of imaging the biliary tree, no patients have subsequently returned with signs or symptoms suggestive of retained stones.

In conclusion, we believe that this technique of intravenous cholangiography should be used as a first-line investigational technique, after ultrasonography, in patients whose clinical, biochemical, or radiological features suggest the presence of common bile duct stones.

REFERENCES

1. Berci G, Sackier JM, Paz-Partlow M. Routine or selected cholangiography. Am J Surg 161:355-360, 1991.
2. McEntee G, Grace PA, Bouchier-Hayes D. Laparoscopic surgery and the common bile duct. Br J Surg 78:385-386, 1991.
3. Begnato VJ, McGee GE, Hatten LE, et al. Justification for routine cholangiogram during laparoscopic cholecystectomy. Surg Laparosc Endosc 1:89-93, 1991.
4. Lees W. Personal communication.

20 *Conditions of and Precautions in Conversion From Surgical Orthodoxy to Laparoscopic Cholecystectomy*

R. Christopher G. Russell

Laparoscopic cholecystectomy is an established technique and is safe when performed by experienced surgeons. It is a preferred procedure in established medical centers in the Western world. The success of this procedure is determined by the surgeon's skill, medical technology, the telescope and video camera, and specialized surgical instruments that must be reliably adapted to the task and in a perfect state of function at all times.

Adequate maintenance and availability of laparoscopic instruments is not possible in all medical facilities. Competent, well-trained surgeons can master the skills necessary for laparoscopic cholecystectomy after having completed some 20 procedures. Skill retention has not been tested, but most procedural complications are experienced by surgeons who are learning to master the technique. Surgeons who use laparoscopic cholecystectomy infrequently will continue to find the procedure a challenge.

One concern in everyday practice expresses the dilemma that if every abdominal surgeon were to be trained in laparoscopic cholecystectomy and be able to then apply the method in every case, the experience would not be regular enough to maintain the necessary skills. Should these techniques therefore be used primarily by the surgeons who perform laparoscopy regularly and frequently? The additional initial costs of laparoscopy may not be justified in smaller hospitals or in developing countries at this stage of an evolving technology. The emerging benefits of laparoscopic cholecystectomy should be compared with those of the established open operation in each individual application as well as in a given overall sound and fiscal environment. "Cholecystectomy" must be carefully defined and the details of its technical execution and innovations in open cholecystectomy should be reviewed and become part of the overall comparison.

OPEN CHOLECYSTECTOMY

New developments of open cholecystectomy have been neglected, and authors of textbooks on the technique have presented traditional surgical methods. However, in 1977 the value of the conventional surgical approach (a large incision, a full exploratory laparotomy, and wide exposure of the anatomy around the porta hepatis) was questioned. In France minicholecystectomy was popularized by Dubois, and in the United States reports of cholecystectomy on an outpatient basis appeared. Articles about the techniques for performing cholecystectomy through a 5 cm incision were published along with these reports.

The standard minicholecystectomy consists of a 5 cm transverse skin incision down to the fascia overlying the abdominis rectus muscle and the oblique muscles. The external and internal oblique and transverse muscles are divided in the line of their fibers; this can be achieved by a splitting technique as opposed to cutting the muscles. Hemostasis must be complete because bruising within the muscle results in postoperative pain.

In open cholecystectomy, the rectus sheath is opened for a short distance, and the rectus muscle is deflected medially without division. The peritoneum is opened by an incision of no more than 6 cm. A retractor (preferably a stabilized ring retractor, so that the assistant's task is made easier or is eliminated) is placed over the edge of the liver, which is retracted upward.[1] A pad is then placed over the hepatic flexure of the colon, and a second retractor blade is positioned to retract the colon downward. A second pad is placed medially to pack away the stomach and to expose the free edge of the lesser omentum. Before these pads can be placed, adhesions should be divided.

When the retractor and the pads are in place, the gallbladder should be exposed and its peritoneal surface traced to the cystic duct. Then the surgeon may perform either a cystic duct or a fundus dissection. Often the fundus dissection is easier to perform first, because the bulky fundus can be held laterally after it has been separated from the hepatic bed. Improved views of the porta hepatis and Calot's triangle result from this technique; however, the surgeon's hand cannot enter the abdomen during the dissection, which must be performed with instruments.

Because hemostasis is important and a bloodless field must be maintained, meticulous technique should be used. The electrocautery hook, which does not obscure vision and facilitates accurate, bloodless dissection, is of great value during fundus dissection. After the gallbladder is separated from the liver bed, the peritoneum over Calot's triangle is divided to expose the branches of the cystic artery, which are then cauterized individually. In an alternative procedure, the main cystic artery vessel can be clipped with an absorbable clip.

The cystic duct is dissected and cholangiography can be performed. Finally, the cystic duct is clipped with an absorbable clip and is divided, and the gallbladder is removed. The absorbable clip should not form a nidus for stone formation and does not appear on subsequent imaging studies.

Drainage is unnecessary. The wound is closed with a purse-string suture of absorbable material (polydioxane [PDS], Ethicon) to the peritoneum. Loosely tied, interrupted large-bite sutures of similar material are placed in the muscles. The fascia is injected with bupivacaine hydrochloride with epinephrine (Marcain) to provide pain relief for 18 hours. The skin is closed with a subcuticular absorbable suture of 5-0 PDS.

The anesthetist should use short-acting anesthetic agents that enable the patient to awake rapidly after operation. The patient should receive intravenous fluids intraoperatively but not during immediate postsurgical recovery. An intravenous cannula should then be used only for access, to administer medication for pain relief. A suppository of diclofenac sodium (Voltarol) will alleviate postoperative pain and can facilitate early mobilization.

A younger patient who has undergone minicholecystectomy could be discharged from the hospital on the day of operation or by 1 to 2 days after operation. The older patient who undergoes that procedure can leave the hospital by the fifth postoperative day.

TECHNIQUES OF LAPAROSCOPIC CHOLECYSTECTOMY
Selection of Cases

The initial success of laparoscopic cholecystectomy has been attributed to the careful selection of patients. However, in current studies,[2-4] the procedure is evaluated in patients with simple and complex cholecystolithiasis. In one such evaluation laparoscopy was successful in 99% of cases.[4] In a study of 75 patients with com-

plicated cholelithiasis, the procedure was successful in 75% of cases; the remainder required laparotomy.[2] No deaths occurred in this series of 75 patients. The conversion rate from laparoscopy to open procedure has received much attention; a 5% conversion rate seems to be standard.

Operative Cholangiography

Most surgeons are undertaking operative cholangiography as indicated by the patient's history, liver function tests, and preoperative imaging, which is usually ultrasonographic. In laparoscopic cholecystectomy and conventional open cholecystectomy, operative cholangiography is possible. In minicholecystectomy, metal trocars do not obscure the image, but the preferable radiolucent instruments are expensive. Stones in the duct can be removed during all techniques of cholecystectomy either by dilating the cystic duct or by choledochotomy, which is much easier to perform during the open techniques (with or without choledochoscopy). If laparoscopic cholecystectomy is chosen, stones in the common bile duct are better managed by upper GI endoscopic sphincterotomy, which should be a separate pre- or postoperative procedure.

Bile Duct Injury

During standard open cholecystectomy, the incidence of bile duct injury varied from 0 to 0.5% (average incidence, 0.2%). In accumulated data a similar percent of injury is found in the results of laparoscopic cholecystectomy. In a study by the Southern Surgeons' Club,[5] seven injuries (0.5%) that resulted from 1518 laparoscopic procedures were cited. Four of these seven injuries were identified during laparoscopy and were repaired after conversion to laparotomy. Three injuries were not recognized until 3, 5, and 14 days after operation, respectively, when patients' liver function tests were abnormal or when an unexplained ileus developed. These three patients required a second operation and Roux-en-Y hepaticojejunostomy. Bile duct injuries were diagnosed during the second, third, tenth, twelfth, thirteenth, twenty-fifth and forty-third procedures performed by various surgeons. In a study by Cuschieri et al.,[6] four bile duct injuries in 1203 patients resulted from laparoscopic cholecystectomy. The incidence of bile duct injuries should be similar in the laparotomy and laparoscopic groups, but most of these injuries occur while the surgeon is learning the laparoscopic technique and in patients whose surgeons perform this procedure only occasionally.

Complications and Mortality

In reports of early experience with laparoscopic cholecystectomy, fewer minor and major complications are cited with laparoscopy. Major complications that occur during the procedure can be immediately recognized and corrected, although some bile duct injuries are noted during the postoperative stages of minilaparotomy or laparoscopic procedures. Fewer and less significant wound problems occur as a result of laparoscopy. Problems in healing such as hernia that develop late are rare after laparoscopy. In comparative studies, laparoscopic procedures result in fewer complications that would delay discharge from the hospital.

Death after laparoscopic cholecystectomy is rare and usually results from unrelated morbidity or preexisting causes. This is also true in patients who have undergone open cholecystectomy. The overall mortality rate for Danish women who underwent cholecystectomy from 1977 to 1981 was 1.2%.[7]

Length of Patient Stay and Procedure Cost

Often the efficacy of surgical procedures is cost-related, and procedure costs are often a function of the length of hospital stay. In the United States the patient stays a shorter period of time in the hospital than does his or her European counterpart; the average American patient's hospital stay is 1.2 days after laparoscopic cholecystectomy.[8] In Europe the length of patient hospital stay is often 3.5 days.[9] The length of time required to perform the procedure in the operating room increases procedural expense. The cost of laparoscopic cholecystectomy can be higher than that of minicholecystectomy,[10] especially if the surgeon uses disposable instruments. However, laparoscopy results in the rapid postoperative recovery of the patient, who often returns to work in an average of 10 days after operation. (After open cholecystectomy, the comparable figure is 41 days.)[10] However, studies from the department of surgery in Vellore in southern India indicate success similar to laparoscopic cholecystectomy with minicholecystectomy. Data related to length of patient stay in the hospital and return to work pertain to culture rather than the patient's medical requirements; this can be changed by encouraging early patient discharge.[10]

CONCLUSION

Two surgical techniques for the management for gallstones are available; each offers advantages and disadvantages. Both procedures are safe and are associated with low patient mortality; both offer rapid recovery and rehabilitation. Laparoscopic cholecystectomy is associated with better patient acceptance because of the cosmetic result, although the wound after minicholecystectomy can be barely visible. Procedural cost, equipment, and the skill required of the surgeon are also important considerations. If many laparoscopic procedures are undertaken at an institution and if a limited range of disposable equipment is used, the cost of laparoscopy is comparable with that of the open procedure. The surgeon who regularly performs laparoscopic procedures attains the skill necessary for success.

Cost reduction can be realized by providing services in medical facilities in which staff specialize in laparoscopic procedures for a high patient volume. Surgeons who perform laparoscopic procedures less frequently may prefer to use open surgical techniques.

REFERENCES

1. Russell RCG, Shankar S. The stabilized ring retractor: A technique for cholecystectomy. Br J Surg 74:826, 1987.
2. Fabre JM, Pyda P, Hons C de S, et al. Evaluation of laparoscopic cholecystectomy on patients with simple and complicated cholecystolithiasis. W J Surg 16:113-117, 1992.
3. Wilson P, Leese T, Morgan WP, et al. Elective laparoscopic cholecystectomy for "allcomers." Lancet 338:795-797, 1991.
4. Martin IG, Holdsworth PJ, Asker J, et al. Laparoscopic cholecystectomy as a routine procedure for gallstones: Results of an "all-comers" policy. Br J Surg 79:807-810, 1992.
5. Southern Surgeons Club. A prospective analysis of 1518 laparoscopic cholecystectomies. N Engl J Med 324:1073-1078, 1991.
6. Cuschieri A, Dubois F, Mouiel, J, et al. The European experience with laparoscopic cholecystectomy. Am J Surg 161:385-387, 1991.
7. Bredesen J, Jorgensen T, Andersen TF, et al. Early postoperative mortality following cholecystectomy in the entire female population of Denmark 1977-1981. W J Surg 16:530-535, 1992.
8. Donohue JH, Farnell MB, Grant CS, et al. Laparoscopic cholecystectomy: Early Mayo Clinic experience. Mayo Clin Proc 67:449-455, 1992.
9. Grace PA, Quereshi A, Coleman J, et al. Reduced postoperative hospitalisation after laparoscopic cholecystectomy. Br J Surg 78:160-162, 1991.
10. Stoker HE, Vose J, O'Mara P, et al. Laparoscopic cholecystectomy—a clinical and financial analysis of 280 operations. Arch Surg 127:589-595, 1992.
11. Saltzstein EC, Mercer LC, Peacock JB, et al. Twenty-four-hour hospitalisation after cholecystectomy. Surg Gynecol Obstet 173:367-370, 1991.

21 Cholecystectomy by the Laparoscopic or Minilaparotomy Approach

John R. McGregor, Patrick J. O'Dwyer, Enda W.N. McDermott, James J. Murphy, and Niall J. O'Higgins

The first cholecystectomy was performed in July 1882 by Carl Langenbuch with a T-shaped incision.[1] Although a variety of alternative treatments have since been proposed, cholecystectomy remains the treatment of choice for patients with symptomatic gallstones. Recent years, however, have witnessed a major change in surgical practice such that the future of traditional laparotomy for cholecystectomy has been called into question. This challenge to conventional surgical teaching has come from the development and increasing popularity of minimally invasive or minimal access operative techniques. Quite apart from any cosmetic advantages these procedures may offer the patient, it is thought that reduced operative trauma encourages a more rapid postoperative recovery, which in turn leads to a shorter hospital stay and promotes an earlier return to normal activity.[2-7]

Minimal access procedures applicable to the surgical management of cholelithiasis are laparoscopic cholecystectomy and the minilaparotomy approach. The purpose of this study was to compare the results of our initial experience with laparoscopic cholecystectomy with findings in a consecutive series of minilaparotomy cholecystectomies performed immediately before.

METHODS

This study was carried out at two university departments of surgery: at Western Infirmary, Glasgow, and St. Vincent's Hospital, Dublin. All data were collected prospectively. No selection criteria were employed in the two consecutive series, and patients were excluded from analysis only if they had preoperative clinical, radiological, or biochemical evidence of common bile duct stones. In such circumstances, open cholecystectomy and common bile duct exploration were carried out through an incision of traditional size (approximately 15 cm).

Laparoscopic cholecystectomy was performed with patients in the supine position in a reverse Trendelenburg tilt. CO_2 pneumoperitoneum was maintained at 15 mm Hg. A nasogastric tube and urinary catheter were routinely inserted. Four ports were employed, and in this series operative cholangiography was not performed. Electrocautery rather than laser was used for dissection, and the use of intraperitoneal drains was at the discretion of the surgeon.

Cholecystectomy by minilaparotomy was carried out through a 5 cm transverse right-sided subcostal incision.[8] The length of the intended wound was accurately measured and the skin marked before incision. In the majority of patients, once the biliary anatomy had been established, the gallbladder was removed from the liver bed from the fundus down before ligation and division of the cystic duct and cystic artery. Operative cholangiography was routinely performed in this series. Just as for the laparoscopic group, there was no strict policy regarding the use of drains. All operations were performed by a consultant surgeon or by an experienced registrar assisted by a consultant.

RESULTS

The laparoscopic cholecystectomy series comprised 91 patients and the minilaparotomy cholecystectomy group 84 patients. As summarized in Table 1, the two groups were highly comparable with respect to preoperative characteristics. Although a higher proportion of patients in the minilaparotomy series were pathologically obese,[9] this difference was not statistically significant.

Laparoscopic cholecystectomy was completed in 85 of the 91 patients in which it was attempted—a success rate of 93.4%. Of the six conversions to open operation, three occurred because of failure to accurately identify the biliary anatomy at laparoscopy. One additional patient required laparotomy to permit removal of a gallstone that was impacted at the junction of the cystic duct and the common bile duct. The remaining conversion was in a patient early in our experience with laparoscopic surgery in whom dense inflammatory adhesions precluded an accurate view of the biliary tree.

Table 1. Preoperative patient characteristics

Characteristics	Laparoscopic Cholecystectomy	Minilaparotomy
Number	91	84
Male/Female	14/77	10/74
Mean age (yr)	52	49
Range (yr)	20 – 75	13 – 87
Obese (%)*	35	45
Acute cholecystitis (n)	23 (25.3%)	24 (28.6%)

*As defined in a report from the Royal College of Physicians.

Table 2. Postoperative complications

Complications	Laparoscopic Cholecystectomy	Minilaparotomy
Bleeding requiring blood transfusion	1	—
Retained gallstones	2	—
Subhepatic fluid collection	1	—
Wound infection	—	2
Pneumonia	—	1
Congestive cardiac failure	—	1
Drain disruption	—	1
TOTAL	4 (4.4%)	5 (5.6%)

In the minilaparotomy series, cholecystectomy was successfully accomplished through a 5 cm incision in 71 of 84 patients (84.5%). The wound was extended by a median 5 cm (range 2 to 8 cm) in the remaining 13 patients. In 11 of these patients, all of whom were obese,[9] wound extension was required because the operating surgeon considered exposure of the biliary anatomy through the 5 cm incision to be inadequate for safe operation. The remaining two wound extensions were required to permit choledocholithotomy in patients in whom common bile duct stones had not been suspected preoperatively.

Minilaparotomy cholecystectomy proved to be a faster procedure than laparoscopic cholecystectomy. The mean operating time was 83 minutes (range 21 to 190) in the laparoscopic series compared with a mean of 58 minutes (range 17 to 120) in the minilaparotomy group ($p < 0.01$; Mann-Whitney U test).

A total of nine significant postoperative complications were recorded, and they are summarized in Table 2. No patient required reoperation. The two patients in the laparoscopic series with retained gallstones had obstructive jaundice—one at 6 weeks and the other at 4 months postoperatively. In each case the common bile duct was successfully cleared by endoscopic sphincterotomy and stone retrieval with no need for further surgery. In the one patient in the minilaparotomy series in whom the drain broke apart during attempted removal, the remainder of the drain was removed under local anesthesia. Finally, there was no difference between the two operations with respect to the hospital stay. The mean duration of the postoperative stay in the laparoscopic series was 3.7 days (range 1 to 17) compared with 4.0 days (range 1 to 12) in the minilaparotomy group.

DISCUSSION

Open cholecystectomy has traditionally been regarded as the treatment of choice for patients with symptomatic gallstones.[10] In experienced hands, it is a relatively simple surgical procedure with proved efficacy and above all it is safe. The incidence of major bile duct injury is estimated at 0.1% to 0.3%[10-14] and operative mortality, at least in patients under the age of 50 years, is negligible.[10,14,15]

In spite of this, recent years have witnessed a dramatic change in the surgical management of cholelithiasis. Throughout the Western world, laparoscopic surgery has rapidly been adopted as the preferred technique for cholecystectomy in a manner unprecedented in modern surgical history. Admittedly the enthusiasm for laparoscopic cholecystectomy can be partly attributed to consumer demand as a result of considerable media attention focusing on the potential advantages of the technique, particularly the earlier return to normal activity. It must be remembered, however, that many of these reported benefits have not been scientifically proved, and it is becoming increasingly clear that the initial quest and desire by the general surgical community to master laparoscopic cholecystectomy exposed patients to an appreciable risk of injury to the common bile duct[4,16-18] or gastrointestinal tract[19] and vascular injury[19] when compared with the traditional open operation.

An alternative method of reducing the trauma associated with surgical access is to shorten the length of the incision used for open cholecystectomy. We have previously reported that in the majority of patients, cholecystectomy can be performed through a 5 cm transverse right-sided subcostal incision.[8] Moreover, in a recent randomized study, we have demonstrated that the length of a subcostal incision may significantly influence patient recovery following cholecystectomy.[5] It is important to note, however, that a reduction in the length of the incision does not appear to increase the risk of major complications associated with gallbladder surgery. In published results of more than 2500 cases of minilaparotomy cholecystectomy[5,8,20-26] there has been only one reported bile duct injury amounting to a 2 mm laceration of the common bile duct,[26] an incidence of 0.04%.

In this report we described our experience with two consecutive series of unselected patients undergoing elective cholecystectomy. Laparoscopic cholecystectomy proved possible in a higher proportion of patients in which it was attempted than did minilaparotomy cholecystectomy through a 5 cm transverse subcostal incision. However, laparoscopic cholecystectomy took significantly longer to perform than minilaparotomy cholecystectomy, even without the use of operative cholangiography. There were no apparent differences between the two series with respect to postoperative outcome.

We conclude that laparoscopic and minilaparotomy cholecystectomy both appear to be safe and effective minimal access procedures when applied to unselected groups of patients. However, a randomized controlled clinical trial is clearly essential to establish the relative roles of each procedure in patient management, and such a study is currently in progress at our institutions. Nevertheless, our preliminary experience would suggest that for centers without the equipment to train personnel in laparoscopic techniques, minilaparotomy cholecystectomy may prove to be an acceptable and cost-effective alternative. Moreover, surgeons familiar with conventional cholecystectomy may find it easier to adapt to a minilaparotomy approach.

REFERENCES

1. Langenbuch C. Ein Fall von Exstirpation der Gallenblase wegen chronischer Cholilithiasis. Heilung Berl Klin Wochenscher 19:725-727, 1882.
2. Holohan TV. Laparoscopic cholecystectomy. Lancet 338:801-803, 1991.
3. Cuschieri A, Dubois F, Mouiel J, et al. The European experience with laparoscopic cholecystectomy. Am J Surg 161:385-387, 1991.
4. Troidl H, Spangenberger W, Langen R, et al. Laparoscopic cholecystectomy: Technical peformance, safety and patient's benefit. Endoscopy 24:252-261, 1992.
5. O'Dwyer P J, McGregor JR, McDermott EWM, et al., Patient recovery following cholecystectomy through a 6 cm or 15 cm transverse subcostal incision: A prospective randomised clinical trial. Postgrad Med J 68:817-819, 1992.
6. Reddick E J, Olsen DO. Laparoscopic laser cholecystomy: A comparison with mini-lap cholecystectomy. Surg Endosc 3:131-133, 1989.
7. Schirmer BD, Edge SB, Dix J, et al. Laparoscopic cholecystectomy: Treatment of choice for symptomatic cholelithiasis. Ann Surg 213:665-677, 1991.

8. O'Dwyer PJ, Murphy JJ, O'Higgins NJ. Cholecystectomy through a 5 cm subcostal incision. Br J Surg 77:1189-1190, 1990.

9. Black D, James WPT, Besser GM, et al. Obesity: A report of the Royal College of Physicians. 1. The health consequences of overweight and obesity. J R Coll Phys Lond 17:6-24, 1983.

10. McSherry CK. Cholecystectomy: The gold standard. Am J Surg 158:174-178, 1989.

11. Morgenstern L, Berci G. Twelve hundred open cholecystectomies before the laparoscopic era: A standard for comparison. Arch Surg 127:400-403, 1992.

12. Ganey JB, Johnson Jr PA, Prillaman PE, et al. Cholecystectomy: Clinical experience with a large series. Am J Surg 151:352-357, 1986.

13. Pickleman J, Gonzalez RP. The improving results of cholecystectomy. Arch Surg 121:930-934, 1986.

14. Davies MG, O'Broin E, Mannion C, et al. Audit of open cholecystectomy in a district general hospital. Br J Surg 79:314-316, 1992.

15. Bredesen J, Jorgensen T, Andersen TF, et al. Early postoperative mortality following cholecystectomy in the entire female population of Denmark, 1977-81. World J Surg 16:530-535, 1992.

16. Traverso LW. Endoscopic cholecystectomy: An analysis of complications—comment. Arch Surg 126:1197, 1991.

17. Shanahan D, Knight D. Laparoscopic cholecystectomy. Br Med J 304:776-777, 1992.

18. Moossa AR, Easter DW, Van Sonnenberg E, et al. Laparoscopic injuries of the bile duct: A cause for concern. Ann Surg 215:196-202, 1992.

19. Deziel DJ, Millikan KW, Economou SG, et al. Complications of laparoscopic cholecystectomy: A national survey of 4,292 hospitals and an analysis of 77,604 cases. Am J Surg 165:9-14, 1993.

20. Morton CE. Cost containment with the use of minicholecystectomy and intraoperative cholangiography. Am Surg 51:168-169, 1985.

21. Ledet WP. Ambulatory cholecystectomy without disability. Arch Surg 125:1434-1435, 1990.

22. Merrill JR. Minimal trauma cholecystectomy (a "no-touch" procedure in a "well"). Am Surg 54:256-261, 1988.

23. Dubois F, Berthelot B. Cholecystectomie par mini-laparotomie. Nouv Presse Med 11:1139-1141, 1982.

24. Goco IR, Chambers LG. Dollars and cents: Minicholecystectomy and early discharge. South Med J 81:161-163, 1988.

25. Russell RCG, Shankar S. The stabilised ring retractor: A technique for cholecystectomy. Br J Surg 74:826, 1987.

26. O'Kelly TJ, Barr H, Malley WR, et al. Cholecystectomy through a 5 cm subcostal incision. Br J Surg 78:762, 1991.

22 *Laparoscopic Cholecystectomy on Unselected Patients*

Thorsten F. Morlang and Wolf J. Stelter

Since 1990 we have performed laparoscopic cholecystectomy as the first-choice treatment for all patients with symptomatic cholecystolithiasis. We do not select our patients, and we accept no primary contraindications to the laparoscopic procedure, for example, acute cholecystitis or prior operation with possible adhesions. If, however, the laparoscopic procedure turns out to be impossible or unsafe, laparotomy is performed without hesitation.

MATERIALS AND METHODS

As part of our preoperative examination we require the following before administering a general anesthetic: chest x-ray evaluation, ECG, and a routine blood work-up. Other specific parameters include patient history, abdominal ultrasonography and specific enzyme determinations. In addition, gastroscopy is considered essential. We require preoperative endoscopic retrograde cholangiopancreatography (ERCP) if there is the slightest suspicion of common bile duct stones. Stones are immediately removed by papillotomy and extraction, and if necessary ERCP is repeated.

We have performed 1000 laparoscopic cholecystectomies in unselected patients (Table 1); in 37 of them conversion to laparotomy became necessary. In six patients with common bile duct stones, laparoscopic exploration of the common bile duct was performed through the cystic duct; it was successful in four.

Table 1. Laparoscopic operations:
April 1990–August 1992

Cholecystectomy	1000
Conversion	37
Exploration of CBD	6
Successful	4
Appendectomy	125
Conversion	22
Diagnostic	55
Conversion	12
Repeat laparoscopy	8
Conversion	1

Table 2. Diagnoses leading to laparoscopic cholecystectomy

Condition	Percent
Cholecystolithiasis	85.6
Acute cholecystitis	8.4
Chronic shrunken gallbladder	4.5
Gallbladder carcinoma	0.7
Gallbladder dysfunction/polyps	0.6

Table 3. Mean operative time

Condition	Time (min)
Cholecystolithiasis	80
Acute cholecystitis	116
Chronic shrunken gallbladder	107

Table 4. Conversions to open procedures

Condition	Percent
Gallbladder dysfunction/polyps	0
Cholecystolithiasis	2.2
Acute cholecystitis	10.5
Chronic shrunken gallbladder	9.4
Gallbladder carcinoma	0.06
TOTAL CONVERSIONS	3.6

Reason for Conversion	No.	Percent
CBD injury	3	0.3
Bowel perforation	4	0.4
Severe adhesions	17	1.7
Technical difficulties	1	0.1
CBD stones after Billroth II	3	0.3
Cystic duct too short	2	0.2
Pneumoperitoneum impossible	5	0.5
Carcinoma	1	0.1
Suspected bleeding	1	0.1
TOTAL	37	

Seventy-five percent of our patients were female, and 25% were male. Most were 50 to 70 years of age (range, 14 to 91 years) (Fig. 1).

Postoperatively, 60% of patients could be discharged within 3 days, and another 28% left the hospital after 4 to 6 days. Others stayed longer, mostly because of age and concomitant medical problems. The average length of postoperative hospitalization was 4 days (range, 1 to 50 days) (Fig. 2).

Our patients had uncomplicated symptomatic cholecystolithiasis in 85% of cases, acute cholecystitis in 8% and a chronic shrinked gallbladder in 4% (Table 2). A few were found to have carcinoma as determined by histological examination; no stones were found in the gallbladder.

Within 2 years we trained a team of 18 surgeons consecutively. The experience of the surgeons varies from just a few to more than 400 cholecystectomies. Our mean operating times were 80 minutes for uncomplicated cholecystolithiasis, 116 minutes for acute cholecystitis, and 107 minutes for chronic shrinked gallbladders (Table 3). An experienced team can perform a normal cholecystectomy in 45 minutes including cholangiography.

Only 2.2% of patients with uncomplicated cholecystolithiasis required conversion to laparotomy. Even in acute cholecystitis and chronic shrunken gallbladders conversion rates were only 10% and 9%, respectively (Table 4). Generally cholecystectomy was completed laparoscopically in more than 96% of cases.

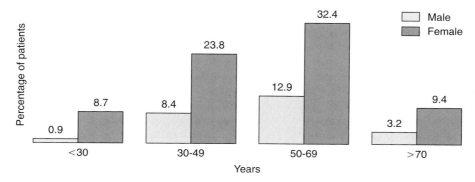

Fig. 1. Distribution of patients by age and sex.

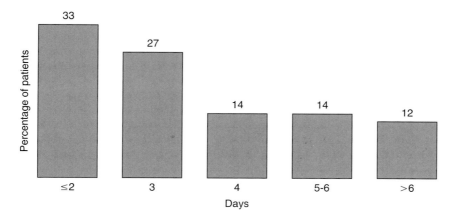

Fig. 2. Average length of postoperative hospitalization (1 to 50 days; average 4 days).

Conversion to laparotomy was necessary as a result of common bile duct injury in 0.3% and bowel perforation in 0.4%.

Laparotomies were done for the following reasons (see Table 4): severe adhesions, defective equipment, common bile duct stones found intraoperatively after a Billroth II procedure, a cystic duct too shrinked to fit for a safe occlusion, inability to insufflate the peritoneal cavity, macroscopic evidence of carcinoma, and suspected massive bleeding which was not confirmed later on. Of the minor complications that occurred (Table 5), the most frequent was perforation of the gallbladder in 16%, followed by minor bleeding that could be controlled laparoscopically in 10%, and loss of stones that were mostly removed in 8%. Liver injuries occurred in 2.5%.

Three patients died perioperatively; one 82-year-old patient died 10 days after an intercurrent Billroth II operation; the cause of death was an infected subhepatic hematoma leading to septic erosion of a larger vessel with massive hemorrhage. A 79-year-old patient with common bile duct stones underwent three ERCPs, nasobiliary drainage, and extracorporeal shock wave lithotripsy before laparoscopic cholecystectomy. She had cardiopulmonary insufficiency and died 12 days later of a myocardial reinfarction. The third patient, 81 years of age, had an intraoperative arterial embolism necessitating lower limb amputation after several embolectomies. After 3 months in the intensive care unit she died of pulmonary complications.

We had four common bile duct injuries. Three were repaired primarily. A stricture developed that required choledochojejunostomy 8 months later in the fourth case. One primary repair was done laparoscopically over

Table 5. Complications in 1000 cholecystectomies

	No.	Percent
Minor Complications		
Biliary fistula	5	0.5
Umbilical fistula	8	0.8
Bleeding	97	9.7
Gallbladder perforation	162	16.2
Loss of stones	78	7.8
Liver injury	25	2.5
Hematoma in abdominal wall	8	0.8
Soft tissue emphysema	4	0.4
Dislocation of jaw	1	0.1
Major Complications		
Perioperative death	3	0.3
Bile duct injury	4	0.4
Bile duct stricture	3	0.3
Biliary peritonitis	3	0.3
Chronic cholangitis	1	0.1
Bowel perforation	4	0.4
Hematoma (relaptm/sc)	8	0.8
Ileus	2	0.2
Postoperative MI	1	0.1
Asystole at anesthesia	1	0.1
Acute renal failure	1	0.1
Pneumothorax	1	0.1
Apoplexy, arterial embolism	1	0.1

Table 6. Incidence of common bile duct stones (n = 1000)

	No.	Percent
Intraoperative cholangiography	645	64.5
Common bile duct stones	75	7.5
Preoperative ERCP	119	
Negative findings	4	
Stones found	59	5.9
Total incidence of CBD stones	134	13.4

an inserted T-tube. Two more biliodigestive anastomoses were necessary after serious strictures from chronic cholangitis and long-term internal biliary fistula after acute cholecystitis. There were four cases of biliary peritonitis from bile leakage; they were treated laparoscopically with abdominal rinsing, occlusion of the leak with a clip, and drainage. Four bowel perforations were repaired and healed without complications, and four cases of early postoperative hemorrhage required repeat laparoscopy or laparotomy. Two cases of bowel obstruction required intervention. We had one patient with a myocardial infarction, one with asystole, and one with acute renal failure. In one patient the diaphragm was perforated by a forceps, which resulted in a pneumothorax. Only three common bile duct injuries occurred in our first 150 cholecystectomies.

CONCLUSION

In our opinion intraoperative cholangiography should remain mandatory before laparoscopic cholecystectomy is performed. We found common bile duct stones in 7.5% of our patients by intraoperative cholangiography, although there was no preoperative suspicion of this (Table 6). If we add those that were found by preoperative ERCP in suspected cases, the total incidence of common bile duct stones in our patients was 13.4%.

23 Laparoscopic Cholecystectomy: Initial Experience and Results in 400 Patients

Virgilio Fresneda Moreno, Jose Fernandez-Cebrian, Isaac Capela Fernandez, Joaquin Perez de Oteyza, Enrique Martinez Molina, Pedro Carda Abella, Vincente Morales Castiñeiras, Eduardo Lobo Martinez, and Pedro Lopez Hervas

The laparoscopic approach is an alternative method to the traditional operative treatment of gallstones; its use and indications are increasing, and it is becoming the first-choice therapeutic approach standard for several surgical teams. New technology presupposes a progressive learning and adaptation process. Sometimes this process exacts a high price: serious and life-threatening complications.

We describe the experience of our surgical team (nine surgeons, each with a different surgical background) in our first 400 patients who underwent laparoscopic cholecystectomy, including morbidity, conversion, and reoperation rates.

PATIENT SELECTION

Indications for laparoscopic cholecystectomy are the same as for standard cholecystectomy (Table 1). Ideal candidates are patients with symptomatic cholelithiasis or symptomatic nonlithiasic gallbladder disease (e.g., polyps, dyskinesia).

The list of contraindications is changing gradually and depends on the experience of the surgical team. In the first 150 patients, those with risk factors (e.g., obesity, acute cholecystitis, chronic liver disease, diabetes,

Table 1. Indications and contraindications for laparoscopic cholecystectomy

Indications

Symptomatic cholelithiasis
Symptomatic gallbladder disease
    Polyps
    Dyskinesia

Absolute Contraindications

Unable to tolerate general anesthetic
Uncorrected coagulopathy
Peritonitis/cholangitis
Biliary fistula
Suspected carcinoma

Relative Contraindications

Acute cholecystitis
Morbid obesity
Previous upper abdominal surgery
Cirrhosis/portal hypertension
Untreated choledocolithiasis
Pregnancy

Table 2. Indications and risk factors: January 1991–September 1992

Indications and Risk Factors	No. of Patients
Indications	
Symptomatic cholelithiasis	
Simple	344 (86%)
Complicated	49 (12.25%)
Acute cholecystitis	
Acute pancreatitis	
Associated choledoco-	15 (3.75%)
lithiasis	
Polyps	7 (1.75%)
Risk Factors	
Diabetes mellitus	13
Obesity	45
Arterial hypertension	40
Chronic lung disease	18
Cardiopathy	26
Chronic hepatopathy	12
Prior surgery	
Upper abdominal	13
Lower abdominal	35
Acute cholecystitis	34

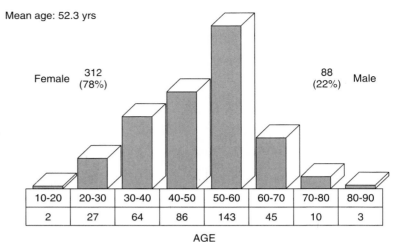

Fig. 1. Patient data by sex and age.

previous upper abdominal surgery, complicated cholelithiasis) were not included, but they were added as we became more experienced (Table 2). The patients' sex-age characteristics are shown in Fig. 1. The study period was from January 1991 to September 1992.

PREOPERATIVE EVALUATION

All patients were evaluated by clinical history, physical examination, and laboratory studies, such as liver function tests, amylase and clotting studies to determine complications of gallstone disease, such as pancreatitis, jaundice, or acute cholecystitis. Ultrasound imaging was used to confirm the presence of gallstones and evaluate the bile ducts for dilation and stones and the pancreas and gallbladder for inflammation. On occasion, oral cholecystograms (8.7%) and intravenous cholangiograms (5.2%) were very useful.

The management of patients with evidence of common bile duct stones remains controversial. Our attitude, similar to that of other investigators,[1] is that preoperatively, in patients with suspected common bile duct stones (e.g., dilated ducts, elevated liver chemistry values, or common bile duct stones demonstrated by ultrasonography), our preference has been to perform endoscopic retrograde cholangiopancreatography (ERCP) with sphincterotomy, delaying laparoscopic surgery for 48 to 72 hours. This protocol was followed in 15 patients (3.75%), with extraction of stones in 14 of them (one false negative). If the diagnosis is made intraoperatively, the procedure is dependent on the size of the stones. For small stones we use ERCP with sphinc-

terotomy in the postoperative period; for large or multiple stones we prefer conversion to laparotomy. Only two patients showed evidence of choledocholithiasis during operation, which had not been suspected previously and was demonstrated by intraoperative cholangiograms. They were suitable candidates for ERCP.

If the diagnosis is made postoperatively, we perform ERCP with sphincterotomy at the time of discovery. Only one patient in our series had residual choledocholithiasis, diagnosed 6 months postoperatively, which necessitated ERCP with sphincterotomy.

All patients were informed of the surgical risks (e.g., conversion, potential common bile duct injuries, bleeding). In addition, all were treated prophylactically with antitetanics, antibiotics (second and third generation cephalosporin), and thromboembolic agents (low-molecular-weight heparin).

SURGICAL TECHNIQUE

Conventional methodology is as follows:

1. Procedures are performed under general anesthesia.

2. The pneumoperitoneum is initiated with a Veress needle (closed method) or with a Hasson cannula (open method), with an upper pressure limit of 12 to 13 mm Hg.

3. Cannulas are placed as follows: umbilical, a 10 mm cannula for the laparoscope; upper midline, a 10 mm cannula is used to dissect the gallbladder; in two lateral sites in the right hemiabdomen, 5 mm cannulas used to expose the gallbladder and hepatic hilus (Fig. 2).

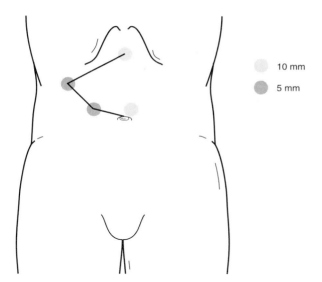

Fig. 2. Sites for cannula placement.

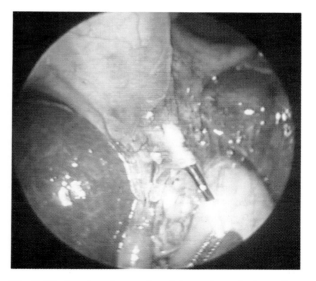

Fig. 3. Cholangiocatheter placed through cystic duct when performing cholangiography.

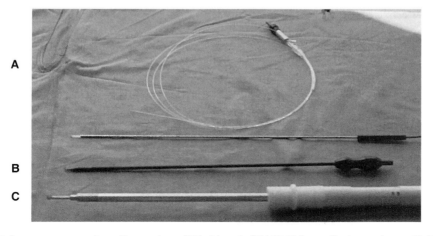

Fig. 4. Instruments used to dissect the gallbladder. **A,** Nd:YAG laser. **B,** Argon laser. **C,** Ultrasonic scalpel.

4. The operative procedure follows the classic steps of a traditional cholecystectomy.

5. For intraoperative cholangiography a clip is placed across the duct adjacent to its junction with the gallbladder. A small incision is made in the anterior wall of the cystic duct. A 5 Fr venous puncture needle is inserted percutaneously under direct vision into the abdomen in the right upper quadrant just below the cos-tal margin. Afterward, a 4 Fr olive-tipped cholangio-catheter is inserted through the venous puncture site into the abdomen, guided by a grasping forceps. The cystic duct is closed slightly with one clip. Gentle flushing with normal saline solution ensures patency (Fig. 3).

6. To dissect the gallbladder, we have used electro-cautery, laser (argon and Nd:YAG), and recently an ul-trasonic (harmonic) scalpel (Fig. 4).

7. The gallbladder is removed through the umbilical port, under visual guidance, with the camera inserted at the upper midline site.

POSTOPERATIVE CARE

The nasogastric tube is removed in the operating room. Patients are monitored in the recovery room for 2 to 3 hours and are then transferred to a regular room. Liquids are offered for dinner. Pirazolone is used for pain relief.

Patients are discharged the following morning. Patients are seen at 7 days, 1 month, 3 months, and 6 months for postoperative follow-up. Liver function tests are often performed during these visits.

RESULTS
Morbidity

Total morbidity was 7% (28 patients) with major complications occurring in 2.5% (10 patients) (Table 3). The principal causes were postoperative bleeding in four patients (from the surface of the liver in two and from the cystic arteries after slippage of the clips in two) and bile leakage from the liver bed in three patients, which was drained successfully; there were two cases of bile duct injury, although one was recognized as being a consequence of necessary suturing over a T-tube. The other injury was discovered postoperatively and required a hepaticojejunostomy with Roux-en-Y. Another complication was a subhepatic abscess (*Staphylococcus aureus* was cultured). If we observe the complications curve (Fig. 5), we can see a progressive decrease after the first

100 patients. Minor complications occurred in 18 patients (4.5%). The primary causes are shown in Table 3.

Analyzing the morbidity rates in the groups with and without risk factors (e.g., obesity, previous upper abdominal surgery, acute cholecystitis, chronic hepatopathy), we observe no statistical differences between them with regard to obesity, chronic hepatopathy and acute cholecystitis; however, there was a significant difference in the prevalence of previous upper abdominal surgery (Table 4). There were no deaths in our series.

Conversion

Conversion was necessary in 17 patients (4.25%), most often because of unclear biliary anatomy (12 patients). Other causes included intraoperative bleeding in two patients, common bile duct injury in one, cholecystoenteric fistula in one, and duodenal injury in one patient with a prior Billroth II gastrectomy (Table 5).

Reoperation

Five patients (1.25%) underwent reoperation for the following reasons: postoperative bleeding in four patients (see above) and inflammatory common bile duct stenosis (Bismuth type I) in one, probably the result of thermic injury from the electrocautery. This patient required a hepaticojejunostomy and Roux-en-Y anastomosis.

Intraoperative Cholangiography

Intraoperative cholangiography was not performed in the first 150 patients because of the meticulous selec-

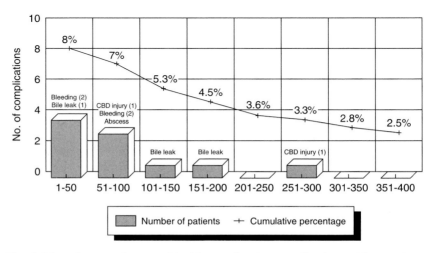

Fig. 5. Note downward curve of incidence of major complications with experience.

Table 3. Postoperative morbidity in 28 patients (7%)

Major Complications (2.5%)	No.	Minor Complications (4.5%)	No.
Postoperative bleeding	4 (1%)	Prolonged ileus	1
Common bile duct injury	2 (0.5%)	Infected wound	3
Biliary leakage	3 (0.75%)	Hematoma	7
Subhepatic abscess	1 (0.25%)	Hernia	1
		Abdominal pain	3
		Subcutaneous emphysema	2
		Unexplained fever	1

Table 4. Morbidity–risk factor correlation

Risk Factors	Morbidity
No risk factors	16 (5.09%)
Risk factors	
Upper abdominal surgery	2 (15.3%)
Chronic hepatopathy	3 (2.5%)
Acute cholecystitis	4 (5.8%)

Table 5. Conversions

Reasons	No. of Patients
Difficulty in visualizing biliary anatomy	12
Duodenal injury	1
Cholecystoenteric fistula	1
Intraoperative bleeding	2
Common bile duct injury	1
RATE	17/400 (4.25%)

Table 6. Intraoperative cholangiography

Cases	No. and Percentage	Attempted Cholangiography	Postoperative Problems
Not attempted	211 (52.75%)	No (211)	Bile leak (2)
First 150 cases (highly selective)			CBD injury (1)
No indications	39 (9.75%)		Residual CBD
Allergy to contrast medium	4 (1%)		stone (1)
Short cystic duct	6 (1.5%)	Yes (189)	
No reason	12 (3%)	Successful	Unsuspected
Attempted	189 (47.25%)		CBD stones (2)
Successful	173 (91.6%)	Unsuccessful	Bile leak (1)
Normal	164 (94%)		
Abnormal	9 (6%)		
Previously unsuspected CBD stones	2		
Abnormal anatomy	3		
Equivocal studies	4		
Unsuccessful	16 (8.4%)		
Unable to cannulate	7		
Extravasation of contrast medium	6		
Breaking cystic duct	3		

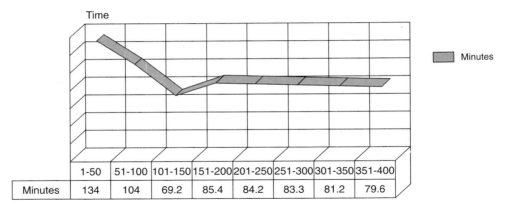

Fig. 6. Duration of operative procedures (average, 90.1 minutes).

tion process. Among the remaining 250 patients, intraoperative cholangiography was attempted in 189 and was successful in 173 (91.6%): 164 patients (94%) were normal and nine (6%) were abnormal, with unsuspected choledocholithiasis in two patients, common bile duct anomalies in three, and uncertain findings in four.

Analyzing the postoperative findings with regard to intraoperative cholangiography, we observed more biliary complications in the group without intraoperative cholangiograms: biliary leakage in three, common bile duct injury in one, choledocholithiasis in one (see Table 6).

Residual Choledocholithiasis

One woman was admitted to the hospital 6 months after surgery because of a residual choledocal stone (intraoperative cholangiography was not performed). She underwent ERCP with sphincterotomy, which was successful.

Operative Time

The duration of the operative procedure (including conventional cholecystectomy after conversion) averaged 90.1 minutes (with a range of 25 to 278 minutes per operation) (Fig. 6).

Laser Versus Electrocautery Versus Ultrasonic Scalpel

A randomized prospective study comparing cut/coagulation capacity, color distortion on the monitor, smoke production, ease of management, and complications (e.g., gallbladder perforation, burning) in 60 patients (20 in each group) showed that the ultrasonic scalpel was superior to the other two instruments (Table 7).

Histopathology

Two patients had carcinoma of the gallbladder, which was not suspected preoperatively (carcinoma in situ in one and stage 5 by Nevins classification in one). Among seven patients with a preoperative diagnosis such as polyps, six had cholesterolosis and one had adenomyomatosis. Among the remaining patients 340 had chronic cholecystitis and 51 had acute cholecystitis.

Length of Hospital Stay

The mean hospital stay for the entire series was 2.1 days (range, 24 hours to 18 days). No outpatient procedures were done.

DISCUSSION

Laparoscopic cholecystectomy is considerably more popular than the classic procedure. However, as with any new surgical technique, we must be aware of any potential complications, particularly in the first patients. The benefits of this approach were well documented by Reddick and Olsen,[2] with a significant reduction in duration of hospitalization and complications.

However, the main concern in laparoscopic cholecystectomy is safety. In 1518 cholecystectomies the Southern Surgeons Club[3] reported a mortality rate of 0.07% and a morbidity rate of 5.1%. In another large series mortality was 0.9% and morbidity 6.4% (Table 8).[4,5] After reviewing these data we must conclude that the total morbidity in our series was higher than that

Table 7. Comparison of dissection instruments

Parameter	Laser		Electrocautery		Ultrasonic Scalpel	
Hemostasis	Good	73.3%		80%		86%
	Med.	20%		20%		6.6%
	Bad	6.6%				6.6%
Color distortion	No	66.6%	No	100%	No	100%
	Yes	33.3%				
Smoke	No	6.4%	No	20%	No	100%
	Yes	93.3%	Yes	80%		
Ease of use	Easy	66.6%	Easy	100%	Easy	100%
Complications						
Gallbladder perforation		—		40%	Any complication	
Burns		20%		20%		

Table 8. Analysis of several series with more than 250 cholecystectomies

Series	No. of Cases	Morbidity	Mortality	Conversion	CBD Injury
Peters (1991)	283	2.1	—	2.8	0.5
Dubois (1991)	330	1.21	—	1	0.6
Soper (1991)	618	1.6	—	2.9	0.2
SSC (1991)	1518	1.5	0.07	4.7	0.5
Cuschieri (1991)	1236	1.6	—	3.6	0.3
SPAW (1991)	500	1	—	1.8	—
Wolfe (1991)	381	3.4	0.9	3	—
Gigot (1991)	3244	6.4	0.2	6.5	0.5
SFCD (1992)	3606	4.3	0.05	7.2	0.78
RyC (1993)	400	2.5	—	4.25	0.5
		(7)			

in other series.[6-9] This may be attributed to the high rate of complications in the first 150 to 200 patients, although they were selected very carefully. It is obvious that the morbidity was influenced by the surgeons' learning curve.

Injury of the common bile duct has been reported in 0.2% to 2%.[10-12] The main causes of injury reported in the literature are misinterpretation of the anatomy and attempts to control hilar bleeding, where adjacent structures can be injured by electrocautery, laser, or he-mostatic clips. In our series injuries included thermic lesions inadvertently produced by electrocautery and small lacerations of the common bile duct caused by scissors. Postoperative bleeding is an infrequent complication, and we believe our cases resulted from technical difficulties during hemostasis and incorrect application of the clips. Another controversial issue is whether to perform routine or selective intraoperative cholangiography. Our data demonstrated a higher rate of complications in the group in which cholangiography was not performed. To reduce the incidence of these complications, we prefer to perform cholangiography routinely, using criteria similar to those of other investigators.[13,14] Thus the management of choledocolithiasis is guided by findings on intraoperative cholangiography and perioperative ERCP disponibility. This is possible because of our low morbidity and mortality rates (ERCP with sphincterotomy, 8.2% and 1.4%, respectively),[15] and to date we believe it is the gold standard for adjunctive treatment of choledocholithiasis.[1] Dissection of the gallbladder from the liver bed is usually performed with electrocautery or laser, although use of these instruments is controversial.[16,17] We conducted a study comparing several characteristics of these instruments with those of the ultrasonic (harmonic) scalpel. The ultrasonic scalpel works by high vibration (55 KHz) of the blade, producing mechanical hemostasis and cutting, denaturing the collagen by vibration; the main advantages are no smoke or heat production since this instrument operates at low temperatures (up to 90° F). In this study the ultrasonic scalpel was preferable to the other two instruments (see Table 7).

Undoubtedly the laparoscopic approach can be used in many cases, elective as well as acute cholecystectomies, but it should only be attempted by surgical teams or surgeons with sufficient experience.[18]

CONCLUSION

The laparoscopic approach is a minimally invasive procedure that offers distinct advantages to the patient although the phenomenon of the learning curve for a new technique is complex and occasionally problems may arise because of early inexperience. Conversion to classical cholecystectomy may be necessary to avoid serious complications.

REFERENCES

1. Thibault C, Mamazza J, Poulin EC. La cholangiopancreatographie rétrograde endoscopique dans le contexte de la cholecystectomie sous coelioscopie. Ann Chir 46:839-844, 1992.
2. Reddick EJ, Olsen DO. Laparoscopic laser cholecystectomy. Surg Endosc 3:131-133, 1989.
3. Southern Surgeons Club. A prospective analysis of 1518 laparoscopic cholecystectomies. N Engl J Med 324:1073-1078, 1991.
4. Gigot JF. Registre Belge des cholecystectomies laparoscopiques. Congress Communication. Second European Congress of Viscerosynthesis. Luxembuorg, 1992.
5. Cuschieri A, Dubois F, Mouiel J, et al. The European experience with laparoscopic cholecystectomy. Am J Surg 161:385-387, 1991.
6. Dubois F, Berthelot G, Lerard H. Cholecystectomie sous coelioscopie. Chirurgie 16:248-250, 1990.
7. Suc B, Fontes Dislaire I, Fourtanier G, Escat J. 3606 cholecystectomies sous coelioscopie. Ann Chir 46:219-266, 1992.
8. Spaw AT, Reddick EJ, Olsen DO. Laparoscopic laser cholecystectomy: Analysis of 500 procedures. Surg Laparosc Endosc 1:2-7, 1991.
9. Schirmer BD, Edge ST, Dix J, et al. Laparoscopic cholecystectomy. Ann Surg 213:665-676, 1991.
10. Peters JH, Ellison CE, Innes JT, et al. Safety and efficacy of laparoscopic cholecystectomy. Ann Surg 213:2-12, 1991.
11. Wolfe BM, Gardiner BN, Leary BF, et al. Endoscopic cholecystectomy: An analysis of complications. Arch Surg 126:1192-1198, 1991.
12. Zucker KA, Bailey RW, Gadacz TR, et al. Laparoscopic cholecystectomy: A plea for cautious enthusiasm. Am J Surg 161:36-44, 1991.
13. Berci G, Sackier JM, Paz-Partlow M. Routine or selective intraoperative cholangiography during laparoscopic cholecystectomies? Am J Surg 161:355-360, 1991.
14. Flowers JL, Zucker KA, Graham SM, et al. Laparoscopic cholangiography: Results and indications. Ann Surg 215:209-216, 1992.
15. Martinez Castro R, Moreira Vicente V, Angel Yepes V, et al. Complicaciones quirurgicas de la esfinterotomía endoscópica. Rev Esp Enf Dig 79:404-410, 1991.
16. Corbitt JA. Laparoscopic cholecystectomy: Laser versus electrocautery. Surg Laparosc Endosc 1:85-88, 1991.
17. Soper NJ. Laparoscopic cholecystectomy. Curr Probl Surg: 00:581, 1991.
18. Martin IG, Holdworth PJ, Asker JK, et al. Laparoscopic cholecystectomy as a routine procedure for gallstones: Results of an "all comers" policy. Br J Surg 79:807-810, 1992.

24 *Laparoscopic Cholecystectomy in the Management of Acute and Chronic Cholecystitis*

Jean-Michel Loubeau and Joseph C. Iraci

Since Carl Langenbuch successfully performed the first cholecystectomy in 1882, laparotomy for removal of symptomatic gallbladders has represented the mainstay of the surgical treatment of cholelithiasis and cholecystitis.

Following the lead of our colleague gynecologists and with the development of highly sophisticated technology in the field of video-assisted surgery, laparoscopic cholecystectomy has become a rapidly expanding alternative form of first-line therapy for diseases of the gallbladder. A recent survey of 1117 hospitals in the United States revealed that 77,604 laparoscopic cholecystectomies had been performed by 1992 at those institutions. In the vast majority of these hospitals, experience with less than 100 operations was reported.

Early in 1990 we made the decision to use endoscopic cholecystectomy as our first choice in the surgical treatment of symptomatic gallbladder disease.

MATERIALS AND RESULTS

As a consequence of our deliberate approach, only seven patients underwent open cholecystectomy as a primary treatment from March 1990 to May 1992, whereas laparoscopic cholecystectomy was undertaken as the initial mode of therapy in 110 individuals. There were 28 males and 82 females (range, 20 to 83 years of age) (Table 1) who underwent a laparoscopic procedure over this 26-month period.

Thirty-two patients (29%) had acute cholecystitis, reflecting the unselected nature of our patient population. The overall mortality of 0.9% (Table 2) was represented by one death in a patient who succumbed from his underlying acquired immunodeficiency syndrome (AIDS). The majority of patients with acute cholecystitis were females, although the number of males in that category was higher than in our overall population with gallbladder disease.

Intraoperative cholangiography was selectively utilized, and we relied primarily on the use of ERCP preoperatively in 16 (15%) of our patients for the confirmation and treatment of suspected common bile duct stones (see Table 2). One patient underwent postoperative endoscopic successful papillotomy for elimination of retained stones several months after laparoscopic cholecystectomy.

In 15 (14%) of the 110 patients in whom laparoscopic cholecystectomy was undertaken as the initial surgical approach, the operation was converted to an open procedure by laparotomy. Ten (67%) of these patients had acute cholecystitis. Therefore, in this unselected group of 110 patients, early in our experience with laparoscopic cholecystectomy, the procedure was successfully car-

Table 1. Patient data: March 1990-May 1992

	No.	Percent	Age (range)
Males	28	25	54 (25-83)
Females	82	75	50 (20-83)
Conventional cholecystectomy	7		
Laparoscopic cholecystectomy	110		

131

Table 2. Pathology found during laparoscopy

	No.	Percent	Females	Males
Chronic	78	71	63 (81%)	15 (19%)
Acute	32	29	19 (59%)	13 (41%)
TOTAL	110	100	82	28
Mortality		1 (0.9%)		
Preoperative ERCP		16 (15%)		
Postoperative ERCP		1		

Table 3. Conversion rate to open procedure

	No. of Patients	Open Procedure	Laparoscopy
Chronic	78	5 (6%)	73 (94%)
Acute	31	10 (31%)	22 (69%)
TOTAL	110	15 (14%)	95 (86%)

ried out in 86% of the patients, that is, 94% of cases of chronic cholecystitis and 69% of cases of acute cholecystitis (Table 3). Three of the five cases of chronic cholecystitis that were converted to laparotomy required an open procedure because of intraoperative events: one each for an inferior vena cava injury, a gastric wall injury, and a filling defect shown on intraoperative cholangiogram where preoperative ERCP had failed. Inability to perform laparoscopic cholecystectomy in cases of chronic cholecystectomy occurred in only 2 of 78 patients (3%).

DISCUSSION

In considering the group of 32 patients with acute cholecystitis, it is interesting to note that those who required laparotomy after an initial attempt at laparoscopic cholecystectomy had been hospitalized for symptoms related to their gallbladder disease for an average of 5 days before the operation. By contrast, the 22 patients with acute cholecystitis in whom the laparoscopic procedure was performed successfully had been in the hospital, on average, less than 2 days before undergoing the surgical procedure (Table 4). Drainage of the subhepatic space was very rarely established, but we relied heavily on intraoperative irrigation of the operative field.

Table 4. Preoperative days of hospitalization in acute cases

Laparotomy (10)	Laparoscopy (22)
5 days	1.9 days

Postoperatively, the average length of stay for patients undergoing laparoscopic cholecystectomy was 1.7 days for chronic cholecystitis and 2.8 days for acute cholecystitis. One 70-year-old female in the latter group who had a previous history of deep vein thrombosis developed recurrent DVT in spite of prophylactic measures and was hospitalized for 10 days following laparoscopic cholecystectomy. Two other significant complications occurred in the chronic group after discharge: one 83-year-old female developed an umbilical hernia and a 63-year-old female was readmitted 3 days after discharge with acute right upper quadrant pain. A hepatobiliary scan in the latter patient suggested a small bile leak, but the symptoms subsided within 24 hours and no further treatment was required.

Table 5. Cases of chronic versus acute cholecystitis

	Chronic	Acute
Females	63 (81%)	19 (59%)
Males	15 (19%)	13 (41%)
TOTAL	78	32

It is interesting to speculate on the relatively higher incidence of acute cholecystitis in males (Table 5). It may be that the disease more readily effects a virulent form in men or, conversely, that warning signals of a chronic nature are ignored in that group reported to have a much lower incidence of gallbladder disease.

CONCLUSION

Although laparoscopic cholecystectomy has gained wide acceptance among surgeons in the treatment of symptomatic gallbladder disease, until recently acute cholecystitis was considered a relatively strong contraindication for laparoscopic surgery. Others have reported on the hazards and safety of laparoscopic cholecystectomy in cases of acute inflammation.[2-4]

In our series of consecutive, unselected cases, conversion to an open procedure was five times more likely in acute than chronic cholecystitis, although it was still successfully carried out in over two thirds of cases of acute inflammation. Furthermore, an analysis of our data suggests that a "golden period" of 48 hours exists after onset of acute symptoms, during which a laparoscopic procedure is much more likely to succeed.

REFERENCES

1. Cooperman A. Laparoscopic cholecystectomy for severe acute, embedded and gangrenous cholecystitis. J Laparoendoscop Surg 1:37, 1990.
2. Peters JH. Safety and efficacy of laparoscopic cholecystectomy: A prospective analysis of 100 initial patients. Ann Surg 213:3, 1991.
3. Ferzli G, Kloss DA. Laparoscopic cholecystectomy in both chronic and acute cholecystitis: A report of 165 consecutive cases. Contemp Surg 40:17, 1992.
4. Deziel DJ, Millikan KW, Economou, SG, Doolas A, Ko ST, Airan MC. Complications of laparoscopic cholecystectomy: National survey of 4,292 hospitals and analysis of 77,604 cases. Am J Surg 165:9, 1993.

25 *Laparoscopic Cholecystectomy in Complicated Gallstone Disease*

Christian J. Lukosch, Andreas Schäfer, and Martin Hürtgen

Laparoscopic cholecystectomy was first performed in France.[1,2] Greater patient comfort, better cosmetic results, a shortened hospital stay, and earlier return to full activity made the laparoscopic cholecystectomy the method of choice for patients with gallbladder disease.[3-5]

Common bile duct injuries during laparoscopic cholecystectomy appear to have a higher incidence than during open cholecystectomy. To avoid this, some authors suggest that intraoperative cholangiography routinely be performed.[6] We routinely perform preoperative intravenous cholangiographies for evaluation of bile duct stones and abnormalities. We perform intraoperative cholangiography only in patients with a cystic duct stone and a high risk of passing the stone into the common bile duct.

Complicated gallstone disease represents a relative contraindication to laparoscopic cholecystectomy.[7] The aim of our study was to evaluate our experiences with the laparoscopic cholecystectomy in complicated gallstone disease and patient safety with this procedure.

MATERIALS AND METHODS

Between January 1990 and August 1992 we performed 319 laparoscopic cholecystectomies at Justus-Liebig

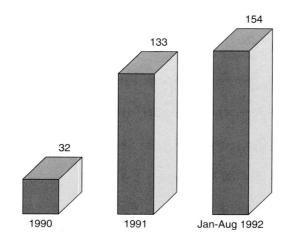

Fig. 1. Number of laparoscopic cholecystectomies per year in our series.

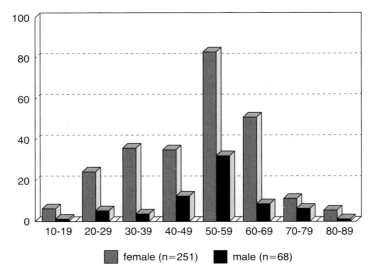

Fig. 2. Distribution by age and sex (n = 319).

University. The number of these procedures we perform has increased steadily: in 1990 we performed 32 procedures, in 1991 133, and in the first eight months of 1992, 154 (Fig. 1). Patients averaged 56.2 years of age (range, 13 to 87); 78.7 percent were women. The highest number of procedures was done in female patients aged 50 to 59 years (Fig. 2).

PREOPERATIVE DIAGNOSIS AND IMAGING

History, physical examination, and a blood chemistry workup are important; ultrasonography, generally performed by the surgeon, was used in all patients for documentation of disease. Preoperative intravenous cholangiography experienced a renaissance; the procedure included 5 mm or thinner tomographies of the bile duct area. It was routinely performed for exclusion of common bile duct stones and to determine anatomical variations. We also performed an upper intestinoscopy. If duct stones are suspected, we proceed to an endoscopic retrograde cholangiography. In the presence of stones, a sphincterotomy and stone extraction are performed. After control ERCP is performed, we proceed with the laparoscopic cholecystectomy.

OPERATIVE TECHNIQUES

After a small skin incision, a Veress needle is introduced percutaneously near the umbilicus. Aspiration of blood, urine, or intestinal contents would indicate improper placement of the needle; however, these complications did not occur. The so-called drop test is performed by placing a drop of saline solution within the open lumen of the insufflation needle. As the needle enters the peritoneal cavity, the relative negative intraabdominal pressure pulls the fluid through the needle. For insufflation we use CO_2 gas, which is relatively innocuous to the patient. The insufflation instrument is usually set at a maximum pressure of 15 mm Hg. After insufflation we verify the degree of pneumoperitoneum by probing with a thin needle in an aspiration-like technique.

The skin incision is enlarged and a 10 mm trocar for the laparoscope with attached camera is inserted. Three additional trocars for various laparoscopic surgical instruments are placed in the right middle abdomen (5 mm), the epigastric region (5 mm) and the left middle abdomen (10 mm). These accessory trocars and sheaths are inserted into the abdominal cavity under direct laparoscopic vision.

After the placement of the accessory trocars and sheaths, the patient is moved to a 30-degree Trendelenburg position and turned to the left. The entire length of the cystic duct and artery are exposed, with special attention to the junction of the common bile duct and any variations of the vessels. We use titanium clips for ligation of the cystic duct and artery, and if possible for the central ligation of the cystic duct we use a resorbable clip. The gallbladder is dissected from the liver bed by monopolar electrocautery or sometimes by laser. The dissection begins near the mobilized gallbladder neck and proceeds superiorly along the medial and lateral attachment to the liver bed. One forceps is placed proximal to the cystic duct clips and is used to retract the gallbladder neck cephalad and anterior. It is important to keep the gallbladder on tension. The gallbladder is routinely removed from the abdominal cavity through the left middle abdominal incision.

RESULTS
Locally Complicated Gallstone Disease

One or more locally complicated findings were present in 169/319 (52.9%) of the patients who underwent laparoscopic cholecystectomy in our series. Chronic inflammation with adhesions to the omentum majus and neighboring organs was present in 101 cases, acute cholecystitis in 39 cases; 25 patients had an occluding stone in the ductus cysticus. In 19 cases hydrops was present

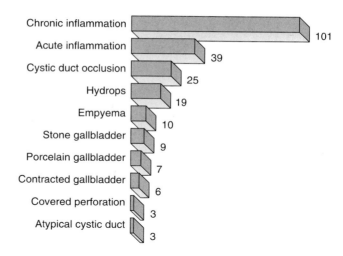

Fig. 3. Locally complicated gallstone disease: distribution of findings.

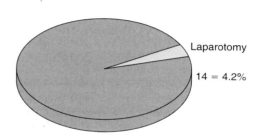

Fig. 4. Conversions to open cholecystectomy.

and in 10 cases an empyema was noted. We encountered a stone gallbladder nine times, a porcelain gallbladder seven times, and an atrophied gallbladder six times. In three cases a covered perforation was seen; three times an atypical form of the common bile duct was found (Fig. 3).

Adhesions

In 73/319 laparoscopically operated patients, we found significant adhesions that had resulted from prior surgery; in 48/73 we performed laparoscopic adhesiolysis. Adhesiolysis was always performed in cases with a history of abdominal pain resulting from adhesions.

Conversion to Open Cholecystectomy

Conversion from laparoscopic to conventional open cholecystectomy had to be performed in 14/333 cases (4.2%) (Fig. 4). The reasons for conversion were gallbladder carcinoma (4), extensive postoperative adhe-

Table 1. Reasons for conversion to open cholecystectomy

Condition	No.
Gallbladder carcinoma	4
Extensive postoperative adhesions	3
Acute cholecystitis	2
Empyematous gallbladder with perforation	2
Gangrenous cholecystitis	1
Injury of the common bile duct	1
Rupture of cystic duct	1
TOTAL	14 (4.2%)

sions (3), acute cholecystitis (2), empyematous gallbladder with perforation (2), gangrenous cholecystitis (1), injury of the common bile duct (1), and rupture of the cystic duct (Table 1).

Complications

A total of 12/319 (3.8 %) complications were reported. No patient died.

Extreme bradycardia during the insufflation procedure was seen in two patients (2/319, 0.06%) with medical histories of cardiac problems. In one of the two cases the procedure had to be interrupted because of this. The patient underwent conventional cholecystectomy 3 days later.

Major complications occurred in one case (1/319, 0.3%), a patient with a shrunken gallbladder. The choledochous duct was completely disrupted. This complication was repaired by a choledochojejunostomy. The patient's postoperative course was without further complications.

Local complications were seen in the area of the gallbladder extraction site, the left middle abdomen, in seven patients (7/319, 2.1%). At the site of trocar incision three patients developed a wound infection, two a seroma, and one a hematoma. In one case a hernia occurred at the site of trocar insertion.

Late complications occurred in two cases (2/319, 0.6%). In one case stones in the common bile duct were found 3 months after laparoscopic cholecystectomy. Prospectively and retrospectively, the preoperative intravenous cholangiography was judged to be normal. This patient underwent an open revision of the com-

mon bile duct at another hospital. One patient with a history of non-Hodgkins lymphoma and who underwent postoperative chemotherapy developed a bilioma 5 months after the cholecystectomy. The bilioma was treated by percutaneous CT-guided drainage.

DISCUSSION

Laparoscopic cholecystectomy has several advantages over traditional laparotomy cholecystectomy. As with any new surgical procedure, there must be critical assessment of the related complications. The rate of bile duct injury during laparoscopic cholecystectomy in our patient group with complicated gallstone disease was 0.6% (1/169); the overall rate of bile duct injury in this series was 0.3% (1/319). The incidence of bile duct injury not recognized at the time of the initial surgery was zero. The exact frequency of bile duct injury as a consequence of conventional cholecystectomy is uncertain, but such injury probably occurs in 0.1% to 0.2%.[8-10] The remission rate was 0.9%. The remission rates in two series of conventional cholecystectomies were 3% and 5%.[11,12]

An important issue for a successful laparoscopic cholecystectomy is high-quality preoperative intravenous cholangiography with thin tomograms of the bile duct. This allows one to rule out the presence of bile duct stones with a high degree of accuracy, and time-consuming intraoperative cholangiography can thus be avoided in most cases. Only in cases of cystic duct stones with a high risk of passing stones into the common bile duct do we conduct intraoperative cholangiography. Another advantage of this approach is the preoperative detection of bile duct anomalies. If bile duct stones are found, we proceed with endoscopic retrograde cholangiography and, if indicated, sphincterotomy. If the control endoscopic retrograde cholangiography shows clear bile ducts, we perform laparoscopic cholecystectomy.

Cautery and laser dissection are equally good methods for removal of the gallbladder from the hepatic bed. Because of the lower cost, we prefer cautery.

We feel that locally complicated gallstone disease is not a contraindication to laparoscopic cholecystectomy. Patients with locally complicated gallstone disease benefit from this new procedure but do not face a considerably higher risk of complications. Nonetheless, laparoscopic cholecystectomy must be considered a major surgical procedure, and the following are requisite: an experienced surgeon, clear exposure of the anatomy, and conversion to cholecystectomy if any doubts arise.

REFERENCES

1. DuBois F, Icard P, Berthelot G, Levard H. Coelioscopic cholecystectomy: Preliminary report of 36 cases. Ann Surg 211:60-62, 1990.
2. Reddick EJ, Olsen DO. Laparoscopic laser cholecystectomy: A comparison with mini-lap cholecystectomy. Surg Endosc 3:131-133, 1989.
3. The Southern Surgeons Club. A prospective analysis of 1518 laparoscopic cholecystectomies. N Engl J Med 324:1073-1078, 1991.
4. Grace P, Quereshi A, Darzi A, McEntee G, Leahy A, Osborne H, Lynch G, Lane B, Broe P, Bouchier-Hayes D. Laparoscopic cholecystectomy: A hundred consecutive cases. Ir Med J 84:12-14, 1991.
5. Klaiber C, Metzger A, Leepin H, Saager C. Laparoscopic cholecystectomy: 100 consecutive cases without postoperative morbidity. Schweiz Med Wochenschr 121:898-902, 1991.
6. Hunter JG. Avoidance of bile duct injury during laparoscopic cholecystectomy. Am J Surg 162:71-76, 1991.
7. Zucker KA. Laparoscopic guided cholecystectomy with electrocautery dissection. In Zucker KA, Bailey RW. Surgical Laparoscopy. St. Louis: Quality Medical Publishing, Inc, 1991, p 143.
8. Viikari SJ. Operative injuries to the bile ducts. Acta Chir Scand 119:83-92, 1960.
9. Raute M, Schaupp W. Iatrogenic damage of the bile ducts caused by cholecystectomy. Langenbecks Arch Chir 373:345-354, 1988.
10. Meyers WC, Jones RS, eds. Textbook of Liver and Biliary Surgery. Philadelphia: JB Lippincott, 1990, p 373.
11. Roos LL Jr, Cageorge SM, Roos NP, Danzinger R. Centralization, certification, and monitoring: Readmissions and complications after surgery. Med Care 24: 1044-1066, 1986.
12. Cohen MM, Young TK, Hammarstrand KM. Ethnic variation in cholecystectomy rates and outcomes. Manitoba, Canada, 1972-1984. Am J Public Health 79:751-755, 1989.

26   *Laparoscopic Cholecystectomy After Previous Laparotomy*

T. Madhusudan and Steven J. Snooks

Many patients requiring laparoscopic cholecystectomy have previously undergone a laparotomy through an upper or lower midline incision with upward extension for a variety of abdominal and pelvic procedures.[1] Intra-abdominal adhesions are a recognized complication of previous laparotomy and pose some degree of difficulty and danger to the performance of laparoscopy.[2] Adhesions can be very vascular and, if injured, can cause intra-abdominal bleeding and impair the surgeon's view.[3] They can also interfere with correct insufflation of the peritoneal cavity and creation of a pneumoperitoneum.[4] Patients with a previous operation have a high likelihood of having intestines adherent to the anterior abdominal wall, thereby making blind trocar insertions and insufflation dangerous.[5]

In 1971 Hasson[6] described the procedure of open laparoscopy using a metallic port. The advantage of the open laparoscopy technique is that access to the peritoneal cavity can be unequivocally established before insufflation, thus avoiding the problems described above.[7]

We present a study of 10 patients in a consecutive series of 80 patients who underwent laparoscopic cholecystectomy and who had previously undergone laparotomy involving a midline incision. The aim of the study was to assess the effectiveness of the Hasson technique of open laparoscopy, using the Hasson laparoscopic cannula (Ethicon), for the creation of a pneumoperitoneum in patients who had undergone previous laparotomy for various procedures with possible intra-abdominal adhesions. In them the blind introduction of a Veress needle is associated with considerable risk.

OPEN LAPAROSCOPY METHOD

Open laparoscopy uses a small 2 cm infraumbilical incision to advance the cannula and laparoscope into the peritoneal cavity under continuous visual control. It does not use a Veress needle to create the pneumoperitoneum or a sharp trocar to introduce the initial laparoscopy cannula.[8]

EQUIPMENT

Standard laparoscopic equipment is used except for the primary laparoscopy cannula. Instead, the Hasson laparoscopic cannula, which is a disposable modification of the one described by Hasson, is used. It consists of a 10 mm trocar and cannula fitted with a cone-shaped sleeve that moves freely but can be locked in any position along the cannula's shaft. A blunt obturator replaces the sharp trocar. Two suture-holder flanges are mounted near the proximal end of the cannula to help retain it on the abdominal wall (Figs. 1 through 5).

TECHNIQUE

After satisfactory anesthesia has been achieved in the patient, a 2 cm infraumbilical transverse incision is made and is extended down to the peritoneum, which is exposed. Two stay sutures are applied to the peritoneum at the 3 o'clock and 11 o'clock positions, and the peritoneum is incised between them. The index finger is introduced into the peritoneal opening and swept around to make sure that no major viscera are adherent just under it.

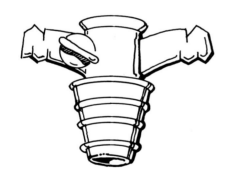

Fig. 1. Hasson cone-shaped sleeve.

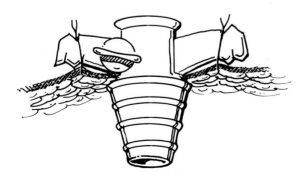

Fig. 2. Hasson sleeve position after fixation on the abdominal wall.

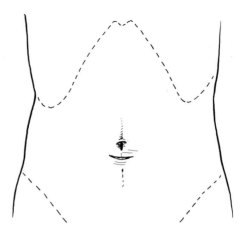

Fig. 3. Infraumbilical transverse incision.

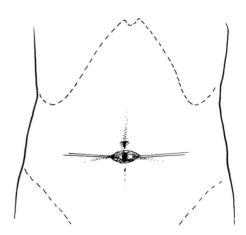

Fig. 4. Stay sutures on peritoneum at the 3 and 9 o'clock positions.

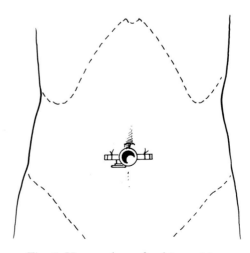

Fig. 5. Hasson sleeve fixed in position.

The cone sleeve is adjusted and locked in an appropriate position on to the shaft to accommodate the thickness of the abdominal wall. The cannula with its blunt obturator is inserted into the peritoneal cavity between the stay sutures. The fascial sutures are pulled snugly into the suture-holder flange. This maneuver pulls the fascia against the cone and provides an airtight seal, thus preventing escape of gas.

The trocar is removed and CO_2 is insufflated through the valve of the cannula to create a pneumoperitoneum. After establishment of adequate pneumoperitoneum, a lighted laparoscope is introduced and the procedure continued as for routine laparoscopy. When laparoscopy has been completed, the instrument is withdrawn, the cavity deflated, and the abdominal wall closed in layers.

RESULTS

In a consecutive series of 80 patients who underwent laparoscopic cholecystectomy in Barking Hospital, Redbridge Health Authority, between August 1991 and June 1992, we used this technique in 10 patients who had undergone a previous laparotomy through a midline or paramedian incision that extended into the upper abdomen.

Of the 10 patients, five had undergone abdominal hysterectomy through an extended midline incision. Three patients had laparotomy for peritonitis of appendicular origin, one patient had a sigmoid colectomy and hepatic resection for carcinoma of the sigmoid with a solitary liver metastasis, and the other patient, apart

from being obese, had previously undergone a bilateral truncal vagotomy and pyloroplasty for peptic ulcer disease (Table 1).

We found the method was successful in all 10 patients, although its use increased the operating time as compared to a routine laparoscopic cholecystectomy. There was no difference in the postoperative morbidity, wound complication, or pain, and the length of stay was not prolonged. There were no signs of any intra-abdominal organ injury either at the time of the procedure or during follow-up postoperatively, which we did up to 3 months.

CONCLUSION

We conclude that laparoscopic cholecystectomy and also other laparoscopic procedures can be very safely performed in patients who have previously undergone a laparotomy and have a high chance of having intra-abdominal adhesions by using the procedure of open laparoscopy as described by Hasson using a modified Hasson open laparoscopic cannula. Thus the need for these patients to undergo open cholecystectomy, as was previously believed, is avoided.

REFERENCES

1. Cuschieri A. Laparoscopy in general surgery and gastro-enterology. Br J Hosp Med 24:252-258, 1980.
2. Cuschieri A, Berci G. Laparoscopic Biliary Surgery. London: Blackwell Scientific, 1990.
3. Berci G, Cuschieri A. Creation of pneumoperitoneum. In Berci G, Cuschieri A, eds. Practical Laparoscopy. London: Baillière Tindall, 1986, pp 44-66.
4. Daniell JF. Laparoscopic enterolysis for chronic abdominal pain. J Gynaecol Surg 5:61-65, 1989.
5. Reddick EJ, Olsen DO, Spain A, et al. Safe performance of difficult laparoscopic cholecystectomies. Am J Surg 161:377-381, 1991.
6. Hasson HM. A modified instrument and method for laparoscopy. Am J Obstet Gynaecol 110:886-887, 1971.
7. Hasson HM. Open laparoscopy versus closed laparoscopy. A comparison of complication rates. Adv Planned Parenthood 13:41-43, 1978.
8. Semm K. Operative manual for endoscopic abdominal surgery. Chicago: Year Book, 1987, pp 95-102.

Table 1. Previous operations with laparotomy

Operation	No. of Patients
Abdominal hysterectomy	5
Appendicular peritonitis	3
Sigmoid colectomy and hepatic resection	1
Vagotomy and pyloroplasty	1

27 Common Bile Duct Examination at Laparoscopic Cholecystectomy

Siegfried Beller, Gerhard Szinicz, and Kurt Erhart

Today laparoscopic cholecystectomy is the surgical treatment of choice for cholecystolithiasis. In many surgical departments, however, minimally invasive surgery of the bile ducts is not yet performed, and the presence of ductal calculi is still regarded as a contraindication for the laparoscopic approach. Over the past years, therefore, numerous authors have dealt with diagnostic imaging of the biliary ducts before or during laparoscopic cholecystectomy.

With such noninvasive methods as history taking, clinical examination, liver enzymes, and ultrasound, biliary duct stones can be detected with a sensitivity of 90%. Routine use of preoperative ERCP can detect ductal stones not diagnosed by noninvasive procedures in another 3% of patients. This benefit, however, is counterbalanced by the risk of iatrogenic pancreatitis (approximately 3% as well) and by the additional stress for the patient.

We have prospectively studied the sensitivity of preoperative intravenous cholangiography and the practicability of operative cholangiography during laparoscopic cholecystectomy.

Preoperative intravenous cholangiography yielded sufficient contrasting of the common bile duct with correct results in only 64 of 100 cases. Intraoperative cholangiography during laparoscopic cholecystectomy, on the other hand, was successful in 95 of 100 cases. Without intraoperative imaging three cases of choledocholithiasis would have been missed.

For these reasons we have discontinued intravenous cholangiography. We routinely perform intraoperative cholangiography instead and have been successful now in 250 consecutive cases with only one exception. The chance to recognize anatomical variations is yet another argument for this strategy, since injuries of the bile duct system can be avoided or diagnosed intraoperatively and then repaired immediately.

We have performed laparoscopic surgery of the common bile duct in 18 patients. In 16 cases choledochal calculi could be removed successfully. The stones were extracted through a choledochotomy in 3 cases, via the cystic duct in 8 cases, and five times they could be pushed into the duodenum with a balloon catheter. In only one case a laparotomy had to be performed, in one other case a stone had to be removed by postoperative ERCP and sphincterotomy.

This success rate of 89% for removal of choledochal calculi by minimally invasive surgical techniques appears to justify the laparoscopic approach to cholecystectomy without prior ERCP, even if there is a suspicion of ductal stones. The advantages of this strategy are evident: the integrity of the sphincter of Oddi can be preserved and the patient does not have to undergo two procedures.

The probability that both laparoscopic and endoscopic techniques fail to remove ductal stones and that open operation will have to be performed is very low. This situation has not yet occurred in our department. We do, however, inform our patients about this remote possibility.

28 *Laparoscopic Intraoperative Cholangiography*

Douglas O. Olsen

Surgical removal of the gallbladder has remained the gold standard for treatment of symptomatic gallstones since it was originally described in 1894. The procedure has been refined over the years to afford a safe and effective means of treating gallbladder disease. Despite this, the search for a less invasive means of treating cholelithiasis has continued. In 1989, our report of laparoscopic cholecystectomy was published describing a minimally invasive technique to remove the gallbladder surgically.[1] This report, along with earlier ones, was confined to select groups of patients and excluded those with common duct pathology. Shortly after the initial report of laparoscopic cholecystectomy, the first technique of laparoscopic intraoperative cholangiography was described, giving the laparoscopic surgeon the option and ability to evaluate a patient's common bile duct intraoperatively.[2] This set the stage for the laparoscopic management of common duct stones.

Intraoperative cholangiography was first described by Mirizzi[3] in 1937 and has been used routinely for evaluation of the common duct prior to biliary surgery. Although many have advocated the use of intraoperative cholangiography as a routine part of cholecystectomy, some would argue that routine cholangiography is not cost effective.[4-10] All surgeons, however, would agree that cholangiography does play some role in the operative management of gallbladder disease. It is therefore a technique that all biliary tract surgeons should have the ability to perform.

TECHNIQUE

The procedure begins after the surgeon has isolated a length of cystic duct high on the neck of the gallbladder. By releasing the serosal attachments of the gallbladder near the infundibulum, the surgeon can make certain that the common duct has not been mistakenly dissected out, confusing it with the cystic duct (Fig. 1). If the cystic duct is markedly shortened, the cholangiogram can be done through the gallbladder itself. Cystic duct cholangiography is generally preferred over gallbladder cholangiography, since the latter may not be possible in as many as 20% to 30% of patients because of acute cholecystitis and hydrops of the gallblad-

der. With the junction of the cystic duct and the neck of the gallbladder identified, a clip is placed across the neck to prevent any stones from passing down into the cystic duct with further manipulation of the tissues. Before placement of the clip, the cystic duct is milked back toward the gallbladder to clear any small stones that might be present in the cystic duct. If the cystic duct is particularly short, the clip can be omitted to allow the cholangiocatheter to be placed as high as possible on the cystic duct. Traction and exposure are maintained on the gallbladder, with one grasper on the fundus and one on Hartmann's pouch. If an Olsen cholangiogram clamp is available (Karl Storz), the approach to the cystic duct is made through one of the lateral ports (Fig. 2). Exposure is maintained with graspers placed through the epigastric port and the remaining lateral port. Scissors are introduced through the same port that will be used to introduce the cholangiogram clamp and are used to make a small incision in the cystic duct. After the incision is made, the clamp is preloaded with a cath-

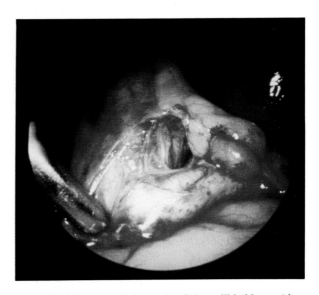

Fig. 1. Mobilization of the neck of the gallbladder to identify its junction with the cystic duct.

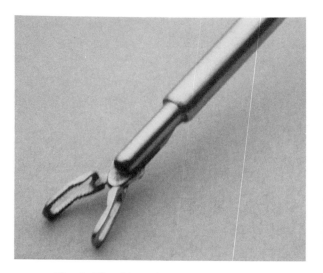

Fig. 2. The Olsen cholangiogram clamp.

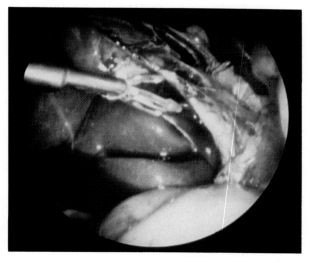

Fig. 3. The catheter is advanced through the clamp and placed in the cystic duct at a right angle.

eter and introduced into the abdomen. Although the clamp can be used with a variety of catheters, we prefer a mushroom-tip catheter such as the Taut catheter (Taut Inc.) or the Cook catheter (Cook Surgical, Inc.). Initially these catheters were available in only one size, which was often too large for some ducts. These mushroom catheters are now available in a smaller size that will fit even the smallest of ducts. The mushroom has the advantage of stabilizing the catheter in the duct, making it less likely to be dislodged during cholangiography. With the clamp introduced into the abdomen, the catheter is advanced just beyond the end of the clamp and placed into the small incision that has already been made in the duct (Fig. 3). Approaching the duct at a perpendicular angle makes the initial introduction of the catheter easier. With the tip of the catheter in the duct, more of the catheter is advanced beyond the clamp, and a slight bend is placed in the catheter allowing the catheter to come into alignment with the duct. This allows the surgeon to advance the catheter further into the duct. The clamp is advanced over the catheter and the jaws are "clamped" over the cystic duct in a perpendicular manner (Fig. 4). This secures the catheter in the duct and prevents any leakage of contrast material. The cholangiogram is shot in the usual manner by means of either a static film technique or fluoroscopy if available. The new digital fluoroscopy units yield high-quality films with the advantage of a dynamic study. Since identification of the ductal anatomy is one

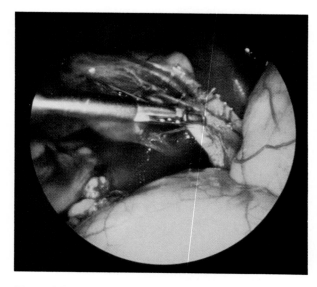

Fig. 4. The catheter is bent into alignment with the cystic duct allowing it to be advanced down the cystic duct and secured with the clamp.

of the advantages of cholangiography, it is important to attempt to fill the common hepatic duct along with the hepatic radicals. A forceful injection of contrast medium is usually sufficient to fill the radicals with little difficulty. When using a static film technique, a two-

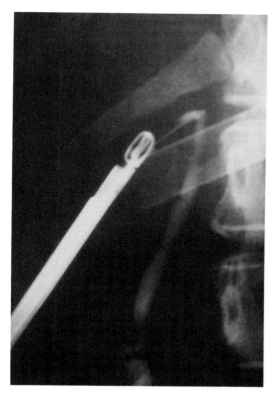

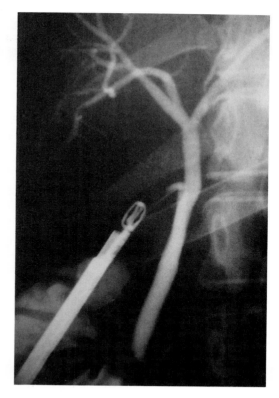

Fig. 5. First shot of a two-shot cholangiogram showing fine filling and detail of the distal common duct.

Fig. 6. Second shot of a two-shot cholangiogram showing anatomy of the biliary tree.

shot cholangiogram is preferred. The first injection is given with approximately 5 ml of full-strength contrast medium followed immediately by a second injection of approximately 12 ml of full-strength contrast medium. The first injection of 5 ml will allow faint visualization of the distal common duct and cystic duct (Fig. 5), providing a good view of fine detail and any small stones that may be present within these structures. The second larger injection fills out the ductal anatomy (Fig. 6), allowing identification of not only the ductal anatomy but any filling defects in the upper system. The use of radiolucent disposable trocars in the midclavicular and epigastric positions will eliminate the problem of obscuring underlying anatomy with overlying hardware.

If a cholangiogram clamp is not available, a percutaneous technique can be used. This entails passing the catheter through a needle sheath as a separate puncture, a *fifth* access site. Since this is made with a 14-gauge needle, trauma to the patient is minimal. The needle is

placed in such a way that the catheter will be entering the abdominal cavity along the same axis as the cystic duct, facilitating passage of the catheter down the cystic duct (Fig. 7). After the catheter is passed through the needle sheath into the abdominal cavity (Fig. 8), scissors are introduced into the abdominal cavity through the epigastric trocar and are used to make a small incision in the cystic duct. Again, the cystic duct is isolated high on the neck of the gallbladder to eliminate the possibility of mistaking the common duct for the cystic duct. A grasper is used to direct the tip of the catheter into the cystic duct incision and advance the catheter down the duct. The catheter is secured with a clip (Fig. 9), taking care not to overcrimp the clip. This is accomplished by injecting saline through the catheter as the clip is closed. Crimping of the clip is discontinued just as resistance to flow is felt. The new Taut catheters have a metal insert at the tip of the catheter that prevents overcrimping from occluding the catheter. The injection sequence is the same as that described previously.

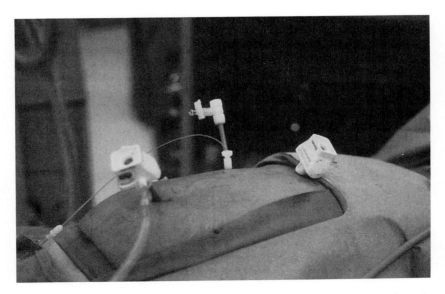

Fig. 7. The catheter is passed through a needle sheath as a *fifth* puncture to introduce the catheter into the abdominal cavity.

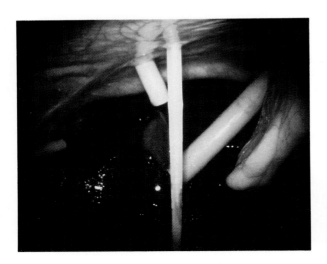

Fig. 8. The catheter is introduced through the needle sheath and manipulated with a grasper within the abdominal cavity to pass the catheter down the cystic duct.

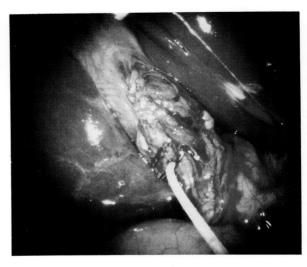

Fig. 9. The catheter is secured in the cystic duct with a partially closed clip.

The clip is easily removed by grasping the hub of the clip and pulling it backward. Once the clip and catheter have been removed, laparoscopic cholecystectomy is carried out in the usual manner.

Other catheters have become available to facilitate laparoscopic cholangiography. The balloon catheter was modified from a vascular irrigation catheter and often will work. Because the balloon catheter relies on the cystic duct to secure the catheter when the balloon is distended, the catheter has its limitations when the catheter cannot be completely passed down the duct or when the cystic duct is short. Ureteral catheters work well, but because of the side hole, the catheter once again is limited in that it must be passed down into the cystic duct far enough to occlude the side hole. The mushroom catheters need only be wedged into the hole in the cystic duct and held in place with either the clamp or a clip. Because of their rigidity, metal catheters are easier to manipulate, but they do not conform easily to the slight variations that often occur with trocar placement or differences in anatomy. This can increase the potential for trauma to the cystic duct.

With the wide variety of catheters and techniques available, all surgeons should be able to find a system that works well for them, allowing cholangiography to be performed whenever indicated.

STRATEGY

When considering the indications for cholangiography, we are first confronted with the issue of a routine versus a selective approach. There are advocates for both views,[4-11] and the issues have been debated since the first description of operative cholangiography. There are both absolute and relative indications for intraoperative cholangiography (see the box). These indications are independent of the issue of a routine versus a selective approach.

The case for selective cholangiography is based to a large extent on the issue of cost effectiveness. This combined with the additional time and skill required to perform cholangiography makes selective cholangiography very appealing. When choosing selective cholangiography on the basis of the clinical and anatomical indicators, the surgeon should be performing cholangiography in at least 10% to 15% of his or her patients. This figure correlates with the incidence of symptomatic common bile duct stones. As patient age increases, so does the incidence of common bile duct stones and likewise the number of cholangiography procedures that should be performed even with a selective approach (see Table 1). If one then considers the degree of uncertainty with clinical indicators, it is easy to see how the number increases to 30% to 40% of patients undergoing cholecystectomy who should undergo selective cholangiography.[4,8] One of the biggest problems with a selective approach is that the surgeon often does not use or ignores clinical criteria and performs cholangiography too infrequently.

There are a number of advantages to performing

INDICATIONS FOR CHOLANGIOGRAPHY

1. Stone in the common duct on ultrasonography or roentgenography
2. Obstructive jaundice
3. Dilation of the common duct more than 1.2 cm
4. Previous cholangitis
5. Preoperative pancreatitis

From Bogokowsky H, Slutzki S, et al. Selective operative cholangiography. Surg Gynecol Obstet 164:124-126, 1987. Reproduced with permission.

Table 1. Incidence of bile duct stones at cholecystectomy according to age

Age (yr)	All Patients/ No. With Stones	Percent
10-20	25/4	16
21-30	92/11	12
31-40	226/21	9
41-50	325/28	9
51-60	473/67	14
61-70	275/85	31
71-80	116/56	48
81-90	11/10	96
TOTAL	1543/282	18

From Hermann R. Surgery for acute and chronic cholecystitis. Surg Clin North Am 70:1263-1275, 1990. Reproduced with permission.

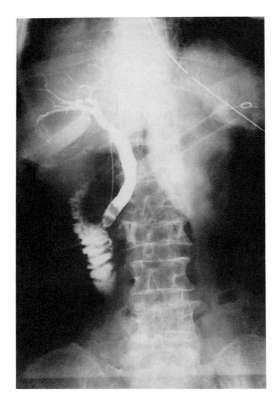

Fig. 10. Cholangiogram showing incidental stones found during routine cholangiography.

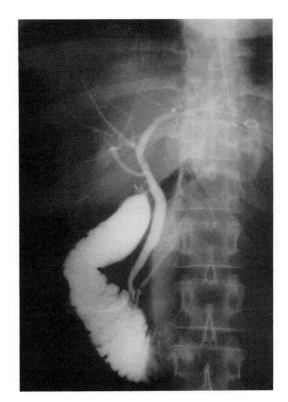

Fig. 11. Cholangiogram demonstrating an accessory right hepatic duct.

routine cholangiography. Classical reasons such as decreased incidence of retained common bile duct stones, decreased negative outcome of common duct explorations, and identification of incidental common bile duct stones should certainly not be forgotten (Fig. 10). Studies suggest that as many as one third of all common bile duct stones will be asymptomatic.[4-6] A policy of selective cholangiography will miss most if not all of these cases. Although as many as 80% to 90%[6-10] of these incidental stones will eventually be passed, a number of them will remain and cause symptoms at a later time. For the laparoscopic surgeon who wishes to examine the common bile duct laparoscopically, routine cholangiography is essential! But even with the importance of locating and diagnosing incidental common bile duct stones, the primary reason for considering routine cholangiography is to avoid injury of the common bile duct. With a policy of dissection high on the neck of the gall-

bladder and then use of cholangiography to verify that the proximal anatomy is normal and free of stones, the surgeon can avoid unnecessary dissection down near the common duct. This will not only reduce the risk of tearing and devascularization injuries of the common duct, but will also decrease the problem of bleeding in an area that can not only be difficult to control but can also lead to injuries in and of itself. If the surgeon loses anatomical orientation and mistakenly dissects out the common duct instead of the cystic duct, the cholangiogram will avoid the devastating injury that would occur if cholangiography were not performed—that is, excision of a segment of common duct. This has been reported to be the most common type of bile duct injury with laparoscopic cholecystectomy.[12] Identification of aberrant anatomy is also a strong argument in favor of routine cholangiography[13] (Fig. 11). Even if the surgeon successfully identifies the cystic duct, the upward traction on the gallbladder that occurs with laparoscopic cholecystectomy puts any structure that is lying in the triangle of Calot in jeopardy as the surgeon begins dissecting the gallbladder off the liver bed. Identifying an anomaly in the anatomy will alert the surgeon and if a question arises, will allow the necessary steps to be taken to avoid an injury.

The real question when considering the issue of selective versus routine cholangiography is whether the one major bile duct injury that may be prevented or the occasional incidental stones that are found with a policy of routine cholangiography makes it worth the extra time and expense. I think it does.

RESULTS

The results of routine cholangiography are very similar to those reported for standard intraoperative cholangiography in open cholecystectomy. In a review of 1059 cases of laparoscopic cholecystectomy, an average of 88 minutes was added to the total operating time, with an 89% success rate in performing the cholangiography. In 5% of patients, unsuspected stones were found by cholangiography. If one considers that these numbers include early experiences when cholangiography had not yet been described, it is easy to see that the technique can be performed even more efficiently with experience. In fact, in a retrospective review of 100 consecutive procedures performed in 1991, we achieved a 97% success rate with cholangiography. With the use of digital fluoroscopy, the average time needed to perform cholangiography was decreased from 20 minutes to less than 10 minutes.

Cholangiography will always play a role in cholecystectomy, and it behooves the surgeon to become proficient in the technique. The *selective* cholangiographer will look for indications to perform the procedure, whereas the *routine* cholangiographer will look for contraindications.

REFERENCES

1. Reddick EJ, Olsen DO, et al. Laparoscopic laser cholecystectomy. Laser Med Surg News Advances 71:38-40, 1989.
2. Reddick EJ, Olsen DO. Laparoscopic cholecystectomy: A comparison with mini-lap cholecystectomy. Surg Endosc 3:131-133, 1989.
3. Mirizzi PL. Operative cholangiography. Surg Gynecol Obstet 65:702-710, 1937.
4. Rolfsmeyer E, Bubrick M, et al. The value of operative cholangiography. Surg Gynecol Obstet 154:369-371, 1982.
5. Hermann R. Surgery for acute and chronic cholecystitis. Surg Clin North Am 70:1263-1275, 1990.
6. Mofti AB, Ahmed I, et al. Routine use of selective perioperative cholangiography. Br J Surg 73:548-550, 1986.
7. Pasquale M, Nauta R. Selective vs routine use of intraoperative cholangiography. Arch Surg 124:1041-1042, 1989.
8. Wilson TG, Hall JC, McWatts J. Is operative cholangiography always necessary? Br J Surg 73:637-640, 1986.
9. Nauta R. Selective vs routine use of intraoperative cholangiography. Arch Surg 124:1041, 1989.
10. Gerber A. A requiem for routine operative cholangiogram. Surg Gynecol Obstet 163:363, 1986.
11. Shively E, Wieman J, et al. Operative cholangiography. Am J Surg 159:380-385, 1990.
12. Davidoff A, Pappas T, et al. Mechanisms of major biliary injury during laparoscopic cholecystectomy. Ann Surg 215:195-202, 1992.
13. Champetier J, Lietoublon C, et al. The cytohepatic ducts: Surgical implications. Surg Radiol Anat 13:203-211, 1991.

29 *Cholecystectomy: Routine Versus Selective Intraoperative Cholangiography*

F. Dubois

Since its introduction by Mirizzi in 1932, intraoperative cholangiography (IOC) has become quite popular. In France it came to be regarded as an essential procedure during open cholecystectomy, since it was found to significantly lower the rate of biliary duct complications. However, since the introduction of endoscopic retrograde cholangiopancreatography (ERCP) and papillotomy, many surgeons, I among them, have become less concerned with the risk of overlooking a common duct stone and have changed this practice; we now perform IOC only in selected patients. In the United States use of IOC has been increasing and it is now almost routine, whereas in France the trend is toward more selective use. The aim of IOC is twofold: to avoid injury to the biliary tract and to avoid overlooking a stone in the common bile duct (CBD).

AVOIDING BILIARY TRACT INJURY

Many surgeons believe that it is imperative to gain precise knowledge of the anatomy of the biliary tree in order to trace the course of the common duct, define the implantation of the cystic duct, and detect possible abnormalities. This can be accomplished by a large dissection of the biliary tree, which is hazardous, or by IOC. In arguing against this practice, it seems that in the case of anatomical abnormalities, congenital or pathological, opening a duct (thought to be the cystic duct) to insert a cholangiocatheter can create unnecessary injuries. The only advantage would be the detection of damage created by the dissection preceding the placement of the cholangiocatheter.

We believe that the technique of dissection close to the neck of the gallbladder, far from the common duct, is preferable. Abnormalities are readily identified and injury is prevented.

The only risk (and it is the same with IOC) is in the event of a major abnormality, that is, if the right hepatic duct or even the entire common duct is adherent along or implanted into the body of the gallbladder.

Fortunately, this is an infrequent occurrence. If during dissection of the neck of the gallbladder such a major duct or even a smaller one is discovered, cholangiography must be performed by puncture of the gallbladder rather than through the cystic duct to determine whether that duct can be preserved or is small enough to be ligated.

AVOIDING RESIDUAL STONES

Since the inception of ERCP, leaving a stone in the CBD at operation is not as hazardous as it once was, when a secondary open biliary operation was imperative. Furthermore, up to 25% of residual stones can migrate spontaneously.

Performing IOC is relatively simple during laparoscopy with newly developed specific cannulas, catheters, or forceps. Nevertheless, it takes at least 15 minutes, even with fluoroscopy, and the rate of failure can vary from 2% to 30%. It is higher in acute cases when the risk of CBD stones is greater.

Clots or bubbles have been found to create false positive results in 2% of patients and false negative results in some. Catheterization of the cystic duct, when difficult, is potentially dangerous and injury to the CBD can occur. The cost, according to Voyles,[3] is between 300 and 500 dollars. It is important to note that IOC is unnecessary in the majority of cases, and risk should be predetermined in selected groups. According to Huguier et al.[5] and Belghiti and Sauvanet,[6] in the absence of jaundice, pancreatitis, infection, or large duct and microlithiasis, the risk of CBD stones is less than 2%. Why then perform routine IOC in 98% of patients, with its inherent risks of false positive and false negative findings and failures?

We are very selective in doing IOC. In the absence of contraindications (mainly allergy to iodine), intravenous cholangiography is performed preoperatively. When the cholangiogram is of good quality, showing either a normal CBD or evidence of stones, we do not perform IOC. In other cases the decision is based on patient history, laboratory findings, and ultrasound images.

If there are no risk factors, we perform laparoscopic cholecystectomy without IOC, using our careful dissection technique. Our choice of procedure—preoperative endoechography, ERCP, or IOC—is based on risk factors and the type of case. This has been our practice in open surgery and since 1988 in more than 2000 laparoscopic cholecystectomies. There have been no cases of primary injury to the CBD and no instances of secondary laparotomy for residual stones; the few abnormalities detected have been treated easily with secondary endoscopic papillotomy.

REFERENCES

1. Berci G, Sackier JM, Paz-Barlow M. Routine or selected intraoperative cholangiography during laparoscopic cholecystectomy. Am J Surg 161:355-360, 1991.
2. Lillemoe KD, Yeo CJ, Talamini MA. et al. Selective cholangiography. Ann Surg 215:669-676, 1992.
3. Voyles CR. In Lillemoe KD, Yeo CJ, Talamini MA, et al. Selective cholangiography. Ann Surg 215:669-676, 1992.
4. Flowers JL, Zucker KA, Graham SM, et al. Laparoscopic cholangiography. Ann Surg 215:209-216, 1992.
5. Huguier M, Bornet P, Charpak Y, et al. Selective contraindications based on multivariate analysis for operative cholangiography in biliary lithiasis. Surg Gynecol Obstet 172:470-474, 1991.
6. Belghiti J, Sauvanet A. La cholangiographie per opératoire at'elle vécue? Actual Dig 12:155-117, 1990.
7. Graves HA, Ballinger JF, Anderson WJ. Appraisal of laparoscopic cholecystectomy. Ann Surg 213:655-664, 1991.

30 Technique and Results of Intraoperative Cholangiography in Laparoscopic Cholecystectomy

Gerhard W. Lotz

One of the most important prerequisites for sensible application of minimally invasive surgery in cholecystectomy is the constant effort to reduce the complication rate. In this effort we advocate obligatory intraoperative cholangiography.

PATIENTS AND RESULTS

From March 1990 to February 1993, we performed 1200 laparoscopic cholecystectomies; 77% of our patients were women, with a mean age of 50.4 years. The histological diagnosis was chronic inflammation or bland gallbladder in 83% and acute cholecystitis, hydrops, or chronic shrinked gallbladder in 16.9%; one patient had adenocarcinoma of the gallbladder. For 13 surgeons the average operating time was 50.2 minutes, and the overall complication rate was 7.9% (Table 1).

The most severe complications were resolved with laparotomy: three cases of postoperative bleeding and three cases of injury to the extrahepatic bile ducts. One patient had a small leak in the common bile duct, which was detected intraoperatively and sutured laparoscopically. In another 45 patients laparoscopic cholecystectomy was not possible and conventional surgery was performed. Five of these patients were treated for lesions in the bile ducts. Thus 0.8% of all patients had biliary tract injuries.

Case Reports

A 27-year-old woman underwent a simple and uneventful laparoscopic cholecystectomy. A Filshie clip was used to clip the cystic duct. During the procedure the wall of the common bile duct was inadvertently grasped, resulting in postoperative jaundice requiring endoscopic retrograde cholangiopancreatography (ERCP) and laparotomy to remove the clip.

A 60-year-old woman had postoperative bleeding, which was treated with repeat laparoscopy and electrocoagulation adjacent to the bile ducts. After 3 unevent-

Table 1. Complications in 1200 laparoscopic cholecystectomies

Complications	No.
Treated by laparotomy	
Bile duct lesion	3
Secondary hemorrhage	3
Laparotomy rate	0.5%
Treated with repeat laparoscopy	
Secondary hemorrhage	4
Choleperitoneum	8
Repeat laparoscopy rate	1.0%
Secondary suturing (after wound infection)	5
Laparotomy rate	0.4%
Conservative treatment	
Intra-abdominal loss of stones	33
Infected subhepatic hematoma	4
Hepatic hematoma	2
Bile secretion	11
Leakage from duodenum	1
Wound infection	13
Pancreatitis	1
Pleural effusion (puncture)	2
Pneumonia	5
Rate	6.0%

ful days, increased bile secretion through the drain necessitated reoperation. Necrosis of the hepatic duct was found and hepaticojejunostomy was performed. After 6 months a stricture developed, necessitating a new biliary intestinal anastomosis in the hepatic porta.

A 33-year-old woman underwent a simple laparoscopic cholecystectomy. Her extrahepatic bile ducts were quite small. The hepatic duct was mistaken for the cystic duct, causing the surgeon to clip and transect the hepatic duct. The error was detected intraoperatively and followed by laparotomy with direct suturing of the bile duct.

DISCUSSION

To date the overall complication rates for laparoscopic cholecystectomy[1-4] have been comparable with those of the standard technique. For conventional cholecystectomy the rate of iatrogenic biliary lesions is 0.06% to 0.03% or one injury per 300 to 500 cholecystectomies.[1-10] In our series of 1200 endoscopic cholecystectomies, bile duct lesions occurred in 0.75%.

Analyzing all nine of our patients with injuries to the bile ducts, we found that the cause of injury was the disease itself, in three, namely, acute inflammation with Mirizzi's syndrome of scleroatrophic cholecystitis. In these cases even with conventional surgery the integrity of the biliary ducts would have been compromised.

In the other six patients iatrogenic injuries may have been prompted by inadequate observation or misinterpretation of anatomical structures. In half of these patients the initial problem was noted postoperatively, whereas in the other three bile duct lesions were recognized at the time of the primary operation and repaired immediately, in one case laparoscopically. Ordinarily these latter cases would not have been included in conventional surgery results.

One third of injuries to the bile ducts are encountered after as many as 500 operations; one case even occurred with a very experienced surgeon who had already performed more than 300 laparoscopic cholecystectomies. Thus the problem of iatrogenic bile duct lesions, in our view, does not arise solely with beginning or inexperienced surgeons.

To avoid this type of complication, starting with operation No. 601, we began using intraoperative cholangiography as a matter of course and increased the rate of x-ray examinations from 30% to 98% in the last 600 operations. As expected, the number of conversions from endoscopic to conventional technique has increased from 2.4% in the first 500 to 4.5% in the last 600.

For intraoperative cholangiography the following instruments were used (Fig. 1), in decreasing order of frequency:

- Modified suction and instillation tube (diameter 1.9 mm)(Wolf)
- Cavafix central venous catheter (1.1 mm)(Braun)
- Injection and puncture cannula (1.8 mm)(Wolf)
- Modified anesthetic cannula (0.7 mm)(Wolf)
- Arrow-Karlan laparoscopic cholangiography catheter (1.2 mm)(Arrow International, Inc.)
- Angiomed puncture needle (1.0 mm)(Angiomed)

Most of these instruments were introduced into the abdomen through a 5 mm trocar sleeve and guided into the cystic duct, which was incised near the gallbladder (Fig. 2). The central venous catheter (Cavafix) and the puncture needle (Angiomed) were inserted directly through the abdominal wall. With some experience, control x-ray examination does not unduly prolong the operation; thus in the last 600 operations, in which intraoperative cholangiography was performed in 98%, our mean operating time was 44.2 minutes.

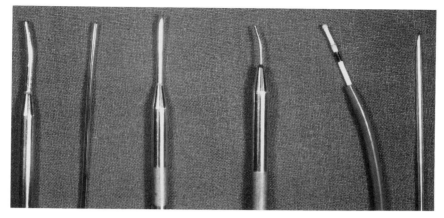

Fig. 1. Instruments used for intraoperative cholangiography.

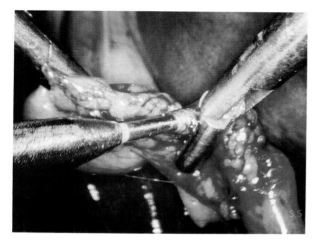

Fig. 2. Modified puncture cannula is guided into the cystic duct and fixed with grasping forceps.

Although there is some debate concerning the need for routine cholangiography in open surgery,[11-14] x-ray examination during laparoscopic cholecystectomy in our view is essential to verify bile duct anatomy. In preparation of the cystic duct there is a significant difference between conventional and endoscopic cholecystectomy; that is, during laparoscopic surgery the cystic duct is often deviated by extreme traction of Hartmann's pouch pulling the common bile duct "tentlike" toward the gallbladder. Thus the common bile and hepatic ducts may be mistaken for the cystic duct, which may be followed by clipping and cutting of these structures.[11]

Of course, intraoperative cholangiography is no substitute for proper identification of the extrahepatic bile ducts, but it may reduce the risk of lesions in the ductal structures. Early recognition of an injury by cholangiography will ensure a proper and prompt response to control the damage.[7,15,16]

In addition, choledocholithiasis was found in 4.6% of patients undergoing x-ray examination despite normal laboratory and sonographic data. All but one of these patients underwent ERCP and stone removal. We performed laparoscopic choledocholithotomy and insertion of a T-tube in one 25-year-old woman.

Whether the number of iatrogenic bile duct lesions may be reduced by control intraoperative x-ray examination and increased familiarity with endoscopic surgery can only be determined by long-term evaluation and more experience.

In this context we would like to emphasize in particular the danger of a chronically atrophied (shrunken) gallbladder, because in most of these cases a good overview of the anatomy cannot be achieved. Conversion to laparotomy is not an indication of failure of the endoscopic technique but rather demonstrates the responsibility and determination of the surgeon.

REFERENCES

1. Cuschieri A, Dubois F, Mouiel J, et al. The European experience with laparoscopic cholecystectomy. Am J Surg 161:385, 1991.
2. Gadacz TR, Talamini MA. Traditional versus laparoscopic cholecystectomy. Am J Surg 161:336, 1991.

3. The Southern Surgeons Club. A prospective analysis of 1518 laparoscopic cholecystectomies. N Engl J Med 324:1073, 1991.
4. Troidl H, Spangenberger W, Dietrich A, et al. Laparoskopische Cholecystektomie: Erste Erfahrungen und Ergebnisse bei 300 Operationen: eine prospektive Beobachtungsstudie. Chirurg 62: 257, 1991.
5. Andrén-Sandberg A, Alinder G, Bengmark S. Accidental lesions of the common bile duct at cholecystectomy. Ann Surg 201: 328, 1985.
6. Cheslyn-Curtis S, Emberton M, Ahmed H, et al. Bile duct injury following laparoscopic cholecystectomy. Br J Surg 79:231, 1992.
7. Garden OJ. Iatrogenic injury to the bile duct. Br J Surg 78:1412, 1991.
8. Gompertz RHK, Rhodes M, Lennard TWJ. Laparoscopic cholangiography: An effective and inexpensive technique. Br J Surg 79:233, 1992.
9. Raute M, Schaupp W. Iatrogene Schäden an den Gallenwegen infolge Cholecystektomie. Behandlung und Ergebnisse. Langenbecks Arch Chir 373:345, 1988.
10. Riggs T, Foshag L, Vargish T, et al. Biliary tract injuries following routine cholecystectomy. Am Surg 52:312, 1986.
11. Berci G, Sackier JM, Paz-Partlow M. Routine or selected intraoperative cholangiography during laparoscopic cholecystectomy? Am J Surg 161:355, 1991.
12. Pier A, Thevissen P, Ablaßmaier B. Die Technik der laparoskopischen Cholecystektomie. Erfahrungen und Ergebnisse bei 200 Eingriffen. Chirurg 62:323, 1991.
13. Reddick EJ, Olsen D, Spaw A, et al. Safe performance of difficult laparoscopic cholecystectomy. Am J Surg 161:377, 1991.
14. Wetter LA, Way LW. Surgical therapy for gallstone disease. Gastroenterol Clin North Am 20:157, 1991.
15. Davidoff AM, Pappas TN, Murray EA, et al. Mechanisms of major biliary injury during laparoscopic cholecystectomy. Ann Surg 215:196, 1992.
16. Moossa AR, Easter DW, van Sonnenberg E, et al. Laparoscopic injuries to the bile duct. Ann Surg 215:203, 1992.

31 Laparoscopic Cholecystectomy and Common Bile Duct Pathology

Paul Sungler, Oskar Boeckl, and M.P. Heinerman

Common bile duct stones and papillary stenosis are still a therapeutic dilemma in laparoscopic cholecystectomy, since laparoscopic choledochotomy and stone extraction require special equipment and a significant amount of time and expertise.[1-5] Overall morbidity and mortality remain to be determined. Open operative common bile duct exploration is the least desirable option when minimally invasive surgery is indicated, although even this procedure is frequently used.[6-9] Several investigators have reported good results with endoscopic retrograde cholangiopancreatography (ERCP) and stone extraction with or without endoscopic sphincterotomy.[4,10-18]

We present the results of laparoscopic cholecystectomy combined with selective preoperative ERCP and stone extraction. We will also discuss the predictability of paraclinical examinations for choledocholithiasis and papillary stenosis and review the literature to evaluate support for our findings.

METHOD

From November 1989 to September 1992, we performed 520 consecutive laparoscopic cholecystectomies. There were 136 men and 384 women, with an age range of 17 to 86 years. Over this same period there were 66 open cholecystectomies because of previous gastric surgery, gangrenous cholecystitis, or gallbladder perforation.

Indications for preoperative ERCP were dilation of the common bile duct on ultrasound examination, a history of jaundice, abnormal liver function tests, and biliary pancreatitis (Table 1). Postoperative ERCP was performed for stones identified intraoperatively on cholangiography, dilation of the common bile duct on ultrasound imaging, or abnormal liver function tests results. During the study 59 patients underwent ERCP preoperatively and two postoperatively. In addition, we performed ERCP in six other patients in this series

152

Table 1. Selection criteria for ERCP

Criteria	Description
Ultrasound examination	Dilatation of CBD >6 mm with/without signs of choledocholithiasis
Laboratory conditions	Elevation of alkaline phosphatase, G-GT, bilirubin (amylase, lipase)
Clinical findings and patient history	Recurrent colicky pain, history of jaundice

CBD = common bile duct.

for indications not related to stones: two for bile leaks, three for suspected common bile duct injury, and one for a double gallbladder. They will be discussed later. Intraoperative cholangiography was performed mainly in patients with preoperative ERCP (n = 49).

RESULTS

ERCP was performed in 59 of 520 patients (11.3%). The following pathological conditions were observed in 91%: stones in the biliary tree in 40 patients—12 with biliary pancreatitis on admission, 10 with severe benign papillary stenosis, three with large duodenal diverticula, and one patient who had just passed a stone with signs of papillitis; ERCP findings were normal in five patients (Table 2). The common bile duct was cannulated and adequately opacified in all patients, endoscopic sphincterotomy was performed in 24 of 28 patients with stones, and the stones were removed by wire basket, stone crusher, and balloon stone extraction techniques in all of them. ERCP was generally performed 2 days before laparoscopic cholecystectomy except in the 12 cases of biliary pancreatitis, where ERCP was performed on admission and laparoscopic cholecystectomy was postponed until liver function test results and pancreatic enzyme levels returned to normal.

There was one complication (1.7%) related to endoscopy and sphincterotomy with postprocedural mild edematous pancreatitis, causing cholecystectomy to be postponed for 5 days; minor hyperamylasemia was noted in four patients, with no delay in discharge from the hospital. In the endoscopic group there were no complications at operation, and in none was a conversion to open cholecystectomy or postlaparoscopic endoscopy necessary.

In the nonendoscopic group there were 16 complications (3.5%) including dissecting problems with duodenal perforation and hemorrhage, technical errors

in clipping the cystic duct and artery, and bile leaks from the liver bed of the gallbladder. None of these complications could have been avoided by more extensive use of intraoperative cholangiography (Table 3).

Eight patients required postlaparoscopic ERCP for a variety of reasons, including common bile duct stones shown by intraoperative cholangiogram (nondilated common bile duct and a narrow cystic duct, thus prohibiting laparoscopic intervention), postoperative dilation of the common bile duct on ultrasound examination, a pain pattern suspicious of a retained stone, elevation of enzyme levels, jaundice in cases of iatrogenic common bile duct injury, leaking cystic stump, and a very rare case of postoperative colicky pain caused by an intrahepatic second gallbladder with stones, necessitating endoscopy to elucidate the anatomy of the biliary tree (Table 4). There were no complications related to postlaparoscopic ERCP, and the conversion rate in the non-ERCP group was 1.9% (n = 10).

The most sensitive and specific indicator for preoperative ERCP was the sonogram followed by abnormal liver function tests and clinical presentation. In the 54 patients (91%) with biliary abnormalities the common bile duct was >6 mm on the sonogram; in two patients with intraoperatively or postoperatively diagnosed duct stones, the common bile duct was <5 mm. Liver function tests only reached a sensitivity of 44.1%, although specificity was 93% (Table 5).

DISCUSSION

This study confirms the value of preoperative ERCP in cases of suspected choledocholithiasis. Endoscopy and stone extraction with or without sphincterotomy can be performed safely with a high degree of therapeutic success. Compared with recent reports, Arregui et al.[1] and Vitale et al.[19] our data show a higher rate of ultimate discovery of common bile duct stones, mainly

Table 2. Use of ERCP in identification and treatment of common bile duct abnormalities

Pathological Conditions	Number	Endoscopic Sphincterotomy	Stone Extraction
Choledocholithiasis	28	24	28
Choledocholithiasis with biliary pancreatitis	12	12	12
Papillary stenosis	10	3	—
Duodenal diverticula	3	—	—
Passed stone, papillitis	1	—	—
None	5		

Table 3. Morbidity of ERCP (n = 59) and laparoscopic cholecystectomy (n = 461)

Laparoscopic Cholecystectomy	Preoperative Endoscopy and Laparoscopic Cholecystectomy
Iatrogenic common bile duct injury (3)	Edematous pancreatitis
Iatrogenic duodenal perforation (2)	Mild amylasemia (4)
Intraoperative hemorrhage (4)	
Postoperative hemorrhage (2)	
Bile leaks (5)	

Table 4. Postoperative endoscopy: indications and procedures (n = 8)

	Number	Endoscopic Sphincterotomy	Stone Extraction
Choledocholithiasis	2	1	2
Iatrogenic common bile duct injury	3	Open reoperation	
Leaking cystic stump	2	Pigtail drain	
Double gallbladder	1	Conventional cholecystectomy	

Table 5. Results of preoperative ultrasound examination: laboratory conditions and pain pattern

	Ultrasound (%)	Laboratory Conditions (%)	Clinical Pain Pattern (%)
Sensitivity	95.5	44.1	69.7
Specificity	99.4	93	94.2
Positive predictive value	95.5	44.4	58.8
Negative predictive value	99.4	94.4	96.3
Accuracy	99	88.9	91.6

related to the stricter indications for ERCP examination by ultrasound. Another study—the multicenter trial with 1983 laparoscopic cholecystectomies[20]—reported a common bile duct stone rate of 3.5%, open common bile duct exploration of 10% versus 90% endoscopic removal, a conversion rate for choledocholithiasis of 52%, and postoperative ERCP in 8%.

A controversy concerning the best management of choledocholithiasis has been raging for decades between "open" and endoscopic surgeons. Some advocate open common bile duct exploration,[21-23] whereas others are proponents of preoperative endoscopy and stone clearance because of reduced morbidity and mortality,[4,24-30] especially since endoscopic sphincterotomy does not destroy the function of the sphincter of Oddi.[29] *Therapeutic splitting*, a procedure in which surgical endoscopy is used in place of surgical open duct exploration, is enjoying tremendous revival in an age of minimally invasive surgery, inasmuch as intraoperative laparoscopic common bile duct exploration is still in the developmental phase and has an overall success rate of only 40%.[1-3,20] Even in combination with postoperative ERCP this results in a high rate of conversion to open common bile duct exploration or, even worse, reoperation, if the stones cannot be removed by ERCP.[2,7,31] Depending on all these factors, in many patients all the benefits of laparoscopic surgery come last. Therefore Reddick et al.[4] and Voyles et al.[17] recommend ERCP as a diagnostic and therapeutic procedure before laparoscopic cholecystectomy, just as Boeckl et al.[24,25] and Heinerman et al.[28] have been doing for conventional cholecystectomy since 1983.

Intraoperative laparoscopic common bile duct exploration is new, delicate, and requires a very high technical standard, including use of fluoroscopes, choledochoscopes, laser lithotripsy, Fogerty catheters, Dormia basket probes, and irrigation catheters in addition to experienced well-trained, and highly skilled surgeons.

Prospective trials will be most useful in ending all the controversy and uncertainty[6-9,31] concerning the best way to manage common bile duct stones. The clinically relevant papillary stenosis with common bile duct dilation, pain, and liver function abnormalities will remain the domain of endoscopy.

To avoid negative ERCP findings, selection criteria are crucial. Ultrasound imaging is an inexpensive, noninvasive method with high sensitivity and specificity, which should definitely be carried out by biliary surgeons.[32,33] In none of our patients did we find any cumulative morbidity with ERCP and laparoscopic cholecystectomy, as was the case with conventional cholecystectomy, according to Neoptolemos.[22]

The management of choledocholithiasis will be dictated by local expertise and feasibility. Of course we will gain experience with all these modalities and will always attempt to clear the duct laparoscopically in cases of unsuspected stones, but we want to emphasize that no conversion was necessitated by choledocholithiasis and postlaparoscopic ERCP was required in only 0.3% in our series. Especially by operating more frequently in older groups of patients with an increased incidence of complicated stone disease, optimum management and skilled laparoscopic surgery in combination with endoscopy will be necessary to facilitate and guarantee minimally invasive surgery.

REFERENCES

1. Arregui ME, Davis CJ, Arkush AM, et al. Laparoscopic cholecystectomy combined with endoscopic sphincterotomy and stone extraction or laparoscopic choledochoscopy and electrohydraulic lithotripsy for management of cholelithiasis with choledocholithiasis. Surg Endosc 6:10-15, 1991.
2. Berci G, Sackier JM. The Los Angeles experience with laparoscopic cholecystectomy. Am J Surg 161:382-384, 1991.
3. Hunter JG. Laparoscopic transcystic common bile duct exploration. Am J Surg 163:53-58, 1992.
4. Reddick EJ, Olsen D, Spaw A, et al. Safe performance of difficult laparoscopic cholecystectomies. Am J Surg 161:377-381, 1991.
5. Spaw AT, Reddick EJ, Olsen DO. Laparoscopic laser cholecystectomy: Analysis of 500 procedures. Surg Laparosc Endosc 1:2-7, 1991.
6. Bailey RW, Zucker KA, Flowers JL, et al. Laparoscopic cholecystectomy. Experience with 375 consecutive patients. Ann Surg 214:531-541, 1991.
7. Blatner ME, Wittgen CM, Andrus CH, et al. Cystic duct cholangiography during laparoscopic cholecystectomy. Am J Surg 161:382-384, 1991.
8. Brandon JC, Velez MA, Teplick SK, et al. Laparoscopic cholecystectomy: Evolution, early results and impact on non-surgical gallstone therapies. Am J Roentgenol 157:235-239, 1991.
9. Smith L, Sackier J, Fitzgibbons R Jr, et al. Scientific session and postgraduate course: Advance in laparoscopic surgery. Surg Endosc 6:205-210, 1992.
10. Akobiantz A, Stoffel U, Wehrli H, et al. Laparoscopic cholecystectomy. Results and experiences 1 year follow-

ing introduction of a new surgical technique (139 cases). Schweiz Rundsch Med Prax 80, 33:821-825, 1991.

11. Cooperman AM, Siegel J, Neil R, et al. Gallstone pancreatitis: Combined endoscopic and laparoscopic approaches. J Laparoendosc Surg 1:115-117, 1993.

12. Cuschiere A. Non-surgical options for the management of gallstone disease: An overview. Surg Endosc 4:127-131, 136-140, 1990.

13. Ferzli G, Kloss DA. Laparoscopic cholecystectomy: 111 consecutive cases. Am J Gastroenterol 86:1176-1178, 1991.

14. Perissat J, Collet D, Vitale G, et al. Laparoscopic cholecystectomy using intracorporeal lithotripsy. Am J Surg 161:371-376, 1991.

15. Ponchon T, Bory R, Chavaillon A, et al. Biliary lithiasis: Combined endoscopic and surgical treatment. Endoscopy 21:15-18, 1989.

16. Van Stiegman G, Pearlman NW, Goff JS, et al. Endoscopic cholangiography and stone removal prior to cholecystectomy. Arch Surg 124:787-790, 1989.

17. Voyles CR, Petro AB, Meena AI, et al. A practical approach to laparoscopic cholecystectomy. Am J Surg 161:365-370, 1991.

18. Wetter LA, Way LW. Surgical therapy for gallstone disease. Gastroenterol Clin North Am 20:157-169, 1991.

19. Vitale GC, Larson GM, Wieman TJ, et al. The use of ERCP in the management of common bile duct stones in patients undergoing laparoscopic cholecystectomy. Surg Endosc 7:9-11, 1993.

20. Larson GM, Vitale GC, Casey J, et al. Multipractice analysis of laparoscopic cholecystectomy in 1,983 patients. Am J Surg 163:221-226, 1991.

21. Föster R, Lindlar R, Vorbeck B, et al. Ist die simultane Cholecystektomie und Choledochusexploration obsolet? Dtsch Med Wschr 115:563-569, 1990.

22. Neoptolemos JP, Carr-Locke DL, Leese T, et al. Acute cholangitis in association with acute pancreatitis. Incidence, clinical features and outcome in relation to ERCP and endoscopic sphincterotomy. Br J Surg 74:1103, 1987.

23. Sackier JM, Berci G, Phillips E, et al. The role of cholangiography in laparoscopic cholecytectomy. Arch Surg 126:1021-1026, 1991.

24. Boeckl O, Heinerman M. ERCP und EPT als prophylaktische Maßnahme in der Gallenchirugie. Acta Chir Austr 15:105, 1983.

25. Boeckl O, Heinerman M, Pimpl W. Einfluß der präoperativen selektiven Endoskopie auf Resultate und Therapiekonzept der Gallengangschirurgie. Dtsch Med Wochenschr 113:1950-1955, 1988.

26. Cotton PB. Endoscopic management of bile duct stones (apples and oranges). Gut 25:587-591, 1984.

27. Heinerman M, Pimpl W, Waclawiczek HW, et al. Combined endoscopic and surgical approach to primary gallstone disease. Surg Endosc 1:195-198, 1987.

28. Heinerman M, Boeckl O, Pimpl W. Selective ERCP and preoperative stone removal in bile duct surgery. Ann Surg 209:267-272, 1989.

29. Heinerman M, Graf AH, Boeckl O. Intraoperative manometric evaluation of sphincter of Oddi function after endoscopic sphincterotomy. SAGES Second World Congress of Endoscopic Surgery. Surg Endosc 4:57, 1990.

30. Soehendra N, Grimm H, Kempeneers I. Choledocholithiasis—Möglichkeiten der Steinextraktion. In Rieman JF, Demling L, eds. Endotherapie der Gallenwegserkrankungen. Stuttgart-Thieme, 1985, p 23.

31. Brodish RJ, Fink AS. ERCP, cholangiography, and laparoscopic cholecystectomy. The Society of American Gastrointestinal Endoscopic Surgeons (SAGES) opinion survey. Surg Endosc 7:3-8, 1993.

32. Sungler P, Waclawiczek HW, Boeckl O. The role of ultrasonography in preoperative evaluation of the common bile duct system. Surg Endosc 2:118, 1988.

33. Sungler P, Heinerman M, Boeckl O. Ultrasonic evaluation of common bile duct pathology: Prospective comparison with intraoperative cholangiography, manometry and ERCP. Hepatobiliary Surg 5:150, 1992.

32 The Role of Modern Radiology in Evaluating Ductal Anatomy, Anomalies, and Injuries

George Berci

Since biliary surgery was first reported by Langenbuch[1] and Kehr,[2] we have been aware of the dreaded complication of ductal injury, the incidence of which (1/500 [0.2%]) is not accurately identified.[3] If this injury is discovered during the primary operation, the patient may benefit from immediate repair and may thus avoid a second or third corrective procedure under more difficult circumstances, such as the occurrence of bile peritonitis, and with the risks of greater morbidity and mortality. Only 10% of all ductal injuries are discovered during the first postoperative week. A majority of patients are readmitted with obstructive or cholangitic symptoms that occur from 3 to 6 months after operation. A few ductal injuries can surface a year or more after the initial procedure. If a patient who has a biloma with biliary peritonitis undergoes operation, there is a high probability that the anastomosis will break down or that a stricture will result.[4]

Endoscopic retrograde cholangiography was a great step forward in anatomical delineation and in dilation of the strictured area, which can help to avoid or to postpone reconstructive surgery. The acute case of ductal injury represents a different level of technical complexity in which anatomical dissection and display are more difficult.

Meticulous dissection and intraoperative cholangiography are important techniques used to help avoid injury. Since intraoperative cholangiography was introduced by Mirizzi,[5] a debate occurred regarding whether the procedure should be used routinely, selectively, or not at all. A more heated debate occurs about its use in relation to laparoscopic cholecystectomy. It is somehow easier to localize the common bile duct during open cholecystectomy with appropriate exploration (even in a difficult case) than it is to do so during laparoscopic cholecystectomy. Another advantage of the standard technique is that an anterograde approach to gallbladder removal can be used; during laparoscopic cholecystectomy, the retrograde technique is used.[5]

INTRAOPERATIVE CHOLANGIOGRAPHY

Several decades ago we realized that some surgeons were reluctant to use intraoperative cholangiography routinely because the equipment available to them was outdated, resulting in undue extension of operating room time. The generator used with these small mobile radiographic units could not produce enough energy to induce rapid penetration in a slightly obese patient; thus many films were underexposed. The injection of contrast material was performed without visual control, and a majority of the two to three films obtained were produced as overfilled completion cholangiograms. A record of the early filling stage was missing as a result of the poorly monitored injection. This is crucial, because in an overfilled duct, the cystic duct configuration or entry into the common bile duct (CBD) is overshadowed and can therefore be misinterpreted, or small stones can be overlooked. The performance of these machines was far from ideal, and many of the films obtained were not informative, so that the procedure must be repeated. In some institutions a lack of collaboration with the radiology department, which results in the delayed appearance of a radiographic technician, had caused many impatient surgeons to discontinue the procedure.

As a result of the review of these disadvantages, we began to use fluorocholangiography in the operating room in 1973.[6] After we had used the technique for two decades, we concluded that the effort and cost would be worthwhile because we could rapidly produce a fluoroscopic image and 6 to 10 films for detailed analysis. Only two cases of ductal injury developed in the last 1200 open cholecystectomies performed with routine intraoperative cholangiography. These procedures were performed before the laparoscopic era. One injury occurred as a complete transection and one as a partial transection. The use of intraoperative cholangiography enabled both injuries to be recognized and repaired immediately.[8]

With the use of fluorocholangiography in the operating room we could immediately see contrast material dispersion with this procedure and could complete an entire study in 3 to 5 minutes, which included fluoroscopy and 6 to 10 films. Because automatic exposure control and a three-phase generator were used, the films were of high quality and were informative, and the early filling stage was documented. This documentation avoided the overshadowing of small stones by contrast material, and we could observe sphincter function and the physiology of the biliopancreatic-duodenal junction.

In our first study (600 cases, 5800 films surveyed), we found that the cystic duct enters only in 17% from the right lateral side of the common duct, in 41% from the posterior aspect; a spiral design was found in 35% of all cases and in 7% the cystic duct was parallel to the common duct.[7] These findings were impossible to see with intraoperative cholangiography, in which the area of the cystic duct drainage into the CBD was flooded with contrast material. This made analysis of the cystic duct anatomy impossible.

There is also a difference between open operation and laparoscopy. During laparoscopic cholecystectomy, the area in question can be observed with only a two-dimensional view. In the early stage of the laparoscopic learning curve, the surgeon must become acquainted with the tactile sensation, working from a television screen, changes in depth of field, and eye-hand coordination. Although there is controversy about when intraoperative cholangiography should be performed, routine use is currently most popular. In an anatomically crowded area, it is important that a "street directory" of the biliary tree be obtained at the beginning of the operation.

Progress in radiation physics and the development of a mobile digital fluoroscope also have facilitated use of radiological techniques in the operating room.[9] These fluoroscopes can be used in several disciplines, such as general, orthopedic, vascular, and thoracic surgery. Thus the cost of equipment purchase, operation, and maintenance can be shared if a larger capital outlay is required. The digital fluoroscopic image is excellent, and pulsed fluoroscopy reduces radiation exposure. The image is instantaneously seen, and interesting images can be stored for analysis after the cholangiographic procedure, which lasts from 3 to 4 minutes. The entire cholangiogram, including positioning, fluoroscopy, and film processing, takes approximately 10 to 15 min-

utes and is a worthwhile extension of a 1- to 2-hour procedure.

The short cystic duct, which occurs in approximately 5% to 6% of cases, is an anomaly that has not been appreciated during open surgery. Two percent of short cystic ducts drain into the right hepatic duct, 1% into the common hepatic duct, and 97% into the distal common duct. If we encounter a short cystic duct during operation, we lift up and identify the CBD as we work from a two-dimensional display on a television monitor. In many cases where traction on a short cystic duct transforms the cystic-common duct junction into a tube the CBD was misidentified as being the cystic duct, and as a result it was inadvertently clipped and divided. During cholangiography, through a short cystic duct held too tightly it becomes immediately obvious if the catheter is inserted into the tented CBD and if contrast enters the CBD directly. If this circumstance is discovered, the patient must undergo exploratory operation, and the hole of the 4 Fr catheter is closed by a suture, or a small T-tube can be inserted below this repair. This management enables patients with this injury to avoid a CBD stricture or a more involved bilioenteric bypass procedure. It is more difficult to liberate and recognize a short cystic duct during laparoscopic cholecystectomy than during open operation.

In the beginning of our experience we limited the use of fluorocholangiography to elective laparoscopic cholecystectomy. As our confidence grew in performing the technique and interpreting the results, we extended the use of fluorocholangiography to acute cholecystectomy. In 1% of cases, accessory or aberrant ducts are found.

Cannulation of the cystic duct is more difficult to perform by laparoscopic cholecystectomy than by open operation, but it can be done. In our hospital in which ten surgeons perform laparoscopic cholecystectomy, the successful cannulation rate is 95%. In cases in which contrast material is not seen in the proximal ductal system, the cholangiogram should be repeated with the patient in the Trendelenburg position, and if the contrast material then does not appear in the proximal ductal system (perhaps there is a clip visible nearby), the patient should undergo an exploratory open operation.

CONCLUSION

We have never seen a faster or more explosive development of a new surgical procedure than that of laparoscopic cholecystectomy. Peer pressure for use of the technique became a significant factor, because many physicians assumed that within 2 years the laparoscopic approach would be used in 80% to 90% of all patients undergoing cholecystectomy. Ductal injuries are one of the most severe complications of biliary surgery, and some patients who experience these injuries become biliary cripples who face repeated exploratory procedures, repeated stricture dilations, portal hypertension, or shortened lifespan.

Biliary duct anomalies of surgical importance occur in 10% of all cholecystectomies and must be recognized early on during the surgical approach. Intraoperative cholangiography is important to avoid and/or identify ductal injuries, as is use of the modern mobile fluoroscopic unit.

Many patients who have CBD stones undergo unnecessary endoscopic retrograde sphincterotomies. Surgeons acquainted with laparoscopic cholecystectomy should learn the extension of that procedure: laparoscopic choledocholithotomy.[10] We are in the early stage of assessing this procedure; in approximately 60% to 70% of patients in our hospital, CBD stones are removed laparoscopically through the cystic duct. In the remaining patients, a direct approach through the CBD is used, or the CBD is explored by open operation.

In the preoperative phase, *only* the high-risk, jaundiced, and/or septicemic patients undergo endoscopic drainage or sphincterotomy. After positive intraoperative cholangiography, appropriate patients undergo laparoscopic removal of the CBD stones. Intraoperative cholangiography is crucial in this removal, because CBD stones cannot be removed laparoscopically without fluoroscopy. The anatomy, the number of stones, the size of the duct, the cystic duct and CBD junction must be known to tailor the approach to the anatomy and to avoid injury. Ductal injury cannot be avoided completely, but every attempt should be made to decrease the incidence of this dreadful complication. The incidence of ductal injury during laparoscopic cholecystectomy in 1990 to 1992 seems to be higher than during cholecystectomy by open operation.[11,12]

The three major steps for avoiding injuries during biliary surgery are meticulous dissection, routine intraoperative fluorocholangiography, and conversion to open operation during the trial dissection if necessary and indicated by technical difficulties and anatomical obstacles or anomalies.

REFERENCES

1. Langenbuch C. Ein Fall von Exstirpation der Gallenblase Wegen Chromischer Cholelithiosis. Hei Lung Berb Klin Wochenschr 19:725, 1882.
2. Kehr H. Chirurgie der Gallenwege. Enke Stuttgart Publishers, 1913.
3. Moossa AR, Mayer DA, Stabile B. Iatrogenic injuries to the bile duct. Arch Surg 125:1028, 1990.
4. Lillemoe KD, Pitt HA, Cameron JI. Current management in benign ductal injuries in advances in surgery. In Cameron JI, ed. St. Louis: Mosby, 1992, p 119.
5. Mirizzi PL. Operative cholangiography. Surg Gynecol Obstet 65:702, 1937.
6. Berci G, Steckel R. Modern radiology in the operating room. Arch Surg 107:577, 1973.
7. Berci G, Hamlin JA. Operative Biliary Radiology. Baltimore: Williams & Wilkins, 1981.
8. Morgenstern L, Wong L, Berci G. 1200 open cholecystectomies before the laparoscopic era. Arch Surg 127:400, 1992.
9. Berci G, Sackier JM. Equipment in operative cholangiography. In Berci G, ed. Problems in General Surgery: Laparoscopic Surgery, special ed. Philadelphia: JB Lippincott, 1991, p 3.
10. Sackier JM, Berci G, Paz-Partlow M. Laparoscopic transcystic choledocholithotomy. Am Surg 571:323, 1991.
11. Way L. Bile duct injury during laparoscopic cholecystectomy [editorial]. Ann Surg 215:195, 1992.
12. Braasch JW. Laparoscopic cholecystectomy and other procedures [editorial]. Arch Surg 127:887, 1992.

33 Diagnosis and Treatment of Complicating Factors in Laparoscopic Cholecystectomy

Joseph C. Iraci and Jean-Michel Loubeau

As laparoscopic cholecystectomy has become the accepted treatment of symptomatic cholelithiasis, the number of patients treated by this modality has risen steadily. It is evident, however, that the procedure is not applicable to all clinical conditions.

METHOD

We will review data collected from the treatment of 131 consecutive patients with symptomatic gallbladder disease (Table 1). Information was collected prospectively over 38 months, March 1990 to May 1993. All patients were treated by a single group of three surgeons working together. These patients were consecutively operated and were not merely deemed to be "good candidates" for laparoscopic cholecystectomy.

Thirty-five (26.7%) of the 131 patients were males and 96 (74.5%) were females. Ages ranged from 20 to 83 years (median age, 51.5).

Seventy patients (53.4%) were admitted on the day of operation; the remaining 61 patients spent from 1 to 11 preoperative days in the hospital. Mean hospital stay was 2.38 days.

RESULTS

In reviewing the data collected, we identified seven factors that complicated the treatment of these patients: previous abdominal operation (6); umbilical hernia (2); acute cholecystitis (28); jaundice or liver function abnormalities (18); unexpected acute cholecystitis (7); defect determined by cholangiography (1); and severe scarring in the operative area (1).

These factors may be divided into preoperative and intraoperative findings. In 42.7% of all the patients, preoperative factors were present such as previous operation, umbilical hernia, acute cholecystitis, and jaundice or liver function abnormalities (Table 2). In 6.8% of patients we discovered intraoperative findings that had not been expected such as acute cholecystitis, defect found at cholangiography, and severe scarring (Table 3).

Of the patients with preoperative factors that complicated the laparoscopic approach, 8 of the 54 patients required conversion to traditional (open) cholecystectomy (Table 4). Patients with previous, unrelated abdominal operations accounted for one of these conversions, while the 28 patients with known acute cholecystitis accounted for 18 of the cases that had to be converted to traditional cholecystectomy.

Of the nine patients with unexpected intraoperative findings, three had to be converted to traditional cho-

Table 1. Patient data: March 1990-May 1993

Number of patients	131
Males	35
Females	96
Ratio of males to females	1:3
Age range (yr)	20-83
Mean hospital stay (days)	2.38

Table 2. Preoperative complicating factors

Complication	No. of Patients
Previous operation	6
Umbilical hernia	2
Acute cholecystitis	28
LFT abnormalities	18

Table 3. Intraoperative complicating factors

Complication	No. of Patients
Unexpected acute cholecystitis	7
Defect seen on cholangiography	1
Severe scarring in operative area	1

Table 4. Results in patients with complicating factors

	Total	Converted	Percent
Preoperative	54	8	14.8
Intraoperative	9	3	33.3

lecystectomy: one patient each with unexpected acute cholecystitis, common duct defect at cholangiography, and scarring in the area of the operation (see Table 4).

Of the 18 patients with either jaundice or liver function abnormalities preoperatively, ERCP was performed before operation. Either a stone was found and extracted or a normal cholangiogram was obtained by ERCP before operation in all of these patients. Overall there were 62 patients in whom these factors were identified (47.3%). Of these, 19.4% were converted to traditional cholecystectomy. This represents 9.2% of the entire patient pool.

Of all complicating factors, 85.5% were seen preoperatively, while only 14.5% were seen intraoperatively. In 12.9% of the patients with preoperative complicating factors, conversion to traditional cholecystectomy was necessary. One third of patients whose complicating factors were diagnosed intraoperatively had to undergo conversion.

CONCLUSION

Most complicating factors were seen preoperatively (over 80%). Therefore most of these can be treated before laparoscopic cholecystectomy. Intravenous antibiotics were given to patients known to have acute cholecystitis. In performing laparoscopic cholecystectomy on patients with acute cholecystitis, the main difficulty we encountered was in grasping and placing traction on the gallbladder. To facilitate this, aspiration of the acutely inflamed gallbladder was routinely performed. In addition, the needle used for aspiration may be left in the gallbladder wall, and this may be used to reflect the gallbladder over the liver laterally or medially.

In patients with umbilical hernia or who had undergone previous abdominal operations, the positions of the Veress needle and trocars had to be variably placed to avoid the problem areas. Most commonly, the Veress needle was placed in the right upper quadrant in patients with umbilical hernias; this area is least frequently involved with adhesions. If previous operations had been performed, the area of the abdomen most removed from the scar was chosen for the initial puncture. Once the pneumoperitoneum had been established in these cases, a 5 mm trocar was initially inserted. Additional trocars were inserted under direct vision using the 5 mm video laparoscope. Once all trocars are safely placed, the 10 mm video laparoscope is substituted for the smaller scope, thus allowing better visualization. Alternatively, an open technique for the placement of the first trocar may be used to avoid the blind placement of a Veress needle into a peritoneal cavity that may potentially be obliterated by adhesions.

ERCP was performed in all patients with preoperative jaundice or liver function abnormalities; in all cases this made successful performance of laparoscopic cholecystectomy possible. If ERCP fails or if there is any question, cholangiography may be performed at the time of laparoscopic cholecystectomy.

Acute cholecystitis complicated the cases of 42 (32.0%) of our patients. Of these, nine (21.4%) were converted to traditional cholecystectomy. Therefore acute cholecystitis is responsible for the greatest number of failed laparoscopic approaches. This factor is important in discussing the planned operation with patients and families preoperatively. It is a factor that one should consider in deciding whether laparoscopic cholecystectomy should be undertaken at all.

Patients with jaundice or liver function abnormalities should have ERCP preoperatively, because almost all of these patients may be managed with this technique, thereby allowing safe laparoscopic cholecystectomy.

If complicating factors are discovered intraoperatively, there is a high probability (one in three) of the need for conversion to traditional cholecystectomy. These numbers will probably diminish with time as new laparoscopic techniques become available.

34 Complications of Laparoscopic Cholecystectomy: Postoperative Hyperbilirubinemia and Small Bowel Gangrene

Enrico Nicolo, Jerome Canady, Biagio Ravo, and John V. Bagnato

Despite its newness, laparoscopic cholecystectomy has replaced open cholecystectomy as the treatment of choice for removal of the gallbladder. Laparoscopic surgery may be associated with some complications related either to the endoscopic procedure or to the operation that is performed through this new approach. The incidence of these occurrences is low and reports from large series are encouraging.[1-5] The experience of the surgeon clearly plays a definite role in reducing the rate of complications.

MATERIALS AND METHODS

Laparoscopic cholecystectomies were performed in 148 consecutive patients from February 1, 1991 to August 31, 1992. All procedures were done at McKeesport Hospital in McKeesport, Pennsylvania. Endoscopic cholecystectomy was the initial procedure, and conversion to open cholecystectomy was at the discretion of the surgeon. All procedures were performed with the patient under general anesthesia, and monopolar electrocautery was the preferred method for dissecting the gallbladder from the liver bed. Average operating time was 1 hour (range 1 to 2 hours). Eleven patients had postoperative hyperbilirubinemia, and two patients had small bowel gangrene secondary to mesenteric ischemia; they are the subjects of this report.

RESULTS

Laparoscopic cholecystectomy was attempted in 148 patients, with a conversion rate of 6% (n = 9). One of these patients required laparotomy for common duct injury, and the remaining eight patients underwent open cholecystectomy because of technical difficulties. Eleven patients had transient postoperative hyperbilirubinemia and two had small bowel gangrene secondary to mesenteric ischemia, which resulted in their deaths.

In the 11 patients who developed postoperative hyperbilirubinemia, preoperative bilirubin and liver function tests were normal. Increased bilirubin levels were observed in six patients on postoperative day 1, and five patients were found to have elevated bilirubin levels on postoperative day 3, after they had been discharged and had returned to the emergency room because of postoperative pain. Bilirubin levels ranged from 2.5 to 6.0 (median 3.5), and peak bilirubin levels were observed on postoperative day 5. Amylase values and liver function test results remained normal, and all patients underwent endoscopic retrograde cholangiography (ERCP) during their hospitalization. ERCP revealed no anatomical abnormalities of the hepatobiliary tree in these 11 patients, and the bilirubin level returned to normal by postoperative day 10.

In the two patients with small bowel gangrene (a 71-year-old man and a 68-year-old woman), laparoscopic cholecystectomy was successful. Medical history revealed that they both had significant diffuse atherosclerotic vascular disease. In addition, they had nausea, fever, diffuse abdominal pain, and leukocytosis (36,000 and 25,000 l ul, respectively) on postoperative day 1. Amylase and bilirubin levels and liver function tests remained normal. On postoperative day 2, leukocytosis and abdominal pain increased. CT scans of the abdomen showed air in the bowel wall suggestive of small bowel ischemia. Each patient underwent exploratory celiotomy. In the male patient, gangrenous bowel was observed from 2 feet beyond the ligament of Treitz to the right transverse colon. The patient underwent small bowel resection, right hemicolectomy, and jejunocolon anastomosis. He did well postoperatively but died on postoperative day 21. Autopsy revealed pulmonary embolus as the cause of death. The female patient had gangrenous bowel extending from the ligament of Treitz to the splenic flexure. The surgeon elected not to proceed any further, and the patient died several hours later.

DISCUSSION

Hyperbilirubinemia after laparoscopic cholecystectomy is a complication highly suggestive of iatrogenic operative injury to the extrahepatic biliary tree; ERCP must be performed immediately for evaluation of injury to the biliary tree. In our series of 11 patients with hyperbilirubinemia after laparoscopic cholecystectomy,

ERCP findings were normal. Bilirubin levels peaked on postoperative day 4 and returned to normal between days 6 and 10. This postoperative increase in the bilirubin level appears to be a benign transient event.

Small bowel gangrene secondary to mesenteric ischemia after laparoscopic cholecystectomy is a catastrophic complication with lethal consequences. Patients with diffuse atherosclerotic vascular disease may have underlying atherosclerotic disease of the splanchnic bed, and the increase in intra-abdominal pressure from the pneumoperitoneum may compromise the splanchnic circulation.

CONCLUSION

Two unusual complications of laparoscopic cholecystectomy are hyperbilirubinemia and gangrene of the small bowel secondary to mesenteric ischemia. Hyperbilirubinemia with a normal ERCP is a benign and transient occurrence. Small bowel gangrene secondary to mesenteric ischemia has a high mortality rate, and surgeons should use caution when performing laparoscopic cholecystectomy as opposed to open cholecystectomy in patients with significant diffuse atherosclerotic vascular disease.

REFERENCES

1. Tomplins RK. Laparoscopic cholecystectomy: Threat opportunity? Arch Surg 125:1245, 1990.
2. Dubois F, Icard P, Beerthelot G, et al. Coelioscopic cholecystectomy: Preliminary report of 36 cases. Ann Surg 211:60-62, 1990.
3. Reddick EJ, Olsen D, Daniell J, et al. Laparoscopic laser cholecystectomy. Laser Med Surg News Adv, Feb. 1989, p 38.
4. Peters J, Gibbons G, Innes J, et al. Complications of laparoscopic cholecystectomy. Surgery 110:769-777, 1991.
5. Peters J, Ellison E, Innes J, et al. Safety and efficacy of laparoscopic cholecystectomy: A prospective analysis of 100 initial patients. Ann Surg 213:3-12, 1991.

---

35   *Postoperative Ileus After Laparoscopic Cholecystectomy*

Manuel Garcia-Caballero, Monserrat Salvi, and Carlos Vara-Thorbeck

We will present a detailed review of postoperative ileus after laparoscopic cholecystectomy and discuss the significance that opening of the abdominal cavity has in the development of postoperative ileus.

A prospective randomized controlled clinical trial was designed in which 80 patients were divided into four groups (n = 20): group 1, patients who underwent conventional cholecystectomy (control group); group 2, those who had conventional cholecystectomy and an injection of 20 ml of 0.5% bupivacaine into the mesentery root; group 3, those who had conventional cholecystectomy and 7.5 mg of propranolol administered intravenously and 0.5 mg neostigmine administered subcutaneously after operation until the first bowel movement; and group 4, those who underwent laparoscopic cholecystectomy.

The shortest period of postoperative ileus was observed in group 4 (36 hours). This period increased in group 2 (72 hours) and in group 3 (84 hours) and was longest in the conventional cholecystectomy (group 1) patients (89 hours). The reduction in postoperative ileus time parallels an improvement in the patients' general comfort and feeling of well-being.

Thus, after laparoscopic cholecystectomy, postoperative ileus is not clinically significant. This study confirms the correlation that exists between reduction of intra-abdominal manipulation and the commensurate evolution of postoperative ileus.

Laparoscopic surgery and its most common application in general surgery—cholecystectomy—have obviated the opening of and manipulation within the abdominal cavity. Both of these, in various combinations, appear to cause postoperative ileus.

The pathophysiological factors of postoperative paralytic ileus remain unclear, in spite of the results of studies[1-5] conducted during the last 20 years. However, some authors agree that the disorder occurs as a result of the triggering of sympathetic inhibitory reflexes originating from receptors in the intestinal wall and in the parietal and visceral peritoneal layers.[6-9] Postoperative intestinal paralysis results from a combination of both these processes.

MATERIALS AND METHODS

Eighty patients who met specific study criteria (Table 1) were evaluated. Each patient had undergone chole-cystectomy for simple cholelithiasis. From this group, 60 patients had undergone conventional cholecystec-tomy, and 20 had had laparoscopic cholecystectomy. The mean age of the patients was 56 (range, 28 to 83 years).

All patients benefitted from routine perioperative preparation, monitoring, and ultrasonography of the bile duct. Patients who were to undergo laparoscopy had intravenous cholangiotomography 24 hours before the operation to diagnosis choledocholithiasis and elimi-nate those patients from the study.

Anesthesia was induced with thiopental (Pentothal, 3-5 mg/kg); atracurium was used to prevent muscular fasciculation during neuromuscular blockade. Anesthe-sia was maintained with N_2O and O_2 and a bolus dose of 0.1 mg of fentanyl followed by a standardized dose of 0.003 mg/kg/hr. At the conclusion of the operation, 0.5 mg of atropine followed by 1 mg of neostigmine was administered to reverse the neuromuscular blockade.

The patients were randomly allocated into the fol-lowing four groups (n = 20), each of which was differ-entiated by the specific postoperative ileus treatment applied:

Group 1: Control group. Conventional cholecys-tectomy, no additional treatment

Group 2: Conventional cholecystectomy, including intraoperative injection of 20 ml of 0.5 bupiva-caine into the mesentery root at the minor curva-ture of the stomach and distal to the ligament of Treitz

Group 3: Conventional cholecystectomy with post-operative administration of 7.5 mg of proprano-lol every 8 hours administered intravenously (or 80 mg administered orally every 12 hours) plus 0.5 mg of neostigmine administered subcutaneously every 12 hours until the first expulsion of gas and feces

Group 4: Laparoscopic cholecystectomy without additional treatment

All patients received the same postoperative analgesic treatment as requested by them (6 g/day of magnesium noramidopirinometasulphate). The pulse rate and ar-

---

Table 1. Exclusion criteria of study patients

Treatment with digitalis or verapamil
Cardiac insufficiency or impairment
Hypotension or bradycardia
Insulin-dependent diabetes
Chronic bronchitis
Obstructive peripheral arteriopathy

---

terial pressure of those patients receiving propranolol were controlled before and after administration of the drug.

The evolution of postoperative ileus was observed according to the protocol (see box) every 6 hours. Pro-gression was determined by registering the first expul-sion of gases and feces after the operation. The degree of patient discomfort was also noted. This observation-al study was concluded for each patient after the first bowel movement.

The data are presented in median, range, and mean values. Group comparisons were performed with ANOVA.

RESULTS

The groups were homogeneous with respect to age and previous clinical and pathological events. Seventy-seven of the 80 patients included in the study were eval-uated at the study conclusion. The remaining three patients, who were in the group treated with propran-olol, had treatment suspended because of bradycardia and/or hypotension, both of which disappeared when the treatment was withdrawn.

Data in Table 2 indicate that efficiency of bowel movements occurred 60 hours after the operation in the control group. The blockade of the sympathetic inhib-itory stimuli (groups 2 and 3) reduced this period only when the sympathetic blockade was performed locally and at the beginning of the surgical procedure.

Avoiding opening the abdominal wall through lapa-roscopic cholecystectomy results in the expulsion of gas-es at a mean time of 12 hours, an improvement when compared with the results from the control group ($p < 0.001$).

A similar result was noted with respect to occurrence of the first bowel movement. The control group (1) and the group treated with inhibitors of the sympathet-ic system plus one stimulant of the parasympathetic sys-

PROTOCOL FOR DATA COLLECTION

Patient

Name _____ Age _____
Diagnosis _____

Surgery

Description:
Level of difficulty (1-10)
Duration: _____ hours _____ minutes
Postoperative day _____ / _____ hours after operation

Postoperative Course

General state   1. severe discomfort   2. nausea   3. tolerable   4. comfortable
Eructation   1. yes   2. no
Vomiting   1. yes   2. no
Feels bowel sounds   1. yes   2. no
Gases   1. yes   2. no
Defecation   1. yes   2. no
Aided or spontaneous   1. yes   2. no
  defecation
Sensation of   1. heaviness   2. discomfort   3. abdominal pain

Postoperative Abdominal Examination

Inspection   1. bloated   2. distended.   3. normal
Palpation   1. involuntary defense   2. voluntary defense   3. soft and depressible
Percussion   1. (+)   2. (++)   3. (+++)
  (resonance)
Auscultation   1. absence of sounds   2. slight sounds   3. normal sounds   4. increased sounds

Additional Postoperative Findings

Alterations of potassium _____
Contents of nasogastric tube _____ ml
Rectal tube _____
Abdominal radiograph _____

Observations

tem (3), produced similar results (see Table 2). However, the early intraoperative blockade of the sympathetic system with bupivacaine in group 2 shortened postoperative ileus after conventional cholecystectomy, which is worth noting ($p < 0.05$) when compared with the results of the control group.

Laparoscopically guided cholecystectomy shortened the postoperative period before defecation when compared with the results of the control group ($p < 0.001$).

The most significant data taken from our protocol on the patients' quality of life after surgical intervention are shown in Tables 3 and 4.

Table 2. Time of expulsion of first gases and feces after surgery

Time (hours)	Group No.			
	1 (n = 20)	2 (n = 20)	3 (n = 20)	4 (n = 20)
Gases				
Median	60	48	48	10
Range	24-90	24-96	45-72	8-14
Mean	60	53	50	12*
Feces				
Median	96	72	96	36
Range	60-125	36-120	45-125	24-40
Mean	89	72†	84	36‡

*$p < 0.01$ (in comparison with control group)
†$p < 0.05$
‡$p < 0.001$ (in comparison with control group)

Table 3. Percentage of patients complaining of general postoperative discomfort

Postoperative Day	Group No.			
	1 (n = 20)	2 (n = 20)	3 (n = 17)	4 (n = 20)
1	45	12	30	0
2	20	12	20	0
3	0	0	10	0

Table 4. Percentage of patients with bowel sounds in the first postoperative days

Postoperative Day	Group No.			
	1 (n = 20)	2 (n = 20)	3 (n = 17)	4 (n = 20)
1	15	41	20	100
2	40	65	90	100
3	70	72	90	100

Analysis of Table 3 data reveals that on the first post-operative day, 45% of the patients who underwent conventional cholecystectomy complained of general discomfort, but none of the laparoscopic cholecystectomy patients suffered discomfort. The two remaining groups registered varying incidences of discomfort (see Table 3). On the second postoperative day the results of both the control group (1) and the groups treated only with postoperative sympathetic blockade (2 and 3) were similar.

One hundred percent of the patients who underwent laparoscopic cholecystectomy experienced bowel sounds after 24 hours (in these patients, the sounds were audible 6 hours after surgical intervention)(see Table 4). However, in 15% of group 1 patients, bowel sounds were detected 24 hours after the operation. Similar figures emerged from the group treated with propranolol and neostigmine (20%). Nevertheless, when an intraoperative sympathetic blockade was performed, an improvement in the incidence of postoperative bowel sounds (41%) occurred.

DISCUSSION

Until this study, no investigators had examined the question of whether laparoscopic surgery reduces the duration of paralytic ileus to a greater extent than does open operation. Despite different studies on the results of laparoscopic cholecystectomy,[10-12] a detailed observation and study of the occurrence and evolution of postoperative ileus in laparoscopic cholecystectomy patients does not exist.

Because electromyography[13] and radiopaque markers[14] have been used to show that no correlation exists between intestinal motility and defecation, we have applied the same protocol used in other clinical studies on the same topic to define the evolution of intestinal ileus after laparoscopic operation.

According to our observations, postoperative ileus after laparoscopic surgery does not exist; this is demonstrated by the recurrence of bowel sounds 6 hours after the operation, the expulsion of the first gases 12 hours post procedure, and defecation between 24 and 36 hours after surgery.

These observations support the view that postoperative ileus occurs as a result of the triggering of inhibitory reflexes caused by the incision and opening of the abdominal wall and by subsequent intra-abdominal manipulation, regardless of the magnitude of the operation.[15] Abdominal opening and manipulation can now

be significantly reduced, because the laparoscopic approach is controlled and targets specific anatomical structures.

When the laparoscopic procedure is compared with open operation, we have noted the following factors:

1. The duration of anesthesia and intra-abdominal manipulation is similar (the mean time of the 20 laparoscopic cholecystectomy operations was 83 minutes).
2. The disease-oriented operative dissections are identical.
3. In the laparoscopic procedure, the various steps can be performed with greater precision than in open surgery. For example, compression and possible injury to the duodenal serosa or the hepatic angle of the colon are avoided during exposure of the operative site.
4. The abdominal cavity is not opened to the outside in laparoscopic surgery, and no pressure is applied to the abdominal wall by the retractors. The peritoneum does not require suturing, which obviates the traction on its edges, necessary to accomplish the closure.
5. The contact made during laparoscopic surgery is from outside the abdomen through the intermediary of long, rigid instruments. Pressurized air for the pneumoperitoneum is introduced first through a Veress needle, and the periumbilical orifice is enlarged to an initial diameter of 10 mm with the passage of the trocar. This orifice is stretched to permit gallbladder extraction at the conclusion of the operation. While direct contact through palpation of the organs is limited in laparoscopy, visual assessment is greatly enhanced because of optical magnification and the detailed exposure made possible of the pneumoperitoneum.

The type of anatomical dissection, the duration of anesthesia, and the intra-abdominal instrumentation are similar to those of conventional cholecystectomy.

However, there are differences between open and closed operations in the degree of compression on the right colon and duodenum and in the potential injury sustained by the serosa as a result of these pressures. The surgical incisions, the pressure exerted by the retractors on the abdominal wall edges, and the peritoneal involvement and cicatrization are different in the two procedures.

Ultrastructural studies can be used to show ways of

avoiding injury to the intestinal wall serosa.[16] This type of injury can induce an inflammatory reaction similar to that caused by a foreign body. The inflammatory reaction occurs in the external layers of the intestinal wall and causes the release of histamine, serotonin, and other substances that activate the free nerve endings of the afferent fibers.[17]

This pathophysiological chain reaction (bowel manipulation, injury to the serosa, inflammatory reaction, and release of inhibitory reflex stimuli) also explains the benefit of the local anesthetics used in our study, benefits recently confirmed[18] by means of a model of aseptic peritonitis in rabbits. In that study, inhibition of the inflammatory response by means of an intravenous application of lidocaine was achieved.

The results of this study suggest that postoperative paralytic ileus does not occur as a result of laparoscopic surgery and that when the abdominal cavity is opened, postoperative ileus is unavoidable. However, the effect of the sympathetic blockade is more beneficial when the blockade is applied to the roof of the mesentery and early in the operative procedure, as opposed to a systemic application postoperatively.

This study also confirms the correlation between gentle and limited intra-abdominal organ manipulation and the duration and evolution of postoperative ileus.

---

36 Percutaneous Management of Postoperative Biliary Strictures

Plinio Rossi, Francesca Maccioni, Roberto Merlino, Franco Orsi, Laura Broglia, Gianluigi Natali, and Vittorio Pedicino

More than 90% of benign biliary strictures occur as a result of surgical trauma to the biliary tree. Cholecystectomy by the traditional open or, more recently, the laparoscopic approach is the primary operation most frequently complicated by bile duct injuries.

Surgical repair of these strictures still represents the treatment of choice: the success rate is 78% to 88% at the first attempt.[1-7] However, recurrence of stricture develops in 15% to 25% of cases, and the surgical success rate decreases with the increase in the number of operations, so that permanent positive results have been reported in less than 61% of patients after the third operation.[1,6] Concomitant biliary cirrhosis and portal hypertension increase operative risk and mortality rates.[6,7]

Recently percutaneous balloon dilation of benign biliary strictures, which is effective and has a low complication rate, has been accepted as a therapeutic alternative to surgery.[8-12] This procedure has been termed *cholangioplasty*. Success rates are comparable with those of surgery, but less morbidity and fewer procedure-related deaths result from cholangioplasty.

The primary clinical problem associated with postoperative strictures is the high rate of recurrence after operation or balloon dilation. Recurrence may develop immediately after the procedure is performed or after several months or years. Recurrence after cholangioplasty may result from chronic inflammation or (possibly) from low compliance of the stricture as a result of an elastic component in the scar tissue. After several attempts of surgical repair or balloon dilation with long-term catheter stenting for recurrent cases, limited therapeutic options remain. Nevertheless, patients with these recurrences must be adequately treated because of the progressive and possible malignant evolution of benign biliary disease to biliary cirrhosis and secondary sclerosing cholangitis.

In the last 4 years a new type of biliary endoprosthesis, the self-expanding metal stent, has become available for clinical use.[13-16] This device, when released at the level of the stricture, spontaneously expands to reach a large final diameter. Good radial force prevents relapse of the stricture. However, the metal stent cannot be removed after placement and often is an obstacle to additional surgery of the biliary tree.

When patients with recurrent strictures are not candidates for surgical repair and do not respond to repeated balloon dilation, self-expanding metal stents may offer a permanent solution: patency of bile duct lumen can be mechanically maintained and elastic recoil and recurrent stenosis can be prevented (at least in part).[17-19]

MATERIALS AND METHODS
Percutaneous Balloon Dilation

Percutaneous biliary dilation may be performed in patients with benign strictures of any cause. Single or multiple strictures and postoperative as well as primary strictures can be successfully treated.

Postoperative strictures may develop at the level of the common bile duct (CBD) after cholecystectomy or at the anastomotic site between a biliary duct and the jejunum or the duodenum, or they may result from surgical intervention in the biliary tree or the liver. A better response to percutaneous dilation is generally obtained in patients with a dominant, single iatrogenic CBD stricture, although a fairly good response may be obtained in patients with anastomotic strictures or intrahepatic ductal stenosis without marked inflammation.

Balloon dilation is also effective in the treatment of primary inflammatory strictures of the biliary ducts, such as sclerosing cholangitis; the success of the procedure depends primarily on the extent of disease. Single or double strictures frequently relapse after dilation.

Since 1983 we have treated 132 cases of benign biliary strictures, many of which were associated with inflammatory changes and infected bile. In 78/132 patients (59%) the biliary stricture was associated with biliary lithiasis. Our protocol for the last few years is as follows: biliary drainage, balloon dilation, and catheter stenting and cholangiographic control.

The most difficult aspect of performing percutaneous balloon dilation is gaining access to the biliary tree to cross the stricture. The manipulations are difficult and often very painful for the patient, who may require neuroleptanalgesia (especially during dilation, which is the most painful phase of the procedure).

When the stricture is crossed, a balloon catheter is inflated at the level of the stenosis. The balloon catheters used for the procedure (those used for angioplasty) can support up to 17 atmospheres of pressure and possess an extremely high radial force, so they can be used in very tight strictures.

The completely inflated balloon is characterized by a "waist" at the stricture site that always disappears as the pressure increases and the stricture gives way (Fig. 1; Fig. 2, *A-C*; Fig. 3, *B*; and Fig. 4, *A*). In some strictures

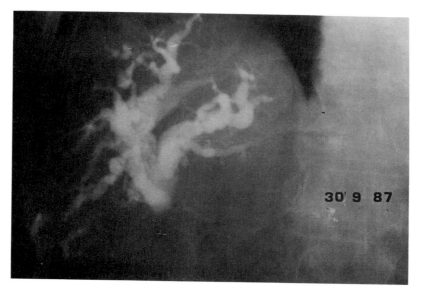

Fig. 1. Seventy-year-old female who underwent cholecystectomy in 1969 and subsequent choledoco-chole docal anastomosis to repair a postcholecystectomy stricture, without success. In subsequent years she had severe episodes of jaundice and cholangitis. She came to our attention in 1987 with a postsurgical CBD stricture, as shown on the cholangiogram. The patient refused further operation.

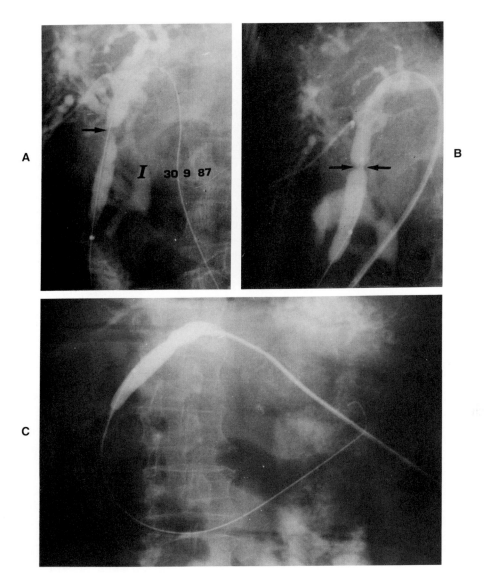

Fig. 2. A-C, Stricture dilation was performed with a 10 mm balloon catheter. The waist on the balloon profile at the level of the stricture *(arrows)* progressively disappears as the pressure increases.

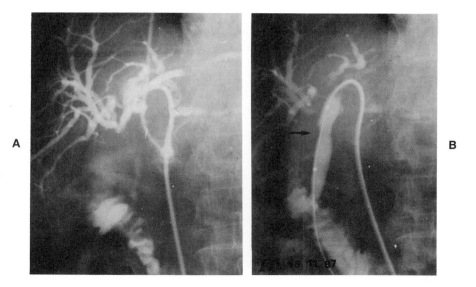

Fig. 3. A and **B,** Two months after balloon dilation, a cholangiogram showed recurrence of the stricture. A second dilation was performed. The stricture showed a lower resistance to dilation, and the waist on the balloon profile was less pronounced and disappeared at lower inflation pressure.

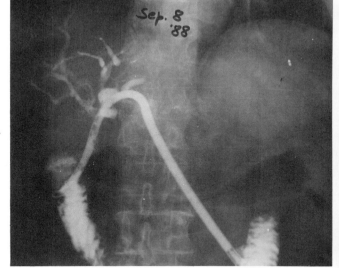

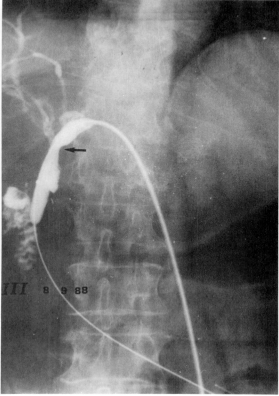

Fig. 4. A and **B,** A large-bore catheter (18 Fr) was left in place to prevent recurrence. Every attempt to remove the catheter was unsuccessful because of persistence of the stricture. A third dilation was performed without permanent success.

this may take only minimal inflation of the balloon for several seconds. In patients who have undergone multiple operations, larger diameter, high-pressure balloons inflated for longer periods of time may be required. Generally, a CBD or an anastomotic stricture requires the use of a 10 mm to 12 mm balloon, but intrahepatic strictures can be inflated with an 8 mm balloon.

After dilation, many authors suggest placing a long-term indwelling stent to reduce the recurrence rate and to provide access to the biliary tree if restenosis occurs (Fig. 4, B). Generally, large-bore catheters ranging from 10 to 20 Fr are preferred. However, the role of stent placement after dilation is controversial, because although stent placement may improve long-term success, the tube may stimulate inflammatory reaction and fibrosis.

When biliary lithiasis is associated with the stricture, the stones are pushed into the bowel after dilation of the stenosis. If the stones are too large and cannot be crushed with a balloon or a basket, they are fragmented with an electrohydraulic lithotriptor and are pushed with a balloon into the bowel. Our success rate in this procedure has been 90%.

The Biliary Metal Stent

The recurrence of the biliary stricture after repeated dilations and long-term catheter stenting is the main indication for the use of metal stents.

Between October 1988 and September 1989, we placed 28 Gianturco Z stents (Cook) and one Wallstent (Medinvent) in 18 patients with recurrent postsurgical strictures (one to four previous interventions per patient). Seven of these patients had a single stricture at the level of the common bile duct, six had one anastomotic stricture, four had intrahepatic strictures associated with an anastomotic stenosis, and one had a biliary-enteric fistula that resulted from iatrogenic closure of the CBD. These patients underwent multiple percutaneous balloon dilations and prolonged catheter stenting without success (see Fig. 1).[18,20] If surgery is contraindicated in these cases, the insertion of metal stents may be beneficial. After several attempts of balloon dilation of recurrent stenoses, limited therapeutic options remain. These options include repeat surgical repair, which is often refused by the patient and is hazardous, additional dilation and long-term catheter drainage. Both options offer no guarantee of permanent patency.

In these cases, metal stents may offer a permanent solution because the patency of the bile duct lumen is mechanically maintained; thus elastic constriction and recurrent stenosis can be prevented. However, if the possibility of surgical repair still exists, metal stent implantation is not indicated. Although cholangioplasty does not negatively affect subsequent operation, the implantation of metal stents might jeopardize future procedures because the stents are difficult to remove.

The best long-term results from metal stent treatment have been obtained in single CBD iatrogenic or anastomotic strictures. Stents placed at the level of intrahepatic strictures have a great tendency to occlude. There are four types of metal endoprostheses commercially available in Europe for use in the biliary tree: Gianturco Z stent, Wallstent (Medinvent), Strecker's Tantalum and Nitinol stents (Elastalloy by Meditech; currently for experimental use only), and Palmaz stent.

All metal stents have similarities in that they are constructed of a thin wire shaped into different designs. Metal stents can be divided into two groups: balloon expandable (Strecker's Tantalum and Palmaz stents) and self-expanding metal stents (Wallstents, Z stents, and Strecker's Nitinol stents). These stents are made of a fine wire mesh that is very flexible (except for the Gianturco stent, which is more rigid because it is made of a stainless steel wire arranged in a zigzag pattern). Experimental developments include silicone-covered stents, or spiral Z stents (made in Japan), which are flexible and easier to introduce.[21]

Z stents seem to be more effective in short fibrotic benign lesions; flexible, fine-mesh longer stents are more suitable for malignant lesions. We have used 28 Z stents (10 single and 8 double) in 17 patients (Fig. 5, B), and we have used a Wallstent in one case.

The Z stents are made of a stainless steel wire, 0.08 mm to 0.1 mm in diameter, according to a modified Gianturco design.[22] The wire is arranged in a zigzag pattern and is tied with a nylon suture that passes through an eyelet at the end of each bend to form a cylindrical structure. The stents are self-expanding, and when they are completely expanded, they have a diameter of 8 to 12 mm and a length of 1.5 cm. When they are compressed, they can be introduced through an 8.5 or 10 Fr delivery catheter. Two or three stents can be linked head-to-tail to dilate long segments.

When Z stents are deployed from the delivery system, they expand to their full size in 12 to 36 hours. Any interventional maneuver through the stent at that point should be avoided to prevent dislodgment or malpositioning.

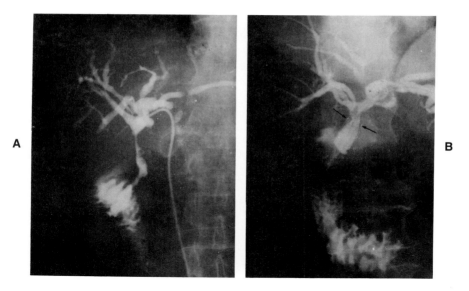

Fig. 5. A and **B,** In October 1988, a single Gianturco Z stent was placed at the level of the stricture. The control shows good stent expansion after release, and normal passage of contrast medium. Every catheter was then removed, and the patient is asymptomatic 54 months after stent placement; she has normal bilirubin levels and normal liver enzyme values.

After stent deployment, a 5 Fr angiographic catheter is left above the stricture to allow for flushing. This catheter is removed when stent expansion is satisfactory (see Fig. 5, *B*).

When multiple stents are necessary, they should be placed in a retrograde manner, with the more distal ones placed first. This is important because it is difficult to pass the introducer through a previously placed stent without causing dislodgment. Moreover, in multiple intrahepatic stenoses, all the ducts in which stents are to be placed should be entered with a guidewire first. This appears to be crucial because a stent, when placed within a major duct opens fully, it may occlude the origin of a smaller duct. Therefore, a guidewire in each branch guarantees an access route after the first stent is opened.

COMPLICATIONS

The primary morbidity and mortality of cholangioplasty relate to biliary drainage, not to actual dilation. The mortality rate of percutaneous transhepatic biliary drainage is very low (approximately 0.5% to 2%) but this rate applies only to neoplastic cases; in patients with benign disease, no procedure-related deaths have been reported.

Major complications include sepsis, which has been reported in 5% to 24% of cases, and bleeding, which occurs occasionally (especially when dilation is performed in large ducts that are full of stones, in cases of tight stenosis, or when there is an arterial injury produced by the passage of the catheter). In most cases, the bleeding is self-limited and does not require blood transfusion or operative control.[23-25]

Complications occurring with metal stents should be classified as early or late complications.

Early complications are similar to those occurring during routine biliary drainage procedures such as those for temporary hemorrhage, sepsis, or pleural effusion. However, the design of metal stents (especially the self-expanding ones) allows for a relatively nontraumatic introduction through the liver in comparison to that of conventional plastic stents, but metal stents are much wider in diameter (10 mm diameter [34 Fr]) than are conventional stents (3 mm to 4.5 mm [10 Fr to 14 Fr]). It is assumed that a large track through the liver tissue results in higher complication rates,[24-27] although this has not been proved. Technical difficulties, such as stent displacement or stent migration in the bowel, during stent insertion, occurred in the early phases of our experience. These are more frequent events when anastomot-

Table 1. Self-expanding metal stents in postoperative biliary strictures: results by type and level of stricture at 48 month's follow-up (range, 43 to 54 months)

Level/ Type	Clinical Results				Stent Status		
	Asymptomatic Patients	Symptomatic Patients		Patient Mortality	Stent Dislodged	Stent Patent	Stent Occluded
CBD	7	5	1	1	0	7/7	0
BEA	6	5	1	0	2	4/4*	0
BEA + IS	4	0	2	2	0	0/4	4/4
Iatrogenic fistula	1	—	1	—	—	0/1	1
TOTAL	18	10	5	3	2/18	11/16*	5/16
PERCENT		55.5%	27.7%	16.6%	11.%	68.7%	31.3%

*Two cases of late stent migration excluded.
BEA = biliary enteric anastomosis; BEA + IS = biliary enteric anastomosis associated with intrahepatic strictures; CBD = common bile duct

ic strictures occur and may be prevented with double-Z stents.[20]

Late complications other than recurrent jaundice rarely occur; they consist of cholecystitis, duodenal ulceration caused by constant pressure of the stent against the mucosa, and CBD perforations. Procedure-related deaths are uncommon; only one case of a lethal complication that resulted from CBD perforation in a patient with cholangiocarcinoma has been described.

In our series, no procedure-related deaths occurred, and no late complications directly related to metal stent implantation occurred.

Late stent occlusion that resulted from hyperplastic mucosal ingrowth associated (in one case) with intrahepatic stones occurred in three patients who were subsequently retreated with balloon dilation and catheter stenting.

RESULTS

The success rate of percutaneous balloon dilation in iatrogenic nonanastomotic strictures (strictures of the CBD after cholecystectomy) is 76% to 88%, a rate comparable to that of surgical results. In anastomotic strictures, the success rate is slightly lower (67% to 73%), as a result of the considerable fibrotic reaction around the stricture,[8,10] but this rate is satisfactory because most patients who undergo the procedure have already undergone at least one or two unsuccessful surgical repairs.

Our experience concerns 132 patients treated for benign strictures in the last 10 years: 24% had iatrogenic strictures; 52%, anastomotic strictures; 17%, inflammatory lesions of the CBD or of the papilla; and 7%, sclerosing cholangitis. We obtained long-term success in 74% of patients, in whom the stricture disappeared and who had no recurrence of symptoms. We obtained best results in single iatrogenic strictures. Anastomotic stenosis had a high recurrence rate, and patients with sclerosing cholangitis had a significantly improved condition but never experienced complete symptomatic relief.[12]

Multiple stones found above the stricture present another difficulty in management. We accomplished complete stone removal in 90% of cases. When the stones were too large to be pushed into the bowel, they were fragmented by means of cholangioscopy and an electrohydraulic lithotriptor.

In two current major works on the clinical use of metal stents in postoperative strictures, long-term results are presented. One of these studies is by our group,[18] the other by Coons.[19] The study results are comparable. We report our experience on 18 patients with recurrent benign biliary strictures (BBS) treated with metal stents.

Table 1 shows the results in 18 patients with BBS. The follow-up ranges from 43 to 54 months, with an average of 48 months. After 3 years of follow-up, 10 patients (55.5%) are asymptomatic and have no signs

Table 2. Forty-eight-months' follow-up patency rate (range 43-53 months)

Level/ Type	Patient Incidence	Percent
CBD	7/7	100%
BEA	4/4	100%
BEA + IS	0/3	0
Fistula	0/1	0
TOTAL	11/16	68.7%

of biliary obstruction; in five patients (27.7%) symptoms recurred and they were eventually treated again; three patients died (two from obstructive jaundice and liver failure and one without jaundice from metastatic gastric cancer).

Recurrence of jaundice resulted from stent occlusion by reactive tissue ingrowth in three cases, to stent migration in one case, and to inflammatory lesion of the papilla of Vater with patency of the metal stent in another case.

The overall 4-year patency rate is 68.7%.[18] In single CBD and anastomotic strictures, no stents occluded (100% patency rate), and all stents placed at the level of intrahepatic stenoses or complicated lesions completely occluded within 4 to 22 months (Table 2).

DISCUSSION

Postoperative strictures are difficult to treat because they are a continuously "fibrosing" disease,[29] the course of which is usually interrupted but is not stopped. The strictures tend to recur.

The success rates of percutaneous balloon dilation vary from 70% to 85%, depending on the series reported. This variability probably reflects the number of patients of each reported series, the different types of patients treated, and the length of follow-up.

Before the clinical introduction of metal stents, no effective alternatives were available with which to treat patients who had recurrent strictures and in whom surgery and bilioplasty had failed. Inadequately treated recurrent biliary strictures may have a progressive and malignant evolution toward secondary sclerosing cholangitis and biliary cirrhosis.

When metal stents became available for clinical use, we believed that they offered a permanent solution to the problem of recurrent strictures. Metal stents are a special type of endoprosthesis designed to relieve vascular stenosis after transluminal angioplasty failure. The positive results obtained in the treatment of vascular lesions induced many clinicians to use these devices experimentally in the management of malignant biliary stenoses.[26,28-30] Although definitive results are not yet available, metal stents seem to offer several advantages when compared with conventional plastic stents in the management of neoplastic biliary strictures.

Because metal stents placed for BBS cannot be removed and because there was no information about long-term patency of the stents, they have been used with some hesitation.[15,17,20,31,32]

In early experimental studies performed on animal models,[13,14] a good biocompatibility of metal stents implanted in biliary ducts was indicated; the limiting factor was that of possible occlusion as a result of the development of sludge and/or papillary mucosal hyperplasia between the struts of the stent within a few weeks. It was also evident that these devices could not be removed even a few days after placement; this is still considered the primary disadvantage of this new generation of biliary stents. Therefore, metal stents were used in experienced centers only and in a limited number of selected patients.[15,20,29]

CONCLUSION

More than 4 years after the placement of the first metal stent, we believe that these stents represent an extremely valid tool in the management of recurrent strictures; they can be used to recanalize the biliary tree when no other procedure is effective. We observed an overall patency rate of 68% at 4-year follow-up.[18] This is a reasonable success rate, because these patients had no therapeutic alternatives. However, the occurrence of late obstructions has been documented, and for that reason metal stent implantation should remain limited to select patients.

We are still convinced that repeated balloon dilation represents the first choice in the treatment of postoperative biliary stenosis when surgical correction is no longer recommended. If balloon dilation fails, the metal stent may be the last resort for recanalization of the biliary tree without the use of a permanent drainage catheter.

Metal stents and balloon dilation are complementary rather than competitive methods; if metal stents are used in patients with failed balloon dilation, an improved overall patency rate may be achieved.

REFERENCES

1. Warren KW, Mountain JC, Midell AI. Management of strictures of the biliary tract. Surg Clin North Am 51:711-730, 1971.
2. Bolton JS, Braasch JW, Rossi RL. Management of benign biliary strictures. Surg Clin North Am 60:313-332, 1980.
3. Glenn F. Iatrogenic injuries to the biliary ductal system. Surg Gynecol Obstet 1978;146:430-434.
4. Way LW, Bernhoft RA, Thomas MJ. Biliary strictures. Surg Clin North Am 61:963-969, 1981.
5. Wright TB, Bertino RB, Bishop AF, et al. Complications of laparoscopic cholecystectomy and their interventional radiologic management. Radiographics 13:119-128, 1993.
6. Pitt HA, Miyamoto T, Parapatis SK, et al. Factors influencing outcome in patients with postoperative biliary strictures. Am J Surg 144:14-19, 1982.
7. Blumgart LH, Kelley CJ, Benjamin IS. Benign bile duct strictures following cholecystectomy: Critical factors in management. Br J Surg 71:836-843, 1984.
8. Mueller PR, Van Sonnenberg E, Ferrucci JT, et al. Biliary stricture dilatation: Multicenter review of clinical management in 73 patients. Radiology 106:17-22, 1986.
9. Moore AV, Illescas FF, Mills SR, et al. Percutaneous dilation of benign biliary strictures. Radiology 163:625-628, 1987.
10. Williams HJ, Bender CE, May GR. Benign postoperative biliary strictures: Dilation with fluoroscopic guidance. Radiology 163:629-634, 1987.
11. Citron SJ, Martin LG. Benign biliary strictures: Treatment with percutaneous cholangioplasty. Radiology 178:339-341, 1991.
12. Rossi P, Salvatori FM, Bezzi M, et al. Percutaneous management of benign biliary strictures with balloon dilation and self-expanding metal stents. CVIR 13:231-239, 1990.
13. Carrasco CH, Wallace S, Charnsangavej C, et al. Expandable biliary endoprostheses: An experimental study. AJR 145:1279-1281, 1985.
14. Alvarado R, Palmaz J, Garcia OJ, et al. Evaluation of polymer-coated balloon-expandable stents in bile ducts. Radiology 170:975-978, 1989.
15. Coons HG. Self-expanding stainless steel biliary stents. Radiology 170:979-983, 1989.
16. Dick R, Gillams A, Dooley JS, et al. Stainless steel mesh stents for biliary strictures. Intervent Radiol 4:95-98, 1989.
17. Rossi P, Bezzi M, Salvatori FM, et al. Recurrent benign biliary strictures: Management with self-expanding metallic stents. Radiology 175:661-665, 1990.
18. Maccioni F, Rossi M, Salvatori FM, et al. Metallic stents in benign biliary strictures: Three years follow-up. CVIR 15:360-366, 1992.
19. Coons H. Metallic stents for the treatment of biliary obstructions: A report of 100 cases. CVIR 15:367-374, 1992.
20. Bezzi M, Salvatori FM, Maccioni F, et al. Biliary metallic stents in benign strictures. Semin Intervent Radiol 8:321-329, 1991.
21. Uchida BT, Putnam JS, Rosh J. Modification of Gianturco expandable wire stents. AJR 150:1185-1187, 1988.
22. Maeda M, et al. Spiral Z-stent—Its mechanical characteristics and clinical use in biliary obstruction. Presented at the Cardiovascular and Interventional Radiological Society of Europe (CIRSE) Annual Meeting. Barcelona, 1992.
23. Adson MA, Berquist TH, Johnson CM. Percutaneous biliary decompression: Internal and external drainage in 50 patients. AJR 136(5):901-906, 1981.
24. Dooley S, Dick R, Irving D, et al. Relief of bile duct obstruction by the percutaneous transhepatic insertion of an endoprosthesis. Clin Radiol 32:162-172, 1981.
25. Mueller PR, Ferrucci JT, Teplick SK, et al. Biliary stent endoprosthesis: Analysis of complications in 113 patients. Radiology 176:531-534, 1990.
26. Lammer J. Biliary endoprostheses: Plastic versus metal stents. Radiol Clin North Am 28:1211-1222, 1990.
27. McLeod G, Armstrong D, McRoss A, et al. Management of malignant biliary obstruction by percutaneously introduced biliary endoprostheses. J Coll Surg Edinburgh 31:210-213, 1986.
28. Lameris JS, Stoker J, Nijs H, et al. Malignant biliary obstruction: Percutaneous use of self-expandable stents. Radiology 179:703-707, 1991.
29. Yoshioka T, Sakaguchi H, Yoshimura H, et al. Expandable metallic biliary endoprostheses: Preliminary clinical evaluation. Radiology 177:253-257, 1990.
30. Mueller PR, Tegmeyer CJ, Saini S, et al. Metallic biliary stents: Early experience [abstract]. Radiology 177:138, 1990.
31. Mueller PR. Metallic endoprostheses: Boon or bust? Radiology 179:603-605, 1991.
32. Mueller PR, Dawson SL. Metallic biliary endoprostheses and biliary stricture dilation. Syllabus: A diagnostic categorical course in interventional radiology. RSNA 111-118, 1991.
33. Adam A, Chetty N. Roddie M, et al. Self-expandable stainless steel endoprostheses for treatment of malignant bile duct obstruction. AJR 156:321-325, 1991.
34. Lammer J. Biliary endoprostheses: Plastic versus metal stents. Radiol Clin North Am 28:1211-1222, 1990.
35. Gillams A, Dick R, Dooley JS, et al. Self-expandable stainless steel braided endoprosthesis for biliary strictures. Radiology 174:137-140, 1990.
36. Irving JD, Adam A, Dick R, et al. Gianturco expandable metallic biliary stents: Results of a European clinical trial. Radiology 172:321-326, 1989.
37. Salomonowitz EK, Antonucci F, Heer M, et al. Biliary obstruction: Treatment with self-expanding endoprostheses. CVIR 3:365-370, 1992.

37 *Laparoscopic Treatment of Large Intrahepatic Cysts*

Volker Lange, Guenther Meyer, Hans-Martin Schardey, and
Friedrich-Wilhelm Schildberg

Ultrasonography and computed tomography have made hepatic cysts a common finding; however, surgical intervention for these lesions is now rarely required, since most such cysts are found incidentally and are asymptomatic. If the cysts are symptomatic, surgical management may be necessary. Several operative procedures have been performed, depending on the nature of the cysts.[1,2] Besides these surgical interventions different percutaneous, nonresective procedures have been described.[3,4,5] We report our experience in the laparoscopic treatment of cysts of the liver.

PATIENTS

All treated cysts in our series were symptomatic and classified as congenital, unilocular or multilocular, solitary cysts of the liver. In nine patients the cysts uniformly presented with such symptoms as a sensation of fullness in the upper abdomen, often increasing in the lateral position, postprandial satiety, recurrent nausea, and in three cases, abdominal pain after little food intake. Only one patient suffered an acute pain episode, leading to hospitalization in another hospital. In this woman (patient 3), we found a pedunculated cyst that might have twisted as reason for the primary admission.

Preoperatively the usual blood chemistry evaluations were obtained, including an *Echinococcus* serology test. The latter test yielded negative results in all patients; otherwise, the patient would have been excluded from the laparoscopic approach. CT scanning was a prerequisite before and 6 weeks after the operation (Figs. 1 through 4). Angiography or ERCP were not done.

Table 1. Clinical data for patients operated on for cysts of the liver

Patient No.	Age	Sex	Location of Cyst	Size (cm)	Follow-up (months)
1	37	F	Left lobe	12.5 × 14	23
2	55	F	Right lobe	4.5 × 8	21
3	59	F	Right lobe	5 × 10	17
			Left lobe	6 × 6	
4	50	F	Right lobe	8 × 10	16
5	56	F	Left lobe	13 × 14	15
6	61	F	Left lobe	10 × 12	12
			Left lobe	7 × 9	
			Right lobe	10 × 12	
7	67	F	Left lobe	10 × 12	11
8	60	F	Right lobe	14 × 17	11
9	58	M	Right lobe	8 × 6	11
			Right lobe	3 × 4	
10	58	F	Right lobe	11 × 9	10

F = female; M = male.

RESULTS

From February 1991 through June 1992, 10 patients underwent laparoscopic operations for symptomatic cysts of the liver (Table 1). Seven patients were operated on for solitary cysts, in two patients there were two cysts, and one patient presented with several cysts, of which three large ones were deroofed. In one case the liver cyst was associated with gallbladder stone disease, so a laparoscopic cholecystectomy was simultaneously performed, because symptoms could not clearly be differentiated. A second patient with concomitant gallbladder stones refused cholecystectomy. She suffered colicky symptoms from these stones for half a year and then was admitted for a laparoscopic cholecystectomy. In one patient, preoperative computed tomography revealed a coin lesion in the lateral aspect of the right lower lobe of the lung. In one session the deroofing was carried out first, and after changing the position of the

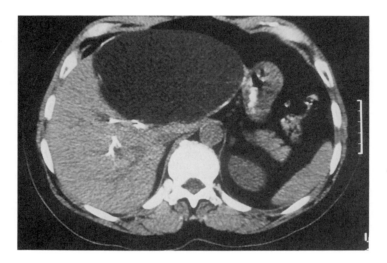

Fig. 1. Large cyst of the left lobe of the liver (patient 5).

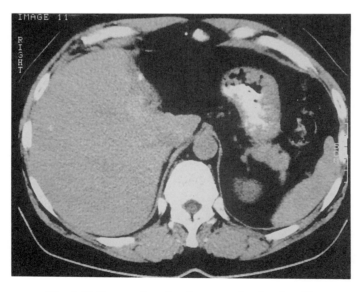

Fig. 2. Follow-up 6 weeks after operation (patient 5).

patient, the pulmonary nodule was removed by thoracoscopic atypical lung resection.

The laparoscopic operations were performed with the patient in reverse Trendelenburg position and under general anesthesia. The ports were placed comparable to the cholecystectomy procedure. A 30- or 45-degree laparoscope (Olympus) was attached to a video camera (Olympus OTV-S2) and a pneumoperitoneum by CO_2 insufflation was established; pressure was maintained at 12 mm Hg. The cysts were punctured and the superficial parts of the wall of the cyst were resected with the electric hook or cautery scissors using monopolar current. The resection line followed the border of the cystic wall to the parenchyme of the liver. Two cysts were located extrahepatically, with a small peduncle to the liver; thus they could be cut off with an EndoGIA (Autosuture) after complete mobilization. The same instrument was used in two cases to resect the fingerlike rest-parenchyme of the left lobe. In another case we used the stapling device to stop bleeding from a major vein of the right lobe of the liver, close to the cava. The vessel was grasped and occluded by forceps, gently elevated, and the tissue of the liver, including the vein, was stapled and cut (Figs. 3 and 4).

Resected specimens were sent for frozen section. The remaining surface of the cyst was inspected for irregularities of the wall or visible bile secretion. Neither finding occurred in our series. In the first three cases we destroyed the remaining wall of the cyst by cautery spatula and in another case by argon beam. We injured a liver vein with a spatula in our very first patient. Bleeding was stopped by injecting fibrin sealant (Tissucol, Immuno) into the surrounding liver tissue, thereby compressing the vessel. Although there was no bleeding, at the end of the operation postoperative oozing was observed. Two units of blood were given to compensate the loss, which could be detected by ultrasound as a hematoma in the operative field. Use of the argon beam required extreme attention by the operator, because the flow of the additional gas immediately led to an elevation of intra-abdominal pressure. By opening one of the trocars, the pressure could be kept in the usual range.

In one cyst protruding close to the gallbladder, an iatrogenic lesion of this organ occurred and therefore we removed it. In all patients but one, Robinson tubes were placed. The other patient, whose operation was fastest (30 minutes), developed an abscess in the former bed of the cyst. The abscess was percutaneously drained under ultrasonographic guidance and healed without complications or bile leakage.

In one patient the surface of the cyst was smaller than presumed preoperatively. In this case only a fenestration of the cyst was possible. By early reunification of the rims of the liver the cyst had half of its former diameter at follow-up 8 weeks after operation. To our astonishment, in further controls the volume of the cyst continuously decreased and presents now 1 year after

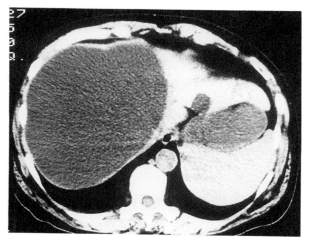

Fig. 3. Giant cyst of the right lobe of the liver (patient 8).

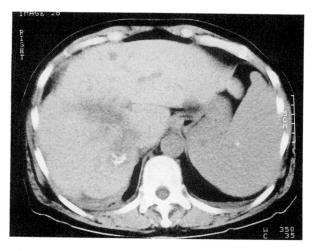

Fig. 4. Follow-up 6 weeks after operation (patient 8). Within the parenchyma of the liver, staples from the EndoGIA are apparent; the EndoGIA was used to stop bleeding from a major liver vein.

the intervention with a diameter of 2×2 cm. The times for the operations ranged from 30 minutes to 3.5 hours in our first patient; on average the procedure lasted 70 minutes. Substitution of blood was never necessary, except in the patient previously mentioned. There was no bile leakage postoperatively. The hospital stay averaged 5 days; the first patients were kept in the hospital longer than absolutely necessary for control. Follow-up was performed by CT scan or ultrasonography.

In the case of the patient who underwent laparoscopic cholecystectomy 6 months later, we found a smooth surface of the liver with no evidence of the previous operation. The only adhesion that could be seen in the abdomen was a thin band from the omentum to one of the 5 mm port incisions.

DISCUSSION

The genesis of nonparasitic, congenital cysts of the liver allows differentiation into two groups: (1) extremely dilated segments of the biliary tree (intrahepatic and extrahepatic manifestation of cysts, as in Caroli's disease) or (2) cystic transformations of tiny clusters of hypoplastic bile ducts (von Meyenburg Complex) that persists from embryonic development. These have no connection to the bile ducts.[6-9] Solitary cysts of the liver belong to the latter group and are, in our opinion, suitable for laparoscopic treatment. These cysts may be uni- or multilocular and are steps on the way leading to polycystic liver disease. They contain straw-coloured, nonbilious fluid and usually become apparent in adults between the third and sixth decade. The cystic wall is lined by cuboidal epithelium.[6,10] Simple puncture of the cysts must fail, because the untreated epithelium continues to secrete fluid.[5] In contrast, cystic formations of the bile ducts were found more often in children or young adults and preferably need resection for the malignant potential of residual cystic tissue.[1,12]

Both types of cysts have to be distinguished from cystadenomas of the liver presenting with or without connection to the biliary tree. They are a rare condition, but transformation into cystadenocarcinoma is proven, so anatomical resection is requested in these cases.[11,12] Preoperative ultrasonography or CT scanning often reveals fine septations and solid papillary invaginations or nodularities of the cyst wall of cystadenomas. Intraoperative dark-colored fluid within the cyst is a suspicious sign and should lead to conscientious inspection of the inner surface of the cyst for detection of wall irregularities.[11] The magnifying lens of the laparoscope may be an advantage for this investigation compared to open surgery. We think that with the lens, unsuspected openings of bile ducts can also be recognized more easily. It is recommended that such a finding be treated by resection or cystoenteric anastomosis,[7,8,10] although oversewing of the biliary radicals has been reported.[2] In solitary cysts following the previous definition, no biliary communication should be expected and could not be seen in our series.

Laparoscopic deroofing of as much of the cyst wall as possible has proven to be a successful procedure in open surgery.[1,10] Meanwhile positive results of the laparoscopic approach are reported by others.[13-15] Because the natural course of congenital cystic disease of the liver is unknown, the parenchyme-saving procedure of deroofing seems to us to be the treatment of choice.[16] After generous anatomical resections of cysts, new cystic formations in the liver remnant finally led to liver transplantation in single cases.[1] Total excision and partial hepatectomy are associated with significant morbidity and mortality.[13] Partial excision or fenestration is associated with a higher percentage of recurrences, even when the cavity is drained for a longer period or packed with omentum.[2,6] Marsupialization and percutaneous interventions bring the potential for infection. Simple puncture is insufficient,[5] and when it is combined with the injection of sclerosing agents, repeated treatments are necessary.[4] The lack of histological and macroscopic examination is also associated with significant morbidity.[3]

Taking all of these considerations into account, laparoscopic deroofing of the cysts has all the advantages of a minimally invasive procedure and seems to yield good results. All our patients are free of complaints. In our first case, follow-up over 2 years showed a constant residual sinus formation 2 cm in diameter in the completely regenerated left lobe of the liver. Whether this resulted from the resorbed hematoma or the remaining epithelium of the cyst cannot be determined. Only one other patient had a cystic cavity of 1 cm after deroofing of a 17 to 14 cm cyst. In the first case we performed electrocoagulation of the remaining epithelium of the cyst, a treatment of doubtful value, which we ultimately abandoned. Subtotal resection of three cysts in a polycystic liver resulted in a slight increase in the size of the remaining cysts. As mentioned earlier, the limited excision in one case was followed by a continuous regression of the cyst, which was reduced 6 weeks after operation to only half of its volume. This finding contradicts the experience of others.[10]

Median follow-up in our series is still short and amounts to 15 months. Wellwood et al.[6] saw five of eight recurrences after limited excision in 10 patients within 1 year, two within 2, and only one within 5 years. We were able to excise more than one third of the cyst wall in all but one patient. Because on average our patients in this series have passed more than a year without relapse, we feel with relative certainty that this technique is successful. The resection of at least one third of the dome of the cyst is recommended as essential by most authors.[2,6,10]

CONCLUSION

Laparoscopic deroofing of congenital, nonparasitic, noninfected, and superficially located liver cysts is a simple technique that yields good results. The indication for operation is only in symptomatic cysts, which as a rule occur with a diameter of more than 10 cm.[2,9] Videoendoscopic intervention offers excellent visualization, can be performed rapidly with some experience, and is a blood-saving procedure.

REFERENCES

1. Lai E, Wong J. Symptomatic nonparasitic cysts of the liver. World J Surg 14:452, 1990.
2. Litwin DEM, Taylor BR, Greig P, Langer B. Nonparasitic cysts of the liver. Ann Surg 205:45, 1987.
3. Gebel M, Schulz M. Ergebnisse der nicht-chirurgischen Behandlung von Leberzysten. Z Gastroenterol 26:252, 1988.
4. El Mouaaouy A, Naruhn M, Lauchart W, Becker HD. Behandlung der symptomatischen, nichtparasitären Leberzysten mittels percutaner Drainage und Spülung mit hypertoner Kochsalzlösung. Chirurgie 62:810, 1992.
5. Saini S, Müller PR, Ferrucci JT, Simeone JF, Wittenberg J, Butch RJ. Percutaneous aspiration of hepatic cysts does not provide definitive therapy. AJR 141:559, 1983.
6. Wellwood JM, Madara JL, Cady B, Haggit RC. Large intrahepatic cysts and pseudocysts. Am J Surg 135:57, 1978.
7. Flanigan DP. Biliary cysts. Ann Surg 182:635, 1975.
8. Klempa I, Menzel J, Kubale R, Brandt G. Zur Problematik der intrahepatischen Gallengangszysten. Chirurgie 57:741, 1986.
9. Schulz F, Függer R, Contreras F, Funovics J. Klinik und Therapie der angeborenen Cystenleber. Chirurgie 55:813, 1984.
10. Edwards JD, Eckhauser FE, Knol JA, Strodel WE, Appelman H. Optimizing surgical management of symptomatic solitary hepatic cysts. Am J Surg 53:510, 1987.
11. Lewis WD, Jenkins RL, Rossi RL, Munson L, ReMine SG, Cady B, Braasch YW, Dermott WV. Surgical treatment of biliary cystadenoma. Arch Surg 123:563, 1988.
12. Hermann RE. Gallengangscysten. Chirurgie 56:193, 1985.
13. Bouillot JL, Salah S, Baccot S, Alexandre JH. Percutaneous surgery of biliary cyst: A case report. J Laparoendosc Surg 2:101, 1992.
14. Fabiani P, Katkhouda N, Iovine L, Mouiel J. Laparoscopic fenestration of biliary cysts. Surg Laparosc Endosc 1:162, 1991.
15. Z'graggen K, Metzger A, Klaiber C. Symptomatic simple cysts of the liver: Treatment by laparoscopic surgery. Surg Endosc 5:224, 1991.
16. Lange V, Meyer G, Rau H, Schildberg FW. Minimalinvasive Eingriffe bei solitären Lebercysten. Chirurgie 63:349, 1992.

38 Technique and Pitfalls of Transjugular Intrahepatic Portosystemic Shunting (TIPS)

D. Azoulay, D. Castaing, A. Dennison, W. Martino, and H. Bismuth

In 1968 Rösch, Hanafee, and Snow[1] pioneered transjugular intrahepatic portosystemic shunting (TIPS) when they inadvertently entered the portal venous system while performing a transjugular cholangiogram. A year later the same authors used a percutaneous approach to create a parenchymal fistula between the inferior vena cava and the portal vein in a dog.

During the 1970s radiologists as well as surgeons investigated this new approach using techniques such as cutting, drilling, and cryotherapy to create parenchymal fistulas.[2] Initially the method used in humans was to repeatedly dilate the created tract using a transjugular approach, and no attempt was made to insert a stent.[3] However, this method resulted in poor patency of the fistulas. Abecassis et al.[4] reported that only 2 of 15 patients had patent shunts 6 months after the procedure. Rösch et al.[5] and Palmaz et al.[6] attempted to solve this particular problem by using stents. Rösch developed the first self-expanding prosthesis and Palmaz created the balloon-expandable prosthesis. In 1900 Richter et al.[7] described the first successful series of TIPS using Palmaz stents in humans. At that time, however, the technique used a combined transjugular and transhepatic route, and it took at least several hours to perform and occasionally much longer (up to 2 days). Since then Ring and colleagues[8] in San Francisco have made technical advances using an expandable metallic stent (Wallstent), resulting in a safer and quicker method of TIPS.

Most "TIPSologists" presently prefer the Wallstent to the Palmaz stent.[9] The advantages and disadvantages of each type of stent are summarized in the box at right.

TIPS TECHNIQUE (Figs. 1-10)

At Paul Brousse Hospital TIPS is performed under full aseptic conditions in the operating theater with the patient under general anethesia. The patient is positioned supine with x-ray and ultrasonographic equipment on the patient's left side. The fluoroscopy equipment has a C arm, which allows views at 90 degrees, and has two screens capable of retaining a fixed image. Computer integration allows at least four images to be maintained at any time. The operating field, which includes the right side of the neck and trunk, is prepared with an antiseptic solution, and the patient is then draped. The surgeon and assistant stand at the head and right side of the patient respectively. There are four stages to the procedure.

Catheterization of the Right Hepatic Vein

The right internal jugular vein is punctured with a 9 Fr catheter with a hemostatic valve (Desivalve, Vygon). Under fluoroscopic guidance, an 8 Fr cholangiography catheter (Catheter Teflon Radiopaque, Cook) is manipulated through the superior vena cava, the right atrium, and the inferior vena cava and into the right hepatic vein.

Text continued on p. 187.

ADVANTAGES AND DISADVANTAGES OF PALMAZ AND WALLSTENT PROSTHESES

Palmaz Prosthesis (balloon expandable, Fig. 9)

Advantages	Can be dilated
Disadvantages	No introducing sheath
	Unique length (30 mm)
	Rigid

Wallstent Prosthesis (self-expanding, Fig. 10, *A* and *B*)

Advantages	Introducing sheath
	Longitudinal flexibility
	Pliability
	Variable length
Disadvantages	Maximum diameter defined in advance
	Compressible

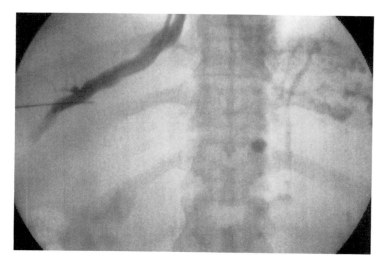

Fig. 1. The right hepatic vein is catheterized and a Chiba needle is placed into the portal vein bifurcation (under ultrasonographic guidance).

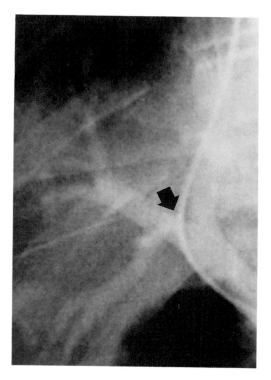

Fig. 2. A fistula is created between the right hepatic and the right portal veins. Note the level of portal vein perforation *(black arrow)*.

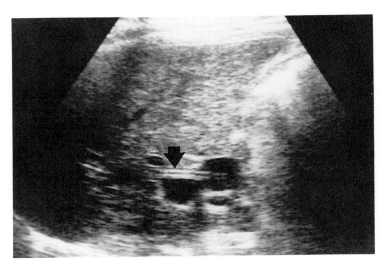

Fig. 3. Venovenous puncture can be performed under ultrasonographic guidance only. Note the Ross needle penetrating into the portal vein *(black arrow)*.

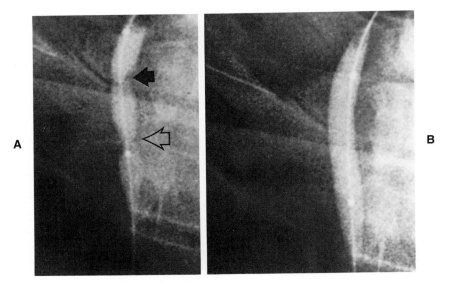

Fig. 4. The venovenous puncture tract is dilated. **A,** With partial inflation, ringlike constriction is present at both hepatic and portal veins perforations *(black* and *open arrows,* respectively). **B,** With full distention, constriction has disappeared.

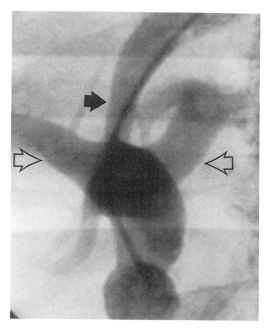

Fig. 5. Stent is deployed *(black arrow)*. Note the persistence of hepatopetal portal flow to the liver *(open arrows)*.

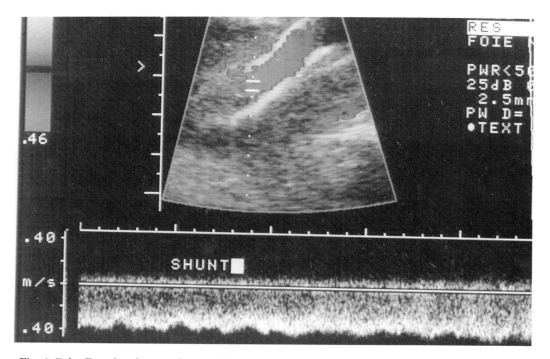

Fig. 6. Color Doppler ultrasound control shows completely expanded stent with good portohepatic flow.

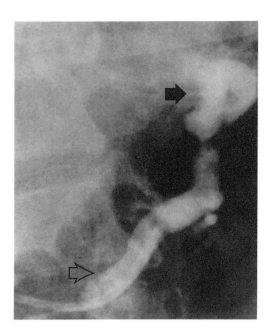

Fig. 7. Retrograde embolization of esogastric varices. Left gastric vein *(open arrow)* is catheterized, and esogastric varices are embolized *(black arrow).*

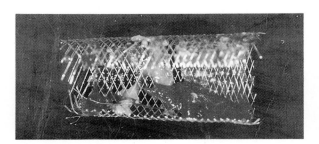

Fig. 8. Stent removed after liver transplantation. Histological examination shows patchy endothelialization.

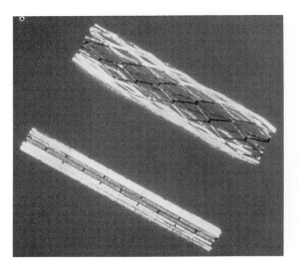

Fig. 9. The balloon-expandable Palmaz prosthesis.

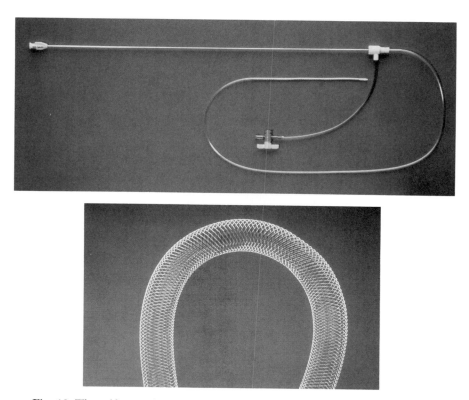

Fig. 10. The self-expanding Wallstent is placed by use of an introducing sheath.

An opacification of the hepatic vein is stored in the memory of the fluoroscopic unit. The free hepatic venous pressure is measured.

Under ultrasonographic guidance, a 0.9 mm Chiba needle (Cook) is placed percutaneously and transhepatically into the main portal vein bifurcation. The latter maneuver enables the surgeon to evaluate, under simultaneous fluoroscopic and ultrasonographic control, the length and direction of the parenchyma separating the right hepatic vein and the right portal vein. The tip of the Chiba needle also delineates the inferior limit of the potential progression of the needle during the venovenous puncture.

Creation of a Parenchymal Fistula Between the Right Hepatic Vein and the Right Portal Vein

Under double control (fluoroscopic and echographic) a 16-gauge modified Ross transjugular needle (Cook) is advanced through the cholangiography catheter and is then directed out of the hepatic vein as close as possible to the origin of the hepatic vein. The needle is guided inferiorly and anteriorly toward the tip of the Chiba needle identifying the portal vein. Once the operator gains experience, it becomes unnecessary to place a Chiba needle into the portal vein, and the entire venovenous puncture procedure can be performed under ultrasonographic guidance only. Free blood reflux through the lumen of the Ross needle indicates portal vein perforation, and then an angiographic image of the portal vein perforation is obtained. A 0.9 mm Amplatz Super Stiff vascular guidewire (Boston Scientific) is passed through the needle and is manipulated across the main portal vein into the splenic or mesenteric vein. The cholangiography catheter is advanced over the guidewire into the portal vein, and the Ross needle together with the guidewire are then removed. The initial baseline portal vein pressure is measured and an image of the portal vein is stored in the memory of the fluoroscopic unit.

Dilation of the Parenchymal Tract

The Amplatz guidewire is inserted again, and the jugular sheath is replaced by another 10 Fr catheter with a hemostatic valve (Check-Flow II, Cook). An 8 mm angiography balloon catheter (Ultra Thin, Boston Scientific) is inflated in the tract between the hepatic vein and the portal vein.

Deployment of the Stent

The balloon catheter is removed and a 2.3 mm Wallstent catheter (Wallstent, Schneider) is introduced. The length of the stent depends on the distance between the two veins. The stent is positioned so that it begins to open into the right portal vein just proximal to its origin, and it is deployed from there through the parenchymal tract toward the hepatic vein. The detached 10 Fr catheter is removed, and a portogram is taken to verify the position of the stent and the direction of the portal flow. If the cephalad end of the prosthesis does not reach the hepatic vein, a second stent is positioned so that it partially overlaps the first one to bridge the additional distance. If portal flow remains hepatofugal, the prosthesis is dilated until the flow becomes hepatopetal.

Measurement of portal pressure enables the operator to evaluate any drop in portal pressure and determine whether the prosthesis should be dilated further.

All material is then removed from the jugular vein. The cutaneous puncture site is sutured and dressed. Heparin is started intraoperatively after portal vein cannulation at a rate of 1 mg/kg/24 hr.

POSTOPERATIVE FOLLOW-UP

The patient is maintained on heparin for 7 days. The dosage of heparin is adjusted to maintain the APTT at 1.5 to 2 times the control. After the patient is discharged, an injection of low-molecular-weight heparin is given daily until day 21 after the operation.

Doppler ultrasonographic examination is performed daily to assess the stent patency until day 7 after the procedure, then at day 14, then monthly. Assessment of esophageal varices is performed on day 14 by endoscopy, and biochemical parameters are measured daily until day 7 after the procedure, then at day 14, and then monthly.

VARIATIONS AND PITFALLS
Use of the Middle or the Left Hepatic Vein

The right hepatic vein is sometimes atrophic or has a sharp angulation that makes the vein almost horizontal. These anatomic variations make catheterization of the right hepatic vein difficult. However, it is possible to position the shunt between the middle or the left hepatic vein and the right or the left portal vein. It is even pos-

sible to position the shunt via a femoral vein approach in case of large inferior right hepatic vein.[10]

Retrograde Embolization of the Esophogastric Varices

It is easy to catheterize the left gastric vein and to embolize the varices through the stent. We prefer to use biodegradable spongel rather than metallic coils.[3]

TIPS in Patients With Portal Vein Occlusion

Radosevitch et al.[11] reported seven successful cases of TIPS placement in 10 patients with portal vein occlusion. Recanalization of the occluded portal vein via the transhepatic approach improved the success of the procedure.

Contraindications to the Use of the TIPS Procedure

Use of the TIPS procedure is currently contraindicated in patients with hepatic neoplasms and spontaneous bacterial peritonitis.

THE PAUL BROUSSE HOSPITAL CENTER EXPERIENCE
Patient Profile

From November 1991 to November 1992, 40 patients underwent 40 TIPS placement attempts at the Paul Brousse Hospital. There were 25 male and 15 female patients who ranged in age from 22 to 74 years. All these patients had biopsy-proven cirrhosis. The type of cirrhosis was alcoholic in 16 cases, posthepatic in 21 cases, and due to other causes in 3 cases. Informed consent was requested and was obtained from all patients included in this prospective uncontrolled trial. The severity of cirrhosis was classified according to our modified Pugh's classification of cirrhosis[12] (Table 1). Eight patients were classified as grade A, 20 as grade B, and 12 as grade C. Indications for the TIPS procedure were sclerotherapy failure in 32/40 cases and/or intractable ascites in 21/40 cases.

Results

The procedure was successful in 35 cases (88%) in a mean time of 112 ± 56 min. The pressure gradient between the right atrium and the portal vein decreased from 20 ± 9 to 9 ± 6 mm HG ($p < 0.02$, paired t-test). Four patients died after the TIPS procedure. However, only one death (a right subclavian artery aneurysm) was directly related to the technique. Five patients presented with an acute and transient episode of encephalop-

Table 1. Paul Brousse classification of hepatocellular function

Criteria

Clinical ascites	1 point
Encephalopathy	1 point
Bilirubin >30 mmol/L	1 point
Albumin <30 gm/L	1 point
(PT + factor II)/2 <60%	1 point
(PT + factor II)/2 <40%	2 points

Classification

Grade A	0 point
Grade B	1-2 points
Grade C	>2 points

PT (prothrombin time) and factor II are given in percent of normal level.

Table 2. Characteristics and results in 35 TIPS procedures in 40 patients at Paul Brousse Hospital

	No. of Patients
Type of cirrhosis	
Alcoholic	16 (40%)
Posthepatic	21 (53%)
Other	3 (7%)
Paul Brousse grade of cirrhosis	
Grade A	8 (20%)
Grade B	20 (50%)
Grade C	12 (30%)
Laboratory data	
Bilirubin	39 ± 29 μmol/L
Albumin	35 ± 7 g/L
Prothrombin index	60 ± 15%
(% of normal level)	
Clinical findings	
Ascites	25 (63%)
Encephalopathy	0
Previous variceal bleeding	37 (93%)
Successful TIPS	35 (88%)
Mortality	
30 day	4 (10%)
Overall	4 (10%)
Control of varices	7/30 (90%)
Control of ascites	15/19 (79%)
Portal pressure (mm Hg)	
Before TIPS	20 ± 9 (p <0.02)
After TIPS	9 ± 6
Encephalopathy (acute only)	5 (14%)
Recurrence of hemorrhage	1/31 (3%)
Thrombosis of TIPS	3/35 (9%)

athy. All of these episodes occurred before day 21 after the TIPS procedure, and all were easily controlled with lactulose. No chronic debilitating encephalopathy occurred.

On postoperative days 2, 3, and 5 three patients had early thrombosis of the shunt, which was diagnosed by Doppler examination. In each of these emergencies the stent was percutaneously reopened and a new stent was deployed into the first one.

Thirty-three cases are available for analysis with TIPS in 28/32 for sclerotherapy failure, 17/21 for intractable ascites.

One patient experienced rebleed on day 9 after the TIPS procedure. Stent thrombosis was diagnosed by Doppler examination, and a second stent was deployed inside the first one concomitant with variceal embolization. No additional bleeding was noted and the patient underwent liver transplantation 27 days later.

None of the remaining patients had any rebleeding. Esophagogastroscopy on day 14 showed shrinkage or disappearance of varices in all cases. Ascites remained unchanged in two cases, improved in six cases who required low dosage of diuretics, and was totally controlled in nine cases.

Nine patients underwent orthotopic liver transplantation after the TIPS procedure. A retrospective comparison with equivalent patients who did not undergo TIPS showed that operative time, blood loss, and the postoperative complication rate were reduced in the

TIPS patients. All nine of the TIPS in place were patent and showed histological endothelialization of the internal lumen of the stents.

COMPLICATIONS

Portosystemic encephalopathy (PSE) has been reported in 10% to 30% of patients[9] following the TIPS procedure. The occurrence of PSE seems to depend on the age of the patient, the diameter of the stent, and the shunt flow.[13] Encephalopathy occurring after TIPS placement tends to be mild and easily controlled.[14]

The lower incidence of PSE after TIPS placement compared with that after surgical portal decompression is most probably related to the small diameter of the stent. A TIPS 8 to 10 mm in diameter, such as a surgical calibrated shunt,[12,15] maintains a mild degree of portal hypertension, this continues portal venous perfusion of the liver and thus alleviates PSE.

Shunt occlusion after PSE is the second most common complication of the TIPS procedure. The incidence of occlusion ranges from 5% to 10%, regardless of the type of prosthesis used. Histopathological studies of the effects of the TIPS has been reported by LaBerge et al.[16] and Vinel et al.,[17] indicating that endothelialization occurs in patches as early as 7 days after TIPS placement. Occlusion of the TIPS may result from thrombosis or pseudo-intimal hypertrophy. TIPS occlusion can be easily corrected by the deployment of a new stent inside the previous one.

Complications related to stent placement can occur at any site from the jugular access to the liver[9]; they include subclavian artery aneurysm,[18] pulmonary embolization of the sent,[19] puncture of the gallbladder,[20] capsule rupture,[21] cardiac puncture,[22] hemobilia, intraperitoneal hemorrhage, contrast-induced transient oliguric renal failure,[23] bacteremia, septic shock and fever,[22] pulmonary emboli and partial venous thrombosis, and intravascular hemolysis.[24]

DISCUSSION

The technical success rate of the TIPS procedure is around 90% in various centers around the world. Approximately 1200 TIPS reports are available in the literature[9]; however, the procedure is complex and those who perform it need advanced technologic skills. TIPS procedures should be performed in units in which high resolution C-arm fluoroscopy, digital subtraction angiographic capability, and high quality ultrasound are available, together with surgeons experienced with catheter guidewire manipulation and angiography techniques and who know intrahepatic anatomy and stent deployment procedures.[25]

TIPS functions as a side-to-side portacaval anastomosis. It reduces portal pressure and thus the risks of variceal bleeding. The TIPS procedure is less invasive, faster, safer, and less expensive than is surgical decompression. TIPS has been performed for active variceal bleeding,[8] prevention of bleeding recurrence (primarily in sclerotherapy failure), intractable ascites[24-28] and acute Budd-Chiari syndrome.[29]

CONCLUSION

Data are not available from prospective clinical trials, but some investigations are currently underway in several centers, including our own. It is important to compare the TIPS procedure with the treatments presently available for acute variceal bleeding and the prevention of recurrent hemorrhage, and also to investigate its place in the management of intractable ascites and hepatorenal syndrome. Because the shunt insertion is relatively noninvasive as well as intrahepatic (it does not compromise subsequent transplantation),[30-33] the TIPS procedure is likely to emerge as an exciting new part of the armamentarium in the treatment of portal hypertension.

REFERENCES

1. Rösch J, Hanafee W, Snow H. Transjugular portal venography and radiological portacaval shunt: An experimental study. Radiology 92:1112-1114, 1969.
2. Reich M, Olumide F, Jorgensen E, et al. Experimental cryoprobe production of intrahepatic portosystemic shunt. J Surg Res 73:14-18, 1977.
3. Colapinto RF, Stronell RD, Gildiner M, et al. Formation of intrahepatic portosystemic shunts using a balloon dilatation catheter: Preliminary clinical experience. AJR 140:709-714, 1983.
4. Abecassis M, Gordon JD, Colapinto RF. The transjugular intrahepatic portosystemic shunt (TIPS): An alternative for the management of life-threatening variceal hemorrhage. Hepatology 5:1032, 1985.
5. Rösch J, Uchida BT, Putnam JS, et al. Experimental intrahepatic portacaval anastomosis: Use of expandable Gianturco stents. Radiology 162:481-485, 1987.
6. Palmaz JC, Garcia F, Tio FO, et al. Expandable intrahepatic portacaval shunt stents in dogs with chronic portal hypertension. AJR 147:1251-1254, 1986.
7. Richter GM, Noeldge G, Palmaz JC, et al. Transjugular intrahepatic portacaval stent shunt: Preliminary clinical results. Radiology 174:1027-1030, 1990.
8. Ring EJ, Lake JR, Roberts JP, et al. Using transjugular intrahepatic portosystemic shunts to control variceal bleeding before liver transplantation. Ann Intern Med 116:304-309, 1992.
9. Conn HO. Transjugular intrahepatic portal-systemic shunts: The state of the art. Hepatology 17:148-158, 1993.
10. LaBerge JM, Ring EJ, Gordon RL. Percutaneous intrahepatic portosystemic shunt created via a femoral vein approach. Radiology 181:679-681, 1991.
11. Radosvich PM, Ring EJ, LaBerge JM, et al. Portosystemic shunts in patients with portal vein occlusion. Radiology (in press).
12. Adam R, Diamond T, Bismuth H. Partial portacaval shunt: Renaissance of an old concept. Surgery 111:610-616, 1992.
13. Sellinger M, Haag K, Ochs A, et al. Factors influencing the incidence of hepatic encephalopathy in patients

with transjugular intrahepatic portosystemic stent-shunt (TIPS) (abstract). Hepatology 16 (suppl):122A, 1992.

14. Somberg KA, Riegler JL, Doherty M, et al. Hepatic encephalopathy following transjugular intrahepatic portosystemic shunts (TIPS): Incidence and risk factors (abstract). Hepatology 16 (suppl): 122A, 1992.

15. Sarfeh IJ, Rypins EB, Conroy RM, et al. Portacaval H-graft: Relationship of shunt diameter, portal flow patterns and encephalopathy. Ann Surg 197:422-426, 1983.

16. LaBerge JM, Ferrell LB, Ring EJ. Histopathologic study of transjugular intrahepatic portosystemic shunts. J Vasc Intervent Radiol 2:549-556, 1991.

17. Vinel JP, Rousseau H, Bilbao JL, et al. Transjugular intrahepatic portosystemic shunts using the Wallstent endoprosthesis: Histological study in animals and in patients (abstracts). J Hepatol 16 (suppl):S9-S10, 1992.

18. Azoulay D, Castaing D, Martino V, et al. Second European Congress of Viscero-synthesis. Minimally invasive surgery and new technology. Luxembourg, September 10-12, 1992.

19. Zemel G, Katzen BT, Becker GJ, et al. Percutaneous transjugular portosystemic shunt. JAMA 266:390-393, 1991.

20. LaBerge JM, Ring EJ, Gordon RL, et al. Transjugular intrahepatic portosystemic shunts (TIPS) with the Wallstent (Rx) endoprosthesis: Results in 100 patients. Radiology (in press).

21. Sanyal AJ, Freedman AM, Shiffman ML. Transjugular intrahepatic portosystemic shunt (TIPS) vs sclerotherapy for variceal hemorrhage: Results of a randomized prospective trial (abstract). Hepatology 16 (suppl):88A, 1992.

22. Davies RP, Hennessy OF, Sissons GRJ, et al. Initial Australian experience of transjugular intrahepatic portacaval shunting (TIPS). Presented at the Annual Meeting of International Hepato-Biliary Pancreatic Association: August 1992.

23. Klastenburg DM, Munoz SJ. Complications of transjugular intrahepatic portal systemic shunting (TIPS) (abstract). Am J Gastroenterol 16 (suppl):88A, 1992.

24. Sanyal AJ, Feedman AF, Purdum PP. Use of transjugular intrahepatic portacaval stent shunt (TIPS) for treatment of intractable ascites: A case report. Am J Gastroenterol (in press).

25. Marks MV, Williams D. Percutaneous transjugular portosystemic shunt: Commentary on this new procedure. Hepatology 15:557-558, 1992.

26. Sanyal AJ, Freedman AM, Shiffman ML. Transjugular intrahepatic portosystemic shunt for ascites: A preliminary report (abstract). Am J Gastroenterol 87:1305, 1992.

27. Ochs A, Sellinger M, Haag K. Transjugular intrahepatic portosystemic stent-shunt (TIPS) for the treatment of refractory ascites and hepatorenal syndrome: Results of a pilot study (abstract). Gastroenterol 102:A862, 1992.

28. Garcia-Villareal L, Zozaya JM, Quiroga J, et al. Transjugular intrahepatic portosystemic shunt (TIPS) for intractable ascites (IA): Preliminary results (abstract). J Hepatol 16 (suppl):S36, 1992.

29. Rossle M, Noeldge G, Ochs A. Feasibility of transjugular intrahepatic portosystemic stent shunt (TIPS) in the treatment of fulminant Budd-Chiari syndrome (BCS) (abstract). Gastroenterology 102:A875, 1992.

30. Brems JJ Hiatt JR, Klein AS. Effect of a prior portosystemic shunt on subsequent liver transplantation. Ann Surg 209:51-56, 1989.

31. Roberts JP, Ring E, Lake JR, et al. Intrahepatic portacaval shunt for variceal hemorrhage prior to liver transplantation. Transplantation 52:160-162, 1991.

32. Mazzaferro V, Todo S, Tsakis AG. Liver transplantation in patients with previous portosystemic shunt. Am J Surg 160:111-116, 1990.

33. Langnas AN, Marujo WC, Stratta RJ. Influence of a prior portosystemic shunt on outcome after liver transplantation. Am J Gastroenterol 87:714-718, 1992.

39 *Laparoscopic Duodenopancreatectomy*

Michel Gagner

In 1935, Whipple et al.[1] successfully resected the head of the pancreas in three patients with ampullary carcinoma. Since then, however, progress has been slow in the development of pancreatic resection techniques because of the anatomical complexies of that area. The most recent technical change has been preservation of the pylorus during duodenopancreatectomy for chronic pancreatitis and periampullary tumors.[2] This procedure is currently indicated for chronic pancreatitis localized to the head of the organ. It provides good long-term relief of pain and, in certain cases, reestablishes pancreatic and biliary flow.[3]

Recently, laparoscopic procedures applied to solid intra-abdominal organs have fostered great enthusiasm for minimally invasive approaches.[4-7] We successfully undertook laparoscopic pylorus-preserving duodenopancreatectomy in a patient suffering from chronic pancreatitis and in another with ampullary adenocarcinoma.

INDICATIONS, CONTRAINDICATIONS, AND PREOPERATIVE CARE

Pylorus-preserving duodenopancreatectomy is indicated in patients afflicted by chronic pancreatitis, recurrent subacute pancreatitis, pancreatic neoplasm of the head and uncinate process, duodenal neoplasms, and primary tumors of the distal common bile duct and the ampulla of Vater. The laparoscopic approach can be used in those patients who are not obese and in whom the mass in the head of the pancreas is small, inflammation surrounding the pathological condition is minimal, the mesenteric vein and artery can be easily dissected from the neck of the pancreas, and blood loss is limited.

Contraindications for this procedure include liver or peritoneal metastasis, positive regional nodes in pancreatic cancer (with other periampullary tumors, survival is substantially better after resection, even though the nodes are positive), mesenteric vessel or vena cava involvement, limited pulmonary reserves, unstable cardiac angina, or previous extensive abdominal surgery with intra-abdominal adhesions.

Preoperatively the bowel is prepared with 4 L of GoLYTELY, and cephalosporin is given on the day of operation. Heparin is administered subcutaneously the day before operation and 4 to 6 units of blood are cross-matched to be used in case of major intraoperative hemorrhage. Appropriate radiological examination by abdominal computed tomography or mesenteric angiography is necessary to exclude extraperiampullary neoplastic extension. Biliary drainage is controversial and is not always necessary preoperatively.

SURGICAL TECHNIQUE

Resection is performed by pylorus-preserving duodenopancreatectomy.[3] The patient is kept in a supine position with both legs abducted; the surgeon stands between the patient's legs and an assistant stands on each side of the patient. CO_2 is insufflated with a Veress needle in the umbilicus at up to 15 mm Hg pressure. After the pneumoperitoneum is established, six 10 mm trocars are inserted (Fig. 1). By means of a 0-degree 10 mm

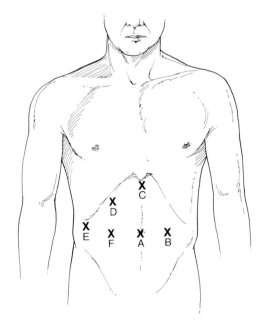

Fig. 1. Sites for trocar insertion: *A*, umbilical; *B*, epigastric; *C*, substernal; *D*, right subcostal; *E*, right flank; and *F*, right iliac fossa.

laparoscope that is inserted in the umbilicus, adhesions of previous cholecystectomy and transduodenal sphincteroplasty are lysed from the right lobe of the liver and the right colon. Finally, the duodenum is dissected free. Diagnostic laparoscopy is performed to rule out metastasis.[8]

The greater curvature of the stomach is grasped and is lifted superiorly and cephalad; an 11 mm Babcock forceps is used from the epigastric port to dissect the gastrocolic ligament and to enter the lesser omentum. This procedure is performed below the gastroepiploic arcade; this provides blood to the preserved pylorus. Clips may be positioned laterally on branches from the gastroepiploic vessels going to the transverse colon. After creation of an 8 to 10 cm window, formal exploration of the lesser sac is undertaken with inspection of the anterior portion of the body and tail of the pancreas, the posterior wall of the stomach (antrum and body), the posterior wall of the transverse colon, and the surrounding mesentery.

When the common bile duct is identified, an intraoperative cholangiogram is obtained with a 22-gauge metallic spinal needle inserted directly into the anterior common bile duct or through the cystic duct to confirm the regional anatomy and to exclude high stenosis or choledocholithiasis. If the gallbladder is present, it is ultimately removed and first used for liver retraction with a grasper on the fundus.

A Kocher maneuver is conducted by upward and medial traction of the duodenum; laparoscopic Babcock forceps are inserted in the epigastric port (Fig. 2). Dissection is performed through the right lateral ports. The retroduodenal areas are dissected anterior to the vena cava and aorta; this frees the head and uncinate process so that suspicious nodes can be identified. The peritoneum covering the common bile duct is opened anteriorly and laterally so that the bile duct can be dissected posteromedially from the portal vein and the right hepatic artery. A suture is then passed with a large curved needle (No. 2 nylon) around the common bile duct through the abdominal wall in the epigastric area so that the bile duct can be suspended and lifted. Next, the common bile duct is transected 2 cm above the duodenum, close to the cystic bile duct junction, with straight endoscopic scissors (Fig. 3). Bile is aspirated under pressure, and a specimen is sent for culture. The anterior pylorus is identified by locating the duodenal veins of Mayo and by endoscopic palpation with a 5 mm metallic probe. A dissector is passed behind the pylorus, and a 3 cm space is created to allow transection of the first portion of the duodenum 1 cm distal to the pylorus (Fig. 4) with a 60 mm endoscopic linear stapler. For this purpose, the 10 mm umbilical trocar is changed to an 18 mm trocar. Reducers from 18 mm to 10 mm or from 18 mm to 5 mm are necessary for continued dissection. The right gastroepiploic vessels are dissected

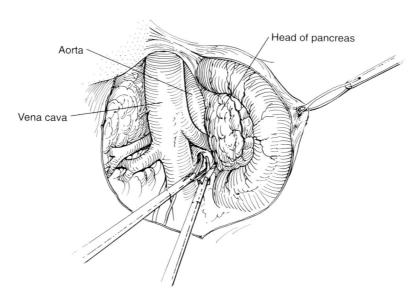

Fig. 2. Laparoscopic Kocher maneuver: 10 mm Babcock forceps inserted via epigastric port are positioned on second portion of duodenum to lift head of pancreas superiorly and medially.

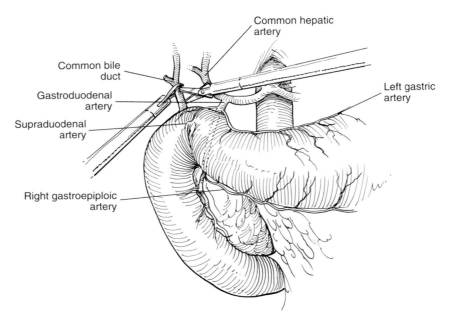

Fig. 3. Common duct is transected with endoscopic scissors just below cystic duct bifurcation and 2 cm above pancreatic superior border.

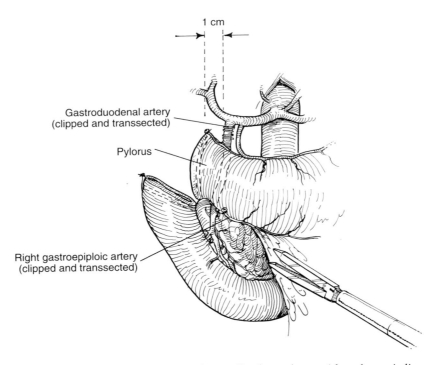

Fig. 4. First portion of duodenum is transected 1 cm distal to pylorus with endoscopic linear stapler.

and clipped at their origin on the gastroduodenal vessels; this frees the inferior stomach. The superior aspect of the stomach is liberated by clipping the right gastric artery close to the superior aspect of the pylorus. When the stomach is free, it is pushed toward the left upper quadrant. The gastroduodenal artery is clipped near its origin from the hepatic artery. The third and fourth portions are mobilized until the ligament of Treitz is well dissected, and the fourth portion of the duodenum at the jejunal junction is transected with two cartridges from a 30 mm endoscopic linear stapler or with one cartridge from a 60 mm linear stapler (Fig. 5). The superior mesenteric and portal veins are then identified and are dissected from the neck of the pancreas by blunt dissection with an irrigation-suction probe.

The pancreas above the mesenteric and portal veins is transected by scissors, and the uncinate process is sectioned with four 30 mm cartridges or two cartridges from a 60 mm endoscopic linear stapler (Fig. 6). Bleeding is controlled with medium- and large-size titanium clips and by hook electrocautery. The pancreatic duct is left open and is cannulated with a 5 Fr pediatric feeding tube. The specimen is then inserted in a 20 × 30 cm sterile plastic bag for later extraction and is retained in the left lower quadrant. For reconstruction, the proximal jejunum is brought behind the colon by creation of a 5 mm window through the mesentery of the middle portion of the transverse colon. The first anastomosis, the pancreaticojejunostomy, is performed with the proximal jejunum in an end-to-side fashion; a 5 Fr diameter pediatric feeding tube is used as an anastomotic stent (Fig. 7). This feeding tube is passed through the abdominal wall next to the umbilicus into the antimesenteric portion of the jejunum and is threaded into the jejunal lumen to the anastomosis. Two 2-0 silk sutures on each side of the pancreas are attached with intracorporeal knots to the antimesenteric serosa of the jejunum. Four sutures of 4-0 absorbable monofilament are applied to the four quadrants of the duct to the jejunal mucosa and are attached around the stent with intracor-

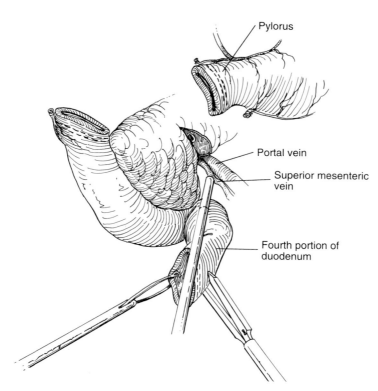

Pylorus

Portal vein

Superior mesenteric vein

Fourth portion of duodenum

Fig. 5. Fourth portion of duodenum is transected with endoscopic linear stapler after mobilization.

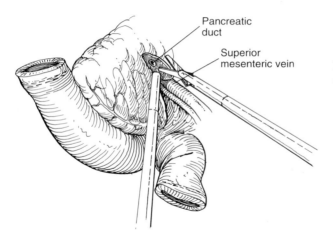

Pancreatic
duct

Superior
mesenteric vein

Fig. 6. Neck of pancreas is transected over mesenteric with scissors to expose main pancreatic duct.

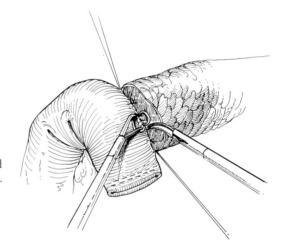

Fig. 7. End-to-side pancreaticojejunostomy anastomosis is performed duct to jejunum with interrupted intracorporeal suturing in all layers.

poreal knots. The anterior side of the anastomosis is further reinforced with a fibrin sealant[9] applied through a long catheter that has been passed through the abdominal wall with a Cordis introducer. Next, hepaticojejunostomy (end to side) is performed distal to this first anastomosis with eight separate sutures of a 4-0 absorbable monofilament tied with intracorporeal knots.

In the first case, the pylorus was anastomosed end to side (distal to the other two anastomoses); the same jejunal loop was used with two 3-0 absorbable monofilament sutures (one posterior and one anterior) running through the epigastric incision. Finally, the completely intact specimen was extracted by means of the epigastric port on the umbilicus, which had been enlarged to 3 cm. In the second case, a complete laparoscopic end-to-end pylorojejunostomy was performed with intracorporeal 3-0 absorbable monofilament sutures running

posteriorly and anteriorly. Fascial incisions were closed with 2-0 absorbable sutures, and pneumoperitoneum was reestablished so that two Jackson-Pratt No. 10 drains could be introduced by means of the left and right trocars (Fig. 8). Finally, the remaining trocars were removed, and the incisions were closed.

Postoperative Care

Morbidity is high after pylorus-preserving duodenopancreatectomy; therefore, postoperative care is extremely important. Jackson-Pratt drains are maintained intra-abdominally for a minimum of 7 days. A nasogastric tube positioned at low suction is left in place for 7 days, after which the patient swallows meglumine diatrizoate (Gastrografin) to permit radiological evaluation for leakage from all anastomoses. If no leaks are apparent and if drainage from the nasogastric tube is

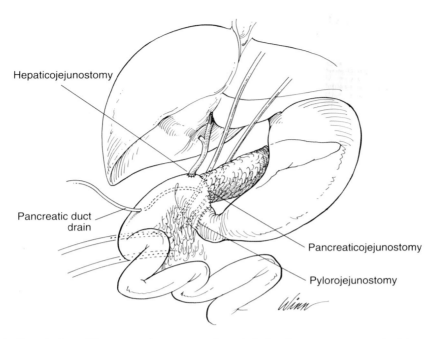

Hepaticojejunostomy

Pancreatic duct drain

Pancreaticojejunostomy

Pylorojejunostomy

Fig. 8. Completion of laparoscopic anastomosis and drain placement: pancreaticojejunostomy, end to side; hepaticojejunostomy, end to side; pylorojejunostomy, end to end; and Jackson-Pratt drains behind and over all anastomoses.

<300 ml per day, the tube is removed, and oral liquids are administered. If leakage is evident from the radiological study or from the Jackson-Pratt drains (high amylase content >2000 IU/ml), the nasogastric tube is left in place until the fistulas and drainage are resolved. We have also used somatostatin analogs (50 μg subcutaneously every 8 hours) to decrease the output of such fistulas. A jejunostomy tube is usually inserted at the time of surgery 30 cm from the last anastomosis through the left paramedian trocar, and enteral feeding is started from the third or fourth day at half dilution at the rate of 20 ml/hr. Increments are progressive according to the clinical status of the patient. Occasionally total parenteral nutrition may be initiated if enteral feedings fail to provide the total amount of daily caloric requirements. With pylorus-preserving modification, 15% to 20% of patients will experience an immediate delay of gastric emptying, which necessitates prolonged placement of a nasogastric tube for an average of 2 to 3 weeks.[3] H2 blockers are administered intravenously postoperatively to decrease the likelihood of anastomotic jejunal ulcers.

Prophylaxis for deep venous thrombosis is initiated in the form of heparin that is administered subcu-

taneously both preoperatively and postoperatively until the patient is fully ambulatory. Serum glucose is measured every 6 hours, and insulin may be given postoperatively, especially during administration of nutritional support. However, some patients will need insulin permanently after more than half of the pancreas has been removed (45% and 69% of patients have required permanent insulin administration at 2 and 5 years after surgery, respectively). Antibiotics (usually cephalosporin) are continued postoperatively for 7 days or until leakage stops. Pulmonary physiotherapy is initiated early to prevent pneumonia and atelectasis. When these measures are used, the range of overall 30-day mortality is 4%.[3] After hospital discharge, the pancreatic stent is removed 6 weeks postoperatively, when the patient should be eating a normal diet.

RESULTS

We have performed this surgical intervention in two patients. A 30-year-old female who was admitted to our service for recurrent continuous upper abdominal pain that had been relieved with narcotics had previously undergone open cholecystectomy and transduodenal sphincteroplasty for pancreas divisum and chronic pancreatitis localized in the pancreatic head. She had also undergone an open ovariectomy for removal of a dermoid cyst.

On admission the patient was cachectic and weighed 45 kg. Other than a right subcostal scar and an infraumbilical midline scar, her physical examination was unremarkable. There were no palpable abdominal masses and no visceromegaly. An abdominal computed tomographic (CT) scan showed a minimally dilated extrahepatic biliary tree with slight enlargement of the head of the pancreas. Endoscopic retrograde cholangiopancreatography (ECRP) failed to opacify either the pancreatic duct or the biliary tree.

On May 25, 1992, surgical laparoscopy was performed. An intraoperative cholangiogram showed a dilated biliary tree without stones. Because of her symptoms and stenosis of Oddi's sphincter, a resection was indicated, and laparoscopic duodenopancreatectomy was performed. Operating time was 10 hours. Pathological examination of the specimen revealed fibrosis and scarring in the head of the pancreas compatible with chronic pancreatitis. The patient received intravenous hyperalimentation during the postoperative period because of her severe protein-calorie malnutrition.

An upper gastrointestinal series was performed on the sixth postoperative day; this showed patent anastomosis with no leaks. A Tc-HIDA scan on the fifteenth postoperative day also gave no evidence of bile leakage. However, the gastrojejunostomy was somewhat small, and the stomach was slow to empty as a result of presumed anastomotic edema. The patient required a nasogastric tube for a prolonged period (20 days), during which she received intravenous hyperalimentation. Her progressive anemia was investigated by upper digestive endoscopy, which confirmed a jejunal ulcer adjacent to and distal to the gastrojejunostomy; the ulcer was treated intravenously with ranitidine.

Another female, 72 years of age, was admitted for jaundice. An abdominal CT scan revealed a dilated biliary tree without a specific mass. Preoperative ERCP showed an ampullar tumor of <2 cm, and biopsy was positive for adenocarcinoma. An angiogram did not divulge mesenteric vessel involvement. The patient underwent a laparoscopic pylorus-preserving duodenopancreatectomy according to the surgical technique previously described; operating time was 8 hours. The pathological specimen showed a 2 cm ampullar adenocarcinoma with adequate resection margins and negative regional nodes. The patient suffered postoperative-

ly from a minor pancreatic leak that was controlled with drainage, somatostatin administered subcutaneously, and antibiotics. She stayed in the hospital for 62 days for social reasons, and there were no signs of recurrence during 9 months of follow-up.

DISCUSSION

Duodenopancreatectomy in specialized centers is associated with <5% mortality and 20% major morbidity. Diagnostic laparoscopy used before the resection of pancreatic cancer may be helpful in the identification of metastasis or tumor extension in the abdominal cavity or adjacent organs. Warshaw et al.[10,11] have had the most extensive experience in the use of laparoscopy for the treatment of pancreatic cancer in North America. In their evaluation of 72 patients, they accurately demonstrated peritoneal seeding in 22 of 23 cases (96% accuracy) and correctly excluded seeding in 24 of 24 cases. When laparoscopy was added to computed tomography and angiography, determination of unresectability was 96% accurate, and resectability was 78% accurate.[10,11]

During laparoscopy, a cholangiogram can be performed if ERCP or a transhepatic cholangiogram failed to opacify the biliary tree. As a result of cholangiogram, choledocholithiasis may be excluded instead of a periampullary tumor. Laparoscopic choledochoscopy may be performed to exclude both choledocholithiasis or a periampullary tumor. If resection is not indicated because of tumor extension or metastasis, a laparoscopic bypass procedure can be performed. Several authors[10] have recommended laparoscopic cholecystojejunostomy or gastrojejunostomy or both. Shimi et al.[12] were successful in performing laparoscopic cholecystojejunostomy for malignant biliary obstruction. Anastomosis, which was 3 cm in length and was made away from the lesion with intracorporeal suturing,[13] was accomplished through a small incision made between the jejunum and gallbladder. Laparoscopic gastrojejunostomy can be performed with the same jejunal loop, side to side with an endoscopic linear stapler.[12] We prefer segment III laparoscopic bile duct hepaticogastrostomy, which combines fluoroscopic, endoscopic, and laparoscopic work for an anastomosis involving the undersurface of the left hepatic lobe and the anterior lesser curvature of the stomach. Local cancer is prevented from invading the anastomosis, unlike in cholecystojejunostomy or choledochojejunostomy.[14]

If the patient is not obese and if the disease is limited to the head of the pancreas, a laparoscopic approach to resection is an option. However, because multiple technical complications are possible (including intra-operative hemorrhage and postoperative anastomotic leaks), the benefit of a laparoscopic approach to surgery of this magnitude may not be as apparent as that of less complex laparoscopic procedures. The greatest problems are the time required to perform anastomoses made by intracorporeal suturing and the difficulty in making the pancreaticojejunostomy water-tight. Future plans include new stapling devices that will be used to perform pylorojejunostomy (and possibly other anastomoses) more quickly.

REFERENCES

1. Whipple AO, Parsons WB, Mullins CR. Treatment of carcinoma of ampulla of Vater. Ann Surg 102:763-779, 1935.
2. Traverso LW, Longmire WP Jr. Preservation of the pylorus in pancreaticoduodenectomy. Surg Gynec Obstet 146:959-962, 1978.
3. Braasch JW, Gagner M. Pylorus-preserving pancreatoduodenectomy: Technical aspects. Langenbecks Arch Chir 376:50-58, 1991.
4. Gagner M, Pomp A. Laparoscopic pylorus-preserving pancreatoduodenectomy. Presented at the Canadian Society for Endoscopic and Laparoscopic Surgery Congress. Ottawa: September 1992.
5. Clayman RV, Kavoussi LR, Soper NJ, Dierks SM, Merety KS, Darcy M, Long SR. Laparascopic nephrectomy. N Engl J Med 324:1370-1371, 1991.
6. Gagner M, Rheault M, Dubuc J. Laparoscopic partial hepatectomy for liver tumours. Surg Endosc 6:99, 1992.
7. Gagner M, Lacroix A, Bolté E. Laparoscopic adrenalectomy in Cushing's syndrome and pheochromocytoma. N Engl J Med 307:1033, 1992.
8. Cushieri A, Hall AW, Clark J. Value of laparoscopy in the diagnosis and management of pancreatic carcinoma. Gut 19:672-677, 1978.
9. Waclawiclek HW, Boeckl O. Die Wertigkeit Der Additiven Anastomosen-62w Nahtversiegelung Mit Fibin Kleber an Gastrointestinal-Trakt. Aktvel Chir 23:17-20, 1988.
10. Warshaw AL, Tepper JE, Shipley WU. Laparoscopy in the staging and planning of therapy for pancreatic cancer. Am J Surg 151:76-80, 1986.
11. Warshaw AL, Fernandez-del Castillo C. Laparoscopy in preoperative diagnosis and staging for gastrointestinal cancers. In Zucker K, ed. Surgical Laparoscopy. St. Louis: Quality Medical Publishing, 1991, pp 101-114.
12. Shimi S, Banting S, Cushieri A. Laparoscopy in the management of pancreatic cancer: Endoscopic cholecystojejunostomy for advanced disease. Br J Surg 79:317-319, 1992.
13. Fletcher DR, Jones RM. Laparoscopic cholecystojejunostomy as palliation for obstructive jaundice in inoperable carcinoma of pancreas. Surg Endosc 6:147-149, 1992.
14. Mouiel J, Katkhouda N, White S, Dumas R. Endolaparoscopic palliation of pancreatic cancer. Surg Laparoscopy Endosc 2:241-243, 1992.
15. Gagner M, Soulez G, Deslandres E, Pomp A. Percutaneous endoscopic hepaticogastrostomy under laparoscopic guidance for malignant biliary obstruction. Presented at the Canadian Society for Endoscopic and Laparoscopic Surgery Congress. Ottawa: September 1992.

VI

Videoendoscopic Techniques in the Diagnosis and Treatment of the Acute Abdomen

40 *Emergency Laparoscopy*

George Berci, Jonathan M. Sackier, and Margaret Paz-Partlow

Laparoscopy has been well known for more than 80 years. Despite excellent reports in Europe and the United States by Ruddock,[1] a surgeon, it was not accepted by general surgeons, and, if a diagnostic dilemma arose, open exploration was preferred. If surgeons had been trained in this important diagnostic and therapeutic modality, many unnecessary operations could have been avoided.

In the United States, gynecologists were more interested and used laparoscopy in the pelvis (pelviscopy), starting with tubal sterilization, diagnostic and staging procedures, and then extending to other miniaccess operations such as oophorectomy, myomectomy, and other procedures previously performed by open surgery. Today, in our institution, approximately one third of all gynecological operations are laparoscopies. Unfortunately, our surgical teaching programs did not include the topic of laparoscopy, and this is another reason that general surgeons are unfamiliar with this procedure.

With the advent of laparoscopic cholecystectomy and the sudden, consequent enormous interest, a huge number of abdominal surgeons are attending training courses. A large number of laparoscopic cholecystectomy cases have already been performed, and this will help to keep laparoscopy in the surgeon's domain. This may encourage other surgeons to use laparoscopy for indications other than laparoscopic cholecystectomy.

In our institution, surgeons trained to perform laparoscopic cholecystectomy are already using laparoscopy for diagnostic purposes in problematic cases, abdominal trauma, or for staging in oncology because of the higher yield compared with other examinations. No one is more familiar with the pathological appearance of intra-abdominal organs and interpretation than the general surgeon. Therefore the good view of an organ at laparoscopy, together with a precise biopsy performed under visual control, is of tremendous help.

Presented as part of a postgraduate course on interventional laparoscopy during the American College of Surgeons 1990 Clinical Congress, San Francisco, California, October 12, 1990. Originally published in Am J Surg 161:332-335, 1991. Reprinted by permission.

BLUNT ABDOMINAL TRAUMA

We live in an age in which frequent motor vehicle accidents and certain types of penetrating injuries cause great problems in establishing an early accurate diagnosis, which is a priority if we are to decrease unnecessary operations in the seriously injured patient. This is especially important in the patient with multiple organ injuries, the elderly patient with severe underlying disease, and the patient with head injury.

The introduction of abdominal lavage improved the diagnosis of intra-abdominal bleeding.[2] Subsequent experience with this test in patients with blunt abdominal trauma has shown that not every positive lavage requires exploration. The incidence of unnecessary diagnostic laparotomies in these types of cases is in the vicinity of 15% to 20%. One in five patients with positive lavage subjected to laparotomy has no visceral injury or continuing significant bleeding sites found at the time of surgery. The introduction of CT scanning has not eliminated the problem of unnecessary laparotomies and their sequelae in terms of increased morbidity and cost of health care.[3]

Laparoscopic inspection of the abdominal cavity in emergencies was advocated by Gazzaniga et al.[4] and Carnevale et al.[5] We have developed a 4 mm miniature laparoscope, which is approximately the same diameter as the lavage catheter and which is easier, faster, and safer to introduce than larger instruments.[6,7] The examination can be performed on a stretcher in the emergency room, in the intensive care unit, or in the operating room. In general, only local anesthesia with intravenous sedation is employed.

INDICATIONS

The following are included as indications for emergency laparoscopy: (1) obscure clinical picture and physical signs with impaired level of consciousness induced, for instance, by head injury, alcoholism, drug ingestion, etc.; in these cases, it is impossible to exclude significant intra-abdominal trauma with certainty on clinical grounds alone; (2) history or evidence of blunt abdominal trauma or stab wounds; (3) unexplained hypotension; and (4) equivocal signs on physical examination in a conscious patient.

A fast and thorough technique allows proper assessment of the extent of injury as well as the assignment of priority of treatment, which influences the eventual outcome of a severe trauma. In our opinion, peritoneal lavage is unduly sensitive and the positive result using the accepted criteria will lead to unnecessary laparotomy in 15% to 20% of patients, since the exposed bleeding will either have stopped spontaneously by the time of surgery or was accidentally created by catheter insertion. Therefore the main value of minilaparoscopy is that it reliably indicates to the surgeon the need for surgical intervention in the trauma patient. In cases in which small amounts of blood are found in the gutters (which would result in a positive lavage), the laparoscopic approach gives the surgeon a larger latitude for decision making.

TECHNIQUE

Local anesthesia (1% lidocaine) is applied in the midline after intravenous sedation (intravenous meperidine and/or diazepam) has been administered according to the patient's condition. The usual site is below the umbilicus, but if the patient has scars from previous abdominal surgery, it can be selected according to need. A set of minilaparoscopic instruments are stored in a mobile cart in a sterile fashion and assembled on a Mayo stand. The basic technique for creating a safe pneumoperitoneum are described elsewhere, as is insufflation by carbon dioxide or nitrous oxide.[8] The abdomen is surgically prepared and draped, and the surgeons should be gloved and gowned. After pneumoperitoneum is obtained, the site of needle insertion is slightly increased and the 5 mm trocar is easily passed through the abdominal wall. A prewarmed minilaparoscope is advanced through the examining trocar sheath.

The abdomen should be systematically examined, including all quadrants, the pelvis, and the suprahepatic spaces. For purposes of retraction, manipulation, suction, or coagulation, the second, smaller, 4 mm trocar and cannula can be introduced under direct vision, generally in the right or left upper lateral quadrants after injecting the site with 1% local anesthetic.

Following the examination, desufflation is performed and stab wounds are closed. No antibiotics are administered unless there is an indication. The entire procedure should not exceed 15 to 20 minutes.

HEMOPERITONEUM

The distribution of blood provides a clue to the location of the bleeding site. A good example is the pelvic fracture where blood is mainly localized in the pelvic area and this is a major source of positive peritoneal lavage. Quantitative assessment is difficult, but an impression can be gained with some experience and the following groups can be identified.

Minimal hemoperitoneum. A small amount of blood is seen in the lateral gutter or streaks of blood are discovered between the intestinal loops. If this small volume remains unchanged and the search for the bleeding site has been negative, the patient can be observed. If the oozing site is found, it may be seen to be oozing minimally or to have stopped. In our series of these types of patients, the bleeding site was discovered in only half the cases. Extremely small volumes of blood in the peritoneal cavity can be sufficient to provide a positive lavage.

Moderate hemoperitoneum. A 5 to 10 mm deep blood level is observed in the paracolic gutters. In this situation, a second trocar is introduced under visual control and the suction cannula is advanced. The hemoperitoneum is evacuated and a systematic search for the injury is begun. The suction cannula itself is used as a palpation probe. Omentum can be elevated or intestinal loops displayed. If the bleeding site is found, for example, a laceration on the anterior surface of the liver, the injury is watched through the laparoscope. If the bleeding is brisk, surgical intervention is indicated. If the bleeding site is not discovered after 5 to 10 minutes of diligent search but the pericolic gutters refill with blood to the previous level, the bleeding vessel is probably not within the range of visualization and surgical intervention is necessary. A small oozing laceration that shows signs of spontaneous hemostasis or a lesion with adherent blood clot without bleeding can be watched. In patients with moderate hemoperitoneum, laparoscopy allows the surgeon to formulate a safe strategy of management. If injuries are found that require immediate attention, a precise location of the injury to a particular quadrant facilitates selection of the optimal incision. The combined suction-coagulation probe may be applied for assessing oozing lesions or, in selected cases, aimed coagulation can be applied provided carbon dioxide has been used for peritoneal insufflation.

Severe hemoperitoneum. If, with the initial aspiration through the pneumoneedle, clear blood is obtained in the syringe, on two or three attempts, the patient should undergo immediate open exploration. If pneumoperitoneum is created and the laparoscopic view demonstrates intestinal loops floating in or surrounded by a pool of blood, the indication for immediate operation is obvious.

Organ perforations. In patients who sustain visceral injury, a yellowish-greenish fluid is observed in the pericolic gutters. The fluid should be aspirated and sent for analysis, but, in general, these findings are indications for open surgery. If several hours have elapsed between the trauma and admission, the injury may not be seen but it may be suspected by indirect findings, such as an omental mass covering a particular region or intestinal loops that appear edematous or hyperemic in certain areas. The palpation probe can be of help by moving such loops or adhered omentum. However, perforation of the retroperitoneal part of the duodenum and pancreatic injuries cannot be visualized by laparoscopy.

Splenic injuries. These are characterized by finding blood in the left paracolic gutter. The omentum covering the spleen is elevated by a pool of blood or blood clot and appears to have a bluish tint. Splenic conservation in suitable cases is desirable. In some cases, the laparoscope reveals only a minimal hemoperitoneum without significant bulging or bluish discoloration of the covering omentum. Even if the spleen scan denotes injury, should the vital signs be stable, the patient can be managed nonoperatively with very careful observation.[9] A normal spleen is usually not seen in the left upper gutter because it is covered by omentum.

Liver injuries. Deceleration injuries are characterized by lacerations on the anterior surface or dome of the liver or under the round and falciform ligaments. These lacerations can be clearly seen using the laparoscope. The undersurface can be inspected with a palpation probe with which the surgeon can gently lift up segments of the right lobe and the entire left lobe. If lesions are discovered, the telescope is advanced and close observation under magnification is performed for a few minutes. In the case of a small oozing laceration, compression or coagulation may be used. If after a prolonged observation time bleeding persists, laparotomy should be considered.

Penetrating injuries. We do not perform laparoscopy on patients who sustain gunshot wounds. However, penetrating stab wounds are an indication for laparoscopy. In a recent review of 89 cases of stab wounds of the abdomen, there had been unnecessary exploration in one third.[10] Our approach to these cases is as follows: The skin wound is temporarily closed to provide a seal for the pneumoperitoneum. The penetration of the parietal peritoneum can be either excluded or confirmed with great certainty. If there has been penetration, the underlying area is inspected using the palpation probe, lifting up the loops of intestine to check for bleeding points, serosal injuries, leakage, or other signs of perforation.

RESULTS (n = 150)

Negative laparoscopy—no exploration. In 56% (n = 84), no hemoperitoneum or other abnormality was discovered. None of these patients subsequently required an exploratory laparotomy.

Positive laparoscopy—no exploration. In 25% (n = 38), a minimal to moderate hemoperitoneum was found but no identifiable injury or only minimal lacerations were discovered. These patients were observed in an intensive care unit. Only one case in this group required laparotomy.

A 35-year-old man in a semicomotose state with a compression skull fracture was admitted after a motor vehicle accident. Laparoscopy revealed a minimal hemoperitoneum in the left lower paracolic gutter without other abnormalities. The patient's condition improved. Oral feeding was started on the third postadmission day. Two days later, the patient developed pain in the left lower quadrant with fever and leukocystosis, and he underwent exploratory surgery on the eighth day. A sealed perforation of the sigmoid colon was found. In retrospect, the minimal hemoperitoneum in the left lower quadrant and the persistent pneumoperitoneum would have been an indication for a contrast enema at an earlier stage.

Positive laparoscopy—exploration. In 19% (n = 28), severe hemoperitoneum was discovered. The laparoscopic findings were confirmed at surgery. In all but one patient, the source of bleeding or organ perforation was located. In this one exceptional case, 700 ml of blood was evacuated during exploration, but no bleeding source was found. The 28 cases included 7 liver lacerations, 11 splenic injuries (in 6 patients the spleen was conserved), 4 organ perforations, and 6 arterial bleeders.

Complications. In one patient, a minimal amount of hemoperitoneum was interpreted as being due to injury to the omentum during the trocar insertion. The patient was kept under observation and made an uneventful recovery.

THE ACUTE, OBSCURED ABDOMINAL DIAGNOSIS

In a majority of cases, the diagnosis of intra-abdominal emergencies is made by clinical assessment, laboratory tests, and radiological and ultrasound findings. Despite this fact, problems are sometimes encountered regarding the exact diagnosis and the need for surgical intervention. In this situation, laparoscopy may provide useful information that could influence the management of the patient. It can be particularly useful in the following situations.

Young female with questionable appendicitis. In female patients with acute onset of right lower quadrant pain, the differentiation between acute appendicitis, ectopic pregnancy, or pelvic inflammatory disease (PID) can be difficult. Diagnosis may be firmly and rapidly established by laparoscopy. In patients with PID, an unnecessary exploration can be avoided and culture material can be obtained and inflammatory fibrinous membranes debrided.

Acute upper abdominal pain. Although differentiation between a perforated peptic ulcer, acute cholecystitis, pancreatitis, or appendicitis is usually obvious from the clinical examination, laboratory results, and plain erect and supine radiography of the abdomen, diagnostic difficulties may be encountered. In practice, the important differentiation is that between acute perforation without obvious subphrenic gas and acute pancreatitis, especially when the serum amylase level is only moderately elevated. This dilemma is easily solved by minilaparoscopy.

Acute appendicitis or organ perforation in the elderly patient. In this type of case, senility (patient obtunded, severe arteriosclerosis evident) may cause significant problems due to difficulty in obtaining an exact history. Abdominal examination and laboratory tests may be noninformative even with severe inflammation or organ perforation. Minilaparoscopy performed with the patient under local anesthesia with intravenous sedation can clarify the situation.

Suspected mesenteric ischemia. In the absence of the full-blown clinical picture, diagnosis of mesenteric vascular insufficiency can be extremely difficult. These patients are old and have coexistent cardiovascular and respiratory diseases, which classifies them as a poor operative risk. Laparoscopy is suitable for the detection of ischemic bowel and for establishing the need for early, active intervention. In this type of patient, we prefer general anesthesia and proceed immediately to laparotomy if the diagnosis is confirmed.

Visualization of the intestines and the colon is facilitated by the use of the secondary trocar inserted in the left upper quadrant along the lateral margin of the rectus muscle for insertion of a palpating probe. The loops must be gently teased by the probe, rather than lifted, and the diagnosis is based on the dusky appearance, lack of serosal sheen, absence of peristalsis, edematous wall, and/or hemorrhagic fluid in the gutter.

CONCLUSION

Laparoscopy has a high diagnostic yield and an excellent safety record. It can verify information obtained by more expensive or time-consuming techniques such as computed tomographic scan and isotope scanning. It is hoped that with more general surgeons trained in laparoscopy, this important procedure will be used more frequently in emergency cases.

REFERENCES

1. Ruddock JC. Peritoneoscopy. Surg Gynecol Obstet 65:523-539, 1937.
2. Root HO, Hauser CW, McKinley CR, LaFave JW, Mendiola RP. Diagnostic peritoneal lavage. Surgery 57:633-637, 1965.
3. Federle MP, Crass A, Brooke J, Trunkey DO. Computed tomography in blunt abdominal trauma. Arch Surg 117:645-650, 1982.
4. Gazzaniga AB, Slanton WW, Bartlett RH. Laparoscopy in the diagnosis of blunt and penetrating injuries to the abdomen. Am J Surg 131:315-318, 1976.
5. Carnevale N, Baron N, Delany HM. Peritoneoscopy as an aid in the diagnosis of abdominal trauma: A preliminary report. J Trauma 17:634-641, 1977.
6. Sherwood R, Berci G, Austin E, Morgenstern L. Minilaparoscopy for blunt abdominal trauma. Arch Surg 115:672-673, 1980.
7. Berci G, Dunkelman D, Michel SL, Snaders G, Wahlstrom E, Morgenstern L. Emergency minilaparoscopy in abdominal trauma. An update. Am J Surg 146:261-265, 1983.
8. Berci G, Cuschieri A. Creation of pneumoperitoneum. In Berci G, Cushieri A, eds. Practical laparoscopy. London: Bailliere-Tindall, 1986, pp 44-66.
9. Morgenstern L, Shapiro SJ. Techniques of splenic conservation. Arch Surg 114:449-454, 1979.
10. Donaldson LA, Findlay IG, Smith A. A retrospective review of 89 stab wounds to the abdomen. Br J Surg 68:793-796, 1989.
11. Berci G, Wahlstrom E. Emergency laparoscopy. In Dent L, ed. Surgical Endoscopy. Chicago: Year Book Medical Publishers, 1985, pp 478-485.

41 · *Laparoscopy in the Management of the Nontraumatic Acute Abdomen*

Benoît Navez

The recent development of laparoscopic cholecystectomy has been further expanded to include additional pathological conditions in the abdomen.

The "acute abdomen" has always been a diagnostic problem; in fact, suspected abnormalities are not always found at the time of laparotomy, and this can lead to a change in therapeutic strategy.

The aim of this study was to examine the diagnostic and therapeutic uses for laparoscopy in acute abdominal pain of nontraumatic origin, once indications for operation are established. Patients in whom the need for urgent operation was uncertain were excluded.

MATERIALS AND METHODS

Emergency laparoscopy was performed in 167 patients (113 women and 54 men). Ages ranged from 13 to 96 years (average 58.1), and operative risk as evaluated by the American Society of Anesthesiology (ASA) classification was as follows: ASA 1 (57), ASA 2 (57), ASA 3 (47), and ASA 4 (6). Risk factors are listed in Table 1. Forty-four percent of the patients had previous abdominal surgery (below the transverse mesocolon in 41% and above the transverse mesocolon in 7%).

A patient presenting with an acute abdomen is examined in the emergency department by a senior resident, and appropriate laboratory investigations are performed, depending on the suspected pathological condition. Once the need for operation has been established, the patient is taken to the operating room and given a general anesthetic; laparoscopy is performed by a trained laparoscopic surgeon before any other surgical procedure. A pneumoperitoneum is established with a Veress needle (maximum pressure 14 mm Hg), and a 10 mm trocar is inserted into the peritoneal cavity, usually through the umbilicus. In the case of significant abdominal distention or previous major abdominal surgery, open trocar placement is performed. If necessary, one or two additional trocars are introduced for examination of the entire peritoneal cavity, depending on the pathologic condition encountered. Once the diagnosis is established, the surgeon decides whether to continue the operation laparoscopically or conventionally.

Patients were not selected on the basis of any pathology, age, or risk factors. The single determining factor in the decision to perform emergency laparoscopy was the availability of a laparoscopic surgeon.

RESULTS

In 90% of the patients (151/167), a complete diagnosis was possible with a laparoscopic approach (Table 2). In 10% of the patients (16/167), laparoscopy yielded only a partial diagnosis (peritonitis or intestinal ischemia) and laparotomy was immediately performed. Intestinal lesions were discovered in most patients (Table 3).

In 34 patients (20%) the preoperative diagnosis suggested by clinical assessment and complementary investigations was revised after laparoscopy (Table 4). Furthermore, this change in the preoperative diagnosis led to a modification of the therapeutic recommendations in 10% of the patients (16/167) (Table 5).

Four patients had normal laparoscopic findings, whereas the preoperative diagnosis had been gastric perforation, intestinal infarction, appendicitis, or acute abdomen of undetermined origin. No other surgical procedures were performed. The postoperative period was uneventful in these four patients with regard to the abdomen. One patient died on postoperative day 12 of an evolutive pleurisy. The final diagnoses in the other three were infectious rectocolitis, renal infarction, and abdominal pain of unknown origin.

In 68% of the patients (113/167), the pathological condition manifested by an acute abdomen was treated exclusively with laparoscopy (Table 6). A conventional surgical approach was chosen in 27% of the patients (45/167) either immediately after diagnostic laparoscopy (28/167) or after a laparoscopic therapeutic procedure was attempted and conversion became necessary (17/167) (Table 7). In two patients a small bowel injury occurred during adhesiolysis for acute obstruction, which necessitated immediate conversion to laparotomy.

Table 1. General risk factors

Risk Factors	Number	Percent
Cardiac	41	25
Vascular	40	24
Pulmonary	19	11
Diabetes	12	7
Other endocrinological diseases	7	4
Obesity	8	5
Neurological disease	7	4
Gastroduodenal ulcer	9	5
Esophagitis	4	2
Immunosuppression therapy (corticosteroids)	3	2
Renal insufficiency	2	1
Other	8	5

Table 2. Complete laparoscopic diagnosis

Diagnosis	Number
Acute cholecystitis	75
Chronic cholecystitis	3
Acute appendicitis	21
Gastroduodenal perforation	10
Small bowel mechanical obstruction (bands-adhesions)	8
Large bowel obstruction	4
Isolated colon perforation (diverticulum-iatrogenic)	2
Intestinal infarction	5
Intestinal ischemia	1
Acute sigmoiditis	1
Incarcerated femoral hernia	1
Mesenteric adenitis	1
Salpingitis	5
Complicated ovarian cyst	3
Omentum necrosis	1
Pelvic abscess	2
Ascite (cardiac, carcinomatosis)	2
Retroperitoneal nodes (+) ileus	1
Negative laparoscopy	4
Bladder perforation	1
TOTAL	151

Table 3. Partial laparoscopic diagnosis

Laparoscopic Diagnosis (n = 16)	Definitive Diagnosis (laparotomy)
Colitis (3)	Ischemic colitis
	Obstructive sigmoid cancer
	Cecal perforated diverticulum
Small bowel obstruction (5)	Incarcerated inguinal hernia
	Small bowel obstruction resulting from bands and/or adhesions (3) (1 ileal necrosis)
	Occlusive metastasis of the ileocecal valve
Peritonitis (7)	Perforated colonic diverticulum (2)
	Perforated sigmoid cancer
	Acute sigmoiditis (2)
	Perforated cholecystitis (ileus+++)
	Perforated colonic infarction
Diffuse adhesions (1)	Ileitis + peritonitis

Table 4. Preoperative diagnosis correction

Diagnosis	Preoperative	Laparoscopy	Laparotomy (after partial laparoscopic diagnosis)
Acute cholecystitis	76	72	
Acute appendicitis	29	19	
Mechanical small bowel obstruction	16	11	1
Large bowel obstruction	4	3	
Gastroduodenal perforation	14	9	
Colonic perforation	3	2	1
Intestinal infarction	9	6	1
Acute sigmoiditis	2	1	1
Acute salpingitis	4	4	
Complicated ovarian cyst	1	1	
Pelvic abscess	3	3	
Incarcerated femoral hernia	1		
Peritonitis	28	20	1

Table 5. Preoperative diagnosis correction with change of therapeutic recommendation

Preoperative Diagnosis	Number	Definitive Diagnosis	Treatment
Acute appendicitis	5	Omentum necrosis	Resection
		Ovarian cyst	Puncture
		Salpingitis	Antibiotics + appendectomy
		Negative exploration	Surgical abstention
		Appendicular peritonitis	Appendectomy (MB) + peritoneal lavage (laparoscopy)
Appendicular peritonitis	2	Perforated peptic ulcer	Laparotomy (suture)
		Acute appendicitis	Laparoscopic appendectomy
Perforated peptic ulcer	2	Acute cholecystitis	Laparoscopic cholecystectomy
		Negative exploration	Surgical abstention
Intestinal infarction	2	Acute cholecystitis	Cholecystectomy (minilaparotomy)
		Negative exploration	Surgical abstention
Biliary peritonitis	1	Ascites, cardiac liver	Surgical abstention
Large bowel obstruction	1	Ascites, peritoneal carcinomatosis	Surgical abstention
Acute abdomen of undetermined origin	3	Acute cholecystitis + peritonitis	Laparoscopic cholecystectomy
		Negative exploration	Surgical abstention
		Bladder perforation	Laparoscopic bladder repair
TOTAL	16/167 (10%)		

Table 6. Laparoscopic treatment

Procedure	Number	Conversions
Cholecystectomy	76	12
Appendectomy	17	2
Repair of perforated peptic ulcer	9	
Adhesiolysis, band section	8	3
Colonic perforation suture	1	
Bladder repair	1	
Puncture—biopsy of ovarian cyst	3	
Peritoneal lavage	4	
Cholecystostomy	1	
Surgical abstention	10	
TOTAL	130	17 (13%)

Table 7. Conventional surgery (open)

Procedure	Number
Appendectomy	4
Intestinal resection	13
Repair of perforated peptic ulcer	1
Adhesiolysis, band section	2
Cholecystectomy	2
Peritoneal lavage	1
Inguinal hernia repair	1
Omentum resection	1
Exploratory laparotomy	2
Ileocolic bypass	1
TOTAL	28

Nine patients underwent a conventional operative procedure assisted by laparoscopy for the following reasons:

- Laparoscopic localization of a colostomy site (four patients) because of a large bowel obstruction as a result of a neoplasm (three patients) or a perforated diverticulum (one patient)
- Laparoscopic peritoneal lavage and conventional appendectomy (three patients) for appendiceal peritonitis
- Laparoscopic liberation and suture of a small bowel perforation associated with conventional repair of a femoral hernia (one patient)
- Laparoscopic peritoneal lavage and small bowel suture by minilaparotomy (one patient) for a pelvic abscess

A total of 11 patients died within 30 days postoperatively (6.6%): seven patients died of spontaneous progression of their disease (four with massive intestinal infarction and three with peritoneal carcinomatosis), and four patients died of cardiac, vascular, or pulmonary causes (two cardiac arrests, one case of pleurisy, and one stroke); three of the deaths occurred after laparoscopic surgery (2.6%).

The overall morbidity rate was 11% (19/157). There were eight abdominal wall complications (seven abscesses and one hematoma), four pulmonary and one cardiac complications, one case of septicemia, one ileus, two spontaneously resolving biliary fistulas, one common bile duct residual stone treated by endoscopic sphincterotomy, one temporary cholestasis (Oddi spasm), and two cases of gallbladder bed hemorrhages, requiring laparotomy in one (Table 8).

For patients treated with laparoscopy only, the average postoperative hospital stay was 5.99 days (range 1 to 28). Among patients treated with conventional surgery assisted by laparoscopy, the mean stay was 9.0 days (range 4 to 15), compared with 18.12 days (range 5 to 58) for conventional surgery. It was estimated that in 133

Table 8. Morbidity

Complications	Laparoscopic Surgery		Conventional Open Surgery	
General				
Pulmonary	2	{ 1 Acute respiratory distress syndrome / 1 Bronchitis	2	{ 1 Pulmonary embolism / 1 Pneumonia
Cardiac failure	1			
Septicemia			1	
Ileus	1			
Local				
Wound abscess, hematoma	5		3	
Gallbladder bed hemorrhage	2			
Temporary biliary fistula	1		1	
Oddi spasm	1			
Common bile duct residual stone	1			
	14/113 (11%)		7/45 (13%)	

patients (79.6%), laparoscopy performed on an emergency basis was beneficial from a therapeutic standpoint (change in therapeutic recommendations, avoidance of laparotomy).

DISCUSSION

The purpose of performing laparoscopy in cases of non-traumatic acute abdomen is to make a diagnosis. Indeed, the diagnosis made after preoperative clinical assessment and complementary investigations is sometimes incorrect, and a different diagnosis is made during surgical exploration of the abdomen.

Until now an incorrect diagnosis of acute appendicitis has generated the most interest in the literature.[1,2,6,8] In 16 cases discovered during laparoscopy by Deutsch et al.,[2] a diagnosis other than acute appendicitis was suspected preoperatively (salpingitis in nine, ovarian cysts in five, a perforated diverticulum of the cecum in one, and normal laparoscopic findings in one). In another study of 86 female patients with suspected acute appendicitis, only 56 cases were confirmed during laparoscopy and 47 on histological examination. With laparoscopy the rate of unnecessary laparotomy decreased from 41% to 19%.[6]

Whitworth et al.[8] noted a 16% incidence of unnecessary laparotomy in combination with laparoscopy versus 68% in the absence of laparoscopy. There were no false negative findings in any of these series.

In cases of acute abdomen (with the exception of obstructions, visceral perforations, and trauma), Paterson-Brown et al.[5] noted that when laparoscopy was used an incorrect therapeutic recommendations were avoided in 25%. Indeed, a precise diagnosis was helpful and could possibly result in a nonsurgical approach. Good results were also reported with a computer-assisted diagnosis.

In our experience, a systematic laparoscopic approach in the presence of acute abdomen allowed us to correct the preoperative diagnostic hypothesis in 20% of patients (34/167). In half of these patients, a revised diagnosis resulted in a modification of the therapeutic recommendations. Sometimes a patient's condition is so serious that any treatment is useless (e.g., massive intestinal infarction). Occasionally the patient can be treated non-operatively (e.g., salpingitis), and in some instances the diagnosis made at laparoscopy can lead to a complete change in the surgical approach.

Under some circumstances laparoscopy cannot provide a precise etiology during the procedure; for example, significant intestinal distention (ileus, large bowel, or distal ileum obstruction), marked adhesions, or deep or posteriorly located lesions. It is sometimes difficult to palpate the lesions with instruments only and the lack of a three-dimensional view make interpretation of images difficult. We do not hesitate to proceed with exploratory laparotomy when we discover peritoneal fluid, pus, signs of intestinal ischemia, or an inflammatory mass with no obvious cause.

In some patients laparoscopic findings were normal. In four patients in our series, no abnormalities were found at laparoscopy. Clinical follow-up confirmed the absence of an evolving intra-abdominal pathological condition that would have been unrecognized at laparoscopy.

After exploratory diagnostic laparoscopy, the surgeon has four therapeutic options:
- Abstention from surgical therapy
- Exclusive laparoscopic treatment
- Open operation assisted by laparoscopy
- Conventional open operative procedure

Surgical abstention. Surgical abstention may be indicated in four situations:

1. Absence of acute progressive pathology, determined after careful examination of all visible abdominal viscera.

2. Disseminated peritoneal neoplasm.

3. Massive intestinal infarction. It is important to examine the entire intestine, sometimes by direct observation without the use of a magnifying lens and video camera, to check coloration. Indeed, partial exploration of the bowel can result in overestimation of the extent of the lesions leading to a decision to abstain from corrective surgery, whereas the patient could perhaps benefit from bowel resection (Fig. 1).

4. Discovery of a disease requiring only non-operative treatment (e.g., acute salpingitis, acute but non-complicated sigmoiditis, mesenteric adenitis, or ileitis).

Laparoscopic surgical treatment. Improvements in the techniques used in laparoscopic surgery currently allow treatment of many acute conditions in the abdomen by laparoscopy only.

Preferential indications are as follows:

1. Cholecystectomy for acute cholecystitis, performed as quickly as possible (72 hours or less) in the course of the inflammatory process, appears to be the treatment of choice, even for high-risk patients. Gangrenous cholecystitis, gallbladder abscess, or gallblad-

der perforation may be treated with laparoscopy, but requires a surgeon experienced in laparoscopic and biliary tract surgery. Of course, the rate of conversion to conventional operation is higher than with elective cholecystectomy.

2. Perforated gastroduodenal ulcer is a good indication for emergency laparoscopic surgery (Fig. 2). The procedure is reported to be safe but nevertheless requires experience with laparoscopic suturing techniques.[4,7] Suturing of the perforation, patching of the omentum, and abundant lavage of the contaminated peritoneal cavity are relatively simple to perform. Associated definitive treatment (vagotomy) of the ulcer disease may be performed in some cases.

3. Laparoscopic appendectomy for acute appendicitis is indicated primarily in cases of obesity, ectopic appendix, and suspected peritonitis and in female patients. In obese patients or in the case of retrocecal appendix, a laparoscopic approach avoids extending the MacBurney incision to gain access to the appendix. In the presence of peritonitis, laparoscopic lavage avoids significant enlargement of the incision or even a median laparotomy. In women with suspected appendicitis, laparoscopy is systematically performed to detect gynecological lesions responsible for symptoms. Excision of a hypertrophic and inflamed appendix by laparoscopy often requires enlargement of the trocar incision and use of wound protection (special pouch, larger trocar). Generally laparoscopic appendectomy requires the use of three trocars: one umbilical trocar (10 mm) for the optic system, one suprapubic trocar (5 mm), and a right lower quadrant trocar (10 mm). In a prospective evaluation comparing laparoscopic and open appendectomy, McAnena et al.[3] found that laparoscopic appendectomy was feasible in the majority of patients. The length of hospital stay and the risk of postoperative wound infection were significantly reduced.

4. Adhesiolysis and/or sectioning of bands in cases of acute small bowel obstruction (Fig. 3) requires extreme caution in laparoscopy. Open trocar placement is advised because of the high risk of bowel injury if the first trocar is introduced blindly. Even after a pneumoperitoneum is established, the distance between the abdominal wall and dilated intestinal loops is small making any blind puncture dangerous and manipulation of loops limited. Moreover, adhesions between the intestine and the abdominal wall are frequently related to previous abdominal surgery. Grasping of the dilated

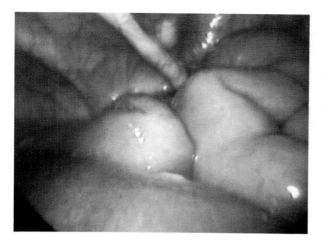

Fig. 1. Segmental intestinal infarction.

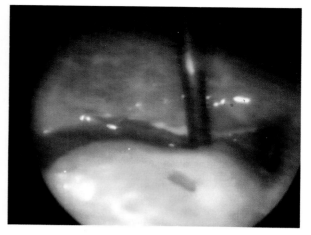

Fig. 2. Perforated peptic ulcer.

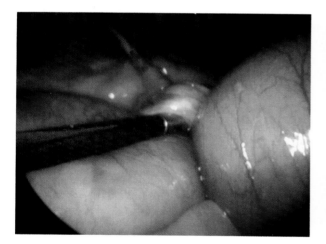

Fig. 3. Small bowel obstruction caused by a thick band.

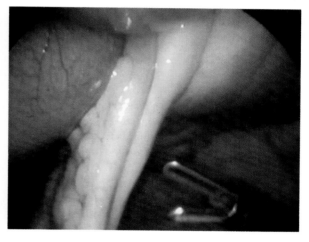

Fig. 4. Small bowel obstruction caused by adhesions to the abdominal wall (dilated and collapsed intestine).

small bowel even with atraumatic clamps should be avoided. The distal flat small bowel can be manipulated and followed proximally to locate the level of obstruction. In the presence of a thick and vascularized band (Fig. 4), sectioning should be done after bipolar coagulation. Adhesiolysis itself should be performed with scissors at a distance from the estimated bowel wall limit. If occlusive adhesions or bands are posterior or access is difficult, it is better to switch to laparotomy.

Finally, the entire small bowel must be examined to detect any other obstruction site. Laparoscopic treatment of small bowel obstruction remains delicate for the surgeon, and caution and experience are required.

5. Other more unusual procedures can also be accomplished with laparoscopy; these include closure of an isolated perforation of the bladder, suturing of a small bowel or colonic perforation without diffuse peritonitis, and bowel resection.

Open operation assisted by laparoscopy. This technique is sometimes an interesting alternative in the following situations: laparoscopic localization of a suitable colostomy site in the case of large bowel obstruction in high-risk patients unable to undergo emergency bowel resection, appendectomy with a MacBurney incision, and peritoneal lavage by laparoscopy.

Open operative procedure. When major lesions are discovered during emergency laparoscopy (e.g., acute perforated sigmoiditis), conventional open operation is the wisest and quickest solution.

In our experience, with the exception of two cases of small bowel injury that occurred during adhesiolysis for obstruction at the beginning of our study, emergency laparoscopy did not cause specific morbidity. It allowed us to determine the exact cause of acute abdomen in 90% of patients and resulted in complete modification of therapeutic recommendations in 10%. Finally, in 68% of patients, acute abdominal pathology was successfully treated with laparoscopy only. Laparoscopy is not only an additional diagnostic procedure but also a new alternative for treating abdominal surgical emergencies.

Admittedly a patient who undergoes laparoscopic surgery exclusively usually enjoys a greater degree of postoperative comfort and achieves a more rapid functional recovery than one who undergoes traditional surgery. However, the surgeon must bear in mind that the only means of visualizing findings and guiding procedures during laparoscopy is by two-dimensional video camera. Instruments used for palpation of organs or intra-abdominal lesions cannot replace the surgeon's hands in assessing volume and consistency. Respect for fundamental surgical principles and the highest degree of caution are required in laparoscopic surgery for acute abdomen. When difficulties arise, conversion to laparotomy is prudent and does not signify failure. Even more so than in elective operations, in an emergency the laparoscopic experience of the surgeon is critical, because he or she is manipulating inflamed and fragile tissues. Thorough knowledge of acute abdominal pathology is also important. Finally, in regard to the learning curve, the surgeon must limit procedures to what can be performed correctly and safely; excessive risk taking, a potential source of accidents, cannot be tolerated.

REFERENCES

1. Dallemagne B, Weerts J, Jehaes C, et al. Douleurs abdominales: Coelioscopie et chirurgie percoelioscopique. Rev Med Liege 45:152-156, 1990.
2. Deutsch AA, Zelikovsky A, Reiss R. Laparoscopy in the prevention of unnecessary appendectomies: A prospective study. Br J Surg 69:336-337, 1982.
3. McAnena OJ, Austin O, O'Connell PR, et al. Laparoscopic versus open appendectomy: A prospective evaluation. Br J Surg 79:818-820, 1992.
4. Mouret P, Francois Y, Vignal J, et al. Laparoscopic treatment of perforated peptic ulcer. Br J Surg 77:1006, 1990.
5. Paterson-Brown S, Vipond MN, Simms K, et al. Clinical decision making and laparoscopy versus computer prediction in the management of the acute abdomen. Br J Surg 76:1011-1013, 1989.
6. Spirtos NM, Eisenkop SM, Spirtos TW, et al. Laparoscopy—a diagnostic aid in cases of suspected appendicitis. Am J Obstet Gynecol 156:90-94, 1987.
7. Sunderland GT, Chisholm EM, Lau WY, et al. Laparoscopic repair of perforated peptic ulcer. Br J Surg 79:785, 1992.
8. Whitworth CM, Whitworth PW, San Fillipo J, et al. Value of diagnostic laparoscopy in young women with possible appendicitis. Surg Gynecol Obstet 167:187-190, 1988.

42 *Appendectomy: Laparoscopic Procedure or Open Surgery?*

Dominique S. Byrne and Graham Bell

Although laparoscopic appendectomy was first described by Semm[1] in 1983, it is still not widely practiced, and many surgeons doubt its value. Various techniques have been described, and case series have been reported,[2-6] but until recently the majority of these appendectomies were elective procedures. However, there is an increasing interest in the use of this approach in acute situations. We have studied the merits of the laparoscopic approach versus those of the open appendectomy in our center during the last 2 years; particular attention was devoted to operating time, length of hospital stay, postoperative analgesic requirements, and surgical complications.

MATERIALS AND METHODS

Data were collected on all patients who underwent appendectomy between August 1990 and July 1992 by means of either a right iliac fossa incision or by laparoscopic technique. The decision to use the laparoscopic approach depended on the availability of a surgeon and theater staff sufficiently experienced in laparoscopic surgery. The only exceptions to these criteria were children under 13 years of age, all of whom underwent open appendectomy.

The indications for surgery were recorded. All patients received prophylactic antibiotics (metronidazole, 1 g administered rectally 1 hour before surgery or 500 mg administered intravenously when anesthesia was induced).

Open appendectomy was performed through a Lanz incision with a gridiron approach to the peritoneum. Four variations of the laparoscopic technique, which fell into two categories, were used:

1. The extra-abdominal excision of the appendix after exteriorization of the appendix and cecal pole through a 10 mm cannula in the right iliac fossa, either (a) with no intra-abdominal dissection and in which only two 10 mm cannulas were used, or (b) after any dissection of intra-abdominal adhesions, peritoneal reflections, and the mesoappendix through a third 5 mm cannula in the suprapubic area or left iliac fossa.

2. The intra-abdominal excision of the appendix, either (a) between preknotted ligatures (the mesoappendix having been secured with ligatures or with diathermy) and in which the same arrangement of cannulas described in 1b was used, or (b) by means of the EndoGIA (Autosuture) stapling device, which was introduced through a 12 mm cannula in the right upper quadrant to divide the mesoappendix and the appendix.

The last three techniques described required the use of three cannulas. Each of these techniques was demonstrated in a short video presentation. The operating time, surgical outcome, duration of postoperative hospital stay, postoperative analgesic requirements, diagnosis, and complications were recorded in all cases.

We also collected data from all patients who underwent emergency appendectomy by means of a paramedian or lower midline laparotomy during the second year of this study in our center and in three neighboring teaching hospitals.

RESULTS

During the study 237 appendectomies were performed (80 laparoscopic and 157 open procedures). The mean age was similar in both groups of patients (laparoscopic procedure patients, 25.2 years [range, 13 to 60 years]; open surgery patients, 25.3 years [range, 2 to 86 years]), and the sex distribution was also similar (laparoscopic, 44 men and 36 women; open, 96 men and 61 women; NS with chi-squared test). The indications for surgery were acute right iliac fossa pain (laparoscopic, 85%; open, 97%), chronic right iliac fossa pain (laparoscopic, 11%; open, 1%), or previous acute appendicitis (laparoscopic, 4%; open, 1%).

Of the 80 laparoscopic procedures performed, 30 were completed by extra-abdominal excision of the appendix; in 15 of these, only two cannulas were used. Forty-two appendectomies were performed intra-abdominally. In 12 of these, the appendix was ligated with preknotted ligatures, and in 30 cases, the EndoGIA stapler was used. The laparoscopic procedure was converted to open surgery in eight cases as a result of technical difficulties (three cases) or because of inflammatory changes resulting in poor visualization of the appendix (five cases).

Diagnoses are listed in Table 1; no significant difference occurred in the two groups of patients, except in the number of cases in which there was evidence of previous appendicitis without ongoing inflammation. This difference is explained by the higher proportion in the laparoscopic group of patients who had chronic right iliac fossa pain or who underwent interval appendectomy.

Details of the operating time, postoperative hospital stay, and postoperative analgesic requirements are listed in Table 2. After the first 20 cases were excluded to allow for the early learning curve, there was no significant difference in operating times in each of the two groups. The laparoscopic approach resulted in significant reductions in the patients' postoperative stays and opiate analgesic requirements. Because some patients failed to participate in follow-up, the data on the time taken to return to full activity are incomplete.

Postoperative complications, which were not significantly different in the two groups, included superficial wound infection (laparoscopic, n = 3; open, n = 7), respiratory infection (laparoscopic, n = 1; open, n = 3), and prolonged postoperative ileus (laparoscopic, n = 2; open, n = 2). Prolonged ileus occurred only in the laparoscopic group in two patients whose operations were converted to open appendectomy.

Between August 1991 and July 1992, 40 laparotomy appendectomies were performed in the four local teaching hospitals. Sixteen of these were performed in a single center. The diagnosis in 11 of these patients was simple acute appendicitis. In two patients, pain was attributed to ovarian disease, two patients had intra-abdominal abscesses secondary to perforated appendicitis, and one patient underwent negative laparotomy. The 13 patients in the first two categories experienced a high postoperative complication rate (wound infection, n = 5; respiratory infection, n = 1; small bowel obstruction requiring a second laparotomy, n = 1; and incisional hernia, n = 1).

Table 1. Indications for surgery in 237 cases

Diagnosis	Open Surgery	Laparoscopic Procedure
Simple acute appendicitis	118	50
Gangrenous appendicitis	5	4
Perforating appendicitis	4	2
Chronic appendicitis	4	5
Previous appendicitis	2	12
Normal appendix	24	7
TOTAL	157	80

*Differences between the open and laparoscopic surgery groups were tested with the chi-squared test: Simple acute appendicitis versus gangrenous and perforating appendicitis, NS; acute appendicitis versus chronic appendicitis and normal appendix, NS; acute appendicitis and chronic appendicitis versus normal appendix, NS; acute appendicitis versus chronic appendicitis, significant ($p < 0.001$).

Table 2. Operative data

	Open Surgery	Laparoscopic Procedure	p^*
Operating time (min)	40 (range, 15-95)	48 (range, 15-135)	<0.05
		45 (range, 15-90) (cases 21-80)	NS
Postoperative hospital stay (days)	4 (range, 1-17)	2 (range, 1-10)	<0.05
Analgesia (doses)			
Opiate	4 (range, 0-9)	1 (range, 0-6)	<0.05
Nonopiate	5 (range, 1-20)	2 (range, 0-25)	NS
Return to activity (days)	26 (range, 10-156)	12 (range, 3-28)	—†

Numerical values are all shown as mean.
*Differences tested by chi-squared tests.
†Data incomplete; statistical test not performed.

DISCUSSION

Our study has demonstrated the feasibility of laparoscopic appendectomy in acute situations. Although we experienced a learning curve effect with respect to operating time and successful procedural outcome, the results of our later cases show that the benefits of laparoscopic appendectomy include earlier hospital discharge, less opiate analgesia, and an earlier return to full activity after surgery. The complication rate did not increase when the laparoscopic approach was used.

After the initial period of our performing laparoscopic appendectomy, the operating time became similar to that required for performing open appendectomy. The last 50 cases in the laparoscopically treated group were completed successfully, and we believe that conversion to open surgery is now rare.

After having used the four techniques described in this chapter, we feel that the choice of technique can be made according to surgical findings. Exteriorization of the appendix is most readily achieved when the appendix is mobile and the inflammatory changes are limited. Intra-abdominal dissection is required to mobilize retrocecal or adherent appendixes. When appendicitis is complicated by friability, gangrene, or perforation or when the base of the appendix and/or the cecal pole is involved, the EndoGIA stapler enables satisfactory excision of the appendix without placing excessive traction on the organ or leaving a diseased stump in situ.

Our study revealed that 40 appendectomies were performed by means of laparotomy in 1 year in an area with a population slightly larger than 700,000. This figure may represent a possible 300 laparotomy appendectomies performed annually in Scotland (population, 5 million). In one center, 13 laparotomies were performed for what proved to be simple appendicitis or simple ovarian disease. We suggest that if laparoscopy had been performed in these cases, laparotomy could have been avoided and the surgery could have been completed either laparoscopically or by means of a right iliac fossa incision, and the high morbidity associated with the procedure could have been reduced.

CONCLUSION

Laparoscopic appendectomy can be successfully performed in almost all cases of acute appendicitis, as well as in nonacute cases. The operation does not take longer than open appendectomy does. Patients can be discharged sooner after laparoscopic surgery, and they require less analgesia. They also seem to experience an earlier return to full activity.

The routine use of diagnostic laparoscopy could reduce the need for laparotomy in cases of lower abdominal peritonitis of unknown cause; thus the high complication rate of laparotomy could be avoided.

REFERENCES

1. Semm K. Endoscopic appendectomy. Endoscopy 15:59-64, 1983.
2. Gangal HT, Gangal MH. Laparoscopic appendicectomy. Endoscopy 19:127-129, 1987.
3. Schreiber JH. Early experience with laparoscopic appendectomy in women. Surg Endosc 1:211-216, 1987.
4. Leahy PF. Technique of laparoscopic appendicectomy. Br J Surg 76(6):616, 1989.
5. Gotz F, Pier A, Bacher C. Modified laparoscopic appendectomy in surgery: A report on 388 operations. Surg Endosc 4:6-9, 1990.
6. Browne DS. Laparoscopic-guided appendicectomy. A study of 100 consecutive cases. Aust N Z J Obstet Gynaecol 30(3):231-233, 1990.

43   *The Operative Technique of Endoscopic Appendectomy*

Kurt Semm

CLASSIC APPENDECTOMY BY LAPAROSCOPY

Since its inception the gold standard for appendectomy was the technique described by McBurney and Sprengel.

In 1980 and 1981 this classical abdominal technique was adapted and transformed into an intra-abdominal, laparoscopic technique (Fig. 1). In Kiel, Germany over the past 10 years this method has proved itself. The indications for appendectomy are as follows: periappendicular adhesions, disease processes affecting the right adnexa, appendicular endometriosis, chronic lower abdominal pain, and early acute appendicitis.

The endoscopic approach, although it has drawn initially much criticism, has gained increasing acceptance over the past 4 years in various surgical centers. The advantages of endoscopic appendectomy are as follows: direct visual diagnosis (thus preventing unnecessary appendectomy and/or hospitalization of the patient for "observation"), immediate postoperative mobilization of the patient, extremely short hospital stay (1 to 3 days), and full recovery after 5 days.

I will review all current technical considerations at issue.

One prerequisite for performing this operation is a full and complete understanding of the pelviscopic surgical technique, which has itself been proved in more than 22,000 pelviscopic procedures performed in Kiel between 1970 and 1993. The safety of this technique is based on many precautions in establishing and maintaining a pneumoperitoneum, and gaining endoscopically and visually controlled entry into the lower abdomen.

ORTHOGRADE AMPUTATION OF THE APPENDIX

Following a modification of appendectomy through laparotomy, orthograde amputation of the appendix, regardless of the degree of infection, may be performed laparoscopically with little blood loss.

Suture and Ligation Technique

As in laparotomy, the safest and most effective method of appendix amputation is the classic suture ligation and transection technique (Fig. 1). Proper placement of trocars is illustrated in Fig. 2. With practice, two trocars offer sufficient freedom of action to ligate, resect, and remove the appendix.

After inspection of the abdominal cavity through a 5 mm 30 telescope, the diagnosis is ascertained and the need for appendectomy verified. The operation is performed through a 10 mm diameter telescope. After exposure of the appendix, a guide suture is placed at the tip of the appendix using a Roeder loop, thus properly

Fig. 1. Classic appendectomy of McBurney and Sprengel modified for use as a pelviscopic technique (according to Semm system). *1,* Placement of a guide ligature at the appendix tip with a Roeder loop. *2,* Suture and ligation of the appendicular artery within the mesoappendix with an endosuture and extracorporeal knotting technique. *3,* Severing of the mesoappendix with hook scissors. *4,* Ligation of the appendix at its cecal end with a Roeder loop. Milking of feces using endocoagulation set at 90° C followed by a second ligation with a Roeder loop. *5,* Removal of crocodile forceps between the double-ligated appendix. *6,* Transection of the appendix with hook scissors and removal through the appendix extractor. *7,* Disinfecting of the appendix stump with iodine. *8,* Placement of purse-string suture with 40-polydioxanone suture material. *9,* Intracorporeal knotting of the purse-string suture. *10,* Invagination of the appendix stump prior to tying the purse-string suture. *11,* Placement of a Z suture using the intracorporeal knotting technique. *12,* Elective placement of a second ligature on the mesoappendix.

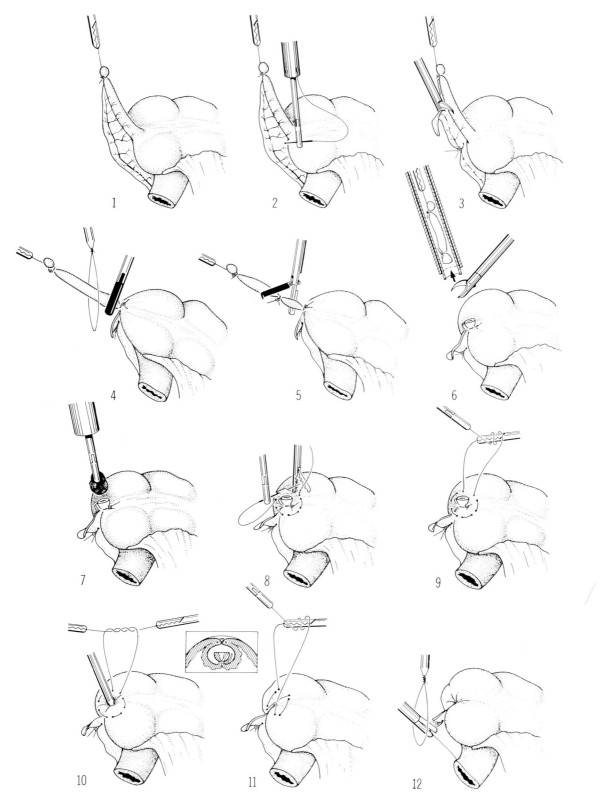

Fig. 1. For legend see opposite page.

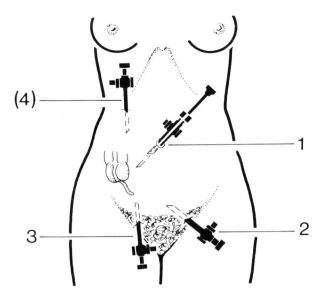

Fig. 2. Sites of trocar insertion for endoscopic appendectomy. *1,* Z puncture within the umbilicus for the endoscope. *2,* Suprapubic Z puncture for the appendix extractor; trocar is 10 mm in diameter. *3,* Suprapubic Z puncture for insertion of instruments. *4,* Upper abdominal puncture (optimal) to simplify intracorporeal knotting.

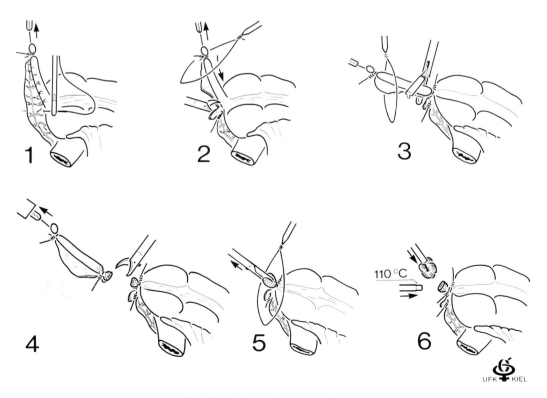

Fig. 3. For legend see opposite page.

displaying the mesoappendix. The appendicular artery is then ligated with an endosuture using the extracorporeal knotting technique, which is performed with instruments introduced through trocars 2 and 3 (Fig. 3, *1*). When adhesions are present an atraumatic bowel grasper introduced through trocar 4 is helpful.

Separation of the mesoappendix follows (Fig. 3, *2*). A Roeder loop is then placed around the entire appendix at the end of the cecum and a second loop is placed 3 cm above this. Between these two Roeder loops the fecal contents are compressed and at the same time sterilized with crocodile endocoagulation forceps at 100° C (Fig. 3, *3*). Transection of the appendix within the coagulated area follows with hook scissors (Fig. 3, *4*).

The appendix is then removed through the appendix extractor (Fig. 3, *5*). A ligature is then placed around the stump for security. The stump is then disinfected with a small iodine swab followed by coagulation of the stump with a point coagulator (Fig. 3, *6*) set at 100° C. As a final step the stump of the appendix is placed posteriorly.

The pneumoperitoneum is then desufflated and the Z-puncture canal is checked for bleeding while simultaneously removing the 10 mm trocar and the telescope. The umbilical wound is closed with skin clips.

Endocoagulation Technique

Endocoagulation is a simpler technique that omits the extracorporeal knotting technique. It is based on the amputation procedure usually used for the retrograde appendix and is illustrated in Fig. 4.

The appendix is first located and isolated by working through trocars 2 and 3 (see Fig. 2). It is then coagulated for 20 seconds with crocodile forceps (with the electrocautery unit set at 120° C) distal to the cecal pole (Fig. 4, *1*). Amputation of the appendix is then performed hemostatically and without contamination

using hook scissors to cut within the coagulated area.

The appendicular mesentery is then inspected with two bowel forceps to ensure proper separation of the cut edges (Fig. 4, *2*). The remaining appendicular stump is ligated close to the cecum with a Roeder loop (when possible with chromic catgut or polydioxanone; Fig. 4, *3*). The loop is introduced through trocar 3 and the biopsy forceps, which pulls the tissue into position, through trocar 2. The entire appendix together with the appendicular omentum is then pulled through a Roeder loop introduced through trocar 3 (Fig. 4, *4*). At the same time the appendicular mesenteric vessels and the appendicular artery, which lie within it, are ligated.

The omentum and the attached appendix are resected with hook scissors introduced through trocar 3 (Fig. 4, *5*). The tissue bundle is then removed through trocar 2, which is either 10 or 15 mm in diameter depending on the size of the appendix and its mesentery. A second ligature is placed around the appendicular stump for security. The wound pedicle is sterilized with the point coagulator set at 110° C and disinfected with an iodine swab (Fig. 4, *6*).

High-Frequency and Laser Coagulation

The difficulties associated with endoscopic intra-abdominal suturing and ligating have caused many investigators to substitute a technique of closing the appendicular artery by means of various coagulation methods. It is important to note that when these coagulation methods are used hemostatic control is not as complete, and there is sometimes significant bleeding during the entire procedure. For this reason these methods may be even more time consuming, since bleeding vessels that are not thoroughly coagulated must be located and controlled. A second ligature is placed around the appendicular stump for security. The stump is sterilized

---

Fig. 3. Endoscopic appendectomy using an endosuture. *1*, Placement of a guide ligature at the appendix tip followed by suture ligation of the appendicular artery using an endosuture with an extracorporeal knotting technique. *2*, Severing of the mesoappendix in the area of the cecal pole using hook scissors followed by transection of the ligated appendicular artery. *3*, Ligation of the appendix at the cecal end using either a chromic catgut or polydioxanone Roeder loop. Milking of feces and simultaneous sterilization of the appendix at the intended site of transection using crocodile forceps. A second distally placed ligation of the appendix. *4*, Following removal of crocodile forceps, transection of the appendix using hook scissors. *5*, Extraction of the appendix through the appendix extractor followed by security ligation of the appendicular stump with a second Roeder loop made of chromic catgut or polydioxanone suture material. *6*, Disinfection of the stump with an iodine swab and coagulation of the stump with a point coagulator set at 100° C.

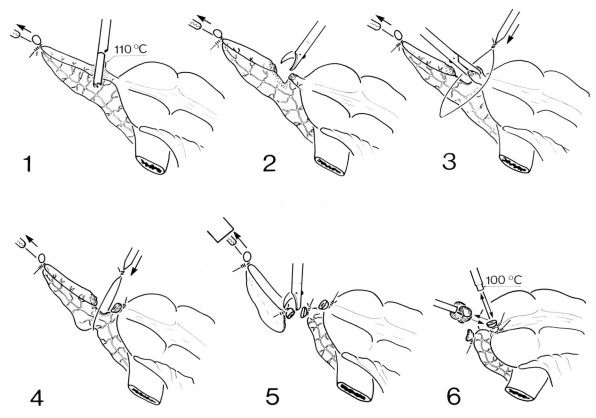

Fig. 4. Endocoagulation technique for appendectomy. *1,* Placement of a guide ligature at the appendix tip after displaying the course of the appendix grasping and coagulated for 20 seconds with crocodile forceps set at 120° C; this is done at least 0.5 cm away from the cecum. *2,* The adherent appendix is transected within the coagulated area using hook scissors. *3,* Following dislodgment of the appendix, the adherent stump is grasped with a blunt instrument and ligated using a Roeder loop made of either chromic catgut or polydioxanone suture material. *4,* The appendix together with the mesoappendix is pulled through a Roeder loop and the appendicular artery is ligated. *5,* Transection of the appendix with the mesoappendix distal to the ligature using hook scissors followed by removal in total through the appendix extractor. *6,* Placement of a second ligature around the appendix stump for security (see Fig. 3, *5*) after coagulation and disinfecting of the stump with iodine.

with the point coagulator set at 110° C and disinfected with an iodine swab (Fig. 4, *6*).

All of the techniques mentioned in this chapter have been used in various centers throughout the world. However, these techniques are neither compatible with the ideals of minimally invasive surgery nor do they save time; their only advantage lies in the fact that intracorporeal and extracorporeal knotting techniques need not be learned. However, this approach is shortsighted, since in an emergency these techniques are irreplac-

able, and a surgeon who is not skilled in them is forced to perform a laparotomy.

High-Frequency Current (Monopolar and Bipolar)

It is also possible to achieve hemostasis by use of uncontrolled destructive heat such as that produced by high-frequency current. After the appendix is isolated the appendicular artery may be coagulated in this way.

NOTE: High-frequency current cannot be controlled,

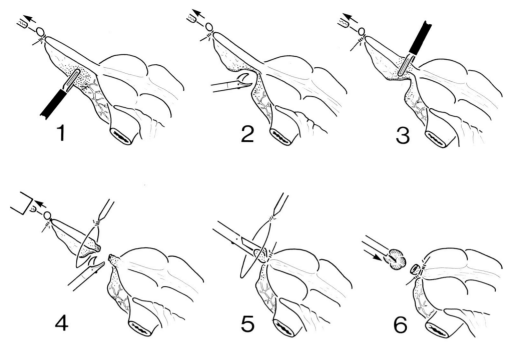

Fig. 5. High-frequency coagulation technique for appendectomy. *1*, Placement of a guide ligature at the tip of the appendix. Careful exposure of the mesoappendix followed by coagulation using bipolar high-frequency current of the appendicular artery. *2*, Severing the mesoappendix at its cecal end using hook scissors. *3*, Coagulation of the appendix at least 1 cm away from the cecum using bipolar high-frequency current. *4*, Resection of the appendix within the coagulated area using hook scissors followed by ligation of the appendix stump using a Roeder loop (see Figs. 3, *4*, and 4, *5*). Removal of the appendix. *5*, Ligation of the appendix stump a second time for security reasons. *6*, Disinfecting of the stump with an iodine swab.

and serious injuries to the cecum and small intestine have been reported in the literature. These complications have over the past decades raised doubts concerning the applicability and acceptance of pelviscopy in general. These problems have been experienced first-hand in Kiel.

Throughout the world the use of high-frequency current has produced complications (bowel and ureter injuries) that have resulted in death after routine gynecological pelviscopic operations. As more general surgeons begin to use pelviscopic operative techniques, it is of the utmost importance to prevent such complications as those encountered in gynecology during the 1960s and 1970s, inasmuch as this could delay the development of new techniques in general surgery.

After the appendicular artery has been thoroughly coagulated with a bipolar instrument (Fig. 5, *1*), sharp dissection of the appendix (Fig. 5, *2*) is performed with hook scissors. To ensure closure of the appendix lumen, bipolar coagulation of the appendix must be performed at least 1 cm away from the cecum (Fig. 5, *3*). A second loop is placed around the free end of the appendix to prevent seepage of intestinal contents from the resected appendix. The appendicular mesentery is pulled into the appendix extractor, and the mesentery is then resected with hook scissors (Fig. 5, *4*). The appendix is then removed through the appendix extractor. The coagulated appendicular stump is grasped and two Roeder loops are placed around it (Fig. 5, *5*). Finally the stump is disinfected with an iodine swab (Fig. 5, *6*).

NOTE: If coagulation with a high-frequency current is performed too close to the cecum itself, necrosis may develop. Each surgeon should note that the elastase enzyme is destroyed at 53° C and the Warburg respiratory enzymes at 57° C. If such high temperatures are applied in the area of the cecal stump, the enzymes are destroyed and the following symptoms may occur: (1) If the temperature-induced damage can be tolerated by the cecal tissue and can be repaired, sharp abdominal pain results typically between the fourth and tenth postoperative days. (2) If the damage caused by high temperature cannot be repaired by the cecal tissue itself, a cecal fistula will develop after a few days. If for some unknown reason unsatisfactory results are achieved too often, some surgeons form a negative opinion of laparoscopic appendectomy and revert to the laparotomy technique. Complications resulting from laparoscopic appendectomy occur only with the use of high-frequency and laser techniques. If only suture techniques are used the postoperative complications of laparoscopic appendectomy are comparable to those encountered in classical laparotomy.

Laser Coagulation

Modern technology has come so far that coagulation of the appendicular artery and transection of the appendix itself may now be performed with lasers. This development, however, neither improves the operative technique nor does it save time. It must be remembered that should hemorrhaging occur, only the methods described under suture and ligation techniques can help

prevent the need for laparotomy. The CO_2 laser is unsuitable for this type of surgery unless the operator is very adept at using a backstop. The Nd-YAG or argon laser is practical only if financial resources are unlimited.

RETROGRADE APPENDIX AMPUTATION

It may be difficult when the appendix lies in the retrograde position and cranially (sometimes as far up as the liver) to locate and dissect out the appendicular artery. This is particularly true when the appendix is acutely inflamed, thickened, and adherent to the lateral pelvic wall. In these cases it is important to immediately ensure a proper view of the operative field by first performing adhesiolysis. Water dissection may be used when necessary. The base of the appendix is exposed (Fig. 6, 1) and the appendix is coagulated as described in earlier sections and illustrated in Fig. 6, 2. Two Roeder loops are then placed around the pedicle for security. The appendicular mesentery is thus free of adhesions (Fig. 6, 3), thereby displaying the appendicular artery. This is either ligated or coagulated after which a Roeder loop should be placed for optimal security. Any gaping peritoneal wounds should be closed with endosutures using intra- or extracorporeal knotting techniques (Fig. 6, 4).

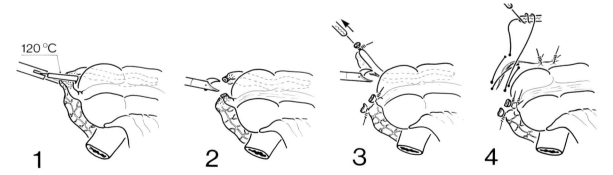

Fig. 6. Retrograde appendectomy. *1*, Careful dissection of the base of the appendix at the cecum. Coagulation of the appendix and any omentum using crocodile forceps set at 120° C. *2*, Resection of the appendix and partial resection of the mesoappendix using hook scissors. *3*, Ligation of both free ends of the appendix as well as ligation of the open end of the mesoappendix. Finally, proper dissection of the retrograde course of the appendix. *4*, A second ligation of the appendix stump for security with closure of any gaping peritoneal wounds using endosutures with either intracorporeal or extracorporeal knotting techniques.

DIFFICULTIES IN ENDOSCOPIC APPENDECTOMY

Only in cases of advanced infection or with perforation and abscess formation is endoscopic appendectomy rendered more difficult. A thickened appendix, such as in a patient with appendix myxoma, may also be problematical.

The Appendicular Abscess

Experience gained by gynecologists in the endoscopic treatment of tubo-ovarian abscess has shown that opening of the ovary or tube allowing pus to drain has not led to the grave consequences that occurred when these structures were opened at laparotomy. The appendiceal abscess should be drained completely and then be irrigated endoscopically. Where required sutures and ligatures should be placed. Essential prerequisites for optimal treatment in such cases are a practiced hand and complete understanding of endoscopic suture and ligature techniques. Tissue trauma is only exaggerated when methods of thermal necrosis are employed. The pus is immediately sent for culture and sensitivity testing, thus ensuring specifically targeted postoperative antibiotic therapy.

The abdominal cavity is then irrigated intraoperatively with 4 to 5 L of normal saline. The value of intra-abdominal administration of antibiotics, for example, Reverin (a tetracycline derivative), has been proved.

The Thickened Appendix

In cases of severe infection, where myxomal changes in the appendix can occur, the appendix may be too thick to remove through the 10 mm trocar. This happens mostly in cases diagnosed with a 5 mm pelviscope at the initial examination of the abdominal cavity. In such instances, therefore, a 10 or 15 mm appendix extractor may be inserted through the puncture wound (site No. 2) (see Fig. 2). When this is not possible, piece-by-piece removal of the appendix does not increase the operative risk to the patient.

Acute Intraoperative Hemorrhage

When despite coagulation or ligation unexpected hemorrhaging occurs—for example, in the case of an aberrant appendicular artery—the bleeding may be stopped by either coagulation or preferably by ligation with a Roeder loop.

INITIAL PREVENTION OF SECONDARY INFECTION

When a classic gridiron incision is used, contamination of the lymphatic vessels with infectious toxins is unavoidable. This can be prevented, however, in pelviscopic appendectomy, since the area of infection is kept within the lymphocytic wall of protection. In cases of severe or advanced infection, antibiotics such as Reverin may be given intra-abdominally at the end of the endoscopic procedure.

NOTE: Systemic antibiotics freely advance from the vascular system into the infected tissue. However, the intra-abdominal fibrin encapsulation around the infected area prevents this, and therefore direct intra-abdominal application is more effective initially.

POSTOPERATIVE THERAPY

After minimally invasive intra-abdominal surgery, it is possible after the initial mobilization to offer the patient tea and on the following day light fluids can be given by mouth. Postoperative therapy is determined by the degree of infection. In the case of severe local infection, drainage to the outside may reduce abscess formation (Fig. 7).

POSTSCRIPT
Warmed Gas

Until now cooled CO_2 gas has been used to insufflate and maintain a pneumoperitoneum in laparoscopic procedures, including appendectomy. After 3 years of clinical research at the University Womens Clinic in Kiel we have found that this reduces body temperature, sometimes to as low as 28° C (Fig. 8). This in turn produces a peritoneal irritation and "catarrh," which causes rather severe postoperative pain. Many surgeons have found that patients have more initial postoperative pain after laparoscopic appendectomy compared with the classic procedure. This problem is attributed to peritoneal irritation and may be resolved by using warmed CO_2 gas (to body temperature), which has an isothermic effect (Fig. 9). The Flow-Therme device (Fig. 10) with its heating cable can be adapted to all types of CO_2 gas insufflators. In clinical studies patients undergoing laparoscopic surgery with warm CO_2 gas required 34% fewer analgesics after the operation compared with a control group and 47% had less shoulder pain. The use of warmed CO_2 gas is now mandatory in pelviscopy.

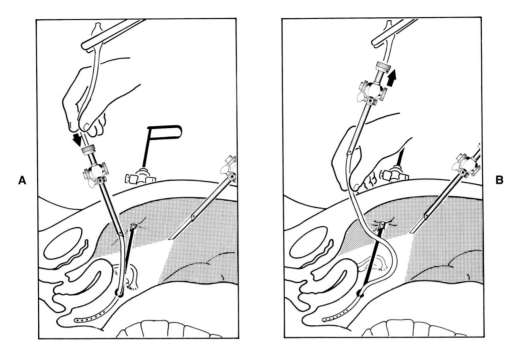

Fig. 7. Pelvic abscess drainage. **A,** A 5 mm diameter silicone Robinson drain (or a 10 mm diameter Easy-Flow drain depending on the size of trocar used) is introduced through trocar 2 (or 3) and is guided into the abscess in the pelvic cavity. **B,** The drain is grasped intra-abdominally using atraumatic grasping forceps and held tight; the trocar is then opened and removed over the drain.

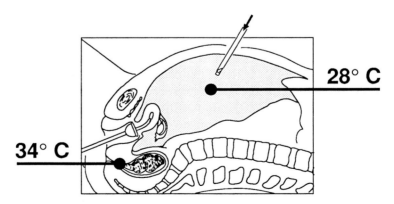

Fig. 8. Body temperature reduced through use of cooled CO_2.

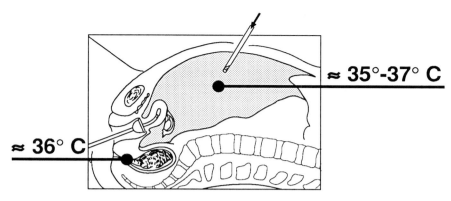

Fig. 9. CO_2 gas warmed to body temperature may counter potential postoperative pain related to peritoneal irritation.

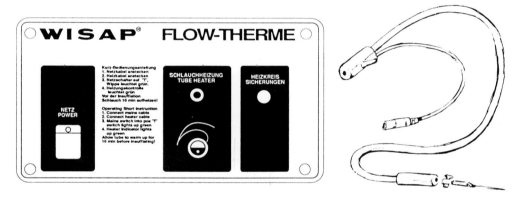

Fig. 10. Flow-Therme warming device can be adapted to all CO_2 insufflators.

CONCLUSION

Compared with classical surgical treatment of appendicitis, the advantages of endoscopic therapy are obvious. The operative procedure has been simplified over the past 10 years. The operating time is short and does not exceed the time required to perform the same procedure by laparotomy. The postoperative therapy, which is dependent on the severity of the inflammation of the appendix, has been standardized. A reduction of 1 to 4 days in the length of hospitalization and a recovery period of days rather than weeks are two of the principal advantages of minimally invasive surgery over laparotomy. There are few contraindications to endoscopic appendectomy, with perhaps advanced gangrenous appendicitis being the only one. However, this is perhaps no longer an absolute contraindication in today's modern medical era.

REFERENCES

1. Götz F, Pier A, Bahcer C. Modified laparoscopic appendectomy in surgery—a report on 388 operations. Surg Endosc 4:6-9, 1990.
2. Hutterer F, Buess G, Theiss T. Fortlaufende und Einzelknopfnaht am Rektum. In Buess G, Unz F, Pichlmaier H,

eds. Endoskopische Techniken. Köln: Deutscher Ärzteverlag, 1988, pp 193-197.

3. Pier A, Götz F, Thevissen P. Laparoskopische Versorgung einer indirekten Inguinalhernie (Fallbeschreibung). Endoskopie Heute 4:5-16, 1991.

4. Pier A. Die laparoskopisch/endoskopische Appendektomie nach Semm in der Modifikation nach Götz: Eine Untersuchung von 255 Fällen Diss i Vorber. Linnich, 1990.

5. Semm K. Advances in pelviscopic surgery (appendectomy). In Current Problems in Obstetrics and Gynecology, No. 10. Chicago: Year Book Medical Publishers, 1982.

6. Semm K. Die endoskopische Appendektomie. Gynäkol Prax 7:131-140, 1983.

7. Semm K. Endoscopic appendectomy. Endoscopy 15:59-64, 1983.

8. Semm K. Technische Operationsschritte der endoskopischen Appendektomie. Langenbecks Arch Chir 376:121-126, 1991.

44 *Laparoscopic Appendectomy: Less and Less Invasive?*

Pierre-Philippe Volkmar, Frédéric Vaxman, Jean Nicolas Boullenois, Franck Gosset, Calin Ionescu, César Solis, Dominique Geiger, Heike Goebel, and Jacques F. Grenier

Laparoscopic cholecystectomies are now performed routinely by many surgeons. However, although appendectomy is the most frequently performed procedure in general surgery and was in fact the first therapeutic gastrointestinal procedure to be performed laparoscopically (Karl Semm, 1983), we are far from consensus regarding the use of this procedure.

We report our experience with two consecutive techniques of laparoscopic appendectomy and compare the results with a retrospective series of conventional appendectomies (see the box on p. 229).

MATERIALS AND METHODS

From November 1989 to May 1992, a total of 122 patients, 30 males and 92 females, with a median age of 24.3 years (range 12 to 63), underwent laparoscopic appendectomy. In the first procedure, called the "out" technique (see the lower box on p. 229), which was performed in 68 patients, we used three trocars: 10 mm in the umbilicus, 11 mm in the right iliac fossa, and 5 mm in the medial suprapubic area, allowing dissection of the appendix with a monopolar hook cannula. After extraction through the 11 mm port, ligation and sectioning of the appendix were performed outside the abdominal cavity.

The second procedure, called the "in" technique, was performed in 54 patients, and required the use of only one 10 mm trocar in the umbilicus, with two 5 mm trocars in the suprapubic area for the surgical instruments. To perform this second procedure, a second 5 mm telescope and preformed ligature loops (Endoloop) were necessary to properly extract the specimen using the umbilical trocar.

Results in these 122 patients were compared with those in a retrospective series of conventional appendectomies, from April 1988 to October 1989, performed before the laparoscopic era in 115 patients, 52 males and 63 females, with a median age of 27.2 years (range 7 to 90).

The following parameters were established for comparison of the series: age and sex, clinical evaluation, operative time, anesthetic time, histological examination, intraoperative diagnosis and associated disease, intraoperative accidents, drainage or not, postoperative flatus transit, postoperative discharge, and postoperative pain (on a scale of 0 to 5). These items were statistically analyzed (descriptive and comparative analysis) with the following tests: control of repartition with confidence intervals, median of dispersion, and skewness and kurtosis.

PATIENT DEMOGRAPHIC DATA

Group 1: Standard Appendectomies, April 1988 to October 1989

115 patients
   52 males
   63 females
Median age 27.2 years (range 7-90)

Group 2: Laparoscopic Appendectomies, November 1989 to May 1992

68 "out" procedures
54 "in" procedures
122 patients
   30 males
   92 females
Median age 24.3 years (range 12-63)

Group 3: Standard Appendectomies (Laparoscopy Contraindicated), November 1989 to May 1992

67 patients
   33 males
   34 females
Median age 28 (range 12-78)
Contraindications to laparoscopy for group 3
   27 Anesthetic considerations
   36 Surgical considerations
   4 Patient refusal

COMPARISON OF TECHNIQUES

"Out" Technique

Two 10 mm trocars placed
   Umbilicus
   Right iliac fossa
One 5 mm trocar placed
   Suprapubically

"In" Technique

One 10 mm trocar placed
   Umbilicus
Two 5 mm trocars placed
   Suprapubically, right and left

RESULTS

Table 1 shows the relevant results concerning age, sex, operative time, anesthetic time, flatus transit, and postoperative discharge. The median ages did not differ in the two groups, but the ranges did. The mean operative time was longer in the laparoscopic group (56 minutes versus 42 minutes) but decreased with the experience of the surgical team. Anesthetic time increased parallel to the operative time. Flatus transit was present 0.9 days postoperatively in the laparoscopic group versus 1.5 days in the standard group. The mean postoperative hospital stay was 2.8 days in the laparoscopic group, ranging from 0 to 11 days: 0 for one ambulatory patient and 11 for an abscess of the pouch of Douglas reoperated on the third postoperative day by median laparotomy. In the standard group, the postoperative hospital stay was 8.3 days.

The majority of women in the laparoscopic group may be attributed to the fact that we chose to examine a greater number of patients with chronic disease by the laparoscopic approach.

Histological examination showed a similar number of acute lesions classified into five types in the two groups (Table 2), but interestingly, there were more normal appendixes in the standard group.

On the other hand, we observed more chronic obliterative appendicitis treated by the laparoscopic procedure, and this again corresponds to the greater number of chronic diseases of the right iliac fossa in women. One case of carcinoid tumor of the appendix smaller than 1 cm and one case of tuberculosis of the appendix were discovered at histological examination.

Contraindications for laparoscopic procedures were as follows:
   Anesthetic considerations (27 cases), including cardiovascular disease and respiratory insufficiency (7 cases) and the lack of a recovery room at night (20 cases)
   Surgical considerations (36 cases), namely a lack of properly trained surgeons, and at the beginning of our experience with laparoscopy because of symptoms of peritonitis at presentation (28 cases), in addition to previous irradiation, multiple laparotomies, digestive fistula, and suspected intra-abdominal tumor
   Patient refusal (4 cases)

For these reasons, during the same period that laparoscopic appendectomies were done, 67 standard appendectomies were also performed by our group. The

Table 1. Relevant surgical data for both groups

Procedure	Sex	Mean Age (yr)	Operative Time (min)	Anesthetic Time (min)	Flatus Transit (postoperative day)	Discharge (postoperative day)
Standard appendectomy (n = 115)	M 52 F 63	27.2	42 (15-110)	59 (20-150)	1.5 (0-4)	8.3 (5-26)
Laparoscopy (n = 122)	M 30 F 92	24.3	56 (20-130)	85 (45-150)	0.9 (0-2)	2.8 (0-11)

Table 2. Results of histological examinations

Procedure	Normal (1)	(2)	Acute (3)	(4)	(5)	(6)	(7)	Chronic (8)	(9)	BK	Carcinoid
Standard appendectomy (n = 115)	27	12	26	17	5	9	2	10	7		
Laparoscopic appendectomy (n = 122)	6	15	28	9	10	4	1	11	36	1	1

(1) Normal; (2) stercoral stasis; (3) catarrhal; (4) phlegmonous; (5) ulcerated; (6) abscess; (7) gangrenous; (8) lymphoid hyperplasia; (9) obliterative.

median age was 28 years (range 12 to 78) in this series. There were no deaths. Morbidity was mainly associated with the pneumoperitoneum as follows:

Shoulder pain (13)
Red face with or without headache (7)
Subcutaneous emphysema (5)
Persistent pain at the puncture site (1)
Urinary retention (1)
Hematoma in the navel (1)
Persistent pneumoperitoneum for 48 hours (1)
Wound abscess (1)
Persistent pain (2) (in one patient large adhesions were removed and in one celiac disease was discovered subsequently)

Drainage was necessary in only two patients in the laparoscopic group, compared with 29 in the standard group.

Conversion to Laparotomy

In four patients (3.27%) the laparoscopic procedure was converted to an open laparotomy (see the box on p. 231). However, the only real operative complication in our series was puncture of the aorta by the Veress needle while attempting insufflation. A median laparotomy was performed to examine the abdominal cavity. No specific treatment was necessary for the injury to the aorta, but two small holes in the same small bowel loop were discovered, requiring a one-stitch suture for each.

CONVERSION TO LAPAROTOMY

Number of Cases Converted

4/122 (3.27%)

Reasons

Two cases converted because of the presence of adhesions (converted to MacBurney approach)
Complications of laparoscopic technique
    One case of bleeding converted to median laparotomy
    One case with associated PCO_2 problem, with transient arrhythmia (converted to MacBurney approach)

In the other laparotomies we employed the traditional MacBurney approach, because in each case the patient's CO_2 level was too high, with transient arrythmia in one instance and strong adhesions in the appendix area in two others.

Postoperative Complications

Only one postoperative complication occurred (0.82%): an abscess of the pouch of Douglas on the third postoperative day, requiring a median laparotomy. It was due to the loss of feces in the abdominal cavity during dissection of the appendix.

DISCUSSION

A balanced evaluation is always necessary after a new procedure is used. On the positive side, we found that with the laparoscopic approach inspection of the whole abdominal cavity is possible, and unnecessary appendectomies can be avoided. In our study one woman was found to have salpingitis; another had an ovarian cyst. Further, postoperative pain is reduced, the length of hospital stay is decreased, wound abscesses rarely occur, and eventration is avoided. The thickness of the abdominal wall does not complicate the operation, and aesthetic results are good.

Negative aspects of the method include the use of gastric tubes and urinary catheters, the fact that operative time can be increased if the surgical team lacks experience, the morbidity that can result from difficulties in establishing the pneumoperitoneum or from the CO_2 that is insufflated. Also, a new procedure requires additional training. At present we are unable to classify the length of time required before the patient's return to work as a negative or positive consideration (it was 10 to 12 days in our series).

Regarding postoperative complications, in the laparoscopic group there were fewer complications (pouch of Douglas abscess in one and wound abscess in one) than with conventional appendectomies (postoperative hypertension crisis in two, pulmonary infection in three, gastric ulcer in one, salpingitis in one, and wound abscesses in three).

CONCLUSION

Laparoscopic procedures are virtually noninvasive, that is, the second technique requires only one trocar in the umbilicus and two small 5 mm trocars in the suprapubic area, which makes it possible to operate on the appendix, pelvic organs, and bowels. These techniques must be performed by properly trained surgeons to achieve optimal results. These techniques enable diagnosis and treatment and greatly benefit the patient, which is the ultimate goal of all new therapeutic procedures.

REFERENCES

1. Bakka A, Reiersten O, Rosseland AR, et al. Laparoscopic appendectomy. Tidsskr Nor Laegerforen 111:1714-1715, 1991.
2. Banerjee AK. Laparoscopic appendicectomy. Lancet 338:893, 1991.
3. Bastien J, LeConte P, LeConte D. Réflexions sur une série homogène de 5000 appendicectomies. Semin Hop 63:285-297, 1987.
4. Batvinkov NI, Garelik PV, Maslakova ND, et al. Diagnostic and therapeutic laparoscopy in surgical practice. Khirugiia (Mosk) 9:42-46, 1990.
5. Bongard F, Landers DY, Lewis F. Differential diagnosis of appendicitis and pelvic inflammatory disease. A prospective analysis. Am J Surg 150:90-96, 1985.
6. Browne DS. Laparoscopic guided appendicectomy. A study of 100 consecutive cases. Aust NZ J Obstet Gynaecol 30:231-233, 1990.
7. Bruhat MA, Dubuisson JB, Pouly JL, et al. Encyc Med Chir Coeliochirurgie 6: 41515, 1989.
8. Bruhat MA, Mage G, Pouly JL, et al. Coelioscopie Opératoire. Paris: Medsi/McGraw-Hill, 1989.
9. Bryson K. Laparoscopic appendectomy. J Gynecol Surg 7:93, 1991.
10. Bruchsbaum HJ, Lifshitz S. Staging and surgical evaluation of ovarian cancer. Semin Oncol 11:227-237, 1984.

11. Buianov VM, Perminova GI, Sokolv AA, et al. Value of laparoscopy in the diagnosis and treatment of appendicular infiltrates. Sov Med 4:98-100, 1989.

12. Christalli B, Cayol V, Izard V, et al. Appendicectomie intra-péritonéale per-coelioscopique. Résultats préliminaires d'une nouvelle technique. J Chir (Paris) 128:302-305, 1991.

13. Christalli B, Ciche R, Izard V, et al. Pelvic pain—evaluation of laparoscopic intraperitoneal appendectomy technique. Ann Chir 45:529, 1991.

14. Chevalier J, Durand A. Réflexions sur une série homogène de 3200 appendicectomies. Lyon Chir 76:251-253, 1980.

15. Dallemagne B, Weerts J, Jehaes C, et al. Douleurs abdominales: Coelioscopie et chirurgie percoelioscopique. Rev Med Liège 45:152-156, 1990.

16. Daniell JF, Gurley LD, Kurtz BR, et al. The use of an automatic stapling device for laparoscopic appendicectomy. Obstet Gynecol 78:721, 1991.

17. Deutsch A, Zelikowski A, Reiss R. Laparoscopy in the prevention of unnecessary appendicectomy: A prospective study. Br J Surg 69:336-337, 1982.

18. Doletskii SI, Shchitinin VE, Dvorovenko EV. Characteristics of surgical tactics in children with acute appendicitis. Khirurgiia (Mosk) 2:93-97, 1990.

19. Engstrom L, Fenyo G. Appendicectomy: Assessment of stump invagination. A prospective, randomized trial. Br J Surg 72:971-972, 1985.

20. Fauque P, Valla (Dir.). Appendicectomie assistée par laparoscopie. Thèsis. Nice: 1990, N° 90, Nice 6542.

21. Flamant Y, Barge J. Questionable appendectomies. Ann Chir 45:284, 1991.

22. Fleming JS. Laparascopically directed appendicectomy. Aust NZ J Obstet Gynaecol 25:238-240, 1985.

23. Gangal HT, Gangal MH. Laparoscopic appendectomy. Br J Surg 76:616, 1989.

24. Gangal HT, Gangal MH. Laparoscopic appendectomy. Endoscopy 19:127-129, 1987.

25. Gans SL, Berci C. Peritoneoscopy in infants and children. J Pediatr Surg 8:399-405, 1973.

26. Godquin B. Le centenaire de l'appendicectomie 1887-1987. Chirurgie 113:336-343, 1988.

27. Gotz F, Pier A, Bacher C. Modified laparoscopic appendectomy in surgery. A report of 388 operations. Surg Endosc 4:6-9, 1990.

28. Gotz F, Pier A, Bacher C. Laparoscopic appendectomy. Indications, technique and results in 653 patients. Chirurg (Berlin) 62:253-256, 1991.

29. Haner C, Inderbitzi R, Kurath J, et al. Appendicitis actua: Vermeidung der unnötigen Laparotomie bei der jungen Frau. Helv Chir Acta 57:33-35, 1990.

30. Hontschik B, Stelter WJ. Comment on the practice of appendectomies. 12:906.

31. Indin IB, Gabinskaia TA, Bukhtiiarov AP. Laparoscopy in the diagnosis of acute appendicitis in children. Khirurgiia (Mosk) 8:26-31, 1990.

32. Jersky J. Laparoscopy in patients with suspected acute appendicitis. S Afr J Surg 18:147-150, 1980.

33. Klaiber C, Metzger A, Zgaggen K, et al. From diagnostic laparoscopy to laparoscopic surgery. Helv Chir Acta 57:693, 1991.

34. Kleinhaus S. Laparoscopic lysis of adhesions for postappendectomy. Pain Gastrointest Endosc 30:304-305, 1984.

35. Laehy PF. Technique of laparoscopic appendicectomy. Br J Surg 76:616, 1989.

36. Leape LL, Ramenofski ML. Laparoscopy for questionable appendicitis. Can it reduce the negative appendectomy rate? Ann Surg 191:410-413, 1980.

37. Leepin H, Klaiber C, Metzger A, et al. Surgical technique in laparoscopic appendectomy (in German). Helv Chir Acta 58:(1-2), Videotape, 1991.

38. Lehmann-Willenbrock E, Mecke H, Riedel HH. Sequelae of appendectomy, with special reference to intraabdominal adhesions, chronic abdominal pain and infertility. Gynecol Obstet Invest 29:241-245, 1990.

39. Mazze RI, Kallen B. Appendectomy during pregnancy—A Swedish study of 778 cases. Obstet Gynecol 77:835, 1991.

40. McAnena OJ, Austin O, Bedermann WP, et al. Laparoscopic versus open appendicectomy. Lancet 338:693, 1991.

41. McKernan JB, Saye PB. Laparoscopic general surgery. J Med Assoc Ga 79:157-159, 1990.

42. McKernan JB, Saye PB. Laparoscopic techniques in appendectomy with argon laser. South Med J 83:1019-1020, 1990.

43. Mounel M, Jaquet A, Mesnard L, et al. La chirurgie per coelioscopique: Ses indications et ses limites. A propos d'une expérience tourangelle. La Revue de Médecine de Tours, 24:9-10, 1990.

44. Mouret P. Cholécystectomie sous coelioscopie. Lyon, 1987 (personal communication).

45. Mouret PH, Marsand H. Appendicectomy per laparoscopy. Technic and evaluation. Presented at the Seccond Congress of Society of American Gastrointestinal Endoscopic Surgeons. Atlanta, March 1990.

46. Mulvihill S, Goldthorn J, Wooley MM. Incidental appendectomy in infants and children. Risk vs. rationale. Arch Surg 118:714-716, 1983.

47. Murat J. Progrès diagnostique et mortalité d'une série de 1400 appendicectomies. Lyon Chir 79:251-254, 1983.

48. Nezhat C, Nezhat F. Incidental appendectomy during videolaseroscopy. Am J Obstet Gynecol 165:559-564, 1991.

49. O'Regan PJ. Laparoscopic appendectomy. Can J Surg 34:256-258, 1991.

50. Orlando R, Lirussi F, Okolicsanyi L. Validity of laparoscopy after abdominal surgery Endoscopy 19:150-152, 1987.
51. Paterson-Brown S, Eckersey JRT, Sim AJW, et al. Laparoscopy as an adjunct to decision making in the "acute abdomen." Br J Surg 73:1022-1024, 1986.
52. Paterson-Brown S, Thompson JN, Eckersley JR, et al. Which patients with suspected appendicitis should undergo laparoscopy? Br Med J 296:1363-1364, 1988.
53. Paterson-Brown S, Vipond MN, Simms K, et al. Clinical decision making and laparoscopy versus computer prediction in the management of the acute abdomen. Br J Surg 76:1011-1013, 1989.
54. Pier A, Gotz F, Bacher C. Die Lasergestütze laparoskopische Appendectomie. Z. Gastroenterol 1991, 29:77-78, 1991; Endoskopie Heute, 3:34-36, 1990.
55. Pier A, Gotz F. Laparoscopic appendectomy. Probl Gen Surg 8:406, 1991.
56. Poole GV. Appendicitis. The diagnostic challenge continues. Am Surg 54:609-612, 1989.
57. Putmant C, Gagliano N, Emmens RW. Appendicitis in children. Surg Gynecol Obstet 170:527-532, 1990.
58. Ragland J, de la Garza J, McKenney Jr. Peritoneoscopy for the diagnosis of acute appendicitis in females of reproductive age. Surg Endosc 2:36-38, 1989.
59. Reddick EJ, Olsen OD. Laparoscopic cholecystectomy and appendectomy. In Laparoscopy for the General Surgeon. Tuttlingen, 1989.
60. Reiertsen O, Rosseland AR, Hoivik B, et al. Laparoscopy in patients admitted for acute abdominal pain. Acta Chir Scand 151:521-524, 1985.
61. Riedel HH, Haag GM. Spätfolgen nach Appendektomie unter besonderer berücksichtigung von Unterbauchverwachsungen, chronischen Unterbauchbeschwerden und Sterilität. Zentralbl Gynäkol 111:1101-1112, 1989.
62. Sackier JM. Laparoscopy in pediatric surgery [Editorial]. J Pediatr Surg 26:1124, 1991.
63. Schreiber JH. Laparoscopic appendectomy in pregnancy. Surg Endosc 4:100-102, 1990.
64. Schreiber JH. Early experience with laparoscopic appendectomy in women. Surg Endosc 1:211-216, 1987.
65. Semm K. Advances in pelviscopic surgery. Curr Probl Obstet Gynecol 15:171, 1982.
66. Semm K. Endoscopic appendectomy. Endoscopy 15:59-64, 1983.
67. Semm K. Operationslehre für Endoskopische Abdominalchirurgie. Stuttgart: Schattauer, 1984.
68. Semm K. Die pelviskopische Appendektomie. Dtsch Med Wochenschr 113:3-5, 1988.
69. Semm K. Technical operative steps in endoscopic appendectomy. Langenbecks Arch Chir 376:121, 1991.
70. Solheim K. Laparoskopisk appendektomi. Tidesskr Nor Laegeforen 111:1707, 1991.
71. Spirtos NM, Eisenkop SM, Spirtos TW, et al. Laparoscopy—a diagnostic aid in cases of suspected appendicitis its use in women of reproductive age. Am J Obstet Gynecol 156:90-94, 1987.
72. Testas P. La chirurgie digestive par voie coelioscopique. Presse Méd 20:301, 1991.
73. Testas P, Delaitre B. Chirurgie digestive par voie coelioscopique. Edition Maloine, 1991.
74. Thomas P. Appendicectomie assistée par laparoscopie : Série personnelle de 212 cas. Thèsis. Lyon: 1988, 88, Lyon M459.
75. Ulitovskii IV. An improved retractor for appendectomy. Vestn Khir 144:111, 1990.
76. Valla JS, Limonne B, Valla V, et al. Appendicectomies chez l'enfant sous coelioscopie opératoire. 465 cas. J Chir 128:306-312, 1991.
77. Vaxman F. Une nouvelle appendicectomie. Gazette Méd 98:40, 1991.
78. Volkmar P, Vaxman F. Minimally invasive surgery and new technology. Presented at the Second European Congress of Viscerosynthesis. Luxembourg, September 10-12, 1992.
79. Waldschmidt J, Schier F. Laparoscopic surgery in neonates and infants. Eur J Pediatr Surg 1:145-150, 1991.
80. Wilston T. Laparoscopically-assisted appendectomies. Med J Aust 145:151, 1986.
81. Whitworth CM, Withworth PW, Sanfillipo J, et al. Value of diagnostic laparoscopy in young women with possible appendicitis. Surg Gynecol Obstet 167:187-190, 1988.
82. Woodward A, Hemingway D, Greaney MG, et al. Which patients should undergo laparoscopy? Br Med J 296:1740, 1988.
83. Zaaf M, Roger B, Vaur JL, et al. Progrès diagnostique et mortalité d'une série de 1400 appendicectomies. Lyon Chir 79:251-254, 1983.

45 *Laparoscopic Peritoneal Lavage Versus Colon Resection by Open Operation in Colon Perforations*

Michael Sean Dudeney, H. Paul Redmond, Orla M. Austin, Paul E. Burke, Austin Leahy, Pierce A. Grace, and David Bouchier-Hayes

The standard treatment for perforations of the colon is surgical intervention and antibiotic therapy.[1-3] However, the surgical procedure that is most appropriate remains controversial.[2,3] Peritoneal lavage is believed to improve survival by reducing peritoneal bacterial cell counts and was effective in some clinical[4-6] and experimental studies.[7] Other studies have contradicted these findings.[8-10] Laparoscopy offers a treatment alternative for perforations of the colon. In this approach a laparoscope is used to confirm the perforation and provide lavage of the peritoneal cavity. Fecal contaminants are aspirated from the cavity, and a large abdominal incision is not necessary. Neither closure of the perforation nor resection of the diseased portion of the colon is performed.

We tested whether laparoscopic peritoneal lavage was as effective as colonic resection in an experimental model of colon perforations, and we examined the effects of those techniques on the intraperitoneal immune system.

MATERIALS AND METHODS

Eighty virus-free female CD-1 mice 6 to 8 weeks old were studied. A regular chow diet was fed for 7 days; then the animals were weighed and randomized for either in vivo mortality analysis or in vivo immunologic studies.

In Vivo Mortality Studies

Sixty mice were anesthetized with ether and were subjected to cecal ligation and puncture that involved a 1 cm abdominal wound, ligation of the base of the cecum with a 3-0 silk suture, and a single puncture of the cecum with a 19-gauge needle. The suture was tied to occlude the passage of feces but was not made tight enough to cause cecal ischemia. The abdominal wall was then closed in two layers with a 2-0 silk suture. After 2 hours, the animals were septic; this was indicated by irregular rippling of fur and decreased activity. Two hours

after the procedure, the animals were randomized into one of three treatment groups.

Group 1 animals (n = 20) underwent laparotomy in which a midline incision 2.5 cm in length was made and the ligated cecum was excised. Group 2 animals (n = 20) underwent peritoneal lavage, which involved the introduction of 9 ml of sterile saline through the abdominal wall in three separate 3 ml aliquots. Three milliliters of saline was required to fill the abdominal cavity without marked distension. Three repetitions of the lavage, for which a 5 ml syringe and a 21-gauge needle were used, produced a clear aspirate. The abdomen was made watertight by application of a small artery clip along the previous abdominal wound. Irrigation fluid was carefully removed. Group 3 animals (n = 20) received a sham laparotomy that involved the insertion of an abdominal suture into the unopened abdominal wall. The skin was cleaned with 70% alcohol before abdominal incisions were made. The animals were then studied for mortality at 6-hour intervals for 5 days.

In Vitro Assays

Isolation and assay of peritoneal macrophages. Peritoneal macrophages were harvested by peritoneal lavage with 5 ml of sterile phosphate-buffered saline (PBS) and were centrifuged, washed, and resuspended in Dulbecco's modified Eagle's medium (DMEM)[11] containing 10% fetal calf serum, 1% glutamine, 1% penicillin and streptomycin, and 0.1% 2-mercaptoethanol. Cells were plated for assays at concentrations of 1×10^6 cells/ml, were allowed to adhere for 2 hours at 37° C, were washed twice in PBS to remove nonadherent cells, and were studied for superoxide (O_2) anion production and tumor necrosing factor (TNF) release.

Peritoneal cell aspirates were also submitted to diff-quick analysis, which was used to calculate macrophage content and neutrophil influx into the peritoneal cavity.

Assay for superoxide anion generation. Superoxide (O_2^-) anion generation was measured as the super-oxide dismutase-inhibitable reduction of ferricytochrome c in response to a stimulus of the phorbol ester, phorbol myristate acetate (1 mg/ml). Results were expressed in nmol $O_2^-/10^5$ cells/90 min.

TNF bioassay. This assay used the L929 mouse fibroblast cells, which were grown to confluency in a 75 cm^2 flask. L929 cells were plated at 5×10^5 cells/well for samples and standard curve analysis. After 24 hours, all wells were aspirated and were replaced with 80 μl of actinomycin D and complete media. Samples and standards were then added in a 20 μl volume and were incubated for 18 hours. For cellular TNF release, peritoneal macrophages were stimulated with LPS (1 μg/ml for 2 hours), and samples were stored at $-70°$C until they were used. 3-[4,5-dimethylthiazol-2-yl]-2,5-diphenyltetrazolium bromide (MTT; 10 ml/well) was then added to each well, and incubation was continued for 4 hours. All wells were then aspirated, and 100 μl of isopropanol and 0.04 NHCl were added. The plate was then incubated for 10 minutes, and 100 ml of distilled water was added to each well. Absorbency was read on a microplate reader (Bio-Tek Instruments, Vermont, USA).

Statistical analysis. Superoxide anion generation and cellular tumor necrosing factor assays were performed on pooled peritoneal macrophages; at least three mice per assay were used. Each experiment was performed three to five times. For in vivo mortality studies, at least 15 mice per group were used. Statistical analysis was performed; the unpaired Student's t-test was used to compare two groups, and ANOVA was used to compare the means of several groups. The chi-squared test was used to assess survival in mortality studies. The level of significance was determined at $p < 0.05$. Data are presented as the mean plus or minus a standard deviation.

RESULTS

Survival at 5 days. The survival rate 5 days following the procedure was significantly higher in the cecectomy group (50%) as compared with that in the peritoneal group (18%) and that in the control group (10%; Fig. 1).

Peritoneal macrophage yield. The peritoneal macrophage yield in animals that had undergone cecectomy was significantly higher (32%) than that of control animals (16%) or that of animals in which lavage was used (6%; Fig. 2).

Neutrophil influx. The neutrophil influx in the peritoneal lavage group was significantly higher (93%) than that in the cecectomy group (64%). Control animals had a yield of 73% (Fig. 3).

Superoxide anion production. Peritoneal macrophages generate superoxide (O_2^-) in response to membrane perturbating agents and phagocytosis. The magnitude of the response correlates with the microbicidal capacity of the activated macrophage. Animals that underwent cecectomy had a yield of 2.8 ± 1.0 nmol.

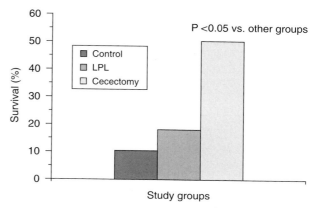

Fig. 1. Survival in each of three groups at 5 days after the procedure. Animals that underwent cecectomy had significantly higher survival rates than did animals in other groups. *LPL* = laparoscopic peritoneal lavage.

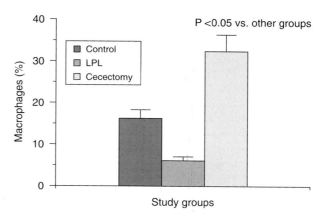

Fig. 2. Peritoneal macrophage yields in each of the treatment groups. The cecectomy group animals had significantly higher macrophage yields than did animals in other groups.

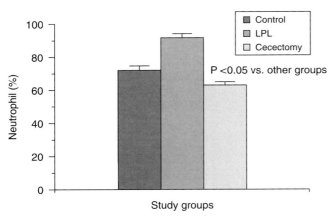

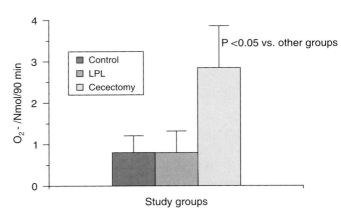

Fig. 3. Neutrophil influx in each study group. Animals that underwent cecectomy had a significantly lower level of neutrophil influx than did animals that underwent lavage or those in the control group.

Fig. 4. Superoxide release in each study group. The cecectomy group animals had significantly higher superoxide release than did lavage group animals or those in the control group.

This level was significantly higher than those of the peritoneal lavage or control group animals, both of which had levels of 0.8 ± 0.5 nmol (Fig. 4).

TNF release. The highest level of TNF release from peritoneal macrophages in response to macrophage secretion of TNF was noted in the cecectomy group (20 pg/ml) as opposed to the lavage group (12 pg/ml) or the control group (3 pg/ml) (Fig. 5).

DISCUSSION

In this study, a significant increase in survival was seen in the cecectomy group, in which the ligated and punctured cecum was excised. The increased survival was accompanied by an increase in peritoneal macrophages, which provide important defense during the initial stage of bacterial contamination.[12,13] Peritoneal macrophages, which are essential in the local immune response to sepsis, were in an increased state of activation indicated by an increase in the levels of TNF and superoxide anions. These anions are inflammatory mediators released by macrophages, and an increase in anion concentration indicates an increase in the macrophage level of activity. The closed peritoneal lavage group failed to show a significant increase in survival when compared with that of the control group. The closed peritoneal lavage group also showed a decrease in macrophage cell number and activation and a decrease in the levels of TNF and superoxide per macrophage.

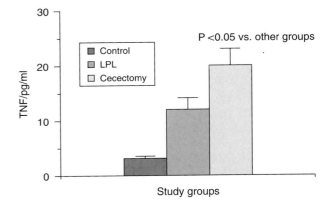

Fig. 5. Tumor necrosis factor (TNF) release in each study group. Cecectomy group animals had significantly higher levels of TNF release than did lavage group animals or those in the control group.

In this model, the intra-abdominal sepsis that results from perforated colonic disease is replicated. Fecal flow was maintained by a ligature at the base of the cecum. If only cecal puncture is performed, death does not result. The ligature around the base of the cecum, even though it is loosely applied, may cause an ischemic condition that would not occur in the patient with perforated colonic disease. In spite of these discrepancies, ours is a model of colonic perforation, and 10% of the animals survived in the control group. Therefore this is a valid model in the comparison of survival that results from various treatments. Any beneficial treatment should increase survival.

The best surgical treatment for acute colonic perforation is controversial.[2,3] Ideally, the diseased portion of colon should be removed; however, the procedure is dependent on whether the septic patient can withstand operation. The safety of colonic anastomosis in a fecally contaminated peritoneal cavity is also controversial. Laparoscopic treatment for that situation can result in rapid, thorough abdominal lavage under direct vision; no large abdominal incision is necessary. This treatment is based on the efficacy of peritoneal lavage, which is widely used in both open abdominal and in laparoscopic surgery in spite of conflicting data[4-10] regarding its effectiveness. A frequent indication for use of the laparoscopic technique is minimal contamination with fecal material, another is any inflammatory process resulting in pus, blood, bile, or other free fluid in the peritoneal cavity. Hemoglobin, for example, in the presence of *Escherichia coli*, significantly increases bacterial proliferation.[14-16] Bile is also an adjuvant in intra-abdominal sepsis.[17]

Several studies have shown that intraoperative lavage offers certain benefits (often when used with antibiotics). The beneficial effects of this combination treatment may be due to antibiotic use rather than to the lavage. Other studies do not indicate benefit from lavage, and few studies have considered its adverse effects. The beneficial effects of lavage are presumed to be due to its decreasing the organisms and inflammatory mediators in the peritoneal cavity. However, the data of Minervini et al.[10] who examined the use of saline lavage in colorectal operations without the use of antibiotics, indicated a marked increase in postoperative septic complications in spite of significant decreases in aerobic and anaerobic bacteria. Edmiston et al.[18] failed to show a decrease in the postlavage peritoneal microbial populations in cecal ligation and puncture in the rat model, and demonstrated the adherence of those organisms to the peritoneal surface and thus their resistance to lavage. In that study, bacterial cell counts returned to prelavage levels within 24 hours after lavage. In this study, we show a significant decrease in macrophages and in antimicrobial activity as a result of lavage. Lavage may be detrimental if it impairs peritoneal immune function. Peritoneal lavage may wash macrophages from the peritoneum; this would compromise the mononuclear phagocyte host defense.

Some studies[4] have indicated the effectiveness of antibiotic lavage, which is a combination of two therapies. In other studies,[9] when the effect of antibiotic lavage is compared in animals given effective systemic antibiotics, no difference is found in the rate of intra-abdominal infection. Antibiotic administration is thus beneficial, but the use of lavage per se may not be.

Dunn et al.[19] showed that intraperitoneal fluid introduction concomitant with infection had a negative effect on outcome. They gave intraperitoneal injections of nonlethal doses of *E. coli* in various volumes of saline; the combination was lethal in direct proportion to the volume of saline infused. This effect was attributed to the dilution of opsonic proteins including complement factors and immunoglobulins. Phagocytic cells need a surface to permit ingestion. If phagocytes float in free fluid, ingestion is inhibited.

Other cells are involved in the host defense against peritoneal infection. Peritoneal mast cells release histamine, which causes vasodilation and increased permeability. They also release leukotriene B_4, a very powerful chemotactic agent. Yong[14] showed that saline lavage depleted mast cells, that the remaining cells were primarily immature, and that regeneration to normal numbers and distribution took 3 to 4 weeks. Bacterial cell numbers returned to prelavage levels within 24 hours.

Cecectomy is effective because it removes the source of sepsis. Animals that undergo cecectomy rely on their immune system for recovery, which explains the significant decrease in the mortality in this group.

Saline lavage without antibiotic therapy confers no significant advantage. Our finding of the failure of saline lavage concurs with the results of other studies. Explanation for saline lavage failure involves the negative effects of lavage (as sole therapy) on the immune system. We show that lavage markedly decreases the number of macrophages, presumably by washing them out of the peritoneal cavity and that it reduces bacterial cell counts for only a brief period. More complex cells such as macrophages require more time than bacteria do to increase the number of mature cells to prelavage levels.

Dilution of chemotactic factors may decrease the rate of recolinization, and dilution of opsonins such as complement factors and immunoglobulins decrease the activity of the immune system.

This study fails to show that minimally invasive peritoneal lavage is an effective treatment for perforated colonic disease in a murine model. We now intend to examine the efficacy of lavage used with antibiotics, a dual treatment that is common in clinical practice.

REFERENCES

1. Way LW, ed. Current Surgical Diagnosis and Treatment, 9th ed. Norwalk, Ct: Lange, 1988, pp 633-680.
2. Finlay IG, Carter DC. A comparison of emergency resection and staged management in perforated diverticular disease. Dis Colon Rectum 30:929, 1978.
3. Ravo B, Mishrick A, Addei K, Castrini G, Pappalardo G, Gross E, Sacker JM, Wood CB, Ger R. The treatment of perforated diverticulitis by one-stage intra-colonic bypass procedure. Surgery 102:771, 1987.
4. Silverman SH, Ambrose NS, Youngs DJ, Shepherd AF, Roberts AP, Keighly MR. The effect of peritoneal lavage with tetracycline solution on postoperative infection. A prospective, randomized, clinical trial. Dis Colon Rectum 29:165-169, 1986.
5. Lygidakis NJ. Surgical approaches to peritonitis. The value of intra- and postoperative peritoneal lavage. Acta Chir Belg 83:345-352, 1983.
6. Stewart DJ, Matheson NA. Peritoneal lavage in appendicular peritonitis. Br J Surg 65:54-56, 1978.
7. Stewart DJ, Matheson NA. Peritoneal lavage in faecal peritonitis in the rat. Br J Surg 65:57-59, 1978.
8. Schein M, Gecelter G, Freinkel W, Gerding H, Becker PJ. Peritoneal lavage in abdominal sepsis. A controlled clinical study. Arch Surg 125:1132-1135, 1990.
9. Lally KP, Shorr LD, Nichols RL. Aminoglycoside peritoneal lavage: Lack of efficacy in experimental fecal peritonitis. J Pediat Surg 20:541-542, 1985.
10. Minervini S, Bently S, Young D, Alexander-Williams J, Burdon DW, Keighly MR. Prophylactic saline peritoneal lavage in elective colorectal operations. Dis Colon Rectum 23:392-394, 1980.
11. Johnston RB Jr, Godzick CA, Cohn ZA. Increased superoxide production by immunologically activated and chemically elicited macrophages. J Exp Med 148:115-127, 1978.
12. Edmiston CE Jr, Goheen MP, Kornhall S, Jones FE, Condon RE. Fecal peritonitis: Microbial adherence to serosal mesothelium and resistance to peritoneal lavage. World J Surg 14:176-183, 1990.
13. Dunn DL, Barke RA, Ahrenholz DH, Humphrey EW, Simmons RL. The adjuvant effect of peritoneal fluid in experimental peritonitis. Ann Surg 199:37, 1984.
14. Yong LC. The regeneration and maturation of mast cells following peritoneal lavage in the rat. Morphol Embryol 31:127-135, 1985.
15. Chong KT. Prophylactic administration of interleukin-2 protects mice from lethal challenge with gram-negative bacteria. Infect Immun 55:668, 1987.
16. Macphee MJ, Zakaleizny I, Marshall J. Mixed lymphocyte culture supernatants provide effective immunotherapy for acute peritonitis in immunosuppressed rats. Surg Forum 37:105, 1986.
17. Yull AB, Abrams JS, Davis JH. The peritoneal fluid in strangulation obstruction: The role of the red blood cell and *E. coli* bacteria in producing toxicity. J Surg Res 2:223, 1962.
18. Hau T, Hoffman R, Simmons RL. Mechanisms of the adjuvant effect of haemoglobin in experimental peritonitis. (Part 1). In vivo inhibition of peritoneal leucocytes. Surgery 83:223, 1978.
19. Hau T, Nelson RD, Fiegel VD, Levenson R, Simmons RL. Mechanisms of the adjuvant effect of haemoglobin in experimental peritonitis. (Part 2). Influence of haemoglobin in human leucocyte chemotaxis in vitro. J Surg Res 22:174, 1977.
20. Andersson R, Srinivas U, Tranberg KG, Benmark S. Effect of bile on peritoneal macrophages in intraabdominal sepsis. Presented at the International Congress on Intraabdominal Infection. Hamburg, 1987.

46   *Simultaneous Videoendoscopic Interventions*

Guenther Meyer, Volker Lange, Hans-Martin Schardey, and Friedrich-Wilhelm Schildberg

A simultaneous intervention is an additional, second operation, with a different indication and tactical approach, that is carried out at the same time as the primary procedure. Multiple interventions simultaneously carried out play an important role in all surgical disciplines. Examples include the combination of carotid endarterectomy with coronary bypass grafting,[1] the simultaneous revascularization of renal arteries with the operation of an abdominal aortic aneurysm,[2] the simultaneous resection of lung and liver metastases,[3] and the repair of multitrauma injuries in one session.[4]

An *absolute* indication for a simultaneous intervention out of necessity results, then, when not performing the intervention would endanger the patient or when the simultaneous intervention could bring about a clear improvement of the surgical result. *Therapeutic* indications are for vital reasons as in the multitrauma patient suffering from splenic rupture and third-degree open femur fracture or in cases of intra-operative iatrogenic lesions to other organs, such as a transection of the ureter. For oncological reasons a simultaneous intervention can be indicated in the presence of an incidentally discovered carcinoma. *Diagnostic* indications include excision biopsies of incidentally discovered or preoperatively recognized lesions of unknown etiology if therapeutic consequences are to be expected. The same holds true for a staging laparotomy in Hodgkin's disease, including therapeutic splenectomy and diagnostic liver biopsy as well as para-aortic, celiac, and mesenteric lymphadenectomy. The repair of a filiform carotid stenosis before cardiac surgery in one session to reduce the potential for intra-operative stroke is an example for a *preventive* indication.

Since every simultaneous intervention represents an expansion of the primary procedure and a concomitant increase in risk proportional to the extent of the operation, a critical attitude with respect to the indication is imperative, especially when an elective operation is planned. The latter case represents a *relative* indication, and the surgeon must carefully weigh the advantages for the patient against the possible increased risk associated with the entire intervention. The advantages should clearly outweigh the increased risk associated with expansion of the procedure. For planned simultaneous interventions, the surgeon must obtain informed consent for the operations.[5] As a rule the indication is seen in view of reducing the overall surgical trauma if a second intervention should be required. A simultaneous intervention avoids additional anesthesia and a second operation. It is generally agreed that the simultaneous intervention should only be carried out if the second procedure by itself is also indicated, as in the case of symptomatic disease. If the simultaneous intervention is more *preventive* in nature, postponement may be advisable.

Interest in performing simultaneous interventions is low among general surgeons, based on the fact that such dual operations are associated with a cumulative postoperative complication rate up to 50% higher and that the mortality of operations with involvement of stomach, duodenum, or colon and gallbladder increases to 30% when simultaneous interventions are performed.[6-8]

In finding an indication for a simultaneous intervention, the main emphasis is put on the individual risk for the patient. Advanced age and associated severe disease are strong arguments against simultaneous interventions for only relative indications, since the cardiovascular risk for simultaneous interventions appears to be increased.[9,10] In addition, one has to consider the magnitude and duration of the interventions to be combined as well as the infectious potential of the underlying diseases. In the literature it has been pointed out that a simultaneous intervention causes an increase in risk if major operations are undertaken or if one of the procedures is for a septic state.[6]

In only 2% to 4% of all laparotomies the primary procedure is combined with a simultaneous intervention.[5] According to a collective review of 4261 simultaneous interventions,[8] the appendectomy is the most common second procedure carried out, followed at a great distance by procedures on the stomach (3%), the biliary

239

Table 1. Overview of 4118 simultaneous operations: incidence of primary and secondary interventions

Primary	Secondary	Number	Percent
Gynecological	+ Appendectomy	3409	82.8
Gallbladder/bile ducts	+ Appendectomy	295	4.7
	+ Stomach	94	2.3
	+ Other abdominal OP	134	3.3
Stomach	+ Gallbladder/bile ducts	78	1.9
Appendectomy	+ Meckel's diverticulum	70	1.7
Herniorrhaphy	+ Appendectomy	10	0.2
Other abdominal procedures	+ Appendectomy	28	0.7

system (2.5%), and Meckel's diverticulum (2%). Much less frequent are gynecological operations (0.4%) and hernia repair (0.2%). According to another collective overview (Table 1), gynecological operations and interventions on the biliary system with appendectomies were the most common combinations of primary and simultaneous interventions. Next in frequency were combined procedures on the gallbladder or biliary system and the stomach.

Minimally invasive surgery has long surpassed the stage at which laparoscopic cholecystectomy was the sole procedure indicated. More and more diseases of the abdomen and thorax are treated laparoscopically or thoracoscopically. Most such procedures involve operations with merely a relative indication. Since reports have been limited to individual cases,[11,12] it remains unclear whether the results obtained in conventional surgery also hold true for simultaneous laparoscopic interventions or whether it is possible to handle the indications in a more liberal way based on the different conditions and reduced overall surgical trauma.

MATERIALS AND METHODS

From July 1991 to August 1992 we carried out simultaneous minimally invasive interventions on 11 patients. There were four men and seven women (average age, 58 years). The youngest patient was 14, the oldest 91 years old.

In seven patients the simultaneous intervention was planned and in four patients unplanned (Tables 2 and 3). Twice the simultaneous intervention was the result of an incorrect diagnosis preoperatively. One female patient (No. 9) presented with a recurrent partial obstruction following abdominal hysterectomy; she was also known to have had endometriosis. Adhesions were assumed to be the cause for the obstruction. Intraoperatively a severe inflammation of the ileocecal area was found, as well as a stricture of the terminal ileum because of kinking. An appendectomy and seromyotomy of the stenotic ileum was carried out. Histologically, endometriosis of the appendix was found, and an excision biopsy from the cicatricial stenosis revealed fibrosis. In another patient (No. 11), laparoscopy was carried out for suspected acute appendicitis. A partial infarction of the greater omentum was found, however, and was treated with partial resection of the greater omentum and an appendectomy. Our youngest patient (a 14-year-old female) had had chronic recurrent lower right abdominal pain since she was 3 months of age. After all diagnostic attempts failed, we decided to carry out a diagnostic laparoscopy. A highly acute phlegmonous appendicitis was found, along with a paraovarian cyst, causing torsion of the fallopian tube without signs of ischemia. With the assistance of our consulting gynecologist, an appendectomy and cyst resection were carried out. In one patient (No. 5) a simultaneous intervention was required for treating an intraoperative iatrogenic lesion to the gallbladder while deroofing a liver cyst, so that a simultaneous cholecystectomy had to be carried out.

In the seven planned procedures two patients underwent herniorrhaphy on both sides for bilateral ingui-

Table 2. Diagnoses in simultaneous interventions

Patient No.	Primary Operation	Secondary Operation
1	Right direct inguinal hernia	+ Left direct inguinal hernia
2	Right direct inguinal hernia	+ Left direct inguinal hernia
3	Right lateral inguinal hernia	+ Cholecystolithiasis
4	Right lateral inguinal hernia	+ Cholecystolithiasis
5	Symptomatic liver cyst	—
6	Symptomatic liver cyst	+ Cholecystolithiasis
7	Symptomatic liver cyst	+ Pulmonary nodule
8	Chronic recurrent duodenal ulcer	+ Cholecystolithiasis
9	Chronic appendicitis	+ Cicatricial ileum stenosis
10	Acute appendicitis	+ Ovarian cyst
11	Omental infarction	—

Table 3. Combination frequency of primary and secondary operations in minimally invasive surgery

Patient No.	Primary Operation	Secondary Operation
1	Herniorrhaphy, right side	+ Herniorrhaphy, left side
2	Herniorrhaphy, right side	+ Herniorrhaphy, left side
3	Herniorrhaphy, right side	+ Cholecystectomy
4	Herniorrhaphy, right side	+ Cholecystectomy
5	Liver cyst deroofing	+ Cholecystectomy
6	Liver cyst deroofing	+ Cholecystectomy
7	Liver cyst deroofing	+ Atypical lung resection
8	Vagotomy	+ Cholecystectomy
9	Appendectomy	+ Seromyotomy terminal ileum
10	Appendectomy	+ Ovarian cyst resection
11	Omental resection	+ Appendectomy

nal hernias; two patients underwent cholecystectomy and right-sided hernia repair. Among the latter was our oldest, a 91-year-old woman. Another woman with symptomatic liver cysts and gallstones was simultaneously treated with deroofing of the liver cyst and cholecystectomy. In one case a vagotomy by the Taylor modification was combined with a cholecystectomy. In another case both a laparoscopic intervention and a thoracoscopic procedure were simultaneously carried out in a patient with a large symptomatic liver cyst in the right lobe of the liver (Fig. 1). Here we incidentally found a solitary pulmonary nodule during preoperative computer tomography in the lateral aspect of the right lower lobe of the lung (Fig. 2). In one session we carried out deroofing of the liver cyst, followed by removal of the coin lesion by thoracoscopic atypical lung resection after changing the position of the patient into left lateral decubitus. After histological examination had revealed a surprising pulmonary adenocarcinoma, the patient underwent lobectomy and mediastinal lymph-

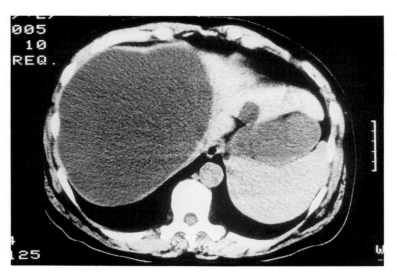

Fig. 1. Solitary cyst (15 × 19 cm) in the right lobe of the liver.

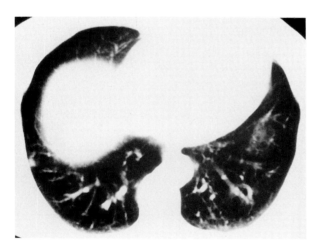

Fig. 2. Same patient as in Fig. 1: small coin lesion in the lateral right lower lobe of the lung. Histologically, pulmonary adenocarcinoma.

adenectomy later on. The specimen was free of tumor tissue, so the carcinoma had been curatively resected by means of thoracoscopy.

RESULTS

In eight cases the primary and secondary interventions were carried out in the same topographic body region (73%); three times the simultaneous intervention was restricted to the upper abdomen and five times to the lower abdomen. Three times different topographic regions were involved (27%): in two patients operations to the upper and lower abdomen were combined, and in one female patient surgery was carried out in both the abdominal and thoracic cavities (Fig. 3). It seems to us that minimally invasive surgery has an advantage in the combination of interventions to different topographic body regions when compared with conventional open surgery, which often leads to (depending on approach) intra-abdominal trauma because of a more difficult exposure as well as soft tissue damage resulting from stronger traction of the laparotomy edges. Different topographic regions can easily be reached by trocar without additional trauma by merely changing the direction of the instruments or by adding small additional trocars through minor stab incisions (Fig. 4).

In only three of our simultaneous interventions were both procedures aseptic (27%). In five cases an aseptic operation was combined with a cholecystectomy, and in two cases with an uncomplicated appendectomy (64%), all of which represent only partially aseptic interventions. In one of our simultaneous interventions an aseptic procedure was combined with an appendectomy for phlegmonous appendicitis, which had to be classified as a septic operation (7%). Intra-abdominal infection-related complications or soft tissue infections were observed in none of the cases. Principally the aseptic intervention was carried out first. In the laparothoraco-

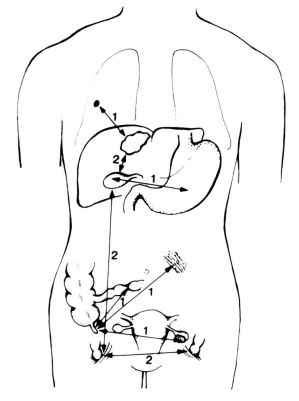

Fig. 3. Incidence of combinations of primary and secondary interventions in minimally invasive surgery (n = 11).

Fig. 4. Combination of a cholecystectomy with a herniorrhaphy as an example of simultaneous interventions in different topographic body regions. Both procedures can be carried out through a 12 mm trocar (endohernia stapler), a 10 mm trocar (for the laparoscope), and a 5 mm trocar (for the grasper). By simply changing the direction of the trocars, the instruments and optics can easily reach distant regions.

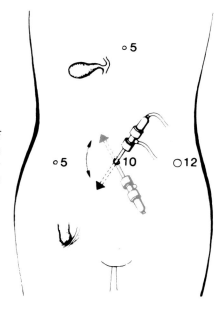

scopic operation the thoracoscopy followed the laparoscopy, because the deroofing of the liver cyst was the larger, primary intervention. Here as well, problems from bile leak were not encountered.

The conclusion, based on experience gained in conventional simultaneous operations, therefore possibly do not hold true to the same degree for minimally invasive simultaneous interventions. In the former, the combination of a septic or partially septic procedure with an aseptic procedure is not advisable,[5,6] because peritoneal complications are more often encountered.[9]

The average duration of operation for all simultaneous interventions was 109 minutes. The shortest was 55 minutes, required for appendectomy and partial omentum resection; the longest time was 210 minutes for a vagotomy combined with a cholecystectomy (Table 4). Severely prolonged operating times were avoided, despite adding secondary procedures. All patients left the hospital by day 7 except for the patient with the simultaneous laparoscopy and thoracoscopy. In the latter case, the reasons for a prolonged stay were the complication of a pulmonary embolism on postoperative day 6 and the therapeutic consequences dictated by the diagnosis of the pulmonary adenocarcinoma (see Table 4). The above-mentioned pulmonary embolism was the only postoperative complication we encountered. It was treated with heparin. No patient died in our series. All patients are presently free of complaint.

Nine of our patients were more than 50 years old; five were older than 60. From conventional simultaneous interventions it is known that the morbidity increases after the age of 60.[8,9] The only complication we observed was an embolism in a 61-year-old female patient. It apparently occurred, however, less as a result of the simultaneous intervention than as a result of an intraoperative complication during deroofing of the liver cyst: after iatrogenic injury to a large hepatic vein at the dorsal aspect of the cystic wall it came to a severe hemorrhage, which we controlled with an EndoGIA stapler. We assume that the embolism that occurred later had its origin at this location.

Similar to reports in the literature about conventional simultaneous interventions,[11,13] procedures on the biliary system and appendix were the leading primary and secondary operations carried out in our patients (see Tables 1 and 3). Unusually high, however, was the number of simultaneous repairs of bilateral inguinal hernias, which we consider to be a good indication. In the evaluation of the overall positive results obtained with the minimally invasive simultaneous interventions we have performed so far, we must keep in mind that it is still a very small group of patients, not allowing us to draw final conclusions. Some of the procedures were minor operations, which in conventional operations have low complication rates.[8,9,14] It is well known, on the other hand, that procedures on the stomach, biliary system, or colon, if combined with simultaneous secondary interventions—independent of the kind or location—represent an increased risk of leading to severe postoperative complications.[8] These procedures constitute about half of the operations we carried out, but we did not observe this increase in risk for minimally invasive interventions.

Several factors may play a role in this seemingly reduced complication rate. One aspect may be similar to single interventions: a clear reduction of approach-dependent trauma. It seems to make a significant difference when results are compared with conventional operations, leading to a major stress reduction for the patient during the postoperative period. Postoperative pain is reduced, pulmonary impairment is less, the patient can be mobilized more quickly, the hospital stay is shorter, and recovery is faster. A more favorable cosmetic result is also obtained. Another advantage of minimally invasive surgical techniques is the more deli-

Table 4. Time-related data for 11 minimally invasive simultaneous interventions

Patient No.	Age (years)	Operative Time (minutes)	Postoperative In-hospital Stay (days)
1	58	100	5
2	50	80	6
3	91	90	7
4	67	70	5
5	65	70	6
6	71	165	5
7	61	180	25*
8	45	210	7
9	50	60	6
10	14	120	4
11	56	55	4
Average	58	109	7

*Postoperative pulmonary embolism occurred; see text.

cate, tissue-sparing preparation made possible by video magnification. Smaller wound surfaces and reduced blood loss are obtained. All this adds up to a definitive reduction of local tissue trauma. The greatly facilitated approach to far distant abdominal organs is another advantage, adding to the effect. The tissue pulling and tearing to improve the surgeon's visibility, which is often encountered in conventional surgery, can be completely avoided. The duration of surgery, averaging about 1.5 hours in our patients (see Table 4), is within the lower range and helps to reduce overall surgical trauma.

CONCLUSION

In summary, the results of our initial experience with minimally invasive simultaneous interventions, in comparison with the conventional approach, seem to indicate an overall reduction in surgical trauma. We therefore believe one can consider a more liberal handling of indications within the frame presented here and that it is possible to expand the spectrum of simultaneous operations to other procedures.

REFERENCES

1. Gugulakis A, Kalodiki E, Nicolides A. Combined carotid endarterectomy and coronary artery bypass grafting. Int Angiol 10:167, 1991.
2. von Segesser LK, Bauer E, Carrel T, Laske A, Turina M. Die simultane Revaskularisierung der Nierenarterien anlässlich der Sanierung von Bauchaortenaneurysmen. Helv Chir Acta 57:771, 1990.
3. Vogt-Moykopf I, Meyer G. Surgical techniques in operations on pulmonary metastases. Thorac Cardiovasc Surg 34:125, 1986.
4. Hansis M, Hoentzsch D, Weller S. Die umfassende Erstversorgung polytraumatisierter Patienten mit dem Fixateur externe—Erstbehandlung und weiteres Vorgehen. Langenbecks Arch Chir (suppl II):525, 1989.
5. Siewert JR, Castrup HJ. Indikationen zu Simultaneingriffen im Rahmen der Abdominalchirurgie. In Heberer G, Schweiberer L, eds. Indikationen zur Operation. Berlin: Springer, 1981, p 125.
6. Esser G, Wirtz G. Indikationen und Prognosen prophylaktischer und simultaner Operationen in der Bauchhöhle. Zbl Chir 112:1099, 1987.
7. Löhlein D, Pichelmayr R. Simultaneingriffe bei Operationen an Magen, Duodenum und dem Gallenwegsystem. Zbl Chir 102:1174, 1977.
8. Reiferscheid M, Langer S. Möglichkeiten und Grenzen des Simultaneingriffs. Langenbecks Arch Chir 333:109, 1973.
9. Löhlein D, Pichelmayr R. Zum Risiko von Simultaneingriffen bei Colon—und Rektumoperationen. Langenbecks Arch Chir 343:205, 1977.
10. Kapral W. Magenresektion und Parallelerkrankung von Gallenblase und Gallenwegen. Chirurgie 39:184, 1968.
11. Bailey R, Flowers JL, Graham SM, Zucker KA. Combined laparoscopic cholecystectomy and selective vagotomy. Surg Laparosc Endosc 1:45, 1991.
12. Ferzli G, Ozuner G, Castellano MR. Incidental appendectomy during laparoscopic cholecystectomy. J Laparoendosc Surg 2:165, 1992.
13. Esser G. Prophylaktische und simultane Operationen im Abdomen. Langenbecks Arch Chir 369 (Kongressbericht 1986):167, 1986.
14. Carstensen G, Hess W. Das Meckel'sche Divertikel, Erfahrungen nach 155 Resektionen. Langenbecks Arch Chir 359:161, 1983.

47 *Mishaps and Risks in Laparoscopic Surgery*

Henning Niebuhr, Ulf Nahrstedt, and Klaus Rückert

At present, laparoscopic surgery is gaining widespread acceptance in clinical practice. Laparoscopic appendectomy and cholecystectomy are beginning to reach gold standard status. Notwithstanding the variety of techniques and results, a number of mishaps, risks, and complications may occur, particularly during the initial stages of learning and early practice experience.

We present our experiences with 71 laparoscopic appendectomies and 395 laparoscopic cholecystectomies and focus on the intraoperative and postoperative complications.

RESULTS

Since the introduction of laparoscopic surgery in our clinic in 1991, we have performed 71 appendectomies (39 in women, 32 in men) and 395 cholecystectomies (307 in women, 88 in men). The average age of the appendectomy patients was 24 years (range 7 to 73) and of the cholecystectomy patients 43 years (range 14 to 91). During the same period we performed 272 conventional appendectomies and 33 conventional cholecystectomies.

We were able to reduce the duration of appendectomy from 70 minutes initially to 37 minutes on average. Cholecystectomy took up to 180 minutes initially. The average duration for intraoperative cholangiography was 38 to 46 minutes. The laparoscopic operations were performed by five surgeons.

Appendectomy

Intraoperative complications. During laparoscopic appendectomy bleeding from the appendicular artery occurred in two cases. In both the bleeding was stopped by laparoscopic techniques. In one patient the appendix was temporarily lost in the abdominal cavity because it was not secured after it had been excised initially. Only after a 1-hour intensive (laparoscopic) search, we were able to remove the appendix from the pouch of Douglas.

Postoperative complications. Postoperatively in two of the patients who had undergone appendectomy, a Douglas pouch abscess developed (in one of them after the aforementioned misplacement of the appendix). Under ultrasonographic guidance, both abscesses were successfully drained transrectally and transvaginally, respectively. One patient had severe diffuse peritonitis that could only be controlled with prolonged lavage. This patient had a subacute inflammation of the appendix with retrocecal adhesions. In four of the patients undergoing appendectomy, wound healing was impaired because of infection, which was managed nonoperatively.

Cholecystectomy

Intraoperative complications. Cystic artery hemorrhage occurred intraoperatively as a result of faulty preparation with hook electrodes in two patients; hemorrhage of the iliac artery was caused by the placement of the first trocar. One bile duct injury was observed because of incorrect use of the electric hook in Calot's triangle in one patient; and accidental opening of the gallbladder during its dissection from the liver bed occurred in two patients.

In the first case of cystic artery hemorrhage, the minor bleeding stopped as we converted to conventional laparotomy. In the second case the bleeding was controlled laparoscopically. Because of acute blood loss, the iliac injury required emergency laparotomy and suture of the puncture wound in the vessel. The bile duct injury was not detected until postoperative day 2, when the serum bilirubin level increased to 9.1.

Endoscopic retrograde cholangiopancreatography (ERCP) showed damage to the bile duct (Fig. 1), necessitating laparotomy and biliodigestive anastomosis. Both accidentally opened gallbladders were removed with no problems. In each case the abdomen was thoroughly irrigated at the conclusion of the procedure.

Postoperative complications. Among the cholecystectomy patients, an umbilical abscess was observed postoperatively in two and a large subcutaneous hematoma in one patient. Both complications were treated nonoperatively. In two patients subhepatic fluid collection was noted 4 days postoperatively. In both of them the fluid was drained percutaneously under ultrasonographic guidance.

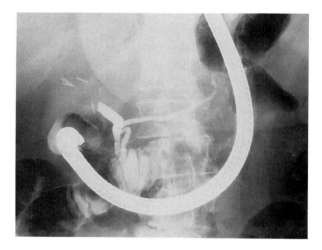

Fig. 1. ERCP shows a damaged common bile duct, delivered postoperatively. Laparotomy and reconstruction by biliodigestive anastomosis were required.

DISCUSSION

New ground is broken with the introduction of video-endoscopic techniques in operative surgery. In contrast to classic operations, the detailed three-dimensional view and the ability to palpate tissues and organs are lost.

Indirect manipulation with elongated instruments guided by a two-dimensional view requires thorough training. Knowledge of other endoscopic techniques is clearly advantageous.

Careless insertion of the first trocar, particularly in a patient with substantial adipose tissue, can lead to injuries to the bowel, bladder, and surrounding vessels, with related consequences. The puncture should be made only when the abdominal walls are distended and sufficiently raised. Gas must enter into the peritoneal cavity freely without obstacles. Saline drop test and trocar puncture should be performed according to the methods of Semm.[17] Trocars should be of sufficient length, particularly in obese patients.

Problems may arise for the anesthesiologist while the pneumoperitoneum is established; the increased CO_2 uptake requires a higher respiratory minute volume for its elimination from the circulation. Uniformly distributed but increased intra-abdominal pressure can lead to pulmonary and cardiac complications that are difficult to overcome, particularly in older high-risk patients. Therefore sufficiently deep anesthesia with corresponding extensive muscle relaxation is essential, since inad-

equate relaxation results in increased intra-abdominal pressure, causing the CO_2-filled and exposed abdominal cavity to shrink from muscle spasm or the intra-abdominal organs to settle precariously deep to the pneumoperitoneum. Under such circumstances, abdominal manipulations can be extremely hazardous.

Appendectomy

Bleeding from the appendicular artery results from vigorous dissection of the mesoappendix with bipolar coagulation forceps and scissors. Usually, however, it can be stopped by laparoscopic techniques.[9,10,16,18] If the appendix is perforated, causing contamination of the abdominal cavity by feces or pus, the consequences (peritonitis, Douglas pouch abscess) should not be underestimated. Delayed necrosis in other areas of the intestine such as the cecum as a result of injury by monopolar electrocautery can be the cause for late postoperative morbidity (or even mortality) if the mishap was not recognized immediately, since the consequences (peritonitis, abscess) develop only postoperatively.[17] Undiagnosed postoperative hemorrhage as a result of inadequate intraoperative care of the appendicular artery and the use of a single proximal Roeder loop or clip have been described and can have serious consequences.

Summary. Careful holding of the appendix and mesoappendix, as well as avoidance of excessive traction, prevents rupture. Meticulous lavage of the appendiceal bed should be part of any appendectomy procedure. Complete drainage of the pouch of Douglas should prevent abscesses.

In this setting it is difficult to insert the irrigation and suctioning tube. It frequently becomes attached to the omentum or the intestinal loops. Thus some type of basket should be used that can be lowered and that can keep the opening of the suction tube away from the organs. Slow suctioning along the parenchymal organs (liver) helps to ensure success.

By using bipolar current exclusively in the area of the appendix, the surgeon can avoid defective currents and dangerous contacts with the bowel.[10,17] However, the bipolar coagulation forceps currently on the market are fragile. As for the hook electrodes, any evidence of defective or worn insulation must be noted and corrected. A possible faulty circuit hooked up at the source of the current by untrained staff may cause burn injuries to tissue. For these reasons we no longer use these electrical devices in appendectomy. Instead, the appendix is prepared by suturing the appendicular artery and closing off the appendix with Roeder loops.

Cholecystectomy

The most serious complications occur during dissection of the structures in Calot's triangle. Dissection too far removed from the gallbladder in the area of the cystic duct and common bile duct junction by means of electrocoagulation can lead to irreversible bile duct injury.* The monopolar hook is a dangerous instrument. The insulation at its tip or back is insufficient, is quickly worn out, and becomes brittle. The degree of temperature remaining in the hook after cautery cannot be appreciated. Both of these factors lead to uncontrollable current and heat effects far from the structure to be dissected, with all of the possible negative consequences.[17]

Careless dissection of the cystic artery and a cautery hook may cause bleeding that cannot be controlled laparoscopically by an inexperienced surgeon. This in turn can necessitate laparotomy. Confusing the right hepatic artery with the cystic artery is always possible and may lead to accidents that will restrict circulation in the liver at least; at other times immediate vascular repair may become mandatory.

Accidental opening of the gallbladder by means of the hook or excessive crushing with forceps can result in pus or bile leakage or release of stones into the abdominal cavity. In addition to observing the operative field such leaks may lead to peritonitis; admittedly a minor risk as initial studies have shown.

Summary. Dissection of the structures in the triangle of Calot should begin close to the gallbladder. In our clinic dissection with a blunt grasper and spatula has proved safe and effective. Thus we are able to keep the use of a hook to an absolute minimum. The cystic duct and the cystic artery must be dissected in their entire circumference; their junctions with parent structures must be satisfactorily exposed and seen on the video monitor. Use of Absolok clips ensures sufficient dissection. The most reliable remedial procedure after the free appearance of bile, pus, or stones is a thorough lavage and aspiration of the irrigation fluid.

STAFF

If the operating room staff is only partly trained, rotates between various rooms, and lacks motivation to master the intricate details of a new technology or has a blasé dilettante's approach to the discipline required in the safe execution of repetitive, at times boring steps on a

daily basis; this can reduce high quality surgical expertise and optimal OR conditions and facilities to near or total failure. In laparoscopic surgery the most difficult tasks no longer rest with the scrub nurse but with the circulating nurse, who must operate the insufflator, the camera, the light source, and the video monitor and recorder and if necessary be able to adjust and repair them adequately. Hence if the staff are not sufficiently trained, considerable problems can arise. Incorrect use of unfamiliar fragile instruments can lead to premature wear of expensive equipment. A surgeon's inability to properly secure the liberated gallbladder or appendix before extraction because of a variety of equipment failures due to staff incompetence may result in time-consuming laparoscopic searches or even laparotomy.

Participation in introductory and developmental in-house courses should be mandatory for all staff. New "recruits"—doctors, nurses, technicians—should be required to assist surgeons who are already well-trained in laparoscopic techniques. For the purpose of a safe yet progressively expanding departmental expertise limiting the number of surgeons to three or four per institution is important initially. These surgeons should have sufficient experience with the techniques of open appendectomy and cholecystectomy and other abdominal operations as a base for the additional training in laparoscopic procedures. This additional experience can be acquired through a variety of educational means: postgraduate courses, laboratory exercises, preceptor- and proctorships, and participation in hospital team efforts with increasing levels of responsibility. After satisfactory credentials have been acquired through these avenues and privileges extended within a given department, the local expertise and mastery of skills can then be expanded as outlined to members of the staff who are willing to learn at their level of participation within the operating team: surgeons, anesthesiologists, assistants, nurses, technicians. These teams must be able to master possible complications such as vascular and visceral injuries.

CONCLUSION

At the outset patients must be carefully selected to prevent unwanted grief. Not every patient is a suitable candidate for laparoscopic surgery. Thus surgeons at the start of a learning curve should have a clear and well defined concept of absolute and relative laparoscopic related and unrelated general contraindications,

---

*References 6, 9, 12, 16, 18, 19, 21.

that changes and hopefully progresses as experience grows.

With increasing experience, the range of indications can be expanded.* However, in our clinic, for instance, the mere suspicion of a malignant growth in the gallbladder is a contraindication to laparoscopic intervention. But the reverse is true of appendectomy. Initially there were numerous indications for laparoscopic appendectomy; perityphlitic abscess and demonstrated perforation were considered the only contraindications.[10,14,16,17] Now, especially after severe septic complications, laparoscopic appendectomy is performed only in obese patients and within the limits of diagnostic laparoscopy to pinpoint pain of unknown origin in the lower right abdomen. When critical intraoperative situations arise, a switch to laparotomy does not indicate failure and indeed suggests an appropriate sense of responsibility. Such an open-minded approach helps avoid complications.[16,19]

---

*References 6, 9, 11, 16, 18, 19, 21.

REFERENCES

1. Buess G. Endoskopie. Von der Diagnostik bis zur neuen Chirurgie. 1.Auflage. Köln: Deutscher Ärzte-Verlag, 1991.
2. Cristalli BG, Izard V, Jacob D, et al. Laparoscopic appendectomy using a clip applier. Surg Endosc 5:176, 1991.
3. Cuschieri A. Endoskopische Mikrochirurgie. Chirurgie 62:248, 1991.
4. Cuschieri A. Variable curvature shape-memory spatula for laparoscopic surgery. Surg Endosc 5:179, 1991.
5. Eigler FW, Walz MK. Laparoskopische Plazierung einer T-Drainage bei Choledocholithiasis. Chirurgie 62:901, 1991.
6. Feussner H, Ungeheuer A, Lehr L, et al. Technik der laparoskopischen Cholecystektomie. Langenbacks Arch Chir 376:367, 1991.
7. Fitzgerald SD, Bailey PV, Liebscher GJ, et al. Laparoscopic cholecystectomy in anticoagulated patients. Surg Endosc 5:166, 1991.
8. Grace PA, Leahy A, McEntee G, et al. Laparoscopic cholecystectomy in the scarred abdomen. Surg Endosc 5:118, 1991.
9. Götz F, Pier A, Schippers E, et al. Laparoskopische Chirurgie. 1.Auflage. Stuttgart: Thieme, 1991.
10. Götz F, Pier A, Bacher C. Die laparoskopische Appendektomie. Chirurgie 62:253, 1991.
11. Ko ST, Airan MC. Review of 300 consecutive laparoscopic cholecystectomies: Development, evolution and results. Surg Endosc 5:103, 1991.
12. Lepsien G, Lüdtke FE, Neufang T, et al. Treatment of iatrogenic common bile duct injury during laparoscopic cholecystectomy through the laparoscopic insertion of a T-tube stent. Surg Endosc 5:119, 1991.
13. Niebuhr H, Nahrstedt U, Rückert K. Protrahierte Blutung und Blutungsschock nach laparoskopischer Appendektomie Vortrag, Tagung der Berliner Chirurgen, October 10-12, 1991.
14. Niebuhr H, Nahrstedt U, Rückert K. Laparoskopische versus konventionelle Appendektomie. Laparoendoskopische Chirurgie 1:90, 1992.
15. Röthlin M, Schlumpf R, Largiadiér F. Die Technik der intraiperativen Sonographie bei der laparoskopischen Cholecystektomie. Chirurgie 62:899, 1991.
16. Rückert K, Niebuhr H, Nahrstedt U. Laparoskopishce Cholecystektomie und Appendektomie. Hamb Ärzteblatt 46:47, 1992.
17. Semm K. Operationslehre für endoskopische Abdominal-Chirurgie. 1.Auflage, Stuttgart: Schattauer, 1984.
18. Stahlschmidt M, Lotz M, Moergel K. Endoskopische Appendektomie und Cholecystektomie. Aerzteblatt Rheinland Pfalz 43:309, 1990.
19. Troidl H, Spangenberger W, Dietrich A, et al. Die laparoskopische Cholecystektomie. Chirurgie 62:257, 1991.
20. Unger SW, Scott JS, Unger HM, et al. Laparoscopic approach to gallstones in the morbidly obese patient. Surg Endosc 5:116, 1991.
21. Woisetschläger R, Wayland W. Laparoscopic cholecystectomy—how does it work and how long does it take? Surg Endosc 5:109, 1991.

VII

Videoendoscopic Techniques in Pediatric Surgery

48 *Laparoscopic Operations in the Neonate and Young Child*

Stanley Scott Miller

Minimally invasive laparoscopic surgical techniques[1] offer several benefits to the patient: reduced postoperative pain, earlier return to normal activities, and reduced cutaneous and intraperitoneal scarring. Concomitant with these developments has been the rapid evolution of electronic equipment and surgical instruments designed for use in laparoscopic surgery.

When training of general and pediatric surgeons in laparoscopic technique is complete, many operations now performed by open methods will be performed endoscopically. Many instruments currently used in open operations have been modified for endoscopic use, and techniques originated for operation within the gas-filled peritoneal cavity have been adapted for use within tissue planes of cleavage. Procedures performed with these modified instruments or techniques include subfascial ligation of perforating veins, inguinal herniorrhaphy, and esophagectomy. Eventually, the term *videoendoscopic surgery* will replace *laparoscopic surgery.*

Laparoscopy has long been used diagnostically in pediatric surgery.[2] However, pediatric laparoscopy was performed less frequently than adult endoscopy because the reduction in size of the instruments for pediatric use resulted in smaller views and poorer images. In 1971, however, Gans and Berci[2] described how technical advances had improved pediatric laparoscopic methods and advocated the use of those techniques in the differential diagnosis of biliary atresia and choledochal cysts, liver biopsy, and the assessment of intersex by the inspection of pelvic organs. Berci et al.[3] reported on 500 diagnostic laparoscopies in a patient population that included children as young as 18 months. Techniques designed for adult general surgery have been applied to pediatric surgical cases in the evaluation of the impalpable or intra-abdominal testis[4,5] and in the assessment of the acute abdomen and possible appendicitis in childhood.[6]

Recently, there has been increasing interest in performing conventional pediatric surgical procedures, such as mobilization of intra-abdominal testis, appendectomy, cholecystectomy, and pyloromyotomy, with laparoscopy. The Fowler-Stephens technique of staged mobilization of the intra-abdominal testis has been adapted so that the first stage is performed laparoscopically. Preliminary clipping of the spermatic vessels leads to augmentation of the collateral vasal blood supply, and the vas-based orchiopexy can be successfully performed through an inguinal incision 6 months or more after the first stage of the procedure.[7] Laparoscopic appendectomy was described by Semm,[8] and several series have reported on the advantage of this technique, even in the management of the acutely inflamed and perforated appendix. Gotz et al.[9] reported on the results of 388 laparoscopic appendectomies, 40% of which were pediatric patients. There were no deaths, and 3% of cases in the first 50 operations had to be converted to open procedures. Two of these were complicated by abscess formation.

Cholelithiasis is not a common condition in childhood, but it does occur in conjunction with sickle cell disease and other hemoglobinopathies. If cholelithiasis causes symptoms, cholecystectomy is required. Laparoscopic cholecystectomy in the pediatric patient has been described primarily as an adult surgical procedure that has been modified for use in a different abdominal cavity.[10] The outcome in pediatric patients is analogous to that in adult patients: reduced hospital stay (mean, 28.5 hours) and earlier return to school (within 1 week).[11] The traditional Fredet-Ramstedt pyloromyotomy has also been modified by laparoscopic incision and spread of the pyloric tumor.[12,13]

Experience with laparoscopic surgery in adults and open surgery in pediatric patients has led us to consider the use of laparoscopy in infants.

A 7-week-old infant was admitted with a 2-week history of vomiting that occurred after each feeding. Minimal weight gain was noted during this period. He was the first-born male of healthy parents by a standard vertex delivery after an uneventful pregnancy of 40 weeks' gestation. His first 2 weeks of postnatal development were unremarkable, and at the time of admission he was not clinically dehydrated. He had had a poor weight gain from birth, and his weight of 4.8 kg on admission placed him below the 50th percentile. A test feeding on admission revealed a palpable pyloric tumor, and electrolyte analysis showed hypochloremic alkalosis. A nasogastric tube was passed, and an intravenous fluid regimen was begun before surgical intervention.

When the infant was under general anesthesia, his general condition was monitored with electrocardiography and blood pressure, transcutaneous PO_2 level, and end tidal CO_2 level evaluations. A nasogastric tube remained in place.

Entry to the peritoneal cavity and establishment of a pneumoperitoneum were made by a small incision in the upper umbilicus that was deepened through the linea alba and peritoneum under direct vision. Stay sutures were placed in the linea alba, and a disposable blunt trocar and cannula (Ethicon) were placed in the peritoneal cavity and were anchored with the stay sutures by the Hasson technique.[14] Insufflation of CO_2 through this cannula was accomplished by connection to an insufflator designed to maintain intraperitoneal gas pressures at a predetermined level that had been set at 6 mm Hg. A 10 mm telescope was inserted and was connected to a video camera and monitor.

After visualization of the pyloric tumor (Fig. 1), secondary 5 mm ports were established under direct endoscopic vision in the left and right subcostal regions. An endoscopic Allis tissue forceps was inserted through the right-sided port and was used to immobilize the tumor. A Beaver scalpel handle and a modified No. 15 blade were inserted through the left subcostal port. Incision of the serosa was performed in the standard fashion (Fig. 2). The scalpel was replaced with forceps, which were used to spread the incision (Fig. 3). Liver retraction was made with the sheath of the left subcostal cannula. There was minimal bleeding, and no hemostasis was required. Saline was instilled into the peritoneal cavity, and air was insufflated through the nasogastric tube to confirm that the mucosa was intact.

The instruments and cannulas were removed under direct vision, and the CO_2 was evacuated. The stab incisions were infiltrated with local anesthetic and were closed with interrupted absorbable suture material.

Normal feeding was instituted 12 hours after the procedure; this is our routine practice after open surgery, and it was well tolerated: no vomiting occurred. The

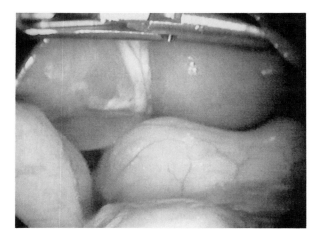

Fig. 1. Pyloric tumor.

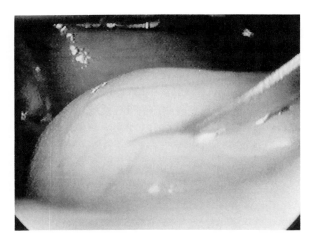

Fig. 2. Incision of pyloric tumor.

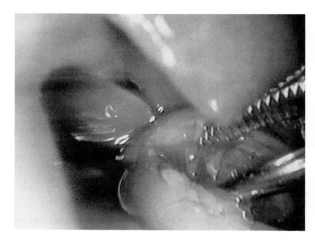

Fig. 3. Spreading of myotomy incision.

infant was discharged on the third postoperative day, although he was well enough to have been discharged earlier. However, because this technique was new, it was thought prudent to have the infant remain in hospital for this time. From our experience with open pyloromyotomies, it seemed that the infant was less distressed and had less postoperative pain than with an open procedure. Review by our surgical outpatient department confirms that satisfactory progress has been maintained.

To date, we have operated on four infants. One of those procedures had to be converted to open pyloromyotomy because of uncertainty about the completeness of the myotomy incision. The results in each case have been completely satisfactory.

Further experience with these techniques is required, but it appears that laparoscopic surgery can be performed safely in infants. Considerable benefits should result from the use of this minimally invasive approach, but careful follow-up is necessary to confirm the advantages of the technique in comparison with those of the traditional approach.

It may appear that the total length of the incisions (2 cm) is equal to that of open surgical incisions. A similar argument is advanced in the comparison of laparoscopic cholecystectomy and minicholecystectomy. Other factors such as minimal tissue handling result in the more rapid return of normal gastrointestinal function after laparoscopic surgery. Improved instrument design should result in fewer stab incisions.

We consider the three main criteria for any laparoscopic operation to be as follows:

1. Establishment of the pneumoperitoneum by a safe technique
2. Adherence (as closely as possible) to well-established techniques that have been proven at open operations (for example, sharp dissection by knife rather than by diathermy)
3. Readiness to convert to the open approach if technical difficulties are encountered or if progress with the procedure is not being made

Establishing an adequate pneumoperitoneum is critical to the success of a laparoscopic operation. The pneumoperitoneum can be established by a closed technique (Veress needle) in one of several standard sites and directions or by the open (Hasson) technique, in which the peritoneal cavity is entered through a small incision, and a blunt trocar and cannula are placed under direct vision and are anchored so that gas leakage is eliminated. We favor the open method because of the proximity of vital structures at the standard sites of needle puncture;

for example, the umbilical vein is relatively larger in an infant, and the liver protrudes further below the costal margin. The telescope is placed through the umbilical or a supraumbilical port, which has served for the initial gas insufflation.

Modern CO_2 insufflators are designed to maintain intraperitoneal gas pressures at a predetermined level. We began the procedure with the lowest possible setting (range, 5 to 6 mm Hg) to ensure clearer visualization of intraperitoneal structures. This produced adequate views without tight abdominal distension. All monitored parameters remained constant throughout the operation.

An awareness of differences between the pediatric and the adult patient is essential. For instance, an unrecognized patent processus vaginalis or hernial sac, which is not uncommon in infants, can lead to a painful scrotal emphysema after operation. Consideration must also be given to the size, placement, and position of the cannulas and to the efficacy and safety of pressures for suction and insufflation during these procedures. However, early experience indicates that laparoscopic surgery in pediatric patients is feasible and that it can be performed safely. However, before these laparoscopic procedures become commonly used in pediatric surgery, appropriate training of surgeons is essential.

It has been predicted that many (if not most) neonatal and pediatric surgical procedures will eventually be performed endoscopically.[15] Benefits to the child include reduced hospital stay, outpatient rather than inpatient treatment in some cases, less pain and resultant distress to child and parents, fewer complications, and improved cosmetic appearance. Other laparoscopic procedures used in the pediatric patient are Nissen fundoplication, lymph node dissections, varicocele ligation, lysis of adhesions, gastrotomies, and enterotomies. Experience with the high-speed electrical tissue morcellator allows removal of solid organs, such as the kidney and spleen, which are divided into pieces and then aspirated.

REFERENCES

1. Reddick EJ, Olsen DO. Laparoscopic laser cholecystectomy. Surg Endosc 3:131-133, 1989.
2. Gans SL, Berci G. Advances in endoscopy of infants and children. J Pediatr Surg 6:199-234, 1971.
3. Berci G, Shore JM, Parrish J. The evaluation of a new peritoneoscope as a diagnostic aid to the surgeon. Ann Surg 178:37-39, 1973.

4. Cortesi N, Ferrari P, Zambarda E. Diagnosis of bilateral crypto-orchidism by laparoscopy. Endoscopy 8:33-34, 1976.

5. Scott JES. Laparoscopy as an aid in diagnosis and management of the impalpable testis. J Pediatr Surg 17:14-16, 1982.

6. Leape LL, Ramenofsky ML. Laparoscopy for questionable appendicitis. Ann Surg 191: 410-413, 1980.

7. Bloom DA. Two-step orchiopexy with pelviscopic clip ligation of the spermatic vessels. J Urol 145:1030-1033, 1991.

8. Semm K. Endoscopic appendicectomy. Endoscopy 15:59-64, 1983.

9. Gotz F, Dier A, Bacher C. Modified laparoscopic appendicectomy in surgery—A report on 388 operations. Surg Endosc 4:6-9, 1990.

10. Sigman HH, Laberge J-M, Croituru D, et al. Laparoscopic cholecystectomy: A treatment option for gallbladder disease in children. J Pediatr Surg 26:1181-1183, 1991.

11. Newman KD, Marmon LM, Attorri R, Evans S. Laparoscopic cholecystectomy in paediatric patients. J Pediatr Surg 26:1184-1185, 1991.

12. Alain JL, Grousseau D, Terrier G. Extramucosal pylorotomy by laparoscopy. J Pediatr Surg 26:1191-1192, 1991.

13. Miller SS, Anderson DN. Case report: Laparoscopic pyloromyotomy in an infant. Min Invasive Ther 1:351-354, 1992.

14. Hasson HM. Open laparoscopy versus closed laparoscopy: A comparison of complication rates. Adv Planned Parent 13:41-50, 1978.

15. Miller SS. Laparoscopic operation in paediatric surgery. Br J Surg 79:986-987, 1992.

49 Laparoscopic Appendectomy in Children: A Report of 1253 Cases

Jean-Stephane Valla

Classic surgical appendectomy in which an incision in the right iliac fossa is used has not changed greatly since its first description a century ago. Open laparotomy and appendectomy, however, have several disadvantages. An ectopic appendix is difficult to find. Abdominal exploration is limited to the region of the right iliac fossa; this prevents thorough examination of the patient with severe abdominal pain and who has an appendix that appears normal. If peritoneal lavage is needed, it is difficult to accomplish it through a McBurney incision in patients with generalized peritonitis. Appendectomy, like any laparotomy, can result in such complications as abscess, evisceration, eventration, or peritoneal adhesions. These complications may lead to subsequent mechanical bowel obstruction, infertility in female patients, and chronic lower abdominal pain.

Laparoscopic appendectomy was developed in the early 1980s by German gynecologists Kurt Semm[1,2] and J. Schreiber.[3,4] The procedure was introduced in 1983 in France by Phillipe Mouret.[5] The appendix is the intra-abdominal organ best suited to resection by laparoscopic technique because of its small size, the ease with which it can be grasped, and its thin mesentery.

Laparoscopic appendectomy offers a means of eliminating many of the disadvantages of classic appendectomy. As a result of recent improvements in video imaging and instrumentation, the promise of laparoscopic appendectomy is now fully realized. We first used this procedure in pediatric patients with suspected acute appendicitis.

We present a retrospective analysis of our initial results with 1253 such procedures and an assessment of the advantages of this minimally invasive procedure compared with those of classic open appendectomy.

MATERIALS AND METHODS

Since the beginning of 1990, we performed 1253 emergency laparoscopic appendectomies. The patients ranged in age from 3 to 16 years (mean, 10 years), and 56% of the children were female. The diagnosis was based on one or more of the following steps: an initial or repeat physical examination, abdominal radiographs, leukocyte blood count, and ultrasonography. Additional routine preoperative studies included an evaluation of hemostasis and a chest radiograph. Prophylactic antibiotics were administered to all patients. General anesthesia with curarization and assisted ventilation was used in all patients.

TECHNIQUE

After anesthesia is induced, the patient is placed with both legs extended, in a dorsal decubitus position. The bladder is catheterized and emptied. The primary surgeon stands on the left side of the patient. To facilitate visualization of the right iliac fossa, the table is tilted into a slight variation of Trendelenburg's position and into the left lateral decubitus position (the left side of the table down). The instruments are the same as those used for operations in adults. The insufflation pressure, which was regulated automatically, is kept < 12 mm Hg. An instantaneous response capnometer is used to monitor end-respiratory PCO_2.

A three-puncture appendectomy technique is used: the video laparoscope is inserted through a cannula positioned in the lower folds of the umbilicus. The trocar and cannula are inserted into the abdomen with the Z-stab technique of Semm, which permits safe passage (usually on the right) through the rectus muscle. The abdominal cavity is explored, and the size and position of the two other laparoscopic cannulas required for appendectomy are determined. Selection criteria are based on organ position and size. The subsequently used trocars and cannulas are inserted under direct vision to avoid injuring underlying structures; the iliac vessels are visible and particularly apparent in children. The appendix is identified and grasped by its distal end to expose the organ and the attached structures. Coagulation of the mesoappendix is started at the organ tip via a hook monopolar instrument or (less often) a bipolar coagulation instrument, or surgical clips may be used to interrupt the vessels.

After the appendix is released from its vascular attachments, it is resected via the "in" technique or the "out" technique. The "in" technique involves ligation with a ligature loop, a surgical clip, or the EndoGIA; resection and appendiceal stump disinfection are performed in the abdominal cavity. The "out" technique involves exteriorization of the appendix through the laparoscopic cannula, which is placed over the cecum. Ligature, resection, and appendiceal stump disinfection are performed outside the abdominal cavity. In patients in whom the out technique is used, the appendiceal stump is then returned to the abdomen, and the trajectory of the abdominal wall puncture is disinfected. The diameter of the cannula (5 to 15 mm) used for organ removal is selected based on the size of the appendix to avoid appendiceal rupture during extraction. In certain cases in our series, retrograde appendectomy or mobilization of the right colon was performed via conventional surgical techniques.

After removal of the appendix, the distal ileum is examined to exclude an associated Meckel's diverticulum. Peritoneal lavage is then performed via a two-way 5 mm (instillation-aspiration) strainer. The insufflated gas is then released progressively, and the skin edges at the incision sites are closed with adhesive strips. In patients with an abscess or generalized peritonitis, antibiotic administration is continued for 5 days; postoperative analgesics can be administered for 24 hours by systemic injection of propacetamol hydrochloride and nalbuphine hydrochloride. After discharge from the hospital, the patients in our study were examined on postoperative days 5 and 15.

RESULTS

Tables 1 through 5 summarize the results of laparoscopic appendectomies for appendiceal and extra-appendiceal lesions, patient mortality (0), surgical fail-

---

Table 1. Anatomopathological lesions diagnosed by pediatric laparoscopic appendectomy

Features	Percent of Cases
Location of Appendix at Surgery	
Normal position	78
Ectopic position	22
Retrocecal	11
Pelvic	6
Subhepatic	3
Mesoceliac	2
Left-sided	1
Gross Pathological Appearance	
Normal appendix	10
Acute appendicitis	62
Appendicitis with peritonitis	16
Scleroatrophic appendix	2
Microscopic Study Results	
Normal appendix	7
Acute appendicitis	67
Appendicitis with peritoneal involvement	26

Table 2. Extra-appendiceal lesions diagnosed during laparoscopic appendectomies

Type of Lesion	No. of Patients
Peritoneal adhesion disease	61
Inguinal hernia	31
Ovarian cyst	16
Parovarian cyst	5
Meckel's diverticulum	5
Salpingitis	5
Primary pneumococcal peritonitis	3
Crohn's disease	2
TOTAL	127

Table 3. Complications

Surgical Result	Percent of Cases
Mortality	0
Surgical failure; laparotomy	0.4
Intraoperative incident	2.2
Postoperative complications	1.7

Table 4. Intraoperative incidents (2.2% of cases)

Type of Incident	No. of Patients
Pneumo-omentum	8
Visceral puncture	12
Appendiceal rupture	18

ure (0.4% of case studies), intraoperative incidents (2.2%), and postoperative complications (1.7%) in 1253 children with acute appendicitis. The mean length of hospital stay was 2 days after removal of a normal appendix or operation for acute appendicitis; the stay was 4 to 5 days after removal of a gangrenous or perforated appendix.

DISCUSSION

Laparoscopy permits exposure of the appendix (regardless of its location), excellent control of hemostasis, and copious lavage of the abdominal cavity in cases of localized or generalized peritonitis. The limitations of the laparoscopic approach are related to the experience of the surgeon, who must recognize when to convert to open laparotomy. In our series we encountered requirements for this surgical conversion in 0.4% patients during our early experience with laparoscopic excision. In those patients, removal of a large, infected appendix required laparotomy; however, initial laparoscopy was used to establish the location of the appendix and mobilization that resulted in a limited abdominal incision. The number of patients requiring conversion to laparotomy is similar to that described in the literature for other laparoscopic appendectomy series.[5-9]

No patients in our series died; this result is consistent with other recent reports of laparoscopic appendectomy[6,8,9] and those of other series of classic appendectomy.[10-12] In our series, a 2.2% incidence of intraoperative and postoperative complications can be classified into complications that result from appendectomy and those that result from a laparoscopic operation.

Intraoperative incidents related to laparoscopy include omental emphysema (pneumo-omentum) and visceral puncture that occurs during insertion of the insufflation needle. Omental emphysema occurs as a re-

Table 5. Postoperative complications (1.7% of cases)

Type of Complication	No. of Patients	Remedial Open Procedure	Repeat Laparoscopy
Omental effusion of serous fluid	3	0	0
Evisceration	2	2	0
Painful hernia	2	0	0
Intestinal obstruction	6	1	1
Residual abscess	4	2	2
Fifth-day syndrome	1	0	0
Wound abscess or hematoma	2	0	0
Abscess and fistula (Crohn's disease)	1	0	0

sult of improper placement of the insufflation needle. Although this may hinder initial abdominal exploration, it usually does not affect the identification and removal of the appendix. In our series the two accidental visceral punctures of the liver and stomach, respectively, resulted in no immediate or late negative consequences. Perforation of the large iliac or aorticocaval vessels is the most serious potential iatrogenic complication; this can be avoided by careful placement of the insufflation needle and laparoscopic trocars. Appendiceal rupture during resection or extraction, which resulted in no sequelae, occurred in 18 patients in our study. This complication is related to the pathological state of the appendix and may also occur during traditional appendectomy.

Another possible intraoperative complication of laparoscopic appendectomy described by Schreiber[4] is thermal injury from the electrosurgical knife; this did not occur in our series.

Only minor postoperative complications were related to the laparoscopic procedure. Isolated incidents of effusion of serous fluid from the puncture sites occurred in three patients, but these episodes were not associated with fever or intestinal transit disorders; effusion stopped spontaneously. Analysis of the serous fluid showed no evidence of microbial infection. In two patients, omental evisceration occurred through one of the puncture sites. The first case involved evisceration of the omentum during removal of a drainage catheter that was placed during operation. The incident appeared to be associated more with the type of drainage catheter used, not the laparoscopic technique. In the second patient, evisceration of an omental fragment occurred after the patient jumped on a trampoline on the sixth postoperative day. (The child was discharged on the second postoperative day.) This evisceration occurred through the umbilical puncture. General anesthesia was induced in this patient; the fascial defect was found to be in continuity with the skin opening (a Z-stab had not been made). If the fascial defect had been closed at the completion of the laparoscopic procedure, this complication would have been avoided.

In two patients with open processus vaginalis, a gas distention of the scrotal area occurred during the procedure, and the patient experienced pain in the inguinal area for 3 days after operation.

Nonspecific complications in this series included intestinal obstruction, residual intraoperative abscess, and "fifth-day syndrome." Early intestinal obstruction occurred on the second postoperative day in four patients with generalized peritonitis. Three patients were managed successfully with nonoperative therapy; however,

one child experienced mechanical intestinal obstruction. In this patient, a "loose" ileoileal intussusception had been reduced during the initial laparoscopic procedure. This finding prompted repeat laparoscopy when postoperative mechanical obstruction was noted. No evidence of intussusception or other causes of mechanical obstruction were found, and the patient's intestinal function returned spontaneously within 48 hours after repeat laparoscopy. In reports of other series of laparoscopic appendectomy, only Mouret and Marsand[5] have described an early obstruction that occurred in one patient on the tenth postoperative day; this was managed by repeat laparoscopy.

Two cases of late intestinal obstruction occurred after initial treatment of appendicitis with generalized peritonitis. A patient with volvulus was treated with conventional surgery (resection); the other patient underwent laparoscopy (lysis of adhesions).

The four cases of postoperative intra-abdominal abscesses in this series appeared to result from different causes. In two patients, a right iliac fossa abscess developed after a purulent appendix was removed. The third right iliac fossa abscess occurred 40 days after laparoscopic appendectomy and Meckel's diverticulum resection using the "out" technique. This abscess, which was not located around the stump of the appendix, was found in the area of the ileoileal anastomosis. The fourth abscess may have resulted from lack of instrument sterilization.

Postoperative intra-abdominal abscess has been described as a complication by Götz et al.,[6] who reported two cases in 388 patients, and by Gilchrist et al.[9] Intestinal obstructions or residual abscesses occurred only in patients with a ruptured appendix.

One patient in our series developed fifth-day syndrome after simple acute appendicitis. Symptoms were typical and resolved with nonoperative management. This complication, which occurs only in children, has not been reported in other series of laparoscopic appendectomies.

In our series, no abdominal wall or wound abscesses occurred in 1052 patients with a normal appendix or simple acute appendicitis; two cases occurred in 201 patients who had appendicitis with perforation. These abscesses are the most common complication that results from standard open laparotomy and appendectomy; some authors[10-13] cite abscess occurrence in from 1.2% to 5.7% of patients who undergo those approaches. Götz et al.[6] reported similar results without routine antibiotic prophylaxis. They described 14 cases of postoperative umbilical cellulitis, which was treated with antibiotic therapy.

The incidence of major postoperative complications in our series (0.7% of patients who required repeat operation) is low when compared with similar reports of the complications of standard open surgery. With laparoscopic surgery, length of hospitalization is shortened, especially in patients with generalized peritonitis (4.5 days in our series compared with 6.9 days for Neilson et al.).[12] Neilson et al. reported an incidence of major postoperative complications in 1.7% of patients who underwent standard appendectomies as emergency procedures in 1988 and 1989; for Putman et al.[10] the incidence was 3.2%; for Chevalier and Durand,[13] it was 4.3%; and in our series, the incidence was 3%. The advantages of laparoscopic surgery in adults and children have been confirmed by other authors.[2,5,7,9]

Although a well-trained laparoscopic surgeon can remove almost any appendix, certain clinical situations require special caution, and indications for laparoscopic intervention can be questioned. Patients presenting with periappendiceal phlegmon and agglutinated loops of bowel may be at risk for iatrogenic intestinal injury if laparoscopic surgery is performed. In young patients (< 5 years of age) with a localized purulent lesion in an otherwise normal abdominal cavity who undergo laparoscopic surgery, an initially localized purulent collection may spread throughout the peritoneal cavity. Initial management of these cases should include an ultrasonographically guided abscess incision centered directly over the palpable purulent mass or percutaneous drainage.[14] Laparoscopic surgery is of immense advantage in patients with generalized peritonitis, because complete abdominal lavage with elimination of false membranes is possible. This type of lavage formerly required extensive enlargement of the right iliac incision or a wide median laparotomy.

Obesity, mental retardation, or the administration of steroids or chemotherapy can obscure a diagnosis of acute appendicitis. If laparoscopy of patients with those factors reveals a normal appendix, other reasons that may have led to operation are more difficult to determine.[15,16] However, laparoscopic appendectomy has been perfected and has proved valuable, so removal of a healthy appendix involves fewer risks. In our series the incidence of diagnostic error was < 10%. In addition, gross examination with the laparoscope can be misleading, because endoappendicitis (inflammation confined to the mucosa) may occur without early evidence of serosa inflammation. This condition occurred in approximately 2% of our patients.

With laparoscopy complete examination of the abdominal cavity is possible; this resulted in the identification of nonappendiceal lesions in 10% of our patients. Many of these lesions might not have been detected by conventional abdominal ultrasonography and limited abdominal exploration through a small McBurney incision. In our series, associated lesions that included small twisted parovarian cysts and peritoneal adhesion disease, as described by Mouret and Marsand,[5] occurred in 61 cases. These adhesions, which occur predominantly in females, are encountered in patients ≥ 10 years of age. The pathogenesis remains unclear; infection by an ascending genital route has been suggested, although peritoneal cultures in our series yielded negative results. Adhesive bands are easily divided with an electrocautery knife, and histological study reveals nonspecific inflammatory fibrous tissue. Although our follow-up is limited, our immediate results indicate that this treatment has eliminated the initial painful symptoms that result from the lesions.

CONCLUSION

The potential disadvantages of laparoscopic appendectomy include the necessity of mastering of a new operative technique, the purchase and maintenance of sophisticated electronic instruments, and the need for backup equipment for the treatment of transient surgical sequelae.

Emergency laparoscopic appendectomy offers advantages when compared with classical laparotomy and appendectomy. With laparoscopy, the appendix is easily and rapidly identified, regardless of its possible ectopic position. Laparoscopy permits complete exploration and saline lavage of the abdominal cavity, wound infection and abscesses are prevented, and cutaneous scarring is reduced. There is also a reduction in the incidence of postoperative intra-abdominal abscesses and postoperative peritoneal adhesions that can cause persistent pain and infertility in females.[17] Length of hospitalization is shortened.

In our experience, the complications resulting from laparoscopic appendectomy were minor; improved surgical skill can eliminate most of those problems.

REFERENCES

1. Semm K. Die endoskopische Appendektomie. Gynäkol Prax 7:131-140, 1983.
2. Semm K. Laparoscopic appendicectomy. Dtsch Med Wochenschr 113:3-5, 1988.

3. Schreiber JH. Early experience with laparoscopic appendectomy in women. Surg Endosc 1:211-216, 1987.
4. Schreiber JH. Laparoscopic appendectomy in pregnancy. Surg Endosc 4:100-102, 1990.
5. Mouret PH, Marsand H. Appendicectomie per laparoscopy. Techniques and evaluation. Presented at the Second Congress of the Society of American Gastrointestinal Endoscopic Surgeons. Atlanta: March 1990.
6. Götz F, Pier A, Bacher C. Modified laparoscopic appendectomy in surgery. A report of 338 operations. Surg Endosc 4:6-9, 1990.
7. Gangal HT, Gangal MH. Laparoscopic appendicectomy. Endoscopy 19:127-129, 1987.
8. Thomas P. Appendicectomie assistée par laparoscopie. Série personnelle de 212 cas. Thesis. University Claude Bernard, Lyon, France, 1988.
9. Gilchrist BF, Lobe TE, Schropd KP, Kay GA, Hixson SD, Wrenn EL, Philippe PG, Hollabaugh RS. Is there a role for laparoscopic appendectomy in pediatric surgery? J Pediatr Surg 27:209-214, 1992.
10. Putman C, Gagliano N, Emmens RW. Appendicitis in children. Surg Gynecol Obstet 170:527-532, 1990.
11. Zaaf M, Roger B, Vaur JL, Bemard JL, Murat J. Progrès diagnostique et mortalité d'une série de 1400 appendicectomies. Lyon Chir 79:251-254, 1983.
12. Neilson IR, Laberge JM, N'guyen LT, Moir C, Doody D, Sonnino RE, Youssef S, Guittman FM. Appendicitis in children: Current therapeutic recommendations. J Pediatr Surg 25:1113-1116, 1990.
13. Chevalier J, Durand A. Réflexions sur une série homogène de 3200 appendiceotomies. Lyon Chir 76:251-253, 1980.
14. Bagi P, Dueholm S. Nonoperative management of the ultrasonically evaluated appendiceal mass. Surgery 101:602-605, 1987.
15. Leape LL, Ramenofski ML. Laparoscopy for questionable appendicitis. Can it reduce the negative appendectomy rate? Ann Surg 191:410-413, 1980.
16. Deutsch A, Zelikowski A, Reiss R. Laparoscopy in the prevention of unnecessary appendectomy: A prospective study. Br J Surg 69:336-337, 1982.
17. Lehmann-Willenbrock E, Mecke H, Riedel HH. Sequelae of appendicectomy with special reference to intra-abdominal adhesions, chronic abdominal pain and infertility. Gynecol Obstet Invest 29:241-245, 1990.

50 *Endoscopic Treatment of Children With Vesicoureteral Reflux Using Teflon: A Summary of Five Years' Experience*

Paul Sauvage

When we decided at the end of 1986 to investigate endoscopic treatment of vesicoureteral reflux in children by the injection of Teflon, we had the impression that the method was not viable. At that time certain authors were introducing, without substantiation, short series with almost 100% success; others, after some brief experiments, were mocking the technique, bolstered by the promoter of the method whose video demonstrations were less than convincing. Having always sought to simplify urological techniques and to shorten hospitalization time, we had to investigate.

The first results were convincing enough for us to pursue the endoscopic treatment despite the conflicting reports about Teflon. After 5 years this is our first statement based on the regular follow-up of children with reflux in all stages whom we have treated at the Service of Pediatric Surgery in Strasbourg, France.

MATERIALS

From January 1987 to December 1991 we operated on 675 children, for a total of 967 refluxing ureters, both primary and secondary, with all stages of reflux (stage I, 113; stage II, 274; stage III, 435; stage IV, 111; stage V, 34) by endoscopy. Reflux in some children in the lesser stages led to treatment after the first infectious episode if it was pyelonephritis or uropathy. The only condition preventing endoscopic treatment was in a young boy whose ureter did not allow the easy passage of a No. 000 cystoscope and use of a 00 Fr needle. (Preliminary inspection of the meatus easily avoids this danger.)

261

METHODS

A frontal oblique view of 30 degrees allows easy inspection and manipulation and is used most often in infants. To facilitate the injection of Teflon, which is delivered in a tube and looks like a thick paste, the needle and the syringe must first be rinsed with glycerin; the glycerin is eliminated during passage of the Teflon paste. The injection is done only if the Teflon appears at the tip of the needle as a very white curl with good consistency. The puncture is made between the ureteral orifice and the inner contour. Before the injection it is important to lift the area with the tip of the needle to look for the apex of the meatus. With the position of the needle checked, the Teflon paste is injected; it preferably produces a cone with abrupt edges (0.5 ml of Teflon are used at the meatus, with half that amount injected in newborns with a 00 Fr needle).

To avoid injection of massive doses, each pressure of the syringe must correspond to a perceptible rise in the rim of the meatus. If the position of the needle tip is faulty, it must be pushed forward or backward while staying in the first point of puncture. If a whitish aspect of Teflon passes under the mucosa, the injection is too superficial, and the needle must be advanced.

In the presence of a double ureter, it is convenient to raise, as much as possible, each orifice separately and to inject the Teflon between the two meatus. The technique is the same as for a patient with one ureter.

When the refluxing orifice is extremely large and occurs anteriorly, the large floor of the meatus must be elevated with two or three injections so that it can lie on the ureteral crest (1.5 ml of Teflon should be injected). After the injection, cystography is performed with the patient under general anesthesia and intubated. One or two x-ray films per micturition will confirm the success of the injection and allow the immediate treatment of a contralateral reflux in case there is more than the initial unilateral reflux.

The next day renal and vesical ultrasonography is performed to show whether the lump of Teflon is swelling and its dimensions and to confirm the absence of dilation of the injected ureters. This examination and culture of the urine are repeated 1 and 3 months after the treatment. In case of failure as shown by cystography after the third month, we limit ourselves to only one reinjection. Further failure requires surgical reimplantation if the reflux is followed by signs of pyelonephritis, or requires simple clinical follow-up if the residual reflux is weak and clinically asymptomatic.

RESULTS

The injection is totally painless. Passage of the cystoscope is acknowledged in young boys by a discrete reaction during general anesthesia, which is very light. That the technique causes very little disability becomes obvious in the recovery room. The first micturition is always painless for girls, but may be painful for young boys during the first 24 hours.

The effectiveness of the method is supported by the 83.5% success rate after one injection and 94.3% after reinjection, with all stages included. The results would have been even better if we had not wanted to treat the worst cases in the same way. In patients with stage IV and V reflux and secondary reflux, the rate of recurrence was 32%.

To date 21 children have benefited from surgical treatment after failure of the endoscopic treatment: 18 with unilateral persistent reflux and three with stenosis. The open surgical treatment did not present any particular difficulty, and the core of Teflon is extracted the same way a pit is extracted from ripe fruit.

Failure is related to the bad position of the core of Teflon at the level of the vesical wall, to its paraureteral location, or to its disappearing in case of multiple punctures. No accident was reported. In one case, excretory anuria in a patient with a functional ureter required use of a ureteral probe for 8 days, with favorable results. Three newborns recovering from severe pyelonephritis with already affected kidneys had a severe recurrence despite the sterility of the urine at the time of the injection. Denseness and some calcifications around the cores of Teflon were noticed nine times without any consequences to the ureters and without clinical manifestation.

DISCUSSION

Our 5 years' experience allows us to confirm the unquestionable advantages of endoscopic treatment with Teflon. For the children and their parents, the technique presents the advantages of a short hospitalization (48 hours), a painless treatment, a very low morbidity rate, and no mortality at all. For the surgeon, advantages are the rapidity, the ease of movement, and the technique's consequences. For the community, the advantages include the technique's very low cost (one fourth that of surgical reimplantation) and the possibility that uninsured families may assume the cost personally.

A disadvantage is recurrence, which results in the need for reinjection in almost 10% of cases—a percentage we view as unacceptable. However, this figure is explained in part by the obligatory learning curve as the method is learned by an entire team and numerous visiting surgeons. Sufficient practice allows improvement in the above-mentioned results, but a percentage of failures will always persist, and this is very frustrating to the surgeon. Indeed, despite perfect technique, the obtained core can disappear completely because it may be composed entirely of glycerin as a result of insufficient rinsing of the injection system.

Movement of the Teflon is the object of some discussion and reservations. In 1984 Malizia, Reiman, and Myers[4] discussed the risks of pulmonary and intracranial migration of the Teflon and the granulomatous reaction resulting from periurethral injection. For more than 30 years, massive doses have been injected in humans into the prostatic lobes, with persistence or recurrence of incontinence as the only known disadvantage. Nor has injection into the vocal cords resulted in any problems.

Since the beginning of our experience, we have wanted to know the reaction of Teflon and its future, so we systematically compiled a video recording and a schema of the endoscopy and the injections and of the doses used, and we followed the cycles of Teflon by a regular echographic control (days 1, 30, and 90 and at 1, 2, 3, and 5 years) and by x-ray films of the abdomen. The echogram revealed a hyperechogenic structure with a cone of posterior shadow at the injection site. This formation is measured, and its flattened or swelling shape is determined. The controls who are older than 5 years confirm that a swelling core of Teflon, when perfectly injected, retains an identical shape and dimension. The shell of the granuloma, which we first described, perfectly limits the injected mass. When the core is no longer found as early as day 30, the Teflon has been eliminated by the natural ways from a superficial injection involving necrosis of the overlying mucous membrane or from points of multiple punctures, allowing the escape of Teflon.

Reflux that persisted after two injections in 18 children and the report of a stenosis in three others led to open surgical treatment. Resection of the Teflon was easily performed in the manner of a pit in a ripe fruit if the core was located parietally or extravesically. A core in the ureteral wall necessitates only resection of the terminal part of the ureter for 2 cm, which does not complicate the reimplantation.

We observed no abnormal adenopathy in the pelvis and no lymphatic migration of Teflon. X-ray films of the abdomen obtained at 1, 3, and 5 years or during a cystography were used to search for possible calcifications. Nine were found, all laterovesical. Calcifications were noticed a few months after the injection in very small newborns. All resulted from generous injections (1.5 to 2 ml) with needles that were too large (5 Fr instead of 3.7 Fr). None of the calcifications caused further problems, and their dimensions did not vary with time. Histologically the calcifications were found at the periphery of the granuloma surrounding the particles of Teflon.

At the present stage of our practice, after spending 5 years and treating more than 750 children, we have found no disadvantage to using this technique—if it were not for the appearance of these calcifications. The analysis of these cases has led us to modify some of our indications. At all stages of reflux the patient can benefit from a Teflon injection, as long as the ureteral orifice is not too big. If the orifice is too big, only one injection must be tried, and in case of failure surgical reimplantation is required. Curiously, although our failure rate in children in stages IV and V is almost 32%, only a very small number of them had to undergo open surgical intervention; the infectious symptomatology softened after the endoscopic treatment.

Contraindications to this technique remain cervical and urethral ectopic implantations and the failures of reimplantations on the vesical dome. (The absence of a real intramural route necessitates using overly large quantities of Teflon and makes the injection ineffective in the short term.)

CONCLUSION

Based on our experience, we can confirm that endoscopic treatment with Teflon injection caused the disappearance of vesicoureteral reflux. In all stages, 83.5% of our cases were corrected after only one injection and 94.3% after reinjection. Observing the patients on the operating table and 3 months after the injection, we did not find any early degradation of our results. The cystographic control we required during the 5 years has so far revealed only two recurrences in absolutely asymptomatic children. The results obtained with the Teflon are 20% superior to those with other products, even when limiting ourselves to only one reinjection.

Laterovesical calcifications in some small newborns occurred in the beginning because of use of an instrument not well adapted to the small size of the orifices and to the thinness of the vesical wall at that age. Those disadvantages are now avoided with the 00 Fr needle, which allows effective injections of 0.2 to 0.3 ml. In older children the doses used diminish with experience, and it is actually rare to exceed 0.5 ml for the ureteral orifice.

This treatment constitutes enormous progress in the treatment of vesicoureteral reflux of children. As long as it is used with care, Teflon should be used until the "perfect product" is developed.

REFERENCES

1. Becmeur F, Geiss S, Laustriat S, et al. History of teflon. Eur Urol 17:299-300, 1990.
2. Geiss S, et al. Multicenter survey of endoscopic treatment of vesicoureteral reflux in children. Eur Urol 17:328-329, 1990.
3. Laustriat S, Geiss S, Becmeur F, et al. Medical history of teflon. Eur Urol 17:301-303, 1990.
4. Malizia AA, Reiman HM, Myers RP. Migration and granulomatous reaction after periurethral injection of polytef. JAMA 251:3277-3281, 1984.
5. Marcellin L, Geiss S, Laustriat S, et al. Ureteral lesions due to endoscopic treatment of vesicoureteral reflux by injection of teflon: Pathological study. Eur Urol 17:325-327, 1990.
6. Sauvage P, Geiss S, Saussine C, et al. Analysis and perspectives of endoscopic treatment of vesicoureteral reflux in children with a 20-month follow-up. Eur Urol 17:310-313, 1990.
7. Sauvage P, Geiss S, Dhaoui R, et al. Analysis and technical refinements of endoscopic treatment of vesicoureteral reflux in children with a 40-month follow-up. Pediatr Surg Int 6:277-280, 1991.

51   *The Potential of Laparoscopy in the Search for the Impalpable Testis*

Philippe Vaysse

The term *impalpable testis* is a clinical diagnosis and the respective diagnostic criteria for the condition should be strict.

In our series we examined children referred to us for impalpable testis. In some cases careful clinical examination led to the discovery of a normally placed gonad that had been missed. The diagnosis of impalpable testis should be made only after clinical examination by an experienced surgeon.

Various authors[1-5] recommend a preoperative examination with the patient under general anesthesia: the relaxation of the abdominal wall might disclose a previously impalpable testis. However, a testis that was palpable during an office visit might be less so when the patient is under general anesthesia, because the testis may have withdrawn into the relaxed abdominal cavity.

Thus clinical evaluations by experienced surgeons might vary. It is important that clinical examinations be repeated with the patient in various positions (squatting, standing, supine), under different conditions (abdominal wall relaxed or tense), and on various occasions (during an office visit, on the day before and the day of operation, when the patient is under general anesthesia). The diagnosis should be determined only after sensitivity to gonadotropins has been evaluated by administration of chorionic gonadotropins, as Naslund et al.[5] have suggested.

The accuracy with which the impalpable testis is defined by various authors results in the wide variation (10% to 20%) with which the condition is reported in the literature.

The accurate diagnosis of impalpable testis depends on the identification of a gonad. No technique is absolutely accurate in gonad identification, but laparoscopy seems reliable. However, analysis of the numerous articles devoted to its use is difficult because of the lack of common terminology. The therapeutic uses of laparoscopy in the management of children with impalpable testis must be evaluated.

LAPAROSCOPIC FINDINGS

Many publications mention the value of laparoscopy in the examination of the inguinal region for impalpable

264

testis.[1-20] It enables visualization of the following conditions:

1. An intra-abdominal gonad near the deep inguinal ring. The gonadal vessels must be identified.[20]
2. An intra-abdominal "vanishing testis" with intra-abdominal blind-ending vas deferens and spermatic vessels. Some authors[2,8] report a blind-ending intra-abdominal vas that is not accompanied by vessels or blind-ending intra-abdominal gonadal vessels with absent vas and epididymis.
3. A complete spermatic cord or gonadal vessels that enter the inguinal canal. If the impalpable testis is unilateral, it is important to compare the constituents of its spermatic cord with those of the other side to determine whether the impalpable testis is normal or hypoplastic. Weiss and Seashore[20] emphasized the importance of determining the patency of the processus vaginalis:
   (a) If the processus vaginalis is patent, a testis that can be maneuvered into an intra-abdominal position may exist beyond the deep inguinal ring.
   (b) If the processus vaginalis is not patent and if the spermatic cord lies in the inguinal canal and no gonad can be palpated, the testis is probably absent. In this situation, the contralateral testis is in the normal position in the scrotum.
4. A spermatic cord that crosses the midline, as in the crossed ectopic testis syndrome.[8,10]
5. In the absence of vas, vessels, and gonad, the diagnosis is testicular agenesis, although the patient should be examined for a high intra-abdominal testis.

Hinman[11] reports that laparoscopy is reliable and that it produces no false positive results and few false negative results.

THERAPEUTIC USES OF LAPAROSCOPY

Laparoscopic findings can be used to avoid unnecessary open operation and to determine the best surgical approach as well as in the treatment of the impalpable testis.

Laparoscopy can be used to avoid open operation in the intra-abdominal "vanishing testis" syndrome[2,3,5-8] and in testicular agenesis.[8] Weiss and Seashore[20] suggested that laparoscopy facilitates the clinical examination of thin young boys who have a closed processus vaginalis and a hypoplastic spermatic cord that slides beyond the internal inguinal ring.

Several publications[11] have presented the value of laparoscopy in determining the best surgical approach for impalpable testis: Pfannenstiel's incision or a high lateral laparotomy is recommended for a high intra-abdominal testis, and a simple inguinal incision is suggested in all other cases. This recommendation is controversial: a high intra-abdominal testis can be reached by an extended classic inguinal incision.[11] Laparoscopy seems particularly appropriate for the management of the crossed ectopic testis syndrome.

Therapeutic uses of celioscopy include the first stage of the Fowler-Stephens operation (ligation of the gonadal vessels), which can be accomplished either by clipping[1,8,21] or with a laser.[19]

The removal of a hypoplastic gonad can also be performed with the laparoscopic technique.[1]

Whether laparoscopy can be used to determine the best surgical approach is controversial. However, the use of laparoscopy can avoid unnecessary open operation and permits the ligation of gonadal vessels in the Fowler-Stephens procedure.

USE OF LAPAROSCOPY IN A CHILD WITH IMPALPABLE TESTIS

The avoidance of open operation as a result of laparoscopy could have benefitted 5% of the children cited by Wright[22] and 9% of the children in our study.[23]

Twenty-eight (13%) of 219 cases we reviewed* could be categorized as having had the intra-abdominal vanishing testis syndrome. The percent is an average that should not mask the great variations among different series (range, 0 to 40%).

The prior ligation of gonadal vessels is justified only in cases on an intra-abdominal testis located far from the internal inguinal ring. Few authors distinguish between the intra-abdominal testis that is near the internal inguinal ring as opposed to being far from the inguinal ring.

Most authors affirm that approximately 60% of intra-abdominal testes are situated high in the abdominal cavity and can be managed by gonadal vessel ligation in the first stage of a two-stage procedure. In the series by Malone and Guiney,[4] three of nine abdominal testes were brought down in a one-stage operation.

It is difficult to evaluate the role of endoscopic orchiectomy in the management of the intra-abdominal testis.

---

*References 2,4,5,8,14,16,20

Because the true impalpable testis is relatively rare, a multicenter prospective study is necessary to evaluate the role of celioscopy in management of the condition. Such a study is under way in France. To date, 53 children and 63 impalpable testes have been treated with celioscopy.

REFERENCES

1. Andze GO, Homsy Y, Laberge I, Desjardins JC, Kiruluta HG. La place de la laparoscopie thérapeutique dans le traitement chirurgical des testicules intra-abdominaux chez l'enfant. Chir Pediatr 31:299-302, 1990.
2. Castilho LN. Laparoscopy for nonpalpable testis: How to interpret the endoscopic findings. J Urol 144:1215-1218, 1990.
3. Lowe DH, Brock WA, Kaplan GW. Laparoscopy for localization of nonpalpable testes. J Urol 131:728-729, 1984.
4. Malone PS, Guiney EJ. The value of laparoscopy in localising the impalpable undescended testis. Br J Urol 56:429-431, 1984.
5. Naslund MJ, Gearhart JP, Jeffs RD. Laparoscopy: Its selected use in patients with unilateral nonpalpable testis after human chorionic gonadotropin stimulation. J Urol 142:108-110, 1989.
6. Abi AA, Wese FX, Opsomer R, Veyckemans F, Van Cangh P. Intérêt de la laparoscopie dans le bilan diagnostic des cryptorchidies avec testicules non palpables. 58:69-78, 1990.
7. Allouch G. Traitement du testicule non palpé. Chir Pediatr 30:161-162, 1989.
8. Bloom DA, Ayers JWT, McGuire EJ. The role of laparoscopy in management of nonpalpable testes. (Paris) 94:465-470, 1988.
9. Cortesi N, Ferrari P, Zambarda E, Manenti A, Baldini A, Pignatti F. Diagnosis of bilateral abdominal cryptorchidism by laparoscopy. Endoscopy 8:33-34, 1976.
10. Gornall PG, Pender DJ. Crossed testicular ectopia detected by laparoscopy. Br J Urol 59:283, 1987.
11. Hinman F. Survey: Localization and operation for nonpalpable testes. Urology 30:193-198, 1987.
12. Kaplan GW. The use of laparoscopy in management of the impalpable testes. Dialogues Pediatr Urol 9:7-8, 1986.
13. Lawson A, Gornall P, Buick RG, Corkery JJ. Impalpable testis: Testicular vessel division in treatment. Br J Surg 78:1111-1112, 1991.
14. Malone PS, Guiney EJ. A comparison between ultrasonography and laparoscopy in localizing the impalpable undescended testis. Br J Urol 57:185-186, 1985.
15. Manson AL, Terhune D, Jordan G, Auman JR, Peterson N, Mac Donald G. Pre-operative laparoscopic localization of the nonpalpable testis. J Urol 134:919-920, 1985.
16. Scott JES. Laparoscopy as an aid in the diagnosis and management of the impalpable testis. J Pediatr Surg 17:14-16, 1982.
17. Silber SJ, Cohen R. Laparoscopy for cryptorchidism. J Urol 124:928-929, 1980.
18. Smolko MJ, Kaplan GW, Brock WA. Location and fate of the nonpalpable testis in children. J Urol 129:1204-1206, 1983.
19. Waldschmidt J, Schier F. Surgical correction of abdominal testis after Fowler Stephens using the neodymium Yag laser for preliminary vessel dissection. Eur J Pediatr Surg 1:54-57, 1991.
20. Weiss RN, Seashore JH. Laparoscopy in the management of the nonpalpable testis. J Urol 138:382-384, 1987.
21. Bloom DA. Two-step orchiopexy with pelviscopic clip ligation of the spermatic vessels. J Urol 145:1030-1033, 1991.
22. Wright JE. Impalpable testes: A review of 100 boys. J Pediatr Surg 21:151-153, 1986.
23. Vaysse P, Galinier P, Guitard J, Moscovici J, Visentin M, Deslaugiers B, Juskiewenski S. Testicules impalpables. A propos de 161 observations. Chir Pediatr 31:345-348, 1990.

52 *Laparoscopic Treatment of Pyloric Stenosis*

Jean-Luc Alain and Dominique Grousseau

Laparoscopy is now used to perform extramucosal pylorotomy in infants with hypertrophic pyloric stenosis. Extramucosal pyloromyotomy was first described by Ramstedt and Fredet in 1907. This operation has not undergone any major modifications since its initial description, and excellent results are consistently achieved, with a very low rate of complications. A slight modification pertaining to access was recently proposed—use of a periumbilical incision. As a result of improvements in anesthesia techniques and monitoring of CO_2 pressures and the development of small-caliber instruments designed for use in the infant abdominal cavity, it is now possible to use the laparoscopic approach.

TECHNIQUE
Anesthesia

It is important that the surgeon be familiar with the ventilatory and hemodynamic complications related to celioscopy in the infant. Alveolar ventilation is proportionally far more important in infants than in adults. Any variation in the concentration of breathing gas levels is automatically reflected at the alveolar and arterial levels. Aspiration of gastric fluids prompted by abdominal hypertension, Trendelenburg position, or incorrect monitoring of airways can promote hypercapnia.

In the infant, shunts are not completely closed for many weeks, and any increase in pulmonary arterial oxygen resistance following hypoxia, hypercapnia, acidosis, or hypovolemia may result in the return of fetal circulation. Thus care must be taken to ensure that there are no contraindications (for example, congenital cardiopathy) or preexisting respiratory problems if the infant is to undergo prolonged assisted ventilation or if relative hypovolemia must first be corrected.

Celioscopy under general anesthesia with assisted ventilation in pure oxygen (without N_2O) should include monitoring of all these parameters, including partial CO_2 pressure through a fast-reading capnometer, which will allow rapid adaptations of the infant's breathing so that normal CO_2 pressure can be achieved.

Laparoscopic Approach (Fig. 1)

The infant is placed on the edge of the table, feet facing the surgeon, who stands between the infant's legs,

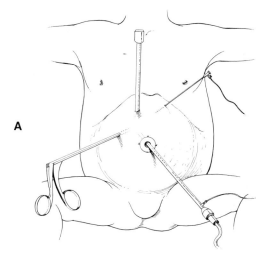
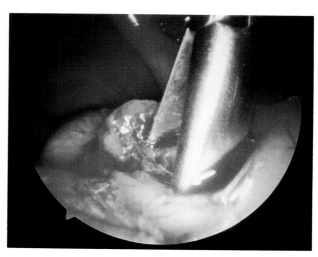

Fig. 1. A, Instrument array for laparoscopic pylorotomy. **B,** Intraoperative view.

which are spread wide apart. The infant's bladder is emptied by manual vesical pressure.

A Veress needle is introduced under the left costal arch within 1 cm of the midline. The rubber-tipped needle is left in place and serves as a palpator, which allows lifting and lowering of the hepatic edge. A pneumoperitoneum is slowly established, taking care not to exceed an insufflation pressure of 8 cm H_2O. To avoid overextension of the pneumoperitoneum after insertion of the trocars, the wall may be suspended by running a thread through it and attaching the thread to a suspension hook placed vertically in the epigastric area.

A 0-degree lens is used and provides a direct view with a 4 mm laparoscope. It is introduced into the well-disinfected umbilicus through a very small aponeurotic and cutaneous incision. Two operational trocars are then placed under videoscopic guidance. The first one, which is 3.5 mm, is placed to the left of the medial line, laterally, for insertion of duodenal prehensile forceps; the second trocar is facing and perpendicular to the previously noted pyloric mass.

After the duodenum is grasped a few millimeters from the pyloric mass, to maintain the duodenopyloric segment during subsequent steps, an incision is made in the mass with a 3 mm diameter bistory with a retractable blade. Care is taken to go from the thickest median portion toward the extremities of the mass. Two potential hazards must be avoided. The blade of the scalpel must not be plunged too deeply because of the risk of perforating the gastric mucosa. Indeed, the incision must remain superficial and allow the introduction first of a spatula to begin, and then of a spreading forceps to complete the separation of the edges.

The separation must be progressive, and the intact gastric mucosa must become visible. The entire length of the mucosa must be verified to detect possible breakage. Some air may then be injected by nasogastric catheter to place the air bubble in a conspicuous position between the edges of the pyloromyotomy. It has even been proposed that this be done with an intragastric endoscope. Above all, if there is the slightest doubt concerning possible mucosal breakage, a laparotomy must be performed. Pyloromyotomy does not lead to any bleeding when performed correctly at the avascular line.

At the end of the operation the trocars are removed after complete desufflation of the abdominal cavity. The tiny cutaneous incisions are closed by a single stitch with thin thread, and no scar is later visible. Mild analgesics are administered during the first 4 hours postoperatively, and feedings are resumed 6 to 10 hours after surgery.

Instrumentation Unique to Pylorotomy

The optical system and the trocars are adapted for use in the newborn infant and as a rule are smaller than 4 mm. A thin scalpel with a retractable blade, a spatula, and spreading forceps, depending on the spreader of Benson, were supplied by Karl Storz and Co.

RESULTS

Since May 21, 1990, our surgical team has operated on 21 newborn infants. The smallest infant weighed 3050 grams. The actual surgery lasted approximately 25 minutes. Accidental perforation of the gastric mucosa occurred in two of the initial cases. These complications were not detected during laparoscopy. The day after surgery, signs of peritonitis appeared, and the infants underwent laparotomy, allowing successful treatment of the perforations. Our first cases were reported in 1991[2] and no other reports of this technique have appeared in the literature.

We conclude that extramucosal pyloromyotomy for hypertrophic pyloric stenosis in the infant is possible with celioscopy. However, extreme caution is required in administering the anesthetic and the instruments must be adapted for use in the newborn infant. The procedure offers the following advantages: ease of postoperative follow-up, less discomfort during follow-up examinations, and no cutaneous scarring. The technique is hazardous, however, in terms of risk of gastric mucosal perforation and should only be performed by surgeons who are extremely skilled and experienced in celioscopic surgery. Classic open pyloromyotomy remains the procedure of choice for the vast majority of infants.

REFERENCES

1. Alain JL, Grousseau D, Terrier G. Laparoscopy and video surgery in surgical treatment of hypertrophic pyloric stenosis in the infant. Press Med 19:42, 1950.
2. Alain JL, Grousseau D, Terrier G. Extramucosal pylorotomy by laparoscopy. J Pediatr Surg 2610:1191-1192, 1991. Surg Endosc 5:174-175, 1991.

VIII

Videoendoscopic Gynecological Surgery

53 Hysterectomy by Laparotomy or Pelviscopy Using a Modified Subtotal Technique Without Colpotomy

Kurt Semm

Until 1960 performance of the supravaginal (i.e., subtotal) hysterectomy was routine. Then, because of the possibility of cervical stump carcinoma (0.3% to 1.8%), total hysterectomy became the method of choice; this represents overtreatment in many instances. In the treatment of benign conditions there is no direct relationship between long-term outcome and some of the steps taken in total hysterectomy such as excision of the broad ligaments, amputation of the cervix with shortening of the vagina, and the violation of pelvic floor nerves resulting from these steps. Yet all of these operative measures will eventually alter sexuality. In the absence of a malignancy, total hysterectomy is advocated as a prophylactic measure to eliminate the endocervical epithelium, because only this tissue can undergo malignant transformation. Until now no malignant degeneration of the pericervical tissue or the broad ligaments has been known. Therefore total hysterectomy is an excessive treatment because of its repercussions on the functions of the pelvic floor in patients with benign disease.

With a simple device known as a *calibrated uterine resection tool* (CURT), we are able to excise the core of the cervix. If benign indications for hysterectomy are present, we can then return to the subtotal technique, which can be performed with greater ease. The ureter and the uterine arteries are not at risk; all the pelvic nerves and the topography of the lower pelvis are preserved.

Tissues that can be removed vaginally can as easily be removed pelviscopically. Big tumors are removed by laparotomy. In cases of uterine prolapse, pelviscopic colposuspension may be performed and replaces the vaginoplasty technique. Therefore in the future we should use only two techniques for hysterectomy: (1) radical hysterectomy for malignant disease and (2) subtotal hysterectomy for benign tumors and irregular or dysfunctional uterine bleeding.

The subtotal abdominal hysterectomy as modified by Semm through a pelviscopic approach is demonstrated in Fig. 1. If open operation is indicated, the same technique is our method of choice in patients with nonmalignant conditions.

In Fig. 1, *A*, the uterus is manipulated and elongated transvaginally with a probe or rod to form a longitudinal muscular tube before perforating the fundus with the pointed endometrial probe, to hold and control the position of the uterine body. This probe is the central component of CURT.

In Fig. 1, *B*, the transvaginal endometrial probe has perforated the uterine fundus and allows it to pivot the uterus on its long axis back and forth and from side to side, to facilitate dissection. The right side shows suture ligation of the fallopian tube and suspension of the ovary in progress using a thread and Swedgedon needle and the extracorporeal knot-tying technique. On the left side the adnexae are already ligated and separated from the body of the uterus, after transection between two single suture ligations, placed and tied extracorporeally as shown on the right side.

All ligaments and adnexae are transected between two single suture ligatures (Fig. 1, *C*). On the right, a hysterectomy with adnexectomy is shown; the left side depicts a hysterectomy without adnexectomy. Sometimes the round ligament and the adnexae are incorporated into a single ligature (Fig. 2). The cardinal ligament is opened, and 10 ml of POR-8 solution (0.05 IU/5 ml) is injected into the cervix bilaterally.

In Fig. 1, *D*, the anterior peritoneum is incised and the bladder flap dissected using aquadissection. Ten to 20 ml of water with 0.05 IU of POR-8/ml is injected subperitoneally. The CURT mounted on the central endometrial probe and guided by it is then advanced with a rotating movement to core out a cylinder of mucosa and surrounding tissues from cervix, uterine body, and fundus until the cutting edges become just visible through the uterine fundus. The POR-8 injection allows performance of this procedure with very little blood loss. The anterior peritoneal and bladder flaps are suspended to the anterior abdominal wall, with special threads that carry a long and a short needle at each end.

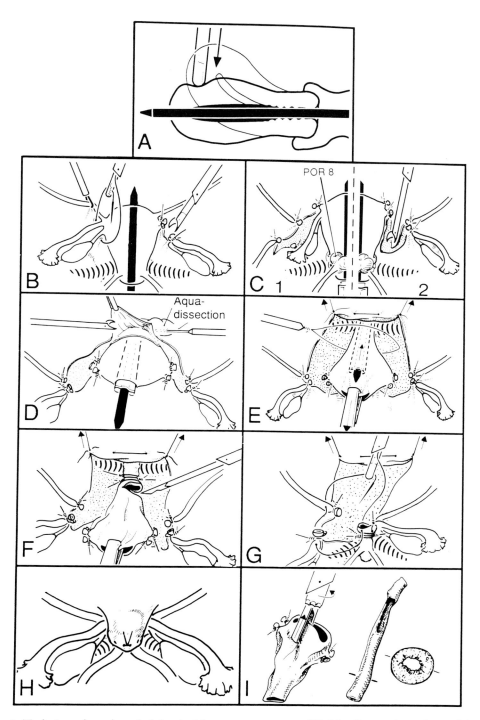

Fig. 1. Technique for subtotal abdominal hysterectomy as modified by Semm through a pelviscopic approach.

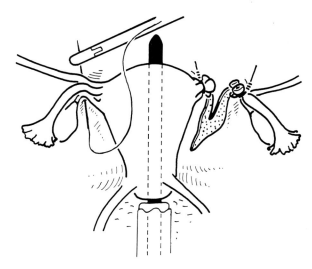

Fig. 2. Round ligament and adnexae are incorporated into a single ligature.

The fundus is grasped with a toothed forceps (Fig. 1, *E*) and is pulled toward the umbilicus. A Roeder loop is placed downward over the elongated cervix before the CURT is taken out through the vagina.

With traction on the uterus in the direction of the umbilicus (Fig. 1, *F*), the uterus is liberated from the paracervical fascial tissue with a scalpel (open technique) or hooked scissors (pelviscopy). After tying down the Roeder loop on the thinned cervix, the body of the uterus is separated through its junction with the cervix **above** the tied loop. Bleeding is stopped with topical hemostatic solutions and with the Erystop probe **(see Fig. 5)** of the Wisap coagulator (see Figs. 4, 5, and 10).

Fig. 1, *G*, shows the cervix sutured to the round ligament (and the fallopian tube) using a swedged-on thread and needle and the extracorporeal knotting technique, as demonstrated on the right. On the left side the round ligament and fallopian tube are already attached to the cervix to elevate the pelvic floor and to allow peritoneal coverage.

After cutting off the long needle of the bladder suspension threads and pulling the short one inside the pelvis, the anterior peritoneal flap is released and sutured to the uterosacral ligaments with the short needles. Like a theater curtain, the peritoneum comes down, and all tissue stumps are located extraperitoneally (Fig. 1, *H*).

Fig. 1, *I*, shows the morcellation of the uterus using the *serrated-edge macro-morcellator* (SEMM) whereby finger-sized pieces are extracted step by step. Shown are the excised cervical cylinder, the incomplete cylinder of the uterus cavity, and the fundus muscle cylinder. On the right are transverse cuts for histological specimens of the cervical cylinder.

The procedure is carried out with an absolute minimum of blood loss (30 to 50 ml). By this method any coagulation using high-frequency current or laser is obsolete. The procedure can, however, be adapted to personal preferences by using staples, clips, cautery, or laser techniques. In minimally invasive surgery the maxim should be: "Blood belongs in the vessels; when it escapes the technique must be changed."

If the cervix and vagina have a diameter larger than that of the uterus because of cervical mucosal prolapse, the technique must be changed as follows (Fig. 3).

First the ectropion of cervical mucosa is demarcated by using Schiller's test. The ectopic cervical glands are clearly demonstrated (Fig. 3, *A*). Bilateral infiltration of POR-8 solution (0.05 IU/ml) follows (Fig. 3, *B*). After introduction of the central probe or rod of CURT, a scalpel is used to cut out the cervical os or ostium as a cone. Because the tip of the knife always touches the central rod or probe as it circumscribes the pointed apex of the cone, there is no danger of opening the pouch of Douglas. This accident is possible only

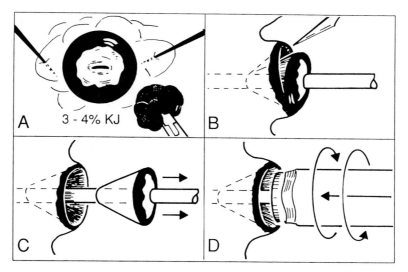

Fig. 3. Modified procedure to accommodate large-diameter cervix and vagina resulting from cervical mucosal prolapse.

when performing the routine scalpel conization without intubating the cervix and the cavity of the uterus with a central rod or probe.

The tissue is removed over the central probe (Fig. 3, *C*). After conization of the large cervical ostium, the calibrated uterine resection tool is advanced over the central rod and rotated manually upward at the appropriate time to excise the muscular cervical canal (Fig. 3, *D*). Should significant bleeding occur, coagulation of the wound for 20 to 60 seconds with a WISAP coagulation probe is performed using the ERYSTOP (see Figs. 4, 5, 10).

After morcellation of the uterus the entire abdomen is irrigated with 5 to 10 L of saline solution using the Wisap CO_2 Aquapurator. Two Robinson drains are introduced through a 5 mm trocar sheath and left in position for approximately 24 hours. This drainage procedure immediately detects any hemorrhage that may occur during the next few hours. If proper ligature material is used, postoperative bleeding seldom occurs.

The whole procedure may also be performed by laparotomy (Figs. 6 and 7). Instead of Roeder loop ligation, the remaining fascial cervical tube ligation of the hollowed cervical stump is performed with two transfixing suture ligatures placed from each side of the cervical cylinder and overlapping each other through the 6 to 12 o'clock axis of the remaining fascial tube or cylinder. These two suture ligatures simultaneously ligate

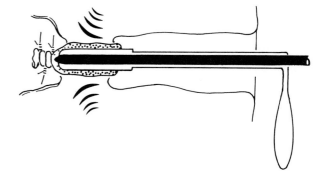

Fig. 4. WISAP coagulation probe.

the ascending branches of the uterine artery on both sides (Fig. 8).

After pelviscopic hysterectomy, the patient can drink fluids on the same day and start a light diet on the next day.

As part of the immediate postoperative treatment, the patient must be monitored for cervical and vaginal bleeding. By using a speculum I designed (Fig. 9), localization of the cervix is easily performed. If a conventional speculum is used, it must be handled very carefully to avoid dislocating the ligatures.

To stop cervical remnant bleeding after hospital discharge, coagulation may be performed in a well-equipped office or minor surgery suite. We recommend

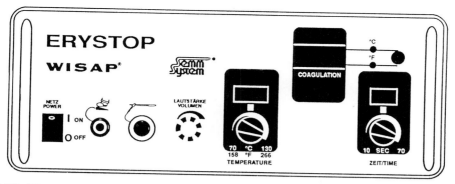

Fig. 5. The ERYSTOP is used to transmit and monitor electrical energy to the WISAP coagulation probe.

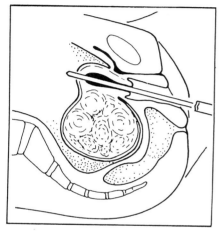

Fig. 6. The subtotal procedure may also be performed by laparotomy, e.g., in case of a large, benign, fibroid tumor.

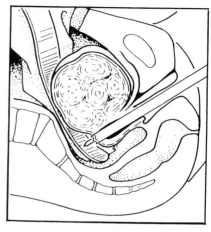

Fig. 7. The CURT device is used to excise the core of the cervix, making a subtotal hysterectomy possible.

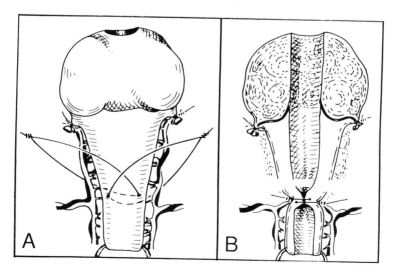

Fig. 8. A, Two transfixing suture ligatures placed via laparotomy simultaneously ligate the ascending branches of the uterine artery on both sides and obliterate the hollow cervical stump. **B,** The uterus is then excised above the closed remaining cervical stump.

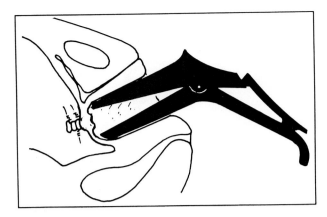

Fig. 9. Semm speculum.

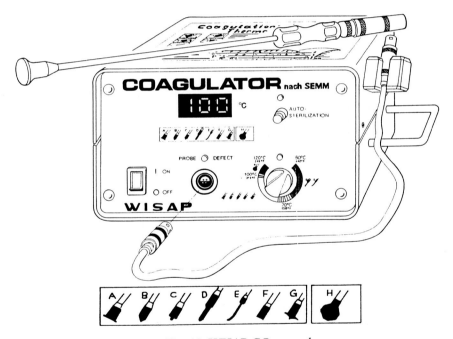

Fig. 10. WISAP CO₂ coagulator.

application for 60 seconds at 100° C using the WISAP coagulator (Fig. 10). For total hysterectomy, the cosmetic results are much better after specimen removal through the vagina.

CONCLUSION

The subtotal hysterectomy as modified by Semm makes it possible once again to perform subtotal hysterecto-

my with all its advantages but with the additional security that a cervical carcinoma can never occur. The function of the pelvic floor remains totally intact. The vagina is not opened, and by conserving the paracervical nerves, we preserve the patient's sexual sensatory function. Subtotal hysterectomy as shown creates a better quality of life for the patient, even after removal of the uterine muscle.

54 The Single Umbilical Puncture Technique in Minimally Invasive Laparoscopic Hysterectomy, Salpingo-oophorectomy, and Appendectomy

Marco A. Pelosi and Marco A. Pelosi III

In 1990 we introduced the single-puncture umbilical technique as an alternative to more invasive multiple-puncture techniques for the performance of laparoscopic hysterectomy, salpingo-oophorectomy, and appendectomy. The term *minimally invasive* implies that the least invasive surgical technique has been selected. The single-puncture concept best fulfills the definition of minimally invasive laparoscopic surgery.[1-3]

The single-puncture modality depends on both simplicity and the surgeon's reliance on his or her skills and dexterity with procedures in which time-honored, standard tools rather than highly technical and costly equipment are used. Our experience indicates that the effectiveness and reliability of the single-puncture approach make it comparable to more invasive and traumatic multiple-puncture techniques. Moreover, the single-puncture technique provides the following additional advantages: expediency, lower cost, avoidance of complications associated with multiple punctures, superior cosmetic results, and the flexibility to be converted to multiple-puncture operation or laparotomy, if indicated.[4]

MATERIALS AND METHODS

The single-puncture laparoscopic technique uses an operative laparoscope and standard nondisposable laparoscopic instrumentation and relies on a minimal number of operating-room personnel. The laparoscopic hysterectomy/adnexectomy and appendectomy are performed with the same basic technique and instrumentation. A general anesthetic is administered in all cases. After the patient is placed in lithotomy position, an indwelling urinary catheter is inserted. The surgical table is then placed in a deep Trendelenburg position. A Veress needle is advanced intraumbilically, and a pneumoperitoneum is created by means of a high-flow CO_2 insufflator. After a vertical intraumbilical stab incision is made, a trocar (enabling the accommodation of a 10

mm operative laparoscope with a 5 mm operating channel) is introduced. We do not routinely use a video system. However, when recording is done, a split-beam video system is attached to the eyepiece of the operative laparoscope (Fig. 1, *A* and *B*). Only three instruments are routinely inserted through the 5 mm operative channel of the laparoscope: bipolar forceps, unipolar scissors, and a high-flow suction-irrigation device (Fig. 2).

LAPAROSCOPIC HYSTERECTOMY

Our indications for laparoscopic hysterectomy are the same as those for abdominal hysterectomy; the laparoscopic approach is used only when we consider a purely vaginal hysterectomy to be contraindicated. Preoperative bowel preparation and prophylactic antibiotics are used routinely. In patients with large myomas we use gonadotropin-releasing hormones preoperatively for 3 months, when feasible, to achieve a reduction in uterine and myoma size and vascularity.

The skillful use of the transvaginal uterine manipulator is critical for the successful performance of laparoscopic hysterectomy. Because no uterine manipulator had been designed specifically for performing laparoscopic hysterectomy, we developed one (NoVA Endoscopy) that has been demonstrated to be effective and versatile regardless of uterine size. The device allows movement of the uterus in any direction and creates maximum uterine anteversion with easy identification of the cul-de-sac, even with a large fibroid uterus extending up to or above the level of the umbilicus. This uterine manipulator can be fitted with a multipurpose laparoscopic illuminator, which allows the performance of a simplified and effective laparoscopically assisted colpotomy. The illuminator lights up the area below the cervix and between the uterosacral ligaments, simplifying both the laparoscopic identification of the cul-de-sac and the creation of the colpotomy incision

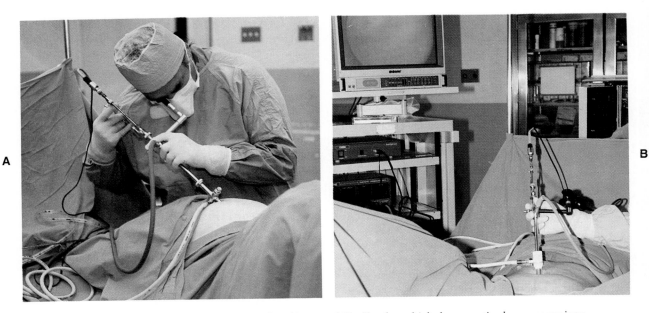

Fig. 1. A, The operative laparoscope is placed intraumbilically after which the operative laparoscopy is to follow. **B,** We do not routinely use video imaging. When recording is done, a split beam video coupler is attached to the laparoscope.

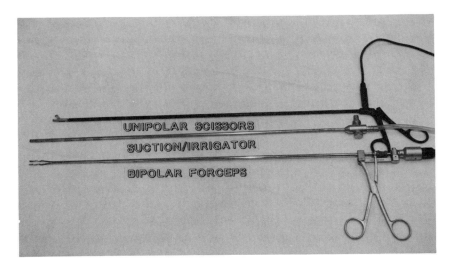

Fig. 2. Only three instruments are routinely used: unipolar scissors, a high-flow suction-irrigator, and bipolar forceps.

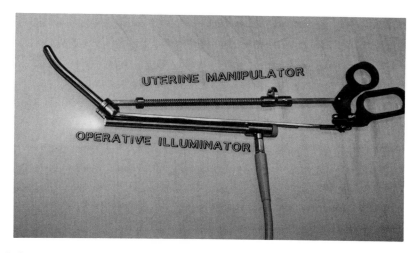

Fig. 3. The Pelosi uterine manipulator with the multipurpose laparoscopic illuminator. The manipulator allows the effective movement of the uterus, regardless of its size, in any direction. The attached illuminator simplifies the creation of a laparoscopic assisted colpotomy.

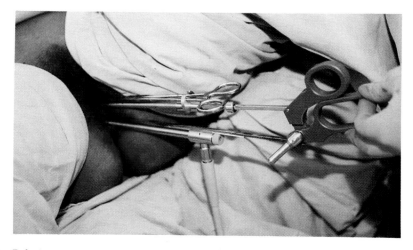

Fig. 4. The Pelosi uterine manipulator and illuminator have been inserted before performance of a laparoscopic single-puncture hysterectomy.

(Figs. 3 and 4). The proper use of the uterine manipulator allows the surgeon to push the uterus upward and laterally, thereby creating adequate tension and exposure of the round, uteroovarian, and infundibulopelvic ligaments, as well as the adnexae. The round ligament is grasped and cauterized at its midportion with electrosurgical bipolar forceps and then cut with scissors (Fig. 5). (Figs. 5 through 13 show a laparoscopic hysterectomy by single-puncture technique.)

A similar procedure is performed on the proximal portion of the fallopian tubes and the utero-ovarian ligament. When salpingo-oophorectomy is needed, the infundibulopelvic ligaments are cauterized and transected instead. The bladder is partially distended with methylene blue solution to aid in identifying anatomical landmarks when dissecting the bladder from the uterus, cervix, and upper vagina. The vesicouterine fold is then opened with scissors (Fig. 6). Although in most cases

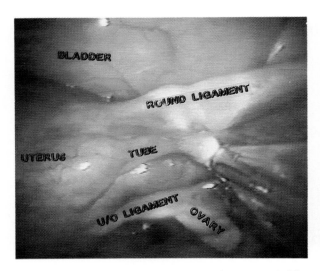

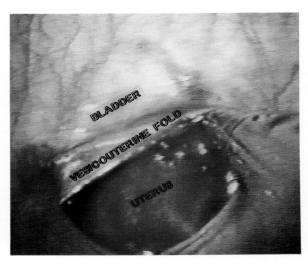

Fig. 5. Laparoscopic hysterectomy (single puncture). The fallopian tube is being cauterized with bipolar forceps. The round and uterovarian *(U/O)* ligaments have already been cauterized before transection.

Fig. 6. Single-puncture procedure. The vesicouterine fold is being opened.

sharp dissection is sufficient to separate the bladder, hydrodissection is occasionally needed. Bleeding in small vessels, if encountered, is easily controlled with unipolar or bipolar coagulation.

Instillation of methylene blue into the bladder offers another advantage in that it enables prompt and easy identification of even pinhole-size bladder injuries that might otherwise go unrecognized during an operation.

In most patients the ureters are easily seen through the intact peritoneum along the lateral pelvic wall. Preoperative ureteral catheterization is also helpful in some instances. When the ureters are difficult to visualize, they are sufficiently dissected so that they may be identified in toto. The integrity of the ureters can be easily tested intraoperatively by an intravenous injection of indigo carmine solution (5 ml). Once the posterior leaf of the broad ligament is incised down to the uterosacral ligament, the uterine vessels are identified and skeletonized with scissors and hydrodissection. The uterine manipulator, by pushing and rotating the uterus, facilitates this step of the hysterectomy.

After the ureters have been identified, the uterine vessels are grasped with bipolar forceps and coagulated. Transection is then performed with scissors. The surgeon must maintain continuous attention to the posi-

tion of the ureters during coagulation and transection (Fig. 7). Following division of the uterine vessels, the dissection is continued with unipolar and bipolar coagulation, and transection of the cardinal and uterosacral ligaments (Fig. 8). The vagina is entered anteriorly by means of unipolar scissors over a sponge placed between the vaginal wall and the cervix (Fig. 9). A laparoscopically assisted colpotomy is then performed. The Pelosi illuminator is attached to the manipulator. The illuminator will light up the area below the cervix and between the uterosacral ligaments, simplifying laparoscopic identification of the cul-de-sac and creation of the colpotomy incision (Fig. 10).

The tissue bridges between the anterior and posterior vaginal openings are cauterized or desiccated and transected with scissors. Areas of bleeding from the vaginal cuff are coagulated. A laparoscopically monitored vaginal delivery of the free uterus is then carried out (Fig. 11). Occasionally, before the uterus is extracted from the vagina, the uterosacral ligaments and the lower portion of the cardinal ligaments are clamped and cut transvaginally. If large myomas are present, a combined laparoscopic and transvaginal bisection, enucleation, or morcellation is performed to safely remove the uterus and myomas through the vagina (Figs. 5, 12, and 13). The vaginal cuff is then closed with absorbable

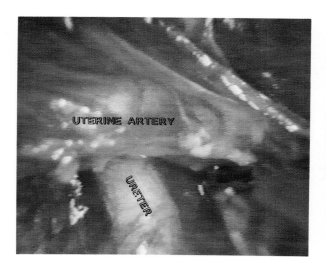

Fig. 7. The dissected right uterine artery and underlying ureter are clearly seen before cauterization and transection of the artery.

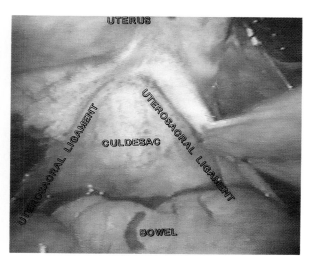

Fig. 8. The right uterosacral ligament is being desiccated. The left uterosacral ligament has already been cauterized and transected.

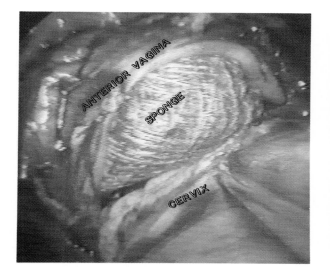

Fig. 9. The vagina has been entered anteriorly using unipolar scissors over a sponge placed between the vaginal wall and the cervix.

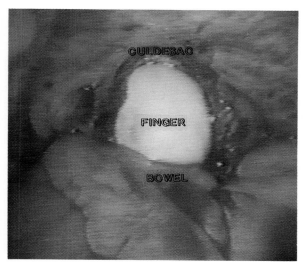

Fig. 10. A laparoscopically assisted colpotomy has been performed.

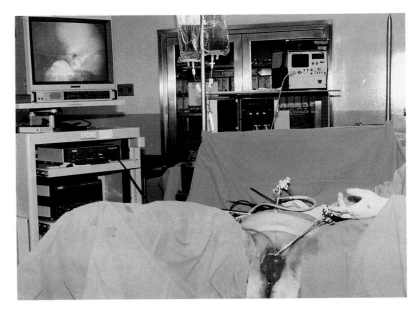

Fig. 11. The tissue bridges between the anterior and posterior vaginal openings were transected and a laparoscopically monitored vaginal retrieval of the uterus and adnexa is being carried out.

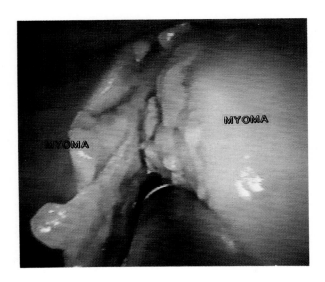

Fig. 12. A large myoma is being bisected to decrease uterine size for easier removal through the vagina.

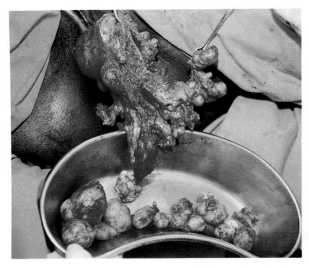

Fig. 13. A combined transvaginal and laparoscopic uterine morcellation and enucleation of myomas is usually needed before the vaginal retrieval of a large fibroid uterus.

sutures, incorporating the uterosacral ligaments and a portion of the cardinal ligaments. After restoration of the pneumoperitoneum, the pelvis is irrigated and hemostasis is ensured. The umbilical puncture site is then closed in layers with absorbable sutures.

LAPAROSCOPICALLY ASSISTED VAGINAL HYSTERECTOMY

It must be emphasized that laparoscopic hysterectomy is a substitute for abdominal hysterectomy and not for vaginal hysterectomy. In our opinion, laparoscopy has no place in the surgical management of patients who are candidates for safe, traditional vaginal hysterectomy except for its possible use in selected cases to inspect the operative field after vaginal hysterectomy has been completed. Under those circumstances, the laparoscope allows easy identification of bleeding sites, achievement of hemostasis, evacuation of blood clots, and the use of copious irrigation and aspiration to reduce the number of vaginally introduced bacteria.

It is important to differentiate between laparoscopically assisted vaginal hysterectomy and laparoscopic hysterectomy. Laparoscopically assisted vaginal hysterectomy indicates that a laparoscopic dissection and transection of the upper uterine pedicles with or without adnexectomy have been performed only up to the level of the uterine arteries, after which a standard vaginal hysterectomy is carried out.[5] Only on rare occasions do we perform laparoscopically assisted vaginal hysterectomy. We have found laparoscopic identification, skeletonization, and division of the uterine vessels and cardinal and uterosacral ligaments to be more efficient than the transvaginal approach in patients undergoing hysterectomy when a purely vaginal hysterectomy is contraindicated.

LAPAROSCOPIC SUPRACERVICAL HYSTERECTOMY

Single-umbilical puncture laparoscopic supracervical hysterectomy is an attractive and effective alternative to total hysterectomy for a select group of well-informed women with healthy cervixes and no associated genital prolapse, and in whom removal of the cervix is not essential to the surgical treatment of the primary gynecological problem.[2,6] When compared with total hysterectomy, supracervical hysterectomy requires less dissection of the bladder from the cervix, which decreases the chances of excessive bleeding and bladder dener-

vation. With abdominal hysterectomy the risk of surgical injury to the ureters, bladder, and lower intestinal tract increases considerably during removal of the cervix. As a result, the supracervical technique decreases the possibility of surgical trauma to those structures. When compared with total hysterectomy, it is apparent that supracervical hysterectomy does not significantly alter the anatomy and integrity of the pelvic floor and vagina. This factor may be responsible for the apparently less compromised bladder and sexual function and decreased long-term morbidity.

Laparoscopic hysterectomy and adnexa removal are carried out, as previously described, up to the level of the cardinal ligaments (cervicoisthmic junction). To remove the endocervical epithelium, supracervical amputation is performed in a *coning-out* fashion. The uterus is then split into symmetrical halves, leaving a portion of the fundus intact so that the uterus can be removed as a single unit through the umbilical puncture site. The ovaries and fallopian tubes are extracted from the same puncture site (Fig. 14). Cauterization of the lower endocervical canal and endocervix is then performed through the vagina.

Uteri considered too large for expeditious removal through the umbilical puncture site are extracted trans-

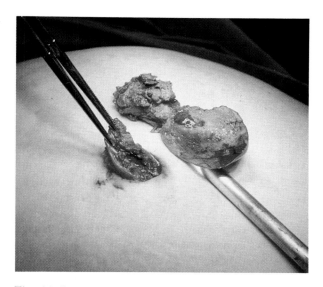

Fig. 14. Laparoscopic supracervical hysterectomy (single puncture). The bisected uterus is being advanced through the umbilical puncture site.

vaginally by means of the recently introduced laparoscopic colpotomy technique. The Pelosi illuminator will light up the area below the cervix and between the uterosacral ligaments, simplifying both the laparoscopic identification of the cul-de-sac and the performance of the colpotomy incision. The colpotomy opening is then closed with absorbable sutures. When feasible, we favor removal of specimens through the umbilical puncture site, since it avoids the need for colpotomy.

The pneumoperitoneum is recreated, the pelvic cavity copiously irrigated, and hemostasis assessed. The cervical stump is not routinely peritonealized. Second-look laparoscopy on several of our postsupracervical hysterectomy patients has revealed complete healing of the cervical stump and no adhesions or distortion of the pelvic anatomy.

The uterine manipulator is then removed, and to further reduce the risk of future development of a malignancy in the retained cervical stump, the lower endocervical canal and exocervix are cauterized transvaginally. Advantages of the technique include the following:

Sexual function
    Orgasmic ability is not compromised
    Undisrupted cervical mobility and secretions
    Less dyspareunia
Urinary tract system
    Fewer long-term urinary symptoms and less bladder dysfunction
Psychological symptoms
    Fewer long-term psychological reactions
Surgery
    Less risk of injury to bowels, ureters, and bladder
    Reduced bleeding and operating time
    Less alteration of the pelvic floor and vagina

COMBINING LAPAROSCOPIC HYSTERECTOMY WITH OTHER LAPAROSCOPIC PROCEDURES

We have successfully combined single-puncture laparoscopic hysterectomy with other laparoscopic procedures: appendectomy, cholecystectomy, herniorrhaphy, and correction of stress urinary incontinence (suprapubic urethropexy and transvaginal needle suspension of the vesical neck). Performing these procedures during laparoscopic hysterectomy does not alter patient outcome or influence the recovery period.

In a large number of female patients, concurrent gynecological and gallbladder abnormalities requiring surgical intervention are present. By use of a combined endoscopic approach, we eliminate the need for cholecys-

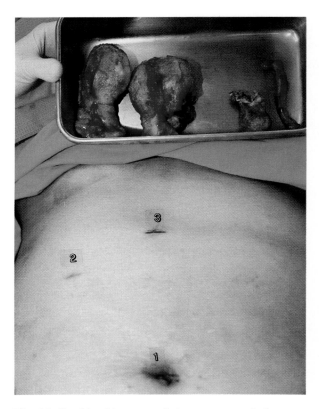

Fig. 15. Combined laparoscopic hysterectomy, cholecystomy, and appendectomy. A single-puncture hysterectomy and an appendectomy were done. Only two additional punctures were used for the cholecystectomy. The uterus, gallbladder, and appendix are shown above the patient's abdomen.

tectomy in the future, thereby effectively reducing hospitalization costs, anesthesia risks, and time away from work. In addition, by performing the hysterectomy and appendectomy with a single umbilical puncture and the cholecystectomy with only two additional abdominal punctures, the combined operation requires a total of only three abdominal punctures[7] (Fig. 15).

LAPAROSCOPIC APPENDECTOMY: SINGLE-PUNCTURE TECHNIQUE

Diagnosis and treatment of appendicitis have been well established for more than 100 years. Until recently the dramatic strides made in the surgical outcome of appendectomy were the result of improved anesthetic agents and methods, the introduction of antibiotics, and the prompt, aggressive management by appendectomy, which had undergone relatively marginal im-

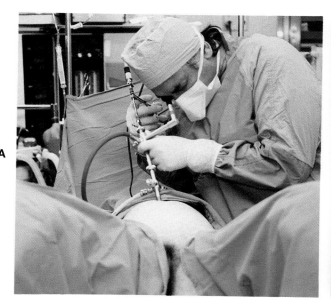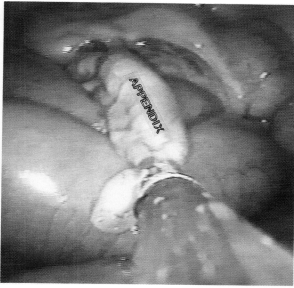

Fig. 16. Laparoscopic appendectomy (single puncture). **A,** Through the operative channel of the laparoscope, the appendix is grasped and its mobility is assessed. **B,** The mobilized appendix and mesoappendix are deflected toward the umbilicus.

provements since its inception. In the early 1980s the first appendectomy solely using laparoscopic techniques was performed by Semm.[8] Despite the successful results achieved by him and his followers in Europe, laparoscopic appendectomy did not gain worldwide acceptance until the advent of laparoscopic cholecystectomy.

We will describe our technique for laparoscopic appendectomy via a single umbilical puncture. Our experience with a single umbilical puncture in more than 120 laparoscopic appendectomies has demonstrated that this simplified, minimally invasive modality is a safe and cost-effective alternative to the multiple-puncture techniques currently in use.

Technique

The appendectomy is performed with an intraumbilically placed operative laparoscope. Unless there is a specific reason to record the laparoscopic procedure, a video system is not used routinely. However, when recording is done, a video coupler is attached to the operative laparoscope. Only three instruments are introduced through the 5 mm operative channel of the laparoscope: bipolar forceps, unipolar scissors, and a suction-irrigation device.

After atraumatic grasping forceps are inserted through the operative channel of the laparoscope, the tip of the appendix is gently grasped to assess the mobility of the organ (Fig. 16, *A*). A prerequisite for successful appendectomy by means of the extracorporeal technique is a mobile appendix. If adhesions are present, they are transsected by sharp dissection. When necessary, bipolar coagulation forceps are used before cutting vascular adhesions. If after these maneuvers are performed the mobility of the appendix is still restricted, the cecum is elevated superiorly and gently pulled toward the umbilicus. Once visualized, the lateral and inferior peritoneal bands of the cecum and appendix are divided to fully mobilize the appendix. The appendix is then grasped and deflected laterally toward the midline to achieve alignment with the umbilicus (Fig. 16, *B*). With the grasping forceps maintained in this position, the cannula and laparoscope are removed as a single unit from the umbilical puncture site (Fig. 17, *A*). The abdomen is then deflated, thereby permitting the appendix to reach the puncture site passively. Pulling of the appendix at this time is avoided to prevent accidental trauma to the organ (Fig. 17, *B*). When the appendix is visualized through the umbilical puncture site, its tip is grasped with a traditional clamp before the

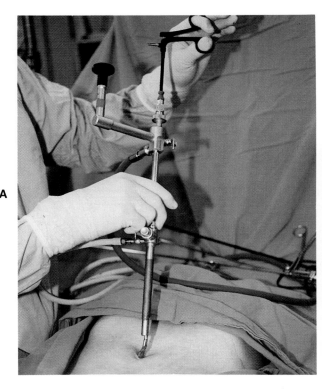

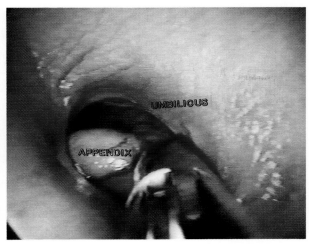

Fig. 17. Laparoscopic appendectomy (single puncture). **A,** The laparoscope and cannula are removed while the grasping forceps maintains its hold on the tip of the appendix. **B,** This maneuver deflates the abdominal cavity, allowing the structure to passively reach the umbilical puncture site.

laparoscopic forceps are released. The appendix in its entirety is then extracted from the abdominal cavity as far as the length of the mesoappendix allows (Fig. 18, *A*). An extracorporeal appendectomy is then easily performed with standard laparotomy techniques (Fig. 18, *B*).

On occasion, because of anatomical or pathological conditions, achieving an adequately mobile appendix is not feasible. Under these circumstances the mesoappendix is systematically coagulated and divided with bipolar forceps and scissors until the base of the appendix is reached. The free appendix is then grasped with forceps, brought to the umbilical puncture site in a manner similar to the one previously described, and the appendectomy is completed extracorporeally. The cannula and the laparoscope are reinserted through the umbilical puncture site and the pneumoperitoneum is re-

stored (Fig. 19, *A*). The appendiceal stump and the mesoappendix are inspected to ensure hemostasis and to confirm the integrity of the ligatures (Fig. 19, *B*).

We have recently developed a single umbilical puncture technique for laparoscopic appendectomy for those infrequent situations in which anatomical or pathological conditions may preclude a safe and effective appendectomy by means of the extracorporeal single umbilical puncture approach. Through the intraumbilically placed operative laparoscope, the appendix and mesoappendix are thoroughly inspected and fully mobilized by adhesiolysis and/or division of the lateral and inferior peritoneal bands. The appendix is skeletonized from the tip to the base by coagulation of the mesoappendix, including the appendicular artery. The coagulated tissue is divided with scissors. Two Roeder loops, made of size 0 catgut, are then used to double-ligate the

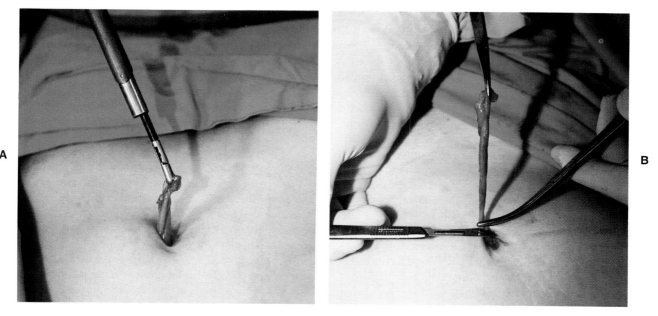

Fig. 18. Laparoscopic appendectomy (single puncture). **A,** The appendix is grasped with a conventional clamp and then extracted from the abdominal cavity, as far as the mesoappendix allows. **B,** Our extracorporeal traditional appendectomy is then easily performed.

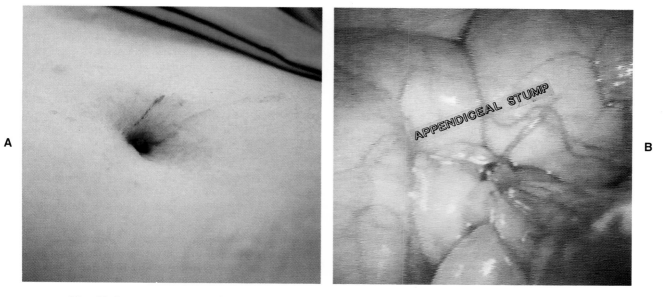

Fig. 19. Laparoscopic appendectomy (single puncture). **A,** The appendiceal stump is pushed back into the abdominal cavity. **B,** The laparoscope is then reinserted, the pneumoperitoneum restored, and the mesoappendix and stump inspected for hemostasis and integrity of the ligatures.

skeletonized appendix. Alternatively, two metallic clips may be used on the organ. Both the Roeder loop and the metallic clip are placed through the operative channel of the laparoscope. The appendix is then transected between the ligatures or the clips and removed through the umbilical cannula.

The anatomical characteristics of the appendix make this structure particularly well suited to the single umbilical puncture laparoscopic technique. In our experience, the average operating time for completion of an appendectomy is 7 minutes. The performance of laparoscopic appendectomy has not altered the outcome or influenced the morbidity or the recovery period of the primary gynecological procedure or cholecystectomy. In the majority of patients, the presence of significant pelvic disease, adhesions, retrocecal appendixes, acute inflammation, and other pathological conditions of the appendix does not present technical difficulties. However, conversion to multiple-puncture laparoscopy or laparotomy in more complicated cases can be easily accomplished.

DISCUSSION

We have presented our comprehensive approach to laparoscopic hysterectomy and appendectomy with the use of a single umbilical puncture. Since our experience illustrates that maximum benefits can be achieved with minimally invasive access, we hope it will stimulate the reader to reconsider the principles of minimally invasive surgery and apply them to his or her own practice of laparoscopic surgery and encourage traditional gynecological surgeons who are still reluctant to use endoscopic surgery to incorporate its philosophy into their surgical management of gynecological conditions.

We find it difficult to justify the routine placement of several surgical ports, which risks potential traumatic complications and results in a less than desirable cosmetic appearance of the abdominal wall. Instead, the number and diameter of the abdominal punctures needed for laparoscopic surgery should be determined on a case-by-case basis and by more efficient use of instrumentation. In most instances the number of punctures can be significantly reduced by more efficient and skillful use of existing instrumentation. Methods include (1) using an operative laparoscope rather than a diagnostic one, since the former contains an operative channel through which instruments may be passed, (2) using multipurpose instruments, (3) placing instruments through an existing surgical port to perform a specific function rather than creating an additional puncture site for the sole purpose of inserting an alternative instrument that cannot be accommodated through the existing smaller ports, and (4) skillfully using the uterine manipulator.

Since we adopted operative laparoscopy into our surgical armamentarium, we rarely perform elective abdominal hysterectomy for benign pelvic conditions. We have successfully performed routine single-puncture laparoscopic hysterectomy in 100 patients in whom the primary indications included symptomatic leiomyomas with uteruses larger than those seen at 16 weeks of pregnancy, advanced endometriosis, and chronic pelvic inflammatory disease with extensive adhesions, and in patients with associated large benign ovarian masses. Some patients had more than one indication. Laparoscopic procedures that are frequently performed at the time of laparoscopic hysterectomy include unilateral/bilateral adnexectomy, extensive adhesiolysis, appendectomy, cholecystectomy, inguinal hernia repair, and vesical neck suspension for urinary incontinence. The patient can resume normal activities within 2 weeks.

At the present time no one is questioning the value of laparoscopic hysterectomy and laparoscopically assisted vaginal hysterectomy in enabling a shortened hospital stay and recovery time in comparison with traditional abdominal hysterectomy. Laparoscopic surgery allows a vaginal approach to be used for many hysterectomies that would otherwise have to be performed transabdominally. However, the increased operating time and equipment costs incurred with laparoscopic hysterectomy and laparoscopically assisted vaginal hysterectomy raise doubts about their cost effectiveness. It is unfortunate that the type of technique used to perform laparoscopic hysterectomy and appendectomy—as complicated and expensive as it may be—is not considered an important issue as long as the current criteria for choosing laparoscopic surgery over laparotomy (shorter hospital stay and faster recovery rate) are met. Presently there are a large number of competing laparoscopic hysterectomy and appendectomy techniques without sufficiently documented data to confirm the superiority of a specific technique's safety, efficacy, and cost effectiveness.

The first extensive study regarding the cost effectiveness of laparoscopy versus laparotomy demonstrated that the use of laparoscopic surgery in all eligible (greater than 80%) patients with an ectopic pregnancy in 1987 in the United States would have resulted in a savings of approximately $138,920 for that year alone.[9] Calculations were based on the utilization of an *ectopic pregnancy laparoscopy tray*. The set consisted of a basic diagnostic laparoscopy tray, an electrosurgical generator (unipolar and bipolar), and a small number of additional instruments (laparoscopic scissors, biopsy and grasping forceps, bipolar forceps, and a unipolar needle). It was assumed that the system would require full replacement every 2 years. An extensive review of the literature regarding laparoscopic treatment of ectopic pregnancy indicated that video imaging, lasers, and stapling-cutting devices were not essential for performing this specific operation.

Our experience further demonstrates that advanced laparoscopic surgery does not require the routine simultaneous use of several instruments and does not necessitate routine use of high technology. Our average material cost per *single-puncture* laparoscopic hysterectomy with *reusable* instruments is $53.40. At our institution the cost per procedure for the *multiple-puncture* technique with *nonreusable* instruments would have been $2,443.75 and the total weight of these disposable instruments would be 7 pounds per case. The cost over 100 cases of our single-puncture technique with nondisposable instruments was $5,340. The cost over 100 cases with a multiple-puncture approach with disposable instruments would have been $244,375, and the total weight of the disposable instruments would have been 700 pounds. Our cost over 120 laparoscopic appendectomies with the single-puncture technique and *nondisposable* instruments was $6,600.

Had we instead used a *multiple-puncture* technique with *disposable* instruments, including a stapling-cutting device, the total cost would have been $138,000, with a total weight of 420 pounds. We strongly believe that because of reduced trauma, simplicity, efficacy, and cost effectiveness, the single-puncture modality best fulfills the concept of minimally invasive surgery.

REFERENCES

1. Pelosi MA, Pelosi MA III. Laparoscopic hysterectomy with bilateral salpingo-oophorectomy using a single umbilical puncture. NJ Med 88:721, 1991.
2. Pelosi MA, Pelosi MA III. Laparoscopic supracervical hysterectomy using a single umbilical puncture (minilaparoscopy). J Reprod Med 37:777, 1992.
3. Pelosi MA, Pelosi MA III. Laparoscopic appendectomy using a single umbilical puncture (minilaparoscopy). J Reprod Med 37:588, 1992.
4. Wolenski M, Pelosi MA. The single puncture approach for advanced pelviscopy surgery. Today's OR Nurse 13:4, 1991.
5. Reich H. Laparoscopic hysterectomy. Surg Laparosc Endosc 2:85, 1992.
6. Semm K. CASH (classical abdominal SEMM hysterectomy). Presented at the AAGL Twenty-first Annual Meeting of the International Congress of Gynecologic Endoscopy, Chicago, September 1992.
7. Pelosi MA, Villalona E. Laparoscopic hysterectomy, appendectomy and cholecystectomy. NJ Med 90:207, 1993.
8. Semm K. Endoscopic appendectomy. Endoscopy 15:59, 1983.
9. Maruri F, Azziz R. Laparoscopic surgery for ectopic pregnancies: Technology assessment and public health implications. Fertil Steril 59:487, 1993.

55 The Pelviscopic Hysterectomy: A Prospective Comparative Study of Sixty Cases

Franz Wierrani, Friedrich Gill, Wolfgang Grin, and Werner Grünberger

Since 1975 we have performed more than 20,000 laparoscopic operations in our department. Initially, laparoscopy was used for diagnostic investigations such as biopsies and for tubal ligations and lysis of adhesions. Later aspiration of cystic fluid and coagulation of endometriosis were performed laparoscopically. With the refinement of microsurgical instruments and the improvement of endoscopic techniques, additional procedures involving tubal, cystic, and myomal resections and tubal sterilization have become possible.

In Austria the first pelviscopic hysterectomy was performed on March 5, 1992. This method is considered minimally invasive; furthermore, it does not alter the topography of the pelvic floor.

At this writing we have performed 30 pelviscopic hysterectomies, some of which involved adnexectomy. In this chapter we review the indications for pelviscopic hysterectomy, duration of the procedure, intraoperative and postoperative complications.

In this prospective 12-week study we compared two groups of patients who all presented with similar indications for hysterectomy. Thirty women (one group) were treated with therapeutic pelviscopy; 30 women (the second group) underwent vaginal hysterectomy.

MATERIALS AND METHODS

The mean age of the patients who underwent pelviscopic surgery was 55.7 years; of those who underwent vaginal hysterectomy, the mean age was 51.2 years (Table 1).

The preoperative evaluation consisted of a Papanicolaou smear, evaluation of secretions, measurement of the cervix and uterine body with vaginal ultrasonography, intravenous pyelography, and determination of possible incontinence with the Gaudenzbogen and perineal ultrasonography with Valsalva's maneuver. Contraindications included suspected cancer, stress incontinence, or a uterus that was too large or immobile.

Twenty-three of the 30 women who underwent pelviscopic surgery had previously undergone one or more laparotomies. In the second group, only 18 had had previous operations (Table 2). In two patients with a history of chronic appendicitis, an appendectomy was performed with the hysterectomy.

A uterus that was too large was a contraindication for a pelviscopic hysterectomy. The weight distribution of the excised organs and tissue of both groups was:

Pelviscopic hysterectomy   390 + 110 g
Vaginal hysterectomy   420 + 165 g

The indications for hysterectomy as a result of bimanual examination, Papanicolaou smear, conization, and curettage were similar for both groups (Table 3). Additional operative procedures performed during hysterectomy were also comparable (Table 4).

To perform a pelviscopic hysterectomy with the surgical technique developed by Semm, we had to devel-

---

Table 1. Patient selection

Type of Operation	No. of Patients	Age Range (yr)	Average Age (yr)*
Pelviscopic hysterectomy	30	45.6 - 72.8	55.7
Vaginal hysterectomy	39	38.72 - 71.5	51.2

*The age of the patient had no influence on the indication for the type of operation.

Table 2. Patient history

Previous Operation*	No. of Patients Who Had Undergone Prior Surgery	
	Pelviscopic Surgery Group	Vaginal Surgery Group
Appendectomy	15	17
Cesarean section	7	6
One adnexal procedure	6	3
Two adnexal procedures	3	3
Stomach bypass	1	0
Pros. select. vagotomy	2	0
Partial intestinal resection	1	0

*Previous operations correlate with 23 of 30 patients in the pelviscopic group and 18 of 30 patients in the vaginal surgery group. Some patients had experienced several illnesses before hysterectomy was performed.

Table 3. Indications for hysterectomy

Condition	Pelviscopic Surgery Group	Vaginal Surgery Group
Uterine leiomyomas	16	9
Chronic recurrent metrorrhagia	7	5
Atypical endometrial hyperplasia	7	4
CIN III with total excision	0	3
Rel. urinary incontinence with uterine vaginal descent	0	9

CIN III = Cervical intraepithelial neoplasia, grade 3 (severe dysplasia and carcinoma in situ).

Table 4. Additional uterine procedures: tubal extirpations

Reason for Surgery	Pelviscopic Surgery Group	Vaginal Surgery Group
Tubal extirpation	13	17
Adhesiolysis	7	2
Ovariectomy	4	9
Cystic excision	6	2

op the following instruments: a cervical-endometrial punch (such as a Gill punch) consisting of a guide rod (5 mm in diameter and 50 cm long), a variable punch cylinder (15 to 20 mm) with a detachable rotation handle, and a uterus morcellator consisting of a cylinder (14.8 mm) with a cutting edge on one end and a rotation handle on the other end.

All procedures were video monitored. Next to the subumbilical incision for the optic trocar, two incisions were made in the upper border of the mons pubis to the left and right of the midline.

After two clamps were applied to the vaginal portion of the cervix at the 3-o'clock and 9-o'clock positions, the guide rod was brought transvaginally into the correct position, and the video monitor was used to guide a targeted perforation of the fundus.

Removal of the adnexa from the uterine superior angles was executed with an EndoGIA stapler or with an Endonaht. If an Endonaht was used, the round ligaments (ligamentia teres uteri) were separated from the tubes, and the suspensory ligaments of the ovaries (infundibulopelvic ligaments) were separated from the uterus. Use of the EndoGIA stapler enabled simultaneous detachment of the ligaments and tubes from the uterus. Adnexectomies were also performed with the EndoGIA stapler and (in some cases) with a preformed loop ligature.

After application of POR-8 (a vasopressor; one ampule diluted in 50 ml NaCl), the broad ligament and the bladder-associated peritoneum in the cervix and isthmus were mobilized and displaced without disturbance of the uterine artery. Finally, after a supracervical seralenloop was placed, punch biopsies were taken from the cervix and the body of the uterus. After the tissue punch was carefully removed, the remaining isolated uterus was ligated supracervically with the seralenloop. Because our technique separates the uterus at the neck-isthmus zone, reperitonealization was not necessary. The excised tissue was removed from the pelvic cavity with the uterus morcellator through the incision enlarged by the trocar.

To monitor possible postoperative bleeding, a Charrier 18 Redondrain that provided continuous suction drainage was inserted through one of the incisions into the pouch of Douglas and remained in position for a maximum of 24 to 48 hours.

RESULTS

The age ranges of our patients who underwent hysterectomy pelviscopically or vaginally were comparable

Table 5. Blood loss

	Pelviscopic Surgery Group (ml)	Vaginal Surgery Group (ml)
Intraoperative	40 (25 - 70)	95 (70 - 200)
Postoperative	20 (15 - 40)	ND

ND = Not determined.

(see Table 1). The average duration of the pelviscopic operation (70 minutes; range, 50 to 95) was notably longer than the vaginal variant (47 minutes; range, 32 to 98).

Extensive lysis of adhesions was necessary in 13 patients before the pelviscopic hysterectomy. In these cases, large areas of the greater omentum and intestines had become attached to the uterine surface.

The average intraoperative blood loss with pelviscopic hysterectomy was less than that of vaginal uterus extirpation, in which postoperative blood loss could not be determined because of the use of gauze strip tamponade (Table 5).

Postoperative complications including bleeding, hematomas, pelviscopic intestinal paralysis, and fever occurred less often when pelviscopic hysterectomy had been performed.

Patients who underwent pelviscopic surgery required a recovery time of 4 days. Those who underwent vaginal hysterectomy remained hospitalized for ≤8 days. One woman was readmitted 1 week after the pelviscopic procedure because of a retrovesical infiltration.

DISCUSSION

The pelviscopic hysterectomy represents a gynecological variation of minimally invasive surgery in which the topography of the pelvic floor remains intact. The sexual life of the patient seems to be less affected by pelviscopic procedures because of minimal damage to the paracervical nerve plexus.

The postoperative morbidity of patients whose uteruses were pelviscopically removed was minimal; the postoperative complication rate was also low. Pelviscopic hysterectomy results in a more rapid postoperative rehabilitation and in a subsequent earlier return to work than does vaginal hysterectomy. All of the patients who underwent pelviscopic surgery were released

Table 6. Postoperative morbidity

	Pelviscopic Surgery Group	Vaginal Surgery Group
Subfebrile temperature	(?)	(?)
Febrile temperature	7	10
Retrovesical infiltration	2	3
Infiltration in vaginal cuff	1	0
Moderate vaginal bleeding	0	6
Abdominal wall hematoma	5	0
Postoperative ileus	0	1

from the hospital on the fourth postsurgical day. Those who underwent vaginal hysterectomy were released, on average, 8 days after surgery. In contrast to the patients who underwent vaginal surgery, the group who underwent pelviscopic surgery did not suffer paralytic ileus (Table 6) and appeared to experience slightly less internal intraoperative bleeding, probably as a result of increased intra-abdominal pressure during the operation and of reduced peritoneal irritation because of the lack of extensive abdominal peritoneal dissection.

The average duration of the pelviscopic operation, 70 minutes, was longer than that of vaginal hysterectomy. However, we continue to reduce the time as we gain experience with the technique.

A particular advantage of the pelviscopic technique is that a transabdominal hysterectomy can often be avoided—even when extensive adhesions occur between the uterus, intestines, and greater omentum.

REFERENCES

1. Aldridge AHS, Meredith S. Am J Obstet Gynecol 59: 52-55, 1950.
2. Korte W. Die Bedeutung der Muskulatur des Collum uteri fur die intraisthmische Technik der Uterusexstirpation, zugleich ein Beitrag zur Vermeidung des Kollumstumpf-Karzinoms. Geburtshelfe Frauenheilkd. 24: 211-218, 1964.
3. Diokno AC. Harninkontinenz—die verschwiegene Behinderung, Part 1. New York: Aufl Acron Verlag, 1988.
4. Kilkku P, Grönross M, Hirvonen T, Rauramo L. Supravaginal uterine amputation vs. hysterectomy. Effects on libido and orgasm. Acta Obstet Gynecol Scand 62:147-152, 1983.
5. Semm K. Operationslehre für endoskopische Abdominalchirurgie—operative Pelviskopie. Stuttgart: Schattauer Verlag, 1984.
6. Nagele F, Husslein P. Zur Frage der inneren Peritonealisierung nach abdominaler Hysterektomie eine retrospektive Pilotstudie. Geburtshelfe Frauenheilkd 11:925-928, 1991.
7. Semm K. Diagnostische und operative Pelviskopie. In Zander J, Graeff W, eds. Kirschnersche allgemeine und spezielle Operationslehre, Bd IX—Gynakologische Operationen. Heidelberg: Springer-Verlag, 1991.
8. Semm K. Hysterektomie per laparotomiam oder per pelviskopiam—ein neuer Weg ohne Kolpotomie Durch CASH. Geburtshlefe Frauenheilkd 12:996-1003, 1991.
9. Semm K. Morzellieren und Nahen per pelviskopiam—kein Problem mehr. Geburtshilte Frauenheilkd 10:843-846, 1991.
10. Semm K. Tissue puncher and loop-ligation—new aids for surgical therapeutic pelviscopy (laparoscopy)—endoscopic intraabdominal surgery. Endoscopy 10:119-124, 1978.

56 Therapeutic Pelviscopy in Suppurative Pelvic Inflammatory Disease

Serge Ginter, Herbert Mecke, and Kurt Semm

Despite the availability of antibiotic treatment, suppurative conditions of the uterine adnexae remain a formidable clinical challenge. The most serious problem is rupture of an adnexal abscess into the free peritoneal cavity, with ensuing peritonitis, a complication that carries a high mortality even in the antibiotic era. Early surgical intervention under the protection of intensive antibiotic therapy has resulted in a dramatic reduction of morbidity and mortality. The intensity of the operative treatment—radical ablation or organ preservation—remains controversial.

In the women's clinic of the University of Kiel we have treated in recent years 66 patients with suppurative pelvic inflammations. For 25 of these patients a laparotomy was indicated, whereas in the remaining 41 patients we were able to proceed with endoscopic surgical techniques in the pelvis.

CLINICAL PRESENTATION

The average age of the patients who were pelviscopically treated was significantly below ($p < 0.01$) the age of patients who required laparotomy (Table 1). Four patients presented with the clinical picture of an acute abdomen, and three of these patients underwent laparotomy. In two patients whose signs and symptoms had subsided, pelviscopy was performed to elucidate the nature of an ill-defined adnexal mass.

Twenty-six patients (39%) presented with a normal WBC on admission ($<10,000/\text{ml}$). However, there was an accelerated sedimentation rate ($>10/20$) in 65 patients (98%).

TREATMENT

Depending on the severity of the clinical picture, patients were either treated first with ampicillin and metronidazole or were given an early operative approach.

The procedures performed during pelviscopy or laparotomy depended on the age of the patient, the severity of the clinical presentation, and the operative findings (Table 2). Elderly patients with adnexal masses or tumors underwent a primary laparotomy with excision of adnexae and total hysterectomy through a classic abdominal approach. In younger patients the diagnosis was usually confirmed by endoscopic pelvic examination. In these patients adhesions between various organs such as bowel, adnexae, and uterus are separated and abscessed membranes peeled off with blunt grasping forceps. If the abscess cavity cannot be entered

Table 1. Patient characteristics

Operative Procedure	Age (years)	Intrauterine Device	Duration of Complaints Before Hospital Admission (days)	Preoperative Antibiotic Therapy
Pelviscopy (n = 41)	33 ± 11* (18-57)	7 (17%)	11 ± 12 (1-60)	15
Laparotomy (n = 25)	41 ± 12* (23-76)	5 (20%)	10 ± 9 (1-38)	8

Ranges are given in parentheses. *p <0.01.

by this approach, the surrounding wall is then incised with hooked scissors—all by pelviscopy. We were able to treat most patients with pyosalpinx by an endoscopic pelvic approach, whereas bilateral tubo-ovarian abscess always required laparotomy and appropriate organ excision. The abscess cavity, pelvis, and entire abdominal cavity are carefully irrigated and all debris and fluid aspirated.

Local and systemic antibiotic coverage is established at the latest after pelviscopic diagnosis and is based on smears and cultures obtained from the pus or inflammatory exudate. Following pelviscopy a suction drain is placed; however, suction is not started until 6 hours after the procedure so as to let the intraperitoneally placed antibiotics take full effect. All patients are seen in follow-up examination within 12 to 24 months and are carefully queried about any abdominal complaints or recurrence of pelvic inflammatory disease.

RESULTS

In nine patients, unilateral or bilateral resection of a fallopian tube or adnexa was required and possible by pelviscopic techniques. Organ-saving minimally invasive surgery was successful in 80% of all patients. In five patients total abdominal hysterectomy and bilateral salpingo-oophorectomy by laparotomy were required, and in another 20 patients unilateral or bilateral salpingectomy or salpingo-oophorectomy through the same approach was indicated to bring the disease under control. The hospital stay and duration of antibiotic therapy were comparable in patients treated pelviscopically and by open procedure (Table 3).

COMPLICATIONS

In a 40-year-old patient with right salpingo-ovarian abscess, it was necessary to create a temporary ileostomy after segmental resection of ileum. A 45-year-old pa-

Table 2. Operative procedure employed in the case of pyo-ovarium, pyosalpinx, and tubo-ovarian abscess

		Pelviscopy	Laparotomy
Pyo-ovarium	Unilateral	6	2
(n = 9)	Bilateral	0	1
Pyosalpinx	Unilateral	12	4
(n = 33)	Bilateral	13	4
Tubo-ovarian abscess	Unilateral	10	8
(n = 24)	Bilateral	0	6
TOTAL (n = 66)		41	25

Table 3. Duration of hospitalization by operative procedure employed

Operative Procedure	Duration of Hospitalization (days*)			Duration of Inpatient Antibiotic Therapy
	Preoperative	Postoperative	Total	
Pelviscopy	3 ± 4	16 ± 8	19 ± 8	13 ± 6
Laparotomy	3 ± 3	18 ± 7	21 ± 7	13 ± 4

*The day of operation is not included in preoperative or postoperative day counts.

Table 4. Incidence of chronic lower abdominal pain and pelvic inflammatory disease following abscess-forming adnexitis

Chronic Lower Abdominal Pain		Recurrent PID	
After Pelviscopic Therapy	After Laparotomy	After Pelviscopic Therapy	After Laparotomy
7 of 26 (27%)	7 of 19 (37%)	2 of 26 (8%)	1 of 19 (5%)

Follow-up period is 1-2 years (n = 45). Organ-preserving surgery was performed in 21 of 26 patients (81%) following pelviscopy and in 3 of 19 (16%) following laparotomy.

tient developed a wound infection and vesicovaginal fistula after open hysterectomy and bilateral salpingo-oophorectomy. A 76-year-old patient with a salpingo-ovarian abscess extending to the right rib cage died 65 days after open hysterectomy and bilateral adnexectomy from coronary and cerebral vascular insufficiencies. The histological diagnosis was ovarian cancer.

Recurrence of PID (Table 4) was observed in two patients and treated by pelviscopic salpingectomy in one patient and by open hysterectomy and bilateral salpingo-oophorectomy in the second patient. A 37-year-old patient, initially treated by diagnostic-therapeutic pelviscopy and high-dose antibiotics for pyosalpinx, had a progressively worsening clinical course that improved dramatically with bilateral pelviscopic salpingectomy. A 44-year-old patient underwent pelviscopic salpingo-oophorectomy for ovarian abscess and was found to have ovarian carcinoma. She was treated by open total hysterectomy and resection of the remaining tube and ovary, as well as appropriate postoperative chemotherapy.

DISCUSSION

Persistent chronic episodes of low abdominal pain were observed in 27% of patients with pelviscopy and in 37% of patients who had been treated through laparotomy. The suspicion of a ruptured tubo-ovarian abscess is a clear indication for operative surgical treatment. Kaplan[4] has even recommended hysterectomy and bilateral salpingo-oophorectomy for nonruptured abscess within 24 to 72 hours of presentation. Other authors find indications for operation only if nonoperative treat-

ment has not resulted in improvement within 24 to 72 hours. For young women it is often possible to remove the affected adnexa only and leave the uterus and a less involved or uninvolved adnexa in place. The total removal of uterus and both adnexae has a high incidence of intraoperative complications; in Kaplan's series,[4] 12 of 71 patients (17%) suffered injuries of the bowel and rectum.

With nonoperative antibiotic treatment and prolonged observation, the danger of rupture of the abscess into the pelvis and peritoneal cavity increases if the clinical picture does not improve. Franklin[11] observed this complication in 15 of 120 patients so treated.

The 2- to 10-year follow-up of patients treated nonoperatively shows the need for operation to clear conditions related to the inflammatory abscess such as adnexal tumors, chronic pelvic pain, or menorrhagia or metrorrhagia in 16% to 31% of patients; pregnancy was possible in 9% to 14% of patients. The preservation of fertility with nonoperative or limited operative treatment is acquired in exchange for a higher incidence of postinflammation adnexal disease and need for corrective operations.

Aducci[15] reported on the first use of pelviscopy in the treatment of suppurative adnexal disease in 1981. Henry-Suchet[16] followed 47 such patients and found that 87% were free of any complaints, whereas 13% had chronic pelvic pain and six of 24 patients who wanted to have children did become pregnant. We found lower abdominal pain in 27% of patients with pelviscopic treatment as compared with 37% of women treated through a laparotomy; however, it should be clear that the more serious and extensive suppurative disease is treated by our open approach.

In addition, it is important to obtain sufficient tissue from the abscess wall, not only for bacterial evaluation but also for histological examination. A tubo-ovarian abscess can hide an ovarian carcinoma, in which case a radical operation—not feasible by pelviscopy—is required. The endoscopic approach to pelvic suppurative disease always results in some degree of peritoneal contamination, a danger that is greatly reduced or even totally eliminated by the open approach.

CONCLUSION

The follow-up findings of a satisfactory incidence of pregnancy and resolved postinflammatory lower abdominal pain with the pelviscopic approach to suppurative disease and tubo-ovarian abscess, are encouraging. Early diagnostic and therapeutic endoscopy for pelvic suppurative disease facilitates the appropriate operative procedure and plays a decisive role in the restoration of reproductive function and reconstruction of anatomical relationships within the pelvis. The approach is therefore especially recommended in younger women who are planning and hoping to have a family as well as in active, mature women to preserve an optimal hormonal equilibrium.

REFERENCES

1. Pedowitz P, Bloomfield RD. Ruptured adnexal abscess (tuboovarian) with generalized peritonitis. Am J Obstet Gynecol 88:721-729, 1964.
2. Mickal A, Sellmann AH, Beebe JL. Ruptured tuboovarian abscess. Am J Obstet Gynecol 100:432-436, 1977.
3. Rivlin ME, Hunt JA. Ruptured tuboovarian abscess—is hysterectomy necessary? Obstet Gynecol 98:482-487, 1967.
4.
5. Landers DV, Sweet RL. Tubo-ovarian abscess: Contemporary approach to management. Rev Infect Dis 5:876-884, 1983.
6. Landers DV, Sweet RL. Current trends in the diagnosis and treatment of tuboovarian abscess. Am J Obstet Gynecol 151:1098-1110, 1985.
7. Scott WC. Pelvic abscess in association with intrauterine contraceptive device. Am J Obstet Gynecol 131:149-156, 1978.
8. Henry-Suchet J, Soler A, Loffredo V. Laparoscopic treatment of tuboovarian abscesses. J Reprod Med 29:579-582, 1984.
9. Mecke J, Semm K. Pelviskopische Behandlung abszedierender Entzündungen im kleinen Becken. Guburtsh Frauenheilk 48:479-484, 1988.
10. Semm K. A new method of pelviscopy (gynecologic laparoscopy) for myomectomy, ovariectomy, tubectomy and adnectomy. Endoscopy 2:85-93, 1979.
11. Franklin EW, Hevron JE, Thompson JD. Management of the pelvic abscess. Clin Obstet Gynecol 16:66-79, 1973.
12. Ginsburg DS, Stern JL, Hamod KA, Genadry R, Spence MR. Tubo-ovarian abscess: A retrospective review. Am J Obstet Gynecol 23:183-189, 1980.
13. Taylor ES. Conservative surgery for pelvic inflammatory disease and endometriosis. Clin Obstet Gynecol 23:183-189, 1980.
14. Friedberg V, Schmidt W. Der Tuboovarialabszess. Gynäkologe 17:143-147, 1984.
15. Adducci JE. Laparoscopy in the diagnosis and treatment of pelvic inflammatory disease with abscess formation. Int Surg 66:359-360, 1981.
16. Henry-Suchet J. Laparoscopic treatment of tubo-ovarian abscesses. Obstet Gynecol 6(suppl 1):60-61, 1986.
17. Egger H, Fleishmann J. Der isolierte Ovarialabszess—zur Klinik, Bakteriologie und Pathogenese. Geburtsh Frauenheilk 37:625-638, 1977.

IX

Videoendoscopic Genitourinary Surgery

57 *Prospects of New Technology in Urological Procedures*

Jens J. Rassweiler, Thomas O. Henkel, Dirk M. Potempa, Reinhold Tschada,
Klaus-Peter Jünemann, and Peter Alken

Within the last 2 years laparoscopic techniques have found increasing use in urological procedures. Laparoscopic pelvic lymphadenectomy[1,2] and varicocelectomy[3] are performed more frequently at various centers, as is laparoscopic nephrectomy.[4,6] However, the frequency with which these procedures are performed cannot be compared with that of laparoscopic cholecystectomy. Most laparoscopic urological techniques require significant expertise and technological improvement. This challenge has inspired urologists to expand the indications for laparoscopic procedures. In addition, new applications of noninvasive extracorporeal techniques for organ ablation have been developed.

PREREQUISITES FOR NEW LAPAROSCOPIC UROLOGICAL PROCEDURES

The success of future laparoscopic procedures is based on the following factors:

- Laparoscopic expertise: Intra-abdominal orientation, dissection, knot tying, and suturing. This expertise can be gained by performing in vitro and in vivo training and an increasing number of clinical laparoscopies.
- Laparoscopic instruments: Endostaplers, clip applicators, needle holders, endoretractors, and tissue morcellators, all of which facilitate performance of new procedures such as laparoscopic anastomosis and organ retrieval.
- New technology: Lasers for simultaneous incision and coagulation or tissue welding, endo-Doppler techniques, and three-dimensional video. These devices may not be essential but will significantly improve the surgeon's ability to perform laparoscopic procedures.

NEW LAPAROSCOPIC PROCEDURES USED IN THE PELVIS

The primary interest in laparoscopic pelvic procedures includes radical prostatectomy and cystectomy with urinary diversion as well as easy techniques such as laparoscopic marsupialization of lymphoceles. Laparoscopic radical prostatectomy has been pioneered by Schuessler et al.[7]; however, endoscopic urethrovesical anastomosis presents many difficulties. Szabo et al.[8] have demonstrated in the canine model that after the surgeon has obtained significant microscopic and endoscopic training such as suturing or knotting, prostatectomy (including water-tight anastomosis) can be performed with acceptable duration of the procedure. Another alternative is to perform the anastomosis by stapling with a biodegradable device with an inflatable anvil, as described for the canine model by Avant.[9] Whether these procedures have clinical application or whether perineal prostatectomy with laparoscopic lymph node dissection is preferable is undetermined.[2]

Simple and partial cystectomy and bladder diverticulectomy have already been performed by some investigators,[10,11] but only in selected cases. Three areas of expertise (listed in order of increasing technical difficulty) are mandatory in laparoscopic radical cystectomy:

- Extended laparoscopic pelvic lymph node dissection (LPLND)
- Cystoprostatectomy
- Urinary diversion

Extended laparoscopic pelvic lymph node dissection has been demonstrated by Schuessler et al.,[1] and a laparoscopic ileal conduit has been performed by Kozminski and Partamian.[12] However, in those studies the ureteral anastomoses were sutured extra-abdominally (the "mini-lap" technique). As a result of extensive training with the pelvitrainer we have performed the entire procedure laparoscopically in the minipig, but we still feel that significant training is necessary before the entire procedure can be performed clinically within acceptable operative times. On the other hand, the laparoscopic reconstruction of a neobladder creates additional difficulties, such as the implantation of the ureters and the operative time necessary for the procedure. Thus widespread use of laparoscopic techniques for radical cystectomy with continent urinary diversion has not been realized.

PROCEDURES USED IN THE UPPER RETROPERITONEUM

Clayman et al.[4] have pioneered transperitoneal laparoscopic nephrectomy (TLN), but the indications for the procedure are restricted to those of benign renal disease. Coptcoat et al.[5] and Rassweiler et al.[6] showed that transperitoneal radical tumor nephrectomy, including en bloc removal of the kidney, Gerota's fascia, and the adrenal gland, is possible for smaller organ-confined tumors when the EndoGIA is used for separate dissection of the hilar vessels and the upper adrenal pole (Fig. 1).

We prefer digital morcellation of the organ within the entrapment sack (Lapsac), which allows classification of the tumor by the pathologist. We feel that laparoscopic technique facilitates dissection and ensures that all criteria of tumor surgery are fulfilled. The respective Lapsac, Espiner bag, or a newly designed organ bag (Fig. 2) are tumor cell impermeable and cannot be injured by digital morcellation. Thus the risk of tumor cell spreading during the procedure is minimal. Long-term studies are necessary to determine the usefulness of laparoscopy for this indication.

TLN can also be combined with antegrade ureteral stripping after transurethral circumcision of the orifice[13] for laparoscopic nephroureterectomy (Fig. 3), for which the primary indication (other than reflux nephropathy) is transitional cell carcinoma of the upper urinary tract. The total operative time of this procedure is approximately 4 hours, which is comparable to that

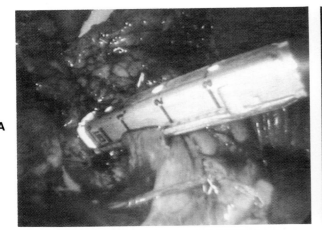

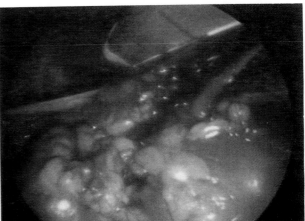

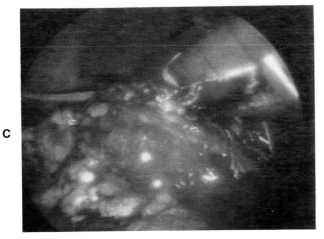

Fig. 1. EndoGIA stapling device for separate dissection of renal hilar vessels. **A,** EndoGIA (white magazine) closed around renal artery. **B,** Open EndoGIA is placed around renal vein. **C,** Dissection of renal vein. Stapler fires six rows of clips and dissects between third and fourth rows.

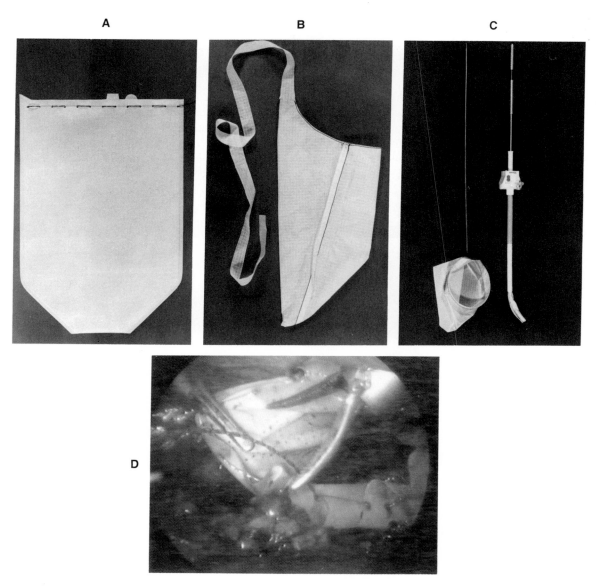

Fig. 2. Available organ entrapment sacks: **A,** (Lapsac, Cook), Self-expanding, closed within abdomen. **B,** Espiner bag, not self-expanding, being pulled out by retrieval string. **C,** Newly designed bag (Angiomed), which can be opened and closed intra-abdominally by special shape-memory ring of nickel-titanium. **D,** Entrapment of kidney, including Gerota's fascia, in Lapsac.

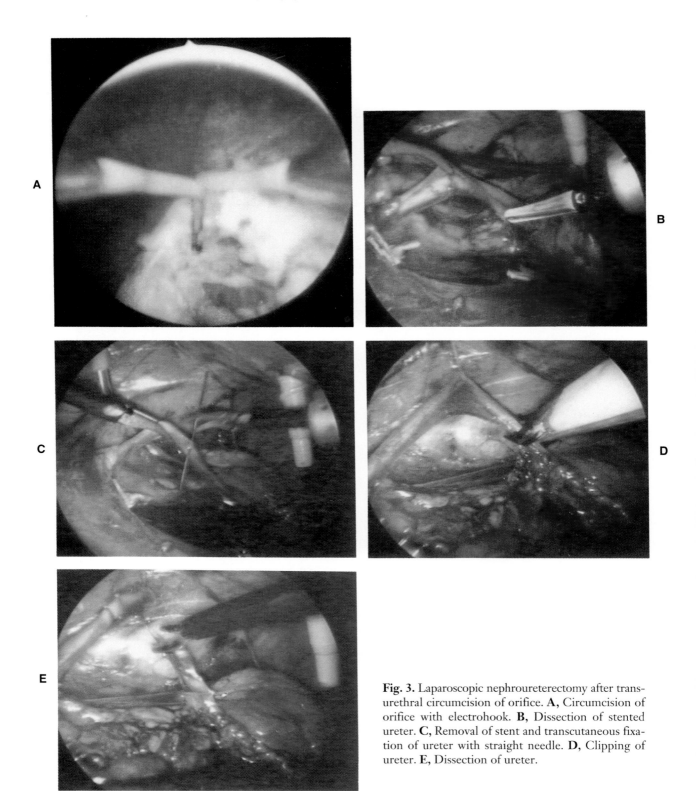

Fig. 3. Laparoscopic nephroureterectomy after transurethral circumcision of orifice. **A,** Circumcision of orifice with electrohook. **B,** Dissection of stented ureter. **C,** Removal of stent and transcutaneous fixation of ureter with straight needle. **D,** Clipping of ureter. **E,** Dissection of ureter.

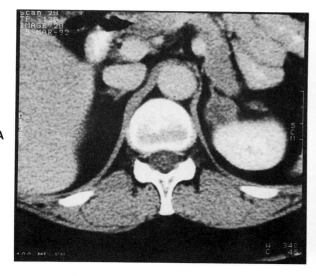
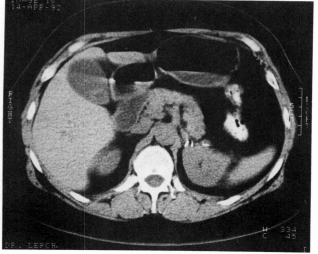

A

B

Fig. 4. Laparoscopic adrenalectomy. **A,** CT scan before procedure shows left-side adrenal tumor. **B,** CT scan after laparoscopic removal of cortical adenoma shows endoclips.

of the standard open surgical technique. Contraindications are a previous operation or radiotherapy in the pelvis. The results of long-term series must be used to determine the value of this technique in tumor removal.

Transperitoneal laterocolic access can also be used in laparoscopic adrenalectomy of a cortical adrenal adenoma (Fig. 4). Kiyotaki[14] has used the operative endoscope of Buess to perform retroperitoneal adrenalectomy, which may be used as an alternative to the transperitoneal approach; however, the size of the endoscope (40 mm) and the restricted view must be considered.

Another useful technique is the modified laparoscopic retroperitoneal lymph node dissection of stage I testicular tumors. Hulbert and Fraley[15] presented first experiences with this approach. Laparoscopy could provide the solution to the conflict of surveillance therapy and diagnostic operative lymphadenectomy in stage I disease of nonseminomatous germ cell carcinoma.

Laparoscopic pyeloplasty, which may be indicated only for primary stenosis, has been performed by Schuessler et al. Reports of long-term series can be used to determine whether the outcome will be superior to those of established percutaneous pyelolysis.

Sound Wave Technology

The improvement of ultrasonic and fluoroscopic localization systems and their use in multifunctional shock wave lithotriptors (third-generation machines) have resulted in the development of new devices that use high-energy ultrasound waves for extracorporeal tissue ablation.[16,17] This new technique is called extracorporeal focused pyrotherapy (Fig. 5). Initial experimental studies and clinical phase I trials have shown that as a result of ultrasonographic localization, a circumscribed coagulation necrosis can be induced. Possible applications, might include small renal cell carcinoma, liver metastases, and benign prostatic hyperplasia. The primary problems include obtaining exact imaging of the organ to be ablated and the monitoring of the procedure.[16,17]

Laser Technology

Modification of different laser systems ensures optimal use of laser technology for the following indications:

- Dye laser with an optical feedback stone detection device (Fig. 6) allows intracorporeal lasertripsy (LISL) of ureteral or bile duct stone.[18]
- Nd:YAG laser probes have been developed for use in the intraluminal[19] or interstitial ablation of prostatic adenomas.
- CO_2 or KTP-532 laser can be used for microsurgical or laparoscopic laser-assisted anastomosis (laser welding[21]).
- KTP laser has been used in simultaneous laparoscopic dissection and coagulation.[2,7,20]

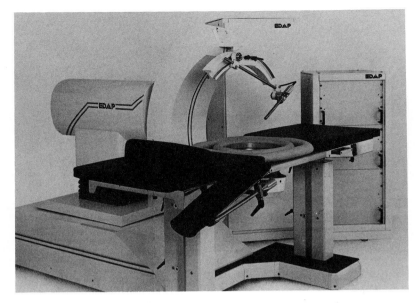

Fig. 5. Clinical prototype for extracorporeal focused pyrotherapy (Edap, France).

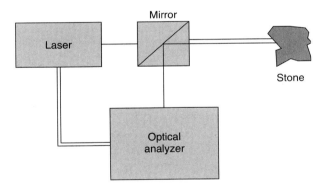

Fig. 6. Principle of optical feedback for stone detection for laser lithotripsy (Telemit). Laser light reflected by the targeted stone or tissue is analyzed. If tissue is targeted, laser release is automatically blocked.

CONCLUSION

Laser technology will have a significant effect on minimally invasive endoscopic urologic procedures. However, it must be determined whether this technical modality can be used cost effectively.

REFERENCES

1. Schuessler WW, Vancaillie TG, Reich H, Griffith DP. Transperitoneal endosurgical lymphadenectomy in patients with localized prostate cancer. J Urol 145:988-991, 1991.
2. Winfield HN, Donovan JF, See WA, Loening SA, William RD. Laparoscopic pelvic lymph node dissection for genitourinary malignancies: Indications, technique, and results. J Endourol 6:103-112, 1992.
3. Hagood PG, Mehan DJ, Worischek JH, Andrus CH, Parra RO. Laparoscopic varicocelectomy: Preliminary report of a new technique. J Urol 147:73-76, 1992.
4. Clayman RV, Kavoussi LR, Soper N, Dierks SM, Mertyk S, Darcy MD, Roemer FD, Pingleton ED, Thomson PG, Long SR. Laparoscopic nephrectomy: Initial case report. J Urol 146:278-282, 1991.
5. Coptcoat M, Joyce A, Rassweiler J, Popert R. Laparoscopic nephrectomy: The Kings and Mannheim clinical experience [abstract]. J Urol 147:433 A, 1992.
6. Rassweiler J, Henkel TO, Potempa D, Günther M, Alken P. Die transperitoneale laparoskopiesche Nephrektomie. Aktuel Urol 23 (in press).
7. Schuessler W, Kavoussi LR, Clayman RV, Vancaillie TG. Laparoscopic radical prostatectomy: Initial case report [abstract]. J Urol 147:246 A, 1992.

8. Szabo Z, Bowyer DW, Moran ME. Operative laparoscopy in urology: Intracorporeal suturing of the lower urinary tract [abstract]. J Urol 147:408 A, 1992.
9. Avant L. Vesicourethral anastomosis stapling technique following radical prostatectomy in the animal. Video presentation at the American Urological Association Meeting, Toronto, 1991.
10. Das S, Creek W. Laparoscopic bladder diverticulectomy [abstract]. J Urol 147:407 A, 1992.
11. Lowe BA, Novy MJ, Strang E. Laparoscopic segmental cystectomy [abstract]. J Urol 147:408 A, 1992.
12. Kozminski M, Partamian KO. Case report of laparoscopic ileal loop conduit. J Endourol 6:147-150, 1992.
13. Bub P, Rassweiler J, Eisenberger F. Harnleiterstripping nach transurethraler Ostium-umschneidung—eine Alternative zur Uretektomie. Aktuel Urol 20:67-69, 1989.
14. Kiyotaki S. Endoscopic adrenalectomy [abstract]. In Proceedings of the Third International Congress of Minimally Invasive Therapy, Boston, November 1991, The Congress.
15. Hulbert JC, Fraley EE. Laparoscopic retroperitoneal lymphadenectomy: Next approach to pathologic staging of clinical stage I germ cell tumors of the testis. J Endourol 6:123-126, 1992.
16. Ter Har G, Sinnett D, Rivens I. High intensity focused ultrasound: A surgical technique for the treatment of discrete liver tumors. Phys Med Biol 34:1734-1750, 1989.
17. Vallancien G, Harouni M, Veillon B, Mombet A, Prapotnich D, Brisset JM, Bougaran J. Focused extracorporeal pyrotherapy: Feasibility study in man. J Endourol 6:173-181, 1992.
18. Rassweiler J, Tschada R, Henkel TO, Jünemann KP, Alken P. Lasertripsy—the importance of an optical feedback-controlled stone detection device in ESWL-resistant ureteral calculi [abstract]. J Urol 147:295 A, 1992.
19. McCullough DL, Roth RA, Babayan RK, Gordon JO, Reece J, Crawford ED, Fuselier A, Krane RJ, Assimos DG, Harrison LH, Elliot JP, Miliam WH, Daniels GF. TULIP—transurethral ultrasound-guided laser-induced prostatectomy—National Human Cooperative Study results [abstract]. J Urol 147:306 A, 1992.
20. Poppas DP, Sutaria P, Sosa E, Mininberg DT, Vaughan ED, Schlossberg SM. Re-establishing continuity of the ureter using laser tissue welding solders for laparoscopic surgery [abstract]. J Urol 147:244 A, 1992.
21. Albala DM, Schuessler WW, Vancaillie TG. Laparoscopic bladder neck suspension. J Endourol 6:137-142, 1992.
22. Rassweiler J, Köhrmann KU, Potempa D, Henkel TO, Jünemann KP, Alken P. Extracorporeal shock wave lithotripsy for renal calculi: Current status and future aspects. Minimally Invasive Ther 1:141-156, 1992.
23. Rassweiler J, Henkel TO, Köhrmann KU, Potempa D, Jünemann KP, Alken P. Lithotripter technology: Present and future. J Endourol 6:1-13, 1992.

58 *Laparoscopic Nephrectomy*

David M. Albala

The earliest recorded renal operations date to 400 BC, with the drainage of abscesses and removal of calculi from patients with renal fistulas. In the early nineteenth century, kidneys sometimes were removed inadvertently during ovarian operations, but doctors observed that the remaining kidney continued to produce normal amounts of urine. In 1869 in Heidelberg, Germany, Gustav Simon reported the first successful nephrectomy in a 46-year-old female with an incurable ureterovaginal fistula.[1] Of the first 10 patients to undergo a nephrectomy, only two survived. Because of the high mortality rate resulting from peritonitis in the early years of renal operations, the extraperitoneal approach became the standard. Surgeons of the late nineteenth century experienced a nearly 50% mortality rate in patients undergoing a nephrectomy. Since then, improvements in instrumentation and aseptic methods have dropped this rate below 2%.[2]

The uncertainty surrounding the feasibility of nephrectomies gradually resolved with the work of a number of investigators of the past century. In 1889 Tuffier noted that experimental animals required a minimum of 1 to 1.5 g/kg body weight of renal tissue to survive. In 1895 Gerota described the anatomy of the renal fascia, and in 1903 Gregoire emphasized the importance of removing malignant kidney tumors en bloc with perirenal fat, the adrenal gland, and lymph nodes. W. J. Mayo, Konig, Kuster, Nagamatsu, and others have since contributed to renal operative technique with a multiplicity of approaches and a greater understanding of diseases involving the kidney.[3]

Despite continued advances, however, significant morbidity can be associated with open procedures on the kidney. For the patient, traditional operative procedures result in significant postoperative pain, hospitalization, convalescence, and disfigurement. As a result, laparoscopy has been used to treat diseases affecting the upper urinary tract. Procedures such as laparoscopic cholecystectomy and dissection of pelvic lymph nodes have confirmed the advantages of the laparoscopic technique when compared with its open-technique counterparts.[4,5] This chapter focuses on the indications, patient preparation, technique, and results of laparoscopic nephrectomy.

INDICATIONS

A laparoscopic nephrectomy may be indicated when a patient's kidney has been irreparably damaged because of long-standing infection, calculus, or obstruction. A laparoscopic nephrectomy may also be indicated in a patient with uncontrollable renovascular hypertension when the patient's general condition is too poor to permit revascularization or when ischemic atrophy is so severe it precludes functional recovery. Irrespective of the indications for nephrectomy in patients with benign disease, a thorough understanding of the patient's disease process and general medical condition, the functional status of the contralateral kidney, and the concurrent regional pathology is necessary before removal of a renal unit.

Although laparoscopic nephrectomy is ideally suited for patients with benign renal disease, several concerns exist regarding its application in patients with renal malignancy. The first of these is the inability to evaluate the patient's intra-abdominal cavity completely for metastatic disease, which can be done by palpation during an open laparotomy. The entire intra-abdominal cavity can be inspected during laparoscopy; however, this process is time consuming.

A second concern is the potential for tumor seeding during renal dissection. Current laparoscopic techniques allow removal of the entire kidney en bloc, including all of Gerota's fascia except for a small portion overlying the adrenal gland. Although the need for an adrenalectomy has been questioned in patients with renal tumors in the lower half of the kidney, it is still recommended for all patients with renal tumors affecting the upper half of the kidney. Robey and Schellhammer[6] have shown that an adrenalectomy is of little or no benefit in establishing tumor-free margins in patients with a lower pole or midportion renal cell cancer.

A third concern is the potential for tumor seeding during morcellation. At present, the kidney is placed in an entrapment sack (e.g., Lapsac, Cook) before morcellation, effectively isolating it from the peritoneal cavity. This sack has been evaluated using dialysis studies and has been shown totally impermeable.

Morcellation is performed completely within the entrapment sack; hence no intra-abdominal contamination occurs. Laboratory testing has shown no flux of electrolytes (sodium, chloride, potassium), glucose, or bacteria (*Escherichia coli, Staphylococcus aureus*) through the sack for up to 24 hours after morcellation. Based on these studies, neither renal dissection nor morcellation should result in tumor spillage.

In patients undergoing laparoscopic nephrectomy, the surgical margins cannot be evaluated fully. And although the histological morphology is unaltered by morcellation, pathological staging is impossible. Debate continues about whether this limited information will alter a patient's treatment because effective adjunct therapy could not be designed to treat patients with advanced disease.

With current laparoscopic techniques, however, large tumors may not be adequately removed because of the limited size of the abdominal cavity, which restricts extended dissection and manipulation into the organ entrapment system. Consequently, the time for applying laparoscopic nephrectomy to include renal cell carcinoma has not yet arrived. At present, laparoscopic nephrectomy and nephroureterectomy should be performed in selected patients with low-grade transitional cell carcinoma confined to the intrarenal collecting system. Overall, performing a laparoscopic ablative operation for renal and ureteral malignancy remains a highly controversial area.

Furthermore, laparoscopic nephrectomy is not indicated in patients with extensive adhesions from multiple, prior open operations, those with a history of sepsis and peritonitis, those with morbid obesity or dilated large bowel, and those with a bleeding coagulopathy. The urine of all patients undergoing a laparoscopic nephrectomy should be free of infection before they undergo the operation.

PATIENT PREPARATION

All patients undergoing a laparoscopic nephrectomy require a mechanical bowel preparation to decompress the intestines and prepare the bowel for inadvertent injury during trocar placement or renal dissection. Broad-spectrum parenteral antibiotics are given 1 hour before the procedure, and all patients are typed and cross-matched for blood transfusion.

LAPAROSCOPIC TECHNIQUE

A general anesthetic is recommended for all patients undergoing a laparoscopic nephrectomy because of the length of the procedure and the patient's position. Controlled ventilation through an endotracheal tube is necessary to ensure adequate oxygenation and avoid hypercarbia. The use of nitrous oxide should be avoided because it may distend the bowel during prolonged laparoscopic procedures.

Under fluoroscopic guidance, the ipsilateral ureter is intubated retrograde with a 7 Fr 11.5 mm ureteral occlusion balloon catheter. The tip of the catheter is placed within the renal pelvis, and the balloon is inflated. The catheter is then pulled downward until it occludes the ureteropelvic junction. A 0.038 inch Amplatz super-stiff guidewire is passed into the catheter and secured in place with a Touhy-Borst adapter. This catheter helps locate the ureter during dissection of the kidney. After the balloon catheter has been positioned, a Foley catheter is placed to allow the bladder to be drained. A nasogastric tube is also placed to keep the stomach and bowels decompressed.

The patient is initially placed in the supine position on a beanbag with sequential compression stockings on the legs to prevent venous thrombosis. The contralateral arm is padded in foam rubber, and an axillary roll is placed to prevent injury to the brachial plexus. The entire abdomen is prepared and shaped all the way to the posterior axillary line on the side of the ipsilateral flank.

A 14-gauge Veress needle is passed through the umbilicus into the peritoneal cavity, and a pneumoperitoneum is established with CO_2. With the patient in a 30-degree head-down position, a midline 11 mm trocar replaces the Veress needle at the umbilicus. Another 11 mm trocar is placed in the midclavicular line 1 cm below the costal margin, and a 5.5 mm trocar is placed in the midclavicular line approximately 5 cm below the level of the umbilicus. At this point, the patient is turned into a full lateral position, and a fourth 5.5 mm trocar

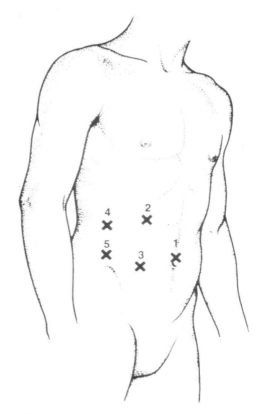

Fig. 1. Port placement for a laparoscopic nephrectomy: 11 mm trocars are placed in positions 1 and 2, and 5 mm trocars are placed in positions 3, 4, and 5.

is placed at the tip of the twelfth rib. A fifth 5.5 mm trocar is positioned 5 cm below this trocar in the anterior axillary line (Fig. 1).

The patient's abdomen is inspected for injuries that may have occurred during trocar placement, and adhesions that could interfere with the renal dissection are taken down. The patient then is placed in a steep Trendelenburg position to help shift the bowels out of the operative field.

The lateral peritoneal reflection of the colon is identified and sharply incised using electrocautery scissors. With gentle traction on the medial edge of the cut peritoneum, the colon can be freed from its retroperitoneal attachments with blunt and sharp dissection. The peritoneal incision should be extended to the level of the iliac vessel. To mobilize the colon adequately, the hepatic and splenic flexure must be taken down on the right or left side, respectively.

The ureteral catheter is then manipulated to help identify the ureter, and blunt dissection is used to isolate the ureter. The ureter is dissected from its retroperitoneal attachments and secured with a 5 mm locking forceps. Care is taken not to transect the ureter; it serves as a crucial landmark in the identification of the renal hilus. As dissection of the ureter continues superiorly, the gonadal vessels can be identified crossing anteriorly. They should be ligated with endoscopic clips and transected.

Following the ureter superiorly, the lower pole of the kidney can be identified and freed from its surrounding tissues. The ureter is then regrasped at the lower pole of the kidney and traction placed inferiorly. The perihilar fat is dissected from the renal vessels; the tissue around each vessel should be carefully dissected to create a free window of adequate length. A multiple-load, single-clip applier is helpful in placing three clips on the proximal end and two clips on the distal end of each vessel, and hook scissors are used to transect each vessel sharply.

Once the hilar vessels have been transected, an incision is made in Gerota's fascia just below the level of the adrenal gland. The upper pole is carefully dissected out, and the remaining posterior and lateral attachments can be dissected free. The ureter is then clipped with the multiple load single-clip applier and transected. The proximal ureter is grasped with a locking forceps, and the entire kidney is repositioned on the surface of the liver. The renal fossa and vascular stumps should be carefully inspected for hemostasis and irrigated with an antibiotic solution. An impermeable nylon entrapment sack is then introduced through the 11 mm subcostal midclavicular trocar site. The mouth of the sack is opened, using grasping forceps, and the laparoscope is moved from the 11 mm umbilical port to the 11 mm superior midclavicular line port. With the use of three grasping forceps placed through the 5 mm ports, the mouth of the sack if held open by the tabs, which are spaced equally around its neck. The kidney, suspended by its ureter, is then removed from the liver and placed in the sack. The grasper holding the ureter is released, and the drawstrings on the sack are grasped with a 5 mm forceps passed through the 11 mm umbilical port. The drawstring around the neck of the bag is tightened, and the neck of the sack is brought out onto the abdominal wall.

An electric tissue morcellator (Cook) is used through the exteriorized neck of the sack to remove the kidney in successive fragments (Fig. 2). The morcellation process is monitored laparoscopically to ensure the morcellator does not perforate the bag, causing loss of tissue and injury to the underlying structures. The tissue is collected in a trap of the morcellator and is sent for histological analysis (Fig. 3). When all the renal tissue has been removed, the empty sack is pulled through the umbilical trocar site.

At the end of the operation, the abdomen is inspected to ensure adequate hemostasis and to identify inadvertent bowel injury. All trocars are removed under direct vision to inspect for abdominal wall bleeding, and the CO_2 is emptied from the peritoneal cavity. The 11 mm trocar sites are closed with a single fascial suture of No. 1 polyglactin, and the skin is closed with a subcuticular suture of 4-0 polyglycolic acid. The 5 mm trocar sites are closed with adhesive strips.

The nasogastric tube is removed from the patient in the recovery room, and a parenteral broad-spectrum antibiotic is administered for 24 hours. The sequential stockings are left in place until the patient is ambulatory, usually on the first postoperative day. Patients are permitted to resume their usual activities as tolerated.

DISCUSSION

In 1990 Clayman et al.[7] successfully carried out the first clinical laparoscopic nephrectomy on an 85-year-old woman with a right lower renal mass measuring 3 cm. Since this initial report, numerous other investigators in both the United States and Europe have performed this procedure.

To date, 18 laparoscopic nephrectomies have been performed at the Washington University Medical Center, the Peter Bent Brigham, and the Loyola University Medical Center in 11 women and 7 men with an average age of 48 years (range, 16 to 85 years). Three of these patients had prior abdominal surgery. The indications for laparoscopic surgery were chronic pain, infection, and a nonfunctioning kidney in 15 patients, renovascular hypertension in one, and a renal mass in two. The kidneys were removed from 17 patients in a transperitoneal manner, and one underwent a complete retroperitoneal procedure. In this latter patient, a Veress needle was placed in the retroperitoneum just below the kidney under fluoroscopic guidance. The area was then insufflated with CO_2. Because of the limited space in the retroperitoneum, a superior trocar was placed in the tenth intercostal space, resulting in a postoperative pneumothorax. Renal dissection was accomplished without problems; however, the limited space caused difficulty in placing the kidney in the retrieval bag.

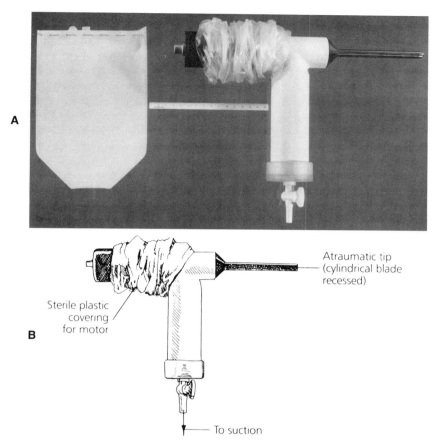

Fig. 2. A, Entrapment sack and high-speed electric tissue morcellator. **B,** Schematic diagram of the morcellator. (**A** from Zucker KA, ed. Surgical Laparoscopy Update. St. Louis: Quality Medical Publishing, 1993; **B** from Clayman RV, McDougall EM, eds. Laparoscopic Urology. St. Louis: Quality Medical Publishing, 1993.)

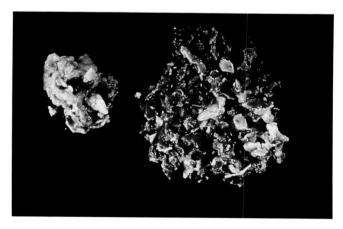

Fig. 3. Gross appearance of morcellated renal tissue.

In the initial eight patients preoperative renal artery embolization was done to help control the renal vessels and decrease hemorrhage. This step has subsequently been abandoned. The average operating time to complete a laparoscopic nephrectomy after retrograde ureteral catheterization was 5½ hours (range, 2½ to 9.2 hours), the bulk of which was spent identifying and dissecting the ureter and the renal vessels. Morcellation was completed in 5 to 20 minutes. Average blood loss was estimated at < 250 ml; no patients received an intraoperative blood transfusion.

The average weight of the kidneys was 150 g (range, 33 to 300 g), and the average length was 11 cm (range, 2 to 18 cm). The pathological process was not altered by morcellation, and most patients demonstrated nephrosclerosis and chronic inflammation. Pathological evaluation of the two patients who had tumors revealed an oncocytoma and a renal cell carcinoma.

Oral intake was begun by the second postoperative day (Table 1). Four early postoperative complications occurred. Transient congestive heart failure developed in the initial two patients because of excessive intraoperative fluid replacement. These two patients also experienced a drop in their hematocrit value and were transfused. No evidence of postoperative bleeding was demonstrated by computed tomography, and the decrease in hematocrit value was likely the result of dilution from fluid overload. To avoid this kind of complication, the intraoperative fluid replacement in patients undergoing laparoscopic procedures should be kept at a maintenance level. The third complication was a pulmonary embolism, which was resolved with anticoagulant therapy. The fourth complication was a pneumothorax, which occurred in the patient undergoing a retroperitoneal approach and resolved after chest tube drainage for several days.

The patients' average hospital stay was 4.3 days (range, 1 to 11 days). The patient with the pulmonary embolism had the longest hospital stay because of the time needed to achieve anticoagulation through oral medication. The average time until patients returned to routine activity was 12 days. In each patient the laparoscopic wounds healed without complication; however, two patients received a 1-week oral antibiotic course to ward off an impending skin infection. Oral pain medication averaged less than two narcotic tablets per patient. Most patients were discharged without any oral narcotic analgesics.

CONCLUSION

At present laparoscopic nephrectomy is a viable procedure in which the entire kidney is dissected free through a videoendoscopic approach. The technique uses entrapment of the specimen by a sack in combination with a recently developed high-speed electrical tissue morcellator for specimen evacuation. This technique should be limited to patients requiring a nephrectomy for benign renal disease. With advances in technology, this technique may some day also have applications in individuals with renal cell carcinoma.

Clearly the laparoscopic procedure is rapidly becoming an alternative to the incisional procedure under the right circumstances. With each day, another standard open operative procedure in urology is being performed with a laparoscope. Although the operative time is lengthy when compared with that of open exploration, increased experience and improved equipment will decrease it. This new technology markedly decreases the patient's need for analgesics, hospital stays, and convalescence. In the future a surgeon will be able to reduce patient discomfort, improve healing of scars, and prevent infection and the disability associated with a large abdominal incision.

REFERENCES

1. Murphy LJT. The kidney. In The History of Urology. Springfield, Ill.: Charles C Thomas, 1972, pp 252-253.
2. Crawford ED. Radical nephrectomy. In Crawford ED, Borden TA, eds. Genitourinary Cancer Surgery. Philadelphia: Lea & Febiger, 1982.
3. Crawford ED. Nephrectomy and nephroureterectomy. In Glenn JF, ed. Urologic Surgery. Philadelphia: JB Lippincott, 1991.
4. Reddick EJ, Olsen DO. Laparoscopic laser cholecystectomy: A comparison with mini-lap cholecystectomy. Surg Endosc 3:131-133, 1989.
5. Schuessler WW, Vancaillie TG, Reich H, et al. Transperitoneal endosurgical lymphadenectomy in patients with localized prostate cancer. J Urol 145:988-991, 1991.

Table 1. Postoperative Course

Activity	Length of Time	Range
Oral intake	1.9 days	1 - 6
Hospital stay	4.3 days	2 - 11
Return to work	1.7 wk	1 - 3

6. Robey EL, Schellhammer PF. The adrenal gland and renal cell carcinoma: Is ipsilateral adrenalectomy a necessary component of radical nephrectomy? J Urol 135:453-455, 1986.

7. Clayman RV, Kavoussi LR, Soper NJ, et al. Laparoscopic nephrectomy. N Engl J Med 324:1370-1372, 1990.

8. Clayman RV, McDougall EM. Laparoscopic renal surgery: Nephrectomy and renal cyst decortication. In Clayman RV, McDougall EM, eds. Laparoscopic Urology. St. Louis: Quality Medical Publishing, 1993.

59 Laparoscopic Pelvic Lymph Node Dissection for Staging of Prostatic Cancer

Jean D. Doublet, Bernard Gattegno, and Philippe Thibault

Assessment of pelvic lymph node status is a major factor in staging or prostatic cancer. Even when an abdominopelvic CT scan examination yields negative results in patients with organ-confined disease, 7% to 30% will have lymph node metastases upon pathological examination and will not benefit from radical prostatectomy.[1-4] Therefore open pelvic lymph node dissection is a mandatory step before radical prostatectomy, but this procedure has its own morbidity.[5] Moreover, frozen section analysis of the lymph nodes is not a totally reliable indicator.[6] Laparoscopy enables minimally invasive pelvic lymph node dissection. We have been using this technique since November 1991 and have evaluated its morbidity, effectiveness, and its place in the therapeutic strategy for prostatic cancer.

MATERIALS AND METHODS

Twenty-five patients underwent laparoscopic pelvic lymph node dissection (LPLND) for staging of prostatic cancer from November 1991 through January 1993. The mean age was 66 years (range, 57 to 77 years). According to the results of clinical examination, endorectal ultrasonography, serum PSA value, chest x-ray evaluation, CT scan, and bone scan, the cancer was initially considered to be stage A1 in three patients, A2 in seven, B1 in ten, B2 in three, and C in two. The Gleason grade was 2 in one patient, 4 in one, 6 in fourteen, 7 in four, 8 in three, and unknown in two patients referred from another center (with cancers described as "well differentiated"). From the results of the CT scan, lymph node metastasis was suspected in three patients. We have no experience with CT-guided needle biopsy. One patient had peritoneal nodes, diagnosed as ectopic splenic tissue. In all patients bone scan was considered as normal. The mean PSA value was 25 ng/ml (range, 2.5 to 135). Seventeen patients had a PSA value of more than 10 ng/ml. One patient had previous cholecystectomy, another had had a laparotomy for an abdominal gunshot wound. Eight patients had had previous appendectomies, and two had had inguinal hernia repairs. One patient had undergone external radiotherapy for prostatic cancer 5 years before laparoscopic surgery and was considered for salvage prostatectomy. All patients were informed of the potential advantages of and inconveniences associated with the technique and about the potential need for a laparotomy; the patients gave their consent for operation. The patients themselves decided if they would have one- or two-step surgery. During the same period, three patients underwent LPLND for staging of bladder cancer, and five underwent miscellaneous laparoscopic procedures.

Technique

No mechanical bowel preparation or preoperative antibiotics were given. LPLND was performed with the patient under general anesthesia. A nasogastric tube and a urethral catheter were placed. A pneumoperitoneum was created through a Palmer needle placed below the umbilical crease after control of the intraperitoneal position by aspiration-injection of air. Four to five liters of CO_2 were insufflated at a maximum pressure of 14 mm Hg. We placed one 10 mm port under the umbil-

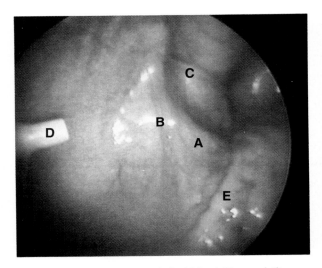

Fig. 1. Preoperative view (left side). *A*, External iliac artery; *B*, spermatic vessels; *C*, vas; *D*, left port; *E*, sigmoid.

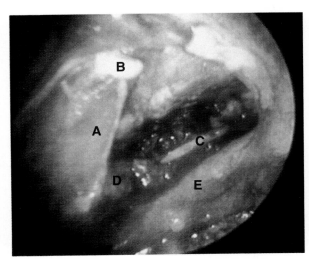

Fig. 2. Peroperative view. *A*, external iliac vein; *B*, vas (transected); *C*, obturator nerve; *D*, lymph node packet; *E*, umbilical fold.

icus for the laparoscope and assessed the correct intraperitoneal position of the port. One other 10 mm port was placed 3 cm above the symphysis pubis, and two 5.5 mm ports (one in each iliac fossa) were placed under laparoscopic control, as previously described.[7] After inspection of the intraperitoneal organs, the operating table was placed in a 20-degree Trendelenburg position, so that the bowel loops migrated to the upper part of the abdominal cavity. The main anatomical landmarks (Fig. 1) are the vas, the umbilical artery, and the external iliac artery. The vas was cut, and then the peritoneal membrane was incised along the external iliac artery. The distal end of the vas was then pulled medially to allow access to the lymph nodes. Dissection of lymphatic and fatty tissue was started just behind the posterior aspect of the pubic bone, which is the second anatomical landmark. The tissue in the area delimited by the external iliac vein, the obturator nerve, the posterior aspect of the pubic bone, and the common iliac bifurcation was removed, using a teasing and cutting technique. The obturator nerve must be clearly seen and preserved (Fig. 2). Hemostasis and obliteration of large lymphatic vessels were obtained by cauterization and clips. The tissue was removed through the lower 10 mm port. The area was then irrigated with saline to control the quality of hemostasis and the other side was dissected. At the end of the procedure the abdominal cavity was in-

spected again to rule out any visceral injury, and the three working ports were removed under laparoscopic control. The laparoscope was then removed and the pneumoperitoneum desufflated. We did not close the fascia. The skin incisions were stapled.

Four patients underwent retropubic radical prostatectomy during the same procedure after frozen section examination of the lymph nodes, and 16 underwent delayed radical prostatectomy after complete pathological examination of the lymph nodes. One patient chose to undergo radiotherapy. Average follow-up after laparoscopy was 7.6 months (range, 1 to 15 months).

RESULTS
Duration

The mean duration of bilateral dissection was 95 ± 45 minutes (range, 35 to 180 minutes); this decreased with surgeon experience. We performed 22 bilateral dissections and two unilateral dissections. We had one technical failure (no lymph node removed by laparoscopy; laparotomy needed). One procedure was interrupted after one side had been dissected because of veinous bleeding and another because one peritoneal node proved to be malignant on frozen section. We had one technical failure and interrupted the procedure after 2 hours because of the poor quality of the pneumoperitoneum.

Mortality

A 66-year-old patient with intraperitoneal metastases died of a stroke on postoperative day 1, without perioperative complication or local delayed complication.

Perioperative Morbidity

One injury of the external iliac vein required laparotomy for control. One ileal injury in a patient with numerous adhesions after appendectomy occurred during adhesiolysis. The lymph nodes were removed and the wound was sutured through a McBurney incision, and the patient was discharged on day 7. He was readmitted 25 days later for an intra-abdominal infected hematoma that required laparotomy with no further complication. In another patient a ureteral injury was diagnosed on day 5, 3 days after the patient had been discharged from the hospital; this was sutured on a double J stent, and no further complications occurred. Three cases of pneumoscrotum were exsufflated at the end of the procedure without further complication.

Postoperative Morbidity

One patient had a transient bilateral obturator nerve paresia, which improved within 1 week. A patient who had previously undergone radiation therapy had a self-resolving perineal lymphedema for 4 weeks. No patient required blood transfusion after LPLND as a single procedure and no deep veinous thrombosis was encountered.

Number of Lymph Nodes

The mean number of lymph nodes removed was 3.7 ± 2.1 (range 1 to 9) on the right side, 4.7 ± 2.1 (range, 2 to 9) on the left side and 8.3 ± 3.1 (range, 4 to 17) for the bilateral LPLND. We checked the obturator fossa in every patient who underwent immediate or delayed laparotomy, and no complementary dissection was needed.

Histological Findings

Four patients had lymph node metastases. PSA value was respectively 12, 35, 60, and 60 ng/ml. Clinical stage was B1, B2, B2, and C, and Gleason score was "well differentiated" for the first patient (referred from another institution), 8, 6, and 7. In one of these cases, metastasis was suspected preoperatively on CT scan. One patient had a negative frozen section examination and underwent subsequent radical prostatectomy. Micrometastases were diagnosed on final pathological examina-

tion. The three other patients did not undergo prostatectomy and received hormonal therapy. One other patient had peritoneal metastases (PSA 47 ng/ml, stage A2, and Gleason grade 6).

Length of Hospitalization

The median length of stay for patients undergoing LPLND as a single procedure was 2 days (range, 1 to 11 days), and the average length of stay was 2.9 days.

Radical Prostatectomy

Five patients underwent perineal radical prostatectomy, and fifteen underwent retropubic radical prostatectomy. One patient received external radiation therapy. The median value for the interval between LPLND and prostatectomy was 20 days.

DISCUSSION

Surgical dissection of the pelvic lymph nodes is necessary. The sensitivity of the CT scan for detection of lymph node metastases ranges from 12.5% to 30%; specificity ranges from 71% to 93%.[8,9] Therefore pelvic lymph dissection is a mandatory step before treatment of prostatic cancer. Frequency of lymph node invasion increases with the Gleason grade, and for tumors of grade 5 to 7 (as for 18 of our 25 patients), the risk of lymph node metastases is as high as 56.3%.[5]

Complete Examination of the Lymph Nodes

Hermansen and Whitmore[6] reevaluated the reliability of frozen section analysis of the lymph nodes in a review of six studies. The false negative rate ranged from 19% to 40.7%; therefore the risk of a nonbeneficial radical prostatectomy is potentially high. In our opinion laparoscopy is a safe procedure, requiring short hospitalization, which can be scheduled before prostatectomy so as to perform a complete analysis of the pelvic lymph nodes on a permanent section. One of our four patients who chose to undergo LPLND and prostatectomy during the same anesthesia had a false negative examination on frozen section.

Mordidity and Mortality

Winfield et al.[10] evaluated the safety of LPLND in 66 patients. Major complications were three cases of hemorrhage and one injury of the external iliac artery; laparotomy was required twice. In 16 patients, Petros et al.[11] reported major complications in 20%. As reported by Kozminsky et al.,[12] among 105 patients who underwent LPLND for prostatic cancer, 12 major complications occurred: two lymphoceles, one obturator nerve injury, one deep vein thrombosis, three instances of postoperative bleeding, two prolonged ileus, one pelvic abcess, one ureteral injury, and one bladder perforation. Laparotomy was necessary in three patients.[12]

The experience of seven institutions over 2 years was reviewed by Kavoussi et al.[13] Forty-two complications were observed in 329 patients, including three bowel injuries, one ureteral injury, one bladder injury, six vascular injuries, one obturator nerve injury, five lymphedemas or lymphoceles, two instances of significant postoperative bleeding, and two bowel obstructions. Ten patients required secondary surgical intervention. These complication rates have to be compared with those of open pelvic lymph node dissection. In 217 patients undergoing this procedure, McDowell et al.[5] noted 48 complications in 42 patients (19.4%), including 10 lymphoceles, 11 wound infections or dehiscences, eight prolonged ileus, two pelvic hematomas, and two lymphatic fistulas. Extraperitoneal pelvioscopy, as described by Mazeman et al.,[14] is an alternative technique for pelvic lymph node dissection. In 101 patients undergoing this operation for bladder (n = 65) and prostatic (n = 36) cancer, there were five cases of lymphorrhea, one injury of the external iliac vein, and one injury of the obturator nerve.

Complications related to laparoscopy occurred mostly at the beginning of our study, i.e., concerning our first nine cases. This has been described by others.[10,13] As with every new technique, LPLND requires practical application, and safety increases with a rigorous standardization of the procedure. No complication related to anesthesia was observed in our series. Pneumoperitoneum pressure was monitored to keep it under 14 mm Hg, thus limiting vena caval compression and hypercarbia. For the same reason we limited the Trendelenburg position to 20 degrees of tilt. In all of our patients, increase in PCO_2 was controlled by hyperventilation of the lungs. Reducing operative time with practice limits the occurrence of such complications.[15] We did not observe any wound dehiscence, despite absence of closure of the aponeurotic incision.

Number of Lymph Nodes

The average number of lymph nodes dissected was 8.3 ± 3.1. Winfield et al.[10] and Kozminsky et al.[12] obtained an average number of 9.6 nodes in 66 patients and 10.8 in 105 patients, respectively. Effectiveness of LPLND and open procedure was compared, and there was no significant difference in the mean number of lymph nodes removed.[10,16] In 36 patients undergoing extraperitoneal pelviscopy for staging of prostatic cancer, the mean number of lymph nodes removed was 6.7.[14] In each of our patients who subsequently underwent laparotomy, we checked the obturator fossa, and no complementary dissection was needed.

Postoperative Hospitalization

Eleven of our patients underwent laparoscopy as a single procedure. The average duration of the postoperative stay was short, in line with French standards. In comparison, postoperative stays reported by American teams ranged from 1.5 days[10] to 1.9 days.[11]

Choice of Approach for Prostatectomy

A retropubic approach enables pelvic lymph node dissection at the same time as prostatectomy. In our opinion, LPLND provides the opportunity to reconsider the perineal approach. Retropubic and perineal prostatectomy have been retrospectively compared in 173 patients with stage A or B prostate cancer. Of these patients, 122 underwent perineal prostatectomy (group 1) and 51 underwent retropubic prostatectomy (group 2). There were no differences in the incidence of positive surgical margins or in complication rate. The median estimated blood loss and the need for transfusion were significantly lower in group 1.[17]

Contraindications

Absolute contraindications are major cardiac or pulmonary diseases and aortic aneurysm greater than 6 cm in diameter. There are relative contraindications, depending on the surgeon's experience, such as previous abdominal surgery, suspicion of bowel adhesions, and a cardiac or pulmonary status that is inconsistent with prolonged pneumoperitoneum and/or the Trendelenburg position.

CONCLUSION

After a learning period, during which the risk of complication was relatively high, we now consider LPLND to be a safe and effective procedure for assessing lymph node status in patients with organ-confined prostatic cancer. LPLND as a single procedure, with complete analysis of the lymph nodes on permanent section and subsequent radical prostatectomy, if beneficial, has become our standard procedure in the treatment of such patients. LPLND is particularly indicated before perineal radical prostatectomy is undertaken.

REFERENCES

1. Gervasi LA, Mata J, Easley JD, et al. Prognosis significance of lymph nodal metastases in prostate cancer. J Urol 142:332, 1989.
2. Oesterling JE, Brendler CB, Epstein JI, et al. Correlation of clinical stage, serum prostatic acid phosphatases and preoperative Gleason grade with final pathological stage in 275 patients with clinically localized adenocarcinoma of the prostate. J Urol 138:92, 1987.
3. Petros JA, Catalona WJ. Lower incidence of unsuspected lymph node metastases in 521 consecutive patients with clinically localized prostate cancer. J Urol 147:1574, 1992.
4. Smith JA, Seaman JP, Gleidman JB, et al. Pelvic lymph node metastases from prostatic cancer: Influence of tumor grade and stage in 452 consecutive patients. J Urol 130:290, 1983.
5. McDowell GC II, Johnson JW, Tenney DM, et al. Pelvic lymphadenectomy for staging clinically localized prostate cancer. Indications, complications and results in 217 cases. Urology 35:476, 1990.
6. Hermansen DK, Whitmore WF Jr. Frozen section lymph node analysis in pelvic lymphadenectomy for prostate cancer. J Urol 139:1073, 1988.
7. Doublet JD, Gattegno B. Curage lymphatique iliaque sous-veineux par coelioscopie. Chirurg Endoscop 3:21, 1992.
8. Bensen KH, Watson RA, Spring DB, Agee RE. The value of computerized tomography in evaluation of pelvic lymph nodes. J Urol 126:63, 1981.
9. Golimbu M, Morales P, Alaskari S, et al. CAT scanning in staging of prostatic cancer. Urology 35:305, 1981.
10. Winfield HN, See WA, Donovan JF, et al. Comparative effectiveness and safety of laparoscopic versus open pelvic lymph node dissection for cancer of the prostate. J Urol 148:244A (124), 1992.
11. Petros JA, Chandhoke PS, Clayman RV, et al. Staging pelvic lymphadenectomy: A comparison of laparoscopic and open techniques. J Urol 148:245A (125), 1992.
12. Kozminsky M, Gomella L, Stone NN, Sosa E. Laparoscopic urologic surgery: Outcome assessment. J Urol 148:245A (127), 1992.
13. Kavoussi L, Loughlin K, Chandhoke PS, et al. Complications of laparoscopic pelvic lymph node dissection (LPLND). J Urol 148:451A (955), 1992.
14. Mazeman E, Wurtz A, Gilliot P, et al. Extraperitoneal pelvioscopy in lymph node staging of bladder and prostatic cancer. J Urol 147:366, 1992.
15. Nyarwaya JB, Samii K. Anesthésie pour la chirurgie digestive coelioscopique. In Testas P, Delaitre B. Chirurgie Digestive par Voie Coelioscopique. Paris: Maloine, 1991, pp 17-30.
16. Parra RO, Andrus C, Boullier J. Staging laparoscopic pelvic lymph node dissection: Comparison of results with open pelvic lymphadenectomy. J Urol, 147:875, 1992.
17. Frazier HA, Robertson JE, Paulson DF. Radical prostatectomy: Pros and cons of perineal versus retropubic approach. J Urol 147:888, 1992.

60 *Laparoscopic Varicocelectomy*

Ara Darzi, P. Declan Carey, N. Menzies-Gow, and John R.T. Monson

Varicocele was noted as a cause of male infertility as early as the 1880s by Barfield.[1] It consists of abnormal venous tortuosities of the pampiniform plexus within the spermatic cord. The incidence of varicocele in the general population ranges from 10% to 20%.[2,3] The majority of varicoceles occur on the left and are believed to be secondary to incompetence of the valvular structures of the internal spermatic vein.

We have used an endosurgical approach to eradicate large varicoceles. Inherent optical magnification and ease of exposure greatly facilitate surgical interruption by clips. In addition, any contribution to the problem from the internal spermatic vein can readily be assessed, as well as the completeness of venous division.

MATERIALS AND METHODS

Laparoscopic varicocelectomy was attempted in 13 patients with a mean age of 37 years. However, one laparoscopic procedure was not possible at the beginning of our study because of pneumoextraperitoneum. All patients had a unilateral left varicocele.

In the subfertile group at least two semen specimens from each patient were checked before surgery; all had varying amounts of oligospermia, severely impaired

317

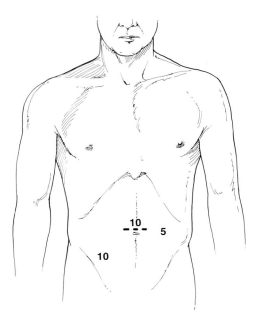

Fig. 1. Position of three trocars for laparoscopic varicocelectomy.

motility, and an increase in immature and tapering forms in the ejaculate. In addition, serum follicle-stimulating hormone, luteinizing hormone, and testosterone levels were within normal ranges. Past surgical histories of the 13 patients revealed no major abdominal operations except for appendectomy in two.

Surgical Technique

With the patient under general anesthesia and muscle relaxation, a pneumoperitoneum was created through a Veress needle introduced into the peritoneal cavity just below the umbilicus. By means of a high-flow CO_2 insufflator, intra-abdominal pressure was maintained between 10 and 14 mm Hg. The peritoneal cavity was insufflated with 3 to 4 L of CO_2. A trocar and cannula (10 mm in diameter) were introduced at the subumbilical region, and the peritoneal cavity was viewed through a 10 mm laparoscope. Two additional ports were placed in the right (10 mm) and left (5 mm) iliac fossa, respectively (Fig. 1). The peritoneum was incised along the internal spermatic vessels for approximately 1 cm with scissors. The internal spermatic veins were dissected off

the spermatic artery and clamped with endoclips (Autosuture). Usually two clips were applied on either side to clamp each vein, and the vein was divided in between.

RESULTS

The internal spermatic vessels were successfully clipped with the laparoscopic procedure in all 12 patients who were able to undergo laparoscopy. Operative time ranged from 35 to 55 minutes with a mean of 40 minutes. Postoperatively, rectal analgesia (Diclofenac) was used for pain relief. All patients were discharged within 24 hours of admission.

Among the 12 successful procedures, there was no intraoperative bleeding or injury to the peritoneal organs. One patient complained of paresthesia along the anterior aspect of the left thigh, which resolved in 6 weeks. No hydrocele of the testis was noted postoperatively.

All varicoceles had disappeared by the first clinical assessment in the outpatient clinic, 3 months after the procedure. Four patients who were operated on for pain and discomfort had symptomatic improvement at their first outpatient visit at 3 months.

The mean follow-up was 8 months, and there has been one recurrence to date. Sperm count improved in seven of the eight subfertile patients to greater than 20×10^6/ml. In addition, sperm motility improved in these patients.

DISCUSSION

Laparoscopic ligation of spermatic veins is a simple and reliable technique for varicocelectomy. In all patients the internal spermatic vessels and vas deferens were easily recognized through the retroperitoneum, and the vessels could be clamped and divided without difficulty.

Current management of varicocele includes percutaneous occlusion[4,5] of the internal spermatic artery and/or vein, as well as surgical ablation.[6,7] There are three distinct approaches to ligation of the internal spermatic vein: scrotal, inguinal, and retroperitoneal.[6] The scrotal approach is used infrequently because of the difficulty in ligating all the veins in the pampiniform plexus, in addition to the risk of damage to the arterial supply of the testis. Inguinal and retroperitoneal approaches are both widely used and accepted.[6,7] At present most large series reviewing the results of varicocele surgery show that approximately 75% of men will have improved semen quality.[4] Pregnancy rates after corrective surgery average 40%.[2,8]

One advantage of laparoscopic surgery compared with an open operation is the use of small stab wounds. This avoids wide dissection along the internal ring or the scrotum. In addition, because of the high magnification provided by video endoscopes it is much easier to identify and preserve the spermatic artery. Although Palomo first reported open high ligation of all internal spermatic vessels at varicocelectomy, in the belief that the testis will survive on the collateral supply from the cremasteric artery and the artery to the vas deferens, it is our belief that the spermatic artery should be identified and preserved.

CONCLUSION

Although follow-up is short, the success rate of laparoscopic varicocelectomy appears to be as good as that of conventional open high ligation. Laparoscopic varicocelectomy offers a number of advantages but is still in its infancy. Studies with long-term follow-up are needed to compare this procedure with surgical ligation and/or balloon occlusion of the internal spermatic veins.

REFERENCES

1. Zorgniotti AW. The spermatozoa count: A short history. J Urol 5:672, 1975.
2. Coolsaet BL. The varicocele syndrome: Venography determining the optimal level for surgical management. J Urol 124:833-840, 1980.
3. Ivanissevich O. Left varicocele due to reflux: Experience with 4470 operative cases in 42 years. J Int Cell Surg 34:742-751, 1960.
4. Getzoff PL. Surgical management of male infertility: Results of a survey. Fertil Steril 24:553-557, 1973.
5. Seyferth W, Jecht E, Zeitler E. Percutaneous occlusion of the varicocele. Radiology 139:335-342, 1981.
6. Dubin L, Amelar RD. Varicocelectomy: 986 cases in a twelve year study. Urology 10:446-452, 1977.
7. Kaufman SL, Kadir S, Barth KH, et al. Mechanisms of recurrent varicocele after balloon occlusion or surgical ligation of the internal spermatic vein. Radiology 147:435-443, 1983.
8. Lipshultz L, Howards SS. Surgical treatment of male infertility. In Lipshultz L, Howards SS, eds. Infertility in Males. London: Churchill-Livingstone, 1983.

X

Videoendoscopic Hernia Repairs

61 Experimental Hernia Repair in Animal and Human Models

Jürgen Schleef, Michael Barthel, Jörg Holste, and Anton Schafmayer

Inguinal hernia repair, which is of major interest to laparoscopic surgeons, is the most common operation performed by general surgeons.[1] This review presents several different techniques as well as a discussion on the value of and approaches used in laparoscopic hernia repairs.

Since 1989 several authors have published their results of laparoscopic inguinal hernia repair.[2-5] Various techniques are described in these articles, and controversy still exists about the best approach to laparoscopic hernia repair. However, in the past 4 years a trend in the choice of techniques can be observed. Although some authors have described hernia repair in which clips and sutures are utilized according to established "open" techniques, most surgeons who perform this operation employ a "mesh" or "plug" repair.[2,8] Clips and sutures are used in a repair technique in which tension is used to approximate tissues; the mesh or plug approach is best described as being tension free. Each type of surgical repair employs different techniques. The plug repair technique of Shulman et al.,[9] used in open surgery, was one of the first operations performed laparoscopically. A smaller patch for closing the defect is used by surgeons, and a combination of these two techniques may also be employed. We utilized this combination technique in patients who had indirect and small direct hernias.[5,10] In patients with large hernias and combined hernias, this approach cannot be performed. Shultz et al.[8] reported on operations in which the plug repair technique was used. They demonstrated that with this technique, which is valuable for correcting an indirect hernia, hernia recurred in patients with a direct hernia.

The most important step in laparoscopic inguinal hernia surgery was the introduction of the large patch repair, which can be performed as a transperitoneal or a preperitoneal procedure.[2] This technique seems to be the best alternative to established open techniques, although long-term results are unknown.

In tension-free repair techniques, mesh is used to close the defect and the inguinal region. For approximately a century, surgeons have been using synthetic materials to support the stability of hernia repair of the abdominal wall.[11-17] In the United States synthetic material is often used, especially in the repair of recurrent inguinal hernias. In Europe the Bassini[18] technique and the Shouldice repair,[19,20] in which synthetic implants are not used, are popular.

The use of resorbable or nonresorbable material is an important consideration in hernia repair.[15,16] Different implant materials are available for surgical use.[21-23]

We performed approximately 140 laparoscopic operations to correct inguinal hernias. In 1991 we used a synthetic nonresorbable implant (Marlex mesh) in a technique that combined small patch repair with plug repair as described by Schultz et al.[8] The initial results were encouraging. After we had performed approximately 20 such procedures, we began to use a resorbable implant (Ethisorb) in a prospective randomized trial that compared the surgical result of nonresorbable and resorbable materials in 60 patients. To obtain additional histological information about resorbable versus nonresorbable materials, we also performed an experimental trial in pigs with inguinal hernias.

In human and animal models, the following questions were addressed: (1) Can inguinal hernia repair be successfully performed via a combined technique that involves prosthetic materials? and (2) Is polypropylene mesh (Marlex) or Vicryl and PDS (Ethisorb) the better implant material with respect to stability, tissue reaction, and clinical result?

EXPERIMENTAL AND CLINICAL TRIALS
Technique

Our trials in animals and initial studies in humans involved a combined technique in which plug repair and a small subperitoneal patch were used.[5]

The operation was performed with the animal or patient under general anesthesia. After the hernia was identified (Fig.1), the hernia sac, which was torn intra-abdominally by forceps, was repositioned. A peritoneal incision approximately 3 cm in length (Fig. 2) was then made ventral and lateral to the hernia. The channel of the hernia was explored toward the external inguinal ring with a preparation forceps. This procedure can be visually controlled with the 45-degree lens. The external ring was left intact and was not opened. Two or three rolls of synthetic mesh 5 mm in diameter and 4 cm in length or Ethisorb hernia cylinders were placed in the defect (Fig. 3). A small 4 × 4 cm patch was placed over the defect, and the peritoneum was closed with titanium clips (Fig. 4).

EXPERIMENTAL STUDIES IN THE PIG MODEL
Materials and Methods

The male pig is an excellent model for experimentation in surgical hernia repair: the pig anatomy is similar to that of humans, and pigs often have large bilateral congenital indirect hernias.

We performed a laparoscopic inguinal hernia repair in six pigs, 10 to 15 kg in weight, that had bilateral hernias.

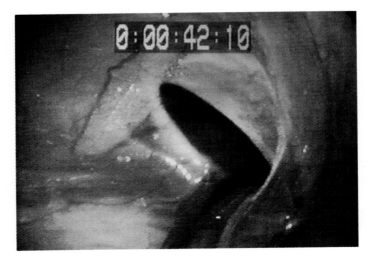

Fig. 1. Indirect inguinal hernia in a male pig.

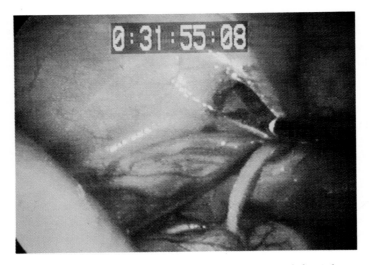

Fig. 2. Peritoneum is incised and preparation of hernia defect is begun.

Three pigs received Marlex implants and three received Ethisorb implants. No major intraoperative complications occurred. Eighty-five days after the repair, the animals were sacrificed and autopsies were performed. Histological examination with various stains provided information about tissue reaction and proliferation.

Results of the Combined Surgical Repair in the Pig Model

In two animals, dislocation of the implants resulted from infection at the site of the operation. In the other animals, no problems occurred and the hernias did not recur. All autopsies revealed no abdominal adhesions in the inguinal region. The defects were found to be closed, and no dislocation of implants was seen in the animals that experienced no infection.

In the area of the transverse muscle and the peritoneal layer, histopathological examination revealed well-developed granulation tissue and fibrosis. The fibers of the implant were surrounded by epithelial cells. Histiocytes and foreign body giant cells indicated focal chronic inflammation. Examination of spermatic cord structures revealed no evidence of compression or reaction to the implanted tissue. The polypropylene

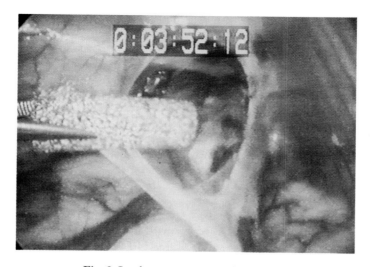

Fig. 3. Implants are positioned in defect.

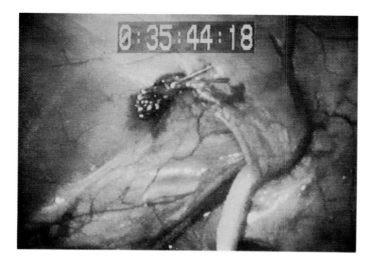

Fig. 4. Inguinal region in male pig after hernia repair.

(Marlex) fibers were intact and were surrounded by fibrous tissue. Ethisorb implants were almost completely resorbed; only a few fibers of PDS could be seen. Fibrosis and granulation were more extensive when Ethisorb implants were used.

CLINICAL STUDY OF HERNIA REPAIR
Materials and Methods

In 1991 we performed a prospective randomized study in which 60 patients with inguinal hernias received either Marlex mesh or Ethisorb mesh and hernia cylinders as part of surgical hernia repair. In each patient the inguinal hernia was identified as either a small direct or an indirect hernia. Larger hernias, combined hernias, or scrotal or incarcerated hernias were contraindications for study participation. Recurrent hernias were not contraindications for a laparoscopic approach.

Patients were informed about the study design; the lack of information about long-term surgical results was emphasized. After laparoscopic exploration, patients were randomized into two groups: those who were to receive nonresorbable implants and those who would receive resorbable implants. The operations were performed with the patient under general anesthesia. A nasogastric tube and a Foley catheter were placed in all patients to avoid stomach or bladder perforation. In all cases, catheters were removed immediately after surgery.[8] On the day after surgery, ultrasonographic evaluation of the abdomen was performed. Patients were discharged from the hospital on postsurgical day 3 or 4. An evaluation of the patient's quality of life and postoperative controls were developed. All patients underwent ultrasonographic and clinical examinations 4, 8, and 12 weeks after surgery. A questionnaire assessing quality of life was distributed to patients.[10,25] Considerations on the questionnaire included physical, functional, psychological, and social characteristics of the patient before and after hernia repair.

Results of Hernia Repair in the Human Model

No patient experienced major complications after surgery. In two cases we converted to the open Shouldice technique because of incarceration and a large combined hernia. Neither implant rejection nor inflammation was noted. In two patients, local hematoma occurred postoperatively, but no surgical intervention was required. Three local wound infections were observed at the puncture site in the abdominal wall. Two patients had periosteal pain in the pubic region because the implants were placed near bone; however, 8 days after surgery both patients were free of pain.

Postoperative examinations performed 5 to 18 months after surgery showed no recurrence of hernia in all patients. Quality-of-life assessments indicated that a majority of patients returned to normal life after surgery. Patients who underwent laparoscopic surgery experienced less pain and less fatigue and returned to work and free-time activities within 2 to 3 weeks after surgery. This recovery period was less than that of patients who underwent the Shouldice technique.

CONCLUSION

Our studies reveal that laparoscopic hernia repair in animal models and humans can be performed without major complications. In some patients this combined method may be a valuable, less invasive approach.

In the pig model, both resorbable and nonresorbable implant materials can be used successfully in hernia repair. In the animal study, no general reaction to synthetic implant material was observed, although granulation and fibrous tissue occurred around the implant. The spermatic structures were intact, and 85 days after surgery, the resorbable implants had almost disappeared. Neither instability nor weakness was noted with either implant.

The randomized and prospective clinical trial in humans indicated similar results. All patients were pain free. No recurrences were noted. Quality-of-life assessments indicated good results and higher satisfaction scores than those of patients who underwent the conventional open technique repair.

At this time, there is no standard laparoscopic technique for hernia repair. Further development of implants, instruments, and additional techniques might result in modification of the principles of laparoscopic hernia repair in the future, but currently, tensionless repair seems the superior technique.

Although hernia repair with resorbable implants must be evaluated in additional studies, preliminary results are encouraging,[12,13,27,28] and use of resorbable material has shown no disadvantages.

The benefits of laparoscopic hernia repair, which can be performed without hospital admission, must be compared with the rate of hernia recurrence, and controlled randomized prospective studies on long-term results must be undertaken. Multicenter studies involving large patient populations would also be of interest.

REFERENCES

1. Sievert JR, et al. Wandel der Eingriffshäufigkeit in der Allgemeinchirurgie. Chirurgie 61:855, 1990.

2. Arregui ME, Davis CD, Yucel O, et al. Laparoscopic mesh repair of inguinal hernia using a preperitoneal approach: A preliminary report. Surg Laparosc Endosc 2:53, 1992.

3. Ger R, et al. Management of indirect inguinal hernias by laparoscopic closure of neck and sac. Am J Surg 159:370, 1990.

4. Ger R. Laparoskopische Hernienoperation. Chirurgie 62:266-270, 1991.

5. Schafmayer A, et al. Endoskopischer Hernienverschluss. Chirurgie 63:257, 1992.

6. Popp LW. Endoscopic patch repair of inguinal hernia in a female patient. Surg Endosc 4:10, 1990.

7. Popp LW. Endoskopische Hernioplastik. Chirurgie 62:336, 1990.

8. Shultz L, et al. Laser laparoscopic herniorrhaphy: A clinical trial. Preliminary results. J Laparoendosc Surg 1:1, 1990.

9. Shulman AG, et al. The "plug" repair of 1402 recurrent inguinal hernias. Arch Surg 125:265, 1984.

10. Schleef J, et al. Die laparoskopische Hernioplastik. Min Invasive Chirurgie 1:35, 1992.

11. Bauer JJ, et al. Repair of large abdominal wall defects with expanded polytetrafluoroethylene (PTFE). Ann Surg 206:765, 1987.

12. Chevalley JP, et al. Entwicklung in der Behandlung der Leistenhernien. Zentralbl Chir 113:36, 1988.

13. Eigler FW, et al. Resorbierbare Kunststoffnetze in der Abdominalchirurgie—Indikationen, Operationsverfahren und Ergebnisse. Chirurgie 56:376, 1985.

14. Nyhus LM. The preperitoneal approach and ileopubic tract repair of inguinal hernia. In Nyhus LM, Condon RE, eds. Hernia. Philadelphia: JB Lippincott, p 154.

15. Goepel R. Über die Verschliessung von Bruchpforten durch Einheilung geflochtener, fertiger Silberdrahtnetze (Silberdrahtpelotten). Verh Dtsch Ges Chir 29:174, 1990.

16. Hamer-Hodges DW, Scott NB. Replacement of an abdominal wall defect using expanded PTFE sheet (Gore-Tex). J R Coll Surg Edinb 30:65, 1987.

17. Willmen HR. Die Wende in der Therapie von Inguinal—und hiatushernien durch Induktion tragfähigen Narbengewebes. Chirurgie 58:300, 1987.

18. Witzel O. Über den Verschluss von Bauchwunden und Bruchpforten durch versenkte Silberdrahtnetze (Einheilung von Filigranpelotten). Zentralbl Chir 27:257, 1900.

19. Bassini E. Nuovo metodo per la cura radicale dell'ernia. Atti Cong Ass Med Ital 2:179, 1887.

20. Schumpelick V. Leistenbruch—Reparation nach Shouldice. Chirurgie 55:25, 1984.

21. Shouldice EE. Surgical treatment of hernia. Ontario Med Rev 11:43, 1944.

22. Usher FC, et al. Polypropylene monofilament: A new biological structure for closing contaminated wounds. JAMA 179:780, 1962.

23. Usher FC. Hernia repair with Marlex mesh. Arch Surg 84:325, 1962.

24. Wolstenholme JT. Use of commercial Dacron fabric in the repair of inguinal hernias and abdominal wall defects. Arch Surg 73:1004, 1956.

25. Usher FC. Hernia repair with knitted polypropylene mesh. Surg Gynecol Obstet 117:239, 1963.

26. Eypasch E, et al. Quality of life and gastrointestinal surgery—a clinimetric approach to developing an instrument for its measurement. Theor Surg 5:3, 1989.

27. Koontz AR. Preliminary report on the use of tantalum mesh in the repair of ventral hernias. Ann Surg 127:1079, 1948.

28. Lam CR, et al. Tantalum gauze in the repair of large postoperative ventral hernias. Arch Surg 57:234, 1948.

62   *Laparoscopic Hernioplasty: Techniques and Results*

Anton Schafmayer, Michael Barthel, Jürgen Schleef, T. Neufang, and G. Lepsien

Inguinal hernia repair is the operation most frequently performed by general surgeons. Different techniques are reported, and a great deal of controversy continues about the value of laparoscopic hernia repair.

In 1989 Bogojavlensky[1] reported on laparoscopic inguinal and femoral hernia repair. In the United States and in Europe, various approaches to laparoscopic hernia repair are used.[2,3] Schultz et al.[4] described the plug repair, which was first mentioned by Schulman et al.[5]

We used the plug repair to correct hernias in 103 patients within a 1-year period.[6] Our results were encouraging; only one recurrence developed in this group of patients. However, plug repair cannot be used for every laparoscopic herniorrhaphy because it has limited applicability. Other authors[7] have described transperitoneal and preperitoneal approaches for the closure of the whole inguinal region with nonresorbable mesh.

Since February 1992, we have used a transperitoneal technique for hernia repair of the inguinal region; a laparoscopic modification of the approach reported by Stoppa et al.[8] In this technique, mesh is used to close the inguinal space, including the direct and indirect compartments of the inguinal region. This technique can be used in the repair of large indirect, direct, or combined "pantaloon" hernias and to prevent new or recurrent hernias. Arregui et al.[9] have reported 105 cases of inguinal hernia repair by a preperitoneal approach.

We shall present our preliminary results with transperitoneal and plug repair during an 18-month period of laparoscopic hernia repair.

TECHNIQUE
Plug Repair

This operation is performed with the patient under general anesthesia, because relaxation of the patient is mandatory. He or she is placed on a normal operating table in a supine position. The pelvis is slightly elevated by an underlying bolster. The evening before operation, the umbilical area is washed and the umbilicus is sponged with an iodine solution to prevent umbilical infection.

After a small stab incision of the skin is made in the lower portion of the umbilicus, a Veress needle is introduced, and the pneumoperitoneum (15 mm Hg) is instilled. Next, two trocars (one 11 mm on the side of the hernia and one 5 mm on the contralateral side) are placed laterally at the level of the umbilicus.

An initial peritoneal incision is made ventral and lateral to the hernia sac, which is everted intra-abdominally by forceps. The incision must be approximately 3 cm in length (Fig. 1). A dissecting forceps is advanced into the channel of the hernia toward the external inguinal ring. The 45-degree telescope can be used to guide this procedure. The external ring should be intact and should not be opened. Two to three rolls of synthetic mesh (5 mm in diameter and 4 cm in length) are then inserted and are placed in the defect (Fig. 2). Finally, a flat mesh (4 × 4 cm) is placed over the opening of the defect, and the peritoneum is closed with titanium clips (Fig. 3). At the end of the operation we perform a final videoendoscopic inspection of the surgical site and external digital control of the correct placement of the rolls of synthetic material from the groin.

We use this procedure to correct small direct or indirect hernias. This technique should not be used to cor-

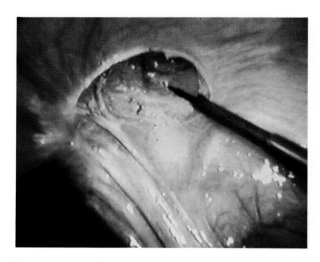

Fig. 1. Peritoneal incision, approximately 3 cm in length, ventral and lateral to hernia sac.

rect large direct inguinal hernias, combined (pantaloon) hernias, or inguinoscrotal hernias.

Transperitoneal Inguinal Laparoscopic Hernia Repair

This procedure, which is a modification of the technique of Stoppa, is also performed with the patient under general anesthesia. After a small stab incision of the skin is made in the lower umbilicus, a Veress needle is introduced and the pneumoperitoneum (15 mm Hg) is instilled. Two 12 mm trocars are placed lateral to the umbilicus and are used to pass variously needed operative instruments in and out under visual control with a 45-degree telescope. An initial peritoneal incision is made at the top of the hernia sac, which is everted intra-abdominally by forceps. The incision should be approximately 6 cm long; this should permit exposure of the complete inguinal region (Fig. 4). The dissection that follows must be carefully performed; the epigastric vessels require special care. After the peritoneal layer is opened, the underlying fatty tissue must be removed (Fig. 5). Normally this procedure is easy. The entire in-

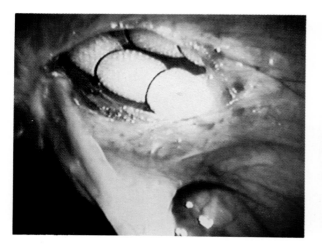

Fig. 2. Two rolls of Marlex mesh are placed in defect.

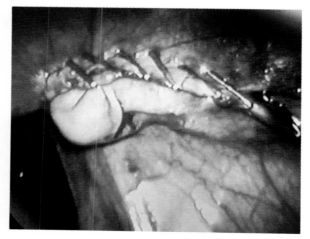

Fig. 3. Peritoneal closure with titanium clips.

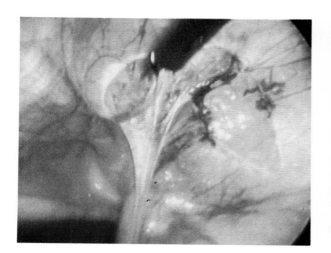

Fig. 4. Peritoneal incision approximately 6 cm in length for modified Stoppa procedure.

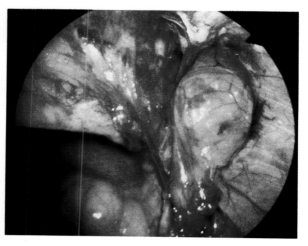

Fig. 5. Fatty tissue underlying peritoneal layer.

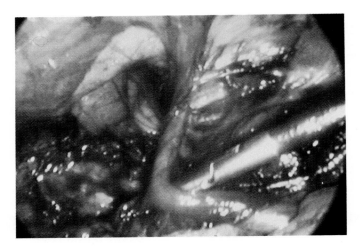

Fig. 6. Preparation of inguinal region; epigastric vessels and spermatic cord (in front of forceps) receive special attention.

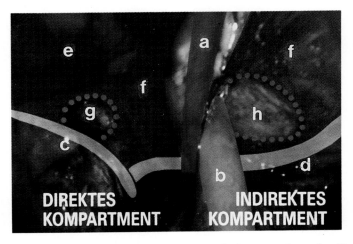

Fig. 7. Anatomy of right inguinal region: *a*, epigastric vessels; *b*, spermatic cord; *c*, Cooper's ligament; *d*, ileopubic tract; *e*, rectus muscle; *f*, transvessel fascia; *g*, defect in direct space; *h*, defect in indirect space.

guinal space can be seen; this facilitates liberation of the herniated structures and of the hernia sac with an atraumatic forceps. The spermatic cord structures and vessels must be carefully protected and preserved (Figs. 6 and 7). After the hernia sac and attached structures have been removed, a 6 × 12 cm Marlex mesh patch is introduced into the abdomen and is positioned to cover the inguinal space from Cooper's ligament to the iliopubic tract (Figs. 8 and 9). A hernia stapler (Autosuture) is used to secure the Marlex mesh in the inguinal area (Figs. 8 and 9). Then the peritoneum is closed over by titanium clips; to reduce tension on the peritoneum, intra-abdominal pressure is reduced (8 to 10 mm Hg). The pneumoperitoneum is completely evacuated, and all trocars are removed under visual control. The skin incision is closed with subcutaneous stitches and is covered with a transparent wound dressing (Coloplast). We have used this technique to correct various types of in-

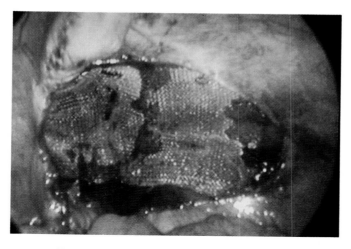

Fig. 8. Marlex mesh patch (6 × 12 cm) in place.

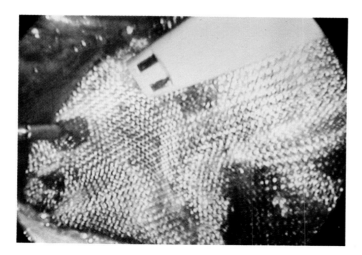

Fig. 9. Fixation of Marlex mesh by hernia stapler.

guinal hernias such as large combined hernias, but it should not be used to repair inguinoscrotal hernias or incarcerated hernias.

RESULTS

From February 1991 to July 1992, in 120 patients we repaired 143 inguinal hernias (114 men and 6 women). In 61 cases the hernia occurred on the right side; 36 patients presented with a left inguinal hernia, and 23 individuals had bilateral hernia. Twenty recurrent hernias were surgically corrected. Patient ages ranged from 18 to 84 years (mean, 49.5 ± 18.9 years). The hospital stay ranged from 2 to 10 days (mean, 3.9 ± 1.8 days). Patients returned to work from 1 to 7 weeks after operation (mean time, 2.8 ± 1.4 weeks). Patients resumed leisure activities after 3.4 ± 2 weeks. All patients were examined 1, 2, 3, 6, and 12 months after surgery; then annual follow-up examinations were necessary (Fig. 10).

Pain

Pain intensity was evaluated by the patient in a quality-of-life assessment each day postoperatively and week-

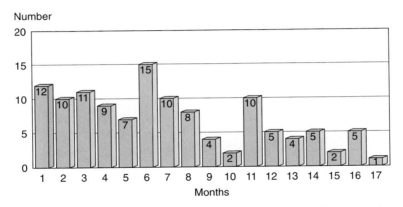

Fig. 10. Follow-up of 120 patients after laparoscopic inguinal hernia repair.

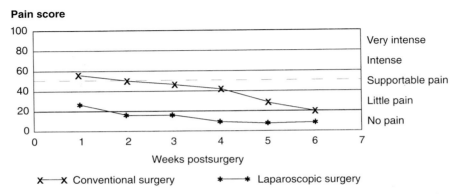

Fig. 11. Postoperative pain intensity in 50 patients with laparoscopic hernia repair and with conventional hernia repair.

ly after week 1. The same follow-up protocol, which had questions regarding the patient's quality of life, was given to 50 patients who underwent the Shouldice technique. Patients indicated a great difference in pain intensity during the first 3 weeks postoperatively (Fig. 11): during the first week, the patients treated by the Shouldice technique required much more pain treatment than did the patients who underwent laparoscopic surgery. Fig. 11 shows the different degrees of patient-perceived pain intensity, which ranged from slight to intense.

Complications

Intraoperative complications. In all patients, operation was performed without major problems. In three cases, the laparoscopic procedure was stopped, and the operation was continued via the conventional Shouldice technique. One patient had a large sliding hernia, and in two cases with incarcerated hernias, reduction of hernia contents was not possible; a dissection could not be performed without endangering the patient.

Postoperative complications. In three patients, postoperative examination revealed an inguinal hematoma. Two patients who underwent plug repair had periosteal pain in the pubic area as a result of implants. All symptoms and findings disappeared within several days, and reoperation was not necessary. In one patient, we observed the dislocation of an implant after plug repair. Laparoscopy was performed in this case, and the implant was removed. The two other mesh rolls were in place, and no evidence of recurrent hernia was seen.

Rate of Recurrence

In an 18-month period, the rate of recurrence was 0.7%. A recurrent hernia was seen 8 weeks after plug repair in a young HIV-infected patient. In this case we performed a plug repair because of the patient's overall poor health. A second laparoscopy was not possible because of the patient's deteriorating condition. No other recurrence has been seen as of this writing. In 22 patients, the observation period after operation has been more than 12 months, and all patients are in good condition.

DISCUSSION

The history of modern inguinal hernia repair dates from the end of the nineteenth century with the first description of techniques by Bassini[10] in Europe and by Halsted[11] in the United States. Since that time, different authors have reported about other hernia repairs.[3,12,13] The common open procedures performed are the Bassini[10] operation and the Shouldice repair.[14] The rate of recurrence is estimated to be between 0.7% and 10% by different study groups.

Laparoscopic hernia repair combines the advantages of a laparoscopic procedure with new technical aspects of inguinal hernia repair. Nevertheless, the results of a new technique must be compared with those of the conventional, established technique. Recurrence rate is the most decisive factor in the evaluation of laparoscopic hernia repair. Studies presented in the literature cannot give precise information about this important aspect because the period of observation has been too short and the number of patients too small. The value of this method can be determined only if larger groups of patients are studied for a longer time. Thus laparoscopic inguinal hernia repair must be performed under standard conditions in a prospective trial. Our patients are constantly controlled, and a quality-of-life assessment is performed to obtain information about subjective effects on the patients.

Our preliminary results are encouraging. The intraperitoneal mesh repair is a procedure that can be performed in a reasonable operative time and without major technical problems. Our modification of the plug repair can be used to repair only small direct or indirect hernias and might not have other applications.

The future of laparoscopic inguinal hernia repair might involve only intraperitoneal mesh repair (a modification of the Stoppa[15] method). Additional study results will indicate whether the preperitoneal approach as described by Arregui as advantageous. These technical aspects will be influenced by new developments in equipment and instruments.

Current laparoscopic hernia repair must be viewed as an alternative technique to that of conventional surgery. It should be performed only by a surgeon who is familiar with advanced laparoscopic operations and only under standard conditions in clinical prospective trials. These conditions are necessary to validate the method.

REFERENCES

1. Bogojavlensky S. Laparoscopic treatment of inguinal and femoral hernia. Presented at the Annual Meeting of the AAGLO, Washington DC, 1989.
2. Arregui ME, et al. Four surgeons describe their separate techniques for performing laparoscopic inguinal hernia repair. Gen Surg News 1:23, 1991.
3. Dion YM, Morin J. Laparoscopic inguinal herniorrhaphy. Can J Surg 35:209, 1992.
4. Schultz L, et al. Laser laparoscopic herniorrhaphy: A clinical trial. Preliminary results. J Laparoendoscopic Surg 1:1, 1990.
5. Schulman AG, et al. The "plug" repair of 1402 recurrent inguinal hernias. Arch Surg 125:265, 1990.
6. Schafmayer A, et al. Endoskopischer Hernienverschluss. Chirurgie 63:357, 1992.
7. Schleef J, et al. Die laparoskopische Hernioplastik. Minimal Invasive Chir 1:35, 1992.
8. Stoppa RE, Rives KL, Warlamount CR, et al. The use of Dacron in the repair of hernias of the groin. Surg Clin North Am 64:269, 1984.
9. Arregui ME, Davis CD, Yucel O, et al. Laparoscopic mesh repair of inguinal hernia using a preperitoneal approach: A preliminary report. Surg Laparoscopy Endosc 2:53, 1992.
10. Bassini E. Nuovo metodo per la cura radicale dell'ernia. Atti Cong Ass Med Ital 2:179, 1887.
11. Halsted WS. Radical cure of hernia. Johns Hopkins Hosp Bull 1:12, 1899.
12. Corbitt J. Laparoscopic herniorrhaphy. Laparoscopy in focus. Newsletter 1:4, 1991.
13. Schultz L, Graber J, Pietrafitta J. Laparoscopic inguinal herniorrhaphy—Lessons learned after 100 cases. Video presented at the Society of Gastrointestinal Endoscopic Surgeons, Washington DC, 1992.
14. Shouldice EE. Surgical treatment of hernia. Ontario Med Rev 11:43, 1944.
15. Stoppa RE. The treatment of complicated groin and incisional hernias. World J Surg 13:545, 1989.

63   *Laparoscopic Herniorrhaphy: A Preperitoneal Approach*

John D. Corbitt, Jr.

Inguinal herniorrhaphy is one of the more common operations performed in the United States, with more than 500,000 of these repairs performed each year. The groin approach, first described by Bassini in 1884, placed emphasis on reconstruction of the inguinal floor. Depending on the literature, this repair is said to have a recurrence rate as high as 10%, which is thought to result from placing tissues on tension that are not normally in opposition to each other.

The recurrence rate has been significantly improved by the development of a tension-free repair using Marlex mesh or prolene to reconstruct the floor through a groin approach, as originally described by Lichtenstein. His latest personal series of 1000 patients shows a recurrence rate of 0%.[4] A previously reported 1- to 6-year follow-up of 1522 patients showed a recurrence rate of only 0.13% (two patients).[2]

Stoppa and Warlaumont[3] and Nyhus[4] have reported their preperitoneal approach, using prosthetic material to cover the floor of the inguinal canal, and an extremely low recurrence rate of 1.4% to 1.7% (in 572 and 203 repairs). Because these repairs have used a groin approach, patients may remain disabled from 1 to 2 weeks, sometimes with significant discomfort and complications such as neuromas, orchitis, epididymitis, and permanent neuralgias.

High ligation of the sac and closure of the internal ring to prevent recurrence was first emphasized by Henry Marcy[5,6] and later modified by LaRoque, who performed 1700 of these procedures. Unfortunately, the follow-up on these procedures is scant, and the exact recurrence rate is unknown.[7-9]

Using the information provided by these surgeons, a laparoscopic repair was originally described using a plug-and-patch method associated with high ligation of the sac, accomplished with Endoloops initially and later by an EndoGIA.[10] After following these patients for 2 years, a greater than 20% recurrence rate was evident. The laparoscopic herniorrhaphy, however, did result in a tension-free, painless repair, and the patient was able to return to normal activity the following day. Patients who did not show early recurrence did well and continue to have an excellent repair. The initially large

recurrence rate is thought to have resulted from the lack of fixation of the mesh to the fascia and use of a small prosthesis.

Using the approach to hernia repair described by Stoppa, Warlaumont, Nyhus and Lichtenstein, a laparoscopic tension-free preperitoneal repair was developed in 1990 that should significantly lower the recurrence rate while still affording the benefits of laparoscopic herniorrhaphy.

MATERIALS AND METHODS

Laparoscopic herniorrhaphies are carried out with the patient under general anesthesia and placed in the Trendelenburg position. A 12 mm incision is made in the umbilicus and an insufflation needle is used to insufflate the abdominal cavity with CO_2 to a pressure of 15 mm Hg. A 12 mm port is inserted through this umbilical incision, and a 10 mm laparoscopic camera with a 30-degree lens is used to observe direct placement of additional ports. All ports are placed at the level of the umbilicus lateral to the rectus sheath. In a tall patient these ports are placed 1 to 2 inches inferior to the umbilicus. These secondary ports are 5 mm ports, minimizing the patient's postoperative pain as well as giving extremely good cosmetic result. (Ten millimeter ports may be substituted if a good 5 mm laparoscope is not available.)

Using the two 5 mm ports, the surgeon, standing on the side opposite the hernia, may now incise the peritoneum anterior to the hernia defect and create a transverse incision, the medial boundary of which is the approximate area of the umbilical ligament, and the lateralmost boundary of which is the anterior superior iliac spine. In cases in which an extremely large indirect sac or direct pseudo-sac exists, the transverse incision is carried across the upper portion of the sac transversely.

An incision is then made around the neck of the sac to allow some redundant peritoneum for future closure. This 360-degree incision is made inside the internal ring to detach the indirect sac completely from the peritoneal cavity. This distal portion of the sac is left intact to prevent injury to the distal cord structures, hematomas, and confusion of the anatomy. In the latter regard, extreme care must be observed in the posterior portion of this incision. The spermatic vessels traverse through the posterior portion of this indirect sac. These vessels, combined with the even more posteriorly located iliac vessels, compose the "triangle of doom," which represents the most dangerous portion of the preperitoneal dissection. If a lipoma is encountered in this dissection, it is removed. It is not necessary, however, to remove all of the fatty tissue in the preperitoneal area before stapling the mesh into place. Amputation of the sac is rarely done in the direct hernia. The direct sac is usually reduced in its entirety. While dissection is more easily performed from the contralateral side of the hernia, after some minimal experience, the surgeon will find that it is easier for a right-handed surgeon to stand on the left side of the patient and the left-handed surgeon to stand on the right side of the patient throughout the entire hernia repair.

The flaps of peritoneum are now developed anteriorly and posteriorly to expose the entire floor of the inguinal canal and/or the direct and indirect defect. Anteriorly the inferior epigastric vessels are left attached to the abdominal wall, and the peritoneum is removed from them. Caution should be used when extending the dissection posteriorly below the level of the inguinal ligament or iliopubic tract, which comprises the pos-

terior portion of the inguinal ring (Fig. 1). The peritoneum is carefully removed from the vas deferens, testicular vessels, and the iliac vessels by traction and countertraction. Again, this "triangle of doom" represents the most hazardous part of the procedure. Injury to these structures is to be avoided by meticulous dissection. No electrocautery is used in this area. After exposing the entire floor, a prosthetic mesh patch is pushed into the abdominal cavity through the 12 mm port. The 10 mm laparoscope is replaced into the 12 mm port. The 3 × 5 inch prosthesis is then placed across the entire floor of the canal to cover the area of both the indirect and direct defect. Although Marlex was originally used as a prosthetic material, this has recently been replaced by SurgiPro mesh, also a polypropylene mesh, because of its property of adhering to the moist surface of the exposed inguinal floor. The graft is initially stapled to the transversalis fascia anteriorly and is then stapled medially and laterally. The graft is also stapled to the inguinal ligament and Cooper's ligament, covering the pubis as well as the transversalis fascia, as indicated in Fig. 2. Cooper's ligament staples are best secured by a stapler specifically designed by U.S. Surgical Corp. to penetrate this hard periosteum. These shorter, stockier 3.0 staples are specifically designed for this area and are not to be used on the anterior and lateral fascia, which requires the longer 3.5 staples for

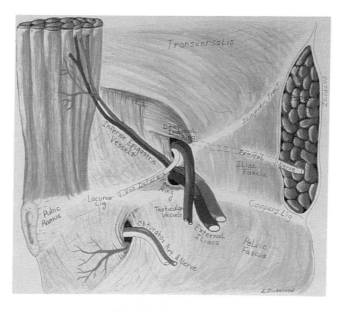

Fig. 1. Pelvic anatomy.

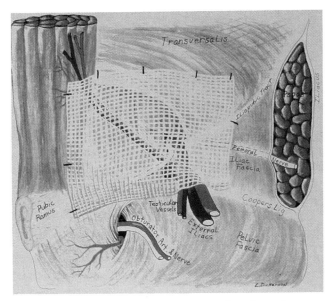

Fig. 2. Placement and fixation of mesh with staples.

deeper penetration to secure the prosthesis. Staples are not placed posteriorly where the iliac vessels and the spermatic vessels can be directly visualized (triangle of doom). Laterally, staples are not placed below the iliopubic tract to avoid injury to the lateral femoral cutaneous nerve. The graft extends medially from the pubis to the anterior superior iliac spine laterally. After the prosthesis is stapled in place, insufflator pressure is reduced to 8 mm Hg, with evacuation of a corresponding amount of CO_2 from the abdominal cavity. This allows relaxation of the peritoneum, which is then clipped together, again utilizing the hernia stapler (U.S. Surgical Corp.). Only the 12 mm incision fascia is closed using a No. 1 PDS suture. The remaining skin incisions are closed with absorbable subcutaneous sutures and Steristrips.

RESULTS

Preperitoneal laparoscopic herniorrhaphies have been successfully completed without major complications in this series. The time necessary for this repair has been greatly reduced by the development of the multifire hernia stapler (U.S. Surgical Corp.). This eliminates time-consuming laparoscopic suturing. Postoperatively patients are allowed to be discharged on the day of their operation and are almost completely free of pain. Cos-

> **PATIENT DATA FOR LAPAROSCOPIC HERNIORRHAPHY**
> (n = 180)
>
> Ages 21-83
> 139 men, 15 women
> 63 right, 65 left
> 26 bilateral
> 26 recurrent
> 68 direct, 95 indirect
> 14 pantaloon
> 3 femoral

metically the 12 mm incision is completely hidden in the umbilicus and the two 5 mm incisions, which are closed with Steristrips, are barely visible after a short time. To date, all 180 patients requesting laparoscopic herniorrhaphy have been repaired including direct, indirect, femoral, and sliding hernias and large scrotal hernias (see box). No hernias have been omitted from our series; however, patients have been carefully screened to ensure they completely understand the procedure and the possibility of recurrence as well as the complications associated with laparoscopy. Follow-up at this time is too short to evaluate the recurrence rate fully; however, early results are promising. Three patients developed transient paresthesia in the distribution of the lateral cutaneous nerve of the thigh. Two resolved in 2 to 3 weeks and the third patient's condition resolved after 6 months. We no longer place staples below the iliopubic tract laterally, which avoids this complication. Postoperative bulges high into the inguinal canal were seen in 13 patients. These were thought to be hematomas, seromas, or reaction to the mesh, but these were not present on examination after 3 months. In the original 180 patients, no recurrences have resulted after as long as 18 months' follow-up. No hydroceles have been noted.

DISCUSSION

Preperitoneal laparoscopic herniorrhaphy results in a tension-free repair with no necessity for groin incision. This repair is almost pain free, and the patient is allowed to return to normal activity on the second postoperative day. Primary indications for laparoscopic herniorrhaphy are the bilateral and the recurrent hernia, although all hernias may be so repaired and patient demand is increasing. Because there is no groin incision and the distal portion of large sacs are allowed to remain in place, neuromas, hematomas, ischemic orchitis, and epididymitis have been eliminated. Using the preperitoneal method we have been able to repair all hernias. Although our follow-up at present is relatively short, the floor of the canal and the repairs appear to be extremely stable and secure, with no recurrences. The time necessary for the preperitoneal repair is initially longer than the laparoscopic hernia repair as originally described.[10] As with laparoscopic cholecystectomy, the learning curve will rapidly decrease operating time to about 30 to 45 minutes. Complete understanding of the anatomy for this new approach is mandatory.

CONCLUSION

Although developmental, the preperitoneal approach to laparoscopic herniorrhaphy appears to be a relatively safe, effective way to repair all inguinal hernias, both direct and indirect, primary and recurrent. The advantage of the laparoscopic approach is a significant reduction in postoperative pain with a rapid return to normal activity. Postoperative complications associated with a groin approach, such as neuromas, neuralgia, epididymitis, ischemic orchitis, hematomas, and seromas, have been eliminated. There have been no major complications associated with laparoscopic preperitoneal herniorrhaphy in this series. At present the only apparent disadvantage is lack of long-term follow-up. However, sufficient information from a transabdominal preperitoneal approach would indicate an extremely low recurrence rate. We are presently using this preperitoneal anatomical repair in all hernias, with the exception of extremely small femoral hernias, which are still repaired by placing a patch over the femoral canal as previously described,[1] or if so desired, may be repaired using this same preperitoneal approach.

REFERENCES

1. Selective data on hospitals and use of services. In Polister P, Cunico E, eds. Socioeconomic Factbook for Surgery. Chicago Am Coll Surg 8:25-42, 1989.
2. Lichtenstein IL. Scientific exhibit ASC meeting, San Francisco, Calif. (Personal communication, October 1990.)
3. Stoppa RE, Warlaumont CR. The preperitoneal approach and prosthetic repair of groin hernia. In Nyhus LM, Condon RE, eds. Hernia. Philadelphia: JB Lippincott, 1989, pp 199-225.
4. Nyhus LM, Pollak R, Bombeck TC, Donahue PE. The preperitoneal approach and prosthetic buttress repair for recurrent hernia. Ann Surg 208:733-737, 1988.
5. Marcy HO. A new use of carbolized catgut ligatures. Boston Med J 85:315-316, 1871.
6. Griffith CA. The Marcy repair of indirect inguinal hernias: 1870 to present. In Nyhus LM, Condon RE, eds. Hernia. Philadelphia: JB Lippincott, 1989, pp 106-118.
7. Marcy HO. The cure of hernia. JAMA 8:589-592, 1887.
8. Marcy HO. Hernia. New York: Appleton, 1892.
9. LaRoque GP. The intra-abdominal method of removing inguinal and femoral hernia. Arch Surg 24:189-203, 1932.
10. Corbitt JD Jr. Laparoscopic herniorrhaphy. Surg Laparosc Endosc 1:23-25, 1991.

64 Preperitoneal Hernia Repair: Comparison of Open and Laparoscopic Techniques

Jose M. Velasco and Van L. Vallina

Although various techniques and approaches are used, the optimal treatment of groin hernia remains elusive, particularly in patients with bilateral, multiple, and/or recurrent hernias. The recurrence rate after conventional anterior repair of groin hernias, particularly recurrent hernias, remains prohibitively high (5% to 30%).[1-3] Although the open preperitoneal approach, first described in 1920 by Cheatle,[4] has been championed for years, it has failed to gain widespread acceptance, partly because of unfamiliarity with the anatomy as seen from a preperitoneal approach and because of reports in the literature about its variable success rate. In addition, hernias may result from an intrinsic or acquired collagen defect.[5] Therefore the use of prosthetic material in hernia repair has gained increased acceptance during the last decade. Ideally, a prosthetic mesh, incorporated into the hernia repair, would provide additional support and strength to otherwise inherently weak tissue. Thus in the past decade we have adopted and further modified the preperitoneal technique with simultaneous prosthetic buttressing of the entire lower abdominal wall for the management of special challenges in hernia repair.[6]

Recent advances in laparoscopic technology have fostered the incorporation and application of laparoscopic techniques to various common surgical problems. Although the majority of current laparoscopic herniorrhaphy methods use some sort of "preperitoneal repair," it is often performed through a transabdominal approach.[7] Precise definition of the preperitoneal anatomy is an absolute requirement for the safe and successful repair of groin hernias (Fig. 1). Ideally, the laparoscopic approach to herniorrhaphy should incorporate and improve the tenets of the conventional repair, which has been considered the gold standard.

In October 1991 we embarked on a prospective feasibility study of a completely extraperitoneal laparoscopic approach to inguinal hernia repair, taking into consideration the principles learned and used in the past 10 years with the open preperitoneal technique.[8]

MATERIALS AND METHODS

The conventional preperitoneal repair of groin hernia is well established. The patient is placed under regional anesthesia. An infraumbilical lower midline incision permits access to both musculopectineal orifices of Brouchard (Fig. 2). Thorough identification of all anatomical landmarks is essential. In addition, a careful, diligent search for both previously diagnosed hernia sacs and unsuspected ones should be made. For bilateral and/or multiple groin hernias, a large prosthetic patch is sutured to Cooper's ligament inferiorly and medially and to the iliopubic tract laterally (Fig. 3). A horizontal keyhole cut of the lateral aspect of the prosthetic material is made to accommodate the cord structures in the male patient (Fig. 4). Alternatively, a 2½ × 4 inch mesh prosthesis is used for unilateral defects. Antibiotic irrigation is applied, and drains are rarely used.

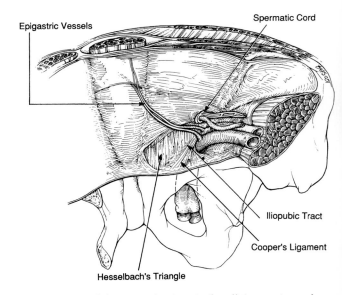

Fig. 1. View of the posterior inguinal wall (preperitoneal approach).

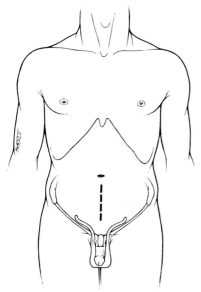

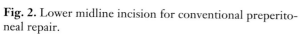

Fig. 2. Lower midline incision for conventional preperitoneal repair.

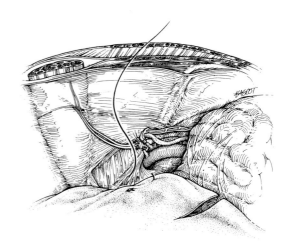

Fig. 3. Suturing mesh prosthesis to Cooper's ligament.

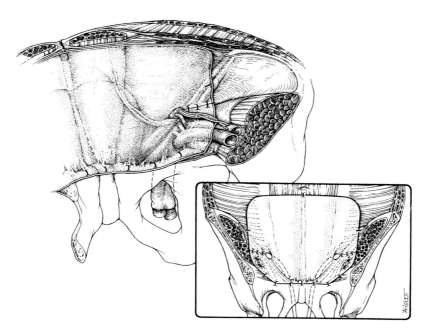

Fig. 4. Mesh prosthesis in place. *Insert*, a bilateral repair.

The laparoscopic approach requires placement of a Hasson trocar into the preperitoneal space just beneath the rectus muscle through an incision made 1 inch below the umbilicus (Fig. 5). Use of a 10 mm operating laparoscope facilitates initial preperitoneal dissection

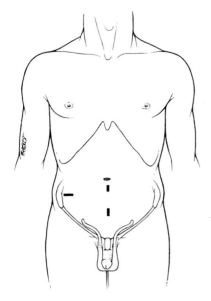

Fig. 5. Incision sites for trocar insertion (right inguinal hernia).

down to the symphysis pubis (Fig. 6). Insufflation is initiated, with a pressure setting of 10 to 12 mm Hg. Once the initial midline dissection is accomplished under direct vision, an 11 mm trocar is inserted in the midline approximately three fingerbreadths above the symphysis pubis. A 30-degree lens is substituted for the operating lens, and further lateral dissection of the peritoneum facilitates identification of the internal ring and the iliopsoas muscle. An additional 11 mm trocar is placed approximately 1 inch medial to the ipsilateral anterosuperior iliac spine. The cord structures are skeletonized, and any existing indirect sac is dissected away or transected, depending on its size. Once all hernia sacs have been reduced or eliminated as a technical concern, a 2½ × 4 inch mesh prosthesis with a precut horizontal keyhole is introduced into the preperitoneal space; the inferior edge of the mesh is stapled to Cooper's ligament and the iliopubic tract (Fig. 7). Care is taken to identify and avoid the lateral femoral cutaneous nerve. The superior edge is stapled to the abdominal wall muscles (Fig. 8). Antibiotic irrigation is applied and proper placement of the mesh verified (Fig. 9). Every laparoscopic procedure was performed with the patient under general anesthesia and on an outpatient basis.

DISCUSSION

The evolution of laparoscopic instrumentation has permitted laparoscopy to emerge as a viable alternative to

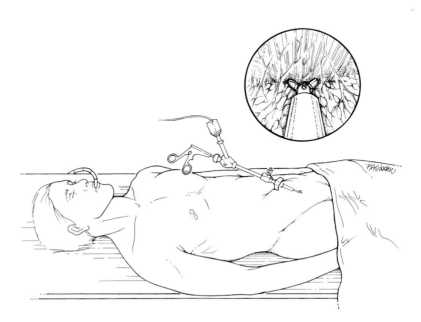

Fig. 6. The operating laparoscope with blunt forceps introduced through the working channel. Dissection of preperitoneal space *(insert)*.

traditional open techniques for the treatment of groin hernias. The preperitoneal approach for correcting difficult hernia problems has received increasing acceptance from the medical community, particularly since the routine incorporation of prosthetic material in the repair has resulted in excellent, short-term follow-up reports.[7-10]

The operative procedure described is a modification of the existing conventional technique popularized by Nyhus[8] and Nyhus et al.[9] and further modified by Stoppa et al.[10] Although a direct comparison of the results between the two patient series is difficult, given the bilateral and/or recurrent nature of the hernias in patients treated with the open technique as compared with both primary and recurrent hernias repaired with the laparoscopic technique. Similarities and differences are apparent when examining advantages and disadvantages of the preperitoneal techniques. The principles of the open preperitoneal technique, as applied to our patients with bilateral and/or recurrent hernias, have resulted in a recurrent hernia rate of 6.2% and a complication rate of 12.4% in the first 4 years of the study. Two patients experienced postoperative urinary retention requiring prolonged catheterization, and two patients experienced paresthesia in the distribution of the lateral cutaneous femoral nerve. One patient's paresthesia lasted 1 week postoperatively, whereas the second patient's paresthesia resolved when the hernia recurred on the same side 6 months later. Both recurrences happened early in the patient series and were secondary to the technical error of using too small a pros-

thesis. Nearly one in three patients undergoing the open technique was ASA Class III, necessitating regional anesthesia in more than one in two patients and general anesthesia in the others. The average operating room time was 61 minutes.

No consensus has been reached by surgeons performing laparoscopic herniorrhaphy about the optimal method of hernia repair. However, there is a belief that it is necessary to perform the herniorrhaphy in the preperitoneal space and that some type of mesh prosthesis

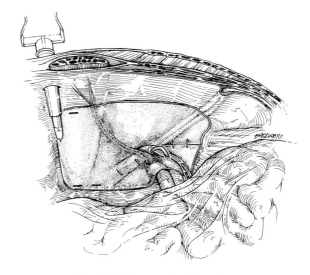

Fig. 8. Mesh prosthesis in place.

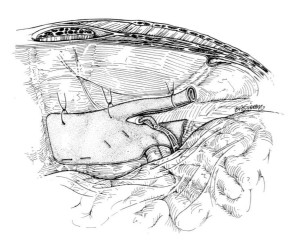

Fig. 7. Mesh prosthesis stapled to Cooper's ligament. Notice upper two thirds of mesh rolled to facilitate insertion, placement, and initial anchoring.

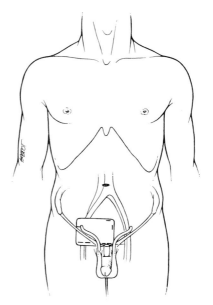

Fig. 9. Anterior view depicting mesh placement.

is always necessary. Access to the preperitoneal space can be achieved laparoscopically either by a transabdominal approach, creating a preperitoneal flap; by a combination of initial transabdominal exploration with identification of potential groin hernia sites and subsequent dissection of the preperitoneal space through extraperitoneal trocar placement; or by a third approach described herein that uses a completely extrapreperitoneal route.

RESULTS

From October 1991 until December 1992, a total of 109 patients underwent laparoscopic herniorrhaphy using these three techniques. The extrapreperitoneal approach was used in 26 patients, with nearly two thirds ASA Class I and the remaining six ASA Class II; general anesthesia was administered in all patients. The average operating room time was 90 minutes (range, 40 to 210 minutes). All patients were discharged within 23 hours. So far no recurrences have been reported in any of these patients. One patient was seen 6 months postoperatively with an incisional hernia at the 11 mm lateral trocar site; the hernia was repaired with the patient under local anesthesia. There was no injury to any nerve structures, and local seroma, which resolved spontaneously, was noticed in four patients.

The open preperitoneal technique affords several advantages over conventional herniorrhaphy, including access to both musculopectineal orifices, identification of unrecognized hernia defects, access to the abdominal cavity if required, easy and complete buttressing of any hernia defects by the use of a mesh prosthesis, and circumvention of scar tissue from previous operations. These advantages are present when laparoscopic techniques are applied to the preperitoneal approach. Additional advantages include improved cosmetic results, possible decreased postoperative pain, and possibly an earlier return to normal activities. Relative disadvantages include the need for general anesthesia and an increased operative time, with an increased cost because of instrumentation needed. However, the completely extraperitoneal technique should lend itself to the use of regional anesthesia to avoid the shoulder pain associated with transabdominal pneumoperitoneum; thus future cases will be performed with the patient under regional anesthesia as warranted.

The completely extraperitoneal technique uses an open approach to enter the preperitoneal space, thus avoiding injuries associated with trocar insertion in the transabdominal technique. Moreover, the completely extrapreperitoneal approach should, theoretically, minimize formation of adhesions by preventing exposure of the prosthetic material to the intra-abdominal contents. Operative times probably will shorten as experience with this technique is gained.

The preperitoneal approach to hernia repair demands thorough familiarity with the anatomy of the inguinal region as seen from the preperitoneal space. Our experience is that education of surgical residents exposed to this technique demands a longer learning period than does the traditional anterior repair. This technique has demonstrated its advocacy in the management of complicated inguinal hernias. Whether or not the laparoscopic preperitoneal approach will provide similar results in the management of all types of hernias will be determined by prospective studies of specific hernia type classifications to provide accurate data for comparison. Currently we are engaged in a prospective examination of the three previously described laparoscopic hernia repairs, for only this type of study will determine the utility of laparoscopic hernia repair and when to use it. This laparoscopic approach may be as ideal for patients with complex hernias in the same way as the open preperitoneal approach. In the repair of primary hernias, this procedure may have the benefits associated with other operative laparoscopic procedures: small incisions, minimal postoperative pain, and a quick recovery and return to work. It is unknown whether insertion of a mesh prosthesis at a young age will have any long-lasting effects. Moreover, long-term follow-up is necessary before conclusions about the procedure's effectiveness and safety can be made.

REFERENCES

1. Ryan EA. Recurrent hernia. Surg Gynecol Obstet 96:343-354, 1953.
2. Glassow F. Recurrent inguinal and femoral hernias. Br Med J 1:215-216, 1970.
3. Thieme T. Recurrent inguinal hernia. Arch Surg 103:238-241, 1971.
4. Cheatle GL. An operation for the radical cure of inguinal and femoral hernia. Br Med J 2:68-69, 1920.
5. Peacock EE, Madden JW. Studies on the biology and treatment of recurrent inguinal hernia. II. Morphological changes. Ann Surg 179:567-571, 1974.
6. Velasco JM, Vallina VL. Scientific exhibit: Bilateral preperitoneal hernia repair with Gore-Tex mesh. Presented at Seventy-Sixth Annual American College of Surgeons Clinical Congress, San Francisco, October 1990.

7. Filipi CJ, Fitzgibbons RJ, Salerno GM, et al. Laparoscopic herniorrhaphy. Surg Clin North Am 72:1109-1124, 1992.
8. Nyhus LM. The preperitoneal approach and iliopubic tract repair of inguinal hernia. In Nyhus LM, Condon RE, eds. Hernia. Philadelphia: JB Lippincott, 1989, pp 154-188.
9. Nyhus LM, Pollak R, Bombeck T, et al. The preperitoneal approach and prosthetic buttress repair for recurrent hernia. Ann Surg 208:733-737, 1988.
10. Stoppa RE, Warlaumont CR, Verhaeghe PJ, et al. Prosthetic repair in the treatment of groin hernias. Int Surg 71:154-158, 1986.

65 *Laparoscopically Controlled Herniorrhaphy for Direct and Indirect Inguinal Hernia: A New Technique*

Hans-Joachim Meyer

Laparoscopic hernia repair preserves the integrity of the anterior abdominal wall. Whether this advantage can compensate for the expense and risks involved in a laparoscopic approach will eventually be determined by assessing long-term results.

Most reports in the literature on methods of laparoscopic hernia repair describe the use of artificial implants, which induce connective tissue proliferation and are used to cover hernial openings. The future of these implants, particularly with respect to infection, is uncertain and the cost of placing them is high. It would therefore be preferable to apply the tried and true principles of conventional hernia repair to laparoscopic operations. Thus far only one laparoscopic method has achieved closure of hernial openings by means of sutures, using the anatomical structures at the level of the transverse fascia.

Many surgeons are unfamiliar with the inguinal anatomy as viewed with a laparoscope. The medial umbilical ligament (obliterated umbilical artery), the spermatic vessels, the round ligament, the vas, and the inferior epigastric artery (which may be localized by diaphanoscopy) serve as laparoscopic anatomical landmarks. After the peritoneum is opened medial to the inferior epigastric artery, mostly by blunt dissection, the following landmarks become visible: the superior pubic ramus with Cooper's ligament, the transverse fascia of the medial wall of the inguinal canal, the iliopubic tract, and the arch.

In indirect inguinal hernias the pneumoperitoneum displaces the transverse fascia of the medial wall of the inguinal canal—which is also the hernial opening—medially. When the abdomen is relaxed the transverse fascia lies in a frontal plane. This displacement by the pneumoperitoneum allows it to appear as the medial side wall of the inguinal canal. Under these conditions the iliopubic tract forms the dorsal wall of the inguinal canal. At the same time it forms the ventral border of the femoral canal. A needle introduced horizontally just lateral to the external inguinal ring at a right angle to the long axis of the inguinal ligament, with the patient in a supine position with a pneumoperitoneum established, therefore passes through the hernial canal and the transverse fascia. The spermatic cord lies dorsally on the floor of the inguinal canal and is not disturbed. After inversion of the hernial sac and dissection of the preperitoneal space, the direct hernial opening becomes visible. The transverse abdominal arch and iliopubic tract are usually forced apart in a ventrodorsal direction leaving a transverse oval slit. After inversion of the hernial sac a cavity lined by rolled-out transverse fascia remains. This rolled-out transverse fascia can also be inverted and when incised the spermatic cord appears to be in an anterior-lateral-caudal position.

Laparoscopic findings suggest that indirect inguinal hernias are a functional disturbance of the transverse fascia, whereas direct inguinal hernias may be considered a structural disturbance of this fascia. Hence hernia repair in indirect hernias should consist of lateral movement of the transverse fascia closing the internal inguinal ring and the inguinal canal. Direct hernia repair should include readaptation of the ventrodorsally parted edges of the iliopubic tract and the transversus abdominis arch. In direct hernias the intra-abdominal pressure supports the lateral fixation of the transverse fascia by pressing against the transverse fascia instead of along the hernial canal. After repair of a direct hernia there is continued intra-abdominal pressure exerted on the weak spot of the transverse fascia (Hesselbach's triangle). This may explain the high recurrence rate in this condition.

With these considerations in mind we developed the following technique of laparoscopic hernia repair in May 1991. It is based on a combination of percutaneously placed U sutures using an awl specifically designed for use outside the abdomen, laparoscopic dissection of the inguinal canal and the preperitoneal space, laparoscopically controlled advancement of the awl, and laparoscopic assistance in the placement of the U sutures. The following setup is preferred: patient with legs spread apart and hip joints hyperextended, monitor placed between the legs, 25-degree laparoscope with a video camera inserted through an infraumbilical incision, a 5 mm cannula for grasping forceps and a 10 mm cannula for dissecting scissors on the left and right of the umbilicus pararectally, and a 12 mm Hg pneumoperitoneum.

INDIRECT HERNIA REPAIR

The peritoneum is incised medially and along the inferior epigastric artery. The peritoneum of the hernial sac is opened in line with the inguinal ligament shining through the peritoneum. Blunt dissection of the hernial sac is carried out until it and the spermatic cord form a rolled-up bundle of tissue on the floor of the inguinal canal. The cremaster muscle is pushed off the free edge of the inguinal ligament. Blunt dissection of the preperitoneal inguinal space is performed until the superior pubic ramus becomes visible. The sites predisposed to femoral and direct hernias are inspected. The transverse fascia and iliopubic tract, which is a dorsal condensation of the transverse fascia and forms the floor of the inguinal canal and at the same time the roof of the femoral canal is exposed. The IEA lying on the transverse fascia at the medial border of the hernial canal is exposed and mobilized. A stab incision is made just lateral to the external inguinal ring over the free edge of the inguinal ligament. The awl is then passed through the stab incision and laparoscopically controlled, and the free edge of the inguinal ligament appears in the inguinal canal. The awl is passed parallel

to the abdominal wall and ventral to the rolled-up bundle of tissue on the floor of the inguinal canal made up of spermatic cord and hernial sac through the transverse fascia. The thread, a nonabsorbable monofilament-strength USP 2 material, is carried along with the awl, which is grasped intra-abdominally, and the empty awl is withdrawn. The long end of the thread remains outside the abdomen, while the short end remains inside.

The same puncture site is used to introduce another awl carrying a thread forming a loop 1 cm ventral and parallel to the path of the first awl. The short end of the first thread is pulled through the loop, the loop is tightened extra-abdominally, and when the awl carrying the tightened loop is withdrawn, it pulls the short end of the first thread outside the abdomen. The U suture with both ends of the thread outside of the abdomen is then complete. The maneuver is repeated in from three or four stab incision sites following lateral to the first. In this way a suture line parallel to the iliopubic tract and ventral to the spermatic cord is generated. When the threads are tied outside the abdomen the knots slide down to the fascia. The transverse fascia is drawn toward the free edge of the inguinal ligament, resulting in closure of the inguinal canal and the deep inguinal ring. The rolled-up bundle of tissue consisting of the hernial sac and the spermatic cord appears as a bulge medially between the ventral suture line and the dorsal iliopubic tract. The medial edge of the peritoneum is drawn behind the internal inguinal ring and sutured to the inguinal ligament using a resorbable U suture introduced by means of the previously described awl technique.

DIRECT HERNIA REPAIR

The hernial sac is grasped intra-abdominally, inverted, and the peritoneum overlying it is incised transversely at its ventral circumference between the medial umbilical ligament and the epigastric vessels. Mostly blunt dissection of the preperitoneal inguinal space is used with exposure of the superior pubic ramus, the iliopubic tract, the hernial opening ventrally with its medial boundary (rectus muscle), its ventral boundary (transverse abdominal arch), and its lateral boundary (transverse fascia of the medial wall of the inguinal canal). All preperitoneal fat is pushed off with a blunt instrument. The rolled-out transverse fascia lining the cavity after removal of the hernial sac is grasped at its deepest point, inverted, and incised transversely. When the dorsal leaf is pulled cranially, its transition into the transverse fascia and the transverse abdominal arch becomes visible. Looking through the direct hernial opening, the outlines of the external inguinal ring and, further ventrally, the skin are visible. The spermatic cord lies just ventral and caudal to the ventral leaf of the incised transverse fascia. It extends laterally where it lies in front of the medial wall of the inguinal canal and is no longer visible. Using curved awls, three to four U sutures are introduced through separate stab incisions and passed through the stout segments of the inverted transverse fascia, the transverse abdominal arch, and the iliopubic tract. The stab incisions lie in a transverse line just cranial and lateral to the pubic tubercle. If closure of the hernial opening is possible only with some tension, the suture line may be protected additionally with a 3×5 cm polypropylene net. The net is held in place with two ventrally placed absorbable U sutures introduced with the awl technique. The net then hangs down over the superior pubic ramus like a curtain. Dorsal fixation is not necessary, because internal abdominal pressure and ventral fixation sutures hold it in place. The peritoneum is again closed using the inverted hernial sac with one or two loosely tied absorbable U sutures, which are also placed with a straight awl.

RESULTS

Since May 1991 we have performed 296 laparoscopic hernia repairs in 266 patients, 200 indirect and 83 were direct.

Complications

The complication rate was 3%. Specific complications included one stab wound infection, three hematomas, and one hematocele (testicular swelling, testicular atrophy, or neurological symptoms were not observed). There was one nonspecific case of postoperative urinary retention. Laparoscopic complications included one enterocutaneous fistula, which healed spontaneously, and two cases of hemorrhaging from port sites.

Contraindications

These included the following: high anesthetic risk, childhood hernias, incarceration, intraoperative irreducibility, adhesions in the lower abdomen, and scrotal sliding hernia with fixation of the intestines.

Recurrences

We observed eight recurrences (4%) among 200 laparoscopically repaired indirect hernias. Since 1992 three recurrences (2.1%) have been observed in 141 indirect hernias. Some of the significant modifications in the development of this new technique were changes in suture materials and the number of U sutures and reinforcement of the posterior wall of the deep inguinal ring. As a result of unacceptable recurrence rates in direct hernia repair, the initially solely intraperitoneal procedure was converted to a technique with preperitoneal dissection. In 30 hernias repaired with the above-described method we observed one recurrence.

Laparoscopically controlled closure by suturing of the inguinal hernial opening is feasible and does not require expensive equipment. Results obtained thus far show few nonspecific complications and no specific complications. Recurrence rates are low but cannot yet be estimated correctly.

66 *Preliminary Results in the Repair of Complex Primary Inguinal Hernias With Expanded Polypropylene Patch*

Josep Domingo Fontanet, Jaume Vall-Llovera Gambus, F. Pi, Jordi Colomer Mascaro, Salvador Navarro Soto, Carles Ortiz Rodriguez, and Enrique Sierra Gil

In this study, the results of the use of an expanded polypropylene patch in the primary repair of complex inguinal hernias were evaluated. A review of 216 inguinal hernioplasties performed with the Bassini method in our department from March 1988 to December 1989 showed a recurrence rate of 7.4%. The Bassini technique requires strong, healthy inguinal structures to ensure lasting closure of the inguinal defect. The high rate of recurrence that we encountered suggested that the inguinal structures in the cases studied were often unsuitable for use in hernia repair.

MATERIALS AND METHODS

Since 1990 we have used the same expanded polypropylene patch that we had been using to repair recurrent hernias for the primary repair of complex inguinal hernias. The patch was implanted when multiple defects in the posterior wall of the inguinal canal were found, if there was a large single defect, or if the surrounding tissues were too weak to hold a sutured repair. We felt that use of the patch would result in a decreased rate of hernia recurrence.

From January 1990 to December 1991, 292 inguinal hernias were repaired in our department. In 281 patients, hernioplasty was performed electively; in 11 cases, it was an emergency procedure. We used the expanded polypropylene patch in 50 patients who underwent an elective operation; the other 231 patients underwent a classic sutured technique (the Bassini method was used in 216 patients, and other techniques were used in 15 patients).

To obtain two homogeneous groups, the hernioplasties performed as emergencies and those in which a sutured technique other than the Bassini method was used were excluded. Only elective hernioplasties in which the Bassini technique was used (216 patients; group A) and those in which an expanded polypropylene patch was used (50 patients; group B) are reviewed.

Group A patients presented with a small defect in the posterior wall of the inguinal canal that could be repaired without apparent tension. Patients in group B had hernias considered to be at high risk of recurrence because a tensionless repair could not be used. In these patients, the expanded polypropylene patch was implanted. Patients in group B were approximately 10 years older than group A patients (59.9 versus 51.3 years), and there were more men in group B (15.6 men/1 woman versus 7.3 men/1 woman in group A).

In group A, 66 patients had a direct hernia, 140 patients had an indirect hernia, and 10 patients had a pantaloon hernia. In group B, 24 patients had a direct hernia, 21 had an indirect hernia, and 5 had a pantaloon hernia.

The polypropylene patch, which was sutured with a continuous silk Polidek suture, was anchored to the pubic tubercle. It was first sutured deep to the inguinal ligament (Cooper's ligament) and then medially to the rectus sheath with a minimum of 5 mm of overlap at that potentially weak site. It was kept taut during the repair but was not sutured under tension. The slit, which was cut to allow the passage of the spermatic cord, was closed by suturing the edges to each other and to the underlying fascia ("patch keyhole"). The wound was closed over a suction drain.

RESULTS

Systemic postoperative complications were noted in two patients: A headache after rachianesthesia and a urinary infection, both of which occurred in group A patients. There were no operative deaths in either group.

Group A patients (10.1%) suffered from 22 local complications: 12 wound hematomas (5.5%), 5 wound seromas (2.3%), 4 wound infections (1.8%), and 1 scrotal hematoma. Local complications occurred in 9 group B patients (18%): A serohematoma superficial to the patch was seen in four patients, a scrotal hematoma occurred in two patients, and three patients had a wound infection.

The mean hospital stay was 4.2 days for group A patients and 7.4 days for group B patients. The mean duration of follow-up was 20 months (range, 8 to 24 months). Seven recurrences (3.2%) were noted in group A and one recurrence (2%) was observed in group B.

DISCUSSION

The postoperative follow-up (20 months) in this series is limited. However, because recurrence after herniorrhaphy as a result of a technical defect usually appears during the first year after surgery, a 20-month follow-up may show findings related to the surgical technique used. The use of an expanded polypropylene patch yielded a recurrence rate of 2%, which was much lower than the approximately 5% rate observed in large series of patients who underwent primary classic hernioplasty.

We emphasize that the hernias in which the patch was used for repair had occurred in a selected group of patients who were at greater risk of complications and recurrence. In spite of this, these patients had a recurrence rate (2%) lower than that of patients whose hernias were repaired with a sutured technique before 1990 (7.4%), and they had a lower rate than did the patients with a lower risk of recurrence who were treated with a suture technique since January 1990 (3.2%).

CONCLUSION

The use of expanded polypropylene patch in the primary repair of complex inguinal hernias was technically easy and resulted in a low recurrence rate.

XI

Videoendoscopic Small and Large Bowel Surgery

67 Percutaneous Management of Postoperative Abdominal Fistulas

Jacques-Henri Boverie, Alain Remont, and Robert F. Dondelinger

Abdominal surgery is the main cause of enterocutaneous fistulas (ENTF), but these can also arise as a complication of inflammatory or neoplastic disease, as well as trauma or radiation injury. ENTF originating from intestinal walls or biliary or pancreatic ducts drain a mixture of digestive secretions and pus or necrotic matter.[1] Low-output fistulas (LOF), draining less than 100 ml/day, become mature with a fibrous tract when initially controlled nonoperatively. Patient morbidity results only from long-term discomfort.[2,3] High-output fistulas (HOF), draining at least 300 ml to as much as 4000 ml/day, cause dramatic morbidity with necrosis perforating the intestinal wall, sentinel abscess at the internal opening, intra-abdominal propagation of sepsis and collections of associated abscesses, and multiple tracts interlaced beneath the skin, leading to external orifices and skin maceration. Nonoperative treatment is given first, except in the most serious cases of peritonitis, which require operative management. Digestive secretions are reduced by antisecretory drugs, especially somatostatin. Parenteral hyperalimentation improves patients' general condition and allows nonseptic fistulas to heal. Operation is indicated when HOF do not show a significant improvement after 6 weeks.[1,2,4]

In the last 10 years, this management has resulted in a decrease in the mortality rate from sepsis from 45% to 67% to 6% to 25%.[2,4] The main causes of treatment failure and a still high surgical mortality rate are emphasized in the surgical literature: "As long as tracts are bathed in digestive secretions abscesses cannot easily heal."[1,4,5] Until recently, radiological studies were limited to the identification of morbid anatomy. Technical advances in interventional radiology have made possible selective catheterization of the most tortuous tracts and drainage of associated abscesses.[3,6-8] The purpose of this report is to describe a radiological method of percutaneous management that allows true controlled external drainage by catheterization of the internal orifice of the bowel, and of the biliary or pancreatic ducts, with diversion of digestive secretions.

MATERIALS AND METHODS

During the past 6 years, of 117 patients treated for ENTF at our institution, 83 (70.9%) had postoperative fistulas. Sixty-eight of these fistulas (81.9%) were HOF and 15 (18.1%) were LOF. Percutaneous management was the therapeutic regimen in all cases. There were 45 men (54.6%) and 38 women (45.4%), ranging in age from 35 to 76 years with a mean of 69 years. HOF usually arose from lesions located between the inferior third of the esophagus and the jejunum, and LOF from the ileum or the colon (Table 1).

Fistulogram and Cannulation

Since the three-dimensional tortuous orientation of tracts was unpredictable, the main tract was identified by injecting a water-soluble povidone-based contrast medium under fluoroscopic control. Fistulograms were obtained directly from the cutaneous opening to demonstrate the main axis and avoid false passage into the subcutaneous tracts at the time of cannulation. Spot films in several projections were taken to delineate the

Table 1. Origin of alimentary tract perforation in relation to high-output and low-output postoperative fistulas

Location	No. of Cases	HOF (%)	LOF (%)
Gastroduodenum	25	30.1	0
Small bowel	17	14.5	6
Bile duct	16	19.3	0
Pancreatic duct	13	15.7	0
Colon	6	0	7.2
Appendix	3	0	3.6
Esophagus and stomach	2	2.4	0
Posthysterectomy	1	0	1.2
TOTAL	83	81.9	18.1

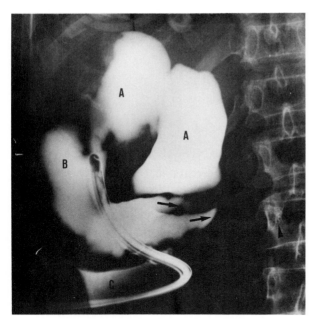

Fig. 1. Post–Roux-en-Y gastrojejunostomy complications. Abscesses are identified on the fistulogram. *A,* Anteroposterior subhepatic spaces; *B,* lateral extension toward the subphrenic recess; *C,* downward spread into the paracolic gutter. Inner branchings point to surgical clips *(arrows).* No connection with bowel lumen is apparent. Abscesses are drained.

anatomy of the deep tracts and communicating abscesses (Figs. 1 and 2).

A 5 to 7 Fr, end-hole, angiographic catheter, narrower than the ENTF and mounted over a 0.89 to 0.97 mm, J-shaped, torquing guidewire, was gently advanced as far as possible into the main tract. Sinuosities were negotiated with the 5 mm J wire protruding from the catheter tip. For LOF the guidewire was anchored directly to the internal opening, and the catheter was advanced over it into the lumen of the bowel. For HOF the guidewire was usually coiled into large abscesses, and the internal orifice was not apparent. All encountered abscesses had to be drained (Fig. 1). The residual ramifications were explored by exchanging catheters and choosing a curvature fitting the anatomy to find a tract that might extend into a collected cavity, the so-called sentinel abscess, near the site of the bowel or duct perforation (Fig. 2, *A*). The catheter was directed into the entrance of the abscess and the guidewire was advanced. Access to the lumen was gained by crossing the sentinel abscess (Fig. 2, *B*).

Draining Modalities

Over a stiff Lunderquist guidewire, the internal-external drainage device was inserted into the lumen of the alimentary tract. The width of the internal openings was

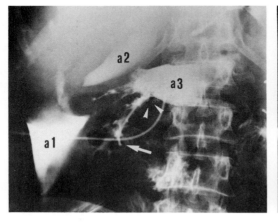
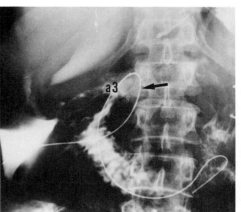

Fig. 2. HOF management sequence. (Same case as in Fig. 1.) **A,** Residual cavities *(a1, a2)* are explored by exchanging catheter. "Sentinel abscess" *(a3)* is discovered near site of bowel perforation *(arrowheads).* Angiographic catheter is passed through it and internal opening is achieved *(arrow).* **B,** Guidewire is introduced deeply into the loop lumen *(arrow).*

estimated from fistulograms and known calibers of withdrawn angiographic catheters. The draining device was to be slightly narrower to avoid enlarging the necrotic internal orifices.

For HOF, 12 to 18 Fr biliary pigtails (Fig. 3) or 20 Fr large-bore T tube (see Fig. 6) catheters were used. For LOF, 6.6 to 12 Fr, multiple side-hole Ring-Lunderquist catheters sufficed to control intestinal contents.

Evacuation of Cavity Contents

Over a guidewire, 8 to 30 Fr surgical sump drains were placed into communicating abscesses and next to the internal orifice to control leakage around the draining device and permit irrigation. Endoluminal drains were set to low suction, and sump drains were set to continuous high suction (Figs. 3 to 6).

RESULTS

The efficacy of the drainage was monitored according to a four-parameter chart (see Fig. 5). Temperature increased on the day after manipulations but returned to normal within 3 days. For HOF, sump drain output decreased with the thermic curve to less than 50 ml after 8 days. Endoluminal tube output reached 3000 ml at the beginning by evacuation of the stasis and then became equal to the normal gastrointestinal tract contents. Skin maceration resolved within 30 days and the external orifice closed around the drains.

An abnormality in the curves indicated bad positioning or a failure resulting from the spread of infection. If only fever persisted, it became necessary to look for another cause (e.g., infection around the parenteral hyperalimentation catheter). As early as the second week after sump drain removal, the fistulogram showed a straight, mature, fibrous tract. The endoluminal drain was removed and a 6 Fr, straight, multiple side-hole catheter was placed in contact with the internal opening. It soon became possible to clamp it without leaks. The ENTF closed spontaneously in approximately 4 to 6 weeks (see Fig. 5).

Of the 68 patients who presented with HOF, 62 (91.2%) were cured in 2 to 7 weeks (mean, 4 weeks), with no need for invasive operative treatment. In six patients radiological management was unsuccessful, with failure of catheterization in two cases (2.9%) and failures of the draining methods in the remaining four cases (5.9%). For the 15 patients with LOF, results were not as good. Only nine of them were cured (60%), and the drainage

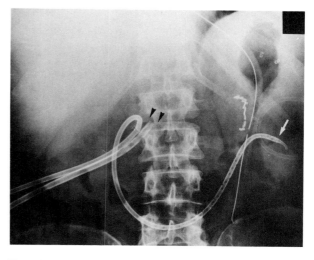

Fig. 3. HOF management sequence. Internal-external drainage and evacuation of cavity contents. (Same case as in Figs. 1 and 2.) An 18 Fr multiple side-hole, biliary pigtail catheter is anchored within the lumen and pushed as far as possible into the afferent loop *(arrow)*. Sump drain is placed next to the internal orifice. After high suction, communicating abscess resolves quickly *(arrowheads)*.

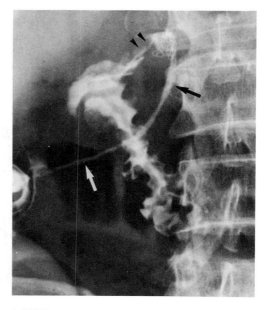

Fig. 4. HOF management sequence. Control. (Same case as in Figs. 1, 2, and 3.) From the third week on, mature tract appears *(arrows)*. Last fistulogram before definitive closure.

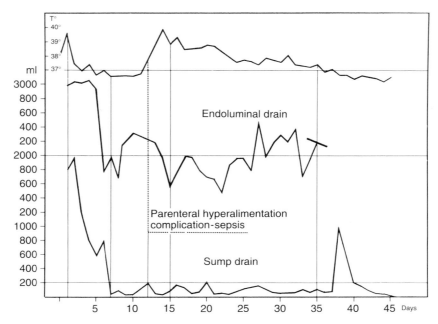

Fig. 5. Drainage monitoring. Typical chart (see text). *1°,* On day 12, output curves remain good while temperature increases (parenteral catheter infection); *2°,* on day 35, endoluminal drain is removed with a concomitant small peak in sump output. Fistula becomes mature and closes spontaneously on day 45.

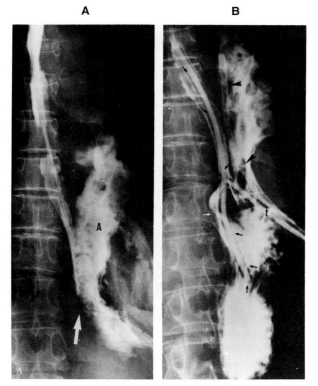

Fig. 6. Lateral site perforation during treatment with T-tube. Emetic esophagogastric rupture. **A,** Initial status. Esophagogastric discontinuity *(arrow)* and large mediastinal abscess *(A).* **B,** T-tube placement. Proximal limb into esophagus *(upper arrows)* and distal limb into stomach *(lower arrows)* are in alignment with the esophagogastric axis, and effluents are drained by the main limb *(t).* Sump drain is in abscess *(arrowheads).*

duration was always longer (mean, 7 weeks). Failure of the draining methods accounted for 23.3% of the unsuccessful outcomes (Tables 2 and 3).

DISCUSSION

No specific premedication was required to perform endoluminal or communicating abscess drainage. Anxiety was the principal cause for patient discomfort. Diazepam was given intravenously as needed. The procedure was performed in all cases during broad-spectrum antibiotic therapy and under intensive medical care for HOF.

Complications were rare and could be avoided by careful manipulation. Bleeding of necrotic ENTF occurred frequently but was transient. False passages were the major risk of sepsis propagation. Pyogenic septa of a collected abscess could also be ruptured if contrast medium was injected too vigorously. The use of a soft, J-shaped guidewire and continuous fluoroscopic control were the safest way to avoid these risks. We encountered no such complications in this series of 83 patients. More recently, however, one patient who presented with HOF associated with two big intra-abdominal abscesses died of sepsis the day after the procedure.

The choice of the draining device depended on the etiology and morphology of the ENTF. HOF in a blind loop occurred after gastrojejunostomy, biliary tract surgery, and pancreatectomy. Perforation resulted from

Table 2. High-output fistulae: Outcome of postoperative percutaneous management

| Etiology | No. of Cases | Successful* | | Drainage Duration (wk) |
		No.	Percent	
Gastroduodenostomy[†]	25	24	96	2-4
Biliary tract surgery[‡]	16	15	93.8	2-6
Pancreatectomy[†,‡]	13	11	84.6	3-6
Intestinal resection[†]	12	10	84.6	2-4
Emetic esophagogastric rupture	2	2	100	6
TOTAL	68	62	91.2	Mean = 4

*Healing without need for surgical treatment.
[†]Failure of draining methods: 4% to 5.9%.
[‡]Failure of catheterization: 2 to 2.9%.

Table 3. Low-output fistulas: Outcome of postoperative percutaneous management

| Etiology | No. of Cases | Successful* | | Drainage Duration (wk) |
		No.	Percent	
Colectomy[†]	6	3	50	4-7
Intestinal resection[‡]	5	4	80	4-7
Appendectomy[†]	3	1	33	6
Hysterectomy	1	1	100	12
TOTAL	15	9	60	Mean = 7

*Healing without need for surgical treatment.
[†]Failure of draining methods: 5% to 23.3%.
[‡]Failure of catheterization: 1% to 6.7%.

stasis in the afferent loop, and the internal opening was terminal because of suture breakdown of the stump. Multiple side–hole, biliary, pigtail catheters provided ideal drainage. The tapered tip facilitated insertion into the axis of the terminal orifice, and the 40 lateral holes allowed the static fluid to be suctioned. In cases of lateral perforation, T tubes were preferred because their horizontal limbs controlled the flow of intestinal contents from above and below the site of perforation (Fig. 6, *A* and *B*). The placement technique was similar to that described by Millan et al.[9] for drainage of the bile duct.

LOF were difficult to cure, particularly those originating from the colon. Fecal matter prevented effective internal-external drainage. Nevertheless, all patients were referred for percutaneous management long after unsuccessful nonoperative treatment. These conditions did not favor radiological drainage.

CONCLUSION

Percutaneous management of HOF is a valuable minimally invasive approach for seriously ill patients. The difficulty does not lie in cannulation or even in the setting of endoluminal drainage but rather in identification and drainage of all associated abscess cavities. Not all patients will respond to minimally invasive treatment. Open operation is indicated after an attempt at closed drainage of at least 8 weeks or for uncontrolled peritonitis. However, in all cases, controlling intestinal output and decreasing the amount of infection will increase the chance of a successful outcome and reduce skin maceration to a minimum. Low-output, long-duration fistulas are also a relative indication.

REFERENCES

1. Fischer JE. The pathophysiology of enterocutaneous fistulas. World J Surg 7:446-450, 1983.
2. Fazio VW, Coutsoftides T, Steiger E. Factors influencing the outcome of treatment of small bowel cutaneous fistula. World J Surg 7:481-488, 1983.
3. Kerlan RK, Jeffrey RB Jr, Pogany AC, et al. Abdominal abscess with low-output fistulae: Successful percutaneous drainage. Radiology 155:73-75, 1985.
4. Harju E, Pessi T, Koikkalainen T, et al. The treatment of high enterocutaneous fistula with surgical drainage and total parenteral nutrition. Int Surg 70:33-38, 1985.
5. Levy E, Parc R, Bloch P, et al. Transorificial intubation with direct neutralisation of digestive juices in cases of gastric or duodenal lesions: Principle and application of a new treatment for severe postoperative peritonitis of gastric or duodenal origin. Ann Chir 36:419-423, 1982.
6. McLean GK, Macki JA, Feiman DB, et al. Enterocutaneous fistulae: Interventional radiologic management. Am J Roentgenol 138:615-619, 1982.
7. Papanicoulaou N, Mueller PR, Ferruci JT Jr, et al. Abscess fistula association: Radiologic recognition and percutaneous management Am J Roentgenol 143:811-815, 1984.
8. Boverie JH, Raimont A. Percutaneous management of fistulas in digestive tract. In Dondelinger RF, Rossi P, Kurdziel JC, eds. Interventional Radiology. Stuttgart: G Thieme Verlag, 1990, pp 746-753.
9. Millan VG, Bramhavar DM, Kwon OJ, et al. Percutaneous replacement of biliary T-tubes. Am J Roentgenol 132:140-141, 1979.

68   *Laparoscopic Techniques Applied to Colonic Procedures*

Morris E. Franklin, Jr., Raul Ramos, Daniel Rosenthal, and William W. Schuessler

As laparoscopy has become an acceptable surgical procedure for the treatment of intra-abdominal disease, it has been adapted for use in bowel surgery. We will review our experience in developing basic techniques in an animal model. We will also review our clinical series of 89 laparoscopic procedures for colonic lesions, both malignant and nonmalignant, and discuss indications, techniques, and results.

ANIMAL STUDIES

In 30 pigs weighing 20 to 30 kg, colon preparation was done with polyethylene glycol solution and parenteral gentamicin (3 mg/kg). After anesthesia was induced endotracheally, sterile technique was used to prepare and drape each animal's abdomen. Pneumoperitoneum was induced by insufflation of CO_2 by means of a Veress needle and an electronic pressure-controlled insufflator. An 11 mm incision was made infraumbilically, and an Endopath (Ethicon) trocar was inserted; a camera-equipped laparoscope was introduced, and a video monitor was used to inspect the peritoneal cavity. Three to five additional ports were placed in the lower abdomen to facilitate the dissection. Adequacy of bowel preparation was confirmed by visualization of the distal colon with a flexible sigmoidoscope. Because to our knowledge these procedures had not previously been performed, we began with simple laparoscopic operations that were used to demonstrate the efficacy of this type of surgery.

A colon wall incision and defect repair were performed in five pigs. A 2 cm full-thickness button of sigmoid colon was then excised with scissors and a KTP 532 laser (Ethicon). The specimen was retrieved through the anus with a snare that was placed through the sigmoidoscope. We used laparoscopic suturing techniques developed in our laboratory to close the colotomy in two layers. The integrity of the suture line was tested laparoscopically by direct visualization after the segment was insufflated with air through the sigmoidoscope. A sigmoid resection with a hand-sewn anastomosis was then performed in five pigs, and a stapled anastomosis was completed in 10 pigs. The initial step

of the colonic resection was the division of the lateral peritoneal attachment of the colon. The vessels were controlled with Endoclips before division. The bowel was transected with the KTP 532 laser at a setting of 12 W. A colonoscopic snare was used to remove the divided segment through the anus. Running inverted 3-0 Vicryl sutures were used to perform an anastomosis in one layer. After this procedure proved feasible, subsequent anastomoses were performed with an ILS circular stapler introduced through the anus. Chromic catgut Endoloops were used as purse-string sutures, the instrument was fired, and the anastomotic integrity was again checked by endoscopy with insufflation pressure.

Results

All pigs survived the operation and were sacrificed 1 to 4 months after surgery. The surgically treated colon segments were examined, and all anastomoses were noted to have healed satisfactorily and to have an adequate luminal diameter. After completion of the animal experiments (a 6-month period), we determined that laparoscopic colotomy, colorrhaphy, colectomy, and restoration of bowel continuity can be safely performed in the porcine model.

CLINICAL EXPERIENCE
Technique

Preoperative bowel preparation consists of administration of oral polyethylene glycol solution or clear liquids with milk of magnesia; standard parenteral and oral antibiotics are also given. General endotracheal anesthesia is used. The patient is placed in the modified lithotomy position with the legs in Lloyd-Davies stirrups. A nasogastric tube and a Foley catheter are placed, and the pneumoperitoneum is created with a Veress needle. An 11 mm incision is then made at the level of the umbilicus, and a 0-degree laparoscope with an attached video camera is introduced through a 10 to 11 mm trocar. The abdominal viscera are carefully inspected. If a tumor is seen in the liver, a biopsy is taken percutaneously with a Tru-Cut needle. Four 10 mm additional ports are introduced under direct laparoscopic visualization:

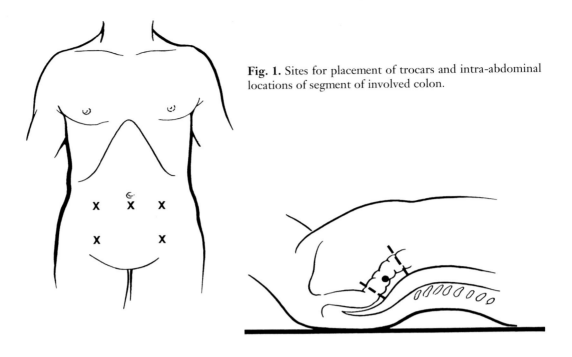

Fig. 1. Sites for placement of trocars and intra-abdominal locations of segment of involved colon.

two in the left lower abdomen and two in the right lower quadrant (Fig. 1). (A suprapubic 5 mm port is placed for introduction of PDS ligature loops.) Additional ports are added as needed.

The patient is placed in a very steep Trendelenburg position with a slight tilt to the right side. Loops of small bowel are gently swept from the left lower quadrant, the right lower quadrant, and the pelvis. Adhesions are frequently encountered and must be transsected sharply or with the laser. The lesion is then assessed laparoscopically and with the flexible sigmoidoscope. The adequacy of the bowel preparation is confirmed with the flexible sigmoidoscope. Any residual intraluminal debris is thoroughly aspirated, and the area is irrigated with a solution of saline and 10% povidone-iodine.

The usual adhesions of sigmoid colon to the pelvic peritoneum in the left pelvic wall are incised, and the colon is mobilized medially; the ureter must be visualized while this maneuver is performed. The extent of the resection is determined by a combined laparoscopic and colonoscopic evaluation that is followed by marking the anticipated proximal and distal lines of resection of the bowel with a small mechanical cut or with

methylene blue that is injected through the flexible sigmoidoscope. These areas are then carefully cleaned of adipose tissue. The mesentery is transected with sharp and blunt dissection and with electrocautery. The mesenteric vessels are either ligated with sutures or are transected after endoclips are applied (Fig. 2). We have developed an extracorporeal ligation technique that can be used to securely ligate vessels as large as the inferior mesenteric artery so that slipping does not occur.

The colon is divided proximally and distally with the KTP laser or with electrocautery, and the specimen removed through the anus with a snare passed by means of the flexible sigmoidoscope (Fig. 3). The proximal end of the colon is controlled, and leakage is prevented by newly developed laparoscopic Glassman clamps. The size of the specimen to be removed is important in the determination of the route of extraction. For small specimens, the transanal route is desirable. However, a large specimen must be placed during the procedure in a specimen bag placed intraperitoneally; at the end of the procedure, the infraumbilical port is enlarged to permit specimen extraction. When the bowel has been transected, the ILS stapler is introduced transanally and is

Cephalad

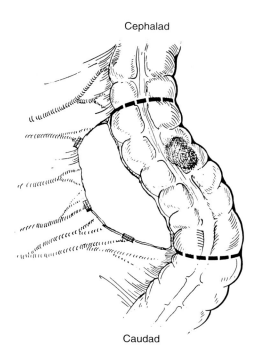

Caudad

Fig. 2. Segment of devascularized bowel (with contained lesion) ready for resection. Mesenteric vessels have been ligated, cauterized, or clipped as required by vessel size.

Cephalad/proximal

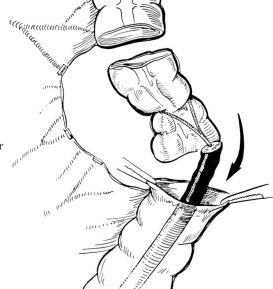

Fig. 3. Divided segment of bowel is removed by colonoscope after capture by endoscopic snare.

Caudad/distal

opened. An Endoloop is positioned over the distal end of the bowel and is tightened to act as a purse-string suture. It is convenient to leave extra bowel in the Endoloop so that slipping is avoided while this suture is tightened. The excess tissue is then removed before the instrument is fired.

The proximal end of the bowel is then placed over the anvil of the stapler and is again secured with an Endoloop. This step is difficult and requires patience as well as coordination among the surgeon, the assistant, and the endoscopist. When the ends of the bowel are secured over the instrument and trimming has been completed, the cartridge is closed, and the ILS is fired under direct vision (Fig. 4). The ILS is removed and the two doughnuts of tissue are inspected. The anastomosis is checked for integrity by saline irrigation of the pelvis and by insufflation of air through the sigmoidoscope to create pressure in the colonic segment. Any air leaks in the defect are repaired with a 3-0 Vicryl suture. The

anastomosis must be rechecked with air insufflation under pressure to ensure the absence of leakage.

Colonic Polypectomy

Colonoscopic localization is mandatory at polypectomy. The standard indications for open polypectomy are also considered to be indications for laparoscopic polypectomy. As many preoperative biopsies as possible should be obtained to identify malignancy.

The patient's position and the insertion sites of working ports depend on the location of the lesion and vary with right, left, sigmoid, or transverse colon lesions. The ports should not be positioned immediately over the lesion but rather at a distant site to provide adequate triangulation and to avoid "dueling" between the instruments. After the patient is positioned and the operating ports and laparoscope are placed, the colonoscope is introduced and the position of the polyp is demonstrated transluminally. This may be difficult; a skilled colonoscopist is required. Continuous communication between the laparoscopist and the endoscopist is mandatory.

Tattooing of the perimeter of the lesion base with methylene blue or india ink is recommended so that the colotomy is performed at the most desirable and convenient level when the lesion is localized and the colon is clean. A colotomy is performed to encompass the thickness of the colon and the base of the polyp. We have found that the KTP 532 laser is ideal for this procedure and that electrocautery and electrosurgical scissors are useful. The specimen is placed back in the lumen of the colon and is retrieved with the colonoscope. Plastic bags can also be used for specimen collection and to reduce the probability of malignant tumor implantation.

The colotomy is then closed with two running layers of 3-0 Vicryl sutures. Intracorporeal instrument knotting is time-consuming and difficult, but it is essential in more difficult and advanced procedures. The use of endostaplers should facilitate these procedures but will never eliminate the need for suturing.

The abdominal wound is then irrigated, and the closure is tested with colonoscopic-induced pressure. The procedure is terminated with the inspection and closure of the ports.

RESULTS

We have performed 15 colotomies (13 polypectomies and 2 full-thickness excisions of endometrial implants), 27 sigmoid colon resections (12 benign and 15 malignant), 19 low anterior resections, 1 high left colon resection at 35 cm (malignant), and 12 abdominal peri-

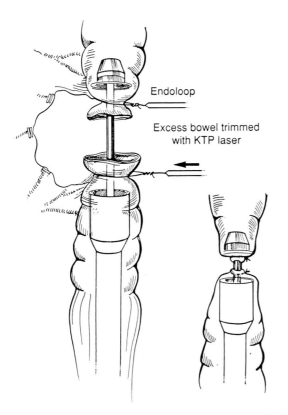

Endoloop

Excess bowel trimmed with KTP laser

Fig. 4. Colon is anastomosed with circular stapler (ILS) introduced transanally. Endoloops are used to secure bowel to stapler.

neal resections (Table 1). The mean hospital stay for all patients was 7.3 days, but the average postoperative stay (with the exclusion of three patients who had extraordinary problems including postoperative stroke, upper gastrointestinal bleeding, and postoperative pneumo-nia) was 3.4 days. The prolonged postoperative stay in the three complicated cases resulted from nonsurgically related problems. One death occurred 21 days after surgery as a result of pneumonia in a 96-year-old patient. Two patients underwent reexploration. One of these pa-

Table 1. Laparoscopic colon operations

Procedure	Pathological Findings	Complications	Coexisting Medical Problems
Polypectomy (15)			
Right colon (7)	Adenomatous polyp	0	Coronary disease
Left colon (2)	Adenomatous polyp	0	0
Transverse colon (2)			
Sigmoid (1)			
Rectum (3)	Endometriosis (2)	0	Arthritis
	Villous adenoma (1)	0	Steroid-dependent arthritis
Sigmoid colon resection (27)			
Benign (12)	Diverticulitis	Cardiovascular accident	Severe peripheral vascular disease
Malignant (15)	Dukes stage B1; 14-44	Postoperative gastrointestinal bleeding	Chronic obstructive lung disease
	Negative lymph nodes		Coronary artery disease
Left colon resection (3)	Dukes stage D with liver metastasis (2)	0	Coronary artery disease
Low anterior resection (19)	Perforated Dukes stage B	0	Prior coronary artery bypass graft
	Adenocarcinoma (2 cases converted to open [extensive carcinoma])		
Abdominal perineal resection (12)	Adenocarcinoma of anus with bleeding (tumor at 10 cm)	Postoperative pneumonia	Severe chronic obstructive lung disease
Transverse colon (1)	Metastatic adeno-carcinoma		
Right colon resection (12)	Adenocarcinoma Dukes stages A-D	2 cases converted to open (extensive carcinoma)	

tients experienced uncontrollable upper gastrointestinal bleeding that resulted from a large gastric ulcer at the gastroesophageal junction; the colonic anastomosis was examined and was found to be intact and healing. The second patient was reexamined for suspected peritonitis; no abnormality was found. There were no wound complications and no episodes of thrombophlebitis or other surgically related complications. No postoperative pulmonary complications occurred, except in the patient in whom pneumonia developed 2 weeks after surgery. In all patients audible bowel sounds were noted in ≤24 hours after surgery; all had had a bowel movement by 30 hours postoperatively, and all tolerated oral liquids by 36 hours. Operative procedures, pathologic findings, and complications are summarized in Table 1.

DISCUSSION

As a result of the laparoscopic treatment of colonic lesions, prolonged ileus, significant postoperative incisional pain, and the morbidity that can result from large abdominal wounds are avoided. The improvement of the quality of life of the patient with metastatic disease and the prevention of ventral hernias are additional benefits. As we began to develop this technique, the amount of time spent to complete the procedure was longer than that required by comparable open procedures. However, the improved patient recovery and diminished physiologic insult to the patient made the laparoscopic approach worthwhile. With improved instrumentation, the procedure can be performed expeditiously. Our later procedures are now completed in time comparable to that for open procedures. Although certain patients in our study had significant postoperative problems, we believe that patients who undergo laparoscopic colon resections fare better than do comparable patients on whom open procedures are performed and that the problems seen here were not a result of the surgical procedure. The duration of hospitalization in patients without major (nonsurgical) medical problems was less, the patients required fewer analgesics, and no procedure-related complications occurred in those who underwent laparoscopic resection.

We have several concerns about laparoscopic colon procedures; these include tumor spillage, retrieval of large segments of colon, and the efficacy of laparoscopic colon resection as a curative procedure for malignancy. Tumor spillage from malignant polypectomy can easily be handled by a primary segmental resection and placement of the specimen in a closed entrapment bag before retrieval. We recommend (and currently practice) this procedure. Large segments of colon removed for benign diseases can be cut and removed piecemeal, or they can be placed in a bag and removed transabdominally.[10] We believe that malignant segments of bowel should always be placed in impervious bags, tied, and removed after creation of the anastomosis. (Exceptions to this procedure are those in which metastasis is established, such as metastasis to the liver.)

The efficacy of laparoscopy as a primary treatment of malignant disease must be determined and we are reluctant to recommend it as such. However, with the laparoscopic approach we were able to identify and to ligate the inferior mesenteric artery at its origin on the aorta and to take the inferior mesenteric vein above that site. We have also found that with the laparoscopic procedure, we retrieve a similar (if not a greater) number of lymph nodes as we do with open procedures. The efficacy of primary laparoscopic treatment of malignancy must be determined and requires extensive study.

CONCLUSION

Laparoscopic techniques for cholecystectomy, bile duct surgery, and gynecological procedures have been successfully performed for several years. The laparoscopic approach results in reduced morbidity, a shorter hospital stay, and less pain, and the outcome is similar to (if not better than) that of open procedures. Our investigations in the laboratory and then in human subjects have expanded our use of this beneficial approach to colon procedures.

REFERENCES

1. Reddick EJ, Olsen D, Alexander W, Bailey A, Baird D, Price N, Pruitt R. Laparoscopic laser cholecystectomy and choledocholithiasis. Surg Endosc 4:133-134, 1990.
2. McKernan JB, Saye WB. Laparoscopic general surgery. J Med Assoc Ga 79:157-159, 1990.
3. McKernan JB. Laparoscopic cholecystectomy. Am Surg 57:309-312, 1991.
4. Perissat J. Laparoscopic cholecystectomy: Gateway to the future [editorial]. Am J Surg 161:408, 1991.
5. Browne DS. Laparoscopic-guided appendectomy. Augt NZT Obstet Gynaecol 30:231-233, 1990.
6. Gotz F, Pier A, Bacher C. Modified laparoscopic appendectomy in surgery. Surg Endosc 4:6-9, 1990.

7. Cuschieri A. The laparoscopic revolution—walk carefully before we run [editorial]. J R Coll Surg Edinb 34:295, 1989.

8. Cuschieri A. Minimal access surgery and the future of interventional laparoscopy. Am J Surg Mar 161(3):404-407, 1991.

9. Cotton PB, Baillie J, Pappas TN, Meyers WS. Laparoscopic cholecystectomy and the biliary endoscopist [editorial]. Gastrointest Endosc 37:94-97, 1991.

10. Clayman RV, Kavoussi LR, Soper NJ, Dierks SM, Meretyk S, Darcy MD, Roemer FD, Pinsleton ED, Thomson PG, Lons SR. Laparoscopic nephrectomy: Initial case report. Urology 146:278-282, 1991.

69 Indications, Advantages, and Technique of Laparoscopically Assisted Segmental Resection for Carcinoma of the Left Colon

Manuel Garcia-Caballero and Carlos Vara-Thorbeck

Because of the good results achieved by the pioneers in laparoscopic cholecystectomy, surgeons began to use this technique in the treatment of other gastrointestinal diseases, such as laparoscopically assisted left colon resection.[1]

Laparoscopic resection of the left colon diminishes operative trauma,[2] with minimal blood loss,[3] and decreases long-term postoperative de novo adhesion formation,[4,5] all of which are advantageous for the patient, as reported in studies of the treatment of benign colonic diseases.[6-9] The experience of most surgeons who perform laparoscopic surgery for colon carcinoma is limited, and those who have treated a larger series of patients stress that "these procedures should not at this time be used as curative procedures for colonic malignancies."[10]

In December 1991 we began to perform laparoscopic colon resection for carcinoma. We intended to add the advantages of this technique to the principles of open colorectal surgery for carcinoma: wide, complete excision of regional nodes, safe anastomosis, low morbidity and mortality rates, and a greater incidence of long-term patient survival.

It is not known whether laparoscopic surgery is curative. Therefore we selected a group of patients who would benefit from the immediate effects of the operation. Patients selected met two criteria: they required palliative surgery as a result of distant metastases, and they were high-risk patients in whom standard surgery would have resulted in high rates of morbidity and mortality.

In this study, we used a detailed protocol to chart the learning curve and to examine the feasibility and practicability of the technique as well as its advantages for the patients (especially with respect to postoperative ileus). We present the results of operation in the first six patients who underwent laparoscopic colon resection.

MATERIALS AND METHODS
Patients

We performed laparoscopic surgery on six patients with colon carcinoma in whom surgical treatment was not curative or on patients >70 years of age who were classified as ASA III or ASA IV. These patients, whose clinical characteristics are summarized in Table 1, underwent laparoscopic left colon resection between December 1991 and February 1992.

Diagnostic Procedures and Surgical Preparation of the Colon

All patients underwent a preoperative examination that consisted of medical history, barium enema, colonoscopy and biopsy, computed tomography to evaluate local and distant metastases, and an evaluation of the patient's general health according to the ASA classification (Table 1).

Table 1. Clinical selection criteria for patients undergoing laparoscopic colon resection

Case No.	Age/Sex	Site	Metastasis	ASA Classification	Associated Diseases	Previous Surgery
1	88/M	Sigmoid	Liver	IV	Chronic renal insufficiency	—
2	68/F	Sigmoid	—	III	High blood pressure, diabetes, cerebral embolism	Cholecystectomy
3	81/F	Sigmoid	—	III	—	—
4	67/F	Cecum	Abdominal wall	IV	High blood pressure	—
5	70/M	Sigmoid	—	III	—	Gastrectomy
6	75/F	Sigmoid	Liver	IV	Myocardial ischemia	—

Colon preparation began at 2 PM on the day before operation with the administration of 3 L of polyethylene glycol (200 ml/10 min). The colon was considered to be clean when the polyethylene glycol solution was excreted without fecal content. This result is normally achieved with 3 L, although the maximum amount used was 5 L. Antibiotic prophylaxis consisted of the administration of three doses of 500 mg of metronidazole on the day before operation at 4 PM and on the day of operation at 8 AM.

SURGICAL TECHNIQUE

The patient is placed in the supine position. The surgeon and first assistant stand on the patient's right side and the second assistant stands between the patient's legs (Fig. 1). Carbon dioxide is insufflated into the abdominal cavity through a Veress needle inserted through the umbilicus. A 10 mm, 0-degree laparoscope is placed through this trocar, replacing the Veress needle.

The peritoneal cavity is then explored visually; special attention is given to metastatic lesions. The other trocars are placed under direct vision (Fig. 2).

The patient is placed in the Trendelenburg position so that the small bowel rests in the upper abdomen. The

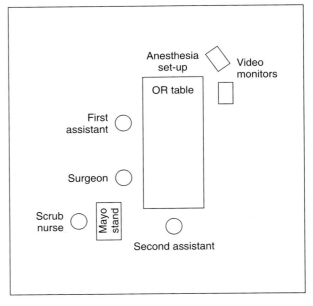

Fig. 1. Operating room for laparoscopic left hemicolectomy. The first assistant, surgeon, and scrub nurse stand on the patient's right side; the second assistant stands between the patient's legs.

table is tilted toward the patient's right side. The peritoneal reflection of the left colon is divided with laparoscopic scissors and electrocautery. When the mesocolon is placed under tension, the mesoperitoneal sheet is opened, and the appropriate vessels are divided with clips. The left colic artery is localized, ligated, and sectioned. Then the colon is transected with an EndoGIA at the distal site, or it is delivered through a transverse muscle-splitting incision of approximately 5 cm made in the left iliac quadrant. Evacuation of carbon dioxide from the abdomen allows the colon to be more easily delivered through the incision. In cases in which that is possible, the ends of the bowel are divided with a gastrointestinal stapler, and an anastomosis is performed (either side to side with the stapler or terminoterminal with a Valtrac ring). After the left iliac quadrant incision is closed, the trocars are reinserted, and carbon dioxide is again insufflated into the peritoneal cavity. The patient is evaluated for hemostasis, and the abdominal cavity is irrigated. The trocars are then removed under direct vision, and the incisions are closed.

When the anastomosis is performed intracorporeally, the stapled end of the specimen is delivered through

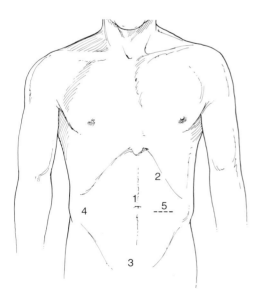

Fig. 2. Left hemicolectomy. *1*, 10 mm umbilical trocar for laparoscope; *2*, left subcostal midclavicular 5 mm trocar for grasping forceps and scissors; *3*, suprapubic 5 mm trocar for grasping forceps and scissors; *4*, right low quadrant 12 mm trocar for EndoGIA and other instruments; *5*, transverse incision for removing specimen.

a 3 cm transverse muscle-splitting incision. The proximal sigmoid vessels are divided extracorporeally, and the proximal site of transection is selected. The bowel is transected with curved Mayo scissors, and the anvil-shaft assembly of the Premium CEEA (PCEEA) stapler with a 31 mm cartridge inserted into the descending colon. The purse-string suture is secured, and this end of the bowel is dropped into the abdominal cavity. After the pneumoperitoneum has been reestablished, the body of the PCEEA stapling device is inserted into the rectum transanally and is advanced to the stapled closure. The trocar and central rod are advanced through the staple line and the trocar is removed through a port. Anvil rod and cartridge shaft are fastened to each other. The mesentery of the descending colon is checked to ensure that volvulus has not been produced. The stapling device is closed and fired. The two doughnuts are examined. Then the pelvis is filled with saline solution, and the rectum is insufflated by means of a Foley catheter to determine whether the anastomosis is airtight.

MONITORING THE POSTOPERATIVE ILEUS, HOSPITAL COURSE, AND LONG-TERM FOLLOW-UP

In our series, after the colon preparation was completed with polyethylene glycol solution at midnight on the day before surgery, each patient was asked to swallow ten 5 mm radiopaque markers to monitor the evolution of postoperative ileus. Patients gave oral consent for participation. The progress of the markers was followed by a radiograph taken on the morning of the surgery and then obtained every 12 hours until the radiopaque markers reached the rectum. This was complemented by a 12-hour delayed examination, as described elsewhere.[11]

In addition to the exact follow-up of postoperative ileus, patients were monitored for analgesic requirement, fever, discomfort, resumption of oral intake and ambulation, postoperative complications, and length of hospital stay.

We examined this group of patients 1, 2, 3, and 6 months after hospital discharge according to the criteria in the box. Ultrasonography, a computed tomographic (CT) scan, and colonoscopy were performed every 6 months. Ultrasonography was performed on patients without previously diagnosed metastasis, and CT scans were performed on patients with known metastasis. Colonoscopy was performed on all patients.

LAPAROSCOPIC COLON RESECTION FOR CARCINOMA: FOLLOW-UP PROTOCOL

General condition	Normal life without complaints
	Normal life and work
	Adequate self-care
	Bed rest required
	Special assistance and care required
Symptoms	Abdominal pain
	Hemorrhage
	Diarrhea
	Constipation
	Weight loss
	Anemia
	Others
Exploratory results	Abdominal mass
	Hepatomegaly
	Ascites
	Other
Laboratory results	Hemoglobin (g%)
	Leukocytes
	Prothrombin
	Proteins (g/L)
	Creatinine (mg%)
	FA (mU/ml)
	GOT (mU/ml)
	LDH (mU/ml)
	CEA (ng/ml)
Ultrasonographic results	Normal results
	Abnormal results (description)
Computed tomographic scan results	Normal results
	Abnormal results (description)
Colonoscopic and biopsy results	Normal
	Residual tumor (intraluminal, mesenteric)
	Primary tumor in other site

FA, fatty acids; GOT, glutamic-oxaloacetic transaminase; LDH, lactic dehydrogenase; CEA, carcinoembryonic antigen.

RESULTS
Perioperative Surgical Findings (Table 2)

In all cases, the tumor was identified by laparoscopy without simultaneous colonoscopy. The overall laparoscopic exploration of the abdominal cavity confirmed suspected metastases. Two patients had liver metastases, and in a third patient, a cecal tumor had invaded the contiguous abdominal wall.

No major intraoperative surgical or anesthetic complications arose—not even the theoretic cardiopulmonary difficulty that can result from the air pressure exerted by the necessary pneumoperitoneum (we always use between 10 and 13 mm Hg in these patients).

No conversion to open surgery was necessary. In all but one case, the resected colon was delivered through the 5 cm transverse incision. In one case (case 3 [see Table 1]), the incision was enlarged to 9 cm to permit the delivery of the tumor.

Two of the patients required a blood transfusion. In case 2, the patient, who arrived at the hospital in an anemic state, required 800 ml of blood before the surgery and the same quantity after surgery. In case 4, 800 ml of blood was transfused postoperatively.

The duration of the procedure ranged from 150 to 180 minutes (mean, 165 min).

The length of the resected colon varied from 13 to

Table 2. Perioperative surgical findings

Case No.	Type of Anastomosis	Surgical Duration (min)	Blood Volume Transfused	Resected Colon (cm)	Nodes/ Total Metastatic	MAC*
1	Extracorporeal	150	—	13	2/8	D
2	Extracorporeal	180	1600 ml	15	0/7	B₂
3	Extracorporeal	180	—	28	1/10	C₂
4	Extracorporeal	180	800 ml	23	3/8	C₃
5	Intracorporeal	150	—	26	1/11	C₂
6	Extracorporeal	150	—	30	2/7	D

*MAC = Modified Astler-Coller system: B_2, primary tumor invades through muscularis propria into subserosa, serosa, or pericolic fat within the leaves of the mesentery; B_3, primary tumor invades through serosa into free peritoneal cavity or into contiguous organ; C_1, C_2, C_3, as in B_1, B_2, B_3, but with positive nodes; D, distant metastasis.

Table 3. Hospital course

Case No.	Analgesics (no. of days)	Antibiotics (no. of days)	Oral Intake (postoperative day)	First Postoperative Defecation	Length of Hospital Stay (no. of days)
1	3	10(M,Cf,Am)	6	6	11
2	3	8 (M, Cf, Am)	3	3	9
3	3	6 (M, AM)	2	4	7
4	6	5 (M, Cf)	5	6	9
5	3	6 (M, Am)	3	5	7
6	3	5 (M, Am)	3	5	7

M = Metronidazole; Cf = ceftriaxone; Am = aminoglycosides.

30 cm. The number of extirpated lymph nodes ranged from 7 to 11, in five patients, ≤ three lymph nodes had evidence of metastasis. In one patient (case 2), no metastatic lymph nodes were detected.

Hospital Course (Table 3)

The use of analgesics (lisine clonixinate [Dolalgial], 400 mg/day) was necessary in five of the six patients for 3 days after surgery. Only the patient in whom the tumor had localized in the cecum required analgesics for 6 days after surgery.

Metronidazole was routinely administered for 3 days after surgery. In all patients, antibiotic treatment was completed with ceftriaxone and/or tobramycin in accordance with the intraoperative findings, the level of contamination, and concomitant diseases.

Oral intake was restored from the second to the eighth postoperative day. The duration of postoperative ileus ranged from 3 to 6 days, and the hospital stay varied from 7 to 11 days. Prolonged hospital stays were related to concomitant diseases or to postoperative complications (Tables 1 and 4).

In spite of the advanced age of the patients, those without metastasis or serious diseases had an uneventful hospital course; intestinal peristalsis and oral intake resumed within 3 days, and hospital discharge occurred

Table 4. Postoperative complications

Case No.	Anastomosis Leak	Wound Infections	Intra-abdomimal Abscess	Cardiorespiratory Disorders
1	—	—	—	Basal left lung atelactasis, decompensated ChRI
2	—	Wound abscess	—	—
3	—	—	—	—
4	—	—	—	Urinary infection
5	—	—	—	—
6	—	—	—	—

ChRI = Chronic renal insufficiency.

7 days after surgery. However, patients with distant metastasis or serious concomitant diseases required a longer hospital stay that did not result from surgery.

Postoperative Complications

Three of the six patients had an uneventful, complication-free hospital course.

In the other three patients, each of whom had metastatic disease, a basal left lung atelectasis and decompensated chronic renal insufficiency, a wound abscess in the umbilical Surgiport, and a urinary infection occurred, respectively (see Table 4).

Chronic renal insufficiency in the first patient occurred during the postoperative period and resulted in a delay in hospital discharge.

Long-Term Results and Quality of Life

The follow-up of these patients included evaluation at 1, 2, 3, and 6 months after surgery. Each follow-up examination was performed according to the protocol outlined in the box on p. 366.

Data on the patients' quality of life after surgery are summarized in Table 5. We can observe how the three patients with metastases presented complaints. Furthermore, only patients 3 and 5 led a normal life after surgery (caring for themselves, going out, etc.) Patient 2, who had hemiplegia, needed bed rest and could not look after herself.

Patient 4 complained of pain during the first month after surgery. Patient 2 had diarrhea for 4 months after surgery, and patients 1 and 6 were constipated for the first 3 months and required laxatives [Duphalac], 5 ml/day).

In postsurgical follow-up (Table 6), patient 1 presented with a crural strangulated hernia and underwent surgery 2½ months after the laparoscopic resection. After 6 months an ultrasonographic exploration of the liver was performed on patients who had had no previous metastatic disease; the results were normal in all cases.

A CT scan was performed on cases with previously demonstrated metastasis; in case 2, an anomalous picture resulted at the surgical site. However, colonoscopy was normal in all six cases.

DISCUSSION

Advances in laparoscopic surgery are extraordinary. Several years ago the introduction of laparoscopic cholecystectomy caused great expectation in some and skepticism in other surgeons. Now the treatment of colorectal cancer by laparoscopy is also controversial, primarily as a result of the disease treated rather than the procedure.

Table 5. Patient quality of life after laparoscopic resection

Patient Condition	Time After Surgery (months)			
	1	2	3	6
General Condition				
Normal life without complaints	3*/6	3/6	3/6	3/6
Normal life and work	2/6	2/6	2/6	2/6
Adequate self-care	5/6	5/6	5/6	5/6
Bed rest required	1/6	1/6	1/6	1/6
Special assistance and care required	1/6	1/6	1/6	1/6
Symptoms				
Abdominal pain	1/6	0/6	0/6	0/6
Hemorrhage	0/6	0/6	0/6	0/6
Diarrhea	1/6	1/6	1/6	0/6
Constipation	2/6	2/6	2/6	0/6
Weight loss	0/6	0/6	0/6	2/6
Anemia	2/6	1/6	2/6	2/6
Other	1/6	0/6	0/6	1/6

*Cases with normal findings.

Table 6. Follow-up findings after laparoscopic resection*

Diagnostic Criteria	Time After Surgery (months)			
	1	2	3	6
Exploratory results	5/6†	5/6	6/6	6/6
Laboratory results	3/6	2/6	3/6	2/6
Ultrasonographic results	—	—	—	3/3‡
Computed tomographic scan results	—	—	—	2/3‡
Colonoscopic and biopsy results	—	—	—	6/6†

* No deaths occurred in the patients studied.
† Proportion of patients with normal findings.
‡ Normal findings or no changes as compared with patient's clinical condition at hospital discharge.

Colon resection by laparoscopy can be accomplished by assisted laparoscopy[12-14] or by total laparoscopy.[10] The many advantages for the patient include reduced discomfort, rapid recovery, and reduced postoperative ileus. Furthermore, the size of the surgical specimen needed and the number of lymph nodes resected are similar to those required in standard surgery, as demonstrated by this study and others.[12-14] However, this new technique must be evaluated in prospective and randomized studies comparing both techniques and their long-term results. Until these studies are conducted, laparoscopic resection cannot be considered curative.[10,15]

Although some surgeons have criticized the laparoscopically assisted procedure as having disadvantages when compared with the open approach, studies conducted in the last 2 years contradict this opinion.[12-14,16] Our experience with laparoscopic cholecystectomy encouraged us to extrapolate the technique to laparoscopic colectomy, which results in less trauma for the patient.

Questions about the technique included the level of skill necessary to perform the procedure, patient selection and randomization, and curative effect. We selected patients who could benefit from the immediate effects of the operation.

Adherence to the rules of randomized trial requires acquisition of a standard skill. However, when the patient requires urgent medical attention, as did the patients we selected, randomization of the first patient (as proposed by Chalmers[16]) is justified to minimize risk.

The alternative is to return to the use of case reports in which technical details are supplied by the authors in their attempt to acquire skills in specific techniques.

CONCLUSION

We used to separate the fiber of the rectus abdominus in our first transverse incision for delivery of the tumor specimen, but we now use a muscle-splitting incision that reduces discomfort from the abdominal wound. Laparoscopically assisted segmental resection is feasible and offers many advantages for the patients, as those presented in this study demonstrate. However, only prospective randomized controlled clinical trials can be used to determine the curative value of the technique.

REFERENCES

1. García-Caballero M. Minimal invasive surgery in the gastrointestinal tract: Challenge for surgeons and new concepts for measuring outcome. Presented at Eurosurgery '92, Brussels, June 1992.
2. Nezhat F, Nezhat C, Pennington E, Ambroz W. Laparoscopic segmental resection for infiltrating endometriosis of the rectosigmoid colon: A preliminary report. Surg Laparosc Endosc 3:212-216, 1992.
3. Kim LH, Chung KE, Aubuchon P. Laparoscopic assisted abdomino-perineal resection with pull-through (sphincter saving). Surg Laparosc Endosc 3:237-240, 1992.
4. Operative Laparoscopic Study Group. Postoperative adhesion development after operative laparoscopy: Evaluation at early second-look procedures. Fertil Steril 55:700-704, 1991.
5. Nezhat C, Nezhat F, Metzger DA, Luciano AA. Adhesion reformation after reproductive surgery by videolaparoscopy. Fertil Steril 53:1008-1011, 1990.
6. Sundin JA, Wasson D, McMillen MM, Ballantyne GH. Laparoscopic assisted sigmoid colectomy for sigmoid volvulus. Surg Laparosc Endosc 4:353-358, 1992.
7. Sharpe DR, Redwine DB. Laparoscopic segmental resection of the sigmoid and rectosigmoid colon for endometriosis. Surg Laparosc Endosc 2:120-124, 1992.
8. Saclarides TJ, Ko ST, Airan M, Dillon C, Franklin J. Laparoscopic removal of a large colonic lipoma. Dis Colon Rectum 34:1027-1029, 1991.
9. Ballantyne GH. Laparoscopically assisted anterior resection for rectal prolapse. Surg Laparosc Endosc 3:230-236, 1992.
10. Franklin ME Jr. Laparoscopic colon resection (letter). Surg Laparosc Endosc 2:183, 1992.
11. García-Caballero M, Vara-Thorbeck C. Evolution of post-operative ileus after laparoscopic cholecystectomy (letter). Surg Endosc (in press).
12. Corbitt JD Jr. Preliminary experience with laparoscopic guided colectomy. Surg Laparosc Endosc 2:79-81, 1992.
13. Jacobs M, Verdeja JC, Goldstein HS. Minimally invasive colon resection (laparoscopic colectomy). Surg Laparosc Endosc 1:138-143, 1991.
14. Fowler DL, White SA. Laparoscopic assisted sigmoid resection. Surg Laparoscopy Endosc 1:183-188, 1991.
15. Orkin BA. Laparoscopic colorectal surgery (letter). Dis Colon Rectum 35:614-615, 1992.
16. Chalmers TC. Randomization of the first patient. Med Clin North Am 59:1035-1038, 1975.

Patrice H. Lointier

The introduction of therapeutic laparoscopy to general surgery has resulted in dramatic changes in the management of a number of common intra-abdominal illnesses. Some recent reports have described segmental colon resections,[1] but the experience with total abdominal colectomy is still in its infancy.[2] However, the mere feasibility of a new technique is no proof of the appropriateness of its application.

We will describe a laparoscopic technique in which the entire colon is removed and a stapled ileorectal anastomosis is created. Our experience in five patients is reported.

MATERIALS AND METHODS

Four women and one man underwent laparoscopically assisted total colectomy. They had not had any previous abdominal operations. Three patients were operated on for familial and nonfamilial polyposis, and two

This work was made possible by Autosuture of France.

had severe chronic constipation caused by colonic dysmotility with no pelvic floor dysfunction.[3,4] Their ages ranged from 19 to 72 years.

A full mechanical and antibiotic bowel preparation was used. Patients were prepared and draped for both laparoscopy and traditional laparotomy. A nasogastric tube and Foley bladder catheter were placed to minimize the risk of trocar injury to the stomach or bladder. A pneumoperitoneum (intra-abdominal pressure, 12 mm Hg) was established. The camera assistant and the nurse stood on the right side of the patient. The monitor was used at the left foot between the patient's legs. The surgical team viewed the operative field on the video monitor. The patient was placed in the lithotomy position (Fig. 1) with the head of the table lowered 15 to 25 degrees (Trendelenburg position). After placement of a 10 mm umbilical port, two 12 mm trocars were placed in the suprapubic position slightly to the left and right of the midline (Fig. 2). A 5 mm trocar was added and placed at the left midclavicular line, slightly superior to the umbilicus. Only the umbilical port was used

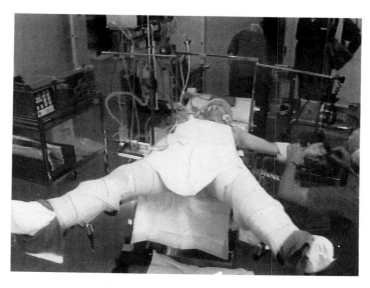

Fig. 1. Positioning of the patient.

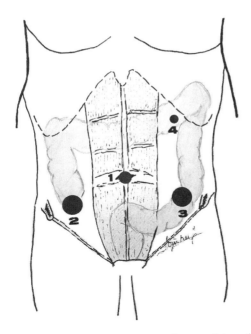

Fig. 2. Four laparoscopic puncture sites used in subtotal colectomy.

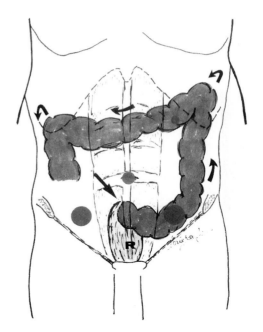

Fig. 3. Colonic dissection beginning at the rectosigmoid junction.

for the video camera and laparoscope. The "operating ports" were the 12 mm sheaths, which permitted maximal surgical flexibility for frequent repositioning of the instruments.

Before colonic mobilization was performed, a thorough visual inspection of the abdominal contents was undertaken. During dissection of the large bowel, table positioning was used to facilitate retraction of loops of bowel from the operative field. The sigmoid colon was first mobilized (Fig. 3) and then lifted with a 10 mm laparoscopic Babcock forceps inserted through the left 12 mm trocar. Pelvic and lateral peritoneal adhesions attached to the colon were sharply divided with a monopolar electrocautery rotating scissors. Using medial traction, the line of Toldt was exposed and divided. The left ureter was easily identified (Fig. 4). An additional grasping forceps was inserted through the 5 mm trocar for better traction and countertraction of the greater omentum and transverse colon. The descending colon was dissected free from the lateral peritoneum and splenic flexure to permit mobilization (Fig. 5). The mesentery was pulled toward the midline to outline the mar-

gins of the mesenteric vessels. The mesenteric vessels were dissected free, clipped, and divided (Fig. 6). To facilitate ligation of the large mesenteric pedicles the vascular EndoGIA 30 stapler was used (Fig. 7). Proximal vascular division and ligation were performed using both these methods.

During mobilization of the left colon, the table was placed in the Trendelenburg position and tilted to the right to help keep loops of small bowel away from the pelvis. When mobilizing the splenic flexure, a reverse Trendelenburg position with table tilt to the right was helpful. At this point of the dissection, when the left colon was mobilized just to the right of the falciform ligament, the laparoscopic dissection was interrupted. A multifiring EndoGIA 30 stapler was used to transect the rectum. We then decided to remove the "freed" colon through a small accessory abdominal incision. The right lower trocar site was enlarged to a 4 cm muscle-sparing incision just above the symphysis pubis (Fig. 8).

The operative dissection approached the hepatic flexure, and a "retrograde" right hemicolectomy was performed (Fig. 9). For this procedure the assistant/

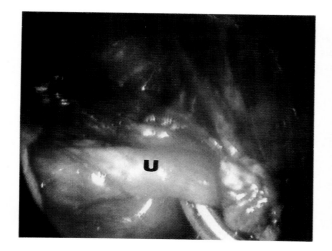

Fig. 4. Left ureter *(U)*.

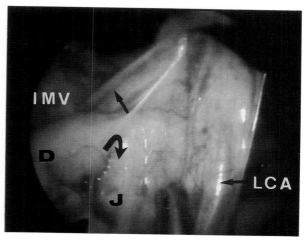

Fig. 5. To mobilize the descending colon, the superior left colonic vascular pedicle is held with an endo-Babcock clamp. (*LCA* = left colonic artery; *IMV* = inferior mesenteric vein; *D* = duodenum; *J* = jejunum.)

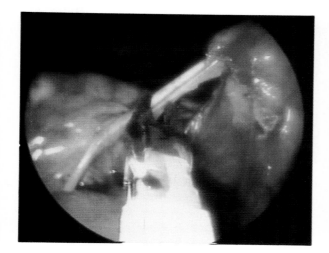

Fig. 6. A clip applier is used to secure the inferior mesenteric vein.

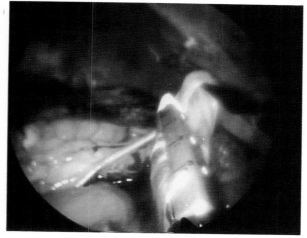

Fig. 7. A multifiring EndoGIA 30 V stapler (using vascular stapler) is used to staple and divide the superior left colonic vascular pedicle at the base of the mesenteric dissection.

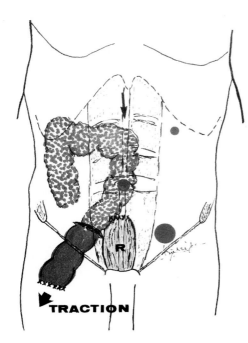

TRACTION

Fig. 8. The right lower trocar site is enlarged to a 4 cm muscle-sparing incision. This technique is used to extract the "freed" left colon and perform a "retrograde" right colectomy without loss of the pneumoperitoneum.

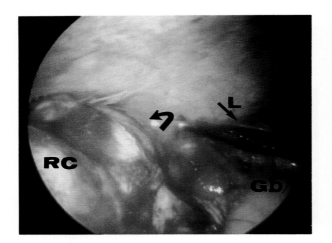

Fig. 9. Toldt's lateral peritoneal reflection along the right colon *(RC)* is incised with scissors and electrocautery. *(L* = liver; *Gb* = gallbladder.)

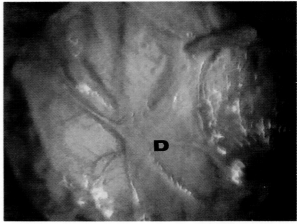

Fig. 10. View of the second portion of the duodenum during right colectomy.

cameraman stood on the right side of the patient. The surgeon and the nurse stood on the left. During extraction the mass of the left colon with its mesentery occluded the skin incision to maintain the pneumoperitoneum. The gastrocolic ligament was transected between surgical clips, and mobilization of the ascending colon and the cecum was completed. The second portion of the duodenum was clearly visible (Fig. 10) dur-

ing this portion of the dissection. The right colon was mobilized laterally along the white line of Toldt. The dissection was continued downward with the patient in a reverse Trendelenburg position and the table at a left lateral tilt (15 degree). This dissection and maneuver were also facilitated by the fact that the left colon was pulled anteriorly through the abdominal incision. The entire colon and the distal ileum were removed from

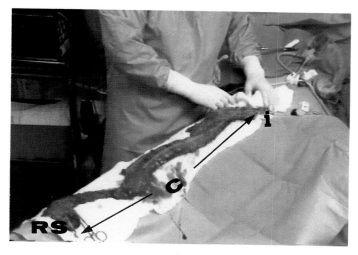

Fig. 11. The resected specimen demonstrates that although the specimen consists of the entire colon and adjacent mesentery, it can be withdrawn easily via the right small skin incision. (*RS* = rectosigmoid; *C* = colon; *i* = ileum.)

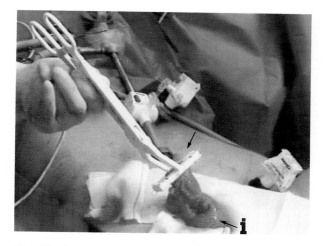

Fig. 12. A purse-string suture is applied to the proximal ileum.

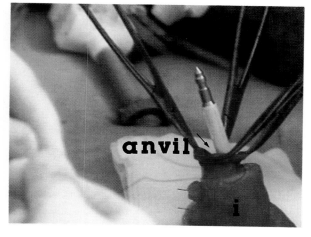

Fig. 13. The anvil of the PCEEA 25 stapler is placed in the ileum.

the abdomen through this incision (Fig. 11). A wound protector was used to prevent bacteria from lodging in the abdominal wall.

The ileum and the colon were separated outside the abdominal cavity. A purse-string suture (Fig. 12) was applied to the ileum to secure the anvil. The anvil of the PCEEA 25 stapler was placed in the proximal ileum and the purse-string tied (Fig. 13). Through the same open-

ing, the anvil of the Premium EEA stapler and the ileum were reintroduced into the abdomen and the pneumoperitoneum was reestablished (Fig. 14). The shaft and cartridge of the PCEEA device was introduced through the anus and maneuvered up to the divided rectum. When the CEEA stapler was satisfactorily positioned in the rectum, the trocar could be advanced through the staple-closed rectal stump into the abdom-

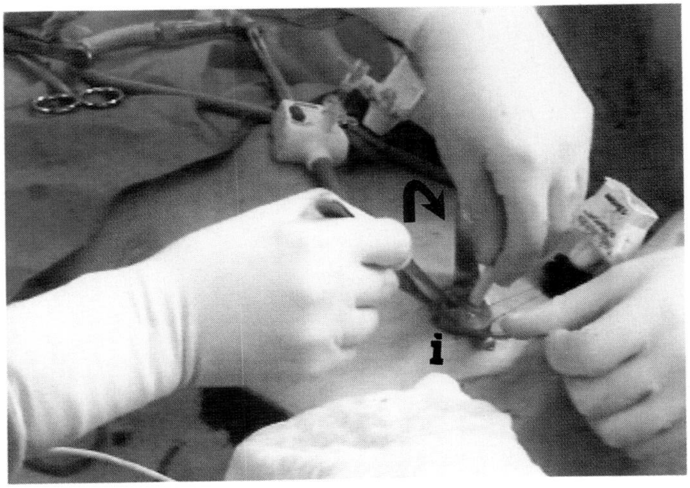

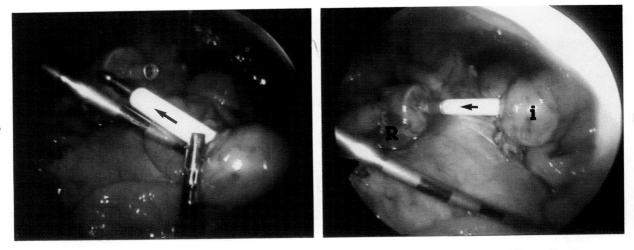

Fig. 14. The ileum ready for the anastomosis is reintroduced into the abdominal cavity.

Fig. 15. A, The body of the PCEEA stapler can be seen pushing on the rectal stump. **B,** The anvil rod is inserted into the shaft of the cartridge of the PCEEA stapler.

inal cavity. The trocar was removed and the anvil rod was inserted into the body shaft of the CEEA stapler (Fig. 15, *A* and *B*). The circular stapler was closed, fired, and then removed through the rectum. In all cases an end-to-side ileorectal anastomosis was created. The staple line could be visually inspected laparoscopically. The two stapled rings of tissue were examined. The pelvis was filled with water and air was injected into the bowel lumen through the anus. No visible intraperitoneal air leakage was detected at the ileorectostomy. A drain was placed in the pelvis for 6 days (Fig. 16). A tempo-

rary clamp was applied across the external portion of the silicone drain to prevent loss of the pneumoperitoneum. The internal portion of the drain was properly positioned utilizing grasping forceps placed through the remaining ports. The procedure was concluded by irrigation and suction as necessary, followed by evacuation of the pneumoperitoneum.

RESULTS

Four patients passed gas on the first postoperative day and one on the fifth day; they were eating by the third

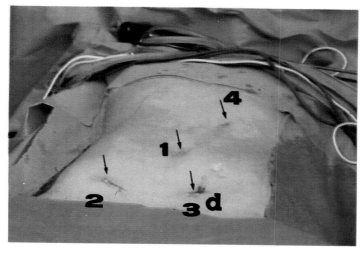

Fig. 16. Final view of the abdominal wall after completion of laparoscopic subtotal colectomy. (*1, 2, 3, 4* = port positions; *2* = small skin incision; *3 d* = drain.)

day. Two patients were discharged on the morning of the seventh day, two on the twelfth postoperative day, and one, a 48-year-old woman, on the sixteenth postoperative day. She had phlebitis 48 hours after operation. Three patients complained of headache and were aching all over for 48 hours. At 3 to 12 months postoperatively, all patients continued to do well, with normal bowel function and total relief of pain and constipation.

Estimated blood loss during the procedures was approximately 200 to 400 ml. The amount was determined using alternating irrigation and suction. All resections included a primary anastomosis. There were no visceral injuries or clinical anastomotic leaks. No closure of the mesenteric defect was performed. No intestinal obstruction was observed. The duration of the procedure was 8 hours for the first patient and 4 hours for the last patient. In each case we used two tissue EndoGIA (Autosuture) linear staplers for rectal transection and five (30 V) vascular staplers to divide the mesenteric vessels (Fig. 17).

DISCUSSION

It is important that patients be carefully selected to identify those most likely to benefit from this new surgical procedure. Indications for a laparoscopic approach to colon surgery are varied, ranging from inflammatory to malignant disease.[5,6] Our indications for laparoscopically assisted total colectomy were benign conditions (i.e., colonic inertia, familial polyposis), but this procedure could be used to treat multifocal small malignant

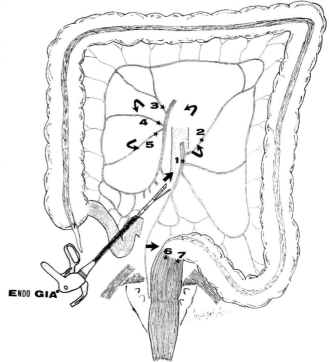

Fig. 17. Seven EndoGIA firings were used to transect the rectum (n = 2) and free the colon (n = 5) from the mesentery and vessels (two tissue and five vascular EndoGIAs).

tumors projecting into the bowel lumen to avoid parietal invasion of malignant cells.[7]

We believed that dissection of the bowel attachments and mesentery could be accomplished safely with "instrumental laparoscopy." The more difficult objective was to free the bowel from the greater omentum by means of electrocautery instruments and clip appliers rather than linear staplers because of the low cost.

Removing the entire nonmalignant bowel by separating it from the mesentery immediately adjacent to the bowel wall is time consuming. Also, attempting to remove a portion of the mesentery made the resection easier. It is possible to remove a great number of lymph nodes, and the extent of the "en bloc" resection appeared identical to that achieved with open laparotomy. The availability of 6 cm endoscopic GIA staplers facilitates both mesenteric dissection and transection of the bowel within the abdomen.

With regard to types of anastomoses and methods of removing specimens, we believe that a small muscle-splitting incision at McBurney's site would allow not only removal of the specimen but also correct insertion of the anvil of the PCEEA stapler, thereby solving both problems at once. Mobilization of the colon can be initiated on either side, but it is preferable to first mobilize the sigmoid colon. Because of the need to prepare the anastomosis with the terminal ileum we can avoid mobilization of too long a segment of the small intestine before the entire colon is extracted. In addition, this procedure is shorter.

Even if a mini-incision is made, it should have a considerable advantage over the larger vertical incision traditionally used. Even if an Endoloop or other tool is placed around the proximal end of the distal and proximal portions of the intestine, when the resected colonic segment is removed through the anus, we believe that bacterial contamination and spillage of malignant tumor cells can occur.[8]

Cleaning fat and mesenteric remnants from the cut edges in preparation for a stapled anastomosis (diameter of the colonic lumen) is time consuming when performed intra-abdominally. Other instruments must be developed for laparoscopic use to further expedite this portion of the operation. Another alternative is perineal resection after ileocolonic intussusception. However, the rectum must be mobilized so that it can be prolapsed through the anal canal with the bowel, incorporating the resected lesions and creating an anastomosis transanally.[9,10]

Because this operation involves dissection on both sides of the abdomen, from the upper regions (splenic and hepatic flexures) down to the pelvis, positioning of the instruments and the surgical team is critical. The patient must frequently be rolled from side to side and placed in both the Trendelenburg and reverse Trendelenburg positions. Although this is a lengthy procedure, it can be performed satisfactorily by a surgeon, an assistant/camera operator, and a nurse. With this technique placement of the trocar does not need to be individualized based on the patient's body shape and the portion of the colon to be resected. We used only four trocars.

It is clear that postoperative pain is decreased and full activity is resumed earlier when segmental colon surgery is performed without an abdominal incision. This was true in our experience for subtotal colectomy.[11] Although 4 to 8 hours were required to complete these resections, this time should decrease as experience is gained. With adequate deep venous thrombosis prophylaxis, pulmonary emboli can probably be prevented as in open procedures. We conclude that major laparoscopically guided bowel surgery is technically feasible and could result in a shorter hospitalization and less patient discomfort with rapid improvements in endoscopic instrumentation.

REFERENCES

1. Corbitt JD. Preliminary experience with laparoscopic-guided colectomy. Surg Laparosc Endosc 1:79-81, 1992.
2. Leahy PF, Pennino RP, Furman RH. Laparoscopically assisted total colectomy. Surg Endosc 6:102, 1992.
3. Dapoigny M, Chaussade S, Lointier P, et al. Apports de l'électromyographie colique dans la constipation de progression par inertie colique [abstract]. Gastroenterol Clin Biol 16:A9, 1992.
4. Pemberton JH, Rath D, Ilstrup D. Evaluation and surgical treatment of severe chronic constipation. Ann Surg 4:403-413, 1991.
5. Fowler DL, White SA. Laparoscopic assisted sigmoid resection. Surg Laparosc Endosc 1:183-188, 1991.
6. Jacobs M, Verdeja JC, Goldstein HS. Minimally invasive colon resection (laparoscopic colectomy). Surg Laparosc Endosc 1:138-143, 1991.
7. Pezet D, Fondrinier E, Rotman N, et al. Parietal seeding of carcinoma of the gallbladder after laparoscopic cholecystectomy. Br J Surg 79:230, 1992.
8. Phillips EH, Franklin M, Carroll BJ, et al. Laparoscopic colectomy. Ann Surg 216:703-707, 1992.

9. Peters WR. Laparoscopic total proctocolectomy with creation of ileostomy of ulcerative colitis: Report of two cases. J Laparoendosc Surg 3:175-178, 1992.
10. Lointier P, Lechner C, Ferrier C, et al. Recto-colectomie gauche périnéale assistée par laparoscopie. Chirurg Endosc 7:10-14, 1992.
11. Wexner S, Johansen OB, Nogueras JJ, et al. Laparoscopic total abdominal colectomy: A prospective trial. Dis Colon Rectum 35:651-655, 1992.

71   *Laparoscopically Assisted Total Abdominal Colectomy*

David G. Jagelman,† Steven D. Wexner, and Juan J. Nogueras

Laparoscopic surgery has evolved from the advances made by gynecological surgery in the past few years, and the advent of videoscope technology. Both have expanded the spectrum of laparoscopic abdominal techniques. Since its inception in 1987, laparoscopic gallbladder surgery has progressed, assisted by industry support and promotion. Today most patients requiring a cholecystectomy can be assured that laparoscopic cholecystectomy is the procedure of choice. The benefits of such minimally invasive surgery have been established, provided the surgeon has the appropriate experience and has the equipment to perform the procedure. It is to be expected that other intra-abdominal procedures might be undertaken by laparoscopic methods. There have been reports of appendectomy, parietal cell vagotomy, hysterectomy, esophageal antireflux procedure, relief of bowel obstruction, and inguinal herniorrhaphy performed by laparoscopic methods plus anecdotal reports of various colon resections performed in a similar manner. The stated advantages of less pain, diminished postoperative ileus, reduced cost, and more rapid postoperative recovery have not been adequately documented for any of these other procedures; however, most reports of laparoscopic colon resection have been small in number and described the initial experience of the operating surgeon. It is also certain that the surgical enthusiasm about performing these alternate procedures laparoscopically with ease has been restricted by the lack of availability of appropriate instrumentation and the limited experience of operating surgeons.

This state of affairs is changing as instrument designers and manufacturers pursue the development and release of newer and better instruments. We still have a long way to go, however, to make laparoscopic colon resection as easy to perform as routine totally open colon resection.

Cumbersome components of laparoscopic colon resection include retraction and mobilization. Vascular ligation of major vessels is still a problem, because most of the clips or sutures available were designed for gallbladder surgery. This is also true for most of the surgical laparoscopic instruments in use. Anastomotic techniques using staples are also inadequate and must be modified to facilitate intra-abdominal anastomosis. Removal of the specimen is an additional problem and at this time essentially involves making an abdominal incision to retrieve it. The concept of transanal evacuation, although attractive, is not appropriate in all cases and may be dangerous. Fecal contamination and tumor spillage may ensue from such attempts, and splitting of the rectum as well as anal sphincter damage may occur. If an incision is required to recover the specimen, the question arises as to whether the incision can also be used to facilitate the anastomosis, thereby eliminating the most difficult component of laparoscopic colon resection.

Our approach to laparoscopic resection is to mobilize the colon by laparoscopic method and to complete the procedure in an assisted way, thereby reducing the size of the incision. Benefits may include the lack of handling of the intestine and the possibility of placing the incision in a more cosmetically acceptable location.

†Deceased.

379

We present our experience with a group of 17 patients requiring total abdominal colectomy with or without ileoanal reservoir. Colonic mobilization was performed initially, and the specimen was removed through a suprapubic, or Pfannenstiel, incision. Prospective assessment of the intraoperative and postoperative complications, the duration of operation, and postoperative hospitalization were recorded. All patients selected for this series had benign disease, because we still have some reservations about the adequacy of laparoscopic resection of malignant colorectal disease.

MATERIALS AND METHODS

All patients undergoing laparoscopic colon resection in our institution are prospectively entered into a surgical registry for analysis and a central registry established by the American Society of Colon and Rectal Surgeons for independent analysis. Data are collected about patients' age, sex, diagnosis, procedure performed, duration of operation, type of incision, type of anastomosis, intraoperative and postoperative complications, and postoperative hospital stay.

All patients in our series underwent a 1-day preoperative bowel preparation consisting of mechanical lavage using 10% mannitol or GoLYTELY. All patients underwent systemic perioperative antibiotic prophylaxis with cefotaxime (Claforan), 2 g IV, and metronidazole (Flagyl), 1 g IV. The antibiotic regimen was discontinued in the recovery room. All patients were positioned in the supine lithotomy position, which allowed access to the anus and provided another point of access to the abdomen for the operating surgeon or assistant.

An infraumbilical incision was made and a Veress needle inserted to inflate the abdominal cavity with CO_2 to a pressure of 15 mm Hg. A 10 or 11 mm trocar (Ethicon) was then inserted by direct puncture.

The camera was advanced through this port and the abdominal contents examined. Two additional 10 or 11 mm trocars were inserted in the suprapubic area to coincide with the anticipated Pfannenstiel incision (Fig. 1). These ports were usually used for retracting the colon with grasping Babcock clamps (Ethicon). A further 10 or 11 mm trocar was inserted in the upper abdomen to the right of the midline, usually for dissection purposes. All of the ports were interchangeable during colon mobilization. With grasping Babcock clamps, the right and left peritoneal attachments of the colon were incised with either electrocautery or scissor dissection to include the terminal ileum and appendix to the hepatic flexure on the right side and the area from the splenic flexure to the sacral promontory on the left. One surgeon performed the dissection and the other surgeon assisted with the retraction. A third experienced assistant was required for control of the camera. Hemostasis was achieved with electrocautery or application of metallic clips. The gastrocolic omentum was dissected by electrocautery dissection and the liberal use of clips. No attempt in this early series of patients was made to ligate the mesenteric vessels. Full mobilization of the colon was achieved in all patients.

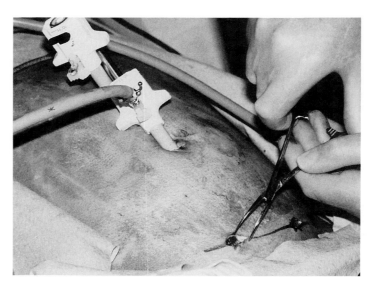

Fig. 1. Laparoscopic trocar insertion.

After full mobilization a classic suprapubic Pfannenstiel incision was made in all patients. The colon was then elevated onto the abdominal wall and the individual colonic vessels were divided between clamps and were ligated (Fig. 2). The terminal ileum was divided at the ileocecal valve. Continuity in patients undergoing ileorectal anastomosis was restored by an end-to-end anastomosis with the use of a transanal circular stapling device (U.S. Surgical Corp.). Patients undergo-

ing an ileoanal reservoir procedure underwent a double-stapled technique. The ileal reservoir (J pouch) of appropriate length was constructed with an ILA 100 stapler (3M Corp.) (Fig. 3).

The rectum was dissected to the levator mechanism through the incision and staple-closed with a PI 30 staple instrument (3M Corp.). The double-stapled ileoanal anastomosis was performed with the CEA 28 mm circular stapler instrument (U.S. Surgical Corp.) (Figs. 4

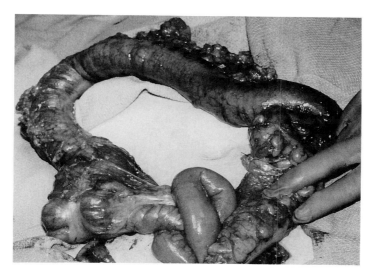

Fig. 2. Colonic specimen removed through Pfannenstiel incision.

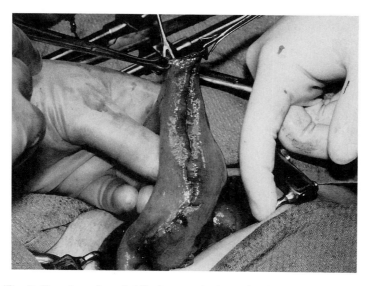

Fig. 3. Creation of stapled ileal reservoir through Pfannenstiel incision.

and 5). One-stage ileoanal anastomosis or the use of a temporary ileostomy was dictated by the patient's condition, nutritional status, and steroid medication and finally by the integrity of the completed anastomosis. An ileostomy, if required, was placed at a preoperative-ly marked site in the right rectus muscle. The Pfannenstiel incision was closed at the completion of the procedure (Fig. 6). All operative manipulations, pelvic dissections, and ileoanal anastomoses were performed through this single incision.

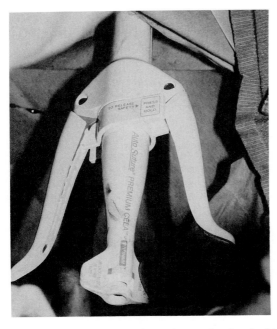

Fig. 4. Transanal insertion of circular stapler for double-stapled ileoanal anastomosis.

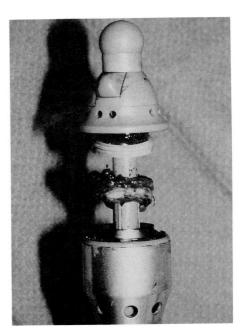

Fig. 5. Two completed doughnuts after firing of circular stapler.

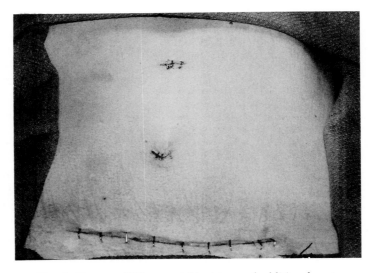

Fig. 6. Closure of Pfannenstiel incision and additional ports.

Patients

Seventeen patients, six males and 11 females with ages from 12 to 54 years (mean, 30), underwent laparoscopically assisted total abdominal colectomy: nine had ulcerative colitis, four had familial adenomatous polyposis, two had colonic inertia, one had Crohn's disease, and one had juvenile polyposis (Table 1). Operative procedures included colectomy and ileorectal anastomosis (3), colectomy with ileoanal reservoir and loop ileostomy (8), and colectomy and one-stage ileoanal reservoir (6) (Table 2).

Results

In our series of 17 patients, all underwent full colonic mobilization without complication. There were no injuries to the intestine during mobilization and no injuries to the spleen during takedown of the splenic flexure.

Table 1. Laparoscopic total abdominal colectomy: diagnoses

Diagnosis	No. of Cases
Ulcerative colitis	9
Familial adenomatous polyposis	4
Colonic inertia	2
Juvenile polyposis	1
Crohn's disease	1
TOTAL	17

Table 2. Laparoscopic total abdominal colectomy operations

Procedures	Cases
Colectomy and ileorectal anastomosis	3
Colectomy, ileoanal reservoir formation, ileostomy	8
Colectomy, one-stage ileoanal reservoir formation	6
TOTAL	17

One patient's epigastric artery was injured during suprapubic trocar insertion that required ligation through the Pfannenstiel incision. No further incisions were required to facilitate removal of the colon or to perform the ileorectal anastomoses, ileal reservoir construction, or ileoanal double-stapled anastomosis.

The length of the procedure from insertion of the Veress needle to closure of the incision ranged from 2 hours 45 minutes to 5 hours (mean length, 3 hours 45 minutes). Postoperative hospital days ranged from 6 to 12 days (mean, 7 days). There was no mortality.

Complications included one injury to the epigastric artery from trocar insertion. One patient developed an intra-abdominal hemorrhage and was returned from the recovery room to the operating room for treatment. The patient with Crohn's disease who received ileorectal anastomosis developed a postoperative anastomotic leak requiring readmission to the hospital, drainage of pelvic abscess, and loop ileostomy. One patient developed upper gastrointestinal bleeding from vomiting that caused a Mallory-Weiss tear.

The postoperative recovery apparently was enhanced by the minimal suprapubic incision, and the return to normal activities seemed more rapid than with a traditional long midline incision. This parameter of recovery is somewhat difficult to measure. All patients, particularly women, were very satisfied with the cosmetic result of the Pfannenstiel incision.

DISCUSSION

The results suggest it is technically feasible to complete such procedures by this method with a low morbidity. The length of hospitalization was acceptably low, but the duration of operation was longer than with traditional methods in our experience. The perceived advantages of reduced hospitalization and rapid recovery to normal activity after laparoscopic colon surgery are still open to discussion. The additional cost of laparoscopic surgery in terms of equipment, prolonged operating time, and training of surgical personnel must be entered into the cost-benefit analysis. It is hoped that pursuing this new and exciting method and the increasing availability of new instrumentation will answer some of the questions about laparoscopic colon resection. Answers can be achieved only by prospective documentation of the cases for review and greater experience of the operating surgeon.

72 Experimental Results of Colon Resection Using the Tübingen Procedure

Marco Maria Lirici, Gerhard Buess, Andreas Melzer, and Horst Dieter Becker

Combining operative laparoscopy and rectoscopy enables the completion of the endoscopic sigmoid resection while eliminating the need for a minilaparotomy to perform the anastomosis or withdraw the specimen. This combined procedure was performed in several variants in a series of 32 animals until the definitive technique was standardized. The technique we describe was developed at the University of Tübingen, Germany.

MATERIALS AND METHODS

The operation was performed on 32 animal models (7 miniature pigs, 9 sheep, and 16 middle-sized pigs). Seventeen animals were operated on to determine the indispensable technology and the definitive operative technique. The procedure we describe in this chapter, an endoluminal or extraluminal variant, was performed in the last 15 animals (all middle-sized pigs) as a standardized trial.

The preoperative protocol consisted of 3 days of fasting and enemas. No antibiotic prophylaxis was given. The animals were operated on while under general anesthesia, with a central venous catheter and electrocardiographic (ECG) monitoring provided. The postoperative protocol consisted of 1 to 2 days of fasting. Forty-eight to 72-hour antibiotic therapy was administered to four animals. The animals were sacrificed during the third postoperative week, and a specimen that included the anastomosis was sent to the pathologist.

OPERATIVE TECHNIQUE

The surgeon and the camera assistant stand on the right and the assistant on the left of the animal. After the pneumoperitoneum is established, four ports are placed in the lower abdomen. A 10 mm cannula is inserted at the right side of the navel. This is the introduction site for a 50-degree laparoscope. An 11 mm cannula and a 5 mm silicone cannula are introduced in the lower right quadrant of the abdomen: the first is an operative port placed 7 cm below and lateral to the navel; the second is a flexible port for a curved grasper designed by Cuschieri and is placed close to the anterior iliac spine. A 5 mm cannula for graspers is placed in the left abdomen opposite the 11 mm port.

The peritoneal cavity is explored, a suprapubic puncture is performed, and a catheter is placed. The table is put in low Trendelenburg, turned right.

The sigmoid colon is grasped and fixed to the abdominal wall by means of two slings. This maneuver is accomplished by passing through the mesocolon with the Cuschieri curved grasper. It permits a clear view of the mesocolon and its vessels. The vessels to the sigmoid colon are freed, ligated (Fig. 1), and divided. The ligature is performed by means of PDS extracorporeal slip knots according to the technique developed by Melzer and Buess for monofilament material. Bipolar coagulation of the vessels on the bowel's side near to the anastomotic line is performed to avoid trouble with threads or clips while preparing the two stumps for the anastomosis. Once the sigmoid colon is prepared, a

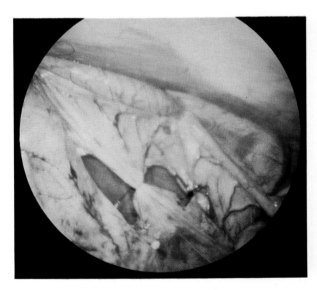

Fig. 1. Vessel ligatures are accomplished by tightening PDS slip knots according to the Melzer-Buess technique.

modified Buess operative rectoscope[1] is inserted into the rectum up to the rectosigmoid junction.

Endoluminal Procedure

The anvil of a 29 mm disposable, curved stapler (Ethicon GmbH) is inserted by means of a specially designed introducer up to the proximal sigmoid. Two 2-0 PDS slip knots are tightened around the bowel with the introducer inside at its proximal and distal levels. The anvil is then fixed to the descending colon or to the proximal sigmoid colon by another PDS slip knot, and the proximal sigmoid colon is divided between the two ligatures. A cable-binding technique has been specially developed to fix the anvil safely. The cable binder is a plastic device provided with ratchets that, when tightened, will not slip back. It is prelocked extracorporeally and tightened around the sigmoid by means of a pusher, thus reinforcing the PDS ligature. The proximal rectum is divided and the specimen fixed around the introducer and withdrawn through the rectoscope. Thereafter the rectoscope itself is withdrawn and changed for the stapler cartridge and shaft under laparoscopic control.

As soon as the cartridge is seen in the monitor, its spike is advanced through the open rectal stump, and another cable binder is tightened around the stump. The colon and rectal stumps are checked and excess tissue resected. The anvil is inserted into the stapler shaft by a special anvil holder (Fig. 2), and the stapler is closed, fired, and carefully removed through the anus.

Extraluminal Procedure

Two 2-0 PDS slip knots are tightened around the sigmoid colon at its proximal and distal levels. A small stab wound is made in the upper rectum just below the distal ligature and in the upper sigmoid colon just above the proximal ligature. The anvil of a 29 mm dividable, curved stapler is inserted into the proximal sigmoid colon by means of the special introducer, passing through the two stab wounds. As the anvil is fixed to the proximal sigmoid colon with a PDS slip knot tightened around its rod, the introducer is withdrawn. The proximal sigmoid colon is now divided, completing the cut between the PDS ligatures. While the upper rectum is held with two forceps, the distal cut also is completed and the specimen removed by pulling it through the rectoscope with a grasper. A prelocked cable binder is then inserted and placed by encircling the rectum. At this moment the rectoscope is changed for the stapler cartridge and shaft. The trocar is advanced and the ca-

ble binder tightened around the rectum down to the central trocar. Another cable binder is tightened around the proximal stump, thus reinforcing the previous ligature and safely fixing the anvil. After closure of anvil to cartridge, while carefully avoiding catching the mesocolon between the two stumps, the stapler is fired. After the surgeon removes the stapler, the anastomosis is

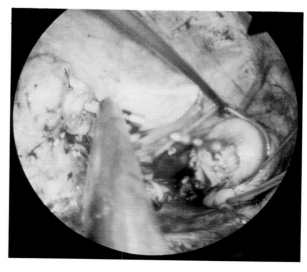

Fig. 2. Anvil is inserted into the stapler shaft by means of the specially designed anvil holder.

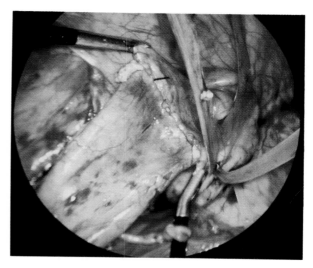

Fig. 3. Endoscopic view of the accomplished end-to-end anastomosis.

checked (Fig. 3) by turning the 50-degree lens looking at both sides of the bowel, and filling the rectum with 50 ml of methylene-blue solution.

RESULTS

The mean length of this operation is 135 minutes (range, 100 to 180 minutes). All the animals that underwent surgery had a problem-free postoperative course: no fever, no rectal bleeding, no signs of sepsis, regular food intake from the second postoperative day, and regular bowel activity.

At the autopsy after the animal's sacrifice, there were few adhesions around the anastomoses, with a localized, encapsulated fluid collection found in one case. The histological findings of the harvested anastomoses showed a good healing process in all cases except for three, in which a small area of dehiscence with histological signs of abscess was found. All the histological alterations were found in the first five animals operated on according to the described technique.

DISCUSSION

The main technical problems of the laparoscopic approach to left colectomy or sigmoidectomy are the anastomosis and the removal of the specimen.[2,3] The combined approach enabled us to set up a completely endoscopic procedure that fit the aim of minimally invasive surgery. Technology allowed us to overcome most of the problems during the research program by developing the anvil introducer, the anvil holder, and the cable-binding technique. These devices enable us to insert the anvil through the rectum up to the proximal sigmoid colon while avoiding any air leak once the bowel is opened and to close the bowel stumps without performing an intracorporeal purse-string suture.

Removal of the specimen may represent a limitation of the method. Because of the diameter of the Buess rectoscope, tumors up to 4 cm can be removed through it, but bigger neoplasms or extremely bulky bowel must be withdrawn through a posterior colpotomy in a female patient or through a minilaparotomy. The combined endoscopic sigmoidectomy is safe and fast. Such a procedure allowed an early recovery of all animals treated. The extraluminal variant avoids any contact between the anvil and the tumor and should be performed in case of suspected or proven malignant neoplasms. This variant is preferred even in the case of stenosing diverticulitis.

Because of the good results of the experimental study, a clinical trial has begun. Benign and malignant tumors and diverticulitis are the main indications for use of endoscopic sigmoidectomy.

REFERENCES

1. Buess G, Kipfmüller K, Hack D, et al. Technique of transanal endoscopic microsurgery. Surg Endosc 2:71-75, 1988.
2. Jacobs M, Verdeja JC, Goldstein HS. Minimally invasive colon resection (laparoscopic colectomy). Surg Laparosc Endosc 1:144-150, 1991.
3. Fowler DL, White SA. Laparoscopy-assisted sigmoid resection. Brief clinical report. Surg Laparosc Endosc 1:183-188, 1991.

73 *Transanal Endoscopic Microsurgery of Rectal Tumors*

Karl Kipfmüller, Manuela DeVos, and Peter Merkle

The theory of the adenoma-carcinoma sequence of large bowel neoplasia is well established. To prevent colorectal carcinoma, an adenoma—when present—must be removed completely. The removal of pedunculated polyps with the electrocautery snare is usually easy. Sessile adenomas must be excised by a mucosectomy that extends to the muscularis propria; a sufficient margin of circumferential clearance must be maintained. This technique ensures accurate histological examination and a low recurrence rate. To accomplish complete removal of large adenomas, a full-thickness excision of the bowel wall should be performed. If an early-stage well-differentiated or moderately differentiated carcinoma (a pT1 tumor) is discovered during operation and if no metastasis to the lymph nodes has occurred, removal with a sufficient margin of clearance can result in cure.

Although local excision is appropriate for benign adenomas, the local treatment of invasive carcinomas can be considered only under certain conditions. For local excision of "early" carcinomas (pT1) ≤ 3 cm that have begun to infiltrate the submucosa, it is essential to remove the tumor with a sufficient margin that can be confirmed by intraoperative histological examination. The degree of tumor infiltration into the muscularis propia (a pT2 carcinoma) that still permits local excision remains to be defined.

This degree of tumor infiltration determines whether local excision can be used. Conventional examination (digital examination, rectoscopy, or barium enema) supplies indirect evidence of the depth of tumor infiltration. However, since 1985, endorectal ultrasonography has provided an objective, documentable definition of tumor infiltration, and all layers of the rectal wall are revealed by this examination. The sensitivity for tumor penetration of the rectal wall ranges from 75% to 95%.[7,11]

Various surgical methods for local excision of rectal tumors are available, such as Parks' transanal technique, in which self-retaining anal retractors and posterior procedures are used either without division of the sphincter (Kraske's technique) or with sphincter division (Mason's transsphincter technique). As an al-

ternative to conventional techniques, transanal endoscopic microsurgery was developed[12] (Fig. 1).

INSTRUMENTATION

The primary instrument used in transanal endoscopic microsurgery is the rectoscope measuring 12 or 20 cm in length and 40 mm in diameter. The instrument choice depends on the tumor site. The insert at the external end of the rectoscope contains ports for the operative instruments and the stereoscopic telescope. Sealing sleeves and caps prevent gas loss when the operating instruments are placed into the rectoscope. The six-fold magnification of the stereoscopic endoscope permits an excellent view during the procedure. The rectal cavity is dilated by pressure-controlled CO_2 insufflation. A roller pump for the suction device and a water rinse to clean the optic front lens are integrated into the unit. Microsurgical instruments designed for endoscopic work, such as a high-frequency cautery knife, forceps, scissors, a needle holder, a clip applicator, and a coagulating-suction device are used.

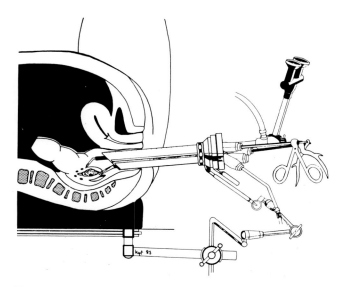

Fig. 1. Transanal endoscopic microsurgery of rectal tumors.

OPERATIVE TECHNIQUE

Patient preparation includes bowel lavage and perioperative antibiotic prophylaxis. Intraoperative positioning of the patient is determined by the tumor site. The lithotomy position is used if the tumor is located posteriorly; the prone or side-lying position is used for tumors of the anterior wall. The operating system is fixed with a double ball-and-socket joint holder (the Martin arm), which is attached to the operating desk. After introduction of the rectoscope, the tumor and surgical field are visualized.

The initial surgical step is to surround the tumor with marking dots (Fig. 2) to define the margin of clearance and the resection line. Electrocautery is used to remove the tumor; a margin of 5 mm of normal mucosa is left to surround an adenoma and a margin of 10 mm is required for carcinoma removal (Fig. 3). Hemostasis is established by use of electrocoagulation. The rectal wall defect is repaired by a continuous transverse suture of a monofilament resorbable thread (Fig. 4). Instead of surgical knots, silver clips are pressed onto the thread. The tumor is then excised and attached in its correct orientation on a cork board for examination by the pathologist (Fig. 5).

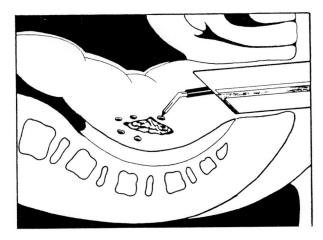

Fig. 2. Tumor is surrounded with marking dots by high-frequency knife.

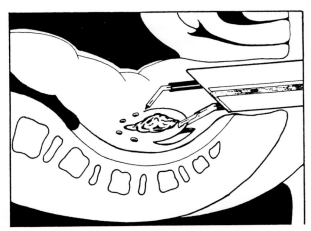

Fig. 3. Tumor is excised along resection line.

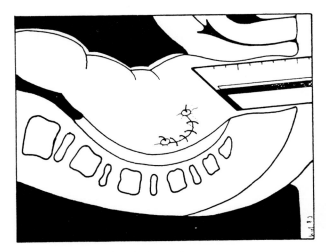

Fig. 4. Defect is closed via continuous transverse suture.

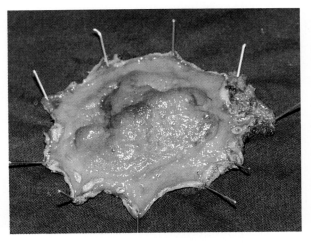

Fig. 5. Sessile adenoma pinned for histological examination.

RESULTS

Since April 1989 we have used the technique of transanal endoscopic microsurgery in 125 patients, 50 of whom had a malignancy (Tables 1 and 2). The average age of the patients was 63.8 years (range, 23 to 89). Eighty-nine of these patients had been diagnosed as having an adenoma, but in 14 of these cases histological examination of the resected specimen revealed focal malignant invasion.

Predominant tumor sites in these patients were the middle third of the rectum (8 to 12 cm from the anal verge; range 4 to 20 cm). The tumors were distributed over the rectal circumference with a slight prevalence at the dorsal rectum. Tumor excision was performed by the full-thickness technique in 80 patients. In seven of these patients, a segmental resection was necessary.

The average area of resection was 32.8 cm²; the average tumor size was 20.1 cm². Intraoperative blood loss was minimal; 12 ml of blood lost during a segmental resection was the maximum. Blood transfusions were not required. Opening of the peritoneal cavity was necessary in seven patients as a result of the excision of tumors near the intraperitoneal part of the rectum. The defects were closed immediately, and no postoperative problems occurred. Operating time depended on the size and site of the tumor. Excision of a small tumor required 30 minutes and removal of large adenomas or those that required segmental resection required 2 to 3 hours.

The histological results are shown in Table 1. Seventy-one patients had an adenoma, and 19 pT1 carcinomas (Fig. 6), 24 pT2 carcinomas (Fig.7), and five pT3 carcinomas were found. One malignant melanoma and one submucosal carcinoid were excised.

The day after operation, patients were ambulatory. Intravenous infusion was carried out for 1 day after mucosectomy. Oral nutrition was begun on the fourth

Table 1. Histological examinations of 125 tumors removed by transanal endoscopic microsurgery

	Number
Adenoma	71
Polyposis	4
pT1 carcinoma	19
pT2 carcinoma	24
pT3 carcinoma	5
Melanoma	1
Carcinoid	1

Table 2. Depth of excision in 125 rectal tumors

	Benign	Malignant
Mucosectomy	20	—
Partial-wall excision	11	2
Full-thickness excision	34	46
Segmental resection	5	2

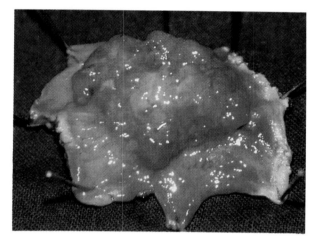

Fig. 6. Polypoid pT2 carcinoma.

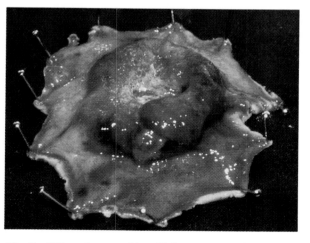

Fig. 7. pT2 carcinoma with sufficient margin of clearance.

postoperative day in patients with full-thickness excision or segmental resection or in those who underwent incision of the peritoneal cavity. The average postoperative hospitalization time was 6.3 days. The rate of complications was reduced. In five patients partial breakdown of the suture line was discovered at rectoscopy on the day of discharge, but these patients had no clinical signs during the postoperative course, and no therapy was necessary. One woman experienced incomplete incontinence that lasted 2 months. Three patients experienced postoperative bleeding (8 to 15 days after surgery), which was managed by suturing with a rigid rectoscope.

Sixteen patients with low-risk pT1 carcinomas underwent local excision and are free of recurrence at the time of this writing. Six patients (three with pT1 carcinomas and three with pT2 carcinomas) underwent radical resection after local excision. No residual tumor was detected. We found one lymph node metastasis in a patient with a high-risk pT2 carcinoma. In two patients with pT2 carcinomas, local recurrence occurred 10 and 12 months, respectively, after local treatment. One local recurrence occurred in a patient who had an adenoma.

DISCUSSION

Initial steps in the diagnosis of a rectal tumor include digital examination and clinical staging.[13,14] Rectoscopy is used to determine the size and tumor site. Additional information is obtained from biopsy results. Digital examination can be used to reach 60% to 80% of rectal tumors. In our study, 79% of the tumors were detected by digital examination, the sensitivity of which was 87% (CS I, 92%; CS II, 67%). These results correspond to the data cited in the literature.[6-8,13,14] The extent of infiltration of tumors of the bowel wall can be predicted. The value of clinical staging depends on the experience of the examiner. Nicholls et al.[14] estimated that the accuracy of an experienced examiner ranges from 67% to 79% and that of an inexperienced examiner from 44% to 83%.

The preoperative staging of rectal tumor infiltration affects therapy. Histologically well-differentiated small rectal carcinomas that have not infiltrated the muscularis propria (low-risk carcinomas) can be treated with local excision that has a sufficient margin of clearance. The indication for preoperative radiotherapy is determined by the depth of infiltration.[15,16]

Since 1985 endorectal ultrasonography has been used for the preoperative staging of rectal tumors (Table 3).[7-9] The accuracy of endorectal ultrasonography in the detection of adenomas (pT0-1 tumors) is greater than 90%.[9-17] With endoluminal ultrasonography rather than digital examination, tumors higher in the rectum can be identified. In our study we estimated the depth of infiltration of all tumors by endoluminal ultrasonography. The results of digital rectal examination and endoluminal ultrasonography are comparable with regard to digitally accessible tumors, but neither method can be used to differentiate sessile polyps from T1 carcinomas. Ultrasonographic endoprobes cannot be used to show the lamina muscularis mucosa (the marginal layer between the mucosa and the submucosa).[9,17] Computed tomography scans (CT) and magnetic resonance imaging (MRI) are used for special examinations, such as advanced tumor growth, in which infiltration of the perirectal fatty tissue (stage pT3) or infiltration of neighboring structures and organs (stage pT4) can be identified. However, CT and MRI are not suitable for the identification of small tumors or for differentiation between stage T1 and stage T2 carcinomas.[11,17-20]

The rate of lymph node metastasis of rectal carcinomas is correlated with tumor infiltration and differentiation. In low-risk carcinomas limited to the submucosa, lymph node metastases are seen in ≤ 3% of cases. There is no cancer-related mortality in patients with low-risk tumors who undergo local excision.[1,3,4,6,23] Cancer-related mortality does increase to ≤ 11% in patients > 70 years of age who undergo radical surgery.[3]

Local recurrences are not seen after anterior resection or abdominoperineal resection of stage pT1 or pT2 carcinomas.[2] The rate of recurrence in patients with low-risk carcinomas who undergo local excision is 0 to 8%; the rate for those with high-risk tumors increases to 20%.[1,3,4,16,23] The 5-year survival rate for patients with stage IA (pT1pN0pM0) is approximately 100% ± 3%;

Table 3. Review of the literature regarding sensitivity of endoluminal sonography to rectal tumors

	Number	Sensitivity
Feifel et al.[7]	42	85%
Glaser[8]	73	87%
Heintz[9]	130	90%
Milsom[10]	52	83%
Kipfmüller et al.[6,17]	107	87%

for stage IB (pT2pNOpMO) it is approximately 78% ± 10%. More than 90% of the patients deemed low-risk survive > 5 years. There is no difference between patients who undergo local or radical excisions.[2,3]

Multivariate data analyses indicate that sphincter function can be preserved with a stapling technique for coloanal anastomosis with a small distal margin of clearance. However, a 5 cm margin in continuity of the operative site is the equivalent of a 3 cm distance in the fixed specimen. Also, low-grade tumors tend to spread by skipping areas. Patients with carcinomas of the lower third of the rectum are at a significantly higher risk of local recurrence if the margin of resection is too small. Thus in 35% of patients with rectal carcinoma, the only viable treatment is abdominoperineal resection and permanent colostomy.[2]

Small, sessile adenomas can be removed by mucosectomy. If tumor size is greater than 3 cm, the risk of malignant transformation increases significantly.[3] In these cases, we perform full-thickness excision. Local excision of pT1 carcinomas, which have a low recurrence rate and a low incidence of lymph node metastasis, can be considered a cure. Even in patients of advanced age, lower postoperative mortality results from local excision. Protocols for treatment of T2 carcinoma are adapted to the individual patient. Those with advanced age and other significant risk factors have a reasonable risk to benefit ratio from local excision.

Transanal endoscopic microsurgery can be used throughout the rectum and the lower sigmoid colon, as opposed to conventional transanal surgical techniques, which can be used only in the lower rectum. Although conventional transanal procedures require mechanical retractors, our technique permits microsurgery through endoscopic magnification of the dilated rectal cavity.[6,12] Parks' transanal technique provides a limited surgical recurrence rate of ≤ 20%.[24] We have seen significantly lower recurrence rates with endoscopic microsurgery.[6,12] Transsphincteric or posterior rectotomy offers a better prognosis than does Parks' technique. However, the required transsection of sphincter structures correlates with a high complication rate: wound infections in 22.2% and fistula formation in 18.8% were reported in the literature.[25] Thus patient stress is clearly increased. Surgical pain, delayed mobilization, and prolonged hospitalization require a long rehabilitation phase. Patients who undergo endoscopic surgery are usually free of complaints, can be mobilized after anesthesia, and quickly recover from physical stress. Complications are rare; death resulting from surgery is uncommon.

CONCLUSION

Limited, sphincter-saving surgery is important in the management of rectal tumors. Benign tumors or early low-risk carcinomas are suited for local excision. Mortality correlates with patients' advanced age. Transanal endoscopic microsurgery affords an almost painless, complication-rare treatment with short-term hospitalization for patients with rectal carcinomas.

REFERENCES

1. Buess G, Kipfmüller K, Hack D, Grüssner R, Heintz A. Junginger Technique of transanal endoscopic microsurgery. Surg Endocsc 2:71, 1988.
2. Gall FP, Hermanek P. Gegenwärtinger Stand der Therapie des Rektumkarzinoms. Zentralbl Chir 112:943, 1987.
3. Gall FP, Hermanek P. Cancer of the rectum—local excision. Surg Clin North AM 68:1353, 1988.
4. Gemsenjäger E, Lokale Excision beim Rektumkarzinom. Schweiz Rundsch Med Prax 76:551, 1987.
5. Heberer G, Denecke H, Demmel N, Wirsching R. Local procedures in the management of rectal cancer. World J Surg 11:499, 1987.
6. Kipfmüller K, Guhl L, Kiehling C, Arlart J, Merkle P. Die präoperative Beurteilung der Infiltrationstiefe con Rektumtumoren—Clinical Staging, Endosonografie und Magnetresonanztomografie. Der Chirurg (in press).
7. Feifel G, Hildebrandt U, Dohm G. Die endorectale Sonographie beim Rektumcarcinom, Chirurgie 56:398, 1985.
8. Glaser F, Kleikamp G, Schlag P, Möller P. Herfarth CH. Die Endosonographie in der präoperativen Beurteilung rectaler Tumoren. Chirurgie 60:856, 1989.
9. Heintz A, Buess G, Junginger T. Endorectale Sonographie zur präoperativen Beurteiling der Infiltrationstiefe con Rektumtumoren. Dtsch Med Wochenschr 115:1083, 1990.
10. Milsom JW, Graffner H. Intrarectal ultrasonography in rectal cancer staging and in the evaluation of pelvic disease. Ann Surg 212:602, 1990.
11. Rifkin MD, Ehrlich SM, Marks G. Staging of rectal carcinoma: Prospective comparison of endorectal US and CT. Radiology 170:319, 1989.
12. Buess G, Heintz A, Kipfmüller K, Ibald R. Transanale Endosckopische Mikrochirurgie beim kleinen Rektumkarzinom. Gastroenterol 24:183, 1989.
13. Mason Y. Rectal cancer: The spectrum of selective surgery. Proc Soc Med 69:237, 1976.
14. Nicholls RJ, Local excision for adenocarcinoma of the rectum. In Mann, CV, ed. Contributions from St. Mark's Hospital. London, 1988, P S.202.
15. Ellis LM, Mendenhall WM, Bland KI, Copeland EM. Local excision and radiation therapy for rectal cancer. Am Surg 54:217, 1988.

16. Minsky BD, Rich T, Recht A, Harvey W, Mier C. Selection criteria for local excision with or without adjuvant radiation therapy for rectal cancer. Cancer 63:1421, 1989.
17. Kipfmüller K, Sauter G, Egner E, Merkle P. Lokale chirurgische Therapie bei Rektumtumoren—unsere Erfahrungen mit der transanalen endoskopischen Mikrochirurgie. Ärzteblatt Baden-Wurttemberg 10:550, 1991.
18. Butch RJ, Stark DD, Wittenberg J, Tepper JE, Saini S, Simenoe JF, Mueller PR, Ferrucci JT. Staging rectal cancer by MR and CT. AJR 146:1155, 1986.
19. Guinet C, Buy J, Sezeur A, Mosnier H, Ghossain M, Malafosse M, Guicarc HM, Vadrom D, Ecoiffier J. Preoperative assessment of the extension of rectal carcinoma: Correlation of MR, surgical, and histopathologic findings. J Comput Assist Tomogr 12:209, 1988.
20. Hodgman CG, MacCarty RL, Wolff BG, May GR, Berquist TH, Sheedy PF, Beart RW, Spencer RJ. Preoperative staging of rectal carcinoma by computed tomography and 0.15 T magnetic resonance imaging. Dis Colon Rectum 29:446, 1986.
21. Lange EE de, Fechner RE, Edge SB, Spaulding CA. Preoperative staging of rectal carcinoma with MR imaging: Surgical and Histopathological correlation. Radiology 176:623, 1990.
22. Hermanek P, Gall FP. Early (microinvasive) colorectal carcinoma. Int J Colorectal Dis 1:79, 1986.
23. Nicholls RJ, Mason AY, Morson BC, Dixon AK, Fry IK. The clinical staging of rectal cancer. Cr J Surg 69:404, 1982.
24. Schiessel R, Wunderlich M, Karner-Hanusch J. Transanale Excision und Anastomosentechnik. Chirurgie 57:773, 1986.
25. Schildberg FW, Wenk H. Der posteriore Zugang zum Rectum. Chirurgie 57:779, 1986.

74 *Transanal Endoscopic Surgery*

Samir Said, Gerhard Buess, and Peter Huber

The transabdominal operations formerly practiced for resection of adenoma have been largely replaced by endoscopic techniques that have a much lower risk of complications. With the advent of the flexible fiberoptic colonoscope, pedunculated polyps can be removed anywhere in the colon (Fig. 1, *A*).

For sessile polyps the use of a diathermy snare is inadequate, since the dysplastic cells of the transitional zone between malignant growth and normal mucosa cannot be removed safely with snare dissection (Fig. 1, *B*). Broad-based tumors (>2 cm) must be removed by surgical excision to prevent recurrences and to avoid perforations and hemorrhages (Fig. 1, *C*). There is general agreement that there is less local recurrence following complete surgical excision of rectal tumors than following transanal fulguration,[1,2] electrocoagulation,[3] tumor ablation by laser,[4,5] and endocavitary radiation as described by Papillon and Berard[6] and Sischy et al.[7]

The principal criticism of these conservative approaches is that tumor destruction is imprecise, no specimen is obtained to evaluate the level of invasion of the rectal wall, and multiple sessions are needed to eliminate the tumor.

The low precision results in part from using the conventional transanal (Parks) technique, with recurrence rates up to 21%,[8,9] the limited area of application (this technique is mainly useful for the lower third of the rectum up to approximately 8 to 10 cm from the anal margin), and the high rate of complications associated with extensive surgical techniques, such as Mason's transsphincteric approach,[10] the Kraske posterior resection,[11] and the standardized transabdominal rectum resections, have all pointed to the necessity of developing an endoscopic minimally invasive approach.

At the Surgical Department of the University of Cologne, an endoscopic system (Fig. 2) has been developed by Buess and co-workers that allows all the conventional surgical techniques to be performed within the whole rectal cavity. The method has been in clinical use since 1983.[12-14]

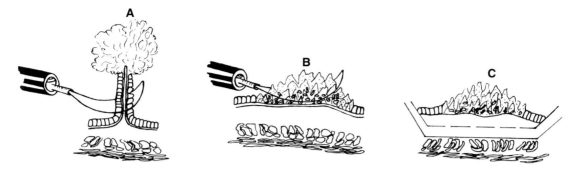

Fig. 1. Appropriate techniques of resecting pedunculated tumors. **A,** Sessile tumors can often not be removed completely and safely with a snare dissection, **B,** and therefore require complete surgical excision, **C,** to prevent recurrence and perforation.

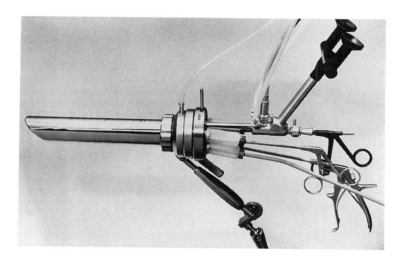

Fig. 2. System for endoscopic operation.

INSTRUMENTS

The operative area is visualized by a rectoscope with an outside diameter of 40 mm (Fig. 3). Depending on the site of the operation in the rectum, either a 120 mm or 200 mm rectoscopic tube, together with its obturator (atraumatic introducer) is used. The tip of the tubes are slanted 45 degrees so that the upper part of the rectoscope protects the telescope; the area underneath the operative field is simultaneously maintained open mechanically. The rear end of the rectoscope's main element can either be attached to an adaptor with a viewing window and illumination insert for the initial survey of the rectal cavity or to a working insert for the telescope and auxiliary instruments.

Loss of gas is prevented by rubber sealing sleeves and caps with different diameters for auxiliary instruments. In addition to the wide-lumen rectoscope, automatic pressure-controlled CO_2 is insufflated to expose the operative area. The combined endosurgical unit (Fig. 4) includes three functions: preselectable pressure-controlled insufflation of CO_2 at a constant pressure of about 10 to 15 mm Hg; rinsing of the lens with distilled water by using a foot controlled switch; and suction of blood, secretions, and coagulating fumes.

The stereoscopic telescope (Fig. 5), with up to six-fold magnification, transmits a three-dimensional image to the surgeon. The assistant, sitting on the left side of the surgeon, can aid in the operation with a semirig-

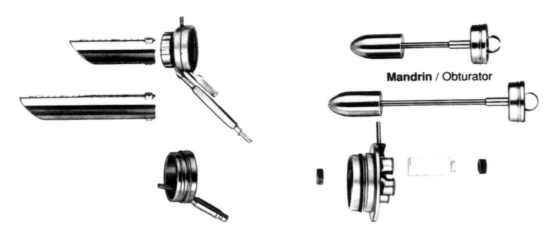

Fig. 3. Wide-lumen endosurgical rectoscope and accessories.

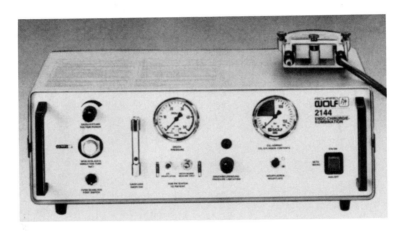

Fig. 4. Combination endosurgical unit.

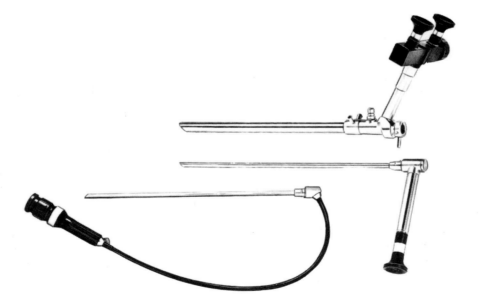

Fig. 5. Stereo telescope, documentation telescope, semirigid telescope.

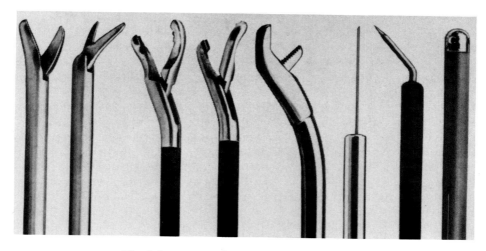

Fig. 6. Instruments for an endorectal procedure.

id (monocular) telescope that is inserted in the probe channel of the stereoscopic telescope, or a video system is used. Automatic gas insufflation to the tip of the optical system prevents clouding over and the lens can be rinsed by water injection. Up to four newly designed instruments (consisting of the HF knife, the combined forceps, the coagulation aspiration-tube, and the needle holder) can be used simultaneously.

Most of the auxiliary instruments (Fig. 6) listed below have angulated tips to enlarge the region to be operated on: a coagulation-suction tube with a monopolar high-frequency connection to perform electrocoagulation of minor bleeding and suction; an almost fully insulated high-frequency knife for partial excision of the bowel wall; a retractable needle for eventual injection of saline solution beneath the tumor; a needle holder with jaws shaped so that the needle automatically aligns when grasped; a high-frequency combination forceps for grasping tissue or holding the needle; scissors for cutting the thread; and stapling forceps for securing the thread used in the continuous suture technique with special silver clips.

OPERATIVE TECHNIQUE

A typical microsurgical procedure using the operative system described would be as follows: The operation is carried out with the patient under general or regional anesthesia. Preoperative patient preparation consists of bowel lavage in accordance with the usual procedure for colonic surgery. Perioperative antibiotic agents are administered. Operative time averages 90 minutes.

The patient is positioned on the operation table in such a way so that the tumor is located below the viewing range of the optical system (in a prone, lithotomy, or lateral position) and the perianal skin is disinfected. A cautious digital stretching of the anus is performed with up to four fingers. After a general visual inspection of the rectum, the rectoscope is fixed to the operating table after focusing on the tumor. The pneumatically distended rectum allows all surgical procedures to be performed endoscopically.

The sessile growth is circumcised with the high-frequency knife so that a 10 mm border of healthy mucosa adherent to the tumor is removed. Next the tumor is excised. Adenomatous tissue does not exceed the muscularis propria, so in these cases a mucosectomy is the appropriate treatment.

In cases of adhesions at the border between submucosa and muscularis propria (e.g., as a result of circatrization following previous polypectomies), partial muscularis propria removal should be carried out. If the tumor lies intraperitoneally, one should refrain from full-thickness removal of the bowel wall, which leads to intraperitoneal leakage of CO_2 gas and potentially to intra-abdominal infection.

Early rectal carcinomas with favorable histological grading (G1 + G2), the so called low-risk carcinomas, are adequately treated by full-thickness excisions. Under palliative conditions, advanced cancers are also treated by full-thickness excision, which averts the need for multiple sessions of cryosurgery, laser tumor ablation, radiotherapy, or other palliative local treatments.

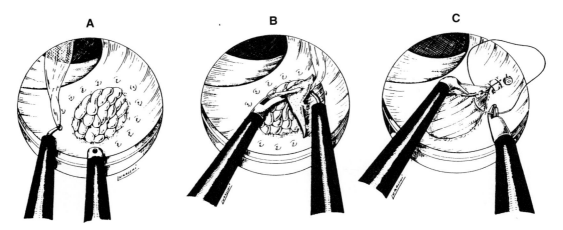

Fig. 7. Endoscopic rectal procedure. **A,** Circumcision of the sessile growth. **B,** Excision of the tumor. **C,** Closure of the defect by a continuous transverse suture.

Minor bleeding points can be coagulated either by the coagulation aspiration tube or by coagulating forceps. Arterial hemorrhages can also be managed by suture ligature. Finally, the mucosal defect is closed by a continuous suture to avert stricture and bleedings. Continuous suturing is done using a transverse direction. The edges of the mucosal defect are thus adapted and the suture is fixed by clamping metal spheres onto both ends (Fig. 7).

POSTOPERATIVE CARE

Intravenous fluids are usually given only for the first postoperative day. Patients generally are able to walk around on the evening of the operation. Pain that necessitates oral analgesic medication for about 3 days will occur if the tumor resection was adjacent to the anus. On average the postoperative stay is 7 days.

INDICATIONS FOR ENDORECTAL SURGERY

The main indication for endorectal surgery is the removal of *broad-based sessile adenomas.* Local excision of *early rectal carcinomas,* defined as a carcinoma that has penetrated only up to submucosa, has been widely accepted.[15,16] Early rectal carcinoma with (1) a favorable histological picture, (2) well or moderately differentiated carcinoma (grades 1 and 2) of the so called low-risk type that did not reveal mucinous adenocarcinoma signet cells, pleomorphic undifferentiated carcinoma, or invasion of lymphatic vessels[17] and in which the probability of regional lymph node metastasis is low (approx-

imately 3%) are therapeutically managed with the endoscopic system by full-thickness disk excision as long as the lesion is located within the extraperitoneal part of the rectum.

Other indications include *palliative excision of advanced cancers* when a contraindication exists for performing radical surgery from a medical point of view or in cases in which the patient is unwilling to undergo extensive surgery. Further indication of endorectal surgery is the *correction of benign rectal strictures* by performing vertical incisions or circular resection of stricture-inducing tissue. Our experience with this technique is limited. The experience we have regarding transanal endoscopic *rectopexy,* which has been performed several times at the University of Tübingen, is at a very early stage.

RESULTS

From July 1983 to December 1992, we performed endoscopic operations on 313 patients at the University of Cologne. Patient ages ranged from 27 to 99 years (average, 65.4 years); 148 were men (47.3%) and 165 women (52.7%). The total number of operations rose to 348 because of recurrences and new tumor formations within the rectum.

POSTOPERATIVE HISTOLOGICAL EXAMINATION

The resected specimen of the tumor is pinned to a cork board with a border of normal mucosa and fixed in formaldehyde solution (Figs. 8 and 9). Adenomas of an area over 200 cm² have been resected, with the resec-

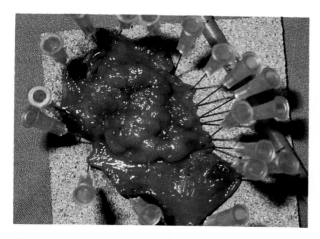

Fig. 8. Specimen excised locally using the disk excision procedure under endoscopic control.

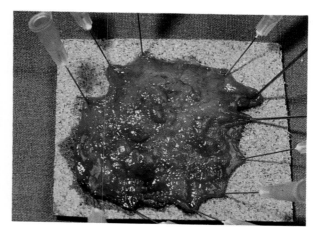

Fig. 9. Disk excision procedure.

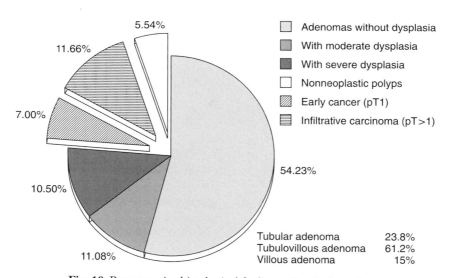

Fig. 10. Postoperative histological findings of excised specimen.

tion line being free from adenomatous tissue. The average size of the resected specimen is 13.3 cm². The precise pathology report is of extreme importance in deciding whether the local excision can be considered adequate or whether further therapy is needed. Therefore histological type, grade of malignancy, depth of invasion in the rectal wall, and absence of neoplastic infiltration in the specimen margins must be evaluated by the pathologist.

Histological Evaluation of the Excised Specimen

Two hundred sixty (75.8%) of the locally excised tumors were adenomas. Sixty-two of these were tubular, 39 villous, and 159 tubulovillous adenomata, indicating that the majority of the removed adenomas were of tubulovillous architecture. Thirty-six (10.50%) of the adenomas contained severe dysplasia, 38 (11.08%) moderate, and 186 (54.23%) did not reveal any dysplasia (Fig. 10).

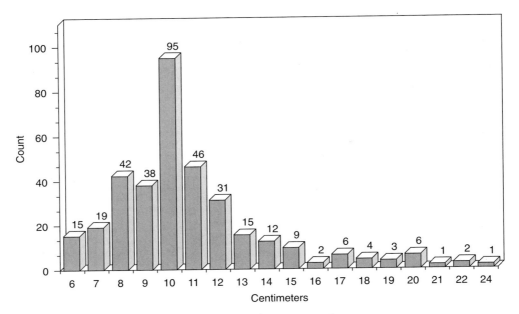

Fig. 11. Tumor distance from anal verge.

Nineteen (5.54%) of the excised polyps proved to be of a nonneoplastic nature, and 24 (7.00%) of the resected tumors were early rectal cancers. All 5 patients with "high-risk early carcinoma" underwent further radical operation, with uneventful postoperative courses. In order to make accurate comparisons with results of other series, a clear distinction has to be made between "malignant polyps," which are adenomas with a focal carcinoma, and those tumors which from the outset of treatment appear as clinical cancer.

Like many other surgical teams, we had initially lacked confidence in the results of local excision of rectal cancer. Therefore most of our patients with rectal cancer, who underwent curative local excision, had large sessile adenomas of the rectum with final postoperative histology containing a focus of invasive carcinoma ("malignant polyps").

Forty (11.66%) of the locally treated tumors were microinvasive cancers that had already penetrated into the muscularis propria (pT > 1). Thus a total of 64 patients with rectal cancer underwent transanal endoscopic excision.

Location of the Tumors in the Longitudinal Axis

The operated tumors were situated in the rectum proper and lower sigmoid (Fig. 11). Excisions were performed within 6 to 24 cm from the anocutaneous line. Most of the locally excised tumors were situated 8 to 10 cm from the anal margin, and their longitudinal extension was up to 11 cm.

Circumferential Extent of the Tumors

Of the 344 tumors located in the rectum (Fig. 12) or lower sigmoid, 4% extended over three quarters of the rectal circumference. Six of them were circumferential, demanding segmental resection; 9% of the tumors included up to three quarters of the rectal circumference, 42% involved more than one quarter and up to half of the circumference, and approximately 45% were determined to be as one quarter of the circumference or less. Major sessile polyps occasionally had to be removed in piecemeal fashion in one session to shorten the operative time.

POSTOPERATIVE COMPLICATIONS

Early postoperative complications occurred as follows:
- Five patients suffered intraperitoneal perforations, which were treated by laparotomy with an uneventful postoperative course.
- Hemorrhage was recorded in four cases and was controlled by using the transanal route.
- Four rectovaginal fistulas occurred. Two of the patients had advanced cancers and they underwent

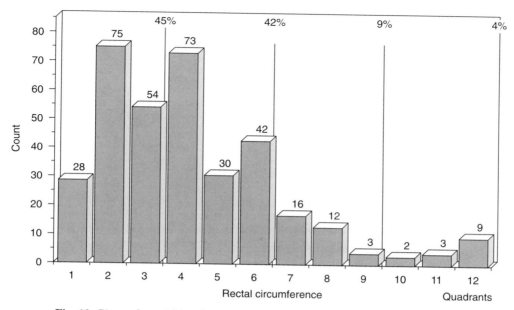

Fig. 12. Circumferential involvement of the endoscopically excised rectal tumors.

Table 1. Long-term follow-up after endorectal microsurgery

	Adenoma and Benign Polyps (n = 196)	Early Rectal Carcinoma (n = 21)	Advanced Carcinoma (n = 32)	Benign Stenosis (n = 3)
Local recurrence	10	1 adenoma + 1 carcinoma	3	1
Tumor progression	—	—	—	—
Stenosis	5	—	—	—
Incontinence	3	—	—	—
Fistula	—	—	—	—
Death from cancer-related causes	—	1 "high risk"	11	—

Follow-up rate, 95.1%; mean follow-up period, 3.3 years.

extensive repairs; the other two had minimal fistulas that were treated nonoperatively.
• There were two postoperative deaths in elderly patients as a result of cardiopulmonary failure. This figure corresponds to a statistically acceptable mortality after conventional transanal local excision.

All complications occurred within the first 3 years of our transanal endoscopic experience.

LONG-TERM RESULTS

Through December 1991, long-term follow-up data have been obtained in 252 of 265 cases, (Table 1). Hence the overall follow-up rate was 95.1%. (The range of follow-up was from 1 month to 8.5 years, with a mean follow-up period of 3.3 years.) Regarding the endoanally removed adenomas and nonneoplastic polyps, 10 patients had recurrences. Thus the recurrence rate was

5.1%. After full-thickness excisions of an early cancer with moderate differentiation, we found 1 local recurrence of an adenoma, which was managed by the transanal endoscopic route, and one Dukes B carcinoma, which was treated by anterior resection.

Among the palliatively treated cases, three patients needed a second transanal endoscopic tumor removal within 6 to 34 months postoperatively. Five slight strictures occurred that did not need any further therapy. Three elderly patients experienced incontinence for gas. Eleven patients with advanced cancer and one patient with high-risk early cancer died within the follow-up period from cancer-related causes.

CONCLUSION

Attempts to employ endoscopic procedures in the treatment of the middle and upper third of the rectum have led to various developments. However, so far no technological development has permitted resection using multiple instruments simultaneously under satisfactory endoscopic control. The endorectal system we employ permits local excision of large rectal tumors with minimal morbidity and excellent presentation of the specimen for complete histological analysis. Although this operation system initially involves relatively high costs, with thorough teaching and training of the surgical team, the obvious advantages of short hospital stays (7 days on average), and the dramatically reduced costs of patient rehabilitation outweigh any financial arguments.

REFERENCES

1. De Graaf PW, Roussel JG, Gortzak E, Hart GAM, Jongman A, van Slooten EA. Early-stage rectal cancer: Electrofulguration in comparison to abdominoperineal exstirpation or low-anterior resection. J Surg Oncol 29:123-128, 1985.
2. Hoekstra HJ, Verschueren RCJ, Oldhoff J, van der Ploeg E. Palliative and curative electrocoagulation for rectal cancer. Cancer 55:210-213, 1985.
3. Eisenstat TE, Oliver GC. Electrocoagulation for adenocarcinoma of the low rectum. World J Surg 16:458-462, 1992.
4. Joffe SN. Contact neodymium-YAG laser surgery in gastroenterology. Surg Endosc 1:25-27, 1987.
5. Mathus-Vliegen EMH, Tytgat GNJ. Nd-YAG laser photocoagulation in gastroenterology: Its role in palliation of colorectal cancer. Arch Surg 37:17-19, 1987.
6. Papillon J, Berard P. Endocavitary irradiation in the conservative treatment of adenocarcinoma of the low rectum. World J Surg 16:452-457, 1992.
7. Sischy B, Remington JH, Sobel SH. Treatment of rectal carcinomas by means of endocavitary irradiation: A progress report. Cancer 46:1957, 1980.
8. Parks AG, Stuart AE. The management of villous tumours of the large bowel. Br J Surg 60:688-695, 1973.
9. Thomson JPS. Treatment of sessile villous and tubulovillous adenomas of the rectum. Dis Colon Rectum 20:467-472, 1977.
10. Schildberg FW, Wenk H. Der posteriore Zugang zum Rektum. Chirurgie 57:779-791, 1986.
11. Westbrook KC, Lang NP, Broadwater JR, Thompson BW. Posterior surgical approaches to the rectum. Ann Surg 195:677, 1982.
12. Buess G, Hutterer F, Theiss R, Böbel M, Isselhard W, Pichlmaier H. Das System für die transanale endoskopische Rektumoperation. Chirurgie 55:677-680, 1984.
13. Buess G, Theiss R, Günther M, Hutterer F, Pichlmaier H. Endoscopic surgery in the rectum. Endoscopy 17:31-35, 1985.
14. Cuschieri A, Buess G, Perissat J, eds. Endoluminal Rectal Surgery. In Operative Manual of Endoscopic Surgery. New York: Springer-Verlag, 1992.
15. Hager T, Gall FP, Hermanek P. Local excision of cancer of the rectum. Dis Colon Rectum 26:149-151, 1983.
16. Graham RA, Garnsey L, Jessup JM. Local excision of rectal carcinoma. Am J Surg 160:306-312, 1990.
17. Hermanek P, Gall FP. Early (microinvasive) colorectal carcinoma: Pathology, diagnosis, surgical treatment. Int J Colorect Dis 1:79-84, 1986.

XII

Lessons Learned From Traditional Techniques in Colorectal Surgery

75   *Perioperative Radiotherapy for Rectal Adenocarcinoma*

Philippe Bérard and J. Papillon†

In the management of rectal adenocarcinoma, the role of perioperative radiotherapy raises a number of questions, many of which may be answered in this report:

- Can patients benefit from radiotherapy?
- Are patients to be selected?
- What are the risks of combined therapy in addition to those of a surgical operation?
- What is the best time in the treatment protocol for radiotherapy?
- What credit can be given to other adjuvant treatments, such as chemotherapy, in this radiosurgical association?

CAN PATIENTS BENEFIT FROM RADIOTHERAPY?

Surgical resection alone has not improved the prognosis of rectal adenocarcinoma with regard to local recurrences, distant metastasis, and long-term survival.[1] Radiotherapy alone can control some rectal adenocarcinomata.[2] This concept is corroborated by the 5% to 15% sterilized specimens found by surgeons after preoperative radiotherapy.[1] These factors favor the use of radiotherapy in the treatment of rectal adenocarcinoma.

PATIENT SELECTION

Patients with T3 tumors and T4 fixed, unresectable cancers are the most suitable candidates for preoperative irradiation[3] because of the high rate of local recurrence. However, T2 tumors (Dukes A) have a local recurrence rate of 7% to 13%.[4,5] This idea argues against restricting the indications for postoperative radiotherapy for Dukes B and C alone and indicates all the more that T2 tumors should not be excluded from a preoperative irradiation protocol. The results that can be offered by endocavitary irradiation[2] for T1 tumors favor the use of radiotherapy in rectal adenocarcinoma regardless of the disease stage. This will be explained further in answers to the questions that follow.

†Deceased.

ADDITIONAL RISKS OF COMBINED THERAPY

The surgeon who is aware of actinic lesions knows the dangers of radiotherapy. Lesions caused by radiation are a side effect of postoperative irradiation given at efficient dosages of 45 to 50 Gy within 4 or 5 weeks. This method has proved less effective in local recurrences when compared with preoperative protocols,[6] which may lead to discontinuation of postoperative radiotherapy in favor of preoperative irradiation, which when carefully planned has no substantial side effects.

TIMING OF RADIOTHERAPY

The lower toxicity of preoperative irradiation and its superiority as far as postoperative local recurrences are concerned are conclusive arguments for preoperative irradiation. In other respects preoperative radiotherapy is always possible, whereas postoperative complications may sometimes preclude some patients from benefiting from early postoperative radiotherapy. We would not discuss this matter if the multiplicity of preoperative irradiation protocols did not call its reliability into question[1]: dosages ranging from 5 to 50 Gy, target volumes varying from the tumor area to the entire pelvis, even spreading to the para-aortic are up to the level of L2, irradiation times varying from 1 day to 4 or 5 weeks, and time of surgery occurring from a few hours up to 6 or 8 weeks after irradiation. Agreement has been reached based on the necessity of giving a "dosage equivalent" of 40 Gy within 4 weeks.

Among all of the protocols, the one we think should be followed is the one we have published previously.[1] It is effective and well tolerated. It consists of giving 30 to 35 Gy within 12 to 15 days using cobalt-60 or photons of 5 to 6 MV in arc therapy though a sacral field. As for adenocarcinoma of the low rectum, in which sphincter preservation is initially considered, a delay of 8 weeks between completion of radiotherapy and surgery seems appropriate to take advantage of tumor regression and to allow a low anterior resection rather than an abdominoperineal resection.

In cases in which sphincter preservation seems possible right away, this delay can be shortened to 3 or 4 weeks, a delay that allows inflammatory reactions to subside. In cases in which an abdominoperineal resection must be performed, the delay will depend on the initial size of the lesion and tumor fixation. In such instances a long delay (8 weeks) is appropriate. We believe the results of this treatment program, in terms of a decrease in local recurrences and an increase in the rate of sphincter preservation,[1,7] are so encouraging that it can be applied safely to our patients on a large scale. Tumor persistence or local recurrences and most of all the inefficacy of preoperative radiotherapy in reducing the rate of distant metastases compel us to consider a combined approach that would include chemotherapy and possibly intraoperative radiotherapy.

THE ROLE OF ASSOCIATED ADJUVANT METHODS
Intraoperative Radiotherapy

The benefits we anticipate when exceeding dosages of 50 to 55 Gy, without harm to the small intestine, bladder, and ureter, lead us to consider using complementary intraoperative radiotherapy in some cases.[8] We do not have sufficient experience in this field to draw any conclusions, but we believe that this association should involve well-trained radiotherapists and well-selected patients only, since the addition of higher dosages is difficult to evaluate. In contrast, in cases of confined local recurrences occurring 18 months after surgery, the addition of 15 to 20 Gy of intraoperative radiotherapy during reoperation for resection of local recurrences to the 30 Gy given previously during preoperative treatment seems to be well tolerated locally,[9] and its efficacy as an adjuvant treatment for resection of local recurrences should be justified.[8]

Chemotherapy

The relative inefficacy of adjuvant radiotherapy, even preoperatively, in the survival of patients with rectal adenocarcinoma is linked to the potential for distant metastasis and presents the opportunity of an association with adjuvant chemotherapy. The efficacy of chemotherapy, as monotherapy, seems to increase when it is combined with radiotherapy, particularly with regard to postoperative irradiation.[10]

Having decided in favor of preoperative radiotherapy, we currently propose to patients with rectal adenocarcinomas T3 and T4 a treatment program of adjuvant chemotherapy using 5-fluorouracil (350 mg/m²/day) and Leucovin (20 mg/m²/day) in six courses of 5 days.[11] The first treatment is given immediately, when the rectal adenocarcinoma is discovered, just before irradiation; the second is given before or after surgical resection, according to the time allowed between completion of irradiation and surgery. The last treatment takes place 6 months after surgery. Such a strategy undoubtedly can improve the prognosis of unfavorable tumors (Dukes B and C). Last, for carcinomas with no extension at all or just a slight extension to the rectal wall, we wonder whether there should be routine preoperative radiotherapy. On this matter we agree with the EORTC investigators,[12] who emphasized the advantage of preoperative radiotherapy in such limited forms only if the risk of local failure must not be underestimated and if they are not prone to distant metastasis.

It is important that all clinicians be aware of these problems if any progress is to be made in the treatment of rectal adenocarcinoma, so that all patients may be given the best chance of cure and anal preservation.

REFERENCES

1. Berard P, Papillon J. Role of pre-operative irradiation for anal preservation in cancer of the low rectum. World J Surg 16:502-509, 1992.
2. Papillon J, Berard P. Endocavitary irradiation in the conservative treatment of adenocarcinoma of the low rectum. World J Surg 16:451-457, 1992.
3. Dubois JB, Rouanet P, Saint Aubert B, et al. La radiothérapie pré-opértiore dans le cancer du rectum. 307 cas évaluables, recul minimum 6 ans. Lyon Chir 87:9-13, 1991.
4. Rich T, Weiss DR, Mies C, et al. Sphincter preservation in patients with low rectal cancer treated with radiation therapy, with or without local excision or fulguration. Radiology 156:527, 1985.
5. Philipshen SJ, Heilweil M, Quan SHQ, et al. Patterns of pelvic recurrence following definitive resections of rectal cancer. Cancer 53:1354, 1984.
6. Glimelius B, Pahlman L. Radiotherapie pré ou post-opératoire dans le cancer du rectum. Résultat d'un essai multicentrique randomisé. Lyon Chir 87:3-8, 1991.
7. Marks G, Mohiuddin M, Eitan A, et al. Conservation sphinctérienne après irradiation pré-opératoire dans le cancer du rectum. L'expérience de l'Hôpital Universitaire Thomas Jefferson. Lyon Chir 87:25-28, 1991.
8. Gunderson LL, O'Connell MJ, Dozois RR. The role of intraoperative irradiation in locally advanced primary and recurrent rectal adenocarcinoma. World J Surg 16:495-501, 1992.

9. Berard P, Gouillat C, Rivoalan F, et al. Traitement chirurgical des récidives pelviennes des cancers rectaux. A propos de 24 exérèses chez 23 patients. Lyon Chir 87:369-372, 1991.
10. O'Connell MJ, Gunderson LL. Adjuvant therapy for adenocarcinoma of the rectum. World J Surg 16:510-515, 1992.
11. Papillon J. Thérapeutique adjuvante et cancer du rectum. Lyon Chir 87:357-359, 1991.
12. Gerard A. Preoperative radiotherapy as adjuvant treatment in rectal cancer: Final results of a randomized study of EORTC. Ann Surg 208:606-614, 1988.

76 Results of Invasive and Noninvasive Treatments for Squamous Cell Carcinoma of the Anal Canal

Philip H. Gordon

In the past decade, management of patients with squamous cell carcinoma of the anal canal has undergone a revolutionary change. What was once believed to be primarily a disease requiring surgical treatment has, for the most part, been handled in a nonoperative manner, especially as the primary form of therapy.

In any discussion on neoplasms of the anal region, one must understand their location and pathology. Unfortunately, confusion exists in this area. The lack of precision in reporting the exact location of a lesion or the inclusion of perianal as well as anal canal malignancies makes it inappropriate to compare the results of different forms of therapy from one series to another, because these series often compare dissimilar lesions. A brief review of the anatomy is indicated.

The anal canal, which extends from the anorectal ring to the anal verge, is lined with different types of epithelium.[1] Below the dentate line is squamous epithelium, and above the dentate line is columnar epithelium. This junction is not abrupt; for a distance of 6 to 12 mm above the dentate line, there is an area where columnar, cuboidal, transitional, or squamous epithelium may be found. This area, often referred to as the cloacogenic zone, has been considered to consist of unstable epithelium, and because of its diversity this epithelium gives rise to an interesting variety of neoplasms. The two areas of the anal canal also have different routes of lymphatic drainage, with neoplasms at or above the dentate line draining cephalad via the superior rectal lymphatic vessels to the inferior mesenteric lymph nodes and laterally along both the middle rectal vessels and the infe-

rior rectal vessels through the ischioanal fossa to the internal iliac lymph nodes. Lymph from the anal canal below the dentate line usually drains to the inguinal lymph nodes. However, if an obstruction is present, lymph can drain to the superior rectal nodes or along the inferior rectal lymphatic vessels to the ischioanal fossa.

For these reasons it seems appropriate to adopt the classification used by the World Health Organization[2]; the following discussion uses their standardized nomenclature. In this classification the anal canal is arbitrarily divided into the area above the dentate line, the so-called "anal canal," and the area below this line, the "anal margin."

HISTOLOGICAL VARIATION

Neoplasms of the anal canal may be classified as carcinoma (squamous cell, basaloid, or mucoepidermoid), adenocarcinoma, (rectal type, arising from the anal glands and ducts, or arising within an anorectal fistula), and malignant melanoma. From a therapeutic point of view, squamous cell, basaloid (cloacogenic), and mucoepidermoid carcinomas can be considered together because of their similar response to treatment.

CLINICAL FEATURES AND DETERMINATION OF DISEASE STATUS

Carcinoma of the anal canal presents at a median age of 60 years and two thirds of the cases are in women.[3,4] In a review of the demographics of anal carcinoma, Wexner et al.[5] have identified a high-risk group consisting of male patients who are admitted homosexuals or bisexuals or have a history of anal condylomata acuminata. A history may elicit symptoms of slight bleeding, discomfort, a lump, or weight loss. Physical examination should include a determination of the location and extent of the carcinoma, which may vary in size, is generally ulcerative, and may occupy varying proportions of the circumference of the anal canal. The relationship to the dentate line should be noted. Anoscopy and proctosigmoidoscopy should be performed. Suspicious inguinal lymph nodes should be biopsied. The liver should be screened for metastases by biochemical function studies as well as ultrasonography. A chest radiograph should be obtained to rule out pulmonary metastases.

At the time of initial diagnosis and treatment of squamous cell carcinoma of the anal canal, pelvic lymph node metastases are present in 30% to 43% of patients, and inguinal lymph node metastases are apparent in 15% to 36% and are unilateral.[6] Lymphatic invasion occurs early, and nodal metastases are present in 30% of patients when smooth muscle is infiltrated and in 58% when the carcinoma has extended to tissues beyond the sphincters.[3] Distant metastases are found at presentation in approximately 10% of patients and usually involve the liver and lungs.[6]

TREATMENT

A review of treatment options has been published previously along with a subsequent update.[6,7] The following discussion draws heavily from those accounts.

Local Excision

In the past this form of treatment was reserved for patients with early lesions or well-differentiated lesions that involved only the submucosa.[8,9] It was also considered for persons who were poor risks for an extensive operation or who refused radical excision. Survival rates following local excision are recorded in Table 1. Today the role of this form of therapy is indeed very limited. The high local recurrence and low 5-year survival rates, combined with the availability of better therapy, favor different treatment options.

Abdominoperineal Resection

For many years, in most centers, squamous cell carcinomas of the anal canal have been treated by abdominoperineal resection. Because of the relatively disappointing long-term survival rates, increasingly radical operations have been advocated. Despite these ag-

gressive approaches, overall survival rates have not improved. Reported 5-year survival rates after abdominoperineal resection have ranged from 24% to 71%, with an average of about 50%, in part reflecting the different referral patterns and extent of disease (Table 2). Some series with better survival rates may have included patients with lesions of the anal margin. Nigro et al.[23] suggested that the anatomic features of the anal canal limit the extent of the operation and that the profuse local blood supply and lymphatic drainage may promote local recurrence secondary to inadequate resection. The perioperative mortality rate is 2% to 6%.[3,4] When synchronous inguinal lymph node metastases are present, the 5-year survival rate after lymphadenectomy and abdominoperineal resection is only 10% to 20%. The reported locoregional recurrence rates after abdominoperineal resection range from 28% to 50% (see Table 2).

As will be discussed subsequently, there is controversy as to whether high-dose radiotherapy or combined chemoradiation is the treatment of choice. What has evolved in the controversy is that abdominoperineal resection should be reserved for residual or recurrent disease or for complications of radiation therapy.

Radical Radiation Therapy

Some centers have for many years preferred primary radiation therapy to abdominoperineal resection for treatment of patients with carcinoma of the anal canal and have reserved radical surgical techniques for those patients with residual carcinoma or serious toxicity from radiation. Reluctance to use radiation therapy has been attributed partly to the failure rates and the incidence of side effects, which are often severe. The techniques used include external-beam radiation alone,[24,25] split-course external-beam, and interstitial radiation.[26] Serious local radionecrosis or anal stricture necessitating operative management has been reported in 5% to 20% of patients, with most recent findings lying at the lower end of this range.[24,26] Approximately three fourths of patients cured by radical radiation therapy or by radiation plus surgery for residual carcinoma retain normal anal function. Papillon and Montbarbon[26] reported local control rates of 90% in patients with primary carcinomas less than 5 cm in diameter and 76% in patients with larger primary carcinomas. They suggested that with appropriate attention to radiation technique chemotherapy is not necessary, except in patients with very advanced lesions. A review by Hintz et al.[27] found a local failure rate of 33% to 42%.

The advantage of interstitial radiotherapy is that it

Table 1. Results of local excision

Reference	Year	No. of Patients	Local Recurrence (%)	5-Year Survival (%)
Golden and Horsley[10]	1976	134	NS	65
Beahrs[11]	1979	21	42	83
Singh et al.[12]	1981	55	20	NS
Greenall et al.[4]	1985	11	64	45
Clark et al.[13]	1986	9	44	NS
Pintor et al.[14]	1989	7	NS	86

NS = not stated.

Table 2. Results of abdominoperineal resection

Reference	Year	No. of Patients	Local Recurrence (%)	5-Year Survival (%)
Golden and Horsley[10]*	1976	487	NS	48
Sawyers[15]	1977	40	NS	52
Welch and Malt[16]	1977	43	37	38
Singh et al.[12]	1981	47	NS	53
O'Brien et al.[17]	1982	21	NS	38
Schraut et al.[18]	1983	24	NS	54
Boman et al.[3]	1984	114	28	71
Frost et al.[19]†	1984	109	27	62
Greenall et al.[4]	1985	103	25	55
Dougherty and Evans[20]	1985	79	43	47
Clark et al.[13]	1986	40	38	NS
Jensen et al.[21]	1988	52	50	NS
Lopez and Kraybill[22]	1988	47	NS	55
Pintor et al.[14]	1989	76	NS	71

NS = not stated.
*Review of the literature.
†May have included some perianal lesions.

provides a high dose over a short time and spares adjacent tissues the harmful effects of irradiation. However, this technique is employed only in specialized centers. Split-course radiotherapy has been used effectively by Papillon and Montbarbon,[26] who found only a 2.5% rate of severe radionecrosis. They reported on a combination of external-beam and interstitial radiation. Of 217 patients followed for 3 years, 68% are alive and well; 19% died of their carcinoma; and 12% had intercurrent disease. Among the 148 patients with complete remission, a remarkable 92.5% had retained anal function. This figure represents 63% of the originally treated patients. Of the 149 patients followed for 5 years, 65% are alive and well.

Treatment with modern, megavoltage, external-beam radiation has resulted in 5-year survival rates of 18% to

Table 3. Results of radical radiation

Reference	Year	No. of Patients	Dose (Gy)	Local Recurrence (%)	Surgery Required for Recurrences and Complications (%)	5-Year Survival (%)
Golden and Horsley[10]	1976	77	NS	NS	NS	26
Beahrs[11]	1979	13	NS	NS	NS	18
Cummings et al.[25]	1982	51	45-50	20	26	59
Frost et al.[19]	1984	11	64-88	18	45	78
Salmon et al.[28]	1984	183	60-65	34	37	59
Eschwege et al.[29]	1985	64	60-65	19	33	46
Doggett et al.[30]*	1988	35	45-75	23	20	92
Otim-Oyet et al.[31]	1990	42†	60-65	31	14 + NR	52
Dubois et al.[32]	1991	28	60-65	18	14	.71

NS = not stated; NR = nonresponders.
*Only included lesions <5 cm (average 3.1 cm).
†Included six anal verge plus six perianal skin carcinomas; four of 42 patients also received simultaneous chemotherapy.

79% (Table 3). Treatment protocols for both dosage and duration differ from center to center. The series with the best survival rate may have included some anal margin carcinomas, which would favorably bias the results. The rates of serious complications (skin radiation necrosis, ulcerations, severe pain, fistulas, or sinus) following external-beam radiation depend on the radiation dosage and techniques and have generally been between 15% and 33%.[6] It is disconcerting to read the report by Frost et al.[19] who, in their small series of patients treated with radiation therapy alone, found a minor complication rate of 33% and a major complication rate of 77%. In their review, Hintz et al.[27] also found a major complication rate of 41% to 72%. In his vast experience, Papillon[33] has demonstrated the split-course regimen of irradiation to be superior to external-beam irradiation alone with regard to tolerance and efficacy and hence favors this form of therapy.

Combination Chemoradiotherapy

In an effort to improve the dismal survival rates with radical surgery alone, Nigro et al.[23] explored the use of preoperative adjuvant chemotherapy and radiotherapy. In this landmark protocol, 5-fluorouracil (1000 mg/m^2/day) was given as a continuous intravenous infusion for 4 days and mitomycin C (15 mg/m^2) as a single intravenous bolus injection, in conjunction with 3000 cGy (200 cGy/day) of external-beam radiation to the pelvis. The 5-fluorouracil infusion was subsequently repeated 1 month later, and 6 weeks following the end of radiation therapy, abdominoperineal resection was performed. In one of their early reports, these investigators noted that at operation, six of nine patients had no residual carcinoma. They suggested that abdominoperineal resection might not be necessary if clinically complete regression of the carcinoma had followed combined radiation and chemotherapy and if a biopsy of the residual scar in the anal canal showed no microscopic disease. In a 1987 update, in which their experience was combined with that obtained by a questionnaire survey of other medical centers, Nigro[34] reported that among 104 patients treated with the combined modality regimen, 31 underwent abdominoperineal resection, with only nine having either gross or microscopic carcinoma. Sixty-two underwent excision of the scar for biopsy purposes only; of these patients, only one had microscopic carcinoma, and 11 had no operative procedure of any kind but had complete clinical regression of their disease. All patients had been followed for a minimum of 2 years, and only 13 of the 104 patients had died of anal canal carcinoma. Other centers have modified the original combined chemotherapy, radiation

Table 4. Results of combination chemoradiation

Reference	Year	No. of Patients	Type of Chemotherapy	Dose (Gy)	Complete Regression (%)	Follow-up (mo)
Cummings et al.[35]	1984	16	5-FU–MTC	50	94	48-84
Cummings et al.[35]	1984	14	5-FU–MTC	25 + 25	100	30-48
Sischy[37]	1985	33	5-FU–MTC	55-65	91	12-108
Meeker et al.[38]	1986	19	5-FU–MTC	30	88	Med 30
Cummings[39]*	1987	18	5-FU–MTC	24 + 24	89	6-30
Flam et al.[36]	1987	30	5-FU–MTC	41-50	87	9-76
Nigro[34]	1987	104	5-FU–MTC	30	93	24-132
Habr-Gama et al.[40]	1989	30	5-FU–MTC	30-45	73	12-60
Sischy et al.[41]	1989	79	5-FU–MTC	40.8	90	20-55
Zucali et al.[42]	1990	38	5-FU–MTC	36 + 18†	84	Med 22

5-FU = 5-fluorouracil; MTC = mitomycin C; Med = median.
*Split-course radiotherapy.
†36 Gy given in 20 fractions and after 2 weeks a booster dose of 18 Gy given to anoperineal area.

therapy, and surgery protocol in various ways, but all have confirmed the success of multimodality therapy in increasing the rate of control of primary malignancies and decreasing the number of patients who require abdominoperineal resection.

The toxicity of the protocol recommended by Nigro[34] has been mild to moderate, with stomatitis, diarrhea, and radiation mucositis and dermatitis being the most common side effects. Approximately 15% of patients developed mild hematologic toxicity. Five percent had severe toxicity associated with acute enterocolitis, but all recovered without long-term complications. Higher rates of toxicity are experienced when chemotherapy is combined with larger doses of radiation.[35,36]

Following the lead established by Nigro,[34] combination chemotherapy and radiotherapy has become a popular and well-accepted form of therapy for squamous cell carcinoma of the anal canal. Deviations from the original radiation doses and the adoption of split-course radiotherapy have been tried. Results of several series are reported in Table 4. Many centers report excellent response rates, mostly in the 90% range. However, follow-up is shorter than for other forms of treatment, often involving only a few months. In 65 patients with a 5-year follow-up, Nigro[34] projected a 5-year sur-

vival rate of 83%, which is for the most part better than the results of abdominoperineal resection or high-dose radiation therapy, although longer follow-up will be required. For many years Papillon and Montbarbon[26] have treated patients with anal canal carcinoma with radiation therapy alone. With the addition of chemotherapy the local failure rate was reduced from 26% to 13%.

Controversy exists as to whether biopsy samples should be taken from the treatment site. Cummings et al.[35] reported only a 6% incidence of local recurrence after patients were deemed to be clinically free of disease. Nigro[34] found only 1 of 62 patients in whom regression was clinically complete to have a positive biopsy. This latter finding suggests that a biopsy may not be necessary.

Inguinal Lymph Nodes

Reports of the incidence of inguinal lymph node metastases vary dramatically from 4% to 40%, with the lower incidence in the more recent reports.[13,19,26,34,43] In the series reported by Stearns and Quan,[43] 60 of 82 patients undergoing prophylactic groin dissections had negative nodes. Based on these statistics, and in view of the high morbidity and mortality rates, the risk of the added procedure outweighs the benefit and prophylactic groin dissection is not recommended. The simultaneous appearance of inguinal metastases is an ominous sign: only 2 of 14 such patients survived 5 years. In contrast, later inguinal metastases carry a better prognosis; after radical groin dissection, 5-year survival rates of 50% to 83% have been documented.[6,44] In the series reported by Clark et al.[13] 10 of 67 patients developed synchronous (two patients) or metachronous (eight patients) lymph node involvement. All 10 patients died including one who was without evidence of disease for 39 months after inguinal dissection for recurrent lymph node metastases. None of the patients in this series underwent prophylactic groin dissection. The median survival of the entire group from the date of the primary operation was 27 months. The median survival from the date of recurrence was 15 months. It would appear that the presence of positive inguinal lymphadenopathy is a harbinger of systemic metastases, since 6 of the 10 patients had evidence of systemic spread. Cummings[39] reported that elective radiation of clinically normal inguinal nodes greatly reduces the risk of late node failure and carries little morbidity. Only 1 of 38 such patients had a late recurrence in the inguinal area after combination chemotherapy and radiotherapy. In series in which the inguinal areas were not treated electively, the late nodal recurrence rate was 15% to 25%.[3,26] For established inguinal lymph node metastases, Nigro et al.[45] use their chemoradiation protocol, which includes the inguinal areas. After 6 weeks, a superficial groin dissection is performed on the affected side if the nodes are not clinically normal. Bilateral inguinal lymph node involvement should be treated with additional radiotherapy, as this is probably only a palliative measure.[45]

CURRENT RECOMMENDATION

Because of the numerous variations in approaches, it is difficult to draw precise conclusions from the literature regarding the best therapy for patients with carcinoma of the anal canal. What has become quite apparent is that radical surgery has been supplanted by radical radiation or combination chemoradiation. There is sufficient evidence favoring chemoradiation administered according to the Nigro protocol[45] as the primary treatment. Multimodality therapy not only achieves excellent short- and long-term results but ultimately improves the quality of life, reducing the need for surgery under most circumstances and minimizing the side effects of high-dose radiotherapy. For patients who do not respond, even more controversy exists. For those with small foci of persistent disease, local excision has been tried as the next line of treatment, whereas other authors have proceeded directly to abdominoperineal resection. Because even the results of abdominoperineal resection have not been dramatic, Nigro et al.[45] have continued with additional courses of chemoradiation therapy. For patients whose carcinoma does not disappear and for all patients whose original lesion was 5 cm or larger, they suggest, beginning 6 weeks after completion of the first course of treatment, a regimen of 2000 cGy over a 2-week period to the local lesion together with an infusion of 5-fluorouracil, 1000 mg/m^2 for 4 days, and on the first day of chemotherapy after appropriate hydration, a single 100 mg/m^2 dose of cisplatin. The 5-fluorouracil and cisplatin are repeated twice at 1-month intervals. If the local lesion persists after the second course of radiation therapy, they suggest application of interstitial implants with the alternative being abdominoperineal resection. For patients with metastatic disease or delayed recurrence, they have used a combination of bleomycin, cisplatin, and VP-16 and more radiation if possible.

A growing number of physicians who treat patients with squamous cell carcinoma of the anal canal recommend combined chemoradiotherapy. To date, a uniform treatment policy has not evolved. A number of questions that are frequently raised include the optimal chemotherapy, the optimal timing of the chemotherapy and radiotherapy, the necessity for synchronous administration of both treatment modalities, and the optimal dose and fields of radiotherapy, in particular the fractionation, total dose, and need for a booster dose to the anal region. Because of the low incidence of this neoplasm, only results from a multicenter trial will help answer these questions.

REFERENCES

1. Gordon PH, Nivatvongs S. The Principles and Practice of Surgery for the Colon, Rectum, and Anus. St. Louis: Quality Medical Publishing, 1992, pp 10-12.
2. Morson BC. Histologic Typing of Intestinal Tumors 62-65. Geneva: World Health Organization, 1976.
3. Boman BM, Moertel CG, O'Connell MJ, et al. Carcinoma of the anal canal: A clinical and pathologic study of 188 cases. Cancer 54:114-125, 1984.
4. Greenall MJ, Quan SHQ, Urmacher C, et al. Treatment of epidermoid carcinoma of the anal canal. Surg Gynecol Obstet 161:509-517, 1985.

5. Wexner SD, Milson JW, Dailey TH. The demographics of anal cancers are changing: Identification of a high risk population. Dis Colon Rectum 30:942-946, 1987.

6. Gordon PH. Squamous cell carcinoma of the anal canal. Surg Clin North Am 68:1391-1339, 1988.

7. Gordon PH. Current status—perianal and anal canal neoplasms. Dis Colon Rectum 33:799-808, 1990.

8. Holm WH, Jackman RJ. Anorectal squamous-cell carcinoma: Conservative or radical treatment? JAMA 188:241-244, 1964.

9. Stearns MW Jr, Quan SHQ. Epidermoid carcinoma of the anorectum. Surg Gynecol Obstet 131:953-957, 1970.

10. Golden GT, Horsley JS III. Surgical management of epidermoid carcinoma of the anus. Am J Surg 131:275-280, 1976.

11. Beahrs OH. Management of cancer of the anus. AJR 133:790-795, 1979.

12. Singh R, Nime F, Mittelman A. Malignant epithelial tumors of the anal canal. Cancer 48:411-414, 1981.

13. Clark J, Petrelli N, Herrera L, et al. Epidermoid carcinoma of the anal canal. Cancer 57:400-406, 1986.

14. Pintor MP, Northover JMA, Nicholls RJ. Squamous cell carcinoma of the anus at one hospital from 1948-1984. Br J Surg 76:806-810, 1989.

15. Sawyers JL. Current management of carcinoma of the anus and perianus. Am Surg 43:424-429, 1977.

16. Welch JP, Malt RA. Appraisal of the treatment of carcinoma of the anus and anal canal. Surg Gynecol Obstet 145:837-841, 1977.

17. O'Brien PH, Jenrette JM, Wallace KM, et al. Epidermoid carcinoma of the anus. Surg Gynecol Obstet 155:745-751, 1982.

18. Schraut WH, Wang CH, Dawson PJ, et al. Depth of invasion, location, and size of cancer of the anus dictate operative treatment. Cancer 51:1291-1296, 1983.

19. Frost D, Richards P, Montague E, et al. Epidermoid cancer of the anorectum. Cancer 53:1285-1293, 1984.

20. Dougherty BG, Evans HL. Carcinoma of the anal canal: A study of 79 cases. Am J Clin Pathol 83:159-164, 1985.

21. Jensen SL, Hagen K, Harling H, et al. Long-term prognosis after radical treatment for squamous cell carcinoma of the anal canal and anal margin. Dis Colon Rectum 31:273-278, 1988.

22. Lopez MJ, Kraybill WB. Squamous cell cancer of the anus. The Ellis Fischel experience and current trends in management. Mo Med 85:669-673, 1988.

23. Nigro ND, Vaitkeviceus VK, Considine B. Combined therapy for cancer of the anal canal: A preliminary report. Dis Colon Rectum 17:354-356, 1974.

24. Cantril ST, Green JP, Schall GL, et al. Primary radiation therapy in the treatment of anal carcinoma. Int J Radiat Oncol Biol Phys 9:1271-1278, 1983.

25. Cummings BJ, Thomas GM, Keane TJ. Primary radiation therapy in the treatment of anal canal carcinoma. Dis Colon Rectum 25:778-782, 1982.

26. Papillon J, Montbarbon JF. Epidermoid carcinoma of the anal canal. A series of 276 cases. Dis Colon Rectum 30:324-333, 1987.

27. Hintz BL, Choryulu KKN, Sudersanam A. Anal carcinoma: Basic concepts and management. J Surg Oncol 10:141-150, 1978.

28. Salmon RJ, Fenton J, Asselain B, et al. Treatment of epidermoid anal canal cancer. Am J Surg 147:43-48, 1984.

29. Eschwege F, Lasser P, Chavy A, et al. Squamous cell carcinoma of the anal canal: Treatment with external beam irradiation. Radiother Oncol 3:145-150, 1985.

30. Doggett SW, Green JP, Cantril ST. Efficacy of radiation therapy alone for limited squamous cell carcinoma of the anal canal. Int J Radiat Oncol Biol Phys 15:1069-1072, 1988.

31. Otim-Oyet D, Ford HT, Fisher C, et al. Radical radiotherapy for carcinoma of the anal canal. Clin Oncol 2:84-89, 1990.

32. Dubois JB, Garrigues Pujol H. Cancer of the anal canal: Report on the experience of 61 patients. Int J Radiat Oncol Biol Phys 20:575-580, 1991.

33. Papillon J. Current therapeutic concepts in management of carcinoma of the anal canal: Recent results. Cancer Res 110:146-149, 1988.

34. Nigro ND. Multidisciplinary management of cancer of the anus. World J Surg 11:446-451, 1987.

35. Cummings BJ, Keane TJ, Thomas GM. The results and toxicity of the treatment of anal canal carcinoma by radiation therapy or radiation therapy and chemotherapy. Cancer 54:2062-2068, 1984.

36. Flam MS, John MJ, Mowry PA. Definitive combined modality therapy of carcinoma of the anus: A report of 30 cases including results of salvage therapy in patients with residual disease. Dis Colon Rectum 30:495-502, 1987.

37. Sischy B. The use of radiation therapy combined with chemotherapy in the management of squamous cell carcinoma of the anus and marginally resectable adenocarcinoma of the rectum. Int J Radiat Oncol Biol Phys 11:1587-1593, 1985.

38. Meeker WR Jr, Sickle-Santanello BJ, Philpott G, et al. Combined chemotherapy, radiation and surgery for epithelial cancer of the anal canal. Cancer 57:525-529, 1986.

39. Cummings BJ. Current management of epidermoid carcinoma of the anal canal. Gastroenterol Clin North Am 16:125-142, 1987.

40. Habr-Gama A, da Silva e Sousa AH, Nadalin W, et al. Epidermoid carcinoma of the anal canal. Results of treatment by combined chemotherapy and radiotherapy. Dis Colon Rectum 32:773-777, 1989.

41. Sischy B, Doggett RLS, Krall JM, et al. Definitive irradiation and chemotherapy for radiosensitization in management of anal carcinoma: Interim report on radiation therapy oncology group study No. 8314. J Natl Cancer Inst 81:850-856, 1989.

42. Zucali R, Doci R, Bombelli L. Combined chemotherapy—radiotherapy of the anal canal. Int J Radiat Oncol Biol Phys 19:1221-1223, 1990.

43. Stearns MW Jr, Quan SHQ. Epidermoid carcinoma of the anorectum. Surg Gynecol Obstet 131:953-957, 1970.

44. Stearns MW, Urmacher C, Sternberg SE, et al. Cancer of the anal canal. Curr Probl Cancer 4:1-44, 1980.

45. Nigro ND, Vaitkeviceus VK, Herskovic AM. Preservation of function in the treatment of cancer of the anus. In Vita V, ed. Important Advances in Oncology. Philadelphia: JB Lippincott, 1989, pp 161-177.

77 Minimal Versus Traditional Access to Colorectal Cancer: The Dilemma of Modern Laparoscopy

R.J. Heald

The value of minimally invasive colorectal surgery for cancer is determined by the quality and completeness of deep pelvic dissection. With conventional techniques, identification of tumor extension and radical excision of neoplasms are difficult; this explains the high rate of local recurrence of rectal cancer and the success rate that varies with surgical expertise.[1] Monson et al. have recently claimed that in their early experience of 10 cases of rectal excision, "The laparoscope afforded unrivaled views . . . permitting very careful radical excisions . . . completely under direct vision."[2] If complete mesorectal excision determines cure, then magnification and greater precision could herald a significant laparoscopic revolution characterized by high cure rates and minimal impairment of sexual and bladder function.[3] State-of-the-art laparoscopic techniques and technology will be necessary to convince the medical profession that such advances are possible and that the operative procedure can be completed expeditiously.

With respect to ablative and reconstructive intra-abdominal surgery, access and exposure are prerequisites of high-quality work. The gallbladder is a simple end-organ that is well situated for laparoscopic access made possible by pneumoperitoneum. Its small artery or arteries and the cystic duct are ideal for occlusion with clips. However, the early massive learning experience required for mastery of this new technique has led to a small but definite rise in common duct injuries, so more complex operative procedures must be approached cautiously. Operations on the colon and rectum demand much greater skill than that required by cholecystectomy.

The large bowel is supported by mesenteries that contain a rich network of blood and lymphatic vessels that receive and may contain the initial spread of the most curable visceral malignancy. Familiarity with the planes around these mesenteries is the principal skill of the colorectal surgeon, and the surgical "cure" of cancer is determined by "clean tumor containment." Thus exposure of the duodenum and pancreatic head or of the inferior hypogastric plexus on the pelvic sidewall are conditions for optimal right hemicolectomy, respectively rectosigmoid or total mesorectal excision. "Anatomical" dissections of "bared" superior mesenteric vessels on the right or of the preaortic region on the left are also hallmarks of high-quality cancer surgery. It is not known whether such dissections can be achieved via laparoscopy.

Surgeons with enduring loyalties to time-honored methods are dismayed to learn that the duodenum and ureter are often not visualized at all during laparoscopy, although some videos demonstrating these new techniques have shown an approach that Sir Stanford Cade would have called "scratching around in the lymph fields."

Another fundamental anxiety relates to the feasibil-

412

ity of cytocidal washouts. Cells shed by the tumor into the lumen can implant into soft pelvic tissues or into the divided bowel ends, and thus the seeds of the patient's destruction are sown.[4,7] If intracorporeal anastomosis is intended (i.e., for rectal and low sigmoid lesions), it is probably impossible to wash out the proximal bowel end, and washing out the distal bowel end below a clamp and before staple application is often omitted. Positioning the anastomosis outside the abdomen (as is possible with surgery for most colon lesions) through a 5 cm incision can obviate this disadvantage, although washout is not mentioned by most surgeons who use laparoscopy. In some video demonstrations, bowel contents from a site near the tumor spilled into the peritoneum during washout. If these occurrences are common and unavoidable with the laparoscopic approach, then both techniques will fall into disrepute.

The use of laparoscopy in the treatment of colorectal cancer is overshadowed by other important issues, such as whether specialization and improved surgical technique can cure more people, how often anal sphincters must be sacrificed,[8] and which patients should receive radiotherapy, and/or postoperative chemotherapy.[9,10] By comparison with these issues, the dream of colectomy without laparotomy is modest, because the 5 cm incision by which it is necessary to deliver the specimen can be almost as painful as a 25 cm incision. The cosmetic benefit provided by laparoscopic colorectal surgery, in addition to that of reduced postoperative pain, may be appreciated more by the younger patient than by the 65-year-old cancer patient. What may be a transient twinge of discomfort to a tough 60-year-old person with cancer may seem unbearable to an adolescent with colitis.

In abdominoperineal excision, extraction of the specimen is possible through the perineum, and this solution would offer aesthetic benefits if the open abdominal component could be avoided. With such an approach the dissection around the tumor is completed from below, the patient is spared an abdominal incision, and the synchronous abdominal and perineal nature of the procedure is preserved by initial laparoscopically guided dissection from above. The perineal incision serves a dual purpose: radical excision and then examination of the specimen.

The use of laparoscopy in surgery for rectal cancer has been inspired by the surgical technology industry, led by patient demand and public pressure, and catalyzed by the competitive nature of surgical practice. Laparoscopy has existed for decades, but recent advances in television technology and in manipulative instrumentation have been critical to the development of the technique. The relationship of surgeons and industry must now move into a new era. Rapid advances are being made in instrumentation for grasping and stapling, and the use of high-definition monitors with laparoscopic systems could herald progress in surgical training and the practice of minimally invasive surgical techniques.

Albert Einstein once commented that "perfection of tools and confusion of aims are characteristics of our time." The goals of cancer surgery must avoid the pitfall of tools over mind and remain true to the ideal outcome: long-term cure, lower locoregional recurrence rates, less anastomotic leakage, fewer stomas, and less autonomic nerve damage.[11] The benefit of a traditional incision is that the tactile and exploratory skills of the participating surgeons are enhanced, whereas visualization is not unless loupes are used by all—somewhat more cumbersome than the laparoscopic magnification. Most of today's surgeons were taught that "big mistakes are made through small holes," that "wounds heal from side to side, not from end to end," and "big surgeon, big incision!"[12]

How should the traditionally trained colorectal cancer surgeon respond to the challenge of new techniques in pelvic surgery? He or she could embrace laparoscopy with enthusiasm, aware of the fact that some skeptics view it as a skill to be learned in defense of livelihood. We believe that those of us who embrace the technique should control their enthusiasm and reserve definitive commitment while leading or participating in the absolutely mandatory prospective, randomized, double-blind studies to assign a rightful place to laparoscopic treatment of cancer, to give our patients the best in long-term survival, and to respect the highest ethical standards while exercising our craft and science—one way or the other.

REFERENCES

1. Fielding LP, Stewart-Brown S, Dudley HAF. Surgeon-related variables and the clinical trial. Lancet 2:778-779, 1978.
2. Monson et al. Lancet (in press).
3. Heald RJ. The "Holy Plane" of rectal surgery. J R Soc Med 81:503-508, 1988.
4. Umpleby HC, Formor BY, Symes MO, Williamson RGN. Viability of exfoliated colorectal carcinoma cells. Br J Surg 71:659-663, 1984.

5. Skipper D, Cooper AJ, Marston JE, Taylor I. Exfoliated cells and in vitro growth in colorectal cancer. Br J Surg 74:1049-1052, 1987.

6. Fermor B, Umpleby HC, Lever JV, Symes MO, Williamson RGN. Proliferative and metastatic potential of exfoliated colorectal cancer cells. J Natl Cancer Inst 76:347-349, 1986.

7. Skipper D, Jeffrey MJ, Cooper AJ, Alexander P, Taylor I. Enhanced growth of tumor cells in healing colonic anastomoses and laparotomy wounds. Int J Colorectal Dis 4:172-177, 1989.

8. Karanjia ND, Schache DJ, North WRS, Heald RJ. "Close shave" in anterior resection. Br J Surg 77:510-512, 1990.

9. Krook JE, Moretel CG, Gunderson LL. Effective surgical adjuvant therapy for high-risk rectal carcinoma. N Engl J Med 324:709-715, 1991.

10. Moertel CG, Flemming TR, MacDonald JS. Levamisole and fluorouracil for adjuvant therapy of resected colon carcinoma. N Engl J Med 322:352-358, 1990.

11. Rectal cancer should be treated by experts [editorial]. Lancet 2:1476, 1986.

12. Norman Tanner. Personal communication.

78 The Influence of Anastomotic Techniques on Prognosis After Operation for Colorectal Cancer

James G. Docherty, Murat Akyol, John R. McGregor, and David J. Galloway

Recurrence of colorectal cancer after a potentially curative operation is a multifactorial phenomenon. Some patients already have occult hepatic metastatic disease[1] or have microscopic deposits of tumor left locally at the time of surgery.[2,3] A number of patients develop recurrence as a result of implantation metastases,[4] and a small number develop metachronous tumors at the site of their anastomosis.[5] In addition, surgical technique is considered important in the pathogenesis of local recurrence,[6] particularly in rectal cancer.[3] However, the influence of anastomotic technique on the incidence of recurrence is controversial. A number of reports have shown high local recurrence rates after stapled curative restorative rectal cancer resections.[7-11] However, other investigators have failed to identify an adverse effect associated with stapling.[12-15] The present study was undertaken to determine the relative frequency of recurrence and disease-free survival rates in a prospectively studied group of patients who underwent colorectal cancer resection and who were randomized to receive either a sutured or stapled anastomosis.

PATIENTS AND METHODS

All patients in this study were the subjects of a previously reported prospective controlled trial comparing sutured and stapled anastomoses throughout the gastrointestinal tract.[16] From the original data base of 1161 patients, 463 consecutive patients underwent a restorative colorectal cancer resection between April 1985 and April 1989 under the care of 13 surgeons in five hospitals in the western and Highland areas of Scotland. Randomization of patients to either a sutured or stapled anastomosis was performed in the operating theater when the surgeon was satisfied that either technique could be undertaken. A stratified randomization technique was used so that each surgeon contributed equal numbers of sutured and stapled anastomoses. Patients were excluded from the analysis for the following reasons: not randomized, 33; palliative resections, 96; postoperative deaths after a curative resection, 12; incomplete follow-up, 28. This left 294 patients who underwent a potentially curative colorectal cancer resection and who were available for study.

Sutured colocolic or colorectal anastomoses were carried out using a single layer of interrupted braided 2-0 polyamide (Nurolon, Ethicon) suture material. Ileocolic anastomoses were fashioned using the same technique or in two layers with a continuous inner layer of 2-0 polyglycolic acid (Dexon Plus, Davis and Geck) and an outer layer of 2-0 polyamide, depending on the sur-

Table 1. Tumor stage by TNM classification

Stage	Tumor	Node	Metastasis
0	Tis	N0	M0
1	T1, T2	N0	M0
2	T3, T4	N0	M0
3	Any T	N1, N2, N3	M0
4	Any T	Any N	M1

Table 2. Patient characteristics

	Sutures (n = 142)	Staples (n = 152)
Sex ratio (M:F)	69:73	69:83
Age (yr)	69.6(11.3)	68.7(11.3)
Weight (kg)	62.5(12.7)	63.7(10.8)
Height (cm)	165.2(10.2)	164.9(8.3)
Hemoglobin (g/dl)	12.7(2.1)	12.8(2.0)
WBC ($\times 10^9$/L)	8.4(2.9)	8.4(2.6)
Albumin (g/L)	37.7(5.1)	38.5(4.6)
Operating time (min)	119.8(40.9)	103.3(41.6)

Values are means (SD).
WBC = white blood cell count.

geon's preference. All stapled anastomoses were fashioned using the TA, GIA, and EEA series of surgical stapling instruments (Auto Suture UK).

The tumor-node-metastasis (TNM) classification was used for tumor staging.[17] Staging was performed after pathological examination of the resected specimen. The stage groupings are shown in Table 1. Potentially curative surgery was defined as removal of all macroscopic evidence of tumor, with tumor-free resection margins on histological examination. Two patients with stage 4 disease were considered to have undergone potentially curative surgery, because both had solitary liver metastases resected. Local recurrence was defined as clinical, histological, or postmortem evidence of recurrent tumor at or in the region of the anastomosis. All other sites of recurrence were classified as distant recurrence.

Disease-free interval and survival time were measured from the time of resection. The estimation of the cumulative probability of recurrence and the cancer-specific mortality rates were calculated by the life-table method of Kaplan and Meier.[18] Comparison of recurrence and cancer-specific mortality rates between sutured and stapled groups was performed by log rank test. Cox's proportional hazards regression model was used for multivariate adjustment for the influence of covariates on recurrence and mortality rates, simultaneously.[19]

RESULTS

The study population consisted of 152 patients who underwent a stapled reconstruction and 142 who received a sutured reconstruction. Patient characteristics for the sutured and stapled groups are detailed in Table 2. Table 3 outlines the anastomotic site and tumor stage in the two groups. Follow-up of the patients ranged from 11 to 54 months, with the median follow-up time in the

Table 3. Anastomotic site and tumor stage

	Sutures (n = 142)	Staples (n = 152)
Anastomoses		
Colorectal	52	57
Colocolic	39	34
Ileocolic	51	61
Tumor Stage		
1	15	20
2	76	88
3	51	42
4	0	2

stapled group 21.2 months and in the sutured group 21 months.

The cumulative probability of tumor recurrence is illustrated in Fig. 1, expressed as the proportion of recurrence-free patients plotted against time during the follow-up period. Of the patients in the stapled group, 19.1% (3.9) had recurrence diagnosed by the end of the second postoperative year, whereas 29.4% (4.4) in the sutured group had developed recurrence ($p < 0.05$). Fig. 2 illustrates the cumulative probability of cancer-specific mortality in the two groups. At the end of a 24-month

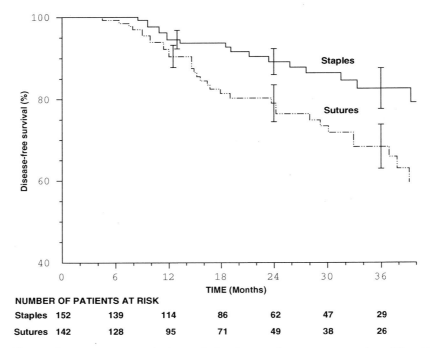

Fig. 1. Incidence of tumor recurrence in the stapled and sutured groups expressed as a life-table curve.

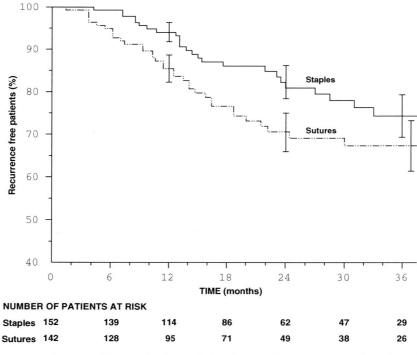

Fig. 2. Cancer-specific mortality rates in the stapled and sutured groups expressed as a life-table curve.

period of follow-up, 10.9% (3) of the stapled group had died as a result of their cancer, whereas 22.3% (4.1) of the sutured group had succumbed to their cancer ($p < 0.01$).

The relationship between site of tumor recurrence and anastomotic technique is detailed in Table 4. Cox's regression analysis was used to identify and adjust for the influence of covariates on outcome. The only independent predictors of recurrence were tumor stage and mode of anastomotic construction (Table 5). With regard to cancer-specific mortality rates, again the only independent predictors were tumor stage and mode of anastomotic construction (Table 6). There was a 42% reduction in the incidence of recurrence with the use of stapling instruments (95%; comparative incidence [CI], 3% to 65%), and there was a 50% reduction in cancer-specific mortality rate, again in favor of stapled anastomoses (95%; CI, 11% to 72%).

Table 4. Number and site of tumor recurrences in sutured and stapled groups tabulated by TNM tumor stage

		Recurrent Tumors		
	Local	**Local and Distant**	**Distant**	**All Recurrences**
Sutured Group				
Stage 1 (15)	2	0	0	2
Stage 2 (76)	7	7	4	18
Stage 3 (51)	7	8	2	17
TOTAL (142)	16	15	6	37
Stapled Group				
Stage 1 (20)	0	0	1	1
Stage 2 (88)	6	6	2	14
Stage 3 (42)	4	1	5	10
Stage 4 (2)	1	0	0	1
TOTAL (152)	11	7	8	26

Table 5. Association between tumor recurrence and perioperative variables (Cox's regression analysis)

Variable	Regression Coefficient	Standard Error	*p* Value
Age			0.60
Sex			0.051
Stage	0.683	0.218	0.001
Grade			0.38
Hemoglobin			0.75
Albumin			0.53
Transfusion			0.93
Anastomotic technique	−0.546	0.263	0.035
Anastomotic site			0.71

Table 6. Association between cancer-specific mortality and perioperative variables (Cox's regression analysis)

Variable	Regression Coefficient	Standard Error	p Value
Age			0.18
Sex			0.06
Stage	0.952	0.249	0.0001
Grade			0.34
Hemoglobin			0.73
Albumin			0.59
Transfusion			0.72
Anastomotic technique	−0.695	0.294	0.015
Anastomotic site			0.75

DISCUSSION

This is the only randomized study of patients undergoing "curative" colorectal cancer surgery that has reported significant reductions in tumor recurrence and cancer-specific mortality rates associated with stapled as compared with hand-sutured anastomoses. In marked contrast, several previous reports have suggested an increased risk of recurrence in association with surgical stapling.[7-11] All of these reports have concentrated on rectal cancers and colorectal anastomoses, whereas this study dealt with all colonic and rectal cancers. A possible explanation for the high recurrence rates in these studies may be that the introduction of the circular stapling instrument allowed performance of restorative surgery for tumors lower in the pelvis than would have been possible with manual suturing techniques[20,21] but only at the expense of adequate tumor clearance.[8] This should not be the case in this study because randomization of the anastomosis to staples or sutures was performed only after the surgeon was satisfied that either technique was feasible.

Previous work from this institution (Western Infirmary, Glasgow) has shown that anastomotic integrity may be critical in the pathogenesis of recurrence of colorectal cancer.[22] In support of this hypothesis is the fact that the reduction in tumor recurrence with the use of staples reported in this study occurred mainly as a result of a reduction in the number of patients with a local component to their recurrence (11.8% for stapled versus 21.8% for sutured). In patients who underwent an anastomosis on the left side and postoperative contrast radiology, we have reported significantly higher local tumor recurrence rates in patients with clinical (46.7%) and radiological (35.3%) anastomotic leaks when compared with patients in whom the anastomosis was intact (12.6%).[23] Similarly, the cancer-specific mortality rate in the anastomotic leak group (clinical and radiological) was three times that of the no-leak group. In this same cohort of patients the incidence of clinical anastomotic leakage was similar between patients with sutured or stapled anastomoses; however, the incidence of radiological leaks was significantly higher for patients with manually sutured as opposed to stapled anastomoses.[22] Our report of the association of increased local recurrence with clinical anastomotic leakage is at variance with the findings of the large bowel cancer project in which the recurrence rates were similar whether the patient had a clinical leak or not.[6] A radiological leak may increase tumor recurrence locally, not only by allowing a greater number of exfoliated intraluminal tumor cells to escape into the perianastomotic area[24] but also by causing a limited inflammatory response in the perianastomotic area, with the concomitant release of growth factors, which have been shown as mitogenic for a number of tumor cell lines in vitro.[25]

In conclusion, these results suggest that the use of stapling instruments in colorectal cancer surgery could be associated with up to a 50% reduction in both tumor recurrence and cancer-specific mortality rates. However, these results were taken from subgroup analysis of a larger trial that was not specifically set up to examine these points; therefore the results require corroboration by further trials. A multicenter study has been set up, coordinated from this department, to examine the effect anastomotic technique and anastomotic integrity have on the long-term prognosis of patients undergoing potentially curative restorative colorectal cancer resections.

The support of Autosuture UK in the conduct of this study is acknowledged. We would also like to thank all the surgeons who contributed patients into the study: S.G. MacPherson, W.R. Murray, and J.A. Bradley (Western Infirmary, Glasgow); B. Sugden and C.G. Morran (Crosshouse Hospital, Kilmarnock); A. Munro, J.R.C. Logie, and P.V. Walsh (Raigmore Hospital, Inverness); G. Bell and J.J. Morrice (Inverclyde Royal Hospital, Greenock); and K. Mitchell (Royal Alexandra Hospital, Paisley).

REFERENCES

1. Finlay IG, McArdle CS. Occult hepatic metastases in colorectal carcinoma. Br J Surg 73:732, 1986.
2. Quirke P, Durdey P, Dixon MF, et al. Local recurrence of rectal adenocarcinoma due to inadequate surgical resection. Histopathological study of lateral spread and surgical excision. Lancet 1:996, 1986.
3. Heald RJ, Husband EM, Ryall RDH. The mesorectum in rectal cancer surgery—the clue to pelvic recurrence? Br J Surg 69:613, 1982.
4. Goligher JC, Dukes CE, Bussey HJR. Local recurrence after sphincter-saving excisions for carcinoma of the rectum and rectosigmoid. Br J Surg 39:199, 1951.
5. Williamson RCN, Davies PW, Bristol JB, et al. Intestinal adaptation and experimental carcinogenesis after partial colectomy. Increased tumour yields are confined to the anastomosis. Gut 23:316, 1982.
6. Phillips RKS, Hittinger R, Blesovsky L, et al. Local recurrence following "curative" surgery for large bowel cancer. I. The overall picture. Br J Surg 71:12, 1984.
7. Hurst PA, Prout WG, Kelly JM, et al. Local recurrence after low anterior resection using the staple gun. Br J Surg 69:275, 1982.
8. Anderberg B, Enblad P, Sjodahl R, et al. Recurrent rectal carcinoma after anterior resection and rectal stapling. Br J Surg 70:1, 1983.
9. Reid JDS, Robins RE, Atkinson KG. Pelvic recurrence after anterior resection and EEA stapling anastomosis for potentially curable carcinoma of the rectum. Am J Surg 147:629, 1984.
10. Bisgaard C, Svanholm H, Jensen AS. Recurrent carcinoma after low anterior resection of the rectum using the EEA staple gun. Acta Chir Scand 152:157, 1986.
11. Rosen CB, Beart RW, Ilstrup DM. Local recurrence of rectal carcinoma after hand-sewn and stapled anastomoses. Dis Colon Rectum 28:305, 1985.
12. Ohman U, Svenberg T. EEA stapler for mid-rectum carcinoma—Review of recent literature and own experience. Dis Colon Rectum 26:775, 1983.
13. Ohman U. Curative potential of EEA stapler in rectal carcinoma. Acta Chir Scand 152:59, 1986.
14. Kennedy HL, Langevin JM, Goldberg SM, et al. Recurrence following stapled coloproctostomy for carcinomas of the mid portion of the rectum. Surg Gynecol Obstet 160:513, 1985.
15. Wolmark N, Gordon PH, Fisher B, et al. A comparison of stapled and handsewn anastomoses in patients undergoing resection for Dukes' B and C colorectal cancer. An analysis of disease-free survival and survival from the NSABP prospective clinical trials. Dis Colon Rectum 29:344, 1986.
16. West of Scotland and Highland Anastomosis Study Group. Suturing or stapling in gastrointestinal surgery: A prospective randomized study. Br J Surg 78:337, 1991.
17. American Joint Committee On Cancer. Manual for staging of cancer, 3rd ed. Philadelphia: JB Lippincott, 1988.
18. Kaplan EL, Meier P. Nonparametric estimation from incomplete observations. Am Stat Assoc 53:457, 1958.
19. Cox DR. Regression models and life tables. J R Stat Soc 34:187, 1972.
20. Goligher JC, Lee PWR, Macfie J, et al. Experience with the Russian model 249 suture gun for anastomosis of the rectum. Surg Gynecol Obstet 148:517, 1979.
21. Heald RJ. Towards fewer colostomies—The impact of circular stapling devices on the surgery of rectal cancer in a district hospital. Br J Surg 67:198, 1980.
22. Akyol AM, McGregor JR, Galloway DJ, et al. Early postoperative contrast radiology in the assessment of colorectal anastomotic integrity. Int J Colorect Dis 7:141, 1992.
23. Akyol AM, McGregor JR, Galloway DJ, et al. Anastomotic leaks in colorectal cancer surgery: A risk factor for recurrence? Int J Colorect Dis 6:179, 1991.
24. Akyol AM. Clinical and experimental studies on gastrointestinal anastomoses and colorectal cancer. Medical degree thesis. Glasgow: University of Glasgow, 1990.
25. Goustin AS, Leof EB, Shipley GD, et al. Growth factors and cancer. Cancer Res 46:1015, 1986.

79 Rectal Prolapse in Adults: Treatment by Anterior Rectal Resection

Olivier Delahaut, Michel Ceuterick, Daniel Jacobs, Martine Goergen, and Juan Santiago Azagra

Rectal prolapse is a condition that is all too often ignored or neglected. Progressing with time, it handicaps the patient's life with constipation, abdominal or perineal pain, incontinence, or a solitary rectal ulcer. For a number of years, especially since the work of Wells,[1] Ripstein and Lauter,[2] Orr,[3] and Loygue et al.,[4] rectopexy, with different variations, has been the most frequently used surgical treatment. The published results are good, but there is a complication associated with this treatment: constipation. It is often present before the operation and becomes more marked afterward.[5-8] Its cause is the dolichocolon that is associated with this pathology.[9] We have abandoned the practice of performing isolated rectopexy and like some other teams have adopted the Fryckman-Goldberg technique[8-12]: anterior rectal resection and fixation.

MATERIALS AND METHODS

Between January 1990 and June 1992, we operated on 14 patients with rectal prolapse: 3 men and 11 women, average age, 56 years (range, 27 to 75). Table 1 lists their symptoms, and Table 2 presents their histories. The clinical workup consisted of a complete physical examination, rectoscopy, barium enema, defecography, anorectal manometry, and cystography. After this workup we divided the patients into subgroups, as shown in Table 3.

Associated rectoceles represent an anterior prolapse. The predisposing mechanisms are common: a deep pouch of Douglas, dolichocolon, and descent of a weak perineal floor. These observations come from different studies and our own experience.[13-18] The barium enema showed the presence of a dolichosigmoid in all patients. In two cases a solitary rectal mucosal ulcer was present. Anorectal manometric measurements and their relation to continence are described in Table 4. Hypertonicity of the internal sphincter is attributed to fibrosis of the anal canal from repeated insults by the prolapse[19] and hypotonicity of the external sphincter to denervation entrapment and stretch injury of the pudendal or perineal nerves.[12,19,20]

Table 1. Patients' symptoms

Symptom	No. of Patients
Constipation	14
Perineal or hypogastric pain	8
Anal continence, after Browning and Parks	14
Grade 1	12
Grade 2	0
Grade 3	1
Grade 4	1
Anal mass	6

Table 2. Patients' medicosurgical histories

Condition	No. of Patients
Diabetes mellitus	1
Chronic obstructive pulmonary disease	1
Hemorrhoidectomy	1
Unsuccessful perineorraphy	2
Childbirth	9

Table 3. Subgroups of rectal prolapse

Classification	No. of Patients
Anorectal prolapse	4
Anorectal prolapse plus internal rectal prolapse	2
Anorectal prolapse plus rectocele	2
Internal rectal prolapse plus rectocele	2
Rectocele	4

Eleven patients were treated by laparotomy and three by a laparoscopic approach. All underwent colonic resection to treat the dolichosigmoid. The anastomosis was carried out using a triple-stapling technique.[21] The resection was completed by fixation of the colorectum at the promontorium with silk sutures. A deep pouch of Douglas and dolichosigmoid were observed in all patients preceding the repair.

RESULTS

No mortality, no fistulas, no anastomotic problems, and no incisional hernias were observed. Among the complications were three noninfected parietal hematomas and one urinary infection. Follow-up is at 6 to 36 months (average, 24 months). Evaluation of the results is based on the patients' complaints and clinical signs. Evaluation was performed at 3, 6, 12 months, and once a year thereafter. Additionally, defecography and anorectal manometry were performed at the third postoperative month.

Thirteen of 14 patients were very satisfied with the treatment. In four out of seven patients, constipation disappeared; it regressed in four. The grade 3 incontinence disappeared. Clinical examination confirmed the disappearance of external manifestations in these 13 patients. Postoperative defecography demonstrated the good physiological mechanism of defecation in the absence of the prolapse. In all patients manometric examination remained unchanged.

In one patient treatment was unsuccessful. The patient had diminished pain, persistent constipation, which regressed partially but was still a handicap, and persistence of preoperative grade 4 incontinence. In this case defecography demonstrated the recurrence of the preoperative rectocele.

DISCUSSION

In our experience colonic resection permits the avoidance of problems linked to isolated rectopexy in which severe constipation persists in 10% to 47% of patients according to different studies.[5-8] The dolichosigmoid is an essential element in the physiopathology of rectal prolapse, along with a weak pelvic floor, a weak anterior rectogenital septum, and the deep configuration of the pouch of Douglas.[9,16]

In our study the results were good in 92% of the patients. Constipation, which was present in 100% of the patients preoperatively, disappeared in 71% and regressed in 29%. Severe preoperative incontinence (grade 4) is an unfavorable prognostic element; it affects the complete elimination of postoperative incontinence and predisposes to recurrence of rectal prolapse. The triple-stapled anastomosis allowed us to achieve maximal security and a reduction in the number of complications.[21] During the last 6 months we have performed our operation by celioscopy.

We are grateful to Drs. F. De Racker, C. Preux, and R. Fritz of the University Hospital Center, Tivoli, for the performance of defecography and manometry.

REFERENCES

1. Wells C. New operation for rectal prolapse. Proc R Soc Med 52:602-603, 1959.
2. Ripstein CB, Lauter B. Etiology and surgical therapy of massive prolapse of the rectum. Ann Surg 157:259-264, 1963.
3. Orr TG. A suspension operation for prolapse of the rectum. Ann Surg 126:833-840, 1947.
4. Loygue J, et al. Complete prolapse of the rectum: A report on 140 cases treated by rectopexy. Br J Surg 58:847-848, 1971.
5. Delemarre JBVM, et al. The effect of posterior rectopexy on fecal continence. Dis Colon Rectum 34:311-316, 1991.
6. McCue JL, Thomson JPS. Clinical and functional results of abdominal rectopexy for complete rectal prolapse. Br J Surg 78:921-923, 1991.
7. Madden MV, et al. Abdominal rectopexy for complete prolapse: Prospective study evaluating changes in symptoms and anorectal function. Dis Colon Rectum 35:48-55, 1992.

Table 4. Anorectal manometry

Finding	No. of Patients
Normal	10
(grade 1)	
Decrease of pressure at the external sphincter	4
<30 mm Hg	1
(grade 4)	
30-50 mm Hg	3
Grade 3	1
Grade 1	2
Increase of pressure at the internal sphincter (grade 4)	1

8. Sayfan J, Pinho M. Sutured posterior abdominal rectopexy with sigmoidectomy compared with Marlex rectopexy for rectal prolapse. Br J Surg 77:143-145, 1990.

9. Watts JD. The management of procidentia. Dis Colon Rectum 28:292-297, 1989.

10. Fryckman HM, Goldberg SM. The surgical treatment of rectal procidentia. Surg Gynecol Obstet 129:1225-1230, 1969.

11. Husa A, Sainio P. Abdominal rectopexy and sigmoid resection. Acta Chir Scand 154:221-224, 1988.

12. Sainio AP, Vantilainen PE, Husa AI. Recovery of anal sphincter function following transabdominal repair of rectal prolapse: Cause of improved continence? Dis Colon Rectum 34:816-821, 1991.

13. Beevors MA. Pudendal nerve function in women with symptomatic utero-vaginal prolapse. Int J Colorectal Dis 6:24-28, 1991.

14. Costalat G. Syndrome de l'ulcère solitaire du rectum: Aspects cliniques, évolutif et bases thérapeutiques. Ann Chir 44:807-816, 1990.

15. Kazuhika Y. Physiologic and anatomic assessment of patients with rectocele. Dis Colon Rectum 34:704-708, 1991.

16. Moshowitz AV. The pathogenesis, anatomy and cure of prolapse of the rectum. Surg Gynecol Obstet 15:7-21, 1912.

17. Parks AG, Porter NH, Hardcastle J. The syndrome of the descending perineum. Proc Soc Med 59:477-482, 1966.

18. Teniere P. La place de l'exérèse colo-rectale pour constipation sévèrè apres promonto-fixation rectale dans le syndrome du périnée descendant. Gastroenterol Clin Biol 13:292-297, 1989.

19. Parks AG, Swash M, Vrich H. Sphincter denervation in anorectal incontinence and rectal prolapse. Gut 18:656-665, 1977.

19a. Williams JD. Incontinence and rectal prolapse: A prospective manometric study. Dis Colon Rectum 32:209-216, 1991.

20. Snooks SJ, Henry MM, Swash M. Anorectal incontinence and rectal prolapse: Differential assessment of the innervation to puborectalis and external anal sphincter muscles. Gut 26:470-476, 1985.

21. Julian TB. The triple-stapled colonic anastomosis. Technical notes. Dis Colon Rectum 32:989-995, 1989.

22. Browning GGP, Parks AG. postanal repair for neuropathic faecal incontinence: Correlation of clinical result and anal canal pressures. Br J Surg 70:101-104, 1983.

XIII

Mechanical and Biological Anastomotic Techniques and Results

80 *Results of 1000 Esophageal Resections With Stapled Anastomoses*

François Fekete, Alain Sauvanet, and Jacques Belghiti

Anastomotic leakage remains a major problem after esophageal resection and is still responsible for most deaths. Manual anastomoses, using one or two layers of interrupted sutures[1] are sometimes difficult to perform at the thoracic level and are associated with a leakage rate of between 10% and 23%.[2-6] Although circular stapling can be associated with stricture formation, numerous studies have reported a dramatic decrease in the leakage rate using this procedure.[7-10]

Between February 1, 1979 and August 1, 1992, in the Department of Surgery for the Digestive Tract at the Beaujon Hospital in Paris, 1000 esophageal anastomoses were performed with a stapler. We report this large experience of using stapling for esophageal anastomosis.

MATERIALS AND METHODS

Of the 1000 patients who underwent esophageal anastomoses in our series, esophageal and/or gastric resection was indicated for carcinoma in 908 patients and for benign esophageal or gastric diseases in 92. The distribution of indications is indicated in Table 1.

Patient ages ranged from 14 to 84 years (median age, 57 ± 9). Cirrhosis, mainly from alcohol abuse, was present in 43 patients. Previous irradiation involving the mediastinal or cervical esophagus was present in 54 patients, including 38 after preoperative radiotherapy (associated with chemotherapy in 26) for nonadjuvant treatment; 10 after head and neck cancers; three after Hodgkin's disease; and three after breast carcinoma. The preoperative mean weight loss was 7 ± 5 kg. An emergency procedure was performed in five patients with a traumatic rupture of the tumor.

Anastomotic procedures performed were esophagogastrostomies in 663 patients; esophagocolostomies in 87; esophagojejunostomies in 249 and esophagoesophagostomy in one. One hundred fifty-eight anastomoses were located in the neck, 696 in the thorax, and 146 in the abdomen (Table 2).

TECHNIQUE

Esophagogastric anastomoses in the thorax were usually done for esophageal carcinoma below the aortic arch using an abdominal and right thoracic approach. During the abdominal stage, a colo-omental detachment was done. The left gastric artery and the short gastric vessels were divided. The gastric tube was created by

Table 1. Indications for esophageal anastomoses in 1000 patients

Malignant Diseases

Esophageal squamous cell cancer	541
Adenocarcinoma of the cardia	227
Carcinoma of the stomach	140
TOTAL	908

Benign Diseases

Caustic stenosis	39
Peptic stenosis	35
Others	18
TOTAL	92

Table 2. Procedures used

		Procedure	No.
Cervical	158	Esogastrostomy	81
		Esocolostomy	77
Intrathoracic	696	Esogastrostomy	580
		Esocolostomy	12
		Esojejunostomy	103
		Esoesophagostomy	1
Abdominal	146	Esojejunostomy	146
	TOTAL		1000

applications of a GIA stapler (Autosuture) starting on the lesser curvature at the junction of the gastric walls served by the right and left gastric arteries, in order to resect all lymph nodes along the left gastric vessels. A Kocher maneuver and a pyloroplasty were routinely performed. During the thoracic stage, a complete posterior mediastinectomy with lymph node dissection was performed respecting the rules of radical surgery. The esophageal transection was done as high as possible if curative resection was attempted, and the anastomosis was performed in the apex of the hemithorax.

An end-to-side esophagogastric anastomosis was done on the posterior wall of the gastric tube (Fig. 1). The size of the stapler was chosen according to the largest inserted Hegar dilator in the esophageal lumen. The staplers most often used were EEA 25 or 28 (Autosuture) or ILS 25 or 29 (Ethicon). Most of the time the stapler was inserted through a vertical anterior gastrotomy at 4 or 5 cm from the apex of the tube (see Fig. 1); the gastrotomy was closed by manual suturing. In case of excessive length and ischemia of the tube, the stapler was inserted through its elbowed top and anastomosis was performed between a healthy posterior gastric wall and the esophagus. The redundant, questionably viable tube

apex, containing the EEA introduction site is then excised proximal to a TA stapled closure placed lateral to the anastomosis (Autosuture). The omentum, brought up into the mediastinum with the stomach, was generally wrapped around the anastomosis and the gastrotomy. More recently anastomoses were sealed with fibrin glue (Tissucol, Immuno Laboratories) during a prospective study. To relieve tension, the gastric walls were sutured to the mediastinal pleura or to the prevertebral fascia.

A left thoracic or thoracoabdominal incision was used for elderly patients with carcinoma of the lower third of the esophagus or of the cardia. The procedure for esophagogastric anastomosis was identical.

Cervical esophagogastric anastomoses were generally performed for carcinoma above the aortic arch. After transthoracic or transhiatal dissection of the mediastinal esophagus, a long gastric tube was fashioned by excising the lesser curvature of the stomach with several applications of the GIA and the tube was lifted into the mediastinum and neck through the esophageal bed. A substernal tunnel was used only for palliative procedures. The circular stapler was inserted through the elbowed apex of the tube and end-to-side esophagogas-

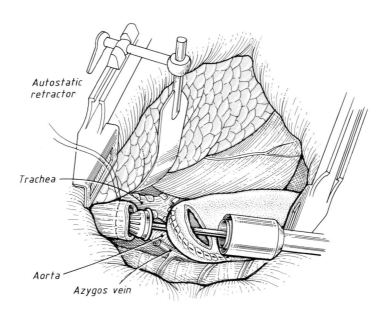

Fig. 1. End-to-side esophagogastric anastomosis placed on the posterior wall of the gastric tube. The circular stapler is introduced through an anterior gastrostomy, some 4 to 5 cm caudad to the suture-closed apex of the tube. Following completion of anastomosis and removal of the instrument, the gastrostomy is closed by manual sutures.

trostomy performed, to preserve the gastric blood supply. The excess gastric tube was excised peripheral to the anastomosis and closure with the TA instrument. The use of a stapler for cervical esophagogastric anastomosis was impossible if the tube was not long enough and a hand-made anastomosis was then performed. We have no experience with oral insertion of the circular, anastomotic stapler.

Esophagojejunal anastomoses were performed after total gastrectomy for carcinoma of the cardia or of the stomach, using an extended total gastrectomy including omental detachment, splenectomy, and celiac lymphadenectomy. An abdominal approach was sufficient for carcinomas of the stomach. For carcinomas of the cardia, a thoracic approach was necessary to perform mediastinal lymphadenectomy and esophageal transection 10 cm above the upper pole of the tumor to avoid microscopic tumor involvement at the level of esophageal transection.

A Roux-en-Y loop was most often used. Greater mobilization of the loop was necessary for thoracic anastomoses and was achieved by dividing the posterior peritoneum of the mesenteric root.

The stapler was inserted through the open end of the jejunal elbow and the anastomosis done end-to-side. The excess jejunum was resected peripheral to a TA-stapled closure, placed lateral to the anastomosis.

Esophagocolic anastomoses were performed for benign disease or for esophageal carcinoma in patients with a previous distal gastrectomy. A transverse isoperistaltic coloplasty was generally used. For cervical anastomoses, a substernal path was created mainly in patients with carcinoma of the esophagus above the aortic arch, or for restoration of the digestive tract after an urgent esophagectomy for caustic burn. Thoracic anastomoses were performed in patients with peptic strictures or esophageal carcinoma below the aortic arch. The cologastric anastomosis was located on the posterior wall of the stomach and the stapler was inserted through an anterior gastrotomy. The coloplasty had to be as straight as possible to avoid swallowing discomfort.

POSTOPERATIVE COURSE AND RESULTS

In 1000 stapled esophageal anastomoses, overall mortality was 7% during the hospital stay. The overall leakage rate was 8.5%. Symptomatic leakage occurred in 5.8% of cases, with a 1.5% mortality related to this complication. Asymptomatic leakage was diagnosed on radiographic examination in 3.7% of cases.

With respect to the underlying disease, the highest rates of leakage and mortality were observed after resection for cancer (Table 3). Only one death from leakage occurred after resection for benign disease.

Viewed from the level of anastomosis, the leakage rate was higher (16%) after cervical anastomoses than after thoracic or abdominal anastomoses (5.9% and 4.7%, respectively). The mortality rate did not differ significantly with anastomotic level (Table 4). For thorac-

Table 3. Results according to the underlying disease

	No.	Mortality (%)	Leakage (%)
Cancer	908	7.4	8.5
Benign lesions	92	2.0	7.5
TOTAL	1000	6.9	8.5

Table 4. Results by anastomotic level

Anastomotic Level	No.	Mortality (%)	Leakage (%)	Mortality Related to Leakage (%)
Cervical	158	8.7	16	1.4
Thoracic	696	6.8	5.9	1.6
Abdominal	146	4.7	4.7	1.4
TOTAL	1000	6.9	8.5	1.5

Table 5. Results by organ anastomosed to the esophagus

Organ	Anastomotic Site	No.	Leakage (%)
Stomach	Cervical	81	18.5
	Thoracic	580	5.9
Colon	Cervical	77	7.8
	Thoracic	12	8.3
Jejunum	Thoracic	103	7.8
	Abdominal	146	4.7
Esoesophagostomy	Thoracic	1	—
TOTAL		1000	

Table 6. Results of fibrin glue with intrathoracic esophagogastrostomies (prospective study)

	No.	Leakage With Fibrin Glue	Leakage Without Fibrin Glue
Intrathoracic esogastrostomy	55	1/28*	3/27*

*$p > 0.5$ (not significant) (chi-squared test).

ic anastomoses, the rate of leakage did not differ significantly with the substitute organ used—stomach, jejunum, or colon. For cervical anastomoses, the rate of leakage was higher when gastroplasty was used (Table 5).

The use of fibrin glue to seal thoracic esophagogastrostomies did not significantly decrease the rate of anastomotic leakage (Table 6).

The overall rate of symptomatic anastomotic stricture was 6%. An anastomotic stricture was observed in up to 15% of cases after use of a small-sized stapler (EEA or ILS 21). Stricture was also frequently observed after healing of anastomotic fistulas.

DISCUSSION

The anastomotic leakage at an esophageal anastomosis may be symptomatic or asymptomatic. Symptomatic fistulas are esophagocutaneous in the neck and esophageal-pleural, -mediastinal, or -aortic in the chest. In our experience, cervical fistulas occurred more frequently, but all healed spontaneously. Leakage of a thoracic anastomosis is less frequent but more harmful, since it can

be responsible for pneumonia and septic shock requiring prolonged respiratory assistance.[11] The risks of thoracic leakage justify a systematic radiographic swallow examination using an iso-osmotic water-soluble contrast medium on the seventh postoperative day, because an asymptomatic fistula may worsen with oral feeding.

Esophageal anastomoses performed with a stapler seemed to be associated with a decreased leakage rate.[7-10] However, a perfect technique is needed to obtain good results. *The purse-string is a key stage:* widely spaced or tearing sutures may lead to incomplete anastomosis. In our experience, the purse-string instruments currently manufactured are not as secure as a hand-made purse-string inserted as an over-and-over whipstitch into the open end of the esophagus. The full thickness of the esophageal wall, particularly the mucosa, must be taken with each suture, which is inserted close to the distal margin to avoid interposition of a thick purse-string margin. When completion of the purse-string is hazardous because of unsatisfactory exposure, the purse-string may be reinforced by passing the string a second time as a whole ligature around the concentrically narrowed "waistline" of the esophagus achieved from the original purse-string, tightened around the center rod of the stapler.

The *degree of tightening* between anvil and cartridge is critical. Both EEA and ILS staplers present markers for levels of tightening. A thickened esophagus above a tumoral obstruction requires careful adjustment to avoid crushing of the esophageal wall.

The amount of tissue *interposition* between the anvil and the cartridge must be carefully planned: a thick purse-string margin or a small cartridge compromise the anastomotic participation of esophageal tissue. It is necessary to release the instrument at times and excise the excess tissue if possible. Sometimes the purse-string must be redone and a larger stapler chosen. If the jejunum is used, a bowel fold may be created and included into the anastomosis on the mesenteric side and close to the efferent loop. Generally, the size of the cartridge must not exceed 25 mm to avoid this problem.

Problems with the introduction and removal of the anvil are avoided by a previous dilatation of the esophagus with Hegar dilatators. The esophagus should not be forcefully dilatated beyond its normal diameter or else the mucosa may split, impairing the safety of the anastomosis.

The *omental graft* seems to prevent diffuse mediastinal infection or rupture into the aorta.[7] However, an important fatty infiltration may require partial omental resection to preserve the vessels of the greater curvature while it avoids compression of the gastroplasty and the thoracic organs. This partial omental resection precludes use of an omental graft around the anastomosis.

In our experience, sealing anastomosis with fibrin glue has not decreased the leakage rate of intrathoracic esophagogastrostomies; however, our prospective study included only 55 patients. Despite these technical precautions, the risk of leakage persists whatever the anastomotic level. In resection of esophageal carcinoma, a cervical site has been advocated to avoid life-threatening effects of a thoracic leakage.[11] In our study, the rate of mortality related to leakage did not differ according to the anastomotic level. This result and the higher rates of leakage and stenosis observed with cervical anastomoses justify the use of a thoracic anastomosis in patients with esophageal carcinoma below the aortic arch.[11]

Strictures have already been reported in both sutured and stapled anastomoses. Mechanisms of stricture are ischemia of the apex of the gastric tube and delayed mucosal healing, particularly after leakage. In our experience, all anastomotic strictures occurred within 3 months postoperatively. Strictures are probably more frequent with stapled inverted anastomoses than after hand-made anastomoses.[12] However, management of these strictures with bouginage is easy and efficient. The higher incidence of strictures does not offset the advantages of staplers for esophageal anastomoses.

REFERENCES

1. Devitt PG, Jamieson GG. Hand-sewn anastomoses of the oesophagus. In Jamieson GG, ed. Surgery of the Oesophagus. Edinburgh: Churchill Livingstone, 1988, pp 703-712.
2. Orringer MB, Sloan H. Esophagectomy without thoracotomy. J Thorac Cardiovasc Surg 76:643-654, 1978.
3. Cooper JD, Jamieson WR, Blair R, et al. The palliative value of surgical resection for carcinoma of the esophagus. Can J Surg 24:145-147, 1981.
4. Maillard JN, Launois B, de Lagausie P, et al. Cause of leakage at the site of anastomosis after esophagogastric resection for carcinoma. Surg Gynecol Obstet 129:1014-1018, 1969.
5. Wong J. Esophageal resection for cancer: The rationale of current practice. Am J Surg 153:18-24, 1987.
6. Chassin JL. Stapling technique for esophagogastrostomy after esophagogastric resection. Am J Surg 136:499-504, 1978.
7. Fekete F, Breil P, Ronsse H, et al. EEA stapler and omental graft in esophagogastrectomy. Ann Surg 193:825-830, 1981.
8. Hopkins RA, Alexander JC, Postlethwait RW. Stapled esophagogastric anastomosis. Am J Surg 147:283-287, 1984.
9. Wong J, Cheung HC, Lui R, et al. Esophagogastric anastomosis performed with a stapler: The occurrence of leakage and stricture. Surgery 101:408-415, 1987.
10. Fabri B, Donnely RJ. Oesophagogastrectomy using the end-to-end anastomosing stapler. Thorax 37:296-299, 1982.
11. Chasseray VM, Kiroff GK, Buard JL, et al. Cervical or thoracic anastomosis for esophagectomy for carcinoma. Surg Gynecol Obstet 169:55-62, 1989.
12. Fok M, Ah-Chong AK, Cheng SWK, et al. Comparison of a single layer continuous hand-sewn method and circular stapling in 580 oesophageal anastomoses. Br J Surg 78:342-345, 1991.

81 Sutureless Compression Anastomosis of the Distal Colon and Rectum With an AKA-2 Instrument

Eberhard Gross and M.O. Köppen

Deficiencies in anastomotic healing after restorative rectal resections still occur frequently. The incidence of clinically apparent leaks after low anterior resection is reported in recent publications to be between 3% and 20%, mostly about 10%.[1-8] If the anastomoses are investigated systematically in the early postoperative period, a high number of additional asymptomatic leaks will be found—two or three times higher than the rate of symptomatic fistulas.[2,6,8] Apart from the morbidity, anastomotic dehiscence is the underlying cause of 30% to 50% of patient mortality following low anterior resection. Therefore research on anastomotic healing is aimed at improving the quality and reliability of the anastomosis.[9]

Halsted's experiments[9] have shown the relationship between anastomotic technique and the healing process, and the results of many animal experiments can be summarized as follows: (1) The healing process shows diminishing inflammatory reaction as the operative trauma is reduced, and (2) biomechanical quality specifications depend on the morphology of the anastomotic healing.

Our own animal experiments have shown that an anastomosis could be created without any foreign material.[10] This sutureless anastomosis is greatly superior to a conventionally sutured anastomosis in terms of biomechanical criteria and morphology, such as microscopic aspects, disturbances of anastomotic healing, histological features, and microangiographic investigations. On the basis of these results, we introduced the compression anastomosis AKA-2 technique in our clinic.[11,12] The sutureless compression anastomosis using no foreign material was first possible only in animal experiments. The compression anastomosis comes closest to the sutureless anastomosis, because the foreign material (the compression rings) remains in the tissue for only a few days. After the rings separate from the anastomotic line, an anastomosis without any foreign body is the result.

MATERIALS AND METHODS

On 147 patients who had been diagnosed with colorectal malignant disease or sigmoid diverticulitis we performed an elective or emergency resection of the distal colon or rectum (Table 1). In most patients a high or low anterior resection or a sigmoid resection was performed (Table 2). For curative operations of cancer of the rectum or in sigmoid cancer cases, the colon and rectum were appropriately resected with high ligation of the inferior mesenteric vessels.

In 24 patients a protective colostomy was performed

Table 1. Indications for resection of the colon and rectum by AKA-2 anastomosis

Condition	Number
Rectal carcinoma	30
Sigmoid carcinoma	34
Adenoma of the rectum and sigmoid	9
Carcinoma of the descending colon	8
Local recurrence	5
Diverticulitis	46
Other	9
Crohn's disease	6
TOTAL	147

Table 2. Operative procedure

Procedure	Number
Low anterior resection	48
High anterior resection	56
Sigmoid resection	37
Ileosigmoidostomy	4
Descending colon-to-rectum pouch and anastomosis (second-stage Hartmann procedure)	2
TOTAL	14

at the time of resection, predominantly in patients with extended or multivisceral resections, in emergency cases, or in patients with serious systemic conditions (Table 3).

The principle of creating a compression anastomosis involves direct contact between two bowel edges, which are compressed by two intraluminal plastic rings (Fig. 1). The plastic rings will be passed with the feces between the fourth and tenth postoperative days.

In its usable and spent configuration, the compression device is composed of three plastic rings. Two rings— base and intermediate—are placed into one bowel end. The third ring (circular anchor, shaped from the periphery of a plastic plate) is placed into the opposing bowel end. The flat base ring carries six blunt pins, each alternating with three ($6 \times 3 = 18$) fishhook-shaped pins. Blunt and hooked pins pass freely through corresponding holes in the intermediate ring. The flat ends of the blunt pins, which are larger than the corresponding holes, keep base and intermediate rings from separating. However, the two rings are held apart by small metal springs surrounding the blunt pins between the two rings. The range of movement of the intermediate ring, along its common axis with the base ring, extends along the length of the blunt pins, minus the space occupied by compressed springs. Both rings can be pushed against each other, but because of the springs, the intrinsic force of the double ring assembly is one of separation and expansion of the intermediate from the base ring (Fig. 2).

The anchor (third) ring is created in the actual process of anastomosis from a plate, fastened to the tip of

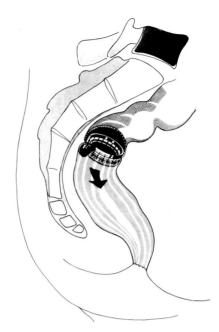

Fig. 1. Coaptation and compression of the two bowel edges by the compression rings, which are placed in the bowel lumen.

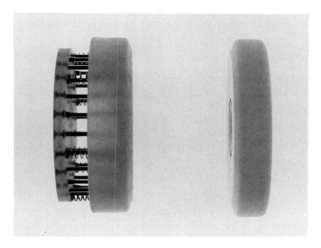

Fig. 2. The distal plastic annular assembly consists of two rings joined together. Metal pins, which are attached to the flat base ring, fit through corresponding bore holes of the second or intermediate ring. In this illustration this ring is hidden inside the outer proximal ring. After activating the instrument, the metal pins pierce through the outer ring and are anchored in that way. Compression is between the intermediate and outer rings.

Table 3. Indications for primary protective colostomy

Indications	Number
Multivisceral resection	10
Large bowel mechanical obstruction	5
Low anterior resection in high-risk patients	3
Crohn's disease with anal fistula	1
Perforated diverticulitis	1
Diverticulitis with fistula	1
Radiologically visible fistula	1
Descending colon-to-rectum anastomosis	1
Immunosuppression	1
TOTAL	24

the central rod of the AKA-2 instrument by a flat metal cone that fits within the circumference of the circular blade. The advancing blade stamps out both purse-stringed bowel walls, contained between the double ring (base and intermediate) and the anchor plate, and then punches out the center of the anchor plate held by the metal cone. This leaves a third ring that serves as an anchoring berth for the hooked pins that advance through both bowel rims to penetrate and hold the anchor ring, slightly ahead of the circular blade (see Fig. 1).

With the distance between base and anchor rings held constant by the safely impaled hooked pins, the intermediate ring is pushed against the anchor (third) ring by the springs and compresses the inverted bowel margins between these two rings. As the union of both bowel ends takes place and their inner rims are sealed by compression necrosis, the entire assembly comes loose as a unit, and is elminated through the anus.

Use of the AKA-2 instrument is similar to that of stapling devices. The steps preceding the actual anastomosis, such as clearing the bowel edges and placing of the purse-string suture, are the same as with stapling techniques. The instrument is introduced transanally. In a high anastomosis, the instrument without the head is guided into position by means of an intestinal tube. The instrument head and magazine are attached onto the instrument shaft, projecting through the rectal stump.

Preoperative patient preparation includes an orthograde bowel lavage on the previous day. The rectosigmoid or rectal stump is irrigated before anastomosis with a disinfective cytocidal solution (povidone-iodine). Perioperative short-term antibiotic prophylaxis is carried out (1 g metronidazole and 2 g cefazolin).

The following investigations were performed prospectively: Intraoperative testing that the anastomosis is leak-proof was performed with the irrigating solution mentioned earlier.

The protocol included a gastrografin enema between the twelfth and fourteenth postoperative days in an otherwise clinically normal course, and endoscopic determination of the anastomosis level was performed between the second and fourth week after operation. In addition, major complications were registered in our research protocols.

RESULTS

Six of 147 patients died (4%) during the hospital stay (Table 4). One female patient developed a leakage and died of septic multiorgan failure despite early reinter-

Table 4. Operative lethality and reasons for mortality

Cause	Number
Anastomotic insufficiency	1
Aspiration pneumonia	1
Bacterial pneumonia	2
Myocardial infarction	1
Septicemia without local complication	1
TOTAL	6/147 (4%)

Table 5. Level of anastomosis and rate of leakage

Level	All Patients (number [%])	Patients Without Primary Protective Colostomy (number [%])
< 5 cm	1/15 (6.6)	1/10 (10.0)
5-10 cm	1/47 (2.1)	1/35 (2.9)
< 10 cm	2/62 (3.2)	2/45 (4.4)
> 10 cm	3/85 (3.5)	3/78 (3.8)
TOTAL	5/147 (3.4)	5/123 (4.0)

vention in which a Hartmann procedure was performed. The cause of the second patient's death was tracheobronchial aspiration; a third patient died of a myocardial infarction. Two very old patients could not be weaned from the respirator and died of pneumonia.

Anastomotic fistulas occurred in five of the 147 patients (3.4%). Of the 62 patients with an anastomosis level of less than 10 cm from the anal verge, two patients developed a fistula (Table 5). In three patients of the 85 with an anastomotic height above 10 cm, a fistula occurred (3.5%). Excluding patients who received a primary protective colostomy, the rate of leakage at an anastomosis level of up to 10 cm is 4.4% (2/45) and at an anastomosis level above 10 cm is 3.8% (3/78).

Two of the five patients with a symptomatic leakage were operated on for a locally advanced rectal carcinoma with liver metastases. One of these two patients was treated with a diverting colostomy, and a Hartmann procedure was performed in the other patient, with recto-pexy and sigmoid resection for associate rectal prolapse. In a patient with chronic renal failure, the symptomatic fistula disappeared spontaneously. In three patients asymptomatic fistulas were detected. In two patients, one of whom had an asymptomatic fistula, an anastomotic stricture occurred and was treated by bouginage. Endoscopic examination between the second and fourth weeks after operation showed anastomoses without epithelial defects in the vast majority of patients. Occasionally the anastomotic line could be identified only from the different colon mucosa folds compared with the rectal mucosa.

DISCUSSION

Anastomosis by compression of the bowel edges is already an accepted principle that has been repeatedly adopted since its first description by Denans.[13] Particularly in recent years, it has been applied in animal experiments and clinically. Because implantation of a foreign material is merely temporary, a less inflammatory reaction could be expected in a compression anastomosis compared with a hand-sutured and stapled anastomosis. After the detachment of the plastic rings and the narrow seam of compressed tissue from the bowel wall on the fourth and sixth postoperative day, the anastomotic line consists merely of a small zone of transition. There are no disadvantages such as those associated with sutures or staples, e.g., disturbed blood supply, necrosis, bacterial transport by threads, infection of the suture of staple tract, or foreign body reaction.

In addition to the low rate of asymptomatic fistulas, the endoscopic observation of early complete epithelialization indicates low-reaction healing of the compression anastomosis. The absence of foreign material a few days after operation makes the compression technique suitable for patients with Crohn's disease, in whom the use of nonabsorbable suture material or even metal clips is contraindicated because of the increased risk of fistula development.

Theoretically, the mechanical relief of the anastomosis by the compression rings in the early postoperative phase may be regarded as an advantage. The width of compression anastomosis exceeds that of a stapled anastomosis, since the external diameter of the compression ring corresponds to the final width of the anastomosis.

A compression anastomosis must be evaluated on the leakage rate following low anterior resection, where anastomosis is always subject to risk. According to the literature, clinically symptomatic leakages occurred in 3% to 30% of patients. In comparison with the anastomotic leakage rates, the factors that influence anastomotic healing, such as the level of the anastomosis and protective measures such as cecal fistula or colostomies are to be considered. Thus the clinical effect of anastomotic fistula is of course less serious than without anastomosis protection, and a higher rate of occurrence of clinically symptomatic fistulas is to be expected in patients who did not undergo a protective colostomy.[14] Analysis of the literature on these criteria reveals that the anastomotic leakage rate after low anterior resection without anastomosis protection is 8% to 30%. Leakage rates in our patients are 4.1% (5/123) and 2.9% in patients with an anastomotic level of up to 10 cm (1/35). The corresponding leakage rates of a group of 140 patients who were operated on in 1989 or before (12 in total) are 4.8% (6/124) and 10.7% (6/56), respectively. The improvement in the results may be a consequence of increasing experience.

Thus the clinical application of the compression anastomosis is established. The rate of symptomatic leaks following restorative rectal resection is not higher than the average rates reported in the literature for anastomoses with sutures and staples. The development of asymptomatic fistulas and stenosis is rare compared with other anastomotic techniques. Favorable results regarding morphological and functional criteria are arguments for the sutureless compression anastomosis of the colon and rectum.

REFERENCES

1. Antonson HK, Kronborg O. Early complications after low anterior resection for rectal cancer using the EEA stapling device. Dis Colon Rectum 30:579-583, 1987.
2. Beard JD, Nicholson ML, Sayers RD, Lloyd D, Everson NW. Intraoperative air testing of colorectal anastomoses: A prospective randomized trial. Br J Surg 77:1095-1097, 1990.
3. Beart WRW, Kelley KA. Randomized prospective evaluation of the EEA stapler for colorectal anastomoses. Am J Surg 141:143-147, 1981.
4. Belli L, Beati CA, Frangi M, Aseni P, Rondinara GF. Outcome of patients with rectal cancer treated by stapled anterior resection. Br J Surg 75:422-424, 1988.
5. Blamey SL, Lee PWR. A comparison of circular stapling devices in colorectal anastomoses. Br J Surg 69:19-22, 1982.
6. Fielding LP, Stewart-Brown S, Blesowsky L, Kearney G. Anastomotic integrity after operations for large bowel cancer: A multicentre study. Br Med 11:411-414, 1980.

7. McGinn FP, Gartell PC, Clifford PC, Brunton FJ. Staples or sutures for low colorectal anastomosis: A prospective randomized trial. Br J Surg 72:603-605, 1985.
8. Theide A, Schubert G, Poser HL, Jostarndt L. Zur Technik der Rektumanastomosen bei Rektumresektionen. Eine kontrollierte Studie: Instrumentelle Naht versus Handnaht. Chirurgie 55:326-335, 1984.
9. Halsted WS. Circular suture of the intestine: An experimental study. Am J Med Sci 94:436-461, 1987.
10. Gross E, Schaarschmidt K, Donhuijsen K, Beyer M, Weidauer T, Eigler FW. Die nahtlose Anastomose: Histologische, biomechanische und mikroangiographische Untersuchungen am Colon der Ratte. Langenbecks Arch 48:156-161, 1986.
11. Eigler FW, Gross E. Die maschinelle Kompressionsanastomose (AKA-2) an Colon und Rektum. Ergebnisse einer porospektiven klinischen Studie. Chirurgie 57: 230-235, 1986.
12. Gross E, Eigler FW. Die nahtlose Kompressionsanastomose am distalen Colon und Rektum. Chirurgie 60:589-593, 1989.
13. Senn N. Enterorrhaphy: Its history, technique and present status. JAMA 21:215-235, 1983.
14. Karania ND, Corder AP, Holdsworth PJ, Heald RJ. Risk of peritonitis and fatal septicaemia and the need to defunction the low anastomosis. Br J Surg 78:196-198, 1991.

82 Suture Technique Without Knot Tying for Colonic Anastomosis

Andreas Imdahl, J. Waninger, Katrin Reichenmiller, and Jörg Haberstroh

Laparoscopic procedures for bowel resections with construction of an anastomosis remain experimental. Suturing and tying are difficult to perform because of the two-dimensional laparoscopic view of the structure and the limitations associated with currently available instruments. Application of clips may replace use of a ligature in many situations. To determine an easy technique for suturing the anastomosis, we compared a clip technique with use of a conventional suturing technique.

MATERIALS AND METHODS

Sixty male Wistar rats weighing 250 to 350 g were divided in two groups, A and B (Fig. 1), and the consent of the German Ethics Committee for Animal Experiments was given. Atropine (50 mg/L) and a solution of ketanest and xylazine (Rompun, 5:1, 1.3 ml/kg) were given for anesthesia. After laparotomy the descending colon was divided without compromising the blood supply, using a surgical microscope with sixfold magnification (Zeiss). A metal rod 2 cm long and 0.5 cm in diameter was inserted into the bowel lumen and later was removed before the last stitches were tied or clipped. Longitudinal lines on the rod, visible through the bowel wall, marked the positions of the knots or clips. A circular engraved scale made it possible to take a bite exactly 2 mm from the wound edge. The operating time was recorded. The construction of an intestinal anastomosis can be confirmed by technical factors such as apposition of the bowel wall, leakage rate, microangiographic investigation of arterial compression, or strength of the anastomosis.

Gambee Suture

In group A the anastomosis was constructed with 10 Gambee stitches using 5-0 polyglactin (Vicryl). A spring balance (Maey) was used to control the tension (0.2 N) while tying the knots.

Clip Technique

In group B eight threads (5-0 polyglactin) were used for the clip technique. A clip (Ti-1, Titan-Ligaclips, Ethicon) was mounted on one end of the thread. After passing the suture through both cut ends, the thread was kept under tension, and a second clip was placed opposite the first clip. The distance between the clips was 3 mm (Fig. 2).

After 4, 7, and 90 days, 10 rats of each group (A, 1 through 3; B, 1 through 3) were sacrificed. The anasto-

Study design

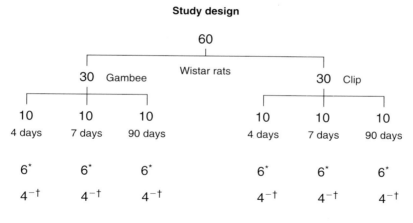

Fig. 1. Study design: 60 rats were divided into two groups.

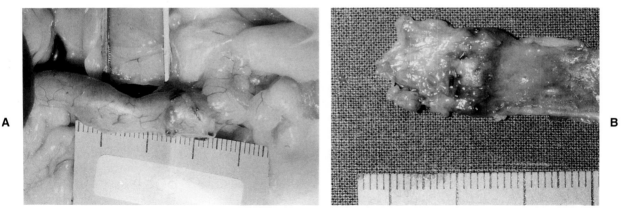

Fig. 2. A, Clip anastomosis after 90 days. Some of the clips are displaced. **B,** Luminal surface of the clip anastomosis after 90 days.

moses were examined macroscopically with regard to stenosis, intra-abdominal abscess formation, and clip loss. The formation of adhesions was graduated: grade 0, no adhesions at all; grade 1, adhesions formed in one fourth the circumference of the anastomosis; grade 2, in one half; grade 3, in three fourths; grade 4, adhesion of the whole anastomosis. The mucosal side of the anastomoses was evaluated for the apposition of the mucosal layer (five grades). Necrotic areas were recorded in square millimeters.

Microangiography

Microangiography was performed in four animals of each subgroup. The abdominal aorta was cannulated (Abbocath, 24 Fr), and the portal vein was opened. The blood vessels were cleaned with 30 ml of heparinized saline solution (20 IV heparin/L). Fifteen milliliters of contrast solution containing Ultravist, Micropaque (Nicholas), and water (1:1:2) were injected. The distal colon was removed, divided along the mesenteric border, and placed on an x-ray film (Cronex 75M, DuPont)

Table 1. Necrosis and apposition

	Postoperative Day	Gambee Suture	Clip
Necrotic area (mm²)	4	10.0 ± 1.6	5.0 ± 3.0
	7	5.9 ± 4.8	5.9 ± 3.9
	90	0.8 ± 1.2*	1.0 ± 1.3*
Apposition (five grades)	4	2.2 ± 0.9	3.1 ± 1.0
	7	2.7 ± 0.8	2.4 ± 1.5
	90	4.0 ± 0.9	4.0 ± 0.8

*$p < 0.05$.

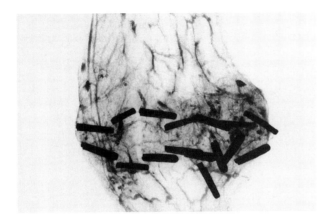

Fig. 3. Microangiogram of a clip anastomosis after 7 days.

for x-ray studies. Slides were taken of the x-ray films and were projected with ×63 magnification. All vessels of the anastomoses were counted (Fig. 3).

Bursting Pressure

To determine the bursting pressure, the anastomoses (5 cm of colon) were fixed on a hollow rod with a central perforation that was connected to a pressure transducer with amplifier and recorder, allowing continuous pressure recording. The colonic segment was filled with saline solution using a perfusion pump (99 ml/hour). A bowel segment proximal of the anastomoses served as control.

Student's *t*-test was used for statistical analysis; *p* values <0.05 were regarded as statistically significant.

RESULTS

Anastomoses were performed more quickly in group B than in group A. There was no difference in the postoperative weight of the animals. One animal in group A died on the sixth postoperative day. A leakage rate of 6.6% was observed in group A on the fourth postoperative day. There was no leakage or death in group B. Small intra-abdominal abscesses were noted in one animal in both groups on the fourth postoperative day and in two of both groups on the seventh day. Forty-three percent of all rats in group B and 53% of group A revealed no stenosis of the anastomoses; 40% of the rats in group B and 23% in group A showed a relative stenosis; and 17% of group B and 24% of group A had almost complete stenosis of the anastomosis. There were no statistical differences in the amount of adhesions and stenosis (Fig. 4).

The extent of necrotic areas was significantly less in both groups after 90 days as compared with the fourth and seventh days. There was no difference between the groups. Apposition of the mucosal layers was better after 90 days without statistical differences between the groups (Table 1).

Microangiography revealed an increase of blood vessels on the seventh and ninetieth days without differences between the groups (Fig. 5). Avascular areas and arterial compression around the sutures of both groups were not observed.

The bursting pressure revealed a marked difference between the fourth and seventh days but without differences between the groups (Fig. 6). After 7 days the bursting pressure exceeded the pressure of the controls. Eighty-five percent of the anastomoses showed a rupture along the suture line.

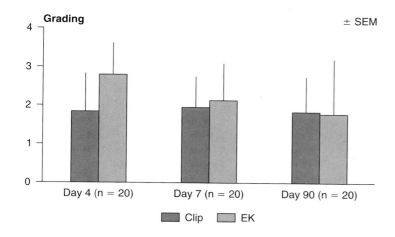

Fig. 4. Grading of adhesions for 10 rats per group on postoperative days. Results are expressed as mean of five grades (0 through 4) ± standard error mean *(SEM)*. The differences were not statistically significant.

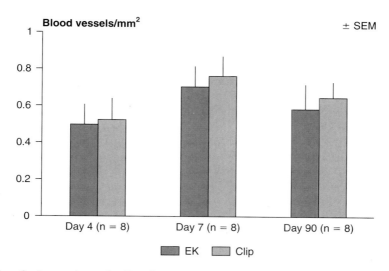

Fig. 5. Results of microangiography. Results are expressed as blood vessel number per square millimeter bowel for four rats per group on postoperative days. Differences were not statistically significant.

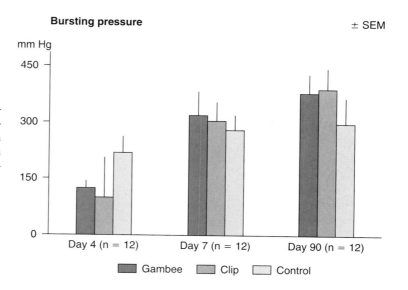

Fig. 6. Results of bursting pressure experiments. Bursting pressure was expressed in millimeters of mercury for six rats per group on postoperative days. The difference between control, clip, and Gambee groups was significant ($p < 0.05$).

DISCUSSION

According to recent publications, laparoscopic bowel resection technically can be performed.[1] The advantages for the patient may be similar to those for laparoscopic cholecystectomy: less pain, shorter hospital stay, better cosmetic results, and quicker return to normal lifestyle. However, performance of the laparoscopic technique is still hazardous and not yet ready for routine application. Suturing the intestinal anastomoses may be influenced by individual factors that require an alternate technique. Experimental studies have investigated the type of approximation, the number of layers, and different suture techniques.[2-5] Experience using a clip technique has not yet been published. The laparoscopic technique of anastomosis should follow the basic principles of intestinal suturing: intact blood supply of the wound edge, approximation without tension, and sealing of the lumen. The technique should be performed within an appropriate time and should be easy to learn.

The quality of wound healing can be assessed by gross appearance. Microangiography detects the regenerating architecture of the vessels.[6] The bursting pressure provides data about the mechanical strength of the anastomoses. Halsted[7] stated that the stitch should not be tied so tight that the tissue looks anemic. Herrmann et al.[5] noted considerable variation between knots tied by different surgeons and even by the same individual. In the present study enough tension was applied to minimize ischemia. Previous experiments had shown that a tension of 0.2 N leads to sufficient apposition of the wound edges using the Gambee stitch without compromise of the blood supply.[2]

The results of our examination demonstrate the feasibility of the clip technique. The operating time with it is reduced compared with that of the Gambee stitch. Although the distance between sutures was greater in group B, a higher leakage rate was not observed.

Microangiography did not reveal differences of the blood supply between the two groups. The clip technique did not lead to compression of blood vessels, although it was difficult to measure the pressure on the tissue between the clips. Bursting pressure reflected the importance of the sutures in the first 4 to 7 days of the healing process.

The clip loss observed at the ninetieth day may have been caused by intraluminal migration of the clips. Clip movements apparently did not influence bowel function or the formation of adhesions.

Clips are often applied in laparoscopic procedures. The clip technique used in this investigation may influence the anastomotic technique for laparoscopic surgery. Further experiments have been designed to apply this technique in laparoscopy.

REFERENCES

1. Jacobs M, Verdeja JC, Goldstein HS. Minimally invasive colon resection (laparoscopic colectomy). Surg Laparosc Endosc 1:144-156, 1991.
2. Waninger J, Kauffmann GW, Shah IA, et al. Influence of the distance between interrupted sutures and the tension of sutures on the healing of experimental colonic anastomosis. Am J Surg 163:319-323, 1992.
3. Herzog B. The one-layer and two-layer intestinal anastomosis in animal experiments. Prog Pediatr Surg 5:27-59, 1973.
4. Ballantyne GH. The experimental basis of intestinal suturing. Effect of surgical technique, inflammation and infection on enteric wound healing. Dis Colon Rectum 27:61-71, 1984.
5. Herrmann JB, Woodward SC, Pulaski EJ. Healing of colonic anastomosis in the rat. Surg Gynecol Obstet 119:269-275, 1964.
6. Jiborn H, Ahonen J, Zederfeldt B. Healing of experimental anastomoses. The effect of suture technique on collagen concentration in the colonic wall. Am J Surg 135:333-340, 1978.
7. Halsted WS. Circular suture of the intestine. An experimental study. Am J Med Sci 94:436-460, 1887.

83   *Unusual Stapling Procedures in the Upper Gastrointestinal Tract*

Louis R.M. Del Guercio

Over the past 25 years the surgical armamentarium has been augmented by the variety of surgical stapling instruments developed through the cooperative efforts of innovative surgeons and persevering engineers at U.S. Surgical Corporation in Norwalk, Conn. Surgeons familiar with the capabilities and proper use of these devices have used them to solve technical problems and expedite operative procedures when confronted by unexpected pathology or anatomical variants during operation.

One example of tactical use of surgical staples is the case of a 28-year-old female police officer severely injured in an automobile crash. She had bilateral tension pneumothoraxes and pulmonary contusions, a sternal fracture, and bilateral Le Fort II fractures. Four days after a difficult endotracheal intubation, she underwent bronchoscopy and esophagoscopy and was found to have a disruption of the posterior trachea at the level of the carina and, at that same intrathoracic level, through-and-through lacerations of the esophagus.[1] She was transferred to the Westchester Medical Center where a right thoracotomy was performed. Fig. 1 illustrates the large tracheal defect revealed after the mediastinal pleura was opened. Ventilation was controlled by guiding the larger endotracheal tube down the left mainstem bronchus and inserting a second smaller endotracheal tube through the tracheostomy and guiding it into the right bronchus. For 7 days postoperatively she was placed on two parallel volume-cycled ventilators and then was jet ventilated through the trache-

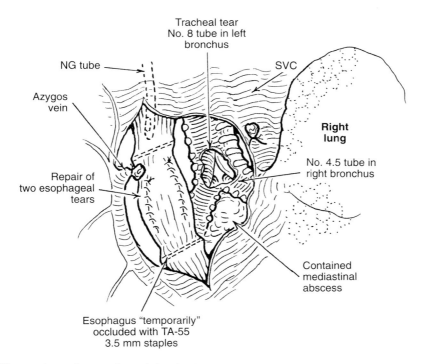

Fig. 1. Traumatic tracheoesophageal fistula showing double-tube ventilation and in-continuity exclusion and repair of esophagus.

439

ostomy until she was weaned to spontaneous respiration 10 days later.[2] Fig. 1 also shows the repair of the two esophageal lacerations with "temporary" segmental exclusion of the esophagus using TA-55 3.5 mm staples. Fig. 2 depicts the mobilization of the excluded esophageal segment and its use as a muscular patch to repair the defect in the membraneous trachea. Bronchoscopy 3 weeks after operation revealed complete reepithelialization of the tracheal defect, and barium esophagography demonstrated free flow into the stomach with only slight narrowing at the site of the injury. The patient recovered completely. This case illustrates the well-known principle that a staple line across a mucosa-lined hollow viscus will disrupt spontaneously because of a lack of fibrotic healing.[3]

Malignant tracheoesophageal fistulas resulting from advanced upper third esophageal cancer's invasion of the trachea are a severe test of palliative skills. Our results over the years with esophageal stents have been dismal, and the best palliation has been achieved with retrosternal reversed gastric tubes anastomosed to the transected esophagus in the neck. A tube is placed in the excluded distal esophagus for decompression and as a conduit for high-intensity intracavitary brachytherapy. GIA stapling instruments applied consecutively several times along the greater curvature of the stomach expedite the operation, which is well tolerated by these debilitated patients. It has not been necessary to reinforce the stapled gastric tube.

In our last 90 patients with esophageal malignancies, my colleagues and I have used transfemoral azygograms for staging. We have found this technique superior to computed tomography or magnetic resonance scanning. When the azygos vein was free of invasion, all of the esophageal cancers were resectable.

Unresectable carcinomas of the distal esophagus or proximal stomach are best palliated through left thoracotomy and diaphragmatic mobilization of the gastric fundus and greater curvature. Esophagogastrostomy for alimentary tract continuity is established either side-to-side, using the GIA instrument, or end-to-side, using the TA-55 and curved end-to-end anastomosis (CEEA) devices. This approach provides good exposure for the brachy-therapists who may prolong life by implanting the cancer with radioactive iodine seeds.

Various mediastinal tumors provide opportunities for novel uses of stapling instruments. Blood loss and air leaks are reduced by stapling across pulmonary adhesions. The vascular pedicles in both curative resections and debulking procedures are best managed using the

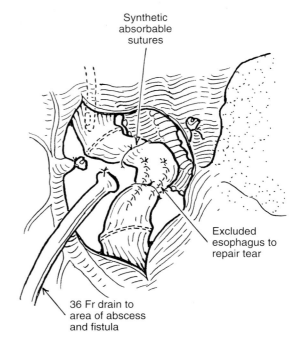

Fig. 2. Use of excluded esophageal segment for repair of membranous trachea.

Roticulator series of staples, which can be maneuvered between the structures of the mediastinum can be dangerous to handle.

Pulsion diverticula of the esophagus and benign intramural tumors lend themselves to resection using the TA instruments. These resections are best performed with a large diameter intraluminal bougie in place.

Chylothorax that does not respond to pleural drainage and total parenteral nutrition can be a difficult problem to manage surgically.[4] Such a case is illustrated by Fig. 3. A 65-year-old man with an epidermoid carcinoma of the right upper lobe had metastases to the chest wall, mediastinum, right lower lobe, and diaphragm. The primary tumor and the metastases to the lower lobe and diaphragm were removed by segmental resection and wedge resection, respectively. Thirty-five iodine-125 seeds were inserted in the areas of pleural and mediastinal involvement. Chylothorax became evident 3 days after operation and was refractory to nitrogen mustard and bleomycin pleurodesis and 2 weeks of total parenteral nutrition. On the thirty-first postoperative day the right side of the chest was reexplored after instillation of 300 ml of olive oil in the stomach. When the pleural space was entered, chyle was seen oozing from

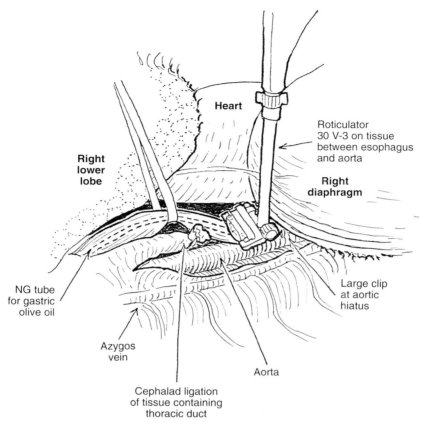

Fig. 3. Roticulator stapling of thoracic duct tissues for persistent chylothorax.

multiple pores on the mediastinal pleura. The distal esophagus was mobilized and the aortic hiatus identified. The spongy, inflamed prevertebral tissue between the aorta and the esophagus was stapled using the 30 V-3 roticulator and transected. The chylous leakage stopped immediately and never recurred. The patient subsequently received 45 Gy of external beam radiation and survived for 2 years.

Few surgeons realize the utility of surgical staples in pancreatic surgery. The TA-55 4.8 mm instrument provides a secure closure across the pancreas in distal pancreatectomies whether or not there is inflammation or chronic scarring. During the performance of Whipple resections the purse-string suture instrument and CEEA anastomotic device speed the reestablishment of gastrointestinal continuity, especially in the pylorus, preserving variation of the pancreaticoduodenectomy. In addition, during the final tedious stages of the pan-

creatic resection, the tissues behind the superior mesenteric vein beyond the uncinate process can be stapled with the TA-55 3.5 mm instrument. When minimal invasion of the portal or superior mesenteric vein is found, the 30 V-3 roticulator can be used for a rapid and safe tangential resection of the involved vein.

Rinecker and Danek[5] and later our group[6,7] have described the use of the GIA instruments without the cutting blade for performing emergency portal azygos disconnections in patients with bleeding gastroesophageal varices. Application of the quadruple line of hemostatic staples to the anterior and posterior walls of the gastric cardia through a gastrotomy high on the lesser curvature is an easier, safer, and more effective procedure than transection and reanastomosis of the distal esophagus using the EEA device. When combined with application of the special GIA stapler across the gastropancreatic fold, which contains the coronary vein and left gastric artery, and with midsplenic artery ligation, this approach to sclerotherapy failures is an effective and fast means of portal azygos disconnection.

With the recent emphasis on minimally invasive surgery, the surgical department at the New York Medical College, Valhalla, working in close cooperation with the interventional radiologists, have developed the following approach to bleeding varices in sclerotherapy failures. First, celiac angiography is performed with occlusion of the midsplenic artery using Gianturco thrombogenic coils. This significantly reduces the splenic contribution to portal flow and pressures.[8] It also reduces the secondary hypersplenism associated with portal hypertension. The next step in the protocol is a minilaparotomy with cannulation of a mesenteric vein for access to the portal vein and the collaterals feeding the gastric and esophageal varices. Absolute alcohol and Gianturco coils are used to clot these coronary and short gastric veins. The long-term rebleeding rate after this angiographic portal azygos disconnection is approximately 30%, but the mortality rate is low.[9] When the recurrent hemorrhage is caused by varices and new collaterals, it is managed by transjugular intrahepatic portacaval shunting (TIPS) using Wall stents.[10]

CONCLUSION

Surgeons today have been blessed with a magnificent variety of diagnostic and therapeutic tools and devices. Surgeons with a thorough knowledge of how and when to use these gifts of modern technology and who are masters of anatomy and physiology can make greater achievements in the treatment of the ill and injured than ever before.

REFERENCES

1. Ladin DA, Dunnington GL, Rappaport WD. Stapled esophageal exclusion in acute esophageal rupture: A new technique. Contemp Surg 35:45-46, 1989.
2. Brimioulle, S, Rocmans R, de Rood M, et al. High-frequency jet ventilation in the management of tracheal laceration. Crit Care Med 18:338-339, 1990.
3. Ravitch MM, Rivarola A, Van Grov A. Studies of intestinal healing. Preliminary studies of the mechanism of healing of the everting intestinal anastomosis. Johns Hopkins Med J 121:343-350, 1967.
4. Robinson CLN. The management of chylothorax. Ann Thorac Surg 39:90-95, 1985.
5. Rinecker H, Danek N. Operative Behandlung blutender Oesophagus-Variceu durch eine subkardiala Blutsperre mittels transmuraler maschineller Klammerung. Chirugie 46:87-93, 1975.
6. Del Guercio LRM, Hodgson WJB, Morgan JC, et al. Splenic artery and coronary vein occlusion for bleeding esophageal varices. World J Surg 8:680-687, 1984.
7. Del Guercio LRM. The esophageal varices problem. In Ravitch M, Steichen FM, eds. Principles and Practice of Surgical Stapling. Chicago: Year Book, 1987, pp 154-162.
8. Del Guercio LRM, Cohn JD, Kazarian KK, et al. A shunt equation for estimating the splenic component of portal hypertension. Am J Surg 135:70-75, 1978.
9. Berman HL, Del Guercio LRM, Hodgson WJB, et al. Minimally invasive devascularization for variceal hemorrhage that could not be controlled with sclerotherapy. Surgery 104:500-506, 1988.
10. Zemel G, Katzen BT, Becker GJ. Percutaneous transjugular porto-systemic shunt. JAMA 266:390-394, 1991.

84 *The Mechanical Colostomy*

G. Chiara, C. Caldato, M. Barban, O. Gualandi, and T. Tommaseo

Although the widespread use of stapling devices in low colorectal surgery has markedly reduced the need for abdominoperineal resection (even in low rectal cancers that might be treated radically by anterior resection with stapled anastomosis), Miles' operation remains the treatment of choice for tumors located <5 cm from the anal verge.

In those patients and in those who undergo Hartmann's operation for palliation or as a temporary solution, the construction of the colostomy, which will continue to affect the patient's well-being, must be accurate. The colostomy technique introduced by Chung and Burke[1] in 1986, which involves the use of a mechanical suture apparatus, reduces the incidence of complications and thus improves the patient's quality of life.

We will report our experience with stapled colostomy.

MATERIALS AND METHODS

From August 1989 to August 1991, 29 patients (18 men and 11 women) underwent mechanical colostomy in the First Department of Surgery at the Regional Hospital of Treviso. In the patients studied (18 of whom underwent Miles' operation and 11 of whom underwent Hartmann's operation), colostomies were performed with a Premium CEEA (PCEEA) circular stapler with a 31 mm cartridge in all except two cases; in those a 28 mm stapler was used because of the small diameter of the colon. Patients were followed regularly every 6 months for 2 years to detect late complications.

TECHNIQUE (Figs. 1 through 3)

When the abdomen was opened and the colon was transected, a purse-string suture was inserted and was drawn around the shaft of the anvil previously introduced into the colonic stump. The parietal peritoneum was then incised from inside the abdomen, the muscular layer of the abdominal wall was split, and the fascia was cut to obtain a space in which the colon could be placed comfortably. Particular care was required while the subcutaneous tissue was dissected up to the dermis. The anvil shaft was then brought through the newly made tunnel into the abdominal wall, and when the skin was perforated, the stapler cartridge was attached from the outside to the anvil shaft, and the instrument was closed and fired, opposing the colonic wall to the dermis. The colon was then anchored by stitches to the parietal peritoneum.[2,3] A sterile adhesive bag was immediately placed on the stoma to avoid contamination of the wound and the abdominal cavity by the feces contained in the colonic loop.

RESULTS

The use of a stapling device in performing a colostomy produces good functional and aesthetic results and a low complication rate. Table 1 shows the complications we

Table 1. Complications of stapled colostomy during 2-year follow-up (n = 29)

Complication	Patient Incidence	Percent of Patients
Parastomal ventral hernia	3/29	10.3
Stenosis	2/29	6.6
Mucosa prolapse	—	—
Partial wound dehiscence	1/29	3.4

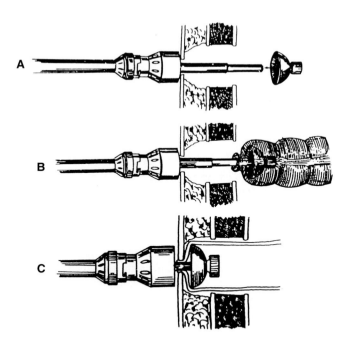

Fig. 1. With the abdomen still open, the peritoneum and abdominal wall are incised from the inside and a funnel is created up to the dermis at the site selected for colostomy. **A,** The central rod of the EEA instrument is advanced inside the abdomen through a stab wound in the skin, and the anvil is attached. **B,** The anvil is advanced into the proximal colon and the purse-string suture is tightened. **C,** The anvil is closed against the cartridge, carrying with it the colon into the abdominal wall funnel and compressing it against the undersurface of the skin. As the EEA is activated, the colon is stapled to the skin, and an ostomy results.

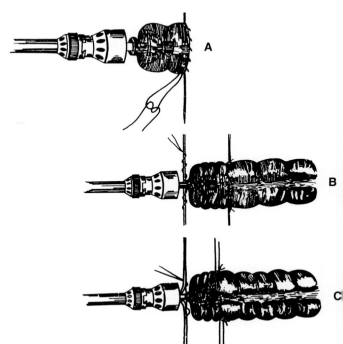

Fig. 2. Technique used when the abdomen is closed first. **A,** The site selected for colostomy is cored out and a purse-string placed in the skin circumference. The proximal colon end is exteriorized and the EEA anvil, attached to the cartridge rod, is placed into the colon end. The colon purse-string is tightened. **B,** The colon end, containing the anvil, is pushed back into the abdomen. To accomplish this step, the anvil is left temporarily at an appropriate distance from the cartridge. After placing colon and cartridge into the abdominal wall funnel, the skin purse-string is tightened. **C,** Cartridge and anvil are closed and the instrument is activated, as in Fig. 1, *C*.

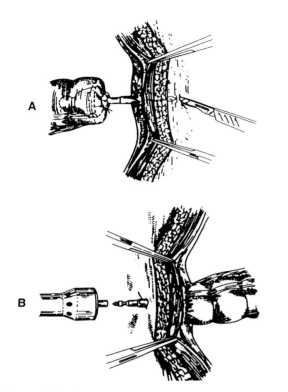

Fig. 3. With the PCEEA instrument the cartridge can be placed into the colon and its trocar used to penetrate through the skin. **B,** The cartridge is then attached and the procedure completed, as in Fig. 1, *C*, and Fig. 2, *C*.

observed during a follow-up period of ≤2 years in the 29 patients who had undergone a stapled colostomy. Of the two patients (6.8%) with stenosis of the stoma, one required reoperation and creation of a new stoma. In both instances, the small caliber of the colon required a 28 mm stapler instead of a 31 mm stapler.

A peristomal herniation, which probably resulted from an excessive opening of the muscular layer, occurred in three of the first patients who underwent mechanical colostomy. A partial suture dehiscence that was observed in one patient on the second postoperative day was closed with interrupted sutures. No patients experienced wound infection in the main incision, or colostomy wound or mucous prolapse.[4]

The two lines of staples usually detach spontaneously within 60 days postoperatively; if this does not happen, the staples must be removed to prevent abnormal tissue reactions that result in stenosis.

DISCUSSION

A stoma may adversely affect the quality of life of a patient to a greater extent than does the disease. The construction of a complication-free colostomy is an essential prerequisite for the psychophysical well-being of the patient.

Complications such as peristomal dermatitis or herniation, retraction, and stenosis result in part from negligence in this phase of intervention.

A stapling device can be used to perform a colostomy easily, quickly, and effectively. The double row of metal staples at the mucocutaneous suture line, which acts as an effective seal may prevent infection of the subcutis and possible peristomal suppuration and fistulas. Less manipulation of the colon stump that is anastomosed to the cutis (as well as the lack of stitches) minimizes tissue trauma, reduces postoperative edema, and permits quick restoration of colostomy function.

The stapled colostomy offers many advantages, including better functional and aesthetic results, reduced operating time, and a low complication rate. The comparatively higher cost of the procedure is the primary disadvantage, but in our opinion, the procedure offers many benefits for the patient, and the speed at which a stapled colostomy can be performed results in cost savings.

Both early and long-term results in our series of 29 stapled colostomies are very encouraging and seem to be satisfactory for the patient as well as for the surgeon.

CONCLUSION

The mechanical colostomy in which a stapler is used is an easily and quickly performed intervention that is well-tolerated by the patient and is almost free of complications.

From August 1989 to August 1991, 29 stapled colostomies were performed at our institution after Miles' and Hartmann's operations were performed for rectal cancer or complicated diverticulitis. We analyzed the complications that occurred from the stapled colostomies and the late functional results. We conclude that as a result of the low complication rate and the slight difference in cost, the mechanical colostomy, when performed with a 31 mm cartridge, is an intervention of choice because it results in reduced operating time, earlier restoration of intestinal function, and a better aesthetic result.

REFERENCES

1. Chung RS, Burke, B. End colostomy and Brooke's ileostomy constructed by surgical stapler. Surg Gynecol Obstet 162:62, 1986.
2. Demma I, Genova G, Agnello G. L'impiego della suturatrice meccanica circolare nel confezionamento delle colostomie terminali. Riv Ital Coloproct 6:87, 1987.
3. Rizzo S, Gubitosi A, Di Giacomo R, Campanile R. La colostomia mediante EEA stapler. Presented at the Atti VI Congresso Nazionale Chir, Naples, 1988.
4. Corno F. Le complicanze degli stomi ed il loro trattamento. Presented at the Atti 91 Congresso, Soc Ital Chir, 1989.

85 *The Double-Stapling Technique in Colorectal Reconstruction*

Charles D. Knight, Sr., F.D. Griffen, and Charles D. Knight, Jr.

The double-stapling technique for colorectal reconstruction after low anterior resection involves closing the lower rectal segment with a linear stapler and performing the anastomosis using a circular stapler across the linear staple row. In 1980 we described this method for stapled low rectal anastomosis,[1] which is a modification of the original technique pioneered by Ravitch and Steichen.[2] Our experience includes 82 primary anastomoses and 11 secondary anastomoses after Hartmann procedures and is the basis for this report.

PRIMARY COLORECTAL ANASTOMOSIS
Materials and Methods

From June 1979 to May 1991, we performed primary colorectal anastomoses in 82 patients using the double-stapling technique. There were 38 men and 44 women. Fifty-seven patients had carcinoma of the colorectum, 20 had diverticulitis, 3 had carcinoma of the ovary, one had sigmoid volvulus, and one had rectal prolapse (Table 1). Among the 57 patients with cancer of the colorectum, 19 had tumors 6 to 8 cm from the anal verge, 13 had tumors 9 to 10 cm from the anal verge, and 25 were above 10 cm (Table 2). Table 3 shows the level of the anastomoses after resection. Twenty-two were below 6 cm.

Technique

The double-stapling technique, as originally described, utilized standard linear and circular staplers. In 1988 U.S. Surgical Corporation modified its circular EEA stapler, the Premium CEEA (PCEEA), and TA-55 lin-

Table 1. Indications for operation

Diagnosis	Number
Carcinoma of the colorectum	57
Diverticular disease	20
Carcinoma of the ovary	3
Volvulus of the sigmoid colon	1
Prolapsed rectum	1

Table 2. Distance of tumor from anal verge

Distance (cm)	Number
6-8	19
9-10	13
11 and above	25

Table 3. Distance of anastomosis from anal verge

Distance (cm)	Number
3-6	22
7-9	21
10-13	39

ear stapler (Roticulator 55), making them even more effective for this procedure. Our current technique using these instruments has been described[3] and is detailed here.

With the patient in the lithotomy-Trendelenburg position, providing for the simultaneous exposure of abdomen and perineum, the abdomen is entered through a low midline incision, and the abdominal cavity is explored. The rectosigmoid colon is mobilized as in any other anterior resection, and if it is determined that a low anterior resection is feasible, the mesorectum is divided below the anticipated lower margin of resection. The 4.8 mm Roticulator 55—a TA-55 stapler modified to rotate at its neck—is placed across the rectum at the distal margin of resection, angled to give optimal ex-

posure and resection margin, closed, and activated (Fig. 1). Pressure can be applied to the perineum by an assistant to elevate the region of dissection, aiding in exposure. A long right-angle clamp is placed proximal to the staple line to prevent soilage, and the rectum is divided along the edge of the stapler. The automatic purse-string instrument is applied at the proximal resection margin. An Ochsner clamp is placed distal to the purse-string instrument, and the colon is transected (Fig. 2). A noncrushing clamp is applied across the proximal colon, and the purse-string instrument is removed. Sizers are passed proximally into the lumen. If only the small sizer will enter, the 28 mm cartridge can be used; if the middle sizer will enter the lumen, the 31 mm cartridge is chosen. We caution against the use of the 25 mm cartridge for this anastomosis; it may be too small to accommodate the doughnut from the thick-walled rectum, and the risk of symptomatic stenosis may be increased.

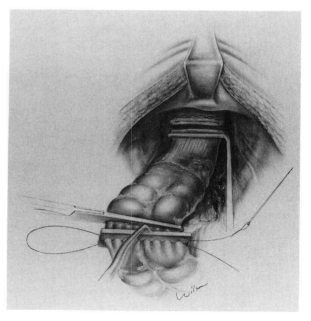

Fig. 1. After the rectosigmoid colon has been mobilized, the Roticulator 55 stapler is applied at the lower limit of the resection and a double row of staples is placed. (From Griffen FD, Knight CD Sr, Whitaker JM, Knight CD Jr. The double stapling technique for lower anterior resection—results, modifications, and observations. Ann Surg 211:745, 1990; with permission.)

Fig. 2. A long right-angle clamp is placed proximal to the staple line, and the rectum is divided along the edge of the stapler. After the upper limit of resection is selected, the mesentery is divided and the colon is incised between the purse-string instrument proximally and an Ochsner clamp. (From Knight CD, Griffen FD. An improved technique for low anterior resection of the rectum using the EEA stapler. Surgery 88:710, 1980; with permission.)

The anvil shaft assembly is then placed in the proximal bowel through the purse-string (Fig. 3), and the purse-string is tied into the groove on the shaft. The intestinal clamp can then be removed. With the edge of the anvil used as the proximal extent of dissection, the fatty appendices and mesentery are removed, allowing approximation of the bowel wall rather than fat at the anastomosis.

Attention is then turned to the perineum. The instrument tray is moved to allow the surgeon access to the anal area. The rectal segment is irrigated transanally with sterile water under pressure using an irrigating syringe to assess for leaks or staple failures (Fig. 4). In high anterior resections, if the distal pouch is too long to distend with 50 ml of fluid, a Foley catheter can be used through the anus to facilitate irrigation with larger quantities of water. Any leaks detected are repaired with sutures.

The PCEEA stapler is introduced into the rectal segment with the center rod retracted within the cartridge. The cartridge is advanced to the Roticulator 55 staple line, and the rod with the trocar attachment is extended a sufficient length to allow transmural visualization anterior or posterior to the staple row. It is then advanced through the rectal wall adjacent to the staple line (Fig. 5). The trocar is removed and the anvil shaft is inserted into the rod (Fig. 6). The PCEEA is closed and activated to make a circular end-to-end inverting anastomosis (Fig. 7). No attempt is made to include the entire circumference of the rectal segment—only that part that matches the proximal colon.

Two or three partial-thickness mattress sutures of 3-0 silk are placed across the anastomosis when technically feasible. The PCEEA is then opened no more than three complete turns and the instrument is removed, using the mattress sutures for countertraction. The tissue in the chamber is checked to ensure that two complete rings or doughnuts are present. A shoestring clamp is placed across the colon above the staple row, and the integrity of the anastomosis is checked by irrigating the rectum with water under pressure (Fig. 8). An alternative is insufflation with air instead of irrigation with water, first filling the pelvic dead space with saline. If leaks are detected, they are repaired with silk sutures. A sump drain, covered with a Penrose drain, is placed deep within the pelvis and brought through a stab wound in the left lower quadrant. The pelvic peritoneum is not sutured. The abdomen is closed in the usual manner.

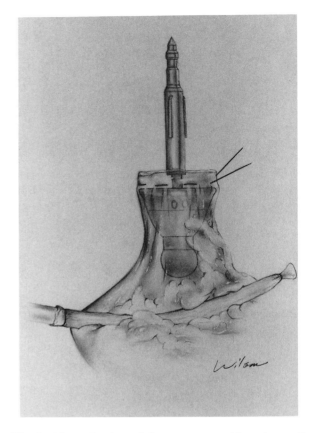

Fig. 3. After selection of the proper cartridge, the anvil shaft assembly is detached from the central rod and placed in the proximal bowel through the purse-string, and the suture is tied into the groove on the shaft. (From Griffen FD, Knight CD Sr, Whitaker JM, Knight CD Jr. The double stapling technique for low anterior resection—results, modifications, and observations. Ann Surg 211:745, 1990; with permission.)

Results

Intraoperative complications were infrequent in our series. All doughnuts were complete. Minor water leaks were noted in four anastomoses; these were repaired with sutures. There was no intraoperative anastomotic disruption. Protective colostomy was not performed in this series. Postoperative complications were also rare: three patients developed an anastomotic leak and each healed without additional surgery for drainage or diverting colostomy. Two patients developed stenosis that required treatment. A benign stricture at 10 cm was

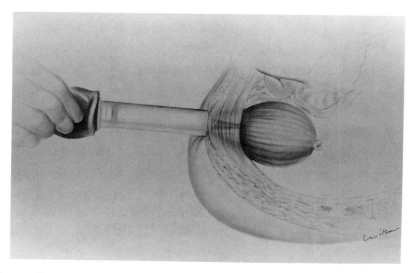

Fig. 4. The rectal segment is irrigated with water under pressure from an irrigating syringe to ascertain leaks or staple failures. (From Knight CD, Griffen FD. An improved technique for low anterior resection of the rectum using the EEA stapler. Surgery 88:710, 1980; with permission.)

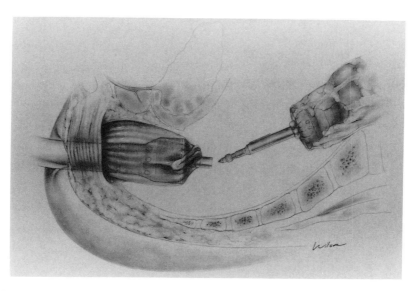

Fig. 5. The PCEEA stapler is introduced into the rectal segment with the anvil shaft assembly removed and the center rod with the trocar attachment retracted within the cartridge. The instrument is advanced, placing the cartridge against the linear staple row. The center rod is extended, passing the trocar into the abdominal cavity adjacent to the staple line; then the trocar is removed. (From Griffen FD, Knight CD Sr, Whitaker JM, Knight CD Jr. The double stapling technique for low anterior resection—results, modifications, and observations. Ann Surg 211:745, 1990; with permission.)

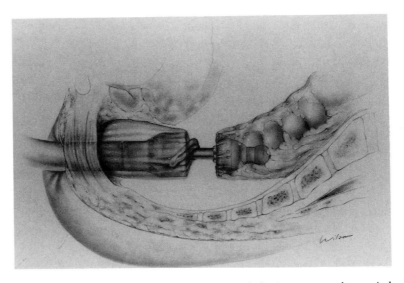

Fig. 6. The anvil shaft is inserted into the center rod and the instrument closure is begun. (From Griffen FD, Knight CD Sr, Whitaker JM, Knight CD Jr. The double stapling technique for low anterior resection—results, modifications, and observations. Ann Surg 211:745, 1990; with permission.)

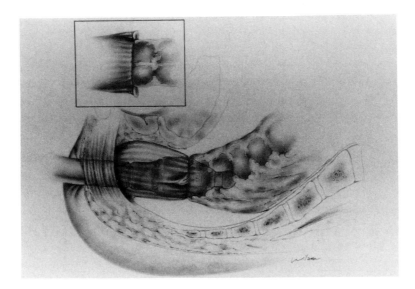

Fig. 7. The PCEEA stapler is closed and activated to make the circular end-to-end inverting anastomosis. No attempt is made to include the entire circumference of the rectal segment; only that part that matches the proximal colon is included. (From Griffen FD, Knight CD Sr, Whitaker JM, Knight CD Jr. The double stapling technique for low anterior resection—results, modifications, and observations. Ann Surg 211:745, 1990; with permission.)

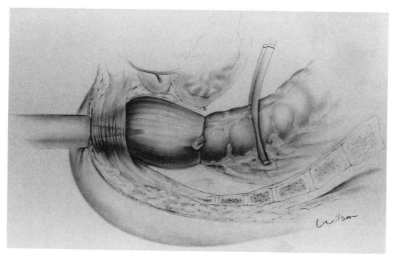

Fig. 8. After the stapler is removed, a shoestring clamp is placed across the colon above the anastomosis, and the integrity of the anastomosis is checked by irrigating the rectum with water under pressure. Leaks are repaired with silk sutures. (From Knight CD, Griffen FD. An improved technique for low anterior resection of the rectum using the EEA stapler. Surgery 88:710, 1980; with permission.)

treated with digital dilation, and a second high stricture required resection using the EEA stapler. One patient had bleeding from a branch of the left superior hemorrhoidal artery, requiring reoperation. Three patients had occasional fecal spotting for 3 weeks, 3 months, and 6 months, but no patient was permanently incontinent. There were no operative deaths. There were 45 patients with cancer who were available for routine follow-up: four had local pelvic recurrence, but data regarding local recurrence are insufficient for statistical evaluation.

Discussion

Circular staplers provide a safe colorectal anastomosis at a lower level than previously possible with other intra-abdominal techniques. The double-stapling technique offers additional advantages: (1) It obviates the technical frustration involved in placing the distal purse-string suture, permitting a lower anastomosis in some patients; (2) the rectal segment is not opened, which minimizes contamination and allows for irrigation of the lower segment; and (3) it avoids gathering on a purse-string the frequently generous circumference of the rectum at the lower margin of resection, which eliminates

puckering and thickness and provides a more precise doughnut and a safer anastomosis.

Clinical anastomotic leak is the chief parameter by which success of colorectal reconstruction is measured. Recent reports[3,4] of circular stapled colorectal anastomoses attest to the safety of the procedure with clinical leak rates of 5% or less. In addition to our series, four other reports of anastomoses performed using the double-stapling technique with appropriate data have been identified.[5-8] Excluding 13 patients with primary diverting colostomies, there are 276 anastomoses with 15 leaks, a rate of 5.4%. This includes our series, with a rate of 3.6% (Table 4).

Stenosis of EEA anastomoses is a concern. We theorize that stricture occurs because mucosa-to-mucosa approximation is precisely prevented by the EEA, which inverts all layers of the proximal colon and distal rectum between the two mucosal edges (Fig. 9). This allows the formation of granulation tissue with delayed mucosal healing, leading to circumferential fibrous contracture. Ischemia caused by the double row of staples and injury caused by compression of tissue between the anvil and cartridge may be potentiating factors. Ana-

Table 4. Incidence of clinical leaks with double-stapled primary colorectal anastomosis without diverting colostomy

Series and Year	Number	No. of Leaks	Percentage of Leaks
Feinberg et al., 1986[5]	72	6	8.3
Griffen et al., 1990[3]	82	3	3.6
Ollier et al., 1991[6]	67	4	6.0
Picciocchi et al., 1988[7]	26	0	0.0
Varma et al., 1990[8]	29	2	6.9
TOTAL	276	15	5.4

Table 5. Incidence of clinical stenosis with double-stapled primary colorectal anastomosis

Series and Year	Number	No. of Stenoses	Percentage of Stenoses
Feinberg et al., 1986[5]	79	0	0.0
Griffen and Knight, 1991	82	2	2.4
Ollier et al., 1991[6]	72	2	2.8
Picciocchi et al., 1988[7]	26	0	0.0
Varma et al., 1990[8]	30	1	3.3
TOTAL	289	5	1.7

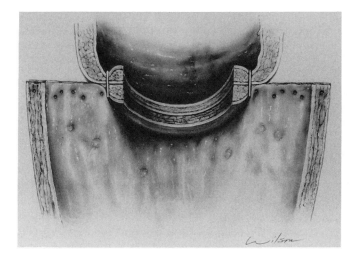

Fig. 9. Hemisection of a double-stapled colorectal anastomosis shows the precise separation of mucosal edges by the other inverted layers of bowel wall characteristic of EEA anastomoses. Healing by second intention causes a circular scar and stenosis, which is later corrected by fecal dilations. (From Griffen FD, Knight CD Sr, Whitaker JM, Knight CD Jr. The double stapling technique for low anterior resection—results, modifications, and observations. Ann Surg 211:745, 1990; with permission.)

tomical stenosis occurs to some degree in most cases and is often sufficient to prevent passage of the endoscope, but this anatomical finding is reversible with fecal dilation, allowing free passage of the endoscope usually within 9 months and always within 2 years in our experience. Stenosis requiring treatment occurred in 5 of 287 patients available for review,[5-8] an incidence of 1.7%, including our series at a rate of 2.4% (Table 5).

Information regarding local recurrence after resection for cancer with stapled reconstruction compared to hand-sewn reconstruction is important. It has been theorized that stapled anastomosis may predispose to local recurrence by causing intraluminal trauma, spilling tumor cells into the pelvis, implanting tumor cells at the staple line, or delaying healing.[9] While some early reports have suggested an increased local recurrence in patients in whom a stapling technique has been employed,[10,11] most others[4,5,12-15] demonstrated no difference between hand-sewn and stapled anastomoses.

The reason for variations in local recurrence in some nonrandomized series may relate to variables in case selection. A basic tenet in curative rectal resection is that the desire to preserve rectal continence should not influence the margins of resection. Assuming that surgeons provide at least a 2 cm distal margin regardless of the method of reconstruction, a more important predictor of local recurrence is the lateral extent of resection. Knudsen et al.[16] and Heald et al.[17] showed a significant reduction in survival in patients with tumors involving the nerves and vessels of the mesorectum; they suggested the complete removal of the mesorectum to improve recurrence rates. The importance of this concept has been emphasized by Fazio et al.,[4] who incorporated it in their technique of low anterior resection with a 2.3% local recurrence rate after curative resection. Rosen et al.[9] pointed out that anatomical variables—width of the pelvis and thickness of the mesorectum—are major factors in the extent of lateral resection and local recurrence. Patients with low tumors share these anatomical limitations and represent a subset of patients best suited for stapled reconstruction. This selection bias in retrospective reviews may affect comparative results. To date there is no evidence that stapled reconstruction affects the rate of local recurrence. Other risk factors for local recurrence after low anterior resection include advanced Dukes staging (B2 to C2 lesions) and poorly differentiated histological grades.[4]

The double-stapling technique has its greatest utility in patients with rectal carcinoma when the need for a low anastomosis is essential. We have returned to hand-sewn anastomosis in some patients with diverticular disease when the proximal bowel for anastomosis is muscular and small or the distal segment is long and tortuous. These circumstances increase the risk for misadventure with staples in a subset of patients who are ideal for sutured anastomosis.

There are three general categories of sphincter-saving procedures to consider when extended low resection with lymphadenectomy is required. These include abdominosacral resection and anastomosis, transabdominal transanal resection with coloanal anastomosis, and extended low anterior resection with stapled anastomosis. Data comparing the relative incidence of stenosis, anastomotic leak, incontinence, and local recurrence are not available. Reasons to expect differences in the incidence of local recurrence have been postulated, but we believe that all options share equally the paramount deterrent to success: the anatomically limited lateral margin of resection. Unique circumstances may occasionally dictate the procedure of choice, but most surgeons will find one approach preferable and almost always applicable. A few surgeons already skilled with the abdominosacral procedure will continue using it. Others comfortable with the ileoanal anastomosis for inflammatory bowel disease will favor the coloanal anastomosis. Many will likely prefer the extended low anterior resection using exposure and dissection with which they are already familiar.

With improved techniques for sphincter preservation after rectal resection, there is an inclination to compromise the lower margin of resection for low anterior resection in patients with carcinoma of the rectum. This should be avoided. If the same strict criteria are observed in selecting candidates for extended low anterior resection with stapled anastomosis that have been followed for low anterior resection with hand-sewn reconstruction, the recurrence and survival rates should remain the same at all levels. Of course, lower lesions still have higher local recurrence rates because of the more limited lateral resection, just as has been observed with abdominoperineal resection for very low lesions. Cure of the patient's cancer should continue to be the overriding objective and preservation of the sphincter a secondary consideration.

DELAYED COLORECTAL ANASTOMOSIS
Materials and Methods

We have utilized the double-stapling technique in 11 patients for colorectal anastomosis following Hartmann procedures. The indication for surgery was diverticulitis with perforation in nine cases, trauma in one, and rectal carcinoma with obstruction in one. The delayed anastomosis was performed in each case without protective colostomy. Our original technique has been described in detail.[18] Modifications since that report include only the improvements allowed by the availability of the PCEEA.

Technique

Patient positioning and preparation are the same as described for primary stapled anastomosis. The previously formed abdominal scar is incised and extended as necessary. Adhesions from the previous operation are divided, but extensive dissection to free up or search for the rectal stump is not necessary. The previously formed colostomy is taken down and the proximal bowel mobilized as necessary for an anastomosis without tension. This proximal stoma is then prepared for anastomosis, and the automatic instrument is used to place the purse-string. After the instrument is removed, the stoma is sized, the appropriate anvil shaft assembly is placed in the proximal bowel, and the purse-string is tied. The assistant surgeon then moves to the perineum and sizers are passed transanally into the rectal pouch. This serves several purposes. First, it dilates the relatively unused pouch so that it will accommodate the cartridge more easily. Moreover, it allows the surgeon to see the optimal site on the rectal stump for anastomosis. It gives the assistant surgeon a feel for the course of the pouch with a smooth, relatively atraumatic instrument that helps later for safely passing the CEEA stapler. Finally, it shows the surgeon where to provide additional but limited dissection on the pouch needed for adequate approximation of the bowel at the time of anastomosis. When the site for anastomosis on the rectal pouch is selected, the CEEA stapler is introduced into the rectum with the trocar recessed into the cartridge. It is cautiously advanced to the anastomotic site, taking care to avoid accidental perforation of the rectum. Then the trocar is passed through the rectal wall, and the anastomosis performed as described for primary stapled anastomosis. When mobilization of the rectum is not required during the primary operation, the long, tortuous segment that results is difficult to negotiate with the CEEA stapler, increasing the risk of rectal injury by the cartridge. We minimize this hazard in these cases by using a catheter passed through the rectal pouch from above to guide the passage of the instrument. This

is accomplished by placing a short stab wound at the proposed anastomotic site, using the sizer in position as a guide. Through this stab wound an 18 Fr rubber catheter is passed into the rectum and retrieved transanally by the assistant surgeon. Its tip is then cut off and the cut end fit snugly over the trocar or center rod. The center rod is then guided by the catheter safely up the rectum through the stab wound. The anastomosis is completed and tested as described for primary anastomosis.

Results

In our series of 11 patients there were no anastomotic leaks and no deaths. One patient developed a clinically significant stricture that was corrected successfully at laparotomy by excising the stricture with the circular stapler introduced transanally, advancing the center rod through the stricture, and applying the anvil shaft through a colotomy above the stricture. After the stricture was excised, it was retrieved transanally as a solitary doughnut with the stapler.

DISCUSSION

Others have reported techniques for double-stapled anastomosis after Hartmann procedures.[19-21] Five additional cases are available for comparison of results from these reports; no anastomotic leak or stenosis occurred.

We believe that secondary circular stapled reconstruction is best used for patients who have Hartmann procedures for obstructive carcinoma of the rectosigmoid colon, and we continue to be enthusiastic about its use in this situation. When surgery is required for diverticulitis, it is our practice to resect only the bowel involved with complications of diverticula. We have noted technical difficulty with performing stapler anastomosis in these patients, who typically have long tortuous rectal segments and small, thick muscular proximal bowel. Eight of our 11 cases were performed by 1984,[18] indicating that we have returned to hand-sewn techniques except for cases with short rectal segments and more normal proximal bowel. For those whose bias is to remove longer segments of diverticula-laden bowel, shorter less tortuous rectal segments and larger less muscular proximal bowel will make both primary and delayed double-stapled anastomosis more useful.

We had early enthusiasm for end-to-side stapled anastomosis when the rectal segment was long and tortuous.[18] We now feel that these anastomoses may be more prone to stricture, are difficult to pass endoscopically should the need arise, and may be difficult to dilate should stricture develop, even with the balloon techniques recently described.[22] A high end-to-side anastomosis resulted in the only stricture in our experience that required operative treatment.

REFERENCES

1. Knight CD, Griffen FD. An improved technique for low anterior resection of the rectum using the EEA stapler. Surgery 88:710, 1980.
2. Ravitch MM, Steichen FM. A stapling instrument for end-to-end inverting anastomosis in the gastrointestinal tract. Ann Surg 189:791, 1979.
3. Griffen FD, Knight CD Sr, Whitaker JM, Knight CD Jr. The double stapling technique for low anterior resection—results, modifications, and observations. Ann Surg 211:745, 1990.
4. Fazio VW, Tjandra JJ. Primary therapy of carcinoma of the large bowel. World J Surg 15:568, 1991.
5. Feinberg SM, Parker F, Cohen Z, Jamieson CG, Myers ED, Railton RH, Langer B, Stern HS, McLeod RS. The double stapling technique for low anterior resection of rectal carcinoma. Dis Colon Rectum 29:885, 1986.
6. Ollier JC, Gavioli-Ferrari M, Adloff M. Abdominal side-to-end colo-rectal anastomosis with circular stapling instruments. In Ravitch MM, Steichen FM, Welter R, eds. Current Practice of Surgical Stapling. Philadelphia: Lea & Febiger, 1991, pp 289-294.
7. Picciocchi A, D'Ugo DM, Duurastante V, Cardillo G. Double stapling technique for low colorectal anastomoses after anterior resection for rectal cancer. Int Surg 73:19, 1988.
8. Varma JS, Chan ACW, Li MKW, Li AKC. Low anterior resection of the rectum using a double stapling technique. Br J Surg 77:888, 1990.
9. Rosen CB, Beart RW, Ilstrup DM. Local recurrence of rectal carcinoma after hand-sewn and stapled anastomoses. Dis Colon Rectum 28:305, 1985.
10. Anderberg B, Enblad P, Sjodahl R, Wetterfors J. Recurrent rectal carcinoma after anterior resection and rectal stapling. Br J Surg 70:1, 1983.
11. Hurst PA, Prout WG, Kelly JM, Bannister JJ, Walker RT. Local recurrence after low anterior resection using the staple gun. Br J Surg 69:275, 1982.
12. Woulmark N, Fisher B. An analysis of survival and treatment failure following Duke B and C rectal carcinoma: A report of the NSABP clinical trials. Ann Surg 204:480, 1986.
13. Ohman U. Curative potential of EEA stapler in rectal carcinoma. Acta Chir Scand 152:59, 1986.
14. Colombo PL, Foglieni CLS, Morone C. Analysis of recurrence following curative anterior resection and stapler anastomoses for carcinoma of the middle third and lower rectum. Dis Colon Rectum 30:457, 1986.
15. Belli L, Beati CA, Frangi M, Aseni P, Rondinara BF. Outcome of patients with rectal cancer treated by stapled anterior resection. Br J Surg 75:422, 1988.
16. Knudsen JB, Nilsson T, Sprechler M, Johansen A, Christensen N. Venous and nerve invasion as prognostic factors in postoperative survival of patients with resectable carcinoma of the rectum. Dis Colon Rectum 26:613, 1983.
17. Heald RJ, Husband EM, Ryall ROH. The mesorectum in rectal cancer surgery—the clue to pelvic recurrence? Br J Surg 69:613, 1982.
18. Griffen FD, Knight CD. Stapling technique for primary and secondary rectal anastomoses. Surg Clin North Am 64:579, 1984.
19. Caracciolo F, Castrucci G, Castigioni GC. Anastomosis with EEA stapler following Hartmann procedure. Dis Colon Rectum 29:67, 1986.
20. Lucarini L, Barigazzi A, Sciandra C, Iannucci P. Restoration of continuity of the large intestine with the Premium CEEA stapler: A new aseptic method. Acta Chir Scand 156:633, 1990.
21. Mittal VK, Cortez JA. Hartmann procedure reconstruction with EEA stapler. Dis Colon Rectum 215:1981.
22. Pietropaolo V, Errara MM, Montori A. Endoscopic dilation of colonic postoperative strictures. Surg Endosc 4:26, 1990.

86 The Triple-Stapled Technique: Further Progress in Colorectal Anastomosis

Juan Santiago Azagra, Martine Goergen, and Michel Ceuterick

First described by F.M. Steichen in 1988 at the First European Congress on stapling in surgery, the triple-stapled (TST) technique is a new, entirely mechanical, end-to-end colorectal anastomosis that eliminates the problem of manipulating the bursa or placing a purse-string suture in one or both extremities of the anastomosis. In this chapter we present our series of 95 patients who underwent colorectal anastomosis using TST technique.

MATERIALS AND METHODS

Ninety-five patients underwent TST technique. The technique associates a circular mechanical suture, using the PCEEA instrument, with two linear staple lines, using either a TA or EndoGIA stapler, according to the approach chosen. This results in an end-to-end colorectal anastomosis that is entirely mechanical.

The steps of TST anastomosis for these two different approaches are compared in the boxes on pp. 456 and 457.

From September 1988 to September 1992 we performed 95 colorectal anastomoses using TST technique on 31 men and 64 women with an average age of 64 years (range, 20 to 84).

Seventy-eight patients underwent anterior resection of the rectum using a classic laparotomy approach, and 17 underwent rectosigmoid colectomy using a strictly celioscopic approach. Forty-seven patients with cancer, 20 with diverticulitis, 15 with rectal prolapse, seven with dolichosigmoid and idiopathic constipation, and six with diverse pathological conditions (three endometrioses, two irradiation stenoses, and one iatrogenic stenosis were treated) (Fig. 1). None of the patients in our series underwent an emergency procedure.

The size of the anastomosis and the instruments used are comparatively presented in Fig. 2 according to the approach used.

None of the anastomoses was protected by colostomy. All of the anastomoses were radiologically controlled using a water-soluble contrast medium at approximately the eighth postoperative day.

Text continued on p.462.

STEPS OF TST TECHNIQUE IN TOTAL LAPAROSCOPIC RECTOSIGMOID COLECTOMY

1. Closure of the distal colon by endo-slipknot.
2. Section of the proximal colon by EndoGIA stapler.
3. Section of the rectum by endoshears.
4. Transanal introduction of PCEEA and intra-abdominal withdrawal of the anvil.
5. Transanal evacuation of the specimen.
6. Closure of the rectal stump by EndoGIA stapler.
7. Partial antimesenteric incision of the proximal colon by endoshears.
8. Introduction of the anvil into the proximal colon anchored by a suture to the anterior colon wall, proximal to its closure.
9. Closure of the proximal colon by EndoGIA stapler.
10. Traction on the anchoring suture advances the pointed anvil stem through the EndoGIA staple line into the abdominal cavity using the Laso to exteriorize the stem of the anvil.
11. Transanal introduction of the PCEEA and trocar perforation of distal staple line.
12. Connection of the anvil stem into the hollow stapler rod.
13. Closing and firing of the PCEEA, creating the totally laparoscopically stapled colorectal end-to-end anastomosis.

STEPS OF TST TECHNIQUE IN ANTERIOR RESECTION OF RECTUM BY LAPAROTOMY

1. Closure of distal end of the rectum with TA-55 (Fig. 3).
2. Anvil stem introduced into the proximal colon (Fig. 4).
3. Closure of colon with TA-55 (Fig. 5).
4. Stem of anvil pushed through center of proximal staple line (Fig. 6).
5. Curved PCEEA with trocar is advanced transanally to pierce the distal staple line (Fig. 7).
6. Anvil stem is connected to the stapler stem (Fig. 8).
7. PCEEA is closed and fired (Fig. 9).
8. Totally stapled colorectal end-to-end anastomosis is created (Fig. 10).

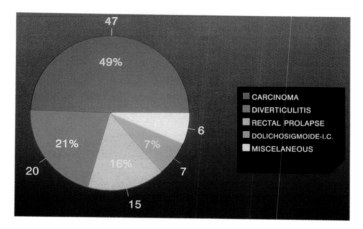

Fig. 1. Pathological factors in 95 cases.

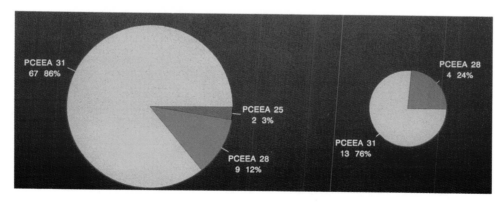

Fig. 2. Size of anastomosis (PCEEA diameter). *ARR* = anterior resection of the rectum, 78 cases; *TLRSC* = totally laparoscopic rectosigmoid colectomy, 17 cases.

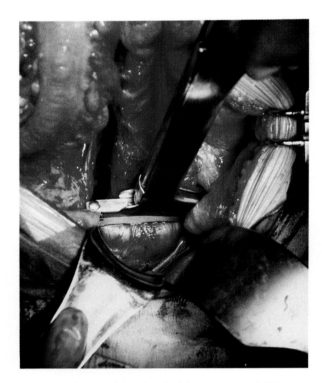

Fig. 3. Closure of distal end of the rectum with TA-55.

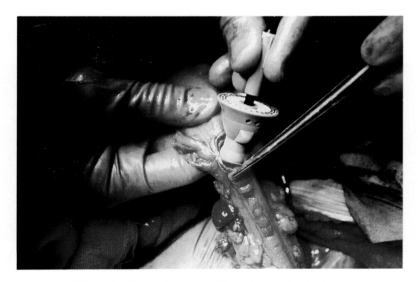

Fig. 4. Anvil stem introduced into the proximal colon.

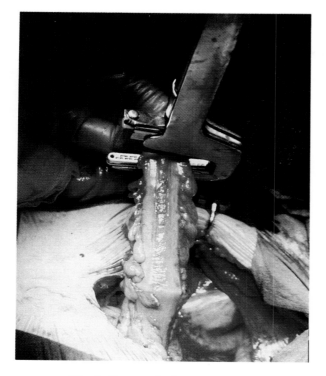

Fig. 5. Closure of colon with TA-55.

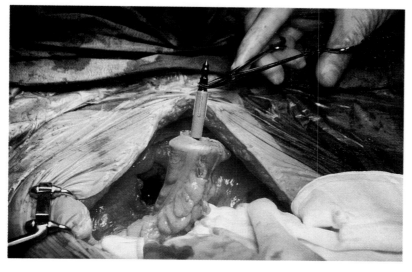

Fig. 6. Stem of anvil pushed through center of proximal staple line.

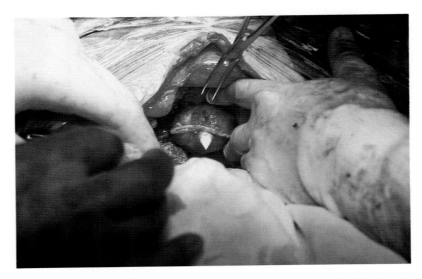

Fig. 7. Curved PCEEA with trocar is advanced transanally to pierce the distal staple line.

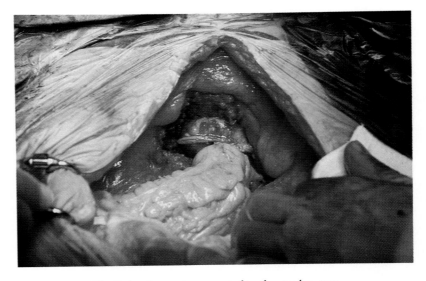

Fig. 8. Anvil stem is connected to the stapler stem.

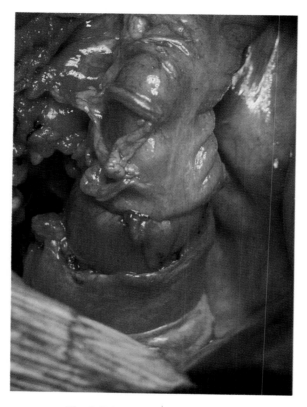

Fig. 9. PCEEA is closed and fired.

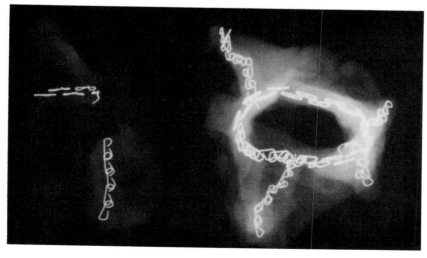

Fig. 10. Totally stapled colorectal end-to-end anastomosis is created.

RESULTS

Mortality, perioperative complications, and complications up to the thirtieth postoperative day are listed in Table 1, late complications in Table 2.

DISCUSSION

Described by Steichen[1] in 1988 at the First Congress on Stapling in Surgery in Luxembourg, the end-to-end colorectal anastomosis using TST technique is simple, rapid, and entirely mechanical, allowing a systematic approach to the placement of "high-risk staples" such as those used in anterior resection of the rectum by completely avoiding the manual or mechanical introduction of a purse-string suture. This type of anastomosis is reproducible from one case to another with no problems arising from colorectal differences in size and wall thickness. This would seem to augment the security of the anastomosis.

Table 1. Perioperative and postoperative complications of TST technique

Complications	"Open Air" Technique (78 cases)	Laparoscopic Technique (17 cases)
Clinical fistula	2 (healing TPN)	1 (using Hartmann's procedure, death from MOF)
Radiological fistula	2	0
Perioperative fecal spill	0	0
Perioperative hemorrhage	0	0
Postoperative hemorrhage	0	1 (medical treatment)
Deep abscess	0	0
Wound infection	6	0
Prolonged ileus	4	0
Lung infection	6	0
Urinary infection	7	0
Methylene blue test	2	0
Intact tissue rings	All	All
Duration of intervention (min)		
Mean	135	240
Range	105 - 200	150 - 330

TPN = total parenteral nutrition; MOF = multiple organ failure.

Table 2. Late complications of TST technique

Complications	"Open Air" Technique (78 cases)	Laparoscopic Technique (16 cases)
Stricture	2 (endoscopic dilations)	0
Wound dehiscence	4	0
Impotence	1	0
Retrograde ejaculation	1	0
Fecal incontinence	0	0

in size and wall thickness. This would seem to augment the security of the anastomosis.

As of 1989 Julian, Kolachalam, and Wolmark[2] reported a series of experimental data that validate TST technique and suggest its high performance in anterior resection of the rectum. We reported our satisfactory preliminary experience with 25 patients in 1990 at the ninety-second French Congress of Surgery in Paris.[3] Mortality and morbidity in our present series corroborate our results. Three patients developed a clinical fistula and two a radiologically proven fistula. The two strictures in our series were found in this group. Two of the clinically proven fistulas healed while the patient received total parenteral nutrition. The two strictures were treated successfully by endoscopic dilation.

The one death in our series occurred in an 83-year-old woman, ASA 3, who had an extensive sigmoid carcinoma and who was operated on using the celioscopic approach. She developed a fistula that was discovered late in her postoperative course and that caused multiple organ failure resistant to treatment.

It appears TST technique is particularly well adapted to celioscopic surgery because it allows performance of rectosigmoid colectomies while avoiding laparotomy.

CONCLUSION

TST technique allows the creation of an entirely mechanical terminoterminal colorectal anastomosis that is systematic and reliable. It does not seem to increase the risk of developing fistulas or stenotic sequelae. TST technique has a choice place in colorectal surgery by celioscopy, allowing us to achieve secure anastomoses while totally avoiding laparotomy.

REFERENCES

1. Steichen FM. Changing concepts in surgical techniques. In Ravitch MM, Steichen FM, Welter R, eds. Current Practice of Surgical Stapling. Proceedings of Second International Symposium and First European Congress on Stapling in Surgery, Luxembourg, 1988. Philadelphia: Lea & Febiger, pp 23-27, 1990.
2. Julian TB, Kolachalam RB, Wolmark N. The triple stapled colonic anastomosis. Dis Colon Rectum 32:989-995, 1989.
3. Azagra JS. Triple suture mécanique termino-terminale dans la résection antérieure du rectum. Techniques et résultats. Presented at 92ème Congrès Francais de Chirurgie. Eurochirurgie 90. Paris: October 1-4, 1990.

---

87 *Comparative Study of Manual Versus Mechanical Sutures in Colorectal Anastomoses and Clinical Consequences*

Arnulf Thiede

Colorectal anastomoses are accomplished by various types of manual sutures, by staples mechanically,[1-3] or by compression rings.[4-5] Comparative examinations in controlled studies showed no basic differences between right- and left-sided colonic resections or between manual suture techniques, stapled anastomotic techniques, and compression anastomoses performed in comparable locations. Among various perioperative target criteria, the rate of leakage has predominated.[6-8] However, when the target criterion of stricture is observed, it tends to occur more often when stapled anastomoses are used,[9,10] compared with other techniques that employ fully absorbable materials such as biofragmentable compression rings.[5,11] We have been conducting trials with stapled anastomoses since 1979 and with biofragmentable compression rings since 1989, in the colorectal region as well as other areas. The boxes on p. 464 summarize our perioperative strategy and the features of stapled anastomoses. I will present and analyze the results of these trials (Table 1).

CURRENT PERIOPERATIVE STRATEGY IN ELECTIVE COLON AND RECTAL SURGERY

- Diagnosis and spread of disease substantiated by:
  Endoscopy and biopsy, contrast enema (Welin)
  External sonography, CT scan
  Clinical staging, endosonography
- Preoperative orthograde lavage, perioperative antibiotic prophylaxis
- Operative technique: high ligation of vessels, systematic lymphadenectomy
- Intraoperative cleansing of bowel stumps with chloramine
- Preoperative, intraoperative, and postoperative measurement of tumor, distance to margins of resection, location of anastomosis from mucocutaneous junction
- Attention to criteria of radical surgery
- Definitive histological diagnosis of tumor type, grade, and stage
- Postoperative control of anastomosis, day 6 to 10, with Peritrast RE enema
- Follow-up examinations at 3-month intervals
- Clinical analysis and manometry of anorectal function before and 3 and 6 months after rectal resection

STANDARD FEATURES OF STAPLED ANASTOMOSES

Domain	Middle and lower third of rectum
Strategy	Transanal end-to-end anastomosis
Technique	Two circles of alternating B-shaped inverting staples
Stapling devices	PCEEA, ILS-stapler
Diameter of rings	33, 31, 29, and 28 mm
Auxiliary tool	Rectal stamp
Advantages	Technical ease (surgeon)
	Expanded indications (patient)
Disadvantages	Cost of operative procedure
	Nonabsorbable metal staples
	Tissue reaction
	CT interference

Table 1. Studies of anastomotic techniques in colorectal surgery

Technique	Period of Study	Form of Study	No. of Patients	Anatomical Region
Stapled	1978-1979	Pilot	82	Colorectal
Stapled versus manual	1979-1982	Controlled	31/29	Rectal
Stapled	1983-1988	Prospective	970	Colorectal
Valtrac ring	1989-	Prospective	152	Colorectal

MATERIALS AND METHODS
Controlled Study 1979 to 1982

Elective colon and rectum resections were guided by strict adherence to the criteria of our current perioperative approach and strategy for such operations. The anastomosis between the colon and rectum was made basically end to end. The rectal purse-string suturing required for the use of the circular anastomosing instrument in the deep pelvis was always performed manually. A rectal stamp (Figs. 1 and 2), centered by the anal canal, allows pressure to be extended onto the perineum and pelvic floor. Depending on the degree of resistance from the perineum, this maneuver elevates the rectal stump by 2 to 4 cm into the pelvis and makes placement

of purse-string sutures safe, even along the edge of short rectal stumps.[27] In hand-sewn anastomoses the posterior wall is created by a double-row technique and the anterior wall by a single row.[2]

Since 1979 this controlled study (stapled versus manual sutures) has been planned and executed as follows (Fig. 3): only those patients were included whose disease was localized in or extended from above into the rectum. With the abdomen opened, a check for resectability was done. Escape cases were defined as those patients who for oncological reasons required abdominoperineal resection or palliative treatment with an endcolostomy. After resection, patients were randomly assigned to one of two groups: group A (hand-sutured

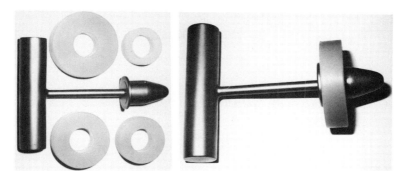

Fig. 1. Rectal stamp made of metal adaptable to four different anatomical dimensions with the use of exchangeable elastic silicon rings of various sizes.

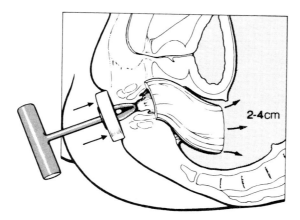

Fig. 2. Schematic illustration of the rectal stamp during application.

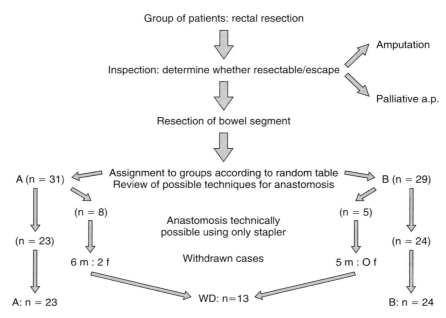

Fig. 3. Planning and execution of the controlled trial. (*A* = hand suture; *B* = planned stapled suture; *WD* = withdrawn cases [operable, continuity restored only by stapler]).

anastomoses; n = 31) or group B (stapled anastomoses; n = 29). At the postresection assessment to determine whether both anastomotic techniques were possible, eight patients in group A and five in group B were eliminated, because in these cases intestinal continuity could only be restored by stapler technique. This third group (n = 13) was designated the withdrawn (WD) group.

In the controlled trial, groups A, B, and WD were analyzed with particular regard to sex distribution. Additional analytic parameters were 6-month mortality, intraoperative and postoperative data, postoperative complications, and the results of 5-year follow-up ending in 1987.

Prospective Study 1983 to 1988

Subsequent to the 1979-1982 controlled study, a prospective trial was conducted in which a stapled anastomotic technique—similar to the one used in groups B and WD of the controlled study—was employed exclusively in 970 patients who required anastomoses to the rectum. The target parameters used in postoperative examinations like frequency of leakage, was subdivid-

ed into primary, secondary, and tertiary leaks (Table 2). Additional target parameters included the following: fistulas, subdivided into presacral, colorectocutaneous, and rectovaginal fistulas; strictures resulting from operative technique; and in-hospital mortality.

RESULTS
Controlled Trial 1979 to 1982

Sixty patients were initially divided randomly into two groups of 31 with sutures (group A) and 29 with staples (group B); however, by the end of the trial this distribution had changed to 23 patients with planned manual sutures and 24 with planned staples, plus a third group of 13 patients who had been withdrawn from groups A and B (group WD). All of the anastomoses in group WD were located in the lower third of the rectum, four at 6 to 8 cm and nine very deep at 3 to 5 cm. The 13 patients in group WD included 11 men and two women (Table 3). Whereas in groups A and B the sex distribution was comparable (about 40% men and 60% women), there was a significant difference in group WD: 85% men versus 15% women (Table 4). In analyzing intraoperative and postoperative data (Table 5), a

Table 2. Anastomotic leaks

Designation	Cause	Evidence	Time of Appearance
Primary leak	Failure of instrument or assembly by OR personnel	Incomplete anastomosis intraoperatively	Intraoperatively
Secondary leak	Anastomotic blood flow	X-ray examination on day 6-10	Postoperative day 6-10
Tertiary leak	Pericolic abscess breaking through anastomosis	Clinical and radiological, from postoperative day 12	From postoperative day 12, first radiological control study before day 12 (no evidence of dehiscence)

Table 3. Distribution of withdrawn cases: controlled trial 1979-1982

Location of Anastomosis	No.	WD Cases*	Males	Females
Middle third of rectum and higher (9 cm and higher)	11	—	—	—
Lower third of rectum				
6-8 cm	28	4	4	—
3-5 cm	21	9	7	2
TOTAL	60	13 (21.6%)	11	2

*Preservation of bowel continuity possible only by use of stapler.

Table 4. Distribution by sex of withdrawn cases: controlled trial 1979-1982

Group	No.	Males	Females	Males	Females
A	23	9 (39.1%)	14 (60.9%)		
B	24	10 (41.7%)	14 (58.3%)		
WD*	13	11 (84.6%)†	2 (15.4%)†	11/30 (36.7%)	2/30 (6.7%)
TOTAL	60	30 (50%)	30 (50%)	Males + females = 21.6%	

*Preservation of continuity possible only by use of stapler.
†WD group differs significantly from groups A and B at the 1% level.

few points must be emphasized. The median for anastomotic locations was deepest with x = 5 cm distance from the mucocutaneous junction in group WD. In 84% of patients the 31 mm PCEEA cartridges (U.S. Surgical Corp.) were used. For the duration of operation, as well as during postoperative hospitalization, both group A (manual sutures) and group WD had a less favorable course than group B (planned staples). Cecal decompression fistulas were left intubated with a Petzer catheter. Spontaneous closure of the cecal decompression fistulas occurred later in the group with manual sutures (x = 24 days) than in both groups with stapled anastomoses (x = 14 days).

Analysis of postoperative complications overall showed more dehiscences of sutures in group A and group WD. Few of these were clinically relevant, and in group B they were not statistically significant (Table 6). Early strictures (radiological evidence) prevailed in group A but with no clinical relevance. The spontaneous closure of cecal fistulas occurred after a median of 24 days in group A (hand sutures) versus only 14 days in both groups B and WD (stapled), which might have been an indication of transitory edema of the manually sutured anastomoses in group A.

The elevated rate of postoperative disturbance of vesical function in group WD (46%) should be considered a consequence of the extensive dissection deep in the true pelvis. In most instances, vesical function returned spontaneously or was restored with nonoperative treatment.

The mortality rate during hospitalization was 1.7%, and the total 6-month mortality rate was 8.3% (for distribution and causes see Table 7). Results of 5-year follow-up in cancer patients showed no significant differences (Table 8). It should be emphasized that the rate of locoregional recurrence—that is, local relapses originating from lymphatic metastases of the lateral pelvic wall—was equal in all three groups. It should also be noted that cancer patients were operated on with strict adherence to the guiding principles of radical surgery. The value of systematic follow-up was confirmed by the early endoscopic removal of polyps in 25% and radically operable secondary carcinomas in 4% (Table 8) of all surviving patients in this controlled study.

The controlled trial confirmed the following:

1. In approximately 22% of rectal resections, intestinal continuity was restored only with the EEA stapler technique.
2. Group A (manual sutures) and group B (staples) remained comparable despite withdrawal of some patients. Group WD differed significantly from groups A and B.
3. The majority of withdrawn patients were men with a narrow pelvis and a firm pelvic floor.
4. In the group with manual sutures, planned cecal fistulas for decompression closed spontaneously with some delay.
5. The stapler offers obvious technical advantages in male patients with a narrow pelvis and a firm pelvic floor.

Table 5. Analysis of intraoperative and postoperative data: controlled trial 1979-1982

Parameter	No.	A	B	WD	Total
Location of anastomosis (cm)	60	x = 3	x = 6	x = 5	x = 6 cm
Staple cartridge	37/60				
% green, 31 mm		—	x = 83	x = 85	x = 84
% blue, 28 mm		—	x = 17	x = 15	x = 16
Duration of operation (hr)	60	x = 3	x = 2.5	x = 3	x = 2.5 hr
Postoperative hospital stay	60	x = 17	x = 15	x = 17	x = 15 days
Cecal decompression fistula (%)	48	74	83	85	80
Diverting colostomy (%)	9	17	13	15	15
Postoperative days with cecal catheter intubation	48	x = 11	x = 11	x = 14	x = 14 days
Spontaneous closure of cecal fistula (days)	48	x = 24	x = 14	x = 14	x = 14 days

Table 6. Analysis of postoperative complications: controlled trial 1979-1982

Complication	No.	Study Groups A (%)	B (%)	WD (%)	Total (%)
Disturbance of wound		4.3	4.3	15.3	6.7
Secondary anastomotic insufficiency					
Total	60	39.1*	12.6	53.9*	31.7
Evident		27.7	8.3	30.8	18.3
Filiform		11.4	4.3	23.1	13.3
Clinically significant	60	8.7	—	15.4	6.6
Colocutaneous fistula	60	4.3	—	23.0	6.7
Stricture (x-ray)					
Total	60	39.1*	—	7.7	16.7
Absolute 0 >1 cm		4.3	—	—	1/7
Relative 0 1-2 cm		34.8*	—	7.7	15.0
Clinically significant	60	4.3	—	—	1.7
None 0 >2 cm	60	60.9*	100.0	92.3	83.3
Postoperative disturbance of bladder function		4.3	4.2	46.2*	13.3

*Highly significant differences.

Table 7. Six-month mortality: controlled trial 1979-1982

Parameter	No.	Study Groups* A	B	WD	Total
Primary mortality (in hospital)	60	4.4%	—		1.7%
Reasons		Peritonitis from suture insufficiency and mitral disease III			
Secondary mortality (within 6 months)		8.7%	8.3%	7.7%	8.3%
Reasons		1X lung embolus	1X cardiac failure		
		1X tumor	1X tumor	1X tumor	

*No significant differences among groups.

Table 8. Follow-up results

Parameter	No.	Group A	B	WD	Total
Diagnosis of carcinoma	54	20	22	12	54
Five-year mortality	60	12	11	2	25/60 (42%)
Independent of cancer	60	5	3	1	9/60 (15%)
Metastases	54	5	6	—	11/54 (20%)
Locoregional recurrence	54	2	2	1	5/54 (9%)
Type of recurrence (pelvic wall)		2	2	1	5
Five-year survival	60	11	13	11	35 (58%)
Polyps removed after first operation	60	6	4	5	15 (25%)
Second operation for carcinoma	54	—	1	1	2 (4%)

6. The location of the anastomosis had a greater influence on continence than the anastomotic technique.

7. With strict adherence to the principles of radical surgery, the type of anastomotic technique does not influence the development of locoregional recurrence.

RESULTS
Prospective Study 1983 to 1988

In the prospective study from 1983 to 1988, a total of 970 patients were treated. Of the anastomoses performed in these patients, 533 were located at 9 cm and higher, 213 at 6 to 8 cm, and 224 at 3 to 5 cm. The finding common to all anastomotic locations was: the deeper the location, the higher the rate of insufficiency (Table 9). For secondary leaks (discovered on days 6 to 10) the clinically relevant rate of insufficiency was only half as important as the radiological evidence (radiological rate of insufficiency, 11%, clinically relevant rate of insufficiency, 5%). Tertiary leaks rarely occurred (1%).

Postoperative anastomotic fistulas were present in 7% of patients. They were subdivided into presacral (5%), colorectocutaneous (1.5%), and rectovaginal (0.5%) types. Presacral fistulas healed after a median of $x = 33$ days and colorectocutaneous fistulas after $x = 18$ days (Table 10). Strictures attributed to technical difficulties were observed in 3.8% (Table 11). They had limited clinical relevance, however. Very deeply located strictures were easily treated by transanal dilation. In rare instances (0.3%) transanal reoperation was required.

The primary mortality rate (Table 12) during hospitalization was low (2.6%). This rate was subdivided into deaths attributed solely to technical problems (0.3%), deaths occurring as a consequence of other existing diseases (1.2%), and deaths resulting from a combination of existing disease and technical difficulties (1.1%). The low rate of complications related to technical mishaps (0.3%) in this large series is evidence of the advantage of high-grade standardization, adherence to sound strategic and technical guidelines, and use of special tools and instruments that create comparable working conditions for surgeons with varying degrees of expertise.

DISCUSSION

With the development of circular stapling instruments based on the original Russian models,[12,13] into practical and reliable devices, the modern stapling instruments produced in the United States have revolutionized the technical steps of gastrointestinal surgery during the past two decades.[14] Modern gastrointestinal surgery without stapling instruments is now a fantasy. The use of staplers may also stimulate completely new surgical strategies, as has already occurred in minimally invasive surgery. A significant advantage for the patient needing rectal surgery[15] is expansion of the indications

Table 9. Anastomotic leaks: prospective trial 1983-1988

Location of Anastomosis	No.	Primary	Secondary		Tertiary
			Radiological	Clinical	
9 cm or higher	533	11 (2%)	32 (6%)	16 (3%)	—
6-8 cm	213	9 (4%)	30 (14%)	11 (5%)	2 (1%)
3-5 cm	224	16 (7%)	47 (21%)	25 (11%)	6 (3%)
TOTAL	970	36 (4%)	109 (11%)	52 (5%)	8 (1%)

Table 10. Fistulas: prospective trial 1983-1988

Location	No.	Presacral	Duration (days) X (range)	Colorecto-cutaneous	Duration (days) X (range)	Rectovaginal
9 cm or higher	533	8	26 (8-53)	8	19 (8-35)	—
6-8 cm	213	9	27 (8-96)	4	17 (8-37)	4
3-5 cm	224	28	38 (8-227)	3	18 (8-45)	2
TOTAL	970	45 (5%)	33 (8-227)	15 (1.5%)	18 (8-45)	6 (0.5%)

Table 11. Strictures caused by surgical technique (partially membranous—of obscure origin): prospective trial 1983-1988

Location of Anastomosis	No.	Temporary	Clinically Permanent	Transanal Reoperation
9 cm	533	8	3	1
6-8 cm	213	8	4	2
3-5 cm	224	9	2	—
TOTAL	970	25 (2.5%)	9 (1%)	3 (0.3%)

Table 12. Primary mortality rate during postoperative hospitalization (n = 25; 2.6%): prospective trial 1983-1988

Location of Anastomosis	No.	Technical Difficulties	Other Existing Disease	Combined
9 cm or higher	533	—	2	3
6-8 cm	213	1	6	4
3-5 cm	224	2	4	3
TOTAL	970	3 (0.3%)	12 (1.2%)	10 (1.1%)

and feasibility of rectal resections that preserve continuity. In addition greater technical ease and functional reliability are provided to the surgeon and his or her team. In very deep colorectal or even coloanal anastomoses, an astonishingly high degree of continence can be achieved after an interval of 3 to 6 months.[16-18]

The higher rate of local recurrence with the use of circular staplers, as reported by Rosen et al.,[19] occurs mainly when the distance between the lower edge of the tumor and the distal line of resection is less than 2 cm.[20] During our operations we took particular care to adhere to the principles of radical surgery and did not allow a distance of less than 2 cm between the lower edge of the tumor and the line of resection. The rate of local recurrence after 5 years observed in our trial was therefore only 9%, a figure that reemphasizes the need to observe the criteria for radical surgery, as was also pointed out by Heald.[21]

The following technical developments should be mentioned briefly: the double stapling technique[22,23,26]; triple stapling technique[14,24]; and the colorectal or coloanal pouch.[1,25]

The primary purpose of the pouch is to replace the rectal ampulla and restore the initially lacking reservoir function after very deep anastomoses. The value of this strategy has not yet been confirmed by long-term studies. On the one hand, in patients with a simple, very deep colorectal anastomosis some reservoir function will return after several months; however, in patients with artificial reservoirs, the possibility of obstipation must be considered.

The purpose of the triple stapling technique is mainly to reduce the rate of contamination in intestinal resections in the true pelvis. Actual findings, however, are limited experimental and modest clinical data.[14,24] Septic complications rarely occur in rectal resections when the following precautions are taken: exact preoperative bowel cleaning, mainly by an orthograde lavage, antibiotic prophylaxis, intraoperative local cleaning and disinfection of the bowel stumps and the true pelvis. The following disadvantages should also be mentioned: they include the higher cost involved in stapling techniques, along with the increased production of collagen in the stapled areas, which might favor the formation of stenoses and strictures.[9]

Larger clinical trials with the double stapling technique have been studied. Knight et al.[23] emphasized the shorter duration of operation, the simple tissue handling, and the low incidence of septic complications, Moritz et al.[26] compared the simple EEA anastomosis with the double stapling technique in a controlled study. Their results favored the double-stapling technique using the target criterion of a secondary anastomosis insufficiency. In relatively small series, however, differences were not statistically significant.

It seems important to mention the rectal stamp,[27] which facilitates essentially every type of suture technique of short stumps in the deep pelvis. This is true for manual and end-to-end stapled anastomosis, as well as for double stapling techniques. In principle, it has the same effect as a fist pushing the pelvic floor into the abdomen, an effect described by Fazio[1] as follows: "Perineal pressure will 'elevate' the low rectal segment to facilitate construction of the anastomosis."

CONCLUSION

In a controlled trial (n = 60), mechanical EEA stapled anastomoses were compared with hand-sutured anastomoses after rectal and rectosigmoid resections. The anastomosis was end-to-end in both groups. The trial demonstrated the practical advantages of staples, including applicability and expansion of the indications for operations to preserve continuity, especially in men. Subsequently the EEA stapled suture technique was examined in 970 patients in a prospective series. The result was a very low rate of complications and secondary anastomotic leaks, with clinical relevance in only 5%, and an equally low mortality rate of 2.6%, with 0.3% attributed to technical difficulties. The incidence of stenoses or strictures was equally low. These results were discussed with regard to the degree of standardization and the guiding principles for choosing a particular technique.

REFERENCES

1. Fazio VW. Circular stapling techniques for low rectal and anal anastomoses. In Ravitch MM, Steichen FM, Welter R, eds. Current Practice of Surgical Stapling. Philadelphia: Lea & Febiger, 1991, pp 273-284.
2. Thiede A, Jostarndt L, Schröder D, et al. Prospective and controlled studies in colorectal surgery: A comparison of hand-sutured and stapled rectal anastomoses. In Ravitch MM, Steichen FM, eds. Principles and Practice of Surgical Stapling. Chicago: Year Book Medical Publishers, 1987, pp 432-436.
3. Wolmark N. Comparison of stapling and manual anastomoses after resection for malignant disease of colon and rectum. In Ravitch MM, Steichen FM, eds. Principles and Practice of Surgical Stapling. Chicago: Year Book Medical Publishers, 1987, pp 463-479.

4. Hardy TG Jr, Aguilar PS, Stewart WRC. Initial clinical experience with biofragmentable ring in sutureless bowel anastomosis. Dis Colon Rectum 30:55-61, 1987.

5. Thiede A, Schubert G, Klima L. Enterale Anastomosen mit dem biofragmentierbaren Valtrac-Ring. Chirurg 62:819-824, 1991.

6. Cahill CJ, Betzler M, Gruwez JA, et al. Sutureless large bowel anastomoses: European experience with biofragmentable anastomosis ring. Br J Surg 76:344-347, 1989.

7. Corman ML, Prager ED, Hardy G, et al., and the Valtrac (BAR) Study Group. Comparison of the Valtrac biofragmentable anastomosis ring with conventional suture and stapled anastomosis in colon surgery. Results of a prospective, randomized clinical trial. Dis Colon Rectum 32:183-187, 1989.

8. Bubrick MP, Corman ML, Cahill CJ, et al., and the BAR Investigating Group. Prospective, randomized trial of the biofragmentable anastomosis ring. Am J Surg 161:136-143, 1991.

9. Dziki AJ, Duncan MD, Harmon JW, et al. Advantages of handsewn over stapled bowel anastomosis. Dis Colon Rectum 34:442-448, 1991.

10. Luchtefeld MA, Milsom JW, Senagore A, et al. Colorectal anastomotic stenosis: Results of a survey of the ASCRS membership. Dis Colon Rectum 32:733-736, 1989.

11. Schubert G, Klima J, Schmidt L, et al. Kolonanastomosen mit dem neuen biofragmentierbaren Valtrac-Ring: Indikation, Technik und erste Erhfarungen mit 151 Anastomosen. Chir Praxis 45:53-64, 1992.

12. Ravitch MM. Historical perspective and personal viewpoint. In Ravitch MM, Steichen FM, Welter R, eds. Current Practice of Surgical Stapling. Philadelphia: Lea & Febiger, 1991, pp 3-11.

13. Steichen FM. Inspiration and rationale for the development of mechanical sutures. In Ravitch MM, Steichen FM, Welter R, eds. Current Practice of Surgical Stapling. Philadelphia: Lea & Febiger, 1991, pp 13-22.

14. Ravitch MM, Steichen FM, Welter R. Current Practice of Surgical Stapling. Philadelphia: Lea & Febiger, 1991.

15. Beart RW, Kelly KA. Randomized prospective evaluation of EEA stapler for colorectal anastomoses. Am J Surg 141:143-147, 1981.

16. Jostarndt L, Thiede A, Lau G, et al. Die anorektale Kontinenz nach manueller und maschineller Anastomosennaht. Ergebnisse einer kontrollierten Studie in der Rektumchirurgie. Chirurg 55:385-390, 1984.

17. Nakahara S, Itoh H, Mibu R, et al. Clinical and manometric evaluation of anorectal function following low anterior resection with low anastomotic line using an EEA stapler for rectal cancer. Dis Colon Rectum 31:762-766, 1988.

18. Beart RW Jr. Coloanal procedure for rectal neoplasms. In Ravitch MM, Steichen FM, Welter R, eds. Current Practice of Surgical Stapling. Philadelphia: Lea & Febiger, 1991, pp 305-310.

19. Rosen CB, Beart RW, Ilstrup DM. Local recurrence of rectal carcinoma after hand-sewn and stapled anastomoses. Dis Colon Rectum 28:305-309, 1985.

20. Rubbini M, Vettorello GF, Guerrera C, et al. A prospective study of local recurrence after resection and low stapled anastomosis in 183 patients with rectal cancer. Dis Colon Rectum 33:117-121, 1990.

21. Heald RJ. Low stapled anastomosis: A means of improving pelvic dissection technique in rectal cancer surgery. In Ravitch MM, Steichen FM, eds. Principles and Practice of Surgical Stapling. Chicago: Year Book Medical Publishers, 1987, pp 499-511.

22. Knight CD, Griffin FD. An improved technique for low anterior resection of the rectum using the EEA stapler. Surgery 88:710-714, 1980.

23. Knight CD, Griffin FD, Whitaker JM, et al. Stapled colo-rectal anastomosis through stapled distal rectum. In Ravitch MM, Steichen FM, Welter R, eds. Current Practice of Surgical Stapling. Philadelphia: Lea & Febiger, 1991, pp 295-304.

24. Julian TB, Kolachalam RB, Wolmark N. The triple-stapled colonic anastomosis. Dis Colon Rectum 32:989-995, 1989.

25. Lazorthes F, Fages P, Chiotasso P, et al. Resection of the rectum with construction of a colonic reservoir and colo-anal anastomosis for carcinoma of the rectum. Br J Surg 73:136-138, 1986.

26. Moritz E, Achleitner D, Hölbling N, et al. Single versus double stapling technique in colorectal surgery. A prospective randomized trial. Dis Colon Rectum 34:495-497, 1991.

27. Thiede A. Rectumstempel. Ein einfaches Instrument zur Erleichterung von Rekonstrucktionen der colorectalen Passage im kleinen Becken. Chirurg 63:72-73, 1992.

88 *Stapled Versus Hand-Sewn Anastomosis for Rectal Cancer*

Gianfranco Fegiz, Marileda Indinnimeo, Stefano Valabrega, Francesco D'Angelo, Giovanni Ramacciato, Luciano Curella, and Paolo Annessi

The advantages of using stapling devices in surgery are still being investigated.[1-3] Nevertheless, almost every surgical team has evaluated these devices and their differences of opinion are significant. Use of stapling devices in colorectal and coloanal anastomosis has been discussed with regard to morbidity and long-term results as compared to hand-sewn anastomosis. Since our experience with these types of anastomoses includes more than 600 patients, we have matched two groups consisting of a total of 247 patients with stapled or hand-sewn techniques and carried out a statistical analysis of clinical and oncological results.

MATERIALS AND METHODS

We evaluated a consecutive series of 247 patients with rectal cancer, who were treated by anterior resection. Ages ranged from 17 to 91 (mean 60) years. Stapled end-to-end colorectal anastomosis or coloanal anastomosis with a double-stapled technique was performed in 162 patients, whereas a double-layer Dexon suture end-to-end colorectal anastomosis was performed in 85 patients.

The two groups of patients were matched with regard to morbidity (clinical follow-up: anastomotic leakage, median hospital stay, and perioperative mortality) and long-term survival (oncological follow-up: local recurrence and 5-year survival). Determination of oncological survival was possible in only 197 patients because of exclusions for perioperative mortality, distant metastases, and patients lost to follow-up (130 had stapled and 67 hand-sewn anastomoses). Statistical analysis was carried out by means of univariate (chi-square) and multivariate (Con model) techniques.

RESULTS

Statistical analysis of morbidity identified significant variables in the verification of statistical homogeneity in the two groups of patients; there was a high incidence of low rectal cancer in the group with stapled anastomoses ($p = K0.0001$). Statistically significant variables included site of tumors ($p = 0.0001$), level of anastomosis ($p = 0.0002$), tumor stage ($p = 0.001$), tumor distance

from the anal verge ($p = 0.002$), and grading ($p = 0.02$). Variables such as age, sex, length of the tumor-free margin, tumor-node-metastasis stage, distant metastases, and nodal involvement were not statistically significant. Data on the tumor site (high, middle, or low rectum) and anastomosis site (less than or more than 6 cm from the anal verge) were matched by univariate analysis in the two groups in terms of clinical leakage, median hospital stay, and perioperative mortality and no statistical significance was found.

A second statistical analysis compared 197 patients who were still alive at 5 years. The following variables were considered in this analysis: tumor site, tumor-free margin, extended surgery, grading, tumor stage, node stage, and tumor-node-metastasis stage. The statistical significance of these variables was evaluated in terms of local recurrence and 5-year survival. Tumor, node, and tumor-node-metastasis stages were statistically significant with univariate analysis ($p = 0.024$, 0.02, and 0.059 for local recurrence, respectively; $p = K0.00001$ for 5-year survival), whereas other variables, particularly the type of anastomosis, were not statistically significant. Multivariate analysis of nodal involvement was significant for local recurrence ($p = 0.04$) and extended surgery and TNM classification for 5-year survival ($p = 0.05$ and 0.00001, respectively); furthermore, the type of anastomosis was not significant.

DISCUSSION

Our data show no differences between stapled and hand-sewn anastomoses in terms of perioperative morbidity and survival. Results of randomized studies on this subject are reported in the literature, but data refer to small series that are not homogeneous and are not exclusively concerned with cancer. Moreover, results are similar to ours[4-6] in terms of morbidity, although clinical leakage was significantly greater in patients with cancer of the middle rectum with hand-sewn anastomosis (24.2% versus 18.1% for stapled anastomosis), which was probably the result of technical difficulties related to the site of the anatomosis (e.g., narrow pelvis in male patients). The need for a diverting colostomy in case of low rectal cancer influences the length of time spent in the hospital, since the colostomy is usually closed during the same hospitalization.

None of the data related to the type of anastomosis were significant in terms of oncological survival: the 5-year survival rates in the two groups were equal (almost 60%). Perioperative staging and correct surgical resection were the most important prognostic factors.[7]

Some technical considerations must be taken into account. Stapling devices permit reduction of the operative time in rectal surgery, allow anastomosis deep in the pelvis, and spare the sphincter muscles in patients with low rectal cancer, resulting in a better quality of life for most patients.

REFERENCES

1. Fazio VW. Cancer of the rectum—a sphincter-saving operation. Stapling techniques. Surg Clin North Am 68:1367, 1988.
2. Fegiz G, Angelini L, Bezzi M. Rectal cancer: Restorative surgery with the EEA stapling device. Int Surg 68:13, 1983.
3. Fegiz G. Manuelle Naht Versus/Sive Maschinernaht (Aus Der Sicht Italiens). Langenbecks Arch Chir 372:93, 1987.
4. McGinn FP. Staplers or sutures for low colo-rectal anastomoses. A prospective randomized trial. Br J Surg 72:603, 1985.
5. Everett WG. Comparison of stapling and hand suture for left-sided large bowel anastomosis. Br J Surg 73:345, 1986.
6. Morano Gonzales E. Results of surgery for cancer of the rectum with sphincter conservation. A randomized study on instrumental vs. manual anastomosis. Acta Oncol 28:237, 1987.
7. Goligher JC. Extended low anterior resection with stapled colo-rectal or colo-anal anastomosis. Ann Chir Gynaecol 75:82, 1986.

89 Results of Stapled Colorectal Anastomosis

Gérard Holbach and Bernward Ulrich

With the increasing frequency of colorectal cancer and the widening interest in sphincter-preserving anterior resection,[1-3] the use of circular staplers to create an end-to-end anastomosis, especially in the lower rectum, has gained in importance.[4] Unfortunately, the clinical use of circular staplers has spread more quickly than the publication of studies proving their advantages. The present study shows the results obtained with circular stapled anastomoses, especially in comparison with hand-sewn anastomoses.

MATERIALS AND METHODS

Between October 1986 and December 1991 the following procedures were performed: 169 circular stapled anastomoses (group A) and 139 hand-sewn anastomoses (group B). The mean age was 68.3 years (range 36 to 95) in group A and 67.1 years (range 12 to 89) in group B (Fig. 1). There were 99 women and 70 men in group A (sex ratio + 1.41/1) and 78 women and 61 men in group

B (sex ratio = 1.28/1). Indications for anastomoses in both groups are shown in Table 1.

In colorectal surgery we are currently using circular staplers almost exclusively for anastomoses through the anus. Thus neoplasia of the rectum and the sigmoid colon accounts for 70% of the indications for this type of anastomosis. During the above mentioned period, 14 anastomoses, all hand-sewn, were performed on emergency basis.

Preoperative Preparation of the Patient

All of the anastomosis procedures except those done on an emergency basis were performed in patients who had been admitted to the hospital the previous day, when colonic irrigation was done. The irrigation volume (lukewarm saline solution) depended on the degree of cleanliness of the washout. When a patient's cardiopulmonary status made washout impossible, a 2-day liquid diet was prescribed, along with laxatives.

475

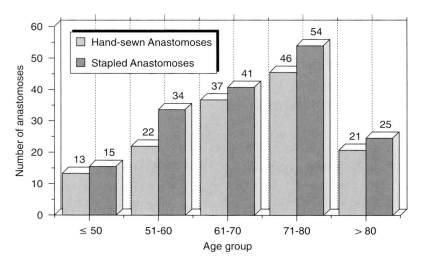

Fig. 1. Number of stapled and hand-sewn anastomoses in each age group from October 1986 to December 1991.

Table 1. Indications for colorectal anastomoses

Group A (Stapled)		Group B (Hand-sewn)	
Cancer of the sigmoid colon	64	Cancer of the right hemicolon	47
Cancer of the rectum	54	Diverticulosis†	21
Diverticulosis*	28	Cancer of the transverse colon	21
Rectal prolapse	5	Cancer of the left hemicolon	11
Cancer of the left hemicolon	4	Cancer of the sigmoid colon	10
Cancer of the transverse colon	1	Other	29
Other	13		
TOTAL	169	TOTAL	139

*Located in the sigmoid colon in 26 and in the left hemicolon in two.
†Located in the right hemicolon in 12 and in the sigmoid colon in nine.

Operative Technique

Perioperative antibiotics were used in both groups (a combination of metronidazole and cefuroxime) for 3 days; the first dose was administered 30 minutes before the surgery was begun. The operations were performed with the patients in a modified Lloyd-Davis position.

For rectal cancer, large mobilization of the organ and surrounding structures is done up to the anorectal ring.[5-11] By straightening the anteroposterior and lateral curves, the rectum can be elevated and stretched, so that the distance from the anal ring to the lower edge of the tumor increases up to 2 or 3 cm. When performed in this manner the sphincter-saving operation becomes possible in many cases, even when tumors are situated in the lower rectum. Furthermore, a coloanal pouch anastomosis is proposed in young patients with good sphincter function and preoperative tumors up to T2 (UICC). In these patients, the so-called double-layer technique is quite satisfactory.[12-16]

In our clinic we prefer the manual purse-string su-

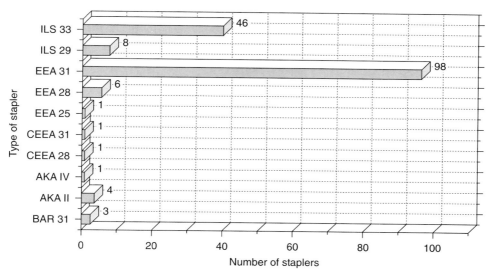

Fig. 2. Stapling devices used from October 1986 to December 1991.

ture to the purse-string clamp technique, because the former allows more tissue to be held—at least when the larger cartridge (31 or 33 mm diameter) is used. In this way the circles or "doughnuts" of tissue are thicker, and thus anastomoses are more secure and the distance from the tumor is lengthened.

Group A consisted of 164 transanal stapled anastomoses; in two patients these anastomoses were done by colotomy, which was then closed with a TA-55 stapler. In three patients we used the biofragmentable anastomotic ring. (Our trial phase included 10 consecutive patients with no postoperative complications in either the small or large intestine; this procedure was abandoned, however, because of the cost.)

Fig. 2 shows the frequency with which circular staplers are used in our clinic. There is a trend toward using the stapling device with the largest diameter (ILS 33), this stapler having been used almost exclusively for the last 3 years. During the same period we performed 70 end-to-end anastomoses, 63 side-to-side anastomoses (always meaning a functional end-to-end anastomosis without a "blind sack," after using the GIA device), and six end-to-end anastomoses.

The circular stapling device was inserted through the anus after anal dilation. The purse-string suture material used was prolene 0. Intravenous application of 1 mg of glucagon was often used to achieve better stretching of the bowel lumen before introducing the anvil into the proximal colon. Far more effective was the injection of 1% xylonest directly into the wall of the proximal colon.[17] The anastomosis was then created in the usual way; while performing this procedure we always closed the stapler completely. As a matter of routine the "doughnuts" of tissue were removed from the cartridge and carefully inspected to ensure that they were complete. Then the competence of the anastomosis was checked by applying a noncrushing bowel clamp proximal to it and injecting a polyvidoniodide solution via a transanal tube. In the presence of a primary insufficiency the anastomosis was repaired with sutures and the competence was rechecked. When there were risk factors such as diverticulosis or stool contamination, we sometimes opted to protect primary, secure anastomoses by reinforcing sutures or epiploic appendices. Where necessary the splenic curve of the colon was mobilized to achieve a tension-free anastomosis.

Hand-sewn anastomoses were all constructed in a single layer. Here only a digital check of the tightness of the anastomosis was done. A suction drain was inserted in the region of the anastomosis. Postoperatively we relied on radiological or endoscopic control of the anastomosis as a matter of course when there was no clinical evidence of complications and when the anastomosis was primarily satisfactory. However, all primarily insufficient anastomoses were examined radiologically. Altogether 10 surgeons participated in the stapled anastomosis procedures described in this report.

RESULTS

In group A there were 11 (6.5%) primary (i.e, intraoperatively detected) leaks and six (3.5%) secondary leaks (Fig. 3). With regard to upper and lower colorectal anastomoses, the incidence of strictly secondary leaks was 3.0% (n = 5 of a total of 165 corresponding operations). The sixth case of secondary insufficiency involved bleeding after a resection for angiodysplasia. The stapled anastomosis was done through a colotomy.

All primary leaks were successfully repaired with sutures. In 2 of the 11 primary leaks the primary insufficiency led to a secondary leak. Reasons for a primary leak included very deep anastomoses performed under difficult anatomical conditions (e.g., a narrow pelvis, or extreme obesity) and a previously damaged wall, especially in combination with a spastic bowel. In one patient despite the use of glucagon, removal of the stapler caused a leak. All 11 leaks were examined radiologically with a water-soluble contrast material during the second postoperative week and were found to be safe.

A protective colostomy became necessary in ten patients in group A for the following reasons: a primary leak (one leak with incomplete "doughnuts" of tissue*) in four and a J-pouch anastomosis in two; other indications included pronounced differences in the diameter of the bowel parts used for the anastomosis, stool contamination; poor blood supply, and protection of a very deep anastomosis. Two patients in group B required protective colostomies because of peritonitis.

In five of the six strictly secondary leaks (stool fistula), a protective colostomy allowed healing of the leak. In one patient a repeat laparotomy became necessary (in addition to the protective colostomy). In one patient (0.6%) a primary leak was observed despite complete tissue rings. The defect was repaired with sutures and then showed anastomotic competence. The anastomosis healed with no complications. Incomplete doughnuts of tissue were present in one patient (0.66%). In five patients both the introduction and especially the removal of the stapling device damaged the seromuscular layers. The defect was repaired with sutures. Table 2 provides the details concerning the 11 primary leaks. The average distance of the anastomoses was 5.67 cm from the anus, and three of the anastomoses were very deep.

---

*Incomplete "doughnuts" of tissue are not an absolute indication of insufficiency; however, they require a protective procedure (e.g., suturing or colostomy). Similarly, complete rings are not always an indication of a secure anastomosis.

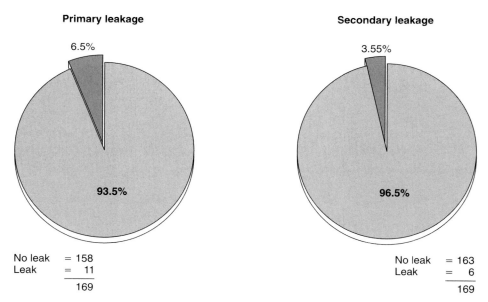

Fig. 3. Primary and secondary leakage rates in colorectal stapled anastomoses from October 1986 to December 1991.

All six exclusively secondary leaks were clinically evident; five were in the form of a stool fistula appearing between the twelfth and the fourteenth postoperative days. One patient had severe bleeding as a result of insufficient closure of the staples (as shown on repeat laparotomy). The bleeding stopped after suturing, and it was decided to perform a protective colostomy. Five of the six secondary leaks were in very deep anastomoses (average = 5.7 cm from the anus). Five of the strictly secondary leaks occurred in male patients whereas there was only one female with this type of leak (Table 3). Radiographic observation showed proper healing of the anastomoses after colostomy; these observations were continued for 3 to 6 months. There were no deaths caused by anastomic insufficiency.

According to Thiede's classification[18] of the anastomotic height of colorectal anastomoses in patients with carcinoma, our study yielded the following results in group A. The following distances were determined intraoperatively by direct measurement: 3 to 5 cm from the anus, 5.36% (n = 6); 6 to 8 cm from the anus, 16.07% (n = 19); and ≥9 cm from the anus, 78.57% (n = 93).

Fig. 4 illustrates the location of deep stapled anastomoses according to the classification for rectal cancer, sigmoid cancer, and rectal prolapse proposed by Thiede et al.[18] The corresponding secondary leaks are also shown. Above 9 cm from the anus, there was one leak among 67 anastomoses (1.5%). Between 6 and 8 cm from the anus, one leak occurred among 12 anastomoses

Table 2. Details concerning primary leakage

Disease	Operative Procedure	Stapler	Anastomotic Height (cm)	TNM Tumor Stage	Colostomy	Secondary Leakage
Rectal carcinoma	Anterior resection	ILS 33	3	I	No	No
Rectal carcinoma	Anterior resection	ILS 33	4	III	Protective	No
Rectal carcinoma	Anterior resection	AKA II	5	II	Protective	No
Rectal carcinoma	Anterior resection	ILS 33	5	II	Protective	No
Ovarian carcinoma (infiltration by)	Anterior resection	ILS 33	5	—	Protective	No
Rectal carcinoma	Anterior resection	EEA 31	6	III	No	No
Rectal carcinoma	Anterior resection	EEA 31	6	IV	No	No
Rectal carcinoma	Anterior resection	ILS 33	8	III	No	Yes
Rectal carcinoma	Anterior resection	ILS 33	>9	IV	No	Yes
Colon carcinoma	Anterior resection	ILS 29	>9	IV	No	No
Colon carcinoma	Anterior resection	EEA 31	>9	I	No	No

Table 3. Details concerning secondary leakage

Disease	Operative Procedure	Stapler	Anastomotic Height (cm)	TNM Tumor Stage	Colostomy	Radiological Control
Rectal carcinoma	Anterior resection	ILS 33	3	III	Yes	Yes
Rectal carcinoma	Anterior resection	EEA 31	3	III	Yes	Yes
Rectal carcinoma	Anterior resection	ILS 33	4	III	Yes	Yes
Rectal carcinoma	Anterior resection	ILS 33	5	II	Yes	Yes
Rectal carcinoma	Anterior resection	EEA 31	7	III	Yes	Yes
Angiodysplasia	Left hemicolectomy	ILS 33	>9	—	Yes	Yes

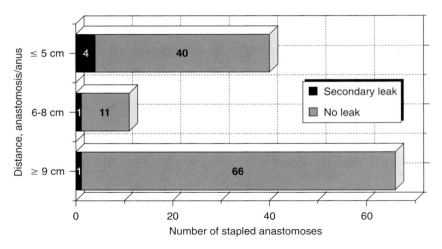

Fig. 4. Leakage rate in stapled colorectal anastomoses in relation to the distance of the anastomosis from the anus.

(8.3%). In the group of very deeply situated anastomoses, there were four leaks among 44 anastomoses (9.1%).

During the previously mentioned period we used the extracorporeal circular stapling technique to treat five cases of rectal prolapse.[19] In four patients we used the ILS 33 stapler and in one we used the EEA 31 stapler. On average, the anastomosis was 2.4 cm from the anus (3 cm from the anus in two patients, 2 cm from the anus in three). There were no secondary leaks and no need for a protective colostomy. No deaths occurred and sphincter function was normal in all patients.

In a group of 139 patients with hand-sewn anastomoses (group B), there was only one secondary leak. It appeared after a right hemicolectomy, performed by a resident in a patient with cancer of the ascending colon. There was no problem in creating a permeable and stress-relieving side-to-side anastomosis (meaning a functional end-to-end anastomosis). The leak resolved spontaneously, and 3 weeks after the operation the patient left the clinic. Unfortunately this multimorbid patient later died of an unrelated tumor.

Six of the 169 patients in group A had wound-healing disorders (rate, 3.55%). Two of them were grossly obese and in one the wound became infected following reestablishment of intestinal continuity (protective colostomy); in the other three patients we were unable to determine the cause of the wound-healing disorder. In group B we noted 11 cases of wound-healing complications (rate = 7.91%). Two patients had diabetes mellitus, and one patient had cachexia. No reason could be

found in the others. No clinically relevant anastomotic strictures were found in either group, and there were no deaths in this series that were related to anastomotic leakage.

DISCUSSION

In 1985 an inquiry among 608 German surgeons concerning the use of staples indicated that 73% of them had experience with this type of device.[20] Today this percentage is undoubtedly higher.[21] We have been using circular staplers since 1978, and from 1986 to 1991 we divided our patients into two groups: one group with stapled and one with hand-sewn anastomoses. A statistical comparison of these two groups was not possible, but we are certain that some of our stapled anastomoses would have been impossible to complete in the traditional hand-sewn manner. For statistical analysis a prospective randomized trial is necessary. In the studies carried out by Thiede et al.[18] there were withdrawn cases, especially in the lower rectum. These withdrawn cases represented patients who were in a randomized group of hand-sewn and stapled anastomoses. However, the realization of a stapled anastomosis only was possible in either group, for technical reasons. Friend et al.,[22] in a 1990 study of 250 patients, demonstrated that eight planned stapled anastomoses could only be completed by hand. In 1986 Everett et al.[23] published similar findings. Aside from the financial advantage of hand-sewn anastomoses, other investigators such as McGinn et al.[24] and Cajozzo et al.[25] could not determine a statistically significant difference between stapled and

Table 4. Leakage rates in stapled colorectal surgery: An international literature review

Reference (year)	No. of Anastomoses	Leakage Rate
Ballantyne and Beart[29] (1985)	107	7.5% (n = 8)
Baran et al.[12] (1992)	104	2.8% (n = 3)
Cutait and Cutait[5] (1986)	140	7.1% (n = 10)
Everett et al.[23] (1986)	44	15.9% (n = 7)
Fazio[6] (1984)	162	3.0% (n = 5)
Fazio et al.[30] (1985)	84	1.2% (n = 1)
Feinberg et al.[13] (1986)	79	7.6% (n = 6)
Gordon and Dalrymple[7] (1986)	143	0.7% (n = 1)
Kennedy et al.[8] (1983)	174	4.6% (n = 8)
Knight and Griffen[9] (1987)	64	1.5% (n = 1)
Griffen et al.[14] (double-layer) (1990)	75	2.7% (n = 2)
Lazorthes and Chiotassol[31] (1986)	82	4.9% (n = 4)
McGinn et al.[24] (1985)	58	12% (n = 7)
Pelissier et al.[32] (1992)	33	6% (n = 2)
Polglase[10] (1987)	120	10.8% (n = 13)
Thiede et al.[18] (1986)	301	5.3% (n = 16)
Ti et al.[33] (1986)	32	10% (n = 3)
Trollope et al.[34] (only deep anterior resection) (1986)	205	1.5% (n = 3)
Wehrli et al.[35] (1989)	169	4.3%
Present study: Holbach and Ulrich (1992)	169	3.5%
TOTAL	2345	
MEAN		5.6%

hand-sewn anastomoses. These discrepancies can be explained by the fact that although there are some surgeons who have a great deal of experience with difficult extracorporeal or supra-anal manual suturing techniques, there are others who do not believe that either a stapled or hand-sewn anastomosis is possible if the remaining rectal stump is very small. Based on local conditions (most often meaning a narrow bowel lumen), we realize that it is sometimes simpler and safer to perform a hand-sewn anastomosis rather than a stapled one.

In our clinic we have been using circular stapling devices, introduced through the anus, to perform sigmoid and rectal resections since 1986. Nearly all of our other colonic anastomoses are hand sewn, not only because of the cost factor but also because ours is a teaching surgical department. The advantages of staplers are as follows: a high degree of reproducible suture safety, a shorter operating time with a simultaneous reduction in the time needed to leave bowel open, less tissue damage and more rapid healing (reduced edema), simple manipulation by using modern staplers, and avoidance of a colostomy. Since the introduction of staplers in 1977, there has been a progressive decrease in the rate of leakage. Unfortunately, it is impossible to determine the exact nature of the importance of the preoperative bowel preparation and antibiotic prophylaxis.

Our secondary leakage rate (3.55%) falls in the upper third of the international average (Table 4). Inasmuch as five of the six leaks were observed in anastomoses situated less than 6 cm from the anus, and the average leakage rate is higher in the international literature, our 3.55% rate is satisfactory (with a total of 10 surgeons).

We believe that among other things our favorable results can be attributed to a delicate operating technique and our considerable experience with staplers. In addition to the fact that the surgical principle of a tension-free anastomosis is still valid, thorough knowledge of the stapler and its limitations is of utmost importance.[26] Injury to the spleen, which often accompanies colorectal surgery (3.44% in our clinic), is a definite indication of how frequently the left colonic flexure is mobilized. Inasmuch as a neat adaptation of the bowel segments without any inclusion of fat (danger of leakage) must be achieved, the bowel stumps must be cleaned up to 2 cm before purse-string sutures can be applied.[27]

By using a purse-string clamp, only a small amount of tissue is inverted onto the rod of the stapling device.[28] This means that the perfusion of the anastomosis could be compromised. The risk can be reduced by using a manual purse-string suture, which is capable of securing a larger amount of tissue. Unfortunately, this technique may squeeze the tissue out of the cartridge, with the risk of a leak at the closure of the stapler (especially with small cartridges). To avoid this danger, we use the largest cartridge available and firmly attach the included tissue with additional ties or sutures onto the rod. It is our opinion that a 31 mm cartridge is the minimum size that should be used; whenever possible we use a 33 mm cartridge. Before introducing the stapler through the anus, it is critical to determine whether the anvil is firmly screwed on; otherwise, the staples do not close correctly (B shape of the staple). The stapler should be removed by the surgeon after three opening half-turns, because only the surgeon can sufficiently control the free removal of the stapler. If the stapler is not free after its firing, either the anastomosis is incomplete or some surrounding tissue is clamped in. In both cases a new anastomosis must be created. Before the introduction of the anvil into the proximal bowel segment, we recommend distending the bowel with forceps (eventually with the help of glucagon or Xylonest). The anvil can also be inserted into a narrow bowel lumen with the aid of a conical metal hat screwed to the anvil (Ethicon ILS).

The fact that no strictures were observed in our patients is evidence favoring the use of the largest diameter cartridge. For safety reasons the stapled anastomosis was protected by reinforcing its front side with sutures, especially when it was situated in the lower rectum. We consider routine intraoperative control of the competence of the anastomosis a must. Primary leaks are repaired with sutures and tested again. Our study confirms the international experience—that is, the lower the anastomosis, the higher the secondary leakage rate. Above 9 cm from the anus, the secondary leakage rate was only 1.5% in our patients; below 5 cm from the anus it was as high as 9.1%. Five (83.3%) of the six sec-

ondary leaks occurred in male patients with an extremely narrow pelvis, and severe technical difficulties were encountered in completing the anastomoses. Thiede et al.[18] claimed an 85% success rate.

In our experience a protective colostomy is indicated to protect a very deep or a technically difficult anastomosis. Furthermore, it is used to protect a pouch or to give safety in the event of stool contamination of the intra-abdominal cavity. As a result of our study procedure (retrospective study), there were no so-called withdrawn or excluded cases. A review of the data available from the international literature comparing hand-sewn and stapled anastomoses yielded no consensus regarding the superiority of any of these procedures.[18,22-25] Up to the present there has been no double-blind study demonstrating any significant differences with regard to mortality and leakage rates.

As a result of the heterogeneous nature of both groups, the results achieved with staplers do not compare with those achieved with manual sutures. Indeed, such a comparison was not the aim of our study. On the contrary, our purpose was to show that both procedures can be justified in colorectal surgery.

CONCLUSION

It is possible to save some time by using staplers. The benefits of a safe deep anastomosis, the avoidance of a protective colostomy, and the decreased operating time, however, must be weighed against the considerable cost and complicated logistics. Nevertheless, hand-sewn anastomosis must be included among the basic techniques that must be mastered by any visceral surgeon. No one technique precludes another, and ideally both should be viewed as complementary to each other.

REFERENCES

1. Fazio VW. Cancer of the rectum—sphincter saving operation. Surg Clin North Am 68:1367-1382, 1988.
2. Goligher JC. Sphinker-erhaltende Resektion bei der radikalen Behandlung des Karzinoms im mittleren Rektum. In Ulrich B, Winter J, eds. Klammernahttechnik in Thorax und Abdomen. Enke: Verlag, 1986, pp 149-158.
3. Goligher JC. Sphincter-saving excision for cancers of the middle and lower parts of the rectum. Ann Gastroenterol Hepatol 22:361-363, 1986.
4. Steichen FM. Die Geschichte und der Einfluss von Klammernahtgeräten in der Chirurgie. In Ulrich B(Hrsg). Klammernahttechnik, Chirurgische Gastroenterologie. Hameln: TM Verlag, 1986.

5. Cutait DE, Cutait R. Stapled anterior resection of the rectum. In Ravitch MM, Steichen FM, eds. Principles and Practice of Surgical Stapling. Chicago: Year Book Medical Publishers, 1987, pp 388-401.

6. Fazio VW. Advances in the surgery of rectal carcinoma utilizing the circular stapler. In Spratt JS, ed. Neoplasms of the Colon, Rectum and Anus, 1st ed. Philadelphia: WB Saunders, 1984, pp 268-288.

7. Gordon PH, Dalrymple S. The use of staplers for reconstruction after colonic and rectal surgery. In Ravitch MM, Steichen FM, eds. Principles and Practice of Surgical Stapling. Chicago: Year Book Medical Publishers, 1987, pp 4902-4931.

8. Kennedy HL, Rothenberger DA, Goldberg SM. Colocolostomy and coloproctostomy utilizing the circular intraluminal stapling devices. Dis Colon Rectum 26:145, 1983.

9. Knight CD, Griffen FD. Techniques of low rectal reconstruction. Curr Probl Surg 20:391, 1987.

10. Polglase MS. Anterior resection for carcinoma of the rectum. In Ravitch MM, Steichen FM, eds. Principles and Practice of Surgical Stapling. Chicago: Year Book Medical Publishers, 1987, pp 373-387.

11. Steichen FM. Changing concepts in surgical techniques. In Current Practice of Surgical Stapling. Philadelphia: Lea & Febiger, 1991, pp 23-37.

12. Baran JJ, Goldstein SD, Resnik AM. The double-staple technique in colorectal anastomoses: A critical review. Am Surg 58:270-272, 1992.

13. Feinberg SM, Parker F, Cohen Z. The double stapling technique for low anterior resection of rectal carcinoma. Dis Colon Rectum 29:885, 1986.

14. Griffen FD, Knight CD Sr, Whitaker JM, et al. The double stapling technique for low anterior resection. Results, modifications and observations. Ann Surg 211:745-751, 1990.

15. Moritz E, Achleitner D, Holbing N, et al. Single vs. double stapling technique in colorectal surgery. A prospective randomized trial. Dis Colon Rectum 34:495-497, 1991.

16. Stahle E, Pahlman L, Enblad P. Double stapling technique in the management of rectal tumours. Acta Chir Scand 152:743-747, 1986.

17. Shlasko E, Gorfine SR, Gelernt IM. Using lidocaine to ease the insertion of the circular stapler. Surg Gynecol Obstet 174:70, 1992.

18. Thiede A, Jostandt L, Hamelmann A. Prospektive und kontrollierte Studien in der kolorektalen Chirurgie—Vergleich von Handnaht und Staplernaht bei Rektumanastomosen. Chirurgische Gastroenterologie mit interdisziplinären Gesprächen: Klammernahttechnik Nr 2 Okt 1986, 91-114.

19. Rötker J, Ulrich B, Kockel N. Extrakorporale Rektumresektion beim Analprolaps mit dem Klammernahtgerät. Chirurg 60:505-508, 1989.

20. Ulrich B, Winter J. Ergebnisse einer Umfrageaktion bei den deutschen Chirurgen betreffs der Klammernahtchirurgie im Herbst 1985. Chirurgische Gastroenterologie mit interdisziplinären Gesprächen: Klammernahttechnik Nr 2 Okt 1986, 9-16.

21. Kockel N, Ulrich B. Gegenwärtiger Stand und Perspektiven maschineller Nahttechniken in der Abdominal-und Thoraxchirurgie. Zentralbl Chir 116:219-241, 1991.

22. Friend PJ, Scott R, Everett WG, et al. Stapling or suturing for anastomoses of the left side of the large intestine. Surg Gynecol Obstet 171:373-376, 1990.

23. Everett G, Friend J, Forty J. Comparison of stapling and hand-suture for left-sided large bowel anastomosis. Br J Surg 73:345-348, 1986.

24. McGinn FP, Gartell PC, Clifford PC, et al. Staples or sutures for low colorectal anastomoses: A prospective randomized trial. Br J Surg 72:603-605, 1985.

25. Cajozzo M, Compagno G, DiTora P, et al. Advantages and disadvantages of mechanical vs. manual anastomosis in colorectal surgery. A prospective study. Acta Chir Scand 156:167-169, 1990.

26. Haschke N, Thiede A. Tricks, Fehler und Gefahren beim Einsatz von Staplern im kolorektalen Bereich. Langenbecks Arch Chir (Suppl Ii Verh Dtsch Ges Forsch Chir): 385-388, 1989.

27. Cohen AM. Purse-string placement for transanal intraluminal circular stapling. Dis Colon Rectum 29:532-533, 1986.

28. Last MD, Fazio VW. The rational use of the purse-string device in constructing anastomoses with the circular stapler. Dis Colon Rectum 28:979-980, 1985.

29. Ballantyne GH, Beart RW Jr. Maschinelle Anastomosen in der kolorektalen Chirurgie. Indikationen und Ergebnisse. Chirurg 56:223-226, 1985.

30. Fazio VW, Jagelman DG, Lavery IC, et al. Evaluation of the proximate-ILS circular stapler. Ann Surg 201:108, 1985.

31. Lazorthes F, Chiotassol P. Stapled colorectal anastomoses: Preoperative integrity of the anastomosis and risk of postoperative leakage. Int J Colorectal Dis 1:96-98, 1986.

32. Pelissier EP, Blum D, Bachour A, et al. Stapled coloanal anastomosis with reservoir procedure. Am J Surg 163:435-436, 1992.

33. Ti TK, Rauff A, Goh HS. Anterior resection using the circular stapling instrument: A Singapore experience. Aust NZ J Surg 56:919-922, 1986.

34. Trollope ML, Cohen RG, Lee RH, et al. A 7 year experience with low anterior sigmoid resections using the EEA stapler. Am J Surg 152:354, 1986.

35. Wehrli H, Koch R, Akovbiantz A. Experiences with 169 mechanical colorectal anastomoses (1981-1984). Helv Chir Acta 55:649-654, 1989.

90 *Compression Anastomosis in Colorectal Surgery*

Riccardo Rosati, Carlo Rebuffat, Uberto Fumagalli, Marco Montorsi, Stefano Bona, Federico Varoli, Giancarlo Roviaro, and Giuseppe Pezzuoli

In the field of digestive tract anastomosis, the concept of compression is very old: it was first introduced by the French surgeon Denans in 1826 and was popularized by John Benjamin Murphy, who presented his "anastomotic button" in 1892.[1] The Murphy button was successfully used to make cholecystoduodenostomies (small bowel anastomoses). Acting as temporary support for the tissues, compression anastomotic devices allow "natural" healing to take place immediately outside the area of compression. After anastomotic healing occurs, the whole compression device detaches from the anastomosis, falls into the intestinal lumen, and is then evacuated.

The main advantages of compression include the following[1-3]:

- Immediate seal of intact tissues at the anastomotic site (because the entire circumference of both bowel ends is held by compression inside the device)
- Anastomotic immobility (the intraluminal apparatus prevents anastomotic distention by gas and feces)
- Absence of foreign bodies at the anastomotic site, thus reducing the likelihood of stenosis and perianastomotic adhesions

However, because of technical problems related to the mechanical inadequacy of compression devices such as the Murphy button and its many modifications, and because of errors in indications for their use, the acceptance, study, and development of sutureless anastomosis was limited.[4]

In recent years interest has been revived in compression devices.[5-7] Russian scientists and surgeons have introduced instruments for compression anastomosis—the AKA-2 and AKA-4—that elicited favorable comments in the Soviet Union and Europe[8-12] but did not gain much popularity in Western countries. Another sutureless anastomotic apparatus called the *biofragmentable anastomotic ring* (BAR-Valtrac, Davis & Geck) was introduced in 1985, and successful animal and clinical trials were reported.[12-16] This is a fragmentable ring made of polyglycolic acid that holds the two intestinal ends to be anastomosed in contact purse-stringed without necrosing the bowel walls. Thus it creates a "juxta-apposition" rather than a compression anastomosis: it detaches from the anastomosis by fragmentation and then passes in the fecal stream, leaving in place the purse-string sutures (which will take longer to be absorbed) in the two inverted anastomotic ends. In the case of a thick intestinal wall, this button acts as a true compression device: the whole button detaches from the anastomosis and is expelled unfragmented. Even if clinical experience is favorable with this instrument, the lack of an applicator precludes its use for low and very low colorectal anastomoses.

At the University of Milan we developed and tested a mechanical device that achieves compression anastomosis by intraluminal placement of an apparatus consisting of three polypropylene rings. The experimental results[17,18] were sufficiently encouraging for us to proceed to the use of the device in humans, as we reported previously.[19,20] Here we will describe our surgical technique and further clinical experience in colorectal surgery with this anastomotic device.

MATERIALS AND METHODS

This compression anastomotic device consists of three interlocking polypropylene rings—an outer, an intermediate, and an inner ring, available in two sizes: 30 mm and 25 mm outer diameters—carried on an instrument very similar to circular stapling devices. The shape of the outer ring, which constitutes the tip of the assembly, allows its easy introduction into the bowel. The carrying instrument first assembles the rings and then separates the button from the instrument.

The technique for using the device is the same as for circular staplers[5]; the surgeon chooses a button smaller than the bowel lumen so as to fit smoothly. The anastomosis will in any case be as wide as the outer circumference of the button, not the size of the circular blade, as with stapling instruments.

The outer ring acts technically as the stapler anvil while the intermediate/inner rings are comparable to the cartridge. Operation of the device is the same as for annular staplers. By operating the carrying instrument, a series of movements is produced that locks the rings and causes the circular blade to cut out tissue doughnuts and a circular dome of the outer ring held by the central shaft and its pressure plate. The carrying apparatus is automatically liberated from the button, which remains at the anastomotic site. The tissue edges are compressed between the outer and intermediate rings, and a "natural" seal occurs outside the area of compression. The tissue doughnuts cut by the circular blade must always be inspected to ensure their completeness. Intraluminal pneumatic control of anastomotic competence can be done as for stapled anastomoses. The rings are inspected for correct assembly from the serosal side and, if possible, also from the mucosal side by digital examination. Digital stretching of the anal sphincters is suggested in all patients at the end of the procedure to allow easier evacuation of the anastomotic rings. Standard postoperative management is followed. Evacuation of feces is not impaired by the presence of the button at the anastomotic site. The button is usually evacuated on about the eleventh postoperative day, painlessly or with very little discomfort; some patients do not even feel its transit through the anus. Patients with protective colostomies may not spontaneously evacuate the button, but it can be easily extracted by digital examination of the rectum.

Ninety-five patients underwent large bowel compression anastomosis with this device at our Institution from May 1986 through June 1990. Clinical findings, indications for surgery, and the type of operation are shown in Table 1. The anastomosis follow-up program consisted of endoscopic control 1 and 3 months after operation, then at 6-month intervals, and a double-contrast enema once in the first year.

RESULTS

Results are summarized in Table 2. One patient (1.0%) died from myocardial infarction on the third postoperative day. At autopsy the gross appearance of the anastomosis was very good: the rings were firmly in place and were gently removed after longitudinal opening of the bowel by cutting the intestinal walls comprised between the buttons. The anastomosis was studied histologically and was at an advanced stage of healing.

As for postoperative anastomotic complications, we observed four (4.2%) subclinical and five (5.2%) clini-

Table 1. Clinical experience with compression anastomosis in surgery of the large bowel: May 1986–June 1990

Patients	95	
Men	55	
Women	40	
Mean age	60.2 (23-82)	
Indications for surgery		
Adenocarcinoma	71	
Diverticulosis	12	
Crohn's disease	5	
Miscellaneous	7	
Operations performed		
Right hemicolectomy	19	
Left colon resection	23	
Left hemicolectomy/anterior resection of the rectum	51	
Total colectomy	2	
Distance of rectal anastomosis from the anal verge		
<4 cm	12	(18.5%)
Between 4 and 8 cm	13	(20.0%)
>8 cm	40	(61.5%)
Protective colostomies	5	(5.2%)

Table 2. Results of clinical experience with compression anastomosis in surgery of the large bowel: May 1986–June 1990

Evacuation of the rings	10.9 days	(5-23)
Postoperative hospital stay (mean)	15.8 days	
Operative mortality (myocardial infarction)	1	(1.0%)
Anastomotic complications		
Subclinical leak	4	(4.2%)
Clinical leak	5	(5.2%)
Hemorrhage	0	0
Stenosis	0	0
Emergency diverting colostomies	5	(5.2%)
Extra-anastomotic complications		
Pulmonary embolism	1	(1.0%)
AAPMC	2	(2.1%)
Diarrhea	6	(6.3%)
Urinary infections	4	(4.2%)

cal anastomotic leaks. Five (5.2%) emergency diverting colostomies were performed. No hemorrhage or other anastomotic complications were observed.

As for extra-anastomotic complications, one patient (1.0%) with intraperitoneal colorectal anastomosis had pulmonary embolism and two (2.1%) had severe antibiotic-associated pseudomembranous colitis (AAPMC); they both recovered with nonoperative therapy without developing any anastomotic complications, as did six other patients with severe diarrhea.

Endoscopic long-term controls showed wide anastomoses with no evidence of stricture. Even the patients who complained of anastomotic leak and the ones with diverting colostomies had wide, nonstenotic anastomoses. The anastomotic line was often difficult to detect even by videoendoscopy. Radiologically the anastomoses were wide and difficult to locate.

DISCUSSION

A sutureless anastomosis is certainly the "ideal anastomosis,"[1,4,6,21] so we tried to combine the old principle of compression with the most recent technological advances. The anastomotic apparatus we describe here consists of an instrument that assembles three molded plastic rings that simply lock together. The metal prototype we employed for this trial was easy to use and reliable, but a completely disposable device has been developed to satisfy the need for reliable and safe proper functioning.

The initial animal trial was very encouraging and confirmed the biological concept of good and quick healing.[17,18] The surgical technique for the anastomosis is even easier than the one usually employed with staplers.[5] The particular shape of the outer ring allows its easy introduction into the proximal bowel lumen. The button size, smaller than the bowel circumference, makes the instrument even easier to introduce. The instrument is automatically extracted on completion of the anastomosis, thus offering an advantage over staplers. The circular blade first cuts the bowel edges held by the two purse-string sutures, then cuts the central dome of the outer ring, automatically separating the button from the carrying instrument.

As with staplers, the tissue doughnuts cut by the circular blade must always be carefully inspected. They must be complete to ensure that the tissue ends are incorporated in the button.

Our initial clinical experience with 75 patients was already reported[19,20]; in an additional 20 patients we observed no fecal impaction at the button site, and thus regular stool evacuation was unimpeded. Even when the smaller button was still in place, evacuation of solid stool was normal. The occurrence of severe diarrhea in some patients, such as the patient with AAPMC, is good evidence of the impermeability of the system, because none of them experienced any anastomotic complications.

The button was evacuated postoperatively at very different intervals (5 to 23 days); since no complication arose in the patient who evacuated it on the fifth day, we believe that button detachment happens only when healing of the anastomosis is complete.[17] In dogs, button detachment does not depend on the amount of compression. Evacuation of the button did not cause problems to any of the patients with regular fecal transit, who often did not even feel its passage. It was extracted manually by digital examination in patients with diverting colostomies.

In this experience the only anastomotic complications were leaks; we observed neither hemorrhage nor stenosis. We observed just one subclinical and one clinical leak in the earlier 75 cases. In the latter 20 cases we employed a button with a different outer ring, so designed to facilitate injection molding. This was followed by an increased number of complications (three-subclinical and four clinical leaks), accounting for a total of four (4.2%) subclinical and five (5.2%) clinical leaks. We recognized the cause of the problem in the drawing of the outer ring profile and, since in the meantime we have developed a fragmentable anastomotic button that gave excellent experimental results (which are as yet unpublished), we decided to interrupt our clinical trials while waiting for the new device to be ready for tests.

As for long-term controls, no stenoses were observed. The anastomoses, which were more often than not difficult to identify, even through accurate endoscopies, were all perfectly healed. Radiologically all the anastomoses appeared to be of very good quality. Moreover, the fact of not having metal foreign bodies such as staples or sutures at the anastomotic site is to be considered a definite advantage if CT scans or magnetic resonance imaging are required for these patients in the future.

CONCLUSION

We believe that a sutureless anastomosis is the "ideal" anastomosis. We also believe that compression is, at the moment, the best method to achieve a sutureless anastomosis, since glues and laser welding do not offer enough guarantees of safety. Once industrially available for clinical use, our instrument can find a definite role in this field.

REFERENCES

1. Murphy JB. Cholecysto-intestinal, gastro-intestinal, entero-intestinal anastomosis and approximation without sutures (original research). Medical Record 42:665, 1892.
2. Juvara E. Un nouveau modèle de bouton anastomotique intestinal avec une nouvelle technique. Arch Sci Med (Bucarest), Paris I:253, 1896.
3. Boerema I. The technique of our method of transabdominal total gastrectomy in cases of gastric cancer. Arch Chir Neerl-Scand 6:95, 1954.
4. Ballantyne GH. The experimental basis of intestinal suturing. Dis Colon Rectum 27:61-71, 1984.
5. Steichen FM, Ravitch MM. Stapling in Surgery. Chicago: Year Book, 1984.
6. Hogstrom H, Haglund U. Postoperative decrease in sutures' holding capacity in laparotomy wounds and anastomoses. Acta Chir Scand 151:533-535, 1985.
7. Jansen A, Brummelkamp WH, Davies GS. Clinical application of magnetic rings in colorectal anastomoses. Surg Gynecol Obstet 537-545, 1953.
8. Knys BI, Capjuk VF, Guskov IA, Sackov AE. Primenenie anastomose "s/pod davleniem" v kirurgieskom lacenii raka tolstoj kiski. Kirurgija, Zurnal imeni NI. Pirogova. Moskva Meditzina 3:107-114, 1984.
9. Liboni A, Mari C, Tartari V, et al. AKA-2: Una nuova suturatrice meccanica circolare introflettente nella chirurgia colorettale. Acta Chir Italica 41:536-538, 1985.
10. Gross E, Eigler FW. Sutureless compression anastomosis of the distal colon and rectum: An expanded report of experience with a total of 140 patients. Chirurgie 60:589-593, 1989.
11. Eigler FW, Gross E. Mechanical compression anastomosis (AKA-2) of the colon and rectum: Results of a prospective clinical study. Chirurgie 57:230-235, 1986.
12. Hardy TG, Pace WG, Maney JW, Katz AR, Kaganov AL. A biofragmentable ring for sutureless bowel anastomosis: An experimental study. Dis Colon Rectum 28:484-490, 1985.
13. Maney JW, Katz AR, Pace WG, Hardy TG. Biofragmentable bowel anastomosis ring: Comparative efficacy studies in dogs. Surgery 103:56-62, 1988.
14. Hardy GT, Aguilar PS, Stewart WRC, Katz AR, Maney JW, Costanzo JT, Pace WG. Initial clinical experience with a biofragmentable ring for sutureless anastomosis. Dis Color Rectum 30:55-61, 1987.
15. Cahill CJ, Betzler M, Gruwez JA, Jeekel J, Patel JC, Zederfeldt B. Sutureless large bowel anastomosis: European experience with the biofragmentable anastomotic ring. Br J Surg 76:334-337, 1989.
16. Dyess DL, Curreri PW, Ferrara JJ. A new technique for sutureless intestinal anastomosis: A prospective randomized clinical trial. Am Surg 56:71-75, 1990.
17. Rosati R, Rebuffat C, Pezzouli G. A new mechanical device for circular compression anastomosis: Preliminary results of animal and clinical experimentation. Ann Surg 207:15-22, 1988.
18. Malthaner RA, Hakki RZ, Saini N, Andrews BL, Harmon JW. Anastomotic compression button: A new mechanical device for sutureless compression anastomosis. Dis Colon Rectum 33:291-297, 1990.
19. Rebuffat C, Rosati R, Montorsi M, Fumagalli U, Maciocco M, Poccobelli M, Rovario GC, Varoli F, Pezzuoli G. Clinical application of a new compression anastomotic device for colorectal surgery. Am J Surg 159:330-335, 1990.
20. Pezzuoli G, Rebuffat C, Rosati R. Clinical use of a new compression anastomotic device in colorectal surgery. In Ravitch MM, Steichen F, Welter R, eds. Current Practices in Surgical Stapling. Philadelphia: Lea & Febiger, 1991.
21. McCue JL, Philips RKS. Sutureless intestinal anastomosis. Br J Surg 78:1291-1296, 1991.

91   *Enteral Anastomoses Using the Biofragmentable Valtrac Ring: A Prospective Study*

Rainer Engemann, Bernd Lünstedt, Siegbert Vogel, and Arnulf Thiede

The first attempts to create seamless bowel anastomoses were made in the early nineteenth century. As early as 1826 Denans[1] was using an anastomotic ring that led to nonirritating healing of end-to-end ileoileostomies in animal experiments. The most celebrated method used the Murphy button, an anastomotic button presented for the first time by Murphy[2] in 1892 to carry out cholecystoduodenal anastomoses.

In Germany, too, experience was gained with the Murphy button and its variations,[3] although neither this button nor its subsequently developed variants found widespread acceptance. Intestinal anastomoses mainly were performed using manual sutures, a situation that did not change until 1967, when stapler instruments with disposable cartridges were developed in the United States. Circular staplers provided surgical advantages, particularly in transdiaphragmatic esophageal and deep rectal anastomoses. However, the full practical advantages of circular staplers cannot be applied at all points of the colon. Thus when the stapling instrument can no longer be introduced transanally, intestinal anastomoses in the region of the colon can be created only with the aid of a separate colotomy. Nor is it always possible to avoid stenoses. To eliminate these disadvantages, attention was directed to the techniques using rings for bowel anastomoses. In 1985 Hardy, Pace, and Maney[4] described a biofragmentable anastomotic ring for bowel compression anastomoses for the first time. This anastomotic ring, marketed under the commercial name Valtrac, consists of fully absorbable polyglycolic acid with barium sulphate as the contrast medium. It allows the creation of inverted serosa-to-serosa intestinal anastomoses. The Valtrac ring does not remain in situ as a foreign body but breaks into fragments. More rarely it is eliminated intact from the body with the passage of stools.

Because initial experimental and clinical studies showed promising results,[4,5] we decided to examine use of this anastomotic ring in a teaching hospital under everyday conditions.

MATERIALS AND METHODS

From March 1989 to December 1991, 234 patients had one intestinal anastomosis using the Valtrac biofragmentable anastomotic ring (BAR); 29 patients had two anastomoses; and four patients had three. Altogether 304 BAR anastomoses were created in these 267 patients—115 men and 152 women, with a mean age of 61.2 years (range, 17 to 90) and 64.2 years (range, 20 to 88), respectively. Only patients selected for elective surgery entered the trial (i.e., patients with obstruction or peritonitis and all nonelective cases were excluded).

TECHNIQUE

The technique for BAR enteral anastomoses using the Valtrac ring has been described.[6] The Valtrac ring is composed of 87.5% polyglycolic acid and 12.5% barium sulphate. The barium sulphate component allows identification of the ring in the single overview radiograph of the abdomen. The polyglycolic acid permits the ring to fragment into parts or to dissolve completely. The ring consists of two mushroom-shaped half rings with a bridge mounted on an applicator. The rings are currently available with four different outer diameters: 25 mm, 28 mm, 31 mm, and 34 mm (in the study presented here, the 25 mm device was not yet available except for single instances). Each ring size is produced in variants regarding the compression zone (i.e., 1.5, 2, or 2.5 mm) (Fig. 1). These sizes refer to the ring distance obtained in the adapted state and must be selected according to the thickness of the bowel wall being compressed.

Design of Operation

Our approach uses the standard preoperative preparation with orthograde bowel enemas, intraoperative ultra-short-term antibiotic prophylaxis, preoperative and postoperative administration of low-dose heparin, parenteral feeding, and visualization of the anastomosis with water-soluble contrast medium on day 7 or 8 after the operation.

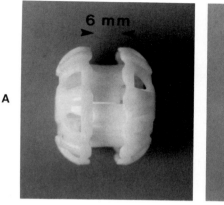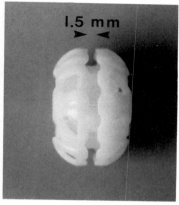

Fig. 1. Valtrac ring in open and closed position.

BAR Anastomosis Technique

The attached adipose and connective tissue in the region of the planned anastomosis is removed approximately 5 mm proximally and distally. Very good circulation in the stumps must be ensured. Any projecting mucosal edge is resected. A continuous, overhand purse-string suture, using 2-0 (rarely 3-0 gauge) Maxon, is performed with either colonic or stomach anastomoses. Alternatively, a purse-string suture clamp can be applied to the small bowel. Before introducing the ring, the opening of the intestine should be dilated gently with a dilation forceps (Fig. 2).

The bridge of the Valtrac ring is then fixed, using specially designed fixation forceps (Fig. 3). The forceps facilitate the introduction of the ring into the distal part of the anastomosis. After sewing this purse-string suture and removing the forceps, the anastomosis can be completed by simple compression. The holding mechanism comes to a stop inside the ring. The surgeon tests the maximal stress of the anastomosis by applying slight traction to the bowel.

The operations were performed by surgeons with various experience according to the training standard of the hospital. Prospectively, the following points were monitored: intraoperative details such as size and type of anastomosis and technical difficulties and postoperative details, including time of the first bowel movement, radiological control of the anastomosis at approximately day 8 by water-soluble contrast medium, and complications such as bleeding, leakage, stenoses, and disturbed motility.

The dissolution of the Valtrac ring was monitored

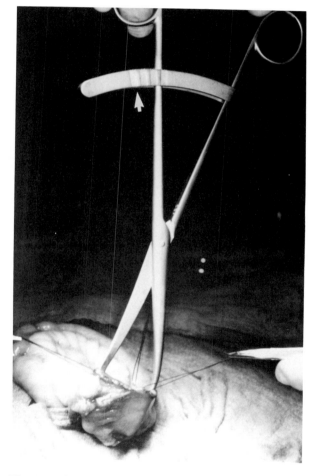

Fig. 2. Dilation of intestinal opening and estimation of adequate ring size *(arrow)*, varying from 25 to 34 mm.

by abdominal x-ray examination between postoperative days 8 and 30. The first 30 patients consecutively operated on were checked between months 6 and 12 after surgery by x-ray contrast visualization or by endoscopy.

RESULTS
Preoperative and Intraoperative Data

Indications for surgery among the 267 patients are shown in Tables 1 and 2. The types and localizations of anastomoses are given in Table 3 (Figs. 4 through 6).

Table 1. Indications for surgery in benign diseases

Diagnosis	Male	Female	Total
Inflammatory bowel disease	3	5	8
Ischemic bowel disease	3	1	4
Ulcer	3	2	5
Pancreatic pseudocyst	2	2	4
Diverticulitis	23	18	41
Elongated sigmoid	1	22	23
Rectal prolapse	4	16	20
Miscellaneous	6	8	14
TOTAL	45	74	119 (44.6%)

Table 2. Indications for surgery in malignant diseases

Diagnosis	Male	Female	Total
Esophageal cancer	2	1	3
Gastric cancer	17	9	26
Colonic cancer	19	31	50
Sigmoid cancer	14	24	38
Rectal cancer	3	5	8
Pancreatic cancer	3	3	6
Intestinal lymphoma	5	3	8
Other malignomas	7	2	9
TOTAL	70	78	148 (55.4%)

Table 3. Type and location of anastomosis in which BAR anastomosis was performed

Location	Total	End-to-End	End-to-Side	Side-to-Side
Colon to colon	155	155	0	0
Small bowel to colon	50	48	0	2
Small bowel to small bowel	75	36	35	4
Stomach to small bowel	14	6	5	3
Miscellaneous	10	1	6	3
TOTAL	304	246	46	12

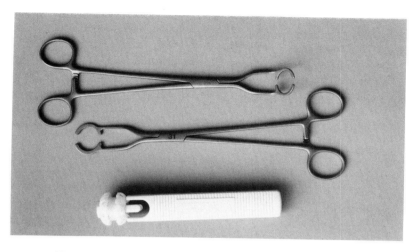

Fig. 3. Valtrac ring mounted on plastic-grip, fixation forceps.

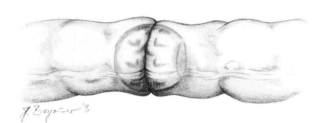

Fig. 4. Colocolostomy.

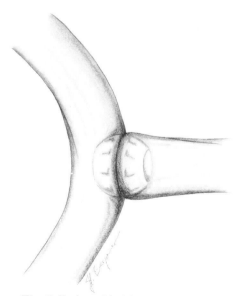

Fig. 5. End-to-side jejunojejunostomy.

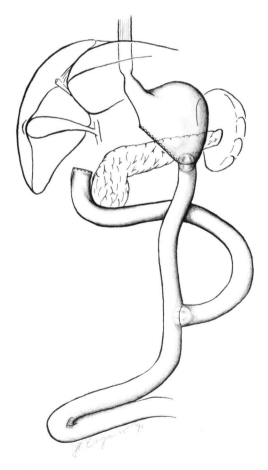

Fig. 6. Valtrac ring for gastrojejunostomy and jejunojejunostomy in Roux-en-Y- reconstruction after partial gastrectomy.

Table 4. Rate of leakage and locations after BAR anastomoses

Location	N	Radiological Leakage (n)	Clinical Leakage (n)
Colon to colon	155	16 (10.3%)	7 (4.5%)
Small bowel to colon	50	2 (4%)	1 (2%)
Small bowel to small bowel	75	1 (1%)	1 (1.3%)
Stomach to small bowel	14	1	1
Miscellaneous	10	0	0
TOTAL	304	20 (6.5%)	10 (3.3%)

Intraoperative Problems

In two instances the ring closure was difficult, probably because the wrong gap size of the compression zone was chosen. In three instances the ring size was not adequate. There were three serosal splits and one primary insufficiency (i.e., the anastomosis was not watertight). In 53 cases an additional suture was needed to correct either the purse-string suture or the anastomosis; in eight cases we used fibrin glue and in nine cases suture and glue. A total of 23% of the patients required intraoperative "corrections" in addition to the standard procedure.

However, comparing the incidence of corrections per anastomosis reveals a learning curve. After establishing the procedure in one hospital,* A. Thiede introduced the technique in another hospital,† so we observed a two-peak learning curve.

Postoperative Data

Postoperatively 6.5% of the anastomoses developed radiologically detectable leakage, with 3.3% of the anastomoses having leakages that were clinically relevant (temperature >38° C, leukocytes >12,000) (Table 4). The rate of leakage was highest in the colocolostomy procedure, followed by small bowel–colon anastomoses. The one insufficient gastrojejunostomy anastomosis was a palliative gastroenterostomy performed in a patient who was severely malnourished as a result of gastric carcinoma.

Problems with other types of anastomoses performed during the same operation included one insuffi-

*Friedrich-Ebert-Krankenhaus Neumünster (FEK).
†Chirurgische Universitätsklinik und Poliklinik Würzburg (CUW).

Table 5. Time table of bowel function after surgery using BAR anastomoses

Activity	Postoperative Days (and range)
First bowel movement	4 days (1-8)
Normal stools	6 days (3-14)
Tea offered	3 days (1-8)
Resorbable diet introduced	6 days (1-14)
Diet progressed as tolerated	8 days (5-18)
Normal food introduced	10 days (7-29)

ciency each with duodenal stump, esophagojejunostomy, J-pouch, colotomy, stapled lower anterior anastomosis, and small bowel perforation after adhesiolysis.

No bleeding episode was caused by a Valtrac anastomosis. However, reasons for bleeding (one instance each) included a stapled J-pouch, splenic artery, esophagitis, and hemorrhoidal bleeding and two instances after gastrectomy.

No intraoperative deaths occurred; however, 14 of 16 deaths occurred postoperatively from severe myocardial insufficiency. Two patients died from a pulmonary embolism.

Table 5 gives information about the return of bowel function and resumption of diet.

DISCUSSION

Since the first publication on BAR anastomoses using the Valtrac device in a clinical study,[5] various studies have been performed experimentally and clinically to investigate this type of anastomosis. Experimental studies in dogs and pigs showed that the creation of colonic anastomoses with the Valtrac ring was faster and simpler than using a running suture or staple technique.[4] Smith, Bubrick, and Mestitz[7] showed that the BAR anastomosis was also as safe as conventional techniques in low anterior resection in dogs irradiated with 5000 rads preoperatively. It was also shown that steroid application did not influence negatively the healing process of the BAR anastomoses in dogs.[8]

Technical Problems

The first clinical studies were undertaken mainly with colonic anastomoses.[5,9,10] Whereas Hardy, Pace, and Maney[4] described no difficulties in creating 27 anastomoses, in the American multicenter study[9] 6% of patients developed a problem or complication during the placement of the device, resulting in its removal. In 4% of the cases the problem could be solved. Similar results were obtained by the European multicenter trial in which 6.9% of patients had problems specific to the BAR.[10] Principally, these problems were that the device was too large to enter the intestine; a serosal tear occurred; and the intestinal wall was too thick for placement between the 6 mm open gap or for closure.

In our own series of 304 anastomoses it was difficult to close the ring in two instances (0.6%) because of choosing the wrong gap size at the compression zone. In three instances the ring diameter was not adequate (1%), and exchanging the ring was necessary. There were three (1%) serosal splits and one primary insufficiency (0.3%), all of which could be corrected. Thus the rate of "major" intraoperative difficulties was 2.9%. In 53 instances an additional suture was needed to correct either the purse-string suture or the anastomosis. Since the first 201 anastomoses were performed in a different institution (FEK) from the last 103 (CUW), we observed a two-peak learning curve concerning the necessary corrections, indicating that with increasing experience with this type of anastomosis, the need for corrections of either the purse-string suture or the anastomosis will diminish. This might also be a bias in the American and European multicenter studies, because the average number of anastomoses per center was low and the experience with this type of anastomosis was not uniform before entering the trial.[11] Because the purse-string suture clamps were not always working properly, we recommend using them only in the small intestine and prefer to use a hand-sewn purse-string suture in colonic or gastric positions. A correct purse-string suture is essential in this type of anastomosis, since in contrast to a circular stapling anastomosis in which the purse-string suture will be cut away during the creation of the anastomosis, in BAR anastomoses the purse-string suture is needed to keep the intestinal wall in the required position.

Leakage

The most significant postoperative complication after intestinal anastomoses is leakage. Rates vary, depending on the site of anastomosis. In the first clinical application by the inventor himself, the rate of leakage was 0 (0/27).[5] The multicenter trials report a rate of 3% without significant difference between the stapled and control groups.[11] In the European multicenter trial the rate was 1.9% (2/101) without difference between the stapled and hand-sewn controls.[10] Our own results show a clinically relevant rate of 3.3% leakage and a radiological rate of 6.5%. Four of the 20 radiologically and 10 clinically insufficient anastomoses required operation, and no death was caused by a Valtrac anastomosis. The 14 deaths resulting from severe cardiopulmonary insufficiency and two from lung emboli, however, reflect the rate of additional coexisting diseases in these patients. The mean age of all patients (63.1 years [range, 17 to 83]) was comparable to that of the multicenter study patients (60.2 years [range, 16 to 89]).[10,11]

Bleeding

The rate of postoperative bleeding complications of the anastomotic region is low in gastrointestinal surgery; however, inverting anastomoses especially must be controlled for bleeding. The rates vary between 0 and 2.7% for colonic and colorectal anastomoses using functional end-to-end techniques and 6% for circular staples.[12] In the American multicenter study there was a gastrointestinal bleeding rate of 1% for the BAR group[11] compared with 0.3% for the combined controls; however, the site of bleeding was not reported in this study. Bleeding was not mentioned in the European report for either BAR anastomoses or the controls.[10] In our own series of 304 BAR anastomoses, no bleeding occurred because of the application of a Valtrac ring.

Stenoses

The first 30 patients (all had colocolostomies) were consecutively followed up by x-ray examination or endoscopy 6 to 12 months after surgery. No clinically relevant stenoses could be observed. Stenosis formation is observed after use of a circular anastomotic technique with placement of circular staples in the high esophagus or deep rectal position. But if no technical errors occur, stricture or stenosis seldom occurs with gastrointestinal anastomoses. Since we did not perform Valtrac anastomoses in these stenosis-susceptible regions we cannot do a final evaluation on this subject.

Bowel Motility

The onset of bowel movements, as monitored in our study, is comparable to the normal time intervals after other techniques.[11] There was no ileus resulting from obstruction of a Valtrac anastomosis, and two gastroenterostomies resulted in delayed emptying of the stomach, as is usually observed in this type of anastomosis. No complication such as trapping dissolved material from a proximal Valtrac ring in a not-yet-dissolved distal one was observed in patients who received multiple BAR anastomoses. However, especially in those patients who had Valtrac rings in a high intestinal position (e.g., with jejunoduodenostomy or gastrojejunostomy), we delayed the onset of ingesting a normal diet 10 days (range, 7 to 29) in the whole group versus 15 days (range, 9 to 20) in the multiple-application group.

CONCLUSION

Enteral anastomoses with the biofragmentable Valtrac ring can be recommended as offering simple-to-learn manipulation and the creation of effectively standardized enteroanastomoses at various bowel sections. Stenoses and postoperative bleeding practically do not occur, and the suture dehiscence rate is comparable to that for stapled anastomoses or manual suture anastomoses at corresponding locations.

The results observed with Valtrac in this prospective study allow the following conclusion: in the colon and the upper and middle regions of the rectum and in the small bowel region, compression anastomoses function excellently and offer an attractive alternative to manual sutures or staples. This is particularly the case in view of the target criteria of standardization, low complication rate, and absence of stenoses. The experience gained in the esophagus, stomach, and bile ducts is currently insufficient to allow an assessment of compression anastomoses in these areas.

REFERENCES

1. Denans FN. Nouveau procédé pour la guérison des plaies des intestins. Recueil de la Société Royale des Médicine de Marseille (Séance du 24 fév. 1826, rédigé par M.P. Roux). Marseille: Imprimerie de'Archard, 1827, pp 127-131.
2. Murphy JB. Cholecysto-intestinal, gastrointestinal, entero-intestinal anastomosis and approximation with sutures (original research). Med Rec 42:665-676, 1892.
3. Czerny V. Über die Verwendung des Murphyknopfes als Erastz für die Darmnaht. Verh Dtsch Ges Chir 25:94-98, 1986.
4. Hardy TG Jr, Pace WG, Maney JW. A biofragmentable ring for sutureless bowel anastomosis. An experimental study. Dis Colon Rectum 28:484-490, 1985.
5. Hardy TG Jr, Aguilar PS, Stewart WRC. Initial experience with a biofragmentable ring for sutureless bowel anastomosis. Dis Colon Rectum 30:55-61, 1987.
6. Thiede A, Schubert G, Klima J, et al. Enterale Anastomosen mit dem biofragmentablen Valtrac-Ring. Chirurg 62:819-824, 1991.
7. Smith AD, Bubrick MP, Mestitz ST. Evaluation of the biofragmentable anastomotic ring following preoperative irradiation to the rectosigmoid in dogs. Dis Colon Rectum 31:5-9, 1988.
8. Maney JW, Katz AR, Li LK, et al. Biofragmentable bowel anastomosis ring: Comparative efficacy studies in dogs. Surgery 103:56-62, 1988.
9. Corman ML, Prager ED, Hardy TG Jr, et al. Comparison of the Valtrac™ biofragmentable anastomosis ring with conventional suture and staple anastomosis in colon surgery: Results of a prospective, randomized clinical trial. Dis Colon Rectum 32:183-187, 1989.
10. Cahill CJ, Betzler M, Gruwez JA, et al. Sutureless large bowel anastomosis: European experience with the biofragmentable anastomosis ring. Br J Surg 76:344-347, 1989.
11. Bubrick MP, Corman ML, Cahill CJ, et al. Prospective, randomized trial of the biofragmentable anastomosis ring. Am J Surg 161:136-143, 1991.
12. Gordon PH, Dalrymple S. The use of staples for reconstruction after colonic and rectal surgery. In Ravitch MM, Steichen FM, eds. Principles and Practice of Surgical Stapling. Chicago: Year Book, 1986, pp 402-431.
13. West of Scotland and Highland Anastomosis Study Group. Suturing or stapling in gastrointestinal surgery: A prospective randomized study. Br J Surg 78:337-341, 1991.

92   *Gastrointestinal Viscerosynthesis With the Biofragmentable Anastomotic Ring*

Tapani Havia

A new anastomotic device, the biofragmentable anastomotic ring (BAR), is based on the old concept of Murphy's button. In its modern version it was introduced by Hardy et al. in 1985. Acceptance of the BAR is increasing. It forms a serosa-to-serosa inverted sutureless anastomosis without tissue necrosis in the anastomotic circumference. No foreign material is left in the bowel wall after ring fragmentation. The anastomosis is also standardized. Murphy's button was originally used in the anastomosis between the gallbladder and the small bowel, but the BAR was designed for large bowel anastomosis.

Our clinical experience with BAR anastomosis consists of having performed 283 compression anastomoses used in gastrointestinal viscerosynthesis procedures since June 1988. Our comparative study of the use of BAR and manual and mechanical sutures in dogs showed no difference in either macroscopic or histological healing of the anastomosis. Our clinical results are presented, with special emphasis on anastomosis-related complications.

MATERIALS AND METHODS

From June 1988 to August 1992 a prospective, randomized trial of the use of BAR was conducted in the Department of Surgery of the University of Turku, Finland. The study randomization was finished in March 1991. Four hundred fifty-nine patients were included in the study. Two hundred eighty-three BAR anastomoses were performed at four gastrointestinal tract sites: stomach-to–small bowel, cholecystojejunal, small bowel–to–small bowel, and colocolic. The remaining 176 procedures were accomplished manually with two-layer anastomoses of the same sites. The patient groups were matched with regard to age, sex, and concomitant disease. Each patient's postoperative course was carefully followed: the number of days of nasogastric drainage was recorded until the volume was < 500 ml/day; the number of days of intravenous therapy, the time required for resumption of an oral diet, and the time un-

til reoccurrence of bowel movements were also noted. All complications and the length of postoperative hospital stay were recorded. The EEA-sizers (for stapling) were also used in end-to-end anastomoses to determine the size of anastomotic ring required in a given case. A slight dilation of the bowel ends was performed. The purse-string suture was usually placed with a purse-string instrument.

The majority of the colonic anastomoses in our study were elective, but many emergency right-sided anastomoses and some acute left colon anastomoses were included. In those cases, the left colon was irrigated intraoperatively. Bowel preparation in patients who underwent the elective procedure consisted of oral bowel irrigation. In the other groups studied (patients who underwent small bowel, stomach, or gallbladder procedures), both elective and acute operations are included.

The focus of this prospective study was the evaluation of anastomosis-related complications and postoperative bowel recovery.

COLONIC ANASTOMOSIS

One hundred twenty-three colonic anastomoses have been created with the BAR technique; these were compared with 71 two-layered manual anastomoses. Ileocolic, colocolic, and colorectal anastomoses were performed. There was no significant difference in the postoperative return of bowel function or in the length of the postoperative hospital stay between the BAR and the suture groups. Six leakages (4.8%) occurred in the BAR group and three (4.2%) were noted in the manual suture group. Three patients with leakage who had undergone BAR anastomosis were very high-risk patients: one was receiving permanent anticoagulant therapy, another had had a severe postoperative myocardial infarction, and the third had had an unprepared left colon before anastomosis. The other three leaks occurred after elective left colon surgery in patients with no known risk factors. All leaks were treated with Hartmann's procedure, and all patients survived.

The long-term follow-up of 30 left colon BAR anastomoses showed one anastomotic stricture that was successfully treated with reoperation.

SMALL BOWEL ANASTOMOSIS

This randomized series consisted of 228 anastomoses, 140 of which were performed with a BAR device and 88 of which were hand-sewn controls. Several types of anastomosis (end-to-end, end-to-side, and side-to-side) were used. In the BAR anastomoses, the purse-string device and 3-0 Maxon monofilament were used. The manually sutured anastomoses were performed with continuous 3-0 Dexon in two layers with the inversion technique. The most common anastomosis performed was a side-to-side jejunojejunostomy after the Billroth II gastric resection (Braun's enteroanastomosis).

One leakage (0.7%) occurred in the BAR group in an end-to-side jejunoileostomy performed for morbid obesity. This leak, which was the only significant anastomosis-related early complication, was successfully treated with a temporary enterostomy that was later closed. Two months after operation, another patient had a jejunal perforation 1 cm from a Roux-en-Y anastomosis. There were possible signs of foreign-body exposure in the bowel wall in this case. A vigorous original snap of the BAR device at the time of coupling may have caused a covered weakness in the jejunal wall that resulted in a "spontaneous" perforation later on.

CHOLECYSTOENTEROSTOMY

In this randomized series, 13 cholecystoenterostomies were performed with the BAR device and 10 were performed by manual suture. This bilioenteric anastomosis was performed primarily to alleviate jaundice in the treatment of pancreatic carcinoma. A purse-string device was used in both the fundus of the gallbladder and in the jejunum. A 28/1.5 mm BAR device was used in all cases. Neither anastomosis-related mortality nor anastomosis complications occurred.

GASTRIC ANASTOMOSIS

Our experience with the use of BAR in gastroenterostomy is limited. Only seven such anastomoses have been performed. One gastroduodenostomy as part of a Billroth I reconstruction was uneventful and did not result in an obstruction. In another (Billroth II) reconstruction, obstruction occurred until the BAR ring was fragmented. Five other anastomoses were performed as palliative gastroenterostomies to relieve duodenal obstruction; four of these were uneventful, but in one very ill patient, a leak developed on the fourteenth postoperative day. Autopsy results on this patient showed that the ring had already fragmented.

CONCLUSION

The biofragmentable anastomotic ring results in a standardized, inverted, sutureless bowel anastomosis. No histological differences were seen in the healing process in the dog model when results of this anastomotic ring were compared with those of the stapled or sutured anastomoses. There were no differences in the recovery of bowel function or in the length of hospital stay when the BAR device was used instead of manually sutured anastomosis in human colonic procedures.

In general, the incidence of anastomosis-related early complications is low and is comparable to that of the two-layer handmade anastomosis in colon, small-bowel, and cholecystoenteric use. The BAR may have advantages in cases in which the healing process is disturbed (e.g., following irradiation).

The long-term follow-up of colonic BAR anastomosis indicated satisfactory results. Although the application of the biofragmental anastomosis ring in gastric surgery requires more investigation, we can recommend the BAR as a safe, reliable alternative to manual anastomosis in colonic, small bowel, and cholecystoenteric procedures.

93   *Treatment of Pancreatic Fistulas Using Biological Sealants*

Vincenzo Costantino and Sergio Pedrazzoli

Fistulas occur as frequent and life-threatening complications of pancreatic surgery; moreover, because they lengthen hospitalization time, they are as costly for the patient as for the health services. This is why some surgeons prefer to perform total or near-total pancreatectomy instead of operations that require anastomosis to the pancreas or pancreatic duct.[1] Precise operative techniques and full preoperative correction of nutritional deficiencies are in themselves considered preventive measures against fistula formation.

Postoperative fistulas may occur early or late. The early type (before the sixth or seventh postoperative day) is usually attributed to errors in surgical technique while creating pancreatic-jejunal anastomosis or suturing the pancreatic stump or to massive necrosis of the anastomosed jejunal loop. This type of fistula does not benefit from the physiological adhesions that occur after all operations; therefore its secretions spread throughout the abdominal cavity, sometimes forming loculations that may become infected. Mortality is high, and these fistulas more frequently require surgical treatment, ranging from simple suture of leaks or peritoneal toilet through drainage to complete excision of the remaining pancreas.

Late fistulas (after the seventh postoperative day) are more common and benefit from physiological scarring of the healing operative site. They usually require only nonoperative treatment, sometimes associated with interventional radiology. Examples of such treatment are as follows:

- Fasting with total parenteral nutrition (TPN), giving sufficient caloric intake for the patient's condition and for the postoperative catabolic phase, thus physiological pancreatic secretions are reduced by this treatment
- Near-total pharmacological suppression of pancreatic secretions by means of somatostatin or analogs
- Neutralizing contamination with antibiotic prophylaxis or, in case of positive cultures, treatment with specific antibiotics for a given bacterial sensitivity
- Compensation for fluid, electrolyte, and protein losses and general conditioning of the patient
- Gentle mechanical debridement of fistula walls and irrigation with acid pH solutions, to clean the fistula and buffer pancreatic secretion
- Protection of the skin against corrosion by secretions, using enterostomal materials around the exit hole of the fistula
- X-ray study check-up of fistula shape and direction and placement or readjustment of drainage tubes to bring pancreatic secretions to the exterior by the shortest and most direct path

We believe this last morphological aspect is very important, since it is the definitive step of all nonoperative treatments. The initial morphological aspect of pancreatic fistulas may influence their healing, according to whether the path is simple and straight or complex and ramified with undrained side collections requiring a series of radiological-surgical maneuvers to drain them. The presence or absence of previously placed drainage tubes, their position with respect to the fistula, type of fistula (ductal or anastomotic), amount of residual pancreas, and the presence or absence of other septic or hemorrhagic complications may all also influence healing and fistula flow itself.

For the pancreatic fistulas we observed, we used all of the nonoperative methods to obtain a low-flow straight fistulous tract small enough to block with human fibrin sealant. This material was deposited with a two-way catheter introduced into the tract and replacing the drainage tube. The sealant was used as a biological glue, allowing the organism to develop normal scarring to repair the lesion[1] (Figs. 1 through 4).

MATERIALS AND METHODS

Our overall experience in the treatment of fistulas with fibrin sealant includes the following locations: nine enteric, two biliary, one vaginal, and twelve pancreatic. Of these pancreatoduodenectomy had been performed in five patients with cancer or a tumor (two for cancer of the pancreas [cases 1 and 11]; one for cancer of the

Text continued on p. 503.

497

Fig. 1. A, B, Pancreatic fistula after left pancreatectomy (case 4). Drainage catheter is not in best sloping position for emptying abscess cavity. **C, D,** Catheter change and complete healing of abscess. Note open communication with Wirsung's duct *(W)*.

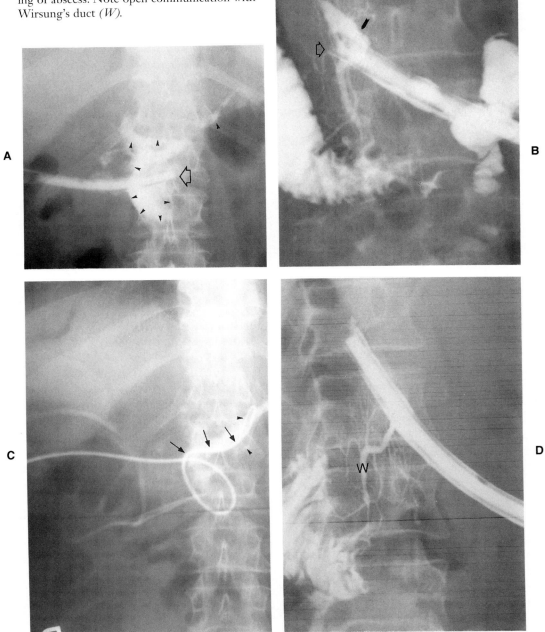

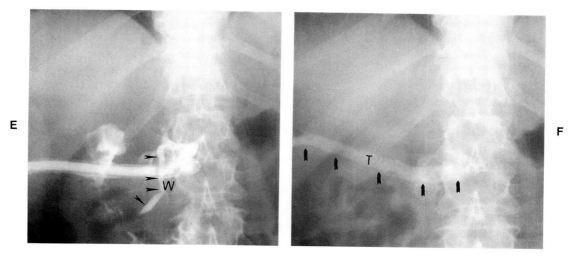

Fig. 1, cont'd. E, Final x-ray examination before sealant injection. Tip of catheter reaches Wirsung duct's opening. **F,** Fistulous tract *(T)* filled with fibrin sealant mixed with contrast medium.

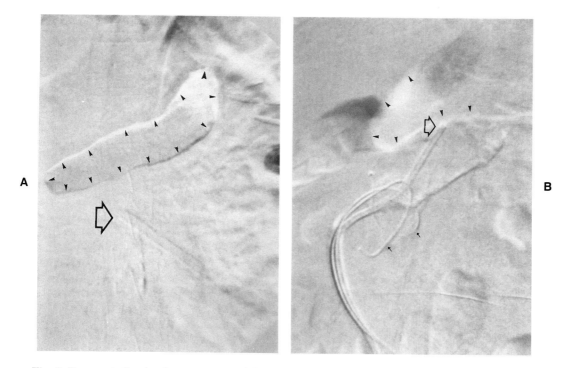

Fig. 2. Pancreatic fistula after acute necrotizing pancreatitis, with drainage and necrosectomy (case 8). **A,** Drainage catheter does not reach cavity. **B,** The drainage tube is pushed along the wire.

Continued.

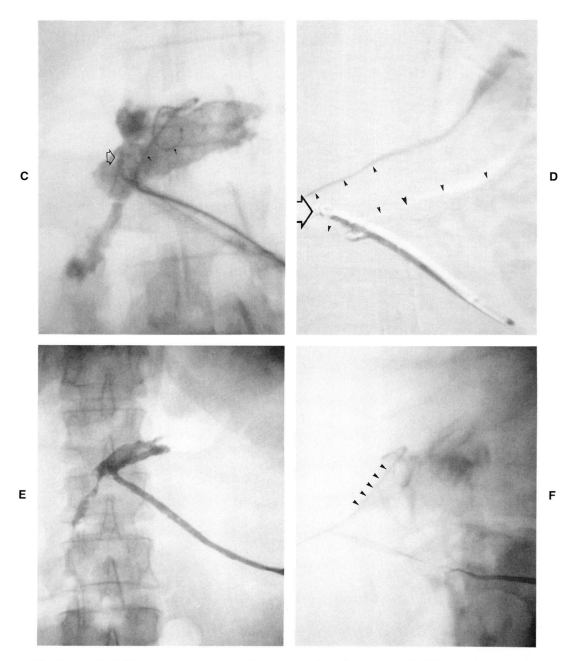

Fig. 2, cont'd. C, Two wires are introduced in better position for drainage. **D,** Tip of catheter reaches abscess cavity. **E,** Reduction of cavity, now suitable for sealant treatment. **F,** After sealant application in fistulous tract, a wire is left in place for future catheter introduction if necessary.

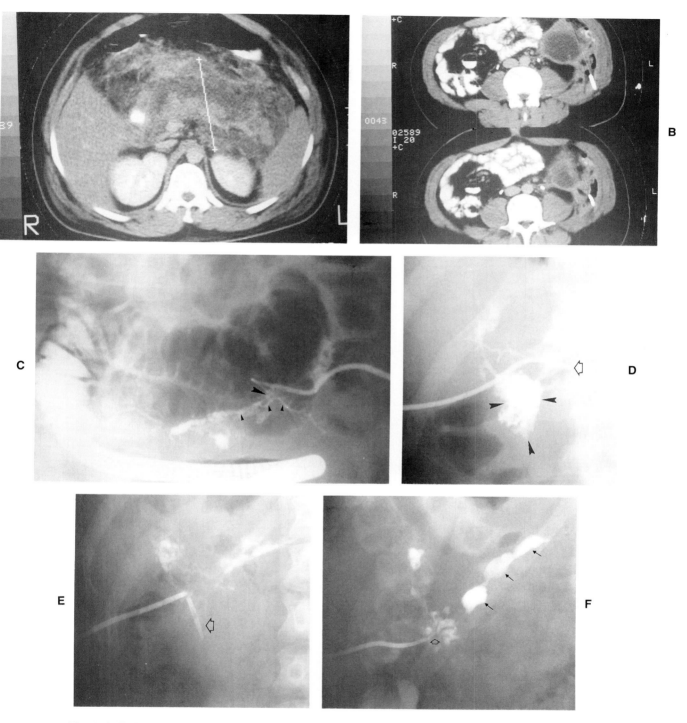

Fig. 3. A, B, Percutaneous drainage of pancreatic pseudocyst after acute necrotizing pancreatitis (case 6). **C,** Retrograde pancreatography shows leakage from Wirsung's duct. **D,** Abscess cavity inadequately drained by catheter. **E,** Correct repositioning of catheter in cavity. **F,** Collections along original fistulous tract are not well drained.

Continued.

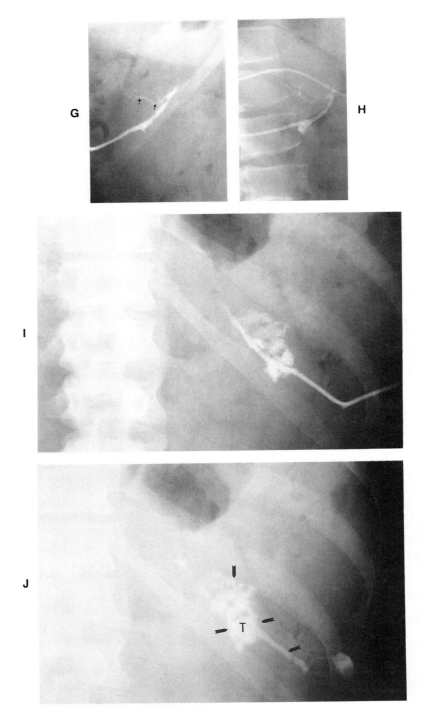

Fig. 3, cont'd. G, H, Further drainage, repositioning, and straightening of fistulous course. **I,** Last fistulography before sealant application under high pressure. **J,** Area of sealant sediment.

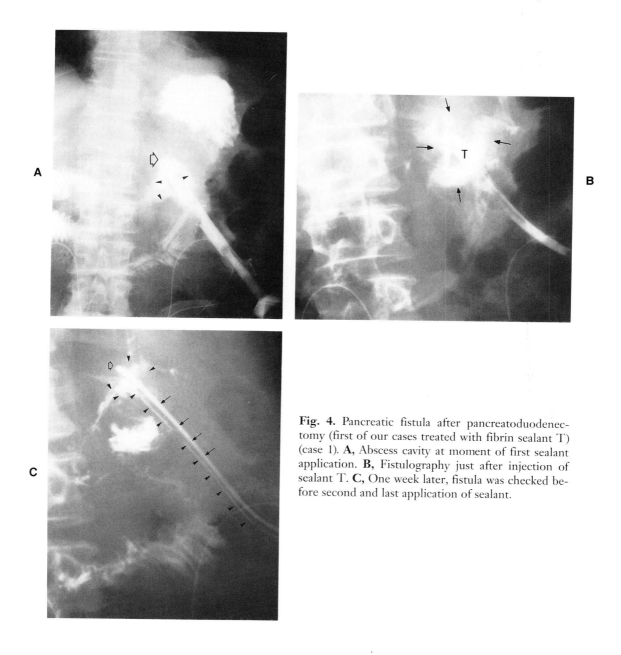

Fig. 4. Pancreatic fistula after pancreatoduodenectomy (first of our cases treated with fibrin sealant T) (case 1). **A,** Abscess cavity at moment of first sealant application. **B,** Fistulography just after injection of sealant T. **C,** One week later, fistula was checked before second and last application of sealant.

papilla [case 7]; and two for endocrine tumors [cases 2 and 12]). Two patients had left pancreatectomy (one for chronic pancreatitis [case 3]; one for cystadenoma [case 4]). One patient underwent pancreatico-jejunal anastomosis for chronic pancreatitis (case 10); one enucleation of an insulinoma of the pancreatic head (case 5). In three patients, operations for acute necrotizing pancreatitis became necessary (one necrosectomy plus drainage [case

8]; one percutaneous drainage of pseudocyst [case 6]; and one cystojejunostomy [case 9]). Two of the above-mentioned patients (cases 6 and 8) had previously been treated in another hospital.

Since 1984 60% of the postoperative patients with pancreatic fistulas observed in our department have been given fibrin sealant treatment. All these patients received TPN and nonoperative treatment (starting with somatostatin or somatostatin analogs), and they all required specific antibiotics.

Morphological study of the tract and assessment of the drainage site with respect to the fistulous abscess were carried out by means of interventional fistulography. This study normally was carried out once a week, in close collaboration between radiologists and surgeons.

The technique is based on the use and fluoroscopic manipulation of angiographic instruments (e.g., wires, preformed catheters, dilators, and cannulas) (Fig. 5). Initial contrast studies reveal the position of the surgical drainage tube in relation to the abscess cavity, its size and shape, the tract, and drainage efficiency during aspiration with a syringe. Procedures vary according to whether the drainage tube must be repositioned, replaced, or a new drainage catheter introduced percutaneously or by open operation at the completion of the contrast study. Badly positioned or ineffective drainage tubes are repositioned after interventional fistulography, with water-soluble contrast media injected through the drainage tube itself, allowing us to choose the best type of wire and/ or most suitably shaped angiographic catheter. The wire and/or catheter (see Fig. 1, *C*) is gently pushed under fluoroscopic control along the fistulous tract to reach possible abscess cavities or the origin of a fistula without a collection. The drainage tube is pushed along the wire to the most suitable point for drainage of all secretions (see Fig. 2, *B* and *C*) or it is removed and replaced by a suitable catheter mounted on the wire left in its original satisfactory

position. If the drainage tube is inefficient in draining secretions, either because of its size or because of the physical composition of the secretions, it is replaced by a larger one, again under fluoroscopic control using an angiographic wire (Seldinger-type method) (see Fig. 1, *A-D*).

To favor washing of the fistulous tract, we use carefully positioned two-way catheters and antibiotic solutions or acid pH solutions to buffer the alkalinity of the pancreatic secretion. When necessary, the skin is protected with enterostomal materials.[2]

In all cases the contrast medium used for fistulography is completely aspirated after the study.

Any side collections are also carefully drained, since they easily become septic and retard healing.

All these radiological procedures aim at creating a straight and narrow path so that the fibrin sealant for complete blockage of the original tract to the skin can be properly applied (see Figs. 1, *F* and 3, *J*).

Fibrin sealant is a combination of two components: a freeze-dried thrombin to which a solution of calcium chloride is added and a freeze-dried protein powder (Tisseel, Immuno AG) dissolved in a solution of fibrinolysis inhibitor (aprotinin, 3000 IU) (Fig. 6). As the two components combine during application, the fibrin sealant consolidates and adheres to the site of application as quickly as the thrombin concentration increases. The thrombin is available in high (Thrombin 500) and low (Thrombin 4) concentrations; by mixing one preparation with the other in the same syringe sealant con-

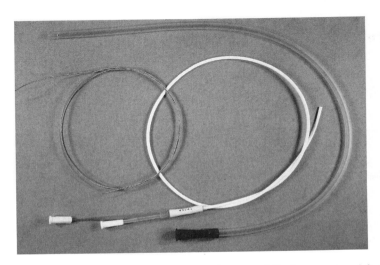

Fig. 5. Wire, silicone drainage tube, and two-way catheter used for interventional fistulography.

solidation is obtained 20 to 30 seconds after injection. Since 1990 a 5 ml solution of aprotinin (20,000 IU) has also been used to reduce the natural fibrinolytic activity. After being prepared properly at 37° C, the two sealant components are separately injected through a two-way catheter (a normal angiographic balloon catheter with the tip cut off) (Fig. 7, *A* and *B*) so they can mix together just outside the tip of the catheter,[4] introduced into the tract through the drainage tube. Mixing starts at the initial point of the fistula, and the catheter is gradually withdrawn until the fistulous lumen is completely filled with sealant.

The persistence of consolidated fibrin sealant in the tract is determined by the following:
- The quantity of fibrin used
- Fibrinolytic activity in the area of the fistulous opening
- The type and quality of fibrinolysis inhibitor added to the sealant or applied to the area of the fistula
- Phagocytosis by macrophages and granulocytes

Fibrinolytic activity in the fistulous area is determined by tissue-bound plasminogen activators. Because it occurs in endothelial cells, fibrinolytic activity is also high in abundantly vascularized areas.[5] High concentrations

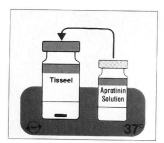
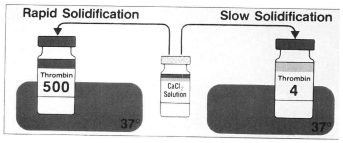

Fig. 6. The fibrin sealant is a combination of two components: a freeze-dried thrombin to which a solution of calcium chloride is added and a freeze-dried protein powder dissolved in a solution of fibrinolysis inhibitor. It adheres to the site of application as quickly as the thrombin concentration increases.

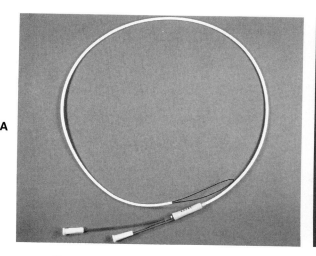
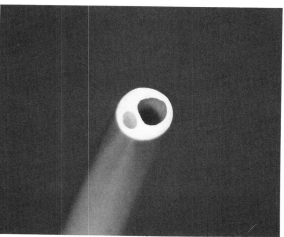

A

B

Fig. 7. A, Two-way catheter (normal angiographic balloon catheter with its tip cut off) used to inject the two sealant components—thrombin and protein—separately, so that they can mix outside the tip of the catheter. **B,** The two channels obtained by cutting off the tip of an angiographic balloon catheter. The catheter is introduced through the fistula drainage tube and the cut-off tip is placed against the fistulous opening. The two sealants are injected simultaneously, one in each channel, and they solidify as they mix at the catheter tip.

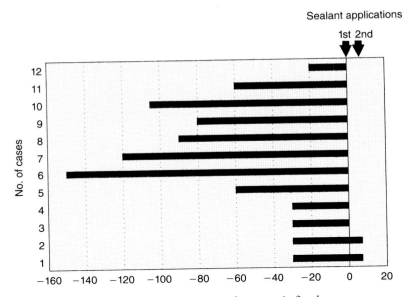

Fig. 8. Duration (in days) of pancreatic fistulas.

of aprotinin retard degradation of the occluding fibrin coagulate.

The two sealant components, in a liquid state, are injected in the two-way catheter at the same time, using two separate syringes. Solidification time depends on the thrombin concentration used. The sealant reaches 70% of its final strength within a few minutes and 100% after approximately 2 hours.

Water-soluble radiopaque medium is added to both sealant components in order not to alter the optimal 1:1 mixing ratio and for better fluoroscopic control of the point of sealant application[2] (see Figs. 1, *F*, 3, *J*, and 4, *B*). In the most difficult cases a malleable wire is left for a few days in the fistulous tract to anticipate possible failure of the sealing treatment by maintaining easy access for a new catheter if necessary[2] (see Fig. 2, *F*).

RESULTS

The results of fibrin sealant treatment are shown in Fig. 8.

Of the 12 patients with pancreatic fistulas, 10 required only one sealant application, which completely and definitively blocked the fistulous tract without complications. In two patients (cases 1 and 2), who had both had previous pancreatoduodenectomies for endocrine and exocrine pancreatic cancer and who happened to be the first patients treated by us, only reduced

fistulous flow and diameter were achieved. A week later the sealant was applied a second time and was fully successful (see Fig. 4, *C*).

DISCUSSION

Pancreatic fistulas may appear after abdominal operation, acute attacks of pancreatitis, or open or closed abdominal trauma. Classification is made after considering not only cause and course but also the nature of the secretion and its flow. Generally accepted treatment includes TPN, pharmacological suppression of secretion, antibiotic therapy, and drainage procedures. X-ray examination and contrast studies are essential to evaluate the effectiveness of treatment. When no healing can be achieved rapidly by nonoperative treatment, drainage procedures must be adopted (Fig. 9, *A* and *B*). They should render the whole fistulous tract straight and smooth so that all secretions and the injected contrast medium can be aspirated easily through the catheter. If collateral branches or fluid collections are detected, additional catheters must be placed in position. Only at this point can fibrin sealant treatment be helpful. Earlier use probably will not be efficacious, whereas much delayed treatment is useless.

Good results have been reported by some authors who used the sealant to tighten pancreatointestinal anastomoses and to protect against leakage of the pancre-

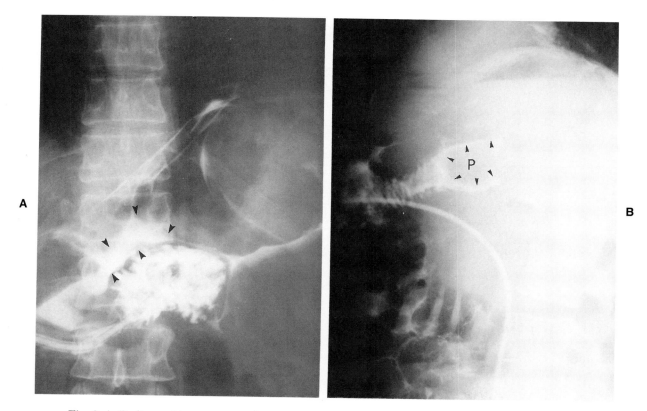

Fig. 9. A, Radiographic contrast studies are essential to evaluate treatment through drainage and the need for readjustments, respectively, in sealant injection. **B,** Drainage procedures should straighten fistulous tracts and give direct access to the fistula to facilitate evacuation of secretions, aspiration of contrast material, and injection of sealants.

atic duct after left pancreatic resection. Nevertheless, the prospective randomized trials that we have conducted since 1986 have failed to reveal the effectiveness of fibrin sealant in preventing fistula formation after primary pancreatic surgery. However, the use of fibrin sealant appears justifiable, since it forms a physiological barrier against organic secretions and also supports an optimal physiological healing mechanism. When the obstructive effect of the sealant ceases with the arrest of the antifibrinolytic action of aprotinin and the degradation of thrombin, new granulating tissue has had time to grow, and the site of injection is gradually completely occluded.

In our experience no complications due to sealing treatment such as local or general infections or allergies have been observed. Only in two cases was a second application needed before the fistula healed. In practice, the technique is simple and easy to repeat. In some cases which would otherwise have required surgical procedures, sealing hastened the healing process. Although the number of treated cases is still relatively low, the results are satisfactory and encouraging for the future.

REFERENCES

1. Gripon S, Bouillot JL, Rolland E, et al. Fistules pancréatiques après duodénopancreatectomie céphalique. Fistulisation dirigée ou totalisation de l'exérèse pancréatique? J Chir (Paris) 3:161-165, 1988.
2. Costantino V, Pedrazzoli S, Miotto D, et al. Trattamento delle fistole con l'uso della colla di fibrina umana (TISSUCOL). Risultati preliminari della nostra esperienza. Acta Chir Ital 41:756-760, 1985.

3. Miotto D, Viglione C, Chiesura-Corona M, et al. La gestione radiologica dei drenaggi chirurgici addominali. Radiol Med 74:13-17, 1987.
4. Pini Prato GP, Cortellini P, Clauser C, et al. Basi biologiche della sintesi tissutale con la colla di fibrina umana. Minerva Stomatol 32:1-5, 1983.
5. The Art of Tisseeling. History Background, Application Technique and Applications of Fibrin Sealing in Modern Surgery. Vienna, Austria: IMMUNO AG, 1988.

94   *Biological Glues and Tissues: Can They Prevent Leakage of an Anastomosis?*

Didier Mutter, Serge Evrard, and Jacques Marescaux

Postoperative anastomosis leakage is a major complication of digestive tract surgery, with a reported incidence of 5% to 30%.[1] This rate is particularly severe in the high-risk anastomosis, such as cervical esophageal anastomosis (26%), and low rectal anastomosis (10% to 30% leaks or fistulas by clinical or radiological diagnosis). Gastrointestinal anastomotic leaks and fistulas continue to cause significant morbidity and mortality in spite of improved preoperative care and the availability of new closure techniques such as stapling and fibrin-based patches. Studies of a new biomaterial for the protective support of anastomotic healing are being evaluated.

STAPLED ANASTOMOSIS

Is stapling superior to simple hand suturing? Staplers are preferred for low colorectal or high thoracoesophageal anastomoses, which are difficult to reach by hand. The anatomical advantages are definite. A stapled suture uses fine, well-tolerated suture material and is immediately leak proof, atraumatic, and well vascularized. Mechanical suturing has led to a significant improvement in the outcome of emergency digestive tract surgery, but it is of negligible value in surgery of the small bowel or intraperitoneal, descending colon compared with hand suturing.

FIBRIN-SEALED ANASTOMOSIS

Fibrin glue is a two-component solution that takes advantage of the final stage of the coagulation process. The main component is human fibrinogen obtained by cryo-precipitation together with fibronectin and factor XIII known to stabilize the fibrin polymers, the clot. The second component is lyophilized thrombin reconstituted in calcium chloride solution. The cohesive elastic sealant adheres to adjacent tissues by physical and chemical bonding in 3 to 5 minutes. Under development since 1970,[2] fibrin glue has been available in France since 1982. It has been studied in vitro and in vivo, in animals and humans, and fibrin sealing is currently an accepted method in operative surgery.

In Vitro Studies

Deposited fibrin stimulates the formation of granulation tissue, including collagen precipitation.[3] Fibrin enhances the cellular growth and mitosis of in vitro fibroblasts. The implanted fibrin clot is rapidly invaded by new capillaries and fibroblasts.[4] Thrombin has mitogenic characteristics in cell culture and affects platelet activation.[5] These characteristics confirm the importance of the fibrin clot in wound repair. The half-degradation time of the glue is only 3 days.[6] Furthermore, when the fibrin glue is immersed in pancreatic juice in vitro, fibrinolysis occurs within 15 hours.[7] This short survival time of the glue makes its use controversial.

Animal Studies

To assess the efficacy of fibrin glue in sealing and preventing leaks from digestive tract anastomoses, healing of different sutured colonic anastomoses in the rat was observed after the addition of biological glue. Heidecke et al.[8] showed an increased bursting-pressure resistance on days 3 and 5, whereas van der Ham et al.[9] concluded that gluing seems to have a negative influence, decreasing the bursting pressure on day 7. In spite of these contradictory results, Giardino et al.[10] and Hjortrup et al.[11] have described nonsutured, glued intestinal anastomoses in pigs that confirm the potentialities of biological glue.

Human Studies

In humans, fibrin adhesives usually supplement sutured or stapled anastomoses to prevent leakage,[12,13] but a reduced leakage rate has not been confirmed. Tashiro et al.,[7] using fibrin glue in patients undergoing pancreatojejunostomy after pancreatoduodenectomy, reported a statistically significant decrease in the incidence of major leaks, but the trial was not prospective. A broad study[14] supporting gluing of anastomoses revealed two major shortcomings: (1) failure to specify the type of anastomosis, hand sewn or stapled, and (2) extreme variations in conditions, that is, type of suture or anastomosis, complications reported without reference to the organ concerned, and absence of criteria for inclusion or exclusion.[14]

THE PATCH

Because neither of these techniques has yet significantly improved anastomosis leakage rates, we have investigated a novel approach to the prevention of anastomotic failure and to the closure of an established fistula. Recent advances in the use of in vitro reconstituted matrices as biological supports for cell culture, as well as the increased frequency of their use in other surgical specialities, suggest that such reconstructed connective tissue might be of value in gastrointestinal surgery.

In this field, the biomaterial actually available is bovine collagen fleece, but there are very few ad hoc reports on the clinical use of artificial connective matrices.[1] Collagen fleece subcutaneously implanted in the rat causes a severe reaction. The possibility of developing antibodies to bovine collagen[15] or thrombin after implantation of fibrin glue[16] is not negligible. New reconstituted connective tissue matrices were developed beginning in 1986. The first, the elastin patch, was fabricated from bovine elastin; the second, the collagen patch, from human placental collagen.

Patch Preparation

For preparation of the first elastin patch,[17] lyophilized powder of cold insoluble proteins was dissolved at 37° C in 6 ml of phosphate buffer, pH 7.4. To a solution containing 40 g/L fibrinogen and 7 g/L fibronectin was added a mixture of 100 mg of human aortic elastin and 0.5 ml of cryoglobulin solution. At this time, 0.1 ml (1000 International units) of Zymofren (Specia, Paris), 1 ml of soluble collagen, and 1 mg thiourea were added. Six units of thrombin were added and stirred. The mixture was then immediately poured into a mold of appropriate shape and kept at 37° C for at least 30 minutes before withdrawal. Excess buffer was removed with blotting paper. The prepared patch was kept until its use in a sanitized package after it had been sterilized by gamma-ray irradiation.

Collagen patches consisted of oxidized collagen of different gallenic forms providing stability of the biomaterial. Collagen (type I + III and type IV) was extracted and purified from placental tissue.[17] This method of human collagen extraction and conditioning has been patented by Imedex.[18,19] Human collagen was prepared[17] from placentas washed with ethanol and neutral and acid buffers to eliminate tissue blood and lipids. The placentas were then digested by pepsin at acid pH to render the collagen soluble. Collagen was recovered by sodium chloride fractionation and acetone dried. Collagen lattices were prepared with sterile collagen powder. Collagen type I + II was mixed with periodic acid, oxidized, lyophilized, and compressed. Collagen type IV was cross linked and oxidized. The oxidized collagen type I + II was lyophilized, and collagen type IV was then poured over the collagen type I + III to form a resistant collagen film coating. The modifications in the successive experimental trials concerned mainly the thickness of the collagen type I + III layer and the importance of the collagen type IV layer.

In Vitro Studies

A prerequisite for a useful digestive tract biomaterial is that it must remain around the digestive anastomosis long enough to allow wound healing, despite aggression by biliary and pancreatic enzymes.[20] The patches were incubated in human bile and pancreatic juice. The elastin patch was quickly lysed in both digestive fluids. The collagen patch was not dissolved after 30 days' incubation with bile and was only partially dissolved after incubation in pure pancreatic juice. In other experiments with bovine collagen fleece they were found to quickly dissolve in pancreatic juice and lose their compact structure following incubation in bile. The human placental collagen patch appears to be the most efficacious in digestive tract surgery (Table 1).

Animal Studies in the Rat

In the second stage of the study, healing of a colon defect covered by the biomaterial in rats was examined. The new reconstituted connective tissue was able to promote healing of normal and pathological digestive tract defects. Wound healing was rapid and without inflammatory reaction. Better adapted biomaterials have been developed following this first prototype. A thick material was resistant and was not assimilated by the host tissues within 30 days, but induced an important inflammatory response leading to stenoses; a thinner material was quickly lysed and inefficient.

Animal Studies in the Dog

Several trials were carried out in dogs, comparing the development of a colonic anastomosis protected with different collagen patches. The patch was modified according to the results of each trial.

Table 1. Degradation times for collagen incubated in bile and pancreatic juice

Collagen	Bile	Pancreatic Juice
Elastin patch	7	<1
Collagen patch	>30	>20
Pangen	8	1
Helistat	>30	2

Results are expressed in days.

In the first trial, which evaluated the ability of the patch to prevent an intentional leak, the healing of transverse colonic anastomoses was compared in 31 dogs. The sutures were deliberately incomplete, with apertures between the knots. They were protected with a glued collagen patch in 11 animals (group A), with a glued and sutured patch in 10 animals (group B), and with epiploplasty in 10 control animals (group C). A barium enema tested the anastomotic permeability at postoperative day 30 (Table 2). The results showed that the biomaterial prevented the occurrence of a colonic fistula under extreme conditions. However, the patch induced anastomotic stenoses and did not integrate with host tissues in 30 days.

In a second trial, the composition of the biomaterial was modified. It was imperative to avoid stricture formation. Ten dogs had a hand-sewn colonic anastomosis protected with a circular patch (group A). In 10 control dogs the anastomosis was protected with fibrin glue alone (group B). The anastomoses were evaluated for gross healing. The colon lumen diameter was measured on radiographs taken after a barium enema. The biomaterial had to be incorporated into the existing tissues within 30 days. In a microscopic study, samples were examined for collagen resorption and histological evidence of healing of the anastomoses (Table 3). Radiographs showed that the biomaterial had no injurious effects. It had been assimilated in 4 of the 10 dogs. Wound healing was not inhibited in the patch-protected group. This already advanced prototype has been proved efficacious for the reinforcement of colonic anastomosis, but we also required that the material be totally absorbed within 30 days.

Table 2. Development of a colonic anastomosis in dogs

Results	Group A (n = 11)	Group B (n = 10)	Group C (n = 10)
Early unsticking and death	3 (27%)	5 (50%)	
Fistulas	2	1	2 (20%)
Nonsignificant stenosis	5 (45%)	4 (40%)	5 (50%)
Significant stenosis	3 (27%)	1 (10%)	3 (30%)

Group A = glued patch.
Group B = glued and sutured patch.
Group C = epiploplasty.

For the third experimental series, the biomaterial was modified and lightened. The different evolution of colonic anastomosis in dogs was then evaluated by two trials. In one, wound healing after 30 days was observed in 20 dogs. The follow-up procedures were the same as in the previous study, with a barium enema radiographic control examination after 30 days and a histological evaluation of the anastomotic samples. Among the 20 dogs, in 10 the anastomosis was reinforced with a patch (group A), and in the 10 control animals the anastomosis was only glued (group B) (Table 4). The development of colonic anastomoses reinforced with the new collagen patch confirmed the favorable results achieved in the previous study. No additional significant stenoses were diagnosed when the patch was used. Microscopic examination of the samples revealed no residual patch material or inflammatory response around the anastomoses. A second long-term trial should confirm these results: 10 anastomoses were controlled in 10 dogs after 6 months and compared with 10 glued anastomoses. The findings were similar in both series.

Table 3. Barium enema control of colonic anastomosis in dogs: importance of the stricture

	Group A (n = 10)	Group B (n = 10)
Radiological stenosis	40.8%	39%

Group A = glued patch.
Group B = control.

Table 4. Barium enema control of colonic anastomosis in dogs: importance of the stricture

	Group A (n = 10)	Group B (n = 10)
Radiological stenosis	36%	57%

Group A = glued patch.
Group B = control.

CONCLUSION

Collagen patches developed over the last 6 years have resulted in improved wound healing without an inflammatory reaction in the absence of retraction and anastomotic stricture; the patch is totally resorbed within 30 days. It is thus an effective approach to the management and prevention of anastomotic leaks and digestive fistulas in humans, and patches could prove to be a valuable addition to the surgical armamentarium for bowel anastomosis.

We have begun the first prospective trial in humans. Hand-sewn colonic anastomoses are secured with a circular glued collagen patch; in a control group the anastomoses are only glued. If this study, which will continue for 1 year, is successful, a multicenter trial will be undertaken.

REFERENCES

1. Marescaux J, Aprahamian M, Mutter D, et al. Prevention of anastomotic leakage: An artificial connective tissue. Br J Surg 78:440-444, 1991.
2. Matras H, Dinges HP, Lassmann HR. Zur nahtlosen interfazikulären Nerventransplantation im Tierexperiment. Wien Klin Wochenschr 37:517-523, 1972.
3. Hedelin H, Lundholm K, Teger-Nilsson AC, et al. Influence of local fibrin deposition on granulation tissue formation. A biochemical study in the rat. Eur Surg Res 15:312-316, 1983.
4. Banerjee SK, Glynn LE. Reactions to homologous and heterologous fibrin implants in experimental animals. Ann NY Acad Sci 86:1054-1057, 1960.
5. Pohl J, Bruhn HD, Christophers E. Thrombin and fibrin induced growth of fibroblasts: Role in wound repair and thrombus organisation. Wien Klin Wochenschr 57:273-277, 1979.
6. Pfluger G, Redl H. Abbau von Fibrinkleber in vivo und in vitro. Zentralbl Urol Nephrol 75:25-30, 1982.
7. Tashiro S, Murata E, Hisaoka T, et al. New technique for pancreaticojejunostomy using a biological adhesive. Br J Surg 74:392-394, 1987.
8. Heidecke CD, Hebeler W, Stemberger A, et al. Experimentelle Untersuchungen von enterotomien des Rattenileums nach Applikation von physiologischen Plasmafraktionen. Zentralbl Chir 105:586-593, 1980.
9. van der Ham WJK, Weijma IM, van den Ingh HFGM, et al. Effect of fibrin sealant on the healing colonic anastomosis in the rat. Br J Surg 78:49-53, 1991.
10. Giardino R, Ussia G, Grilli-Cicilioni C, et al. Colorectal anastomosis with fibrin sealant and transanal approaching device in pig. Eur Surg Res 18:S1-129, 1986.

11. Hjortrup A, Nordkild P, Kiaergaard J, et al. Fibrin adhesive versus sutured anastomosis: A comparative study in the small intestine of pigs. Br J Surg 73:760-761, 1986.

12. Petrelli NJ, Cohen H, De Risi D, et al. The application of tissue adhesives in small bowell anastomoses. J Surg Oncol 19:59-61, 1982.

13. Thorson GK, Perez-Brett R, Lillie DB. The role of tissue adhesive fibrin seal in oesophageal anastomoses. J Surg Oncol 24:221-223, 1983.

14. Schlag G, Redl H. Fibrin sealant and its modes of application. In Schlag G, ed. Fibrin Sealant in Operative Medicine. Berlin: Springer-Verlag, 1986, pp 6, 13-26.

15. Charriere G, Hartmann DJ, Vignon E, et al. Antibodies to types I, II, IX, and XI collagen in the serum of patients with rheumatic diseases. Arthritis Rheum 31:325-332, 1988.

16. Lawson JH, Pennel BJ, Olson JD, et al. Isolation and characterization of an acquired antithrombin antibody. Blood 1990, 76:2249-2257, 1990.

17. Tiollier J, Dumas H, Tardy M, et al. Fibroblast behavior on gels of type I, III and IV human placental collagens. Exp Cell Res 191:95-104, 1990.

18. Tardy M, Tayot JL. Imedex US Patent 4, 1986, 931 546.

19. Tardy M, Tayot JL. European patent application, 1986, 86 401 794.

20. Scheele J. Grundlagen der anastomosenheilung. In Scheele J, ed. Fibrinklebung. Berlin: Springer-Verlag, 1984, pp 115-119.

95 Oncological Aspects and Consequences of Laparoscopic Versus Open Techniques in Colon Resection

Anton Jansen

Since surgeons discovered the therapeutic potential of the laparoscopic approach to gallbladder surgery, that technique has been applied to other procedures. The development of a stapling apparatus for endoscopic use has made intracorporeal reconstruction of the gastrointestinal tract possible. Surgeons subsequently began to apply the laparoscopic approach to colon surgery.

"Keyhole" surgery has a negative connotation for surgeons.[1] Wide access, especially in colon surgery, is still regarded as a valid axiom and is thought to be essential to adequate tumor control, so laparoscopic colon resection has been received with skepticism in the surgical community. In addition, serious complications that were reported after laparoscopic gallbladder surgery[2] have dampened the initial enthusiastic reports of the pioneer laparoscopic surgeons.[3] The use of an unproven laparoscopic technique to treat colonic malignancies has caused concern among oncologic specialists because radical surgery offers the best therapeutic option for patients with colon cancer. One concern is that laparoscopic colon resection may be performed less radically than open operation and that as a result, the survival rate may not be as good.

In our view, the laparoscopic approach is justified in patients with colon cancer if the technique used is essentially identical to that of the current open surgical technique and if the laparoscopic procedure is performed according to current principles of oncologic colon surgery. Those principles include high and early ligation of the main vascular pedicle, extensive dissection of the adjacent mesentery with its lymph nodes, minimal manipulation of the tumor, preoperative and intraoperative sterilization of the colonic contents with distilled water to prevent tumor cell seeding. In October 1991, we successfully performed the first laparoscopic colectomy in our hospital.

In the Netherlands we have started a randomized, prospective, coordinated study involving seven hospitals. In the second phase of the study, other centers will join our study group. We shall train the newly admitted surgical teams in the laparoscopic techniques that we have used.

In our first laparoscopically treated patients, the indications for surgery were colon carcinoma with curative intent in two patients and a palliative resection in a patient whose cancer had metastasized. Postoperative recovery in these patients was quick and uneventful. The pathology reports showed adequate margins of all resection sites in all three patients. This early experience encouraged us to continue to apply this technique in colon cancer patients. We remained aware of the possible limitations of the technique, but we were convinced that a radical resection could be successfully performed laparoscopically as well as by open operation.

The short- and long-term effects of laparoscopic techniques applied to colonic resection are not known. Reports of laparoscopic colon resection are scarce in the world literature. In addition, the indications and contraindications for laparoscopic colon surgery are not yet defined, and the operative techniques are not standardized. Results of prospective clinical trials in colon cancer patients are not yet available; however, reports have been published from a smaller series by enthusiastic endoscopic surgeons.[4,5] Prospective multicenter trials evaluating the possible benefits of this new method are in early stages.[6]

In this chapter we shall discuss the current status and the future of laparoscopic treatment in patients with colon cancer. First, we shall evaluate the course and characteristics of colorectal carcinoma. Second, we shall investigate current surgical therapeutic options. Third, we shall review the indications for the use of laparoscopic surgery in the treatment of colon cancer.

LOCAL GROWTH OF COLON AND RECTAL CARCINOMA

Carcinoma of the colon is characterized by relatively slow growth; the doubling time of the tumor is estimated to be approximately 660 days (2 years).[7] The doubling time of colon tumor metastasis, however, is estimated to be between 50 and 116 days.[8,9] The difference between the rate of colon carcinoma growth and the speed of increase in metastasis has not been clarified.

A colon tumor rises gradually from a polypoid or ulcerating lesion and grows circumferentially as a result of the intramural circular lymphatic network within the bowel wall. This growth may lead to stenosis and ultimately to bowel obstruction. Surprisingly, the growth does not extend in a longitudinal direction: The extent of microscopic disease in that direction is limited to a maximum of 12 mm.[10] As a result, the small distal resection margin in colon carcinoma can be confined to 2 cm of the tumor in histologically well-differentiated to moderately differentiated lesions.

Except for its annular growth, the tumor penetrates in a radiating fashion through the bowel wall from the muscularis mucosa through submucosa and muscular layers into and through the subserosa. Ultimately the growth extends into the pericolonic or perirectal fat and mesentery. In more advanced stages, the growth invades the adjacent structures of the small bowel, bladder, uterus, and ovaries and the retroperitoneal tissues. Therefore lesions involving only a portion of the bowel circumference and lesions confined within the bowel wall are in an earlier stage of the disease process than are the circular growing tumors that have extended through the bowel wall.

Lymph Node Metastasis

Lymph node metastasis means that the carcinoma is in an advanced stage. Lymph node involvement in lesions limited to the inner layer of the bowel wall is seen in <3% of cases, depending on the degree of tumor differentiation.[11] Lymph node metastasis occurs in an orderly fashion in well-differentiated or moderately differentiated tumors.[12] In poorly differentiated tumors, hematogenous metastasis, which may be the first indication of distant disease, occurs without lymph node involvement.

Metastatic disease progresses from the epicolic nodes to the paracolic nodes, the intermediate nodes, and finally the principal nodes located at the base of the inferior mesenteric artery (Fig. 1). Metastasis to more centrally located nodes without involvement of the earlier lymph node stations is rarely seen.[13] Retrograde lymphatic drainage caused by blockage of the lymphatic system by tumor occurs in <4% of patients.[14] Metastasis to the internal iliac lymph nodes from rectal tumors that occur below the peritoneal reflection may be found at a relatively early stage of the disease. In these cases, the margins between the tumor and the pelvic wall are

Metastatic site

Epicolic nodes on bowel wall
↓
Paracolic nodes along marginal artery
↓
Intermediate nodes along colic arteries
↓
Principal nodes at base of supplying arteries

Fig. 1. Progression of lymphatic metastasis.

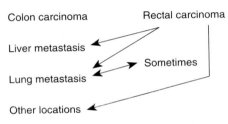

Fig. 2. Hematogenous spread.

small, and the possibility of residual disease after operation is greater than it is after the removal of colonic tumors.

Hematogenous Metastasis in Colorectal Carcinoma

Hematogenous metastasis occurs in advanced stages of disease usually at a later stage than does lymph node metastasis. In 25% of patients, hematogenous metastases are present at initial presentation. Hematogenous metastasis also follows an orderly progression (Fig. 2). In colon carcinoma, the first metastatic site is the liver, the second is the lung. In more advanced disease, metastasis to other organs is possible.[15] In rectal carcinoma, the lung can be the first metastatic site. Primary hematogenous metastasis to other locations is rare.

There is a positive correlation between the hematogenous spread of colon carcinoma and positive lymph nodes, stenosing tumors, perineural and intravascular tumor invasion, and poorly differentiated and mucus-containing tumors.

Histological Grading

Patients with ulcerating and polypoid-growing tumors have a better prognosis than do those with circular-growing tumors; patients with well-differentiated and moderately differentiated tumors have a better prognosis than do those with poorly differentiated, mucinous, or scirrhous forms of cancer.

Factors Influencing the Prognosis of Patients With Colorectal Carcinoma

There is a negative correlation between survival rates and depth of bowel wall penetration by tumor. There is also a negative correlation between nodal involvement and survival. Although colorectal carcinoma is considered to be treatable, the prognosis of the patient with a colorectal carcinoma is uncertain. August et al.[16] studied the outcome of 100 surgically treated patients with colon carcinoma. Only 51% of the patients were cured by surgery. Thirty percent of the patients studied were incurable at time of surgery, and 25 of the 70 patients (36%) who underwent a "curative" operation had recurrent disease. Four of these 25 patients survived. These figures demonstrate that recurrent disease is frequently fatal.

Studies in which routine second-look operations were performed 6 to 12 months after the primary operation showed that in 50% of patients with recurrent disease, recurrence was local, but in the remaining group of patients, a combination of local and distant metastasis was found.[17] Several hypotheses can be used to explain the causes of recurrence:

1. Residual tumor in lymph nodes and lymph channels is not recognized during the operation.
2. Tumor cell emboli are drained by veins *before* or *at the time of* resection.
3. Tumor cells on a serosal surface, in an interstitial space, or in lymphatic channels are dislodged by intraoperative manipulations.
4. Tumor cells persist at the margins of the resection.

These hypotheses allude to oncological rules for colon cancer surgery.

Survival rates and morbidity and mortality rates for open operation may vary considerably.[18] Postoperative mortality may vary as much as 20% in the reported literature. Reports of the incidence of local recurrence may vary as much as 21%, intraperitoneal sepsis as much as 17%, and anastomotic leakage as much as 25%. Survival rates 10 years post surgery vary from 20% to 63%. These figures show that the survival of a patient undergoing surgery for colorectal carcinoma is most influenced by the skill of the surgeon.

STATUS OF SURGICAL TREATMENT OF COLORECTAL CANCER

Surgery for colorectal cancer should prevent local recurrence of the tumor. In surgery for colorectal carcinoma, wide removal of the tumor and its mesentery with good lateral margins is advocated.[19]

The no-touch technique described by Turnbull et al.[20] remains attractive, although it is unproven. In this technique, before the tumor is manipulated, the surgeon divides the supplying blood vessels, veins, and arteries first. Turnbull stated that by doing this, venous embolization of tumor cells to the portal circulation was prevented. He also recommended high ligation of the vessels to remove the principle lymph node stations, which are the highest lymph nodes at the apex of the mesentery. Because of this high ligation, wide resection of the adjacent bowel is necessary to obtain good circulation at the remaining bowel segments. Thus high ligation also includes wide resection of the bowel and mesentery. Manipulation of the tumor must be prevented for the reasons mentioned earlier.

Some surgeons emphasize avoidance of dislodgement of tumor cells and prevention of tumor cell seeding in the suture line and peritoneal cavity.[21] They recommend preoperative and intraoperative irrigation of the colon with cytocidal solutions such as Dakin's solution or povidone-iodine (Betadine), or with distilled water so that any superficially lying tumor cells dislodged during the procedure will be killed by these substances. However, this effect (especially on suture line recurrence) has not been proven. In growths involving the serosal surface, some surgeons advocate covering the tumor with gauze drenched in Dakin's solution to prevent intraperitoneal seeding. The effect of this technique on recurrence is unknown.

An equally important principle is to avoid cutting through tumorous tissue during the procedure and to prevent perforation of the intestine, both of which result in local recurrence. The necessity for high or low ligation of the vessels is discussed by several authors.[22] In randomized studies,[22] there seems to be no difference in patient survival whether high ligation or low ligation was used. Other authors[23,24] who conducted relevant studies concur.

In survivors of colorectal carcinoma, only 3% of 442 patients had more than five positive lymph nodes, which were all clustered near the tumor.[23] This implies that extensive lymph node metastasis is associated with a poor prognosis. No patients with positive principal nodes (at the base of the inferior mesenteric artery) survived.[24] These facts support the hypothesis that patients with advanced disease (including extensive lymph node involvement) will die regardless of the extent of the surgical procedure performed. However, patients with limited disease including growths limited to the inner layers of the bowel wall and without lymph node metastasis are more likely to survive, regardless of the extent of the operation performed.

Only a small subgroup of colon cancer patients with positive lymph nodes clustered near the tumor and involving epicolic and marginal and/or intermediate nodes may benefit from extensive resection. This is also true for patients with carcinomas that have invaded other organs but that show no lymph node involvement.

Those patients also benefit from extensive dissection and resection.

THEORETIC ADVANTAGES AND DISADVANTAGES OF LAPAROSCOPIC COLECTOMY

Theoretically, the laparoscopic technique has advantages when compared with open surgical technique. The main advantage of laparoscopy is diminished trauma to the abdominal wall, which facilitates early recovery and physical activity with less chance of pulmonary and thromboembolic complications and infections (Fig. 1). Because good magnification is possible in laparoscopy, the procedure can be performed with great precision, and essential structures such as the ureters and larger blood vessels can be identified.

In laparoscopic surgery prevention of intra-abdominal bleeding is essential for success. Gross bleeding necessitates conversion to open operation. A moderate quantity of oozing blood leads to diminished ability to identify anatomical structures, and to cumbersome and time-consuming suction and irrigation. Precise hemostasis interferes with the speed of the operation, but blood loss is reduced. Surgical trauma and blood loss may have an adverse effect on the long-term results of oncological procedures.[25]

The diminished possibility of direct palpation may lead to underestimation of the extent of disease, but as a compensation for this, surgical trauma by manipulation is reduced.

QUESTIONS CONCERNING LAPAROSCOPIC SURGERY IN COLON CANCER PATIENTS

Whether patients with colon carcinoma benefit from laparoscopic surgery is unanswered. Large colon resections can be performed laparoscopically [26,27] so usually only a small abdominal incision is necessary for specimen extraction. Postoperative recovery is easier, and complaints of pain are typically fewer in these patients. Quick postoperative recovery is important, especially for the patient who undergoes palliative surgery, but for patients in whom surgery is curative in design, survival remains the most important issue. Early recovery from the procedure is important but is secondary to the ultimate result.

The essential question—whether a resection can be done as radically with the laparoscopic approach as with open surgery—is still unproved. Also unproved is the question of whether perioperative staging can be determined as satisfactorily by laparoscopy as by open surgery, and if not, what the consequences are for the patient. Whether the laparoscopic approach is less disturbing to the immune response system because of diminished trauma and blood and fluid loss is unknown. These questions will remain unanswered until the results of clinical trials are known. The first important question is whether the laparoscopic approach is as *safe* as open surgery for the patient.

Experience with laparoscopic colon resection is still limited. Only a few pioneering surgeons can be considered experts in that field. A majority of surgeons have no experience or relatively limited experience in performing laparoscopic colon resection. Because colon cancer occurs less frequently than does gallbladder disease and because of the greater complexity of laparoscopic colon resection, the learning curve for laparoscopic colon resection requires more time than that of gallbladder surgery. In addition, mortality and morbidity rates of open procedures are still high. Therefore surgical training to ensure proper, safe performance of laparoscopic colon resection is of utmost importance.

TECHNICAL POSSIBILITIES AND LIMITATIONS OF LAPAROSCOPY IN ONCOLOGIC COLON RESECTION FOR MALIGNANT DISEASE
Possibilities and Limitations of Diagnostic Laparoscopy

In colorectal carcinoma, laparoscopy can be used diagnostically to assess the extent of local disease: whether a growth is limited to the bowel wall or has penetrated the serosal layers can be easily determined. With laparoscopy, the invasion of other organs, peritoneal and liver metastases, and enlarged lymph nodes can be easily identified. Intra-abdominal anatomy and the position of the tumor can be assessed; this is essential in determining the best treatment. The main disadvantage of laparoscopy is the lack of palpation. This can be partially overcome by the use of dissectors or graspers as palpation instruments and by endosonography, a diagnostic tool that is of value only in the detection of liver metastases. However, the sensitivity and specificity of endosonography in the detection of lymph node metastases are low, so even with this evaluation the extent of disease is difficult to assess. However manual palpation as performed in open surgery, is also not entirely accurate. In our view the loss of ability to palpate does not seem to be important in the perioperative staging of carcinoma. A palliative smaller resection is performed only when liver metastases occur. In all other situations a wide resection will be performed with curative intent. In our view, surgery for colorectal carcinoma should begin with laparoscopy, after which a decision between a closed or open therapeutic approach can be made.

Possibilities and Limitations of Therapeutic Laparoscopy

Laparoscopic technique has several applications in bowel surgery. In open bowel surgery, a large abdominal incision is indicated because mobilization of the peritoneal attachments over a long area is required for resection and for a tension-free anastomosis. The extent of the abdominal incision can be diminished if mobilization is performed with the laparoscopic approach. Thus laparoscopic assisted colectomy may be beneficial, especially if radical resection is not mandatory, as in patients whose disease has metastasized. In those patients, only segmental resection is necessary to prevent intraluminal bowel obstruction.

A laparoscopic assisted colectomy begins with laparoscopic mobilization of the colon. The location of the tumor determines the site of incision for local resection. The abdominal wall incision is kept as small as possible, but it must accommodate extracorporeal resection and anastomosis. The anastomosis can be made with sutures or staples, depending on the operative findings and the surgeon's preference.

If a *radical resection* is undertaken, a different approach is necessary (Fig. 3). It should be emphasized that the laparoscopic approach should never interfere with the current oncologic principles described previously. Thus radical laparoscopic colectomy must be performed in a standardized manner according to existing

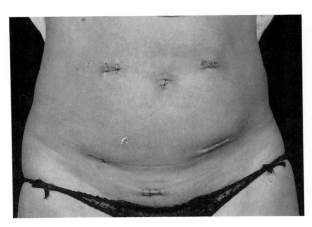

Fig. 3. Patient 4 days after radical low anterior resection.

rules of radical cancer control. The following aspects are important in radical laparoscopic resection for colon cancer:

1. The main vascular pedicle must first be ligated at its origin.
2. A wide mesenteric dissection must be performed and safe longitudinal margins obtained.
3. The lateral resection margins, especially in the pelvis, must be as large as possible.
4. Intraperitoneal and intraluminal cell seeding must be prevented.

The main vascular pedicle can always be identified laparoscopically. When the vascular pedicle is identified, a "window" can be created by incising the visceral peritoneum medial to and beneath the vascular pedicle. When the vascular pedicle is lifted and stretched, the pedicle can be freed up to its origin from or to the parent vessels. For endoscopic ligation of these larger vessels, we use an occlusive stapler (EndoGIA) with a vascular cartridge. In our experience, the pedicle can be freed laparoscopically just as well as in open operation, and the EndoGIA ligation can be performed at the same level laparoscopically as it would be in open operation with vascular clamps.

Next, the proposed resection lines through the mesentery are defined. Usually only one or two arteries and veins are encountered. These structures can be identified, clipped, and cut. Because a small abdominal incision is always made for specimen removal, the part of the mesentery near the colon can be divided extracorporeally.

The bowel must be transsected to extract the specimen. In left-sided lesions, the rectum is transsected. The videocolonoscope is then used to determine the line of transsection, which should be at least 2 cm beyond the tumor distally. In right-side lesions, the ileum proximal to the tumor is transsected. Lateral resection margins should be kept as large as possible, especially in the pelvic region. This can be accomplished easily by videolaparoscopic guidance. We think that pelvic dissection is performed more accurately with laparoscopy than with open surgery. The pelvic wall is the lateral border of the dissection; therefore, the resection should be performed as close as possible to the pelvic wall.

To prevent intraluminal and peritoneal cell seeding, distilled water should be used for preoperative cleansing of the rectum and during intraoperative colonoscopy. Care should be taken not to touch the tumor during laparoscopic mobilization to prevent peritoneal cell seeding. Careful positioning of grasping instruments above or below the tumor is therefore very important.

If these principles are followed, we feel that laparoscopic dissection can be performed as radically and with as much oncologic success as can be accomplished by open operation.

The limitations of radical laparoscopic colectomy are as follows:

1. Adhesions from previous operations or peritonitis may result in a cumbersome, time-consuming dissection and possible intestinal damage; open operation may be easier and safer to perform.
2. In patients with intra-abdominal obesity, the laparoscopic approach may be difficult. In the beginning of the learning experience, conversion to an open approach should be liberally instituted.
3. A tumor located very low in the pelvis may preclude radical laparoscopic colectomy. There are no angulating or roticulating stapling instruments with which to perform adequate transsection of the rectum at this moment of technological development.

In our opinion, two laparoscopic techniques are useful in the treatment of colorectal carcinoma. In a palliative resection, laparoscopic mobilization is undertaken to diminish the necessity for a large abdominal incision. This approach may contribute to the early recovery of an already debilitated patient. In a radical resection (radical laparoscopic colectomy), laparoscopic ligation of the vascular pedicle and its mesentery, as well as laparoscopic anastomosis, must be undertaken.

Indications for Laparoscopic Colectomy in Colorectal Carcinoma

Palliative resections. In patients with proven metastatic disease, laparoscopic assisted colectomy is the surgical technique of choice. The laparoscopic approach is complementary to open operation. This technique can be applied to malignancies of the cecum and the ascending sigmoid, and descending colon because after laparoscopic mobilization, extracorporeal resection and anastomosis can easily be performed. In lesions situated lower than these sites, laparoscopic mobilization alone is insufficient to permit resection and anastomosis. In these cases, radical laparoscopic colectomy or open operation should be considered.

Laparoscopic abdominoperineal resection for palliation seems a good alternative to open treatment. With this approach, only a circular abdominal wall incision is used for the colostomy, thus an abdominal midline incision is avoided. In carcinomas of the transverse colon, which occur less frequently, open operation should be considered because the colon is mobile and an extended hemicolectomy may be preferable.

Resections with curative intent. The laparoscopic approach is an alternative to classic colon resection and should be used only after careful evaluation during initial exploratory laparoscopy. Laparoscopic colectomy can be performed in all stages of the disease except in locally advanced invading cancers. In that case, removal of the specimen requires a large abdominal incision. In low anterior resection in a small pelvis, the laparoscopic approach should be undertaken only after assessment of the technical feasibility of transsecting the rectum with the currently available stapling apparatus. In the case of gross intra-abdominal obesity or when inflammatory adhesions are present, an open procedure should be considered. The majority of carcinomas in the colorectum can be resected with the laparoscopic approach used according to current oncologic rules for resection of colorectal carcinoma and with proper technique.

Various procedures for laparoscopic colectomy are listed in Table 1. More extensive colon resections, such as extended right or left hemicolectomy or total colectomy for multiple adenomas and carcinomas, require a large dissection in several abdominal sites. Although laparoscopic resection might be possible, we prefer the classic open approach.

Until the results of prospective clinical trials are available, laparoscopic colectomy is not a widely accepted procedure. Laparoscopic colon resection with curative intent should be performed only according to a strict protocol, which should include standardization of the laparoscopic technique and careful documentation of the operation, including operating time, intraoperative complications, postoperative complications, and short- to long-term follow-up. The patient should receive a letter for informed consent and be given general information about the procedure and its presently unproven status.

Laparoscopic Surgical Techniques for Cancer Resection With Curative Intent

Laparoscopic right hemicolectomy. The patient is positioned on a straight operating table that is rotated with the right side upward. This permits the small bowel to fall to the left side of the abdomen, and the right colon is exposed.

The surgeon stands on the patient's left side opposite the video monitor, which is placed on the patient's right side. The nurse also stands on the patient's right side; the camera assistant is next to and on the right side of the surgeon. The position and use of the four trocar ports are demonstrated in Fig. 4.

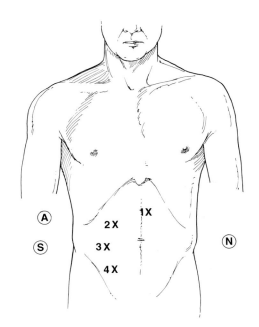

Fig. 4. Positions of the trocar ports in left hemicolectomy

Trocar 1	Right hand of assistant	Grasper
Trocar 2	Left hand of assistant	Camera
Trocar 3	Right hand of surgeon	Scissors
Trocar 4	Left hand of surgeon	Dissector

A = assistant; S = surgeon; N = nurse.

Table 1. Indications for laparoscopic colectomy

Location of Carcinoma	Laparoscopic Operation
Cecum and ascending colon	Right hemicolectomy
Descending colon	Left hemicolectomy
Sigmoid colon	Sigmoid resection
Rectosigmoid	Rectosigmoidectomy
Rectum	
Upper rectum	Low anterior resection
Midrectum	Open operation
Lower rectum	Abdominoperineal resection

After the pneumoperitoneum is established and the video laparoscope is inserted, the first intra-abdominal inspection is performed. If the surgeon then decides to proceed laparoscopically, the other three trocar ports are inserted. The dissection is started with the identification of the right ureter, which is visible through the peritoneum at its crossing over the iliac vessels. The cecum is grasped and is pulled upward and to the left, and the dissection of the parietal attachments is begun with the Endograsper-clinch or endo-needle-nose dissector in the left hand and Endoscissors in the right hand. The hepatic flexure is then mobilized as much as possible, although a part of the mobilization of the flexure can be performed later through the minilaparotomy.

The retroperitoneal attachments of the mesentery are freed by identifying the right ureter and the duodenum as protected landmarks. Adhesions between the omentum and right colon and at the hepatic flexure are freed. The visceral peritoneum is cut medially down to the ileocolic artery, which can be easily identified. A mesenteric window is created by lifting and stretching the vascular pedicle with a grasping instrument. The ileocolic artery and vein can be dissected free to their levels of origin.

At this stage the vascular pedicle is divided as close to its origin as possible with the vascular EndoGIA (U.S. Surgical Corp.). Then the right colic vessels are identified and transsected between vascular staples or clips. Next, the mesentery is divided toward the proposed ileal resection site. Usually, only two or three arteries and veins are encountered and divided in the mesentery. The ileum is then transsected 15 cm from the ileocecal valve with an EndoGIA 30 or 60. At that stage, the distal resection site can be stapled closed at the transverse colon with an Endo-TA 60 (U.S. Surgical Corp.).

A transverse minilaparotomy is made in the right hypochondrium, sufficient in size to allow easy extraction of the specimen. To prevent cell seeding, the wound is protected by a makeshift plastic sleeve fashioned from an empty IV fluid bag. As the specimen emerges from the abdomen, terminal ileum first, the proximal ileum is also brought to the surface and the mesentery of the transverse colon, including the marginal artery, is ligated and divided (Fig. 5).

The transverse colon is transsected between the previously placed Endo-TA staple lines and a proximal bowel clamp placed to prevent spillage. Alternatively, and for greater safety, the bowel may be transsected and closed at both ends beyond the Endo-TA staple lines

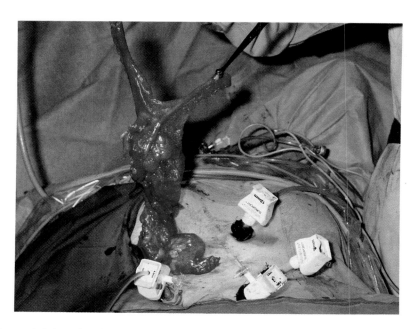

Fig. 5. Dissected right colon delivered by small transverse abdominal incision. Note length of vascular pedicle, which is grasped with Babcock clamp. Specimen includes appendix, cecum, and ascending and part of transverse colon including adjacent mesentery. Note position of trocar ports.

with the GIA-80 instrument. Ileocolic anastomosis is made with the GIA and TA instruments by using the functional end-to-end technique. The mesentery can be closed at this stage or can be left open, but the bowel must be replaced carefully into the proper posterior position in the abdomen to prevent small bowel herniation. The abdominal wall incision is then closed, and a pneumoperitoneum is reestablished with careful inspection of the resection site. No rotation of the small bowel should occur. A suction drain is left behind for 24 hours. The trocars are removed, and skin and fascia openings are closed.

The resected specimen includes the distal ileum; the cecum; the ascending colon; the hepatic flexure; and part of the transverse colon with its adjacent mesentery including the epicolic, paracolic, and principal lymph nodes at the bases of the ileocolic and the right colic vessels.

Laparoscopic Low Anterior Resection

The patient is placed into modified lithotomy and Trendelenburg positions, with the left side rotated upward. These maneuvers make the small bowel fall away from the sigmoid colon to the right and upper abdominal cavity. The video monitor is placed at the caudal side of the patient. The surgeon stands on the patient's right side, as does the assistant. The nurse stands on the patient's left side.

After a pneumoperitoneum is established, three trocar ports are inserted at the right side of the abdomen, and one trocar is inserted at the left side. The exact positions are shown in Fig. 6.

The videocolonoscope is used to assess the location of the tumor. At that stage, the distal resection line can be marked with clips or thermocautery. First, the left ureter is identified. Then the sigmoid colon is grasped with the left trocar port and is pushed in a right and upward direction to create tension. The resection is then begun: The parietal peritoneal attachments are cut with the Endoshears until the splenic flexure is reached.

If additional mobilization is needed to obtain adequate length for a tension-free anastomosis, the operation may be continued with further mobilization of the splenic flexure. The posterior attachments are then divided; the left ureter is used as a landmark. The dissection is performed from the left lower gutter in an upward direction. This is the easiest way to keep the right plane of separation between the colon, the mesentery,

and Gerota's fascia. Then the visceral peritoneum is incised in front of and below the aortic bifurcation and below and medial to the superior hemorrhoidal vessels. Windows are opened at this level around the hemorrhoidal vessels to the posterior retroperitoneal space by lifting and stretching the hemorrhoidal pedicle with a grasper. At first the mesentery is elevated from the posterior surface anterior to the bed of the left iliac artery and vein. The left ureter can then be identified again through the mesocolic window. The dissection of the hemorrhoidal vascular pedicle is carried out in a cranial direction to its origin from the inferior mesenteric vessels, which are freed up circumferentially at this level. The artery and vein are sometimes situated close together; at other times, there is a distance between them. The EndoGIA is used to ligate and divide the artery and (if possible) the vein in one stage; otherwise, the vein must be clipped and transsected separately. The left colic vessels are then dissected and transsected with

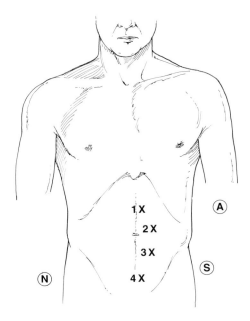

Fig. 6. Positions of trocar ports in right hemicolectomy and rectosigmoid resection

Trocar 1	Left hand of assistant	Grasper
Trocar 2	Right hand of assistant	Camera
Trocar 3	Left hand of surgeon	Dissector
Trocar 4	Right hand of surgeon	Scissors

A = assistant; S = surgeon; N = nurse.

a clip applier (or with the EndoGIA in more difficult situations). The avascular part of the mesentery is further divided until the marginal vessels are reached.

Then the dissection is continued in a caudal direction within the pelvis, close to the pelvic walls, first on the right side and then the left side of the rectum, which is then elevated posteriorly from the sacral hollow with ease. The dissection is carried down until the proposed distal level of resection is reached. The rectum and mesorectum are then transsected with one or two applications of the EndoGIA 60 under direct visualization with the videocolonoscope.

A small transverse muscle-splitting incision is made in the left lower quadrant, and the colon is brought outside the abdomen with the distal resection site first. After the rectosigmoid, still attached to the proximal colon, has been brought outside the abdominal cavity (Fig. 7), the proximal resection site is defined, and the mesentery—including the marginal artery and vein—is divided. At this stage, adhesions left after the laparoscopic dissection can be freed through the mini-incision. The purse-string instrument is then applied on the proximal colon, and a bowel clamp is placed opposite the purse-string device on the specimen, which is then transsected between device and clamp and is removed. The appropriate cartridge of the PCEEA instrument

is chosen, and the anvil is placed into the proximal descending colon, and the purse-string is tightened (Fig. 8). With a long rectal stump the PCEEA cartridge is placed transanally into the rectum, cartridge and anvil are assembled through the minilaparotomy, and the instrument is fired. If the rectal stump is short, the proximal colon carrying the anvil is again placed into the abdomen and the abdominal wall incision is closed.

The pneumoperitoneum is reestablished. The PCEEA cartridge is placed again transanally and the central hollow rod and trocar of the cartridge are advanced through the previously stapled rectal closure. The trocar is removed through one of the operating laparoscopy ports and the central rod of the anvil is joined into the hollow rod or shaft of the cartridge. The PCEEA instrument is closed, activated, and removed through the anus, with the anvil attached to the cartridge.

The anastomosis can be inspected with the videocolonoscope. A suction drain is left in the pelvis, and the trocar openings are closed.

The resected specimen includes a part of the rectum at least 2 to 3 cm below the tumor and the sigmoid and includes the epicolic paracolic, intermediate, and principal lymph nodes up to the origin of the inferior mesenteric artery and vein (Fig. 9).

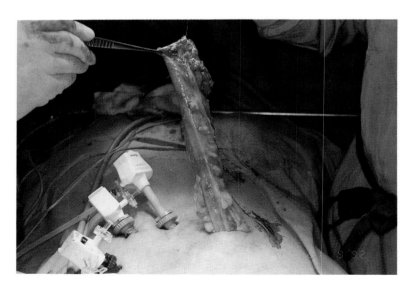

Fig. 7. Rectosigmoid colon is extracted with small incision. Note length of specimen and positions of trocars.

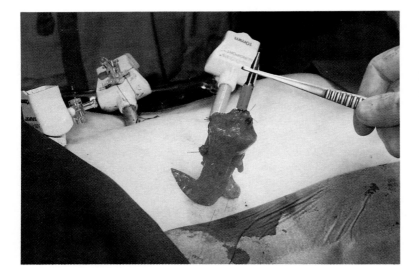

Fig. 8. Positions of trocars and abdominal incision in left colon resection. Anastomosis is performed with PCEEA.

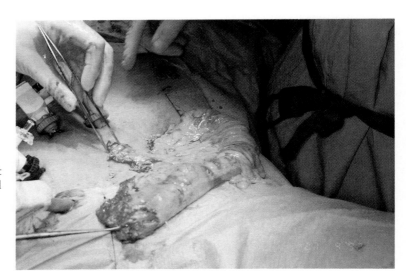

Fig. 9. Resected rectosigmoid. Note extent of mesenteric dissection including principal lymph nodes at apex of specimen.

LAPAROSCOPIC ABDOMINOPERINEAL RESECTION

In laparoscopic abdominoperineal resection, the rectosigmoid colon is dissected with the method described for low anterior resection. The inferior mesenteric pedicle is divided near its origin and the mesentery is skeletized.

The pelvic dissection begins with the lateral sides of the pelvis and continues with the dissection of the meso-rectum from the hollow of the sacral space. This is accomplished by elevation of the rectum with a grasper or retractor and by dissection with the Endoshears or the EndoCusa, which facilitates separation of the posterior attachment while continuous suction of the accumulated blood in the pelvis is provided. The anterior dissection plane is easily opened with this apparatus, and the collateral ligaments can be dissected precisely. The middle hemorrhoidal vessels can be clipped or coagulated as determined by their sizes. The dissection is continued as far down as possible until the pelvic floor is reached. Then the colon is transsected and closed on both sides of the proximal resection line at the border between the descending colon and the sigmoid colon with an EndoGIA 30 or 60. A circular colostomy incision is made in the mid-upper left lower quadrant by excision of an annular disk of skin and subcutaneous tissue, and a vertical linear incision of the abdominal wall between lateral rectus sheath and flat abdominal muscles. The proximal colon is then brought through this abdominal incision. The perineal part of the operation is performed in a traditional fashion; the patient is placed in a lithotomy position. The specimen is extracted by means of the perineal incision, which is then closed. A drain is inserted into the pelvis to prevent accumulation of pelvic clots. The proximal bowel is opened, and an end colostomy is fashioned in the usual way.

The resected specimen includes the sigmoid colon, the rectum, and the anus, as well as the sigmoid mesocolon to the origins of the inferior mesenteric artery and vein with the mesorectum and the perirectal lymph nodes.

RESULTS

From October 1991 to February 1993, 116 laparoscopic colectomies were performed in a pilot study by members of the Dutch Coordinated Study Group for Laparoscopic Colon Resection. The indications for laparoscopic colon surgery are described in Table 2. In 67 patients, the operative indication was colon cancer. In a majority of cases (58 patients), a radical laparoscopically assisted colectomy was performed, but in nine cases a laparoscopically assisted colectomy was performed for palliative resection.

The surgical procedures accomplished are listed in Table 3. For colorectal cancer, 35 laparoscopic rectosigmoidectomies, 23 right hemicolectomies, and 8 low anterior resections were performed. Laparoscopic sigmoid resection, right hemicolectomy, and low anterior resection were the most frequently performed operations for colorectal cancer.

Mean operating time was 4 hours for laparoscopic sigmoid resection, 3.5 hours for laparoscopic right hemicolectomy, and 4.15 hours for low anterior resection.

One patient died 3 weeks after operation of multiorgan failure primarily caused by exsanguination that

Table 2. Indications for laparoscopic colon resection

Indication	No. of Resections Performed
Diverticulitis	33
Cancer	
Palliative resection	9
Curative resection	58
Tubulovillous adenoma	13
Crohn's disease	2
TOTAL	115

Table 3. Laparoscopic colon procedures, October 1991–February 1993

Procedure	No. of Procedures Performed
Sigmoid resection	68
Low anterior resection	8
Reconstruction after Hartmann's procedure	9
Right hemicolectomy	26
Ileocecal resection	5
TOTAL	116

was unrecognized after trocar injury to the epigastric artery. Another patient died as a result of anastomotic leakage.

In this series, the conversion rate to open operation was 17%, primarily as a result of intra-abdominal adhesions and obesity. The postoperative complications are listed in Table 4. Major complications requiring repeat laparotomy occurred in four cases: in two cases as a result of anastomotic dehiscence (1.7%); in one case, because of torsion of the small bowel; and in one case as a deep abdominal abscess.

Late complications were encountered in five patients with anastomotic stricture. In these patients, the stricture was treated successfully with balloon dilation. In the patient group without major complications, postoperative recovery was remarkably fast; the average hospital stay was 7.1 days.

Histologic examination of the cancer specimen revealed clear margins of the proximal, distal, and lateral resection sites in all patients treated with curative intent. The extent of the mesenteric dissection was determined by the number of lymph nodes removed with the specimen. The number of lymph nodes examined was 9.2 ± 2.5, which is not different from that obtained in open operations. The current follow-up period is too short for the analysis of long-term results.

My experience in laparoscopic colectomy for colon cancer includes 32 patients. Except for one repeat operation for a deep abscess, no major complications have occurred. In all specimens, clearance of the proximal, distal, and lateral margins was obtained. My operations averaged 5 hours in the first five patients and 3 hours 15 minutes in the last five patients treated laparoscopically (Fig. 10). No local recurrences have been detected.

Table 4. Complications of laparoscopic colon resection

Type of Complication	No. of Patients With Complications	Percent
Minor		4.3
Thrombosis	1	
Urinary infection	1	
Wound infection	2	
Major (laparotomy required)		3.4
Torsion, small bowel	1	
Deep abdominal abscess	1	
Anastomotic leakage	2	
Late		
Anastomotic strictures	6	5.2
TOTAL	14	12.9

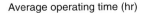

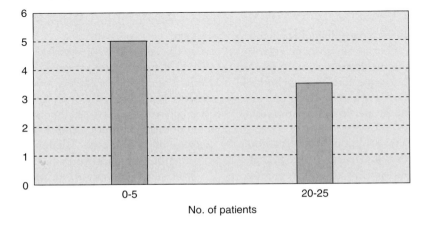

Fig. 10. Learning curve in laparoscopic sigmoid resection (operating time).

CONSIDERATIONS FOR LAPAROSCOPIC TREATMENT OF COLORECTAL CARCINOMA

Patients with colon cancer have a poor prognosis: Only 50% survive. Approximately one of three patients admitted for operation has metastases and will die from the disease regardless of operative technical modality. The extent of local disease defines the fate of patients without metastases. In patients with limited disease (partially circumferential histologically well-differentiated to moderately differentiated tumors with growth contained within the bowel wall and without lymph node metastasis), surgical therapy is almost always curative, regardless of how the resection is performed.

In advanced cases with gross lymph node involvement, distant metastases, and poor histopathologic factors including intravascular and perineural invasion, the prognosis is poor regardless of the extent of resection. In locally advanced disease that is limited to the region with extension of growth beyond the bowel wall and some lymph node involvement that is near the tumor, wide resection may be more beneficial than limited resection, but the long-term outcome is uncertain. If local growth is extensive, with involvement of other organs, radical resection may provide cure.

The surgical options in treatment of colorectal carcinoma are influenced by the extent of disease. In patients with metastasis, resection almost always provides the best palliation. It restores the continuity of the gastrointestinal tract, prevents obstruction and ileus, and reduces pain (especially that resulting from rectal cancers) caused by invasion of the neural structures. Palliative resection should be performed with the least surgical trauma in these already debilitated patients.

The extent of the abdominal wall incision for palliative resection can be reduced by mobilizing the colon with laparoscopic assisted colectomy.

Our experience with right-sided and left-sided lesions shows that after laparoscopic mobilization in the majority of cases, a small abdominal incision (approximately 7 cm) is necessary for resection. Postoperative recovery is facilitated. These patients can begin chemotherapy within 2 weeks after operation.

In our opinion, there is no doubt that laparoscopic assisted colectomy is the best approach for this category of patients. In resection with curative intent, the role of laparoscopic colectomy is not yet defined. Our results of the pilot study and those reported by other surgeons show that the operation can be performed safely. A mortality rate of 1.7% occurred in our first

116 patients (2/116) who underwent laparoscopic assisted colectomy; this rate is comparable with that of conventional surgery.

However, mortality and morbidity are surgeon-dependent, and the complexity of laparoscopic colon resection creates a learning curve that is much longer than that of other laparoscopic procedures. That complexity is demonstrated by the long operating time required in the initial phase of the learning curve, as well as by the high conversion rate.[28] In our opinion, these procedures should be performed only by a highly motivated surgical team and by surgeons experienced in both laparoscopic and open surgery. The operations must be performed regularly and according to the established protocol. Results of the procedures must be carefully recorded to benefit scientific analysis.

As mentioned earlier, operations intended to provide cure begin with laparascopy. To prevent a high late intraoperative conversion rate, a decision is made after diagnostic laparoscopy to proceed with operative laparoscopy or to perform an open operation. In cases in which difficult anatomy is encountered, open operation is preferable to laparoscopy, which may require late intraoperative conversion if the decision was initially delayed. Laparoscopic colectomy may be time-consuming or impossible in cases of gross intra-abdominal obesity or adhesions or low-situated rectal cancers. For low resections, an angulating or roticulating EndoGIA instrument is required for adequate rectal transection. The longer, stronger, curved instruments that are needed to perform these resections in difficult circumstances will soon be available.

CONCLUSION

We think that current oncologic principles should be applied to laparoscopic colon surgery, although controversies still exist about the best method of surgical treatment. Our results and those of other authors[28] have shown that a resection as radical as or more radical than that of open operation can be performed. In our histologically examined specimens, the resection sites were free of tumor, and our pathologists were unable to detect which approach had been used. The number of lymph nodes obtained for examination was the same as that obtained in open operation.

Thus we strongly believe that it is worthwhile to continue our efforts. However, we must await the results of randomized prospective studies to demonstrate the possibilities and limitations of laparoscopic colon surgery. It will also be interesting to clarify the effect of the limited blood and fluid loss during the laparoscopic procedure on the patient's long-term survival.

Furthermore, the economic benefits, which are now of great importance, must be assessed. Our preliminary results showed a shortened length of hospital stay and a quicker postoperative recovery in laparoscopically treated patients, in whom the return to normal activity after the operation was also shortened. We expect that laparoscopy will enable a significant decrease in the mean hospital stay. Our current operating time for laparoscopic rectosigmoidectomy is 3 hours and 15 minutes. Although this time is acceptable, we believe that in the next 2 years, significantly less time will be required to perform the procedure as a result of new and improved instruments and imaging and retraction systems. As a result of increasing experience and careful patient selection, surgeons will perform the procedure more quickly.

If we consider the progress that we have made during the past 2 years in the development of laparoscopic colon surgery, we can expect application of this new technique to surgery for colorectal carcinoma.

REFERENCES

1. Taylor I. Keyhole colon surgery [editorial]. Can Top 9:1, 1993.
2. Meyers WC, Branaum GD, Farouk M, et al. A prospective analysis of 1518 laparoscopic cholecystectomies. N Engl J Med 324:1073-1078, 1991.
3. Smith R. Injuries to the common bile duct during laparoscopic cholecystectomy. Br Med J 303:1475, 1991.
4. Jacobs M, Verdeja JC, Goldstein HS. Minimally invasive colon resection. Surg Laparosc Endosc 1:144-150, 1991.
5. Monson RT, Darzi A, Carey PD, et al. Prospective evaluation of laparoscopic assisted colectomy in an unselected group of patients. Lancet 2:831-833, 1992.
6. Go Pmnyh, Jansen A, et al. A prospective, randomised, multicenter, cost-effectiveness study of conventional versus laparoscopic colectomy for colorectal carcinoma (in preparation).
7. Spratt JS, Ackerman LV. The growth of colonic adenocarcinoma. Am Surg 27:23-28, 1961.
8. Collins VP, Loeffler RK, Tivey H. Observations on growth rates of human tumors. AJR 76:988-1000, 1956.
9. Finlay IG, Brunton GF, Meek D, et al. Rate of growth of hepatic metastasis in colorectal carcinoma. Br J Surg 69:789, 1982.
10. Black WA, Waugh JM. The intramural extension of carcinoma of the descending colon, sigmoid, and rectosigmoid: A pathologic study. Surg Gynecol Obstet 87:457-464, 1948.
11. Grinnell RS. The grading and prognosis of carcinoma of the colon and rectum. Ann Surg 109:500-533, 1939.
12. Gilchrist RK, David VC. Lymphatic spread of carcinoma of the rectum. Ann Surg 108:621-642, 1938.
13. Stearns MW, Deddish MR. Five-year results of abdominopelvic lymph node dissection for carcinoma of the rectum. Dis Colon Rectum 2:169-172, 1959.
14. Grinnell RS. Lymphatic block with atypical and retrograde lymphatic metastasis and spread in carcinoma of the colon and rectum. Ann Surg 163:272-280, 1966.
15. Brown CE, Warren S. Visceral metastasis from rectal carcinoma. Surg Gynecol Obstet 66:611-621, 1938.
16. August DA, Ottow RT, Sugarbaker PH. Clinical perspective of human colorectal cancer metastasis. Cancer Metastasis Rev 3:303-324, 1984.
17. Gunderson LL, Sosin H. Areas of failure found at reoperation (second or symptomatic look) following "curative surgery" for adenocarcinoma of the rectum. Cancer 34:1278-1292, 1974.
18. McArdle CS, Hole D. Impact of variability among surgeons on postoperative morbidity and mortality and ultimate survival. Br Med J 302:1501-1505, 1991.
19. Stearns MW, Schottenfeld D. Techniques for the surgical management of colon cancer. Cancer 28:165-169, 1971.
20. Turnbull RB, Kyle K, Watson FR, et al. Cancer of the colon: The influence of the no-touch isolation technic on survival rates. Ann Surg 166:420-427, 1967.
21. Cole WH, Roberts SS, Strehl FW. Modern concepts in cancer of the colon and rectum. Cancer 19:1347-1358, 1966.
22. Surtees P, Ritchie JK, Philips RKS. High versus low ligation of the inferior mesenteric artery in rectal cancer. Br J Surg 77:618-621, 1990.
23. Harvey HD, Auchincloss H. Metastases to lymph nodes from carcinomas that were arrested. Cancer 21:684-691, 1968.
24. Grinnell RS. Results of ligation of inferior mesenteric artery at the aorta in resection of the descending and sigmoid colon and rectum. Surg Gynecol Obstet 120:1031, 1965.
25. Foster RS, Costanza MC, Foster JC, et al. Adverse relationship between blood transfusions and survival after colectomy for colon cancer. Cancer 55:1195-1201, 1985.
26. Wexner SD, Johansen OB, Hoqueras JJ, et al. Laparoscopic total abdominal colectomy: A prospective trial. Dis Colon Rectum 35:651-655, 1992.
27. Jansen A. Laparoscopic gastro-intestinal and gallbladder surgery: Will the promise be fullfilled? Scand J Med (Suppl; in press).
28. Falk PM, Beart RW Jr, Wexner SD, et al. Laparoscopic colectomy: A critical appraisal. Dis Colon Rectum 34:1030-1031, 1991.

XIV

Videoendoscopic Techniques in Operations on the Esophagus

Jean-Marie Collard, J.B. Otte, and P.J. Kestens

Over the last 200 years, numerous surgical techniques have been described and used for the management of hypopharyngeal diverticulum.[1] Only a few of these have withstood the test of time: resection of the pouch by left cervicotomy; diverticulopexy into the posterior pharyngeal wall or prevertebral ligaments by left cervicotomy, each with or without concomitant myotomy of the cricopharyngeus muscle and the muscle layers of the proximal esophagus; cricomyotomy alone; and endoscopic sutureless division of the common wall between the esophageal lumen and the diverticular pouch by electrocautery or laser coagulation.

We describe a new endoscopic suturing technique with which we have recently experimented and propose guidelines for choosing the most appropriate surgical technique according to the size of the diverticulum.

ENDOSCOPIC SUTURING TECHNIQUE

Through a double-lipped Weerda endoscope (Karl Storz Instruments), the two lips of which may be approximat-

ed and angulated according to each patient's own pharyngeal anatomy, an EndoGIA 30 stapler (U.S. Surgical Corp.) is introduced into the pharynx and placed across the spur between the esophagus and the diverticulum, one fork into each lumen (Fig. 1).

Closure and activation of this instrument allows forward displacement of a median knife and concomitant delivery of three rows of staples to each side of the transection line. In this way the esophageal and the diverticular walls are stapled together, and the visceral lumen is not opened during the entire procedure. After the stapler is removed, the cricopharyngeal muscle, which has just been divided, acts on the two wound edges so that they retract laterally to create a common cavity (Fig. 2). A large diverticulum requires a second placement of the stapler on the distal part of the diverticular spur.

PATHOPHYSIOLOGY

The pathogenesis of hypopharyngeal diverticulum remains controversial in spite of the numerous radiological,

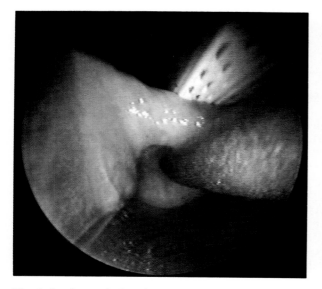

Fig. 1. Stapler ready for placement across the spur.

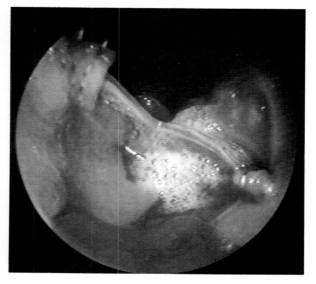

Fig. 2. The two wound edges retract laterally by the action of the cricopharyngeal muscle.

manometric, and histological studies that have been performed to understand the mechanisms leading to the development of the diverticular pouch from the posterior pharyngeal wall proximal to the cricopharyngeus muscle.

The main hypotheses include the following: megapharynx requiring more than one swallow to empty,[2] insufficient attachment of the hypopharyngeal wall to the prevertebral ligaments resulting in impairment of the cricopharyngeal stretch and relaxation when the larynx moves forward during swallowing[3]; high resting pressure of the upper esophageal sphincter (UES)[4]; normal UES resting pressure[5]; UES hypotonia,[6-8] UES achalasia[9]; and lack of pharyngoesophageal coordination.[6,8,10] More recent studies in patients with a cricopharyngeal bar have introduced a new concept on which esophageal physiologists will probably agree: despite complete manometric relaxation of the UES at swallowing, low compliance of the cricopharyngeus muscle prevents complete anatomical relaxation of the esophageal mouth and creates a resistance to flow, resulting in an increase in hypopharyngeal pressure so that the weak posterior wall of the pharynx proximal to the sphincter is pushed backward, giving rise to a diverticular pouch.[11,12] Impairment of cricopharyngeal muscle compliance can be ascribed to histopathological changes such as myositis.[13,14] According to Ferguson,[1] "The presence of demonstrable cricopharyngeal dysfunction is underscored in the majority of patients with pharyngoesophageal diverticula. The small percentage of patients with apparently normal function emphasizes our failure to completely understand the underlying pathophysiological mechanisms in every individual."

It appears that the diverticular pouch is only a consequence of the disease, and not the disease itself. Thus misunderstanding the critical role played by the UES theoretically exposes the patients to postoperative fistula or recurrence that may occur after resecting of the pouch without myotomy.[9,15]

CHOICES IN SURGICAL TREATMENT

The following strategies are proposed for surgical management of hypopharyngeal diverticulum (Table 1): Transcervical myotomy of the cricopharyngeal muscle and the muscularis of the proximal esophagus alone is the technique of choice for small diverticula (< 2 cm). Because of this sole muscular section, the mucosa of the small pouch realigns itself with that of the cervical esophagus below.

Transcervical diverticulopexy plus myotomy is indicated in medium-sized diverticula (2 to 3 cm). In such cases myotomy that could be achieved by endoscopic sectioning of the common wall would be limited to the proximal portion of the UES, leaving the distal portion functioning. The main advantage of diverticulopexy plus myotomy over other techniques is that the pharyngeal lumen is never opened and the esophageal mucosa is never cut during the entire procedure, which allows early oral feeding. For this reason this technique should be used in debilitated patients with hypoproteinemia or in those taking medications such as steroids since both of these conditions carry a risk of postoper-

Table 1. Comparison of the most common surgical techniques

	Myotomy Alone	Diverticulopexy Plus Myotomy	Endoscopic Methods	Resection Alone
Type of diverticulum				
Small	+	−	−	−
Medium	−	+	(+)	(+)
Large	−	(+)	+	(+)
Aesthetic sequelae	(+)	(+)	−	(+)
Risk of fistula	−	−	(+)	+
Risk of recurrence	(+)	(+)	(+)	+
Postoperative fasting period (days)	1	1	3	7

ative fistula from the suture line after resectioning of the pouch. Very large diverticula (6 cm or more) are best managed by other techniques, because there may not be enough room for placement of the large pouch behind the pharynx.[16]

Large diverticula (4 cm or more) may be managed with endoscopic techniques.[17] By creating a common cavity between the diverticulum and the proximal esophagus, they abolish stasis of food and prevent regurgitation into the mouth and respiratory passages. Division of the common wall also allows sectioning of the muscular structures that form the UES. The procedure is quick and simple, and there are no cosmetic sequelae even though the latter are usually of minimal importance, because hypopharyngeal diverticulum occurs mostly in elderly persons in whom the postcervicotomy scar and lines in the cervical skin merge with time.

Endoscopic procedures that were used until now were sutureless electrocautery or laser coagulating techniques[18,19] that could theoretically expose the cervical spaces adjacent to the transection line to septic contamination from the digestive lumen. This was suggested by the low-grade fever that was reported by Van Overbeek and Hoeksema[18] and experienced by some of our patients in the early postoperative period. Impelled by recent developments in celioscopic devices, we have experimented with the stapling technique, described previously. Possible advantages of the latter over the coagulating methods include:

- Suturing of the two wound edges resulting in optimal hemostasis and no septic contamination of the neck
- Prevention of perforation of the bottom of the diverticulum, since the course of the knife ends a few millimeters proximal to the distal end of the stapler
- No need for any expensive equipment such as a laser source

Regarding resectioning of the diverticulum, the only residual indication is a large diverticulum in a patient with a narrow oropharyngeal channel. In this instance, there is not enough room in the neck for diverticulopexy. It can make introduction of the endoscope into the hypopharynx impossible. In other cases, the 5- to 7-day fasting period required for healing of the esophageal suture prolongs the postoperative hospital stay and increases the patient's discomfort. Moreover, postoperative fistula and late recurrences are far from being the exception.

CONCLUSION

There is more than one surgical modality to management of most of the benign esophageal diseases. Hypopharyngeal diverticulum is one of them. It is essential for the surgeon to be able to practice any of these techniques correctly and to choose the most relevant procedure according to the clinical presentation of the disease, its stage, the patient's own anatomical specificity, and concomitant general conditions.

REFERENCES

1. Ferguson MK. Evolution of therapy for pharyngo-esophageal (Zenker's) diverticulum. Ann Thorac Surg 51:848-852, 1991.
2. Wilson CP. Pharyngeal diverticula: Their cause and treatment. J Laryngol Otol 76:151-180, 1962.
3. Dohlman G, Mattsson O. The role of the crico-pharyngeal muscle in cases of hypopharyngeal diverticula. Am J Roentgenol 81:561-569, 1959.
4. Hunt PS, Connell AM, Smiley TB. The crico-pharyngeal sphincter in gastric reflux. Gut 11:303-306, 1970.
5. Henderson RD, Hanna W, Marryatt G, et al. Crico-pharyngeal dysphagia secondary to gastro-esophageal reflux: Clinical investigative and pathologic findings. In DeMeester TR, Skinner DB, eds. Esophageal Disorders: Pathophysiology and Therapy. New York: Raven Press, 1985, pp 169-175.
6. Ellis FH, Schlegel JF, Lynch VP, et al. Crico-pharyngeal myotomy for pharyngo-esophageal diverticulum. Ann Surg 170:340-349, 1969.
7. Knuff TE, Benjamin SB, Castell DO. Pharyngo-esophageal (Zenker's) diverticulum. A reappraisal. Gastroenterology 82:734-736, 1982.
8. Duranceau A, Rheault MJ, Jamieson GG. Physiologic response to crico-pharyngeal myotomy and diverticulum suspension. Surgery 94:655-662, 1983.
9. Belsey R. Functional disease of the esophagus. J Thorac Cardiovasc Surg 52:164-188, 1966.
10. Lichter I. Motor disorder in pharyngo-esophageal pouch. J Thorac Cardiovasc Surg 76:273:275, 1978.
11. Cook IJ, Dodds WJ, Dantas RO, et al. Opening mechanisms of the human upper esophageal sphincter. Am J Physiol 20:G748-759, 1989.
12. Dantas RO, Cook IJ, Dodds WJ, et al. Biomechanics of crico-pharyngeal bars. Gastroenterology 99:1269-1274, 1990.
13. Cruse JP, Edwards DAW, Smith JF, Wyllie JH. The pathology of a crico-pharyngeal dysphagia. Histopathology 3:223-232, 1979.
14. Lerut T, Vandekerkhof J, Leman G, et al. Crico-pharyngeal myotomy for pharyngo-esophageal diverticula. In DeMeester TR, Matthews HR, eds. Interna-

tional Trends in General Thoracic Surgery, vol. 3. Benign Esophageal Disease. St. Louis: CV Mosby, 1987, pp 351-363.

15. Nicholson WF. The late results of operations for pharyngeal pouch. Br J Surg 49:548-552, 1962.

16. Hauters P, Segol P, Leroux Y, et al. Place de la myotomie du crico-pharyngien associée a une diverticulopexie dans le traitement du diverticule de Zenker (quinze années d'expérience). Ann Chir 42:726-730, 1988.

17. Hains JD. Internal pharyngo-oesophagotomy (Dohlman procedure). In Jamieson GG, ed. Surgery of the Oesophagus. Edinburgh: Churchill-Livingstone, 1988, pp 457-459.

18. Van Overbeek JJM, Hoeksema PE. Endoscopic treatment of the hypopharyngeal diverticulum: 211 cases. Laryngoscope 92:88-91, 1982.

19. Knegt PP, de Jong PC, Van der Schans EJ. Endoscopic treatment of the hypopharyngeal diverticulum with the CO_2 laser. Endoscopy 17:205-206, 1985.

97 *Laparoscopic Staging of Cancer of the Esophagus*

John R. Anderson

Carcinoma of the esophagus is associated with distressing dysphagia, and resection involves great operative risk. The prognoses for squamous carcinoma of the esophagus and adenocarcinoma of the cardia are poor, especially when these diseases are disseminated. Resection should be reserved for those cases without metastatic disease. Adequate palliation of malignant dysphagia in patients with widespread disease can now be achieved with a variety of nonoperative methods. The accurate and reliable detection of intra-abdominal metastatic disease is important in avoiding unnecessary radical operations.

Hepatic metastases are associated with poor prognosis. Methods for the preoperative detection of hepatic metastases include biochemical tests, isotope liver scanning, ultrasonography, and computed tomography (CT). Each of these methods has its limitations and drawbacks.

Laparoscopy has been evaluated in the assessment of intra-abdominal malignant dissemination in patients with carcinoma of the stomach,[1,2] pancreas,[3] biliary tract,[4,5] and in those with nongastrointestinal malignancies.[6-10] There are few studies on the role of laparoscopy in the preoperative assessment of patients with malignant dysphagia.[1,11] Dagnini et al.,[11] who studied 369 patients with carcinoma of the esophagus and cardia, found liver metastases in 10% of those cases, peritoneal metastases in 4.9%, and omental metastases in 1.6%. False negative results occurred in only 4.4% of the 250 patients who underwent operation in that study.

We present a prospective comparative evaluation of the accuracy of laparoscopy, ultrasonography, and CT in the detection of intra-abdominal metastasis in this study.

MATERIALS AND METHODS

During a 30-month period, 90 consecutive patients treated for malignant dysphagia at Glasgow Infirmary were studied. All had biopsy-proven carcinoma of the esophagus or cardia, but patients with proximal gastric cancer involving the cardia and esophagus were excluded from the study. All patients underwent abdominal ultrasonography with a real-time ultrasonographic scanner, contrast-enhanced CT by an EMI 005 whole-body scanner (EMI Ltd), and laparoscopy. During laparoscopy, patients received a general anesthetic with intermittent positive pressure ventilation. An Olympus oblique viewing laparoscope was used with an Eder Insumat Insufflator. The laparoscope was inserted subumbilically, except in nine patients who had undergone previous abdominal surgery. In some cases a liver biopsy was obtained under direct vision. Instruments for laparoscopic manipulation and punch biopsy were not available. Each procedure was performed by a single investigator who had no knowledge of the results of the ultrasonography and CT scan investigations. The results of all three investigations were considered with other data when decisions regarding individual patient management were made.

Intra-abdominal metastases were considered to be

present only when histological confirmation was obtained from the results of laparotomy and biopsy, laparoscopy and biopsy, or autopsy.

The sensitivity, specificity, and accuracy of each technique was calculated. The sensitivity of the investigation is defined as the proportion of positive test results in all patients with proven disease; the specificity is the proportion of negative test results in all patients who did not have disease; and the accuracy is the ratio of the corrected results (true positive plus true negative) to the total number of tests. Statistical analysis was performed using the Yates corrected chi-squared test.[2]

RESULTS

Fifty-five of the 90 patients studied were men, and 35 were women. There was a mean age of 64 (SD, 11.7; range, 40 to 93 years). Thirty-six patients had squamous carcinoma, and 54 had adenocarcinoma. Of those patients with squamous carcinoma, 11 cases involved the upper third of the esophagus; 19, the middle third; and six, the lower third. Thirty-nine of the adenocarcinomas involved the cardia but were primarily located in the esophagus rather than in the stomach, and 15 carcinomas were confined to the esophagus (three in the upper third and 12 in the middle third [Table 1]).

Thirty-eight of the 65 patients who underwent laparotomy had resection of the primary tumor. Fifteen of the remaining 27 patients received traction prosthet-

ic tumor intubation either as a planned procedure (eight cases) or because the guidewire failed to pass during attempted endoscopic intubation (seven cases). Of the remaining 12 patients who had advanced disease at laparotomy, three underwent pulsion tumor intubation with a prosthesis at the time of laparotomy, eight were subsequently treated by laser recanalization, and one was treated with chemotherapy. Open operation was not undertaken in 25 patients because of widespread metastatic disease (20 patients) or because the patients were considered unfit for major operation (five patients). Twelve of the 25 patients were managed by pulsion intubation, 11 by laser therapy, and two by radiotherapy.

Table 2 shows the number distribution and origin of the intra-abdominal metastases. Intra-abdominal disease occurred in 23 (51%) of the 45 patients with upper- or middle-third lesions of the esophagus and in 27 (60%) of the 45 patients with tumors involving the lower third of the esophagus or the cardia.

Twenty-five patients had hepatic metastases that were confirmed histologically by laparotomy and biopsy or by laparoscopy and percutaneous biopsy under direct vision. None of these patients had hepatomegaly or abnormal liver function tests. Seventeen metastases (68%) occurred in patients with adenocarcinoma and eight (32%) occurred in patients with squamous carcinoma. Seven metastases (28%) occurred in patients who had lesions of the upper or middle third of the esophagus and 18 (72%) occurred in those with lesions of the lower third of the esophagus or the cardia.

Thirty-five patients had histologically proven nodal metastases at the time of laparotomy; 22 of these metastases (63%) were in patients with adenocarcinoma, and 13 (37%) were in patients with squamous carcinoma. Seventeen nodal metastases (49%) were associated with upper- or middle-third lesions of the esophagus and 18 (51%) with lesions of the lower third of the esophagus or cardia. Nine patients had peritoneal metastases at laparotomy: five in patients with adenocarcinoma and four in those with squamous primaries. Four nodal metastases were found in conjunction with middle- or upper-third lesions of the esophagus and five were associated with lower-third lesions or cardia.

All 90 patients investigated were used to calculate the sensitivity, specificity, and accuracy of the three investigative modalities with respect to hepatic metastases. Metastases could be confirmed histologically via laparoscopy and needle biopsy and without laparotomy. However, because peritoneal and nodal metastases could only be confirmed via histological evaluation after lapa-

Table 1. Clinical data (n = 90)

Patient Characteristic	No. of Patients
Age (yr)	
Mean	64
Range	40-93
Sex	
Men	55
Women	35
Diagnosis/location	
Squamous cell carcinoma	
Upper third	11
Middle third	19
Lower third	6
Adenocarcinoma	
Cardia/lower third	39
Middle third	12
Upper third	3

Table 2. Intra-abdominal metastases by site of tumor and pathological factors

Tumor Site	No. of Patients Diagnosed	Intra-Abdominal Metastases		
		Hepatic	Nodal	Peritoneal
Squamous cell carcinoma of the esophagus				
Upper third	11	2	0	0
Middle third	19	4	9	4
Lower third	6	2	4	0
Adenocarcinoma of the esophagus				
Upper third	3	0	0	0
Middle third	12	1	8	0
Lower third	39	16	14	5
TOTAL	90	25	35	9

Table 3. Hepatic metastases (n = 25)

Test Results	Technique Used		
	Laparoscopy	Ultrasonography	CT Scan
Positive sensitivity	22 (88%)	12 (48%)	14 (56%)
Negative specificity	65 (100%)	63 (97%)	63 (97%)
False positive	0 (0)	2 (2%)	2 (2%)
False negative	3 (3%)	13 (14%)	11 (12%)
Accuracy	96%	83%	85%

rotomy, only the 65 patients who underwent laparotomy were considered when the sensitivity, specificity, and accuracy of the investigative modalities in detecting these metastases were calculated.

Laparoscopy correctly identified 22 of the hepatic metastases; there were three false negatives and no false positives. These results give a sensitivity of 88%, a specificity of 100%, and an overall accuracy of 96% (Table 3). Of the three false negatives, two resulted from failure to visualize one lobe of the liver as a result of intra-abdominal adhesions from previous operations, and one resulted from the posterior location of a metastatic deposit. Ultrasonographic examination identified 12 of the hepatic metastases; 13 false negatives and two false positives occurred. These results indicate a sensitivity of 48%, a specificity of 37%, and an accuracy of 83%. In 14 patients, hepatic metastases were identified via CT. Eleven false negatives and two false positives

occurred; these results show a sensitivity of 56%, a specificity of 97%, and an accuracy of 85%. Laparoscopy was significantly more sensitive than was ultrasonography ($p < 0.01$) or CT scan ($p < 0.02$) in the detection of hepatic metastases; it was also more accurate than both techniques ($p < 0.01$ for both modalities). There were no statistical differences between the results of ultrasonographic scan and CT scan in the detection of hepatic metastases. Twelve of the hepatic metastases were detected by all three tests; two were detected by laparoscopy and CT. Three were missed by all three tests, and eight were detected only by laparoscopy. The false positive results of ultrasonography and CT occurred in four different patients, and subsequent follow-up by repeated CT has failed to show metastatic deposits that might have indicated occult hepatic metastases on the first investigation.

Peritoneal and nodal metastases were confirmed his-

Table 4. Nodal metastases (n = 35)

Test Results	Technique Used		
	Laparoscopy	Ultrasonography	CT Scan
Positive sensitivity	18 (51%)	6 (17%)	11 (31%)
Negative specificity	29 (97%)	28 (98%)	26 (87%)
False positive	1 (1.5%)	2 (3%)	4 (6%)
False negative	17 (26%)	29 (45%)	24 (37%)
Accuracy	72%	52%	57%

Table 5. Peritoneal metastases (n = 9)

Test Results	Technique Used		
	Laparoscopy	Ultrasonography	CT Scan
Positive sensitivity	8 (89%)	2 (22%)	0 (0)
Negative specificity	56 (100%)	56 (100%)	56 (100%)
False positive	0 (0)	0 (0)	0 (0)
False negative	1 (1.5%)	7 (11%)	9 (14%)
Accuracy	98%	89%	—

tologically only if laparotomy was performed. Of the 65 patients who underwent open operation, 35 had histologically confirmed intra-abdominal nodal metastases (Table 4). In 21 of these patients (60%), the nodes involved occurred around the celiac axis. Laparoscopy identified 18 of the 35 patients with nodal disease; 17 false negatives and one false positive occurred. Ultrasonography detected only six nodal metastases; there were 29 false negatives and two false positives. CT detected 11 nodal involvements; 24 false negatives and four false positives occurred. The sensitivities were therefore 51%, 17%, and 31%; the specificities, 97%, 93%, and 87%; and the overall accuracy, 72%, 52%, and 57% for laparoscopy, ultrasonography, and CT results, respectively. Laparoscopy was more sensitive ($p < 0.01$) and more accurate ($p < 0.05$) than was ultrasonography in the detection of nodal metastases. The difference between laparoscopy and CT, however, failed to reach statistical significance at the 5% level. There were no differences between the results of ultrasonography and CT in the sensitivity or accuracy of detecting nodal metastases.

Nine patients had peritoneal metastases proven at laparotomy (Table 5). Before operation eight of these patients were correctly identified by laparoscopy; there were no false positive results, but the one false negative examination occurred in a patient with a metastatic deposit on the inferior surface of the transverse mesocolon. In these nine cases, the sensitivity of laparoscopy was 89%; the specificity 100%; and the accuracy 98%. Ultrasonographic examination demonstrated free intra-abdominal fluid in two patients who had ascites but no definite metastatic deposits, and CT failed to detect peritoneal disease. Neither morbidity nor mortality was associated with laparoscopy.

DISCUSSION

To plan proper treatment for patients presenting with malignant dysphagia, one must determine the extent of metastasis. This is especially true in cases of intra-abdominal metastasis. Much attention has been given to preoperative detection of hepatic metastases. Biochemical tests of liver function are relatively easy to perform and have become widely available as a result of increased automation in testing. The role of biochemical tests in the accurate assessment of liver metastases may seem limited however.[12-14] Isotope scanning has shown promise in the detection of liver metastases, but the results of scanning conflict. In 1982, Lamb and Taylor[15] found that liver scintigraphy and ultrasonography were 97% accurate in the identification of liver metastases in 100 patients with colorectal cancer; 15 of these patients had liver metastases. Most other authors, however, have reported accuracies of approximately 65% to 80%.[8,16-18]

Ultrasonographic scanning (and gray-scale ultrasonography in particular) is now widely available. Although in the work of Lamb and Taylor[15] a 97% accuracy was indicated for ultrasonography, other authors have not been able to reproduce these results, and figures of 75% to 80% accuracy are usually reported.[1,14,16]

Several studies[14,16] have now shown that CT is only slightly more accurate than ultrasonography in the detection of liver metastases; CT accuracy rates of 80% to 85% are reported. Smith et al.[16] compared the accuracy of scintigraphy with that of ultrasonography and CT in patients who had a variety of primary tumors and potential hepatic involvement. They found little difference in the accuracy of the three techniques; scintigraphy and ultrasonography were 80% accurate, and CT was 84% accurate. In the study by Smith et al.,[16] lesions <3 cm in diameter were likely to be missed by all three techniques; the researchers concluded that direct visualization and biopsy were the only methods of definitive diagnosis of hepatic metastases. Studies by Kemeny et al.[14] indicated a sensitivity of 87% for CT results combined with evaluation of carcinoembryonic androgen levels, but the overall accuracy was only 64% for this combined method of assessment.

Laparoscopy is widely used as a diagnostic and therapeutic tool in gynecology, and its use in general surgery is rapidly increasing. Complications in patients who received local or general anesthetic have been relatively few,[1,4,5,9] and diagnostic accuracy has been high. The staging of pancreatic tumors and other intra-abdominal tumors has been improved with laparoscopy,[3,10] and the accurate evaluation of the liver in patients with primary bronchial, breast or lymphoid tumors has been well documented.[6,8] One major benefit of laparoscopy is that tissue samples can be obtained accurately under direct vision, not only from the liver but also from node and peritoneal metastases. This technique often can be used to confirm or refute the results of other noninvasive investigations.

Few studies have evaluated the role of laparoscopy with respect to tumors of the esophagus or cardia,[1,11] and there are no comparative studies of the effectiveness of ultrasonography, CT, and laparoscopy in the evaluation of this group of patients. In our study, the results of ultrasonography and CT in the detection of liver metastases were similar to those reported by others.[1,14,15,16] Laparoscopy was the significantly superior technique; overall accuracy was 96%, and histological confirmation of the metastatic disease was possible. The three false negative results of laparoscopy in this study resulted from inadequate visualization as a result of intra-abdominal adhesions in two patients and from the posterior location of metastases in the third patient. Although some of these problems might have been resolved by insertion of the laparoscope in different quadrants of the abdomen or with the use of instruments to break down adhesions, we must accept that laparoscopy and scanning techniques may fail. The liver metastases in these three cases were also missed by both ultrasonographic and CT techniques. In 12 of the 25 patients with liver metastases, disease was detected by all three modalities. CT and ultrasonography have equally high specificities (97%); therefore, positive results can be relied upon. Laparoscopy is probably not required when CT or ultrasonographic results have shown metastatic disease to the liver unless histologic confirmation is desired. However, in all eight patients with negative ultrasonographic and CT results, laparoscopy revealed hepatic metastases. This number of patients constitutes 32% of all cases with proven liver metastases studied. Laparoscopy is a useful additional investigation in patients who may undergo open operation if either of the scanning techniques yields normal results.

Both scanning techniques generated poor results with regard to identification of nodal metastases. Laparoscopic results were better than those of ultrasonography but were not significantly superior to those of CT. Metastatic deposits may occur in nodes that are only slightly enlarged; thus the metastases might not be visible on scans at the present resolution. Usually, smaller nodes can be identified via laparoscopy, but they may or may not contain tumor. Because a significant proportion of these nodes may be located around the celiac axis, they may not be visible via standard laparoscopic techniques. Nodal metastases are of less importance than metastases of the liver or peritoneum in determining the resectability of tumors of the esophagus and cardia, but knowledge of nodal metastases may be important in staging the disease of patients who are refused operative treatment on other grounds. Appropriate palliative therapy can then be planned as a result of accurate staging.

Peritoneal metastases preclude curative resectional surgery. In this study, free peritoneal fluid was revealed via ultrasonography in two cases, but peritoneal metastases in nine patients were not revealed by either CT or ultrasonography. If punch biopsy had been available, histological proof of peritoneal disease could have been obtained and may have obviated laparotomy in some of these patients. The metastatic deposits missed by laparoscopy were located on the inferior surface of the transverse mesocolon in one patient. These deposits might have been detected via the techniques described by Cuschieri and Berci.[19]

In this study, 51% of patients with upper- and middle-third lesions of the esophagus had evidence of intra-abdominal metastases similar to those of the 60% of patients with lower-third lesions of the esophagus and the cardia. Searching for intra-abdominal metastases is important even in patients with upper-third esophageal lesions, because unnecessary operation can be avoided.

In patients with carcinoma of the esophagus or cardia, laparoscopy offers a safe, accurate, reliable method of assessing the abdomen for metastatic disease. In a significant proportion of patients with malignant dysphagia, unnecessary open operation can be avoided and palliation can be more carefully planned when laparoscopy is used with nonoperative palliative methods.

REFERENCES

1. Shandall A, Johnson C. Laparoscopy or scanning in oesophageal and gastric carcinoma. Br J Surg 72:449-451, 1985.
2. Gross E, Bancewicz J, Ingram G. Assessment of gastric cancer by laparoscopy. Br Med J 288:1577, 1984.
3. Cuschieri A, Hall AW, Clark J. Value of laparoscopy in the diagnosis and management of pancreatic carcinoma. Gut 19:672-677, 1978.
4. Irving AD, Cuschieri A. Laparoscopic assessment of the jaundiced patient: A review of 53 patients. Br J Surg 65:678-680, 1978.
5. Hall TJ, Donaldson DR, Brannan TG. The value of laparoscopy under local anaesthesia in 250 medical and surgical patients. Br J Surg 67:751-753, 1980.
6. Bleiberg H, Rozencweig M, Mathein M, et al. The use of peritoneoscopy in the detection of metastases. Cancer 41:863-867, 1978.
7. Friedman IH, Grossman MB, Wolff WI. The value of laparoscopy in general surgical problems. Surg Gynecol Obstet 144:906-908, 1977.
8. Margolis R, Hansen HH, Muggia FM, Kantouwa S. Diagnosis of liver metastases in bronchogenic carcinoma. Cancer 34:1825-1829, 1974.
9. Lewis A, Archer TJ. Laparoscopy in general surgery. Br J Surg 68:778-780, 1981.
10. Sugarbaker PH, Wilson RE. Using celioscopy to determine stages of intra-abdominal malignant neoplasms. Arch Surg 111:41-44, 1976.
11. Dagnini G, Caldironi MW, Marin G, Buzzaccarini O, Tremolada C, Ruol A. Laparoscopy in abdominal staging of esophageal carcinoma. Gastrointest Endosc 32:400-402, 1986.
12. Baden H, Andersen B, Augustenborg G, Hanel HK. Diagnostic value of gamma-glutamyl transpeptidase and alkaline phosphatase in liver metastases. Surg Gynecol Obstet 133:769-773, 1971.
13. Ranson JHC, Adams PX, Localio SA. Preoperative assessment for hepatic metastases in carcinoma of the colon and rectum. Surg Gynecol Obstet 137:435-438, 1973.
14. Kemeny MM, Sugarbaker PH, Smith TJ, et al. A prospective analysis of laboratory tests and imaging studies to detect hepatic lesions. Ann Surg 195:163-167, 1982.
15. Lamb G, Taylor I. An assessment of ultrasound scanning in the recognition of colorectal liver metastases. Ann R Coll Surg Engl 64:391-393, 1982.
16. Smith TJ, Kemeny MM, Sugarbaker PH, et al. A prospective study of hepatic imaging in the detection of metastatic disease. Ann Surg 195:486-491, 1982.
17. Castagna J, Benfield JR, Yamada H, Johnson DE. The reliability of liver scans and function tests in detecting metastases. Surg Gynecol Obstet 134:463-466, 1972.
18. Lunia S, Parthasarathy KL, Bakshi S, Bender MA. An evaluation of ^{99m}Tc-sulfur colloid liver scintiscans and their usefulness in metastatic work-up: A review of 1424 studies. J Nucl Med 16:62-65, 1975.
19. Cuschieri A, Berci G. Practical Laparoscopy. Eastbourne: Baillière Tindall, 1986.

98 *Minimally Invasive Techniques in Esophageal Surgery*

Alberto Peracchia, Ermanno Ancona, Alberto Ruol, Romeo Bardini, Andrea Segalin, and Luigi Bonavina

Minimally invasive procedures have recently been used in the surgical treatment of various diseases of the esophagus,[1] e.g., carcinoma, leiomyomas, pharyngoesophageal and thoracic diverticula, gastroesophageal reflux disease, motor disorders of the body of the esophagus, and achalasia.

In the near future minimally invasive procedures will be used more and more frequently in esophageal diseases, paralleling technological improvements, the development of specific instruments, and increasing specific expertise. However, it should always be remembered that minimally invasive procedures represent only a new alternative in the approach to well-standardized surgical procedures, that they are delicate operations despite the minimal invasiveness, and that they require the observance of correct indications and traditional therapeutic standards. Furthermore, these operations should be performed only by surgeons with a wide open surgery experience in the same diseases to minimize intraoperative and long-term complications and to reduce treatment failures. To assess the results obtained with minimally invasive procedures, it is of utmost importance, especially in this initial phase, to evaluate the results by means of objective tests. To summarize, it should be remembered that the technique has to serve the therapeutic goals, not vice versa.

CANCER OF THE THORACIC ESOPHAGUS

The standard approach to cancer of the thoracic esophagus is represented by transthoracic esophagectomy, since it allows an optimal exposure of the tumor and a sound lymph node dissection in the mediastinum. Transhiatal esophagectomy without thoracotomy is indicated when preoperative staging suggests that the tumor is resectable but the patient is unfit for thoracotomy because of concomitant medical conditions. Another indication is represented by tumors of the cervical esophagus without involvement of the intrathoracic esophagus and by selected tumors of the gastric cardia, both requiring removal of the thoracic esophagus in continuity.

Minimally invasive techniques can now be used to perform esophagectomy for cancer[2-5] when thoracotomy is contraindicated. These techniques are indicated when preoperative staging suggests that the tumor is suitable for transhiatal esophagectomy without thoracotomy (T1 to T3, possibly N0, M0), and the patient is unfit for thoracotomy. The first technique is thoracoscopic esophageal dissection (see the box), the sec-

---

CARCINOMA OF THE THORACIC ESOPHAGUS
Pros and cons of thoracoscopic esophageal dissection in comparison with standard transhiatal esophagectomy

Pros

Easy and safe dissection of the esophagus from adjacent structures

Indicated even in bulky tumors of the upper and middle thoracic esophagus

Sampling and standard dissection of mediastinal lymph nodes possible

Effective hemostasis with reduced risk of bleeding

Reduced risk of lesioning the thoracic duct, tracheobronchial tree, recurrent laryngeal nerves, and pulmonary branches of the vagus nerve

Reduced risk of intraoperative cardiac dysrhythmias

Reduced postoperative thoracic pain

Reduced postoperative stay in the ICU

Reduced postoperative pulmonary complications

Cons

Longer operating time

Sectioning of the azygos vein cross indicated to facilitate esophageal dissection

Selective bronchial intubation with one-lung ventilation required

Contraindicated in the presence of massive pleural adhesions

ond technique is esophageal dissection with "scopic" devices through the hiatus and a cervical incision (see the box). Both techniques allow the surgeon to perform accurate mediastinal dissection, lymphadenectomy of periesophageal nodes, and reduce the risk of injury to recurrent laryngeal nerves, thoracic duct, tracheobronchial tree, and azygos vein. When the thoracoscopic approach is used, esophageal dissection is made easier by dividing the azygos vein and sectioning the esophagus at the apex of the chest. At present, videoendoscopically assisted esophageal dissection through the hiatus and the cervical incision seems to be more precise; however, the thoracoscopic approach will probably become safer, allowing performance of a more accurate mediastinal lymphadenectomy, with the development of specific instruments. It is likely that even enlarged lymphadenectomy will become possible. In selected cases it may be advantageous to use a combination of the two techniques.

CARCINOMA OF THE THORACIC ESOPHAGUS
Pros and cons of transhiatal-transcervical microsurgical dissection of the esophagus in comparison with standard transhiatal esophagectomy

Pros

Easy and safe dissection of the esophagus from adjacent structures
Sampling of mediastinal lymph nodes possible
Effective hemostasis with reduced risk of bleeding
Reduced risk of lesioning the azygos vein, thoracic duct, tracheobronchial tree, recurrent laryngeal nerves, and pulmonary branches of the vagus nerve
Reduced risk of intraoperative cardiac dysrhythmias
Reduced postoperative thoracic pain
Reduced postoperative stay in the ICU
Reduced postoperative pulmonary complications

Cons

Indicated only in small tumors, especially when located at the thoracic inlet or in the lower thoracic esophagus
Lymphadenectomy long and difficult; almost impossible in the upper mediastinum and along the tracheobronchial tree

---

To date, we have operated on 10 patients with thoracic esophageal cancer using minimally invasive techniques. No intraoperative or postoperative complications related to the procedure were recorded.

ESOPHAGEAL LEIOMYOMA

Transthoracic extramucosal enucleation represents the standard treatment for esophageal leiomyoma. Symptomatic leiomyomas of the thoracic esophagus can now be enucleated through a thoracoscopic approach.[6] In our opinion, intraoperative videoesophagoscopy is mandatory, since it can assist the thoracoscopic dissection of the tumor from the esophageal mucosa. Furthermore, it is important to verify the integrity of the mucosa from inside. After enucleation of the leiomyoma, the muscular layer has to be approximated with a running suture or with interrupted stitches.

Four patients were operated on with no intraoperative or early postoperative complications. During follow-up, a patient in whom the muscular layer had not been approximated showed pseudodiverticular bulging of the mucosa and mild dysphagia to liquids.

In two more patients the thoracoscopic approach had to be converted to open thoracotomy. In one patient a small mucosal perforation was done during thoracoscopic dissection, and we preferred to repair the tear immediately through a minithoracotomy. The second patient had a bulky plunging goiter that did not allow us to perform a selective bronchial intubation with right lung exclusion; during thoracoscopy it was impossible to obtain satisfactory collapse of the lung and we preferred to shift to a safer open chest enucleation of the leiomyoma through an open thoracotomy.

THORACIC ESOPHAGEAL DIVERTICULA

The standard treatment for epiphrenic diverticula of the esophagus consists of transthoracic (left thoracotomy) diverticulectomy, extramucosal myotomy of the lower esophageal sphincter, and an anterior fundoplication according to Belsey's technique.

Recent advances of minimally invasive surgery have made possible the thoracoscopic resection of symptomatic pulsion diverticula of the thoracic esophagus using endostaplers.[1]

We have undertaken a pilot study of thoracoscopic diverticulectomy. The protocol consists in pretreatment barium swallow x-ray examination, endoscopy, 24-hour esophageal pH monitoring, and manometry: if the lower esophageal sphincter is hypertensive and/or does not relax on swallowing, we perform a pneumatic dilation of the cardia using low-compliance balloons inflated at 10 PSI for 1 minute. Seven days after this procedure a gastrografin swallow is performed. A manometric and pH study is performed a month later. Follow-up consists in repeated esophagograms, endoscopy, and esophageal function studies.

Five patients have been treated so far by means of pneumatic dilation of the lower esophageal sphincter followed by right thoracoscopic diverticulectomy. Intraoperative esophagoscopy was very helpful in assisting the dissection of the diverticulum and to verify from inside the integrity of the mucosa and the stapled suture. The muscular layer should be approximated with sutures.

Four patients had an uneventful postoperative course, and are doing well 6 to 10 months after operation. The control barium swallow x-ray examination showed a regular profile of the esophagus, and there is no evidence of reflux on 24-hour esophageal pH monitoring. The fifth patient had a leakage at the level of the suture line that required transthoracic repair.

PHARYNGOESOPHAGEAL (ZENKER'S) DIVERTICULA

The usual treatment for pharyngoesophageal diverticula consists in the myotomy of the pharyngoesophageal sphincter and diverticulectomy, through a left cervical incision. Some authors consider that myotomy of the pharyngoesophageal sphincter and diverticulopexy is an effective approach as well.

We have operated on an elderly patient with Zenker's diverticulum (4 cm in diameter) and a long history of dysphagia and aspiration pneumonia, using the minimally invasive surgical approach proposed by Collard and Kestens.[7] An EndoGIA stapler was inserted through the patient's mouth, and the stapler's jaws were positioned, one anteriorly in the esophagus and the other posteriorly in the pouch. Two applications of the EndoGIA were necessary to divide the septum between the esophagus and the diverticulum. We emphasize that the sectioned septum included the fibers of the pharyngoesophageal sphincter, and therefore a myotomy was performed. The postoperative gastrografin swallow showed no leakage. It was shown that a widely communicating space was created between the diverticulum and the esophagus, which allowed easy passage of the food bolus. Postoperative manometry showed that the pressure of the upper esophageal sphincter was satisfactorily reduced. The patient resumed oral feeding

7 days after operation and has no complaints after 6 months.

MOTOR DISORDERS OF THE BODY OF THE ESOPHAGUS

A long esophageal myotomy is indicated in few selected patients with motor disorders of the esophageal body, such as diffuse esophageal spasm and the "nutcracker esophagus." The operation is generally performed through a thoracotomy, but good results have been recently reported using a thoracoscopic approach.[8]

ACHALASIA

The standard surgical treatment for achalasia of the esophagus consists in the myotomy of the lower esophageal sphincter (Heller's procedure) combined with an antireflux repair. Besides the transabdominal and the transthoracic approaches, a laparoscopic approach has also been recently proposed.[9]

In four patients we performed this operation through a laparoscopic approach: after the extramucosal myotomy, an anterior Dor hemifundoplication was fashioned. Laparoscopic myotomy was assisted by videoesophagoscopy and a balloon dilator within the esophageal lumen. This provided satisfactory exposure of the anterior aspect of the esophagus without the need of a circumferential dissection. The clinical, radiological, endoscopic, manometric, and pH monitoring results confirmed that, at least in the short-term follow-up the minimally invasive approach is safe and effective.

GASTROESOPHAGEAL REFLUX DISEASE

Nissen antireflux repair is the most widely used operation in patients with gastroesophageal reflux disease. It should be performed after a complete preoperative workup consisting of an esophagogram, endoscopy, manometry, 24-hour esophageal pH monitoring, and scintigraphic gastric emptying scan. The technical principles and details of the Nissen operation are well standardized. A laparoscopic approach has been recently proposed for this operation.[10-12]

We have performed a Nissen-Rossetti antireflux repair using a laparoscopic approach in three patients. In these patients the fundoplication was calibrated over a 60 Fr Maloney dilator. A posterior crural repair was routinely performed. No intraoperative difficulties were encountered. The short-term follow-up of our patients is satisfactory, both subjectively and on the basis of endoscopy, manometry, and pH measurements.

CONCLUSION

Minimally invasive procedures represent a promising surgical approach in selected patients with malignant and benign diseases of the esophagus. There is no doubt that the operative trauma and postoperative pain are markedly reduced in comparison with standard procedures. However, further experience and longer follow-up will define the precise indications, merits and limits of this approach. If good results are to be obtained, it should always be remembered that although minimally invasive procedures are appealing they should never twist the sound principles of open surgery. Surgeons facing minimally invasive surgery should have a wide experience in the traditional surgical techniques and should be aware of the fact that when the intraoperative technical result is not satisfactory, quick conversion to open surgery is mandatory. It should never be forgotten that postoperative complications can be prevented in the operating theater.

REFERENCES

1. Peracchia A, Ruol A, Bardini R, Segalin A. Mini-invasive procedures in esophageal surgery. In Proceedings of the Third World Congress of Endoscopic Surgery, Bordeaux, 1992.
2. Naruhn MB, Buess GF, Becker HD, Mentges BR. The endoscopic microsurgical dissection of the esophagus in the treatment of esophageal carcinoma: Technique and preliminary clinical results. Eur Surg Res 23:1-5, 1991.
3. Bumm R, Hoelscher AH, Feussner H, Tachibana M, Siewert JR. Endoscopic esophageal dissection: Indications, techniques and clinical results. In Proceedings of the Fifth World Congress of the International Society for Diseases of the Esophagus, Kyoto, 1992.
4. Dallemagne B, Weerts JM, Jehaes C, Markiewicz S, Bona S, Hosselet JL, Vadhat O, Lombard R. Case report: Subtotal oesophagectomy by thoracoscopy and laparoscopy. Min Invas Ther 1:183-185, 1992.
5. Cuschieri A, Shimi S, Banting S. Endoscopic oesophagectomy through a right thoracoscopic approach. J R Coll Surg Edinb 37:7-11, 1992.
6. Bardini R, Segalin A, Ruol A, Pavanello M, Peracchia A. Thoracoscopic enucleation of esophageal leiomyomas. In Proceedings of the Third World Congress of Endoscopic Surgery, Bordeaux, 1992.
7. Collard JM, Kestens PJ. Endoscopic suture of the hypopharyngeal diverticulum: A new technique. In Proceedings of the Fifth World Congress of the International Society for Diseases of the Esophagus, Kyoto, 1992.
8. Shimi SM, Nathanson LK, Cuschieri A. Thoracoscopic long oesophageal myotomy for nutcracker oesophagus: Initial experience of a new surgical approach. Br J Surg 79:533-536, 1992.
9. Pinotti HW, Domene CE, Nasi A, Santo MA, Libanori H. Surgical treatment of achalasia through myotomy and fundoplication by videolaparoscopy: Early follow-up. In Proceedings of the Fifth World Congress of the International Society for Diseases of the Esophagus, Kyoto, 1992.
10. Hill LD, Kraemer JM, Kozarek RA, Aye RW. The laparoscopic Hill repair: A definitive laparoscopic antireflux procedure. In Proceedings of the Fifth World Congress of the International Society for Diseases of the Esophagus, Kyoto, 1992.
11. Pinotti HW, Domene CE, Nasi A, Santo MA, Libanori H. Surgical treatment of reflux esophagitis through partial fundoplication by videolaparoscopy: Early follow-up. In Proceedings of the Fifth World Congress of the International Society for Diseases of the Esophagus, Kyoto, 1992.
12. Gagea T. Laparoscopic Nissen's fundoplication: Preliminary report on ten cases. Surg Endosc 5:170-173, 1991.

99 Thoracoscopic Approach to Esophagectomy and Removal of Esophageal Benign Tumors: Technique, Initial Results, and Prospects

D. Gossot and M. Celerier

Decreasing the mortality and morbidity rates of esophageal surgery remains one of the goals for surgeons. Avoiding the consequences of thoracotomy in fragile patients might be the first step toward this goal.[1] For the time being, two new techniques have been developed using the thoracoscopic[2] and the mediastinoscopic[3] routes. We describe a thoracoscopic technique we first tested in animals[2] and recently applied to humans.

ESOPHAGECTOMY
Technique

The preparation and draping for the thoracoscopic technique are done as for a usual open procedure. The double-lumen endotracheal tube must be placed in perfect position. If not, an incomplete lung collapse will result, making exposure of the mediastinum difficult. Unless the esophageal tumor stenosis is too tight, a nasogastric (NG) tube is introduced to help identify and grasp the esophagus. The patient is in the left lateral position, right side up. The right arm must be pulled up to free the axilla for eventual insertion of additional trocars. There is no need to arch the patient.

The telescope is introduced into the seventh intercostal space (ICS) in the midaxillary line. Two lung retractors (Fig. 1) are introduced in the anterior axillary line, usually in the fourth and sixth ICS. Time must be taken for correct exposure of the mediastinum. Gently flattening the lung with the retractor while the anesthesiologist aspirates the right bronchus helps keep the lung deflated. The esophageal dissection may be started only if the view of the mediastinum is clear. If oozing or hemorrhage occurs, hemostasis will be very difficult to achieve if vision is hindered by the lung.

Once exposure of the posterior mediastinum is complete (i.e., when the esophagus can be clearly identified), two additional 10 mm ports are introduced, one in the fifth ICS in the posterior axillary line or even more posteriorly and one in the sixth ICS in the anterior axillary line for dissecting instruments and a clip applier.

Even if one of the retractors is a 5 mm one, it is more convenient to use only 10 mm trocar tubes, giving the surgeon the choice to change the position of the instruments or of the telescope during the procedure. Through the posterior trocar tube, a grasping forceps is introduced. The mediastinal pleura is grasped, elevated, and opened with scissors. The pleural incision is continued from bottom to top, with or without cautery, depending on the degree of mediastinal inflammation. The lateral sides of the esophagus are loosened using the blunt tip of closed scissors or a dissector.

After it is partly freed, the esophagus is grasped with esophageal forceps (Fig. 2) and is pulled upward and backward. The position of the forceps can be shifted along the length of the esophagus, and its use offers more versality than a more or less stationary vesseloop or tape passed around the esophageal body to expose it. The hemostasis of esophageal vessels is achieved with cautery and clips. The use of curved scissors and curved forceps is very helpful for dissection of the mediastinal side of the esophagus. This stage of the procedure is sometimes made difficult by a minor and permanent oozing, which requires frequent suction. To avoid an awkward inflation of the lung during suction, short aspiration periods must be used. Keeping one or two trocars vacant is also an efficient solution, making it possible to keep a permanent suction device in place.

When the esophagus has been mobilized up to the upper third level, the azygos vein must be divided. The blunt-tipped scissors are gently slipped under the mediastinal pleura, which is divided up to the top of the chest. The back side of the vein is dissected using scissors and a dissector. Before engaging the endostapler, confirmation that the dissector tip is visible at the superior edge of the vein and that 2 cm of the azygos are totally free (Fig. 3) is necessary. The vein is then divided using the vascular endostapler, which must be introduced perpendicular to the vein (i.e., through the port used for the telescope). Thus the telescope must be moved to another port, and the previous 10 mm tro-

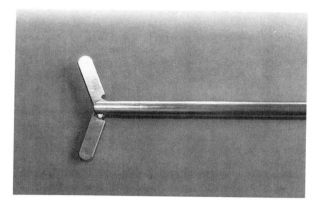

Fig. 1. Lung retractor (Olympus) used for thoracoscopic esophageal surgery.

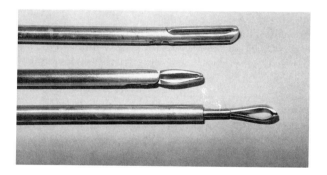

Fig. 2. Esophageal grasping forceps (Olympus).

car of the telescope must be exchanged with a 12 mm one. When the vein is completely held between the stapler's jaws, the stapler can be fired. The division of the azygos vein allows complete dissection of the upper third of the esophagus.

The esophageal dissection then is continued downward to the diaphragm. The dissection of the lower third can be left incomplete if the creation of a substitute organ is conducted through a laparotomy, because the lower part of the esophagus is easy to mobilize via laparotomy. However, if esophageal replacement is conducted laparoscopically, it is easier to dissect the esophagus as far as possible through the thoracoscopy. Once the esophagus is totally free, the esophagectomy can be completed superiorly through the cervicotomy and inferiority through the abdomen (Fig. 4). A chest tube is placed in the esophageal bed.

The esophageal reconstruction is made using either the colon or the stomach, according to the surgeon's preference and the availability of either organ and the surgical team's expertise. A gastric esophageal substituted can be created and placed laparoscopically, as described by Dallemagne and Weerts.[4] However, this technique is time-consuming and its benefit, compared with the open technique, has not yet been demonstrated.

Initial Results

Twelve attempts at esophagectomy have been made using a right thoracoscopic approach in ten men and two

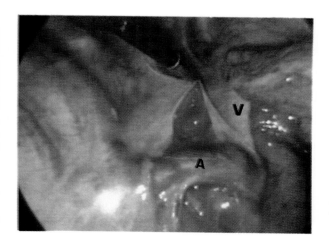

Fig. 3. Azygos vein is totally dissected. (A = azygos vein, V = vena cava).

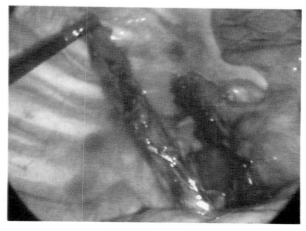

Fig. 4. View of the esophagus (caustic stenosis) after complete mobilization and division via cervicotomy.

women with an average age of 45 years. The indication for surgery was squamous cell carcinoma in seven patients, an adenocarcinoma in one, and a caustic stricture in four. The whole esophagus was mobilized thoracoscopically, and the esophagectomy was completed through the abdomen. The reconstruction was achieved using a gastric substitute and mediastinal pull-through technique performed by laparotomy. The esophago-gastric anastomosis was made in the neck.

Three failures resulted for the following reasons: a large tumor, making a thoracoscopic dissection unsafe (one case) and incomplete lung collapse, making the exposure of the posterior mediastinum difficult (two cases). These three cases were converted to thoracotomy. In the remaining eight patients, the thoracoscopic dissection was successful. The average procedure time was 85 minutes. The postoperative course was uneventful in six patients. Two patients had a left atelectasis, and one had a right pleural effusion.

Discussion

Until recently there were only two ways to perform an esophagectomy: either through thoracotomy or through a transhiatal approach from the abdomen. The respiratory morbidity rate of open esophagectomy is high, ranging from 6% to 10%.[1] This high morbidity rate is partly responsible for the 6% to 15% mortality rate of esophagectomy. Many techniques of esophagectomy without thoracotomy have been described since the report of Orringer and Sloan.[6] With some particular conditions such as caustic necrosis, transhiatal liberation can be performed easily without danger or risk of hemorrhage.[7] However, in many cases this technique does not allow suitable adjustments in the dissection of a crowded anatomical area, and the middle third of the esophagus remains hidden, even when using a large phrenotomy.[8] Although the blood vessels to the esophagus are small,[9] there is an indisputable hazard of hemorrhage. In Orringer and Orringer's report,[10] the average blood loss was 900 ml. In a review of the literature, Liebermann-Meffert et al.[9] have noted a fatal hemorrhage rate of 1.6% (most often as a result of an injury of the azygos vein) and a tracheal tear rate of 3%. The advantage in terms of respiratory morbidity has not been demonstrated. In a series of 304 esophagectomies without thoracotomy (EWT) collected by Perrachia and Bardini,[11] the pulmonary complications were as follows: tracheobronchial tear (1.5%), pleural effusion (17.8%), and operative mortality rate 10.3%, Shahian et

al.[12] have reported a higher respiratory morbidity rate (although not significant) after EWT than after open esophagectomy.

For 3 years Buess et al. improved the technique of EWT by the use of an endoscopic microsurgical dissection of the esophagus through mediastinoscopy.[13] The operating mediastinoscope is introduced into the posterior mediastinum through a left cervicotomy. It has a central working channel, and its optics offer an image enlarged two to four times, thus allowing accurate dissection of vessels and nerves. The esophagus is dissected downward and removed transhiatally through a laparotomy. After this method was demonstrated as efficient and safe in an animal model,[13] Buess et al.[3] reported a series of 17 human cases with no operative mortality and with minimal blood loss (<200 ml).

The thoracoscopic approach for esophagectomy is another way of trying to reduce, if not solve, the problem of respiratory morbidity. The technique is too recent and our series too short to form an opinion about the results. Compared with the mediastinoscopic approach, the thoracoscopic approach has the advantage of giving a wider view of the pleural cavity and of the mediastinum. Thus it allows a more extended excision than that of mediastinoscopy. Evaluation of both techniques is necessary to determine whether these methods are complementary or opposed to one another.

THORACOSCOPIC REMOVAL OF BENIGN TUMORS OF THE ESOPHAGUS
Technique

The preparation and first stages of thoracoscopic removal of benign esophageal tumors are similar to those of thoracoscopic esophagectomy. The approach is a right thoracoscopy, with double-lumen endotracheal intubation and an NG tube placed into the esophagus. The procedure is easy in the case of a small tumor located on the right side of the esophagus. It can be more problematic if the tumor is large or located on the left side of the esophagus. In such a case the esophagus must be almost completely mobilized lengthwise to allow rotation, thus exposing the tumor to the right side of the mediastinum.

Difficulty results because the tumor is usually not clearly visible on the esophageal wall and the surgeon is not able to use manual palpation. It can be helpful to perform an intraoperative endoluminal esophagoscopy to locate the limits of the tumor precisely by transillumination and observation through the thoracoscope. These limits are then marked on the esophageal wall using thoracoscopically guided electrocautery.

The muscular layer is then opened with blunt-tipped scissors, with their direction perpendicular to the esophageal wall. Once the tumor appears between the muscular fibers, it is caught with a grasping forceps or a su-

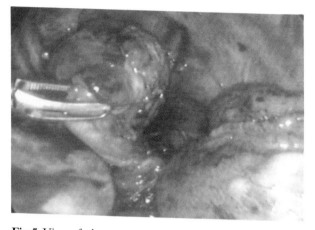

Fig 5. View of a large squamous cell carcinoma of the esophageal upper third. The esophagus was previously divided via cervicotomy.

ture is passed through it using a straight needle. The tumor is pulled upward, and the dissection is continued using the same principles as in open surgery (Fig. 5).

Compared with open chest surgery, the main problem is not to lacerate the muscle fibers, since the esophagus can not be firmly held as in conventional surgery. The esophagus has a tendency to slide and twist under the scissors tips. Laceration of the muscular fibers may result in a difficult repair if the edges of the tumor excision are not clean. Once the tumor has been removed, an examination to determine whether or not the mucosa has been opened can be performed by injecting methyl blue through the NG tube. However, positive results of this test make the repair of the mucosal wound difficult by giving a blue coloration to the whole operating field. Thus it is more convenient to inject gas through the esophagoscope and ask the endoscopist to look carefully at the mucosa (Fig. 6). Then the muscular layer is closed with a continuous suture (Fig. 7). At the end of the procedure, the tumor is removed through a short counterincision in the axilla. A chest tube is placed in the posterior mediastinum.

Initial Results

Four patients have been operated on for a leiomyoma of the esophagus through right thoracoscopy. The tumor was located on the right side of the esophagus in three cases and on the left side in one case. The size of

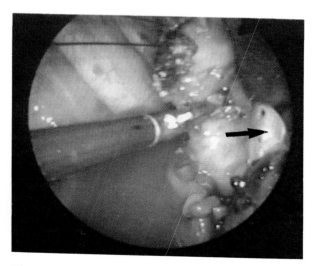

Fig. 6. Removal of a large leiomyoma of the esophagus. Mucosa is transilluminated (*arrow*) through esophagoscopy.

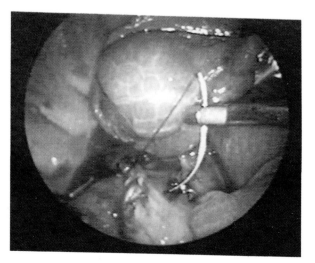

Fig. 7. Closure of the esophageal wall after removal of a leiomyoma.

the tumor ranged from 2 to 8 cm. The limits of the tumor and the integrity of the esophageal mucosa were checked during the procedure using transillumination through the esophagoscope. It was necessary to divide the azygos vein in three cases to expose the tumor. After removal, the muscular layer was sutured.

In one case the dissection was very difficult because of a preoperative attempt to remove the tumor through esophagoscopy. In two cases an opening in the mucosa was made, resulting in a small fistula in one case. The tumor was easily removed in the remaining cases.

Discussion

Benign tumors of the esophagus (i.e., mainly leiomyomas and cysts) are rare. They seldom give rise to symptoms (approximately one third of the patients[14]); thus their surgical treatment may seem out of proportion with their benign nature.[15] However, complications such as an increase in size, causing obstruction and pulmonary disorders or even malignant forms, have been reported.[14] So unless to do so is contraindicated, these tumors are usually removed. Generally a small lateral thoracotomy does not allow sufficient control of the esophagus, in which case a large thoracotomy is performed. The thoracoscopic approach is well suited to the benign nature of these tumors.

PROSPECTS IN ENDOSCOPIC ESOPHAGEAL SURGERY

Although thoracoscopic treatment of esophageal diseases is quite new, numerous applications will probably soon be found.

Endoscopic transthoracic surgery of the esophagus is in its first stages of development. Articles on clinical cases are being published now that it has been demonstrated that its use is definitely feasible in animals.[2,3] It is too early to have an opinion about the benefits in terms of morbidity and survival. However, the morbidity-to-benefit ratio favors this approach: avoiding the consequences of thoracotomy in fragile patients is already progress. Nevertheless, the following questions must be answered in the near future.

What are the respective indications for the mediastinoscopic and thoracoscopic approaches? The mediastinoscopic technique has been demonstrated as a safe method, especially with regard to the control of perioperative hemorrhage.[3] There is no need for selective tracheal intubation, thus decreasing the risk of atelectasis. However, the technique does not allow a view of the surrounding mediastinal structures, thus making carcinologically sound operations almost impossible. Buess et al.[3] justify their approach by the fact that the surgical resection of esophageal cancer is primarily palliative. This opinion is supported by others.[16] But some surgeons have shown a significant benefit in en bloc esophagectomy for early stage (N0 and N1) carcinomas.[17] Although extensive node dissection has been shown as feasible through thoracoscopy in animal models,[2] it is not known whether such a dissection can be performed safely on humans.

Is there a place for thoracoscopy in preoperative staging? As far as lymph node involvement is concerned, no ideal preoperative examination has been found. Endosonography is more accurate than computed tomography.[18] Tio et al.[19] have demonstrated that endoscopic ultrasonography can detect periesophageal nodes in most cases (95%). Nevertheless, the specificity is poor: 50% of the nodes are in fact only inflammatory nodes. Tio et al.[19] have suggested performing sonographically guided biopsies to enhance the accuracy of endosonography. Thoracoscopic node picking might give the best results—laparoscopic staging has already been shown very effective in treating cancer of the cardia[20]—but the procedure is more invasive than endosonography. However, in some cases in which the tumoral stenosis is too tight to allow the passage of the sonographic probe or in case of doubt, thoracoscopy may be indicated.

REFERENCES

1. Nishi M, Hiramatsu Y, Hioki K, et al. Risk factors in relation to postoperative complications in patients undergoing esophagectomy or gastrectomy for cancer. Ann Surg 207:148-154, 1988.
2. Gossot D, Ghnassia MD, Debiolles H, et al. Thoracoscopic dissection of the esophagus: An experimental study. Surg Endosc 6:59-61, 1992.
3. Buess GF, Becker HD, Naruhn MB, et al. Endoscopic esophagectomy without thoracotomy. Probl Gen Surg, 8:478-486, 1991.
4. Dallemagne B, Weerts GM. Subtotal esophagectomy by thoracoscopy and laparoscopy. Minimally Invasive Ther 1:320, 1992.
5. Akiyama H, Tsurumaru M, Ono Y, et al. Transoral esophagectomy. Surg Gynecol Obstet 173:399-400, 1991.
6. Orringer MB, Sloan H. Esophagectomy without thoracotomy. J Thorac Cardiovasc Surg 76:643-654, 1978.
7. Gossot D, Sarfati E, Celerier M. Early blunt esophagectomy in severe caustic burns of the upper digestive tract. Report of 29 cases. J Thorac Cardiovasc Surg 94:188-191, 1987.

8. Goldberg M, Freeman J, Gullane PJ, et al. Transhiatal esophagectomy with gastric transposition for pharyngeal malignant disease. J Thorac Cardiovasc Surg 97:327-333, 1989.

9. Liebermann-Meffert DAI, Luescher URS, Neff UR, et al. Esophagectomy without thoracotomy: Is there a risk of intramediastinal bleeding? Ann Surg 206:184-192, 1987.

10. Orringer MB, Orringer JS. Esophagectomy without thoracotomy: A dangerous operation? J Thorac Cardiovasc Surg 85:72-80, 1983.

11. Peracchia A, Bardini R. Total esophagectomy without thoracotomy: Results of a European questionnaire (GEEMO). Int Surg 71:171-175, 1986.

12. Shahian DM, Neptune WB, Ellis FH, et al. Transthoracic versus extrathoracic esophagectomy: Mortality, morbidity and long-term survival. Ann Thorac Surg 41:237-246, 1986.

13. Kipfmüller K, Naruhn M, Melzer A, et al. Endoscopic microsurgical dissection of the esophagus. Results in an animal model. Surg Endosc 3:63-69, 1989.

14. Arnorsson T, Aberg C, Aberg T. Benign tumors of the esophagus and esophageal cysts. Scand J Thorac Cardiovasc Surg 18:145-150, 1984.

15. Gossot D, Sarfati E, Celerier M. Faut-il opérer les tumeurs bénignes de l'oesophage? Med Chir Dig 16:483-484, 1987.

16. Barbier PA, Becker CD, Wagner HE. Esophageal carcinoma: Patient selection for transhiatal esophagectomy. A prospective analysis of 50 consecutive cases. World J Surg 12:263-269, 1988.

17. Skinner DB, Ferguson MK, Soriano A, et al. Selection of operation for esophageal cancer based on staging. Ann Surg 204:391-400, 1986.

18. Ziegler K, Sanft C, Semsch B, et al. Endosonography is superior to computed tomography in staging tumors of the esophagus and the cardia [abstract]. Gastroenterology 94A:51-57, 1988.

19. Tio TL, Coene PPL, Luiken GJ, et al. Endosonography in the clinical staging of oesophago-gastric carcinoma. Gastrointest Endosc 36:2-10, 1990.

20. Watt I, Stewart I, Anderson D, et al. Laparoscopy, ultrasound and computed tomography in cancer of the esophagus and gastric cardia: A prospective comparison for detecting intra-abdominal metastases. Br J Surg 76:1036-1039, 1989.

---

100 Thoracoscopic Esophagectomy: Minimally Invasive Direct-Vision Esophageal Mobilization for Cancer

A.D.K. Hill, Ara Darzi, and John R.T. Monson

Total esophagectomy is traditionally performed using either a full thoracotomy or a transhiatal approach. Thoracotomy is highly invasive and is associated with considerable morbidity. Orringer first popularized blunt transhiatal esophagectomy[1-4] for both benign and malignant disease. Its main advantage over the two-stage Lewis-Tanner procedure[5,6] or the three-stage esophagectomy[7] is the avoidance of a thoracotomy. The disadvantages of a blunt esophagectomy include blood loss and trauma to the azygos vein, bronchus, and recurrent laryngeal nerves. In addition nodal dissection is not possible with this technique. Mobilization of the esophagus using a mediastinoscope has been described by Beuss et al., but this is associated with limited node dissection and difficulty in dissecting the lower end of the esophagus.

We will describe a technique that we have performed in six patients in whom thoracic mobilization of the esophagus is undertaken thoracoscopically using a series of ports placed in the right side of the chest.

OPERATIVE TECHNIQUE

The operation is performed with the patient under general anesthesia; a double-lumen endotracheal tube is placed to enable collapse of the right lung during the endoscopic dissection. The first part of the operation consists of the endoscopic dissection of the thoracic esophagus in the right thorax with the patient in the semiprone position. In the second stage of the operation the stomach is mobilized through an upper midline incision with the patient supine, while the cervical esophagus is dissected through an incision anterior to

547

the left sternocleidomastoid muscle in the neck. The cervical esophagus is divided and the esophagus and tumor are delivered through the abdominal wound. The "tubulized" stomach is then pulled through into the neck to be anastomosed to the cervical esophagus.

To facilitate collapse of the right lung, an electronic pressure-controlled CO_2 insufflator (Storz) is operated at a setting of 1 to 3 mm Hg. This pressure is used to avoid cardiac arrhythmias and mediastinal shift. Dissection of the esophagus can be facilitated by the placement of a flexible endoscope. This aids the surgeon in identifying the esophagus at the start of the procedure by visualising the light within the lumen of the esophagus. Movement of the endoscope within the esophagus can be used to facilitate dissection. Four thoracoscopic ports are used. The upper two (one 5 mm and one 10 mm) are placed in front and behind the lower angle of the scapula. The lower two (both 12 mm) are placed several interspaces below these just above the diaphragm. The procedure is commenced with the camera in the lower anterior port.

The thoracoscopic dissection begins at the level of the azygos vein, irrespective of the tumor site. The pleura is divided above and below the vein which is then dissected free from the underlying esophagus. We routinely divide the azygos vein using an EndoGIA (Autosuture) linear stapler. The mediastinal pleura over the entire esophagus from the thoracic inlet to the inferior pulmonary vein is then divided. Above the azygos vein the dissection plane is between the esophagus and the superior vena cava and trachea. An articulated dissector (Endodissect; Autosuture) can be used for the dissection and separation of these structures from the esophagus. Any nodes encountered in this region can be dissected and removed separately. Complete mobilization of the posterior aspect of the esophagus is greatly facilitated by use of a variable curvature–shaped memory dissector.[8] Alternatively, a soft rubber sling may now be passed around the mobilized upper esophagus.

The middle third of the esophagus is mobilized by moving the rubber sling in a caudal direction. Any large arteries feeding the esophagus from the aorta can be clipped and divided under direct vision. Separation of the esophagus from the tracheal bifurcation, the pericardium, pericardiophrenic vessels and phrenic nerves is also completed under direct vision. Care must be taken in the use of diathermy to avoid thermal injury to the thoracic duct and trachea. Again, enlarged lymph nodes may be dissected with the esophagus or separately. On occasion it is useful to carry out this dissection using the harmonic scalpel (Ultracision, Inc.), which produces less thermal damage to surrounding tissues than does diathermy.

For dissection of the lower third of the esophagus, the camera port should be moved to the upper anterior porthole. The inferior pulmonary ligament is divided with scissors (Autosuture) after electrocoagulation of the vessels within its fold. After mobilization of the thoracic esophagus, a single chest tube is inserted, and the abdominal and cervical stages of the operation are performed simultaneously.

The stomach is mobilized through an upper midline incision using the orthodox technique, with preservation of the right gastroepiploic arcade and division of the left gastric artery. The cervical esophagus is mobilized through an incision along the anterior border of the sternocleiodomastoid muscle. The carotid sheath is retracted laterally. The esophagus is mobilized after identification of the recurrent laryngeal nerve. The cervical esophagus is divided and a Penrose drain is anchored to the distal port. The esophagus is then delivered through the abdominal wound. The gastric fundus is then anchored to the Penrose drain, and a cervical gastric pull-through is performed, followed by an anastomosis between the proximal esophagus and the fundus of the stomach using a single layer of simple, interrupted polydioxamine suture. The cervical and abdominal wounds are then closed in a standard fashion.

DISCUSSION

This approach to esophageal mobilization is safe and feasible; further experience will be needed before its place in esophageal surgery is determined. The benefits of this procedure include better visualization and better nodal clearance. It also obviates the need for a thoracotomy. Whether this approach can permit radical esophageal dissection is unclear at this time. Avoidance of a thoracotomy leads to improved postoperative respiratory function, with early discharge from the intensive care unit. The risks of injury to intrathoracic structures and cardiac arrhythmias encountered with blunt transhiatal esophagectomy are largely obviated. Further developments in instrumentation may make this operation technically easier. Such developments might reduce the longer operative time currently associated with this procedure. Finally, the role of preliminary thoracoscopy in staging of esophageal cancer is an intriguing possibility.

REFERENCES

1. Godfaden D, Orringer MB, Appelman BD, Kalish R. Adenocarcinoma of the distal oesophagus and gastric cardia: Comparison of transhiatal oesophagectomy and throacoabdominal oesophagectomy. J Thorac Cardiovasc Surg 91:242-247, 1986.
2. Stewart JR, Sarr MG, Sharp KW. Transhiatal (blunt) oesophagectomy for malignant and benign oesophageal disease: Clinical experience and technique. Ann Thorac Surg 40:343-348, 1985.
3. Orringer MB. Transhiatal oesophagectomy for benign disease. J Thorac Cardiovasc Surg 90:649-655, 1985.
4. Orringer MB. Transthoracic versus transhiatal oesophagectomy: What difference does it make? Ann Thorac Surg 44:116-118, 1987.
5. Tanner NC. The present position of carcinoma of the oesophagus. Postgrad Med J 23:109-139, 1947.
6. Lewis I. The surgical treatment of carcinoma of the oesophagus with special reference to a new operation for growths of the middle third. Br J Surg 34:18-31, 1946.
7. McKeown KC. Total three stage oesophagectomy for cancer of the oesophagus. Br J Surg 63:259-262, 1987.
8. Cuschieri A. Variable curvature shape memory spatula for laparoscopic surgery. Surg Endosc 5:179-181, 1991.

101 Esophagectomy by Right Thoracoscopy: Feat of Skill or Real Breakthrough?

Jean-Marie Collard, J.B. Otte, and P.J. Kestens

During the last 2 years we have seen extraordinarily rapid developments in endoscopic surgery. More and more surgical procedures that had been carried out exclusively by conventional laparotomy and thoracotomy are now performed through minimally invasive approaches: cholecystectomy, common bile duct stone extraction, appendectomy, antireflux procedures, proximal gastric vagotomy, Heller myotomy, and even more complex operations, such as esophagectomy or colon resections.

We report our early experience with thoracoscopic esophagectomy to begin to define, if possible, the place of this new surgical approach in the management of the esophageal diseases.

PATIENTS

From September 1991 to April 1992, we performed right thoracoscopy on seven patients to remove the diseased esophagus (Table 1).

Patient 1. Patient 1 presented with a middle third tumor located just below the carina and multiple metastatic nodes in the upper abdomen and the neck. A palliative esophagectomy was carried out close to the esophagus itself. By combined laparotomy and left cervicotomy, the entire stomach, which was lengthened by denudation of the lesser curvature[1] was pulled up to the neck retrosternally. The patient's postoperative recovery was good.

Patient 2. Patient 2 had previously been admitted to our institution following caustic injury to the esophagus and stomach. He had been treated nonoperatively, but a long esophageal stricture developed from the cricopharyngeal muscle down to the lower third of the esophagus, as well as a stricture of the antrum. Esophagectomy was carried out by right thoracoscopy close to the esophagus. By laparotomy and cervicotomy, the proximal two thirds of the stomach could be pulled up to the left pyriformis sinus after resection of the antrum and gastrojejunostomy between the remaining portion of the stomach and a Roux-en-Y loop, as described by Ioshida et al.[2] Postoperative recovery was good.

Patient 3. Patient 3 was very thin with a lower third tumor. The esophagus itself, the adjacent mediastinal lymph nodes, and the fatty and fibrous sheath covering the aorta, the pericardium, the pulmonary veins, the trachea, and the main stem bronchi were removed en bloc by thoracoscopy. Neither the azygos vein nor the thoracic duct were included in the resection bloc. At laparotomy, the neoplastic spread into the proximal stomach along the lesser curvature led us to perform a total gastrectomy and to restore digestive tract continuity using a colon segment.[3] Postoperatively the patient developed hepatic failure with ascites, which justified a second laparotomy. Hepatic failure was caused by ligation of a left hepatic artery 2 mm in diameter that in retrospect was the only artery to the liver. The large artery that had originally been seen in the hepatic pedicle was, in fact, an aberrant splenic artery originating from the superior mesenteric artery. Although microscopic repair of the injured left hepatic artery was successful, the patient developed abdominal sepsis and died several weeks later.

Patient 4. Patient 4 presented with a large lower third tumor. Videoendoscopic inspection of the right pleural cavity revealed tumor invasion of the lower lobe of the right lung and a minimal pleural effusion that had not been evidenced by preoperative CT scan of the chest. The esophagus was bypassed using the Postlethwait technique[4] by laparotomy and cervicotomy.

Patient 5. Patient 5 had a lower third tumor. Extensive en bloc esophagectomy including resection of the azygos vein and the thoracic duct was attempted by right thoracoscopy. Accidental injury of right-sided intercostal artery flush with its aortic origin required thoracotomy to maintain hemostasis. The en bloc resection was completed conventionally. Mediastinal fibrosis was found while performing further esophageal dissection, which might explain the accidental arterial injury. The entire stomach was then pulled up to the neck by laparotomy and cervicotomy. A bilateral pulmonary infection developed on the third postoperative day, but further postoperative course was uneventful.

Patient 6. Patient 6 had a lower third tumor. Extensive en bloc resection could be completed by right thoracoscopy. The right-sided intercostal veins were sev-

Table 1. Experience with thoracoscopic esophagectomy at the University of Louvain

Patient No.	Esophageal Lesion	Surgical Procedure	Operating Time in Minutes (thoracic step)	Intraoperative Complication	Postoperative Outcome
1	Middle third tumor	Subtotal esophagectomy flush with the esophagus	310	—	Good
2	Caustic esophagitis	Subtotal esophagectomy flush with the esophagus	190	—	Good
3	Lower third tumor	Minimal en bloc esophagectomy	157	—	Death from hepatic failure
4	Lower third tumor	Exploratory thoracoscopy	30	—	Good
5	Lower third tumor	Extensive en bloc esophagectomy	60* + 120†	Intercostal artery injury flush with the aorta, leading to thoracotomy	Patient 5 developed bilateral pulmonary infection, with eventual good outcome
6	Lower third tumor	Extensive en bloc esophagectomy	390	—	Good
7	Lower third tumor	Extensive en bloc esophagectomy	390	—	Good

*Thoracoscopy time.
†Thoracotomy time.

ered close to the azygos vein, which was included in the resection bloc, as were the right hemiazygos vein and thoracic duct. Postoperative recovery was uneventful. Thirty-three lymph nodes were found at postoperative histological examination of the resected specimen.

Patient 7. This patient was 74 years old and had a lower third tumor. Similar to patient 6, an extensive en bloc esophagectomy including resection of the azygos vein, the thoracic duct, and mediastinal lymph nodes was performed. Postoperative recovery was good.

TECHNIQUE

With the patient under general anesthesia and one-lung ventilation, he is turned on his left side. Five trocars are inserted into the right pleural cavity: one in the fourth intercostal space, two in the sixth, and two in the eighth. This allows introduction of the videoendoscope, a lung retractor, a Johan or Babcock endoscopic clamp to grasp the mediastinal tissues, and various instruments such as an insulated electrosurgical hook knife, a clip applicator, or scissors for dissection. The mediastinal pleura is incised down to the right sympathetic nerve, the azygos vein, the descending aorta, or the esophagus itself, depending on the extent of the resection. In an extensive esophagectomy, the right-sided intercostal veins are divided between clips from the apex of the chest down to the hiatus. The thoracic duct may be individualized just above the diaphragm and divided between clips as well. The mediastinal pleura alongside the pericardium and the hiatus is incised to initiate dissection on the left side of the mediastinum. After completion of the posterior-inferior dissection, a Penrose drain is placed around the esophagus, which greatly facilitates further dissection up to the pulmonary veins, the subcarenal area, and the main stem bronchi. The two vagus nerves are identified and divided distal to the recurrent nerves. The azygos arch is transected using an EndoGIA 30 stapler (U.S. Surgical Corp.), which has been inserted into the right side of the chest through a 12 mm trocar. Dissection is then completed upward alongside the trachea and the right hemiazygos vein, the latter being included in the resection bloc when esophageal resection is extensive. The freed esophagus is abandoned in the chest, the five trocars are removed, and two chest tubes are inserted into the right pleural cavity through two of the five small incisions. The three other openings are closed. The patient is placed in the recumbent position for laparotomy and cervicotomy. The esophagus is then dissected and transected in the neck and pulled down to the abdomen.

DISCUSSION

Evaluation of the merits of this new surgical approach must be made in reference to those of more conventional techniques of esophagectomy that are routinely performed, taking into account that there will be further improvements of the procedure itself, as well as developments in thoracoscopic devices.

Open en bloc resection of the esophagus for cancer, including the soft tissues covering the organs adjacent to the esophagus and the potentially involved lymph nodes in the posterior mediastinum and the upper abdomen, has been shown to provide long-term survival and cure for 30% to 60% of the patients with normal lymph nodes, and for 15% to 20% of those with a small number of metastatic lymph nodes.[5-8] Therefore we agree with DeMeester that after resection limited to the esophagus itself, "cure is relegated to a chance phenomenon, occurring when existing lymph node metastases are inadvertently taken with the specimen."[9] Moreover, recent data published by Japanese surgical teams[10-12] stress the importance of systematically adding a radical neck dissection to the posterior mediastinectomy and the extensive lymphadenectomy in the upper abdomen, whatever the location of the tumor in the esophagus. Even though substantial improvement in survival rates has not yet been proved by any well-conducted prospective randomized study, systematic extension of the thoracic and abdominal lymphadenectomy to the neck in patients who are eligible for potentially curative surgery will be a critical matter for discussion in the future.[13]

Consequently, critical questions concerning esophagectomy by thoracoscopy are:

1. Is en bloc resection of the esophagus feasible by thoracoscopy?
2. If so, what conditions are necessary for safety?
3. Is esophagectomy by thoracoscopy indicated in cancer palliation and in benign diseases?
4. What are the advantages of this new approach over conventional techniques of esophageal resection?

En bloc resection of the esophagus including the adjacent soft tissues, the locoregional lymph nodes (subcarinal, periesophageal, periaortic, perihiatal), the azygos vein, and the lower segment of the thoracic duct could be achieved on patients 6 and 7. However, it appeared clear from these cases that thoracoscopic peritracheal lymph node dissection was hazardous to perform and that there was a need for grasping the periphery of the resection bloc with forceps, which might theoretically result in inadvertently crushing potentially involved lymph nodes. Such technical problems will probably be solved in the future with further experience with this type of procedure. If not, it puts into question the concept of a resection carried out through normal tissues beyond the limits of the neoplastic process by using gentle manual handling of the mediastinal tissues, made possible through a conventional thoracic incision.

In our opinion, this new approach addresses small tumors of the lower two thirds rather than those developed in the proximal third of the esophagus close to the trachea in a space where there are less soft tissues around the esophagus than in the lower two thirds of the mediastinum. The latter tumors as well as those big ones that are suspected of adhering to adjacent organs such as the main stem bronchi or the aorta on preoperative CT scan should be treated by a more conventional approach.

Safe performance of en bloc resection of the esophagus for cancer by thoracotomy requires great experience with esophageal surgery and good knowledge of the surgical anatomy of the mediastinum. This is even more true for esophageal surgery by thoracoscopy. For instance, it is obvious that untoward injury to any esophageal, bronchial, or right-sided intercostal artery, which commonly and inconsequently occurs when performing en bloc esophagectomy by thoracotomy, is much more difficult to control and repair through trocars than through a thoracic incision. In such an instance, the surgeon has to open the chest without any hesitation, as we did in patient 5. Moreover, conventional surgical instruments must be available on a table inside the operating room, ready to use at any time.

Palliative resection of esophageal cancers may classically be achieved either by thoracotomy or by a combined transhiatal and transcervical approach without thoracotomy. The former is best indicated in upper third tumors, whereas the latter is usually employed for tumors located at thoracic inlet level or in the lower two thirds of the esophagus. These conventional techniques are likely to be replaced either by right thoracoscopy, as in patient 1, or by a technique of transhiatal mediastinal videoendoscopy, as already performed by other teams. Anyway, palliative thoracoscopic esophagectomy made close to the esophagus is a much less hazardous procedure than thoracoscopic en bloc resection of the esophagus. On the other hand, our experience with patient 4 emphasizes the fact that thoracoscopy will be an excellent alternative to exploratory thoracotomy in the future.

Esophageal resection for benign disease is much less commonly needed than in the past, especially for gastroesophageal reflux. The best indication for esophagectomy by thoracoscopy should be a long caustic stricture similar to that described for patient 2. Although resection of such a stricture instead of a bypass operation remains controversial, fibrous esophageal adhesions that may develop after initial nonoperative management of a caustic burn are more safely dissected off the adjacent organs under video control by thoracoscopy than by transhiatal blunt esophagectomy without thoracotomy.

Although there has been great improvement of postoperative analgesic techniques over the past decade, an advantage of the thoracoscopic approach over conventional thoracotomy should be reduction of postoperative discomfort, especially pain related to the thoracic incision and its repercussions for respiratory function. In addition, respect of the technical rules for proper thoracic incision and closure does not prevent residual thoracic pain in some patients. Finally, avoidance of cosmetic sequellae is, of course, not a primary concern with esophageal cancer management.

REFERENCES

1. Collard JM, Otte JB, Jamart J, Reynaert M, Kestens PJ. An original technique for lengthening the stomach as an oesophageal substitute after oesophagectomy: Preliminary results. Dis esophagus 2:171, 1989.
2. Ioshida M, Iwatsuka M. Separated and pedicled wide gastric tube as an esophageal substitute. In Siewert J, Hölscher A, eds. Diseases of the Esophagus. Berlin: Springer Verlag, 1988, p 451.
3. Otte JB, Lerut T, Collard JM, Brecx JF, Gruwez J, Kestens PJ. Les plasties coliques de l'oesophage. Acta Chir Belg 82:389, 1982.
4. Postlethwait R. Technique for isoperistaltic gastric tube for esophageal by-pass. Ann Surg 189:673, 1979.
5. Akiyama H, Tsurumaru M, Kawamura T, Ono Y. Principles of surgical treatment for carcinoma of the esophagus: Analysis of lymph node involvement. Ann Surg 194:438, 1981.
6. Skinner DB. En bloc resection for esophageal carcinoma. In Delarue N, Wilkins E, Wong J, eds. International Trends in General Thoracic Surgery. Vol 4, Esophageal Cancer. St Louis: CV Mosby Co, 1988, p 193.
7. Collard JM, Otte JB, Reynaert M, Fiasse R, Kestens PJ. Feasibility and effectiveness of en bloc resection of the esophagus for esophageal cancer: Results of a prospective study. Int Surg 76:209, 1991.

8. Collard JM, Otte JB, Reynaert M, Fiasse R, Kestens PJ. Five year survival after subtotal esophagectomy for cancer (in press).

9. DeMeester TR, Barlow AP. Surgery and current management for cancer of the esophagus and cardia. Parts I and II. Current Problems in Surgery. Chicago: Year Book Medical Publishers, 1988, XXV:510.

10. Yoshida M, Murata Y, Yamamoto M. Surgical treatment for thoracic esophageal cancer. Presented at the Sixth World Congress of Bronchoesophagology, Tokyo, 1989 (abstract).

11. Tsurumaru M, Akiyama H, Udagawa H, Ono Y, Suzuki M, Watanabe G. Colo-thoraco-abdominal lymph node dissection for the intrathoracic esophageal cancer. Presented at the Fourth World Congress of the I.S.D.E., Chicago, 1989 (abstract).

12. Kato H, Watanabe H, Tachimori Y, Itzuka T. Evaluation of neck lymph node dissection for thoracic esophageal carcinoma. Ann Thorac Surg 51:831, 1991.

13. Skinner DB. Cervical lymph node dissection for thoracic esophageal cancer. Ann Thorac Surg 51:884, 1991.

XV

Videoendoscopic and Traditional Techniques in Operations on the Gastroesophageal Junction

102 Diagnosis of and Operative Indications for Gastroesophageal Reflux

Tom R. DeMeester

DEFINITION OF GASTROESOPHAGEAL REFLUX

Gastroesophageal reflux is a common disease that accounts for approximately 75% of esophageal pathology. Despite its common occurrence, a definition of the disease has been difficult to formulate.[1] The disease may be defined by its symptoms; however, this can be misleading, because symptoms thought to indicate the disease, such as heartburn and acid regurgitation, are common, and many individuals consider them normal and do not seek medical attention. Even when these symptoms are excessive, they are not specific to gastroesophageal reflux. They can be caused by other diseases, such as achalasia, diffuse spasm, esophageal carcinoma, pyloric stenosis, cholelithiasis, gastritis, gastric ulcer, duodenal ulcer, or coronary artery disease. Gastroesophageal reflux is often associated with other foregut disorders (such as duodenogastric or esophagopharyngeal reflux) that can preoccupy the patient, who may then disregard the complaints of heartburn and regurgitation that are key elements of gastroesophageal reflux. In addition, gastroesophageal reflux can cause chest pain that may suggest heart disease. Finally, a symptomatic definition of the disease does not provide the incentive to pursue the evaluation of patients who have difficulty expressing their health complaints. Consequently, patients with poorly understood symptoms may be dismissed erroneously as not having the disease.

Endoscopically diagnosed esophagitis is another definition for gastroesophageal reflux disease, but this also may be misleading. That patients with esophagitis, found on endoscopy, have excessive regurgitation of gastric juice into the esophagus is implied if these terms are used synonymously. This is true in 90% of patients, but in 10% the esophagitis has another cause, the most common of which is unrecognized chemical injury from drug ingestion. The definition of gastroesophageal reflux as endoscopically diagnosed esophagitis leaves undiagnosed those 40% of patients with proven reflux who have symptoms of gastroesophageal reflux not evident as esophagitis upon endoscopic evaluation. Obtaining an esophageal biopsy is of little help, because the sensitivity and specificity of an esophageal biopsy in the absence of endoscopically evident esophagitis are 0.75 and 0.9, respectively, and because the accuracy of the biopsy interpretation depends on the skill of the pathologist. Consequently, many patients whose severe symptoms require medical attention but who do not have endoscopic esophagitis are treated expectantly. Viewing gastroesophageal reflux as endoscopic esophagitis classifies the reflux as a sequela of esophagitis. Esophagitis, however, is a tissue injury that occurs as a consequence of gastroesophageal reflux but that is not synonymous with the disease. Defining the disease by its complication is not sound reasoning.

Another definition of gastroesophageal reflux disease refers to its basic pathophysiological abnormality: increased esophageal exposure to gastric juice. Twenty-four-hour esophageal pH monitoring with a pH probe that is placed 5 cm above the lower esophageal sphincter is used to quantitate the time during which the esophageal mucosa is exposed to gastric juice.[2,3] This exposure is expressed by measuring the cumulative time during which the esophageal pH is <4, the number of episodes in which the pH drops to <4, and the duration of each of these episodes. These measurements are the components used to express the results of esophageal pH monitoring. A computer program called the ESOpHOGRAM summarizes the results of pH monitoring with a mathematical formula in which the overall esophageal acid exposure is expressed as a composite score.

The upper limits of normal for each of these components and the composite score were established at the 95th percentile of 50 normal subjects who were free of symptomatic or objective evidence of a foregut abnormality (Table 1). Symptomatic patients in whom either the composite score or the percent total time pH of <4 exceeds the 95th percentile of normal subjects are considered to have increased esophageal exposure to gastric juice. Typical symptoms or complications of the disease are not essential for diagnosis. Extensive clinical

Table 1. Normal values for pH <4 (50 normal subjects)

Component	Mean ± SD	95% Confidence Interval
Total time (min)	1.51 ± 1.36	4.45
Upright time (min)	2.34 ± 2.34	8.42
Supine time (min)	0.63 ± 1.0	3.45
No. of episodes	19.00 ± 12.76	46.90
No. >5 min	0.84 ± 1.18	3.45
Longest episode (min)	6.74 ± 7.85	19.80
Composite score	5.95 ± 4.43	14.72

experience has shown that 24-hour esophageal pH monitoring, when analyzed according to the above principles, has the highest sensitivity and specificity in the detection of gastroesophageal reflux disease. However, this monitoring does not determine the reason for the increased exposure.

THE ANTIREFLUX MECHANISM

The antireflux mechanism in humans consists of a valvular cardia and the propulsive pumplike action of the body of the esophagus. Mechanical or functional failure of either the organ or the action may lead to abnormal esophageal exposure to gastric juice, but the function of one may compensate for the failure of the other. Failure of both, however, leads to abnormal esophageal acid exposure. Approximately 60% of patients with documented reflux have mechanical failure of their distal esophageal sphincter; in the remaining 40%, reflux is caused by esophageal or gastric pathologic factors. Mechanical failure of the sphincter is diagnosed by esophageal manometry in which the absence of adequate mechanical components of the sphincter (Fig. 1), such as a sphincter pressure of ≤6 mm Hg, a segment of sphincter of <1 cm in length that is exposed to the positive pressure environment of the abdomen, and/or an overall resting sphincter length of <2 cm. If one (or a combination) of these findings is present, the patient is diagnosed as having a mechanically defective sphincter. Failure of one or two components of the sphincter may be compensated for by the clearance function of the esophageal body. Failure of all three components leads to increased esophageal exposure to gastric juice.[4]

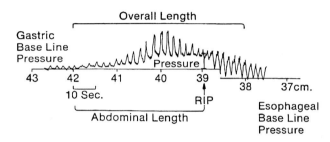

Fig. 1. Sample manometric measurement of the lower esophageal sphincter. (*RIP* = respiratory inversion point.)

Recently it has been shown that the resistance of the sphincter to reflux of gastric juice is determined by the integrated effects of radial pressures exerted over the entire length of the sphincter. The distribution of these pressures can be quantitated by three-dimensional computerized imaging of sphincter pressures and by calculating the volume of this image, which is called the sphincter pressure vector volume (SPVV) (Fig. 2). A calculated SPVV <5th percentile or <1212 is an indication of a mechanically defective sphincter.[5]

In a study of 50 normal volunteers and 150 patients with increased esophageal exposure to gastric juice and with various degrees of esophageal mucosal injury,[3] calculation of the SPVV increased the accuracy of manometry in the identification of a mechanically defective sphincter when compared with the accuracy of standard techniques. The superior results of manometry were par-

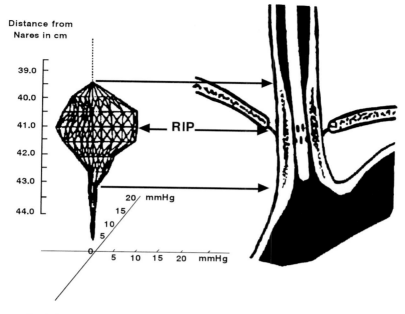

Fig. 2. Computerized three-dimensional imaging of lower esophageal sphincter. A catheter with four to eight radial side holes is withdrawn through the gastroesophageal junction. For each level of the pullback, the radially measured pressures are plotted around an axis representing gastric baseline pressure. When a stepwise pullback technique is used, the respiratory inversion point (*RIP*) can be identified.

ticularly evident in patients without mucosal injury who had subtle sphincter abnormalities. Three-dimensional lower esophageal sphincter manometry and calculation of the sphincter pressure vector volume should, therefore, become the standard techniques for assessment of the barrier function of the lower esophageal sphincter in patients with gastroesophageal reflux disease (Fig. 3).

In the past, refluxed acid gastric juice was usually regarded as the major damaging agent of gastroesophageal reflux disease. Current studies [4,18] show that the prevalence and severity of the complications of gastroesophageal reflux disease (such as esophagitis, stricture, and Barrett's esophagus) are related to increased esophageal exposure to both acidity and alkalinity (Fig. 4). Combined esophageal and gastric pH monitoring showed that the alkaline component in patients with gastroesophageal reflux resulted from excessive reflux of duodenal contents through the stomach into the distal esophagus. These findings indicate that the mechanical characteristics of the lower esophageal sphincter and

reflux of acid gastric juice contaminated with duodenal contents are the most important causes of mucosal injury in patients with gastroesophageal reflux disease (Fig. 5). These results also explain why some patients, particularly those with severe esophagitis, do not heal while they are receiving acid suppression therapy, and when a complication such as a stricture or Barrett's esophagus may develop.[1]

The incidence of a mechanically defective sphincter was positively correlated with increasingly severe complications of gastroesophageal reflux disease. Although it is tempting to attribute the loss of sphincter function to inflammation or tissue destruction, the identification of a defective sphincter in patients with gastroesophageal reflux disease without mucosal injury suggests that the mechanical defect of the sphincter is primary and is not due to inflammation or tissue damage.[1] It is important to identify the patients with gastroesophageal reflux disease who have a mechanically defective lower esophageal sphincter before complications develop to avoid the loss of esophageal body function

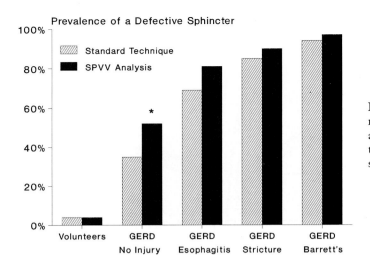

Fig. 3. Comparison of standard manometric techniques and SPVV analysis in the identification of a mechanically defective lower esophageal sphincter. *$p < 0.05$ versus standard manometry. (*SPVV* = sphincter pressure vector volume.)

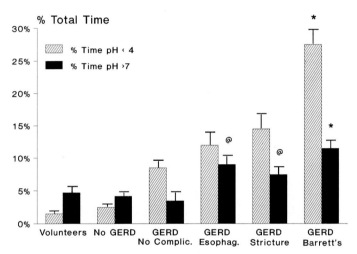

Fig. 4. Esophageal acid and alkaline exposure in study groups expressed as percent of total time pH <4 and pH <7. (*GERD* = gastroesophageal reflux disease. *$p < 0.01$ versus GERD patients with no complication; @$p < 0.05$ versus GERD patients with no complications.)

Fig. 5. The prevalence of complications in patients with gastroesophageal reflux disease and acid reflux or acid/alkaline reflux with or without a mechanically defective lower esophageal sphincter (LES). (*$p < 0.01$ versus patients with normal LES; @$p < 0.05$ versus patients with acid reflux and a defective LES.)

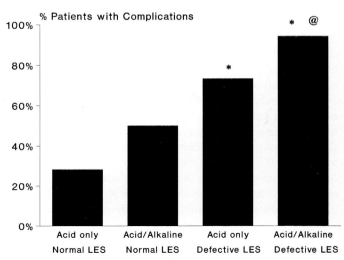

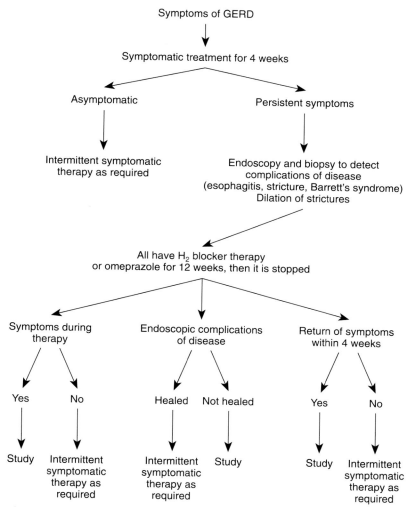

Fig. 6. Management (organigram) of gastroesophageal reflux.

that occurs as mucosal injury progresses.[6] In such patients, operative treatment should be performed before the loss of esophageal body function occurs. Measurement of the sphincter pressure vector volume is superior to standard manometric techniques in the identification of a mechanically defective lower esophageal sphincter as the cause of increased esophageal acid exposure, particularly in patients who have no mucosal injury.

In patients with increased esophageal acid exposure that results from a mechanically defective lower esophageal sphincter, reconstruction of a functional sphincter by an antireflux procedure provides the only ration-

al therapy: Reflux of gastric contents in >90% of patients is eliminated. This control of gastric contents is achieved by increasing the total and abdominal sphincter pressure vector volume to normal. Failure to restore the three-dimensional sphincter pressure profile to normal has been associated with persistent or recurrent reflux. The management of gastroesophageal reflux is shown in Fig. 6. It consists of dietary, postural, and antacid therapy. If there is no improvement in 2 weeks, endoscopy is performed and an 8- to 12-week course of H_2 blockers is initiated, after which all medication is stopped and the patient is reevaluated.

A patient with symptoms that indicate gastroesophageal reflux disease should be studied if those symptoms persist after 8 to 12 weeks of acid suppression therapy, if complications of the disease are unimproved, or if symptoms recur within 4 weeks of the cessation of therapy. An antireflux procedure is indicated if there is increased esophageal exposure to gastric juice on 24-hour pH monitoring and if a mechanically defective sphincter is identified by motility testing. Before a Nissen fundoplication is performed, the patient must be evaluated to determine the amplitude of esophageal contractions, the degree of esophageal shortening, gastric pathology, and whether a hiatal hernia or an adenocarcinoma has developed. These abnormalities may contraindicate the procedure, or the repair may need to be modified to include a gastroplasty, partial fundoplication, vagotomy, or bile diversion procedure.

The procedure by which to construct a competent, permanent antireflux mechanism with Nissen fundoplication is as follows:

1. Expose the esophageal hiatus and cardia.
2. Restore the lower esophageal sphincter pressure to a level two to three times that of the resting gastric pressure and its overall length to 3 cm by a method that allows the sphincter to respond to changes in intra-abdominal pressure. This can be accomplished by placing a 1 to 1.5 cm fundoplication around the distal esophagus.
3. Ensure that the fundoplication is around the distal esophagus rather than the stomach and that the fundoplication is not too long or too tight; those conditions cause dysphagia. An appropriate fundoplication can be accomplished by constructing a wrap over a No. 60 Fr bougie and by placing the wrap between the right vagus and the esophageal wall (Fig. 7).
4. Ensure relaxation of the lower esophageal sphincter to facilitate normal swallowing after surgery. This can be accomplished by use of only the fundus of the stomach in construction of the wrap.
5. Ensure that the resistance of the fundoplication does not exceed the peristaltic power of the esophagus. This can be accomplished by avoiding a total fundoplication if esophageal peristalsis is absent or is of low amplitude.
6. Ensure that the fundoplication remains in the abdomen by approximation of the crura and by use of gastroplasty when the esophagus is short and the repair is under tension. Laparoscopic and endoscopic techniques are providing new methods of accomplishing this procedure with a limited incision or through separate ports.[7]

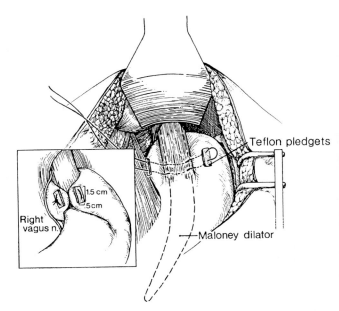

Fig. 7. Construction of the fundoplication by the transabdominal approach. Note the placement of the horizontal mattress stitch and the positions of the pledgets. The wrap is formed over a 60 Fr bougie; enough space is left to allow passage of an index finger through the wrap adjacent to the bougie. *Inset:* The completed fundoplication (*n* = nerve).

The actuarial success rate of a Nissen fundoplication in the control of reflux symptoms in a personal series of 100 consecutive patients with uncomplicated conditions over a 10-year period is 91% (Fig. 8). Eighty-three percent of these patients felt that they had been cured, and 10% felt that their condition had improved as a result of the operation.[8] Ninety-two percent would have operative treatment again if that were necessary. A multi-institutional randomized study of medical and surgical therapies that involved 248 patients showed that the results of a Nissen fundoplication as described above were superior to those of nonoperative medical therapy after 2 years of follow-up in which symptom score, endoscopic results, 24-hour esophageal pH monitoring, and patient satisfaction scores were used as end points.

OTHER PREOPERATIVE CONSIDERATIONS

Before an antireflux repair is performed, the following factors that may contraindicate the procedure or that may suggest modification of the repair should be considered:

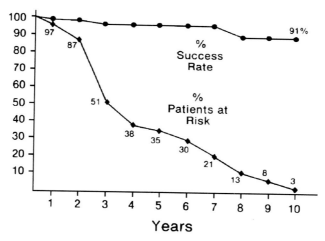

Fig. 8. Actuarial success rate of Nissen fundoplication in the control of reflux symptoms. The numbers on the lower curve represent the patients at risk for each subsequent yearly interval from which the actuarial curve was calculated.

1. The propulsive force of the body of the esophagus should be evaluated by esophageal manometry to determine whether it has sufficient power to propel a bolus of food through a newly reconstructed valve.[6]

2. Anatomic shortening of the esophagus can defeat any attempt at an adequate repair and leads to increased recurrence. This shortening is suggested radiographically by a sliding hiatal hernia that will not reduce in the upright position or that measures >5 cm between the diaphragmatic crura and gastroesophageal junction on endoscopy. Motility findings must be carefully evaluated, and gastroplasty (in addition to fundoplication) must be performed.[9]

3. Nausea, epigastric pain, and loss of appetite, which we have accepted as part of the reflux symptoms complex, can be caused by duodenogastric reflux that occurs independently or in association with gastroesophageal reflux. This reflux is often (although not always) seen in patients who have had previous upper gastrointestinal surgery. In those patients, the correction of only the incompetent cardia will result in a disgruntled individual who continues to complain of nausea and epigastric pain on eating. Twenty-four-hour pH monitoring of the stomach in these patients can be used as a method of demonstrating duodenogastric reflux. To further substantiate the diagnosis, a Tc-HIDA scan can be performed to demonstrate reflux of bile from the duodenum into the stomach. Sucralfate may relieve the symptoms. If operation is indicated to control gastroesophageal reflux and if severe bile reflux is pres-

ent, concomitant bile diversion procedure should be considered.[10,11]

4. Gastric hypersecretion and associated gastric or duodenal ulcer disease should be identified. Approximately 30% of patients with proven gastroesophageal reflux on 24-hour pH monitoring have hypersecretion on gastric analysis, and in 2% to 3% of patients who have had an antireflux operation, a gastric or duodenal ulcer will develop. As a result of these factors, the proposed antireflux procedure may be modified by the addition of a gastric resection or a highly selective proximal vagotomy.[12]

5. Patients with dysphagia and chest pain should be evaluated for a hiatal hernia. In some patients, hernia-related symptoms account for the failure of nonoperative therapy.[13]

6. Although delayed gastric emptying is not a major pathophysiological factor in gastroesophageal reflux disease, it can contribute to postoperative symptoms after antireflux repair—and to a patient's disgruntlement.[14]

7. A stricture that may result from reflux or drug ingestion (or from a combination of these factors) should be identified. A stricture also indicates a loss of esophageal contraction and may affect the choice of repair.[15,16]

8. The cause of chest pain in one out of two patients is gastroesophageal reflux disease.[17]

9. An occult adenocarcinoma should be excluded before surgery is performed in patients with Barrett's esophagus.[18]

REFERENCES

1. DeMeester TR, Stein HJ. Gastroesophageal reflux disease. In Moody FG, Carey LC, Jones RS, et al., eds. Surgical Treatment of Digestive Disease, 2nd ed. Chicago: Year Book, 1989, pp 65-108.

2. DeMeester TR, Wang CI, Wernly JA, et al. Technique, indications and clinical use of 24-hour esophageal pH monitoring. J Thorac Cardiovasc Surg 79:656-667, 1980.

3. DeMeester TR, Johnson LF, Guy JJ, et al. Patterns of gastroesophageal reflux in health and disease. Ann Surg 184:459-470, 1976.

4. Zaninotto G, DeMeester TR, Schwizer W, et al. The lower esophageal sphincter in health and disease. Am J Surg 155:104-111, 1988.

5. Stein HJ, DeMeester TR, Naspetti R, et al. Three-dimensional imaging of the lower esophageal sphincter in gastroesophageal reflux disease. Ann Surg 214:374-384, 1991.

6. Stein HJ, Bremner RM, Jamieson J, et al. Effect of Nissen fundoplication on esophageal motor function. Arch Surg 8:20, 1990.

7. Richardson JD, Larson GM, Polk HC. Intrathoracic fundoplication for shortened esophagus: Treacherous solution to a challenging problem. Am J Surg 143:29-35, 1982.

8. DeMeester TR, Bonavina L, Albertucci M. Nissen fundoplication for gastroesophageal reflux disease: Evaluation of primary repair in 100 consecutive patients. Ann Surg 204:9-20, 1986.

9. Pearson FG, Cooper JD, Patterson GH, et al. Gastroplasty and fundoplication for complex reflux problems: Long-term results. Ann Surg 206:473-481, 1982.

10. DeMeester TR, Fuchs KH, Ball CS, et al. Experimental and clinical results with proximal end-to-end duodenojejunostomy for pathologic duodenogastric reflux. Ann Surg 206:414-426, 1987.

11. Fuchs KH, DeMeester TR, Hinder RA, et al. Computerized identification of pathologic duodenogastric reflux using 24-hour gastric pH monitoring. Ann Surg 213:13-20, 1991.

12. Barlow AP, DeMeester TR, Ball CS, et al. The significance of the gastric secretory state in gastroesophageal reflux disease. Arch Surg 124:937-940, 1989.

13. Kaul BK, DeMeester TR, Oka M, et al. The cause of dysphagia in uncomplicated sliding hiatal hernia and its relief by hiatal herniorrhaphy: A roentgenographic, manometric, and clinical study. Ann Surg 211:406-410, 1990.

14. Hinder RA, Stein HJ, Bremner CG, et al. Relationship of a satisfactory outcome to normalization of delayed gastric emptying after Nissen fundoplication. Ann Surg 210:458-465, 1989.

15. Bonavina L, DeMeester TR, McChesney L, et al. Drug-induced esophageal strictures. Ann Surg 206:173-183, 1987.

16. Zaninotto G, DeMeester TR, Bremner CG, et al. Esophageal function in patients with reflux-induced strictures and its relevance to surgical treatment. Ann Thorac Surg 47:362-370, 1989.

17. DeMeester TR, O'Sullivan GC, Bermudez G, et al. Esophageal function in patients with angina type chest pain and normal coronary angiograms. Ann Surg 196:488-498, 1982.

18. DeMeester TR, Attwood SEA, Smyrk TC, et al. Surgical therapy in Barrett's esophagus. Ann Surg 212:528-542, 1990.

103 *Laparoscopic Antireflux Procedures*

Karl-Hermann Fuchs, Johannes Heimbucher, Stephan M. Freys, and Arnulf Thiede

PATHOPHYSIOLOGICAL ASPECTS

Gastroesophageal reflux is one of the most common functional abnormalities of the GE junction in Western countries. Years ago symptoms of gastroesophageal reflux were associated with hiatal hernia.[1] This led to the conclusion that the hernia itself must be the cause of the symptoms. It seemed reasonable to attempt to correct these symptoms by surgically reducing the hernia with simple closure of the hiatal crura.[2] The result of these first surgical efforts was uniform failure.[3] At the time, however, the reason for these failures was not evident. There is a definite association between reflux disease and the presence of hiatal hernia. However, this relationship is still not fully understood.[4] It has been shown that simple correction of hiatal hernia to a normal anatomical state improves gastroesophageal reflux in only a few patients.

A number of operations were designed to restore normal anatomy, such as the Hill operation, the Allison repair, and the Lortat-Jacob procedure.[2,5-7] The design of these gastropexy operations put the stomach and esophagus under continuous tension as a result of normal respiratory and swallowing movements. Consequently there was a high incidence of dislodgments, which resulted in loss of the intra-abdominal position of the cardia and the return of reflux symptoms. The most popular of these operations, the Hill procedure, anchors the gastroesophageal junction posteriorly to the median arcuate ligament. With the exception of the Hill procedure, these early operations did not withstand the test of time and were gradually abandoned.

As a result of studies of gastrointestinal function, it became evident that the lower esophageal high-pressure zone is a major factor in this disease.[8,9] It is now known that the most common cause of gastroesophageal reflux is mechanical and functional failure of the lower esophageal sphincter. It has also been shown that other factors can be involved, such as insufficient esophageal clearance function and gastric abnormalities. The basic pathophysiological abnormality of gastroesophageal reflux disease is excessive exposure of the esophagus to gastric juice, resulting in damage to the mucosa.

Currently three main causes are known, which can occur singly or in combination.[4] They are (1) a mechanically defective lower esophageal sphincter, (2) inefficient esophageal pump function, and (3) abnormalities of the gastric reservoir, such as increased gastric pressure, excessive gastric dilation, delayed gastric emptying, and/or increased gastric acid secretion.

PREOPERATIVE FUNCTION TESTING

Mechanical failure of the antireflux barrier is diagnosed by measuring inadequate mechanical characteristics of the lower esophageal sphincter by manometry. This criterion was defined as having any one or a combination of the following: an average lower esophageal sphincter pressure of less than 6 mm Hg, an average lower esophageal sphincter length exposed to the positive pressure environment of the abdomen of 1 cm or less, and an average lower esophageal sphincter overall resting length of 2 cm or less.[9] The most common cause of a mechanically incompetent cardia is inadequate lower esophageal sphincter pressure, but the efficacy of a normal lower esophageal sphincter pressure can be nullified by an inadequate intra-abdominal length or an abnormally short overall resting length of the lower esophageal sphincter.

Increased esophageal exposure to gastric juice can also be caused by a failure of the propulsive pumplike function of the body of the esophagus, resulting in inefficient esophageal clearance of refluxed gastric juice.[10,11] This can be due to damage of the esophageal wall by noxae such as excessive reflux, a myogenic abnormality, a motility disorder, or a reduction in salivary flow.

Increased esophageal exposure to gastric juice, secondary to a gastric disorder, has not been recognized as a cause of the disease for a long time. Clinical studies have indicated that up to 30% of patients with gastroesophageal reflux have a disturbance of upper gastrointestinal motility that is manifested by delayed gastric emptying.[12] This results in gastric retention and an increased probability of reflux through a normal sphincter. Gastric distention can result in shortening of the length of a normal sphincter, similar to the shortening of the neck of a balloon on inflation. With excessive distention the sphincter is shortened, resulting in low resistance to prevent reflux. There is evidence that increased gastric acid secretion can lead to increased esophageal acid exposure.[13,14] This is most likely caused by augmentation of physiological reflux by increased gastric volume and the high acidity of that volume.

INDICATIONS FOR OPERATIVE THERAPY

Antireflux surgery is symptom driven, and the indication for surgery is the presence of uncontrolled symptoms of heartburn or regurgitation. Since operation is a mechanical therapeutic approach to gastroesophageal reflux disease, patients with a mechanically incompetent cardia will benefit the most from it. Consequently an antireflux procedure should be considered only for those patients who have (1) uncontrolled symptoms of increased esophageal acid exposure as a result of increased reflux of gastric juice, that is, heartburn, regurgitation, chest pain, chronic cough, wheezing, or dysphagia; (2) an increase in esophageal exposure to gastric juice as documented by 24-hour esophageal pH monitoring; and (3) a documented mechanical defect of the lower esophageal sphincter.[4]

However, these clear indications are not fully accepted by gastroenterologists. At present, potent medication is available to reduce gastric acid secretion, which allows for successful reduction of reflux symptoms, as well as pathological acid exposure of the esophageal mucosa, as long as the medication is taken by the patient. But long-term use of these drugs can cause side effects, and patient compliance can be a problem. Many gastroenterologists no longer discuss with their patients the possibility of surgical treatment. With the advent of minimally invasive surgery, surgeons have an opportunity to deserve renewed confidence from their gastroenterology associates and their patients.[15]

Because of the high prevalence of gastroesophageal reflux in Western populations, optimal treatment of this disease is very important. Most patients with reflux, especially those with borderline incompetence of the lower esophageal sphincter, will be treated with a high rate of success by nonoperative antisecretory therapy with H_2 blockers, antacids, or omeprazol. In these patients the existing usually minor esophagitis will be reduced quickly, and they will be free of symptoms within a few weeks. However, in many patients compliance can be problematic. In young patients an unwillingness to undergo long-term medical treatment—in many cases lifelong—still leads to requests for surgery to achieve permanent resolution of this disease. On the other hand, it must be emphasized that in a large group of patients with a defective antireflux mechanism, treated unsuccessfully with medical therapy over a long period of time, complications such as ulcers, bleeding, strictures, and even cancer will develop.

Therefore there is a need for definitive surgical treatment of the functional defect. The procedure must be safe, with minimum morbidity. It is obvious that the new laparoscopic techniques should be applied under these conditions. Looking at the design of 180-degree hemifundoplication, it is evident that this operation can be done laparoscopically with very limited risk in a reasonable amount of time.

Before a surgical antireflux repair, two important factors must be considered.[16] First, the patient should be questioned regarding complaints of epigastric pain, nausea, vomiting, and loss of appetite. These symptoms can be caused by bile reflux gastritis, which occurs independent of or in association with gastroesophageal reflux. The problem is usually seen in patients who have had previous upper gastrointestinal surgery, although this is not always the case. The correction of only the incompetent cardia in such patients will result in patient dissatisfaction and continued complaints of nausea and epigastric pain made worse by eating. Gastric function tests such as 24-hour gastric pH monitoring and gastric emptying scintigraphy will reveal underlying gastric causes of reflux. Second, the propulsive force of the body of the esophagus should be measured. There should be sufficient force to propel a bolus of food through the newly constructed valve. This is determined by stationary and 24-hour ambulatory esophageal manometry or a radioisotope esophageal transit time study.[17] Failure to recognize inadequate esophageal contractility can lead to postoperative dysphagia.

AVAILABLE ANTIREFLUX PROCEDURES

Currently Nissen fundoplication, the Belsey Mark IV operation, Toupet posterior hemifundoplication, Watson anterior fundoplication, Hill posterior gastropexy, and the Angelchik prosthesis are reported to be the most widely used antireflux procedures.[18-24]

The Belsey Mark IV procedure is, in essence, a partial fundoplication or a 240-degree gastric wrap around the distal esophagus, whereas the Nissen technique is a complete fundoplication, or a 360-degree gastric wrap.[18,20] Of the two operations, the Nissen procedure has become the most popular, and variations of the operation are now used by the majority of surgeons worldwide for treatment of reflux.[19] Hill[7] has added a degree of fundoplication to his operation, which improves the results of the procedure to nearly the same extent as the Nissen technique. Angelchik and Cohen[23] have designed a silicone prosthetic collar that can be easily placed around the abdominal esophagus as an antireflux device. Despite controversy regarding complications with the Angelchik prosthesis, there have been increasing reports of its safety and efficacy in the control of reflux.

Aware of the complications and troublesome side effects of the full-wrap Nissen fundoplication technique, investigators have searched for better alternatives.[22,24,25] The hemifundoplication procedures of Watson et al.[24] and Toupet[22] involve a 180-degree wrap with a less-obstructing effect on the distal esophagus, causing less gas bloating and persistent dysphagia. Critics comment that there is a higher risk of reflux recurrence because of the limited sphincter augmentation and a possible higher risk of wrap breakdown.

The primary goal of all antireflux operations is to mechanically augment the high-pressure zone in the distal esophagus to improve the resistance of the lower esophageal sphincter. However, extensive augmentation has side effects. Simple gastropexy or fundopexy has not been successful in open operations to sufficiently correct pathological gastroesophageal reflux. On the basis of the pathophysiological background of gastroesophageal reflux disease, it is known that partial and especially 360-degree fundoplication techniques can control pathological gastroesophageal reflux completely, since their effect on augmentation of the distal esophageal high-pressure zone is greatest. Troublesome symptoms resulting from mechanical problems with total 360-degree fundoplication, such as gas-bloat phenomenon or persistent postoperative dysphagia, have been reported and are the main reasons that most gastroenterologists object to this type of operation.[3,4,19] However, in the past few years surgeons have, with increasing understanding of the pathophysiology, attempted to limit the size of the fundoplication and successfully reduce postoperative persistent dysphagia.[19]

LAPAROSCOPIC TECHNIQUES

Undoubtedly the 360-degree Nissen fundoplication is the most popular antireflux operation among surgeons. However, the original version has been greatly modified. We believe full 360-degree Nissen fundoplication is indicated for patients with clear incompetence of the lower esophageal sphincter, with severe symptoms, and/or with severe reflux esophagitis refractory to nonoperative treatment. We perform the laparoscopic Nissen procedure in the same way we perform the open 360-degree wrap in laparotomy, according to the DeMeester-Nissen sandwich technique. In patients with concomitant esophageal pump failure, we prefer hemifundoplication. In addition, as an alternative to long-term treatment for reduction of gastric acid secretion with H_2 blocker or omeprazol therapy, especially in patients with borderline incompetence of the lower esophageal sphincter, we recognize the usefulness of 180-degree partial fundoplication or hemifundoplication.

The technique involves the usual instruments used for laparoscopic surgery. The procedure can be facilitated by a number of special instruments, such as curved dissection forceps for work behind the esophagus and special grasping forceps for the stomach, but it also can be done with regular instruments. It must be emphasized that a laparoscopic Babcock clamp is best suited for holding the distal esophagus and stomach to optimally dissect the target area. After a proper pneumoperitoneum is established, a 10 mm trocar is inserted into the abdominal cavity through a supraumbilical incision, and a 30-degree 10 mm laparoscope is inserted. In addition, 10 mm trocars, preferably with automatic valves, are brought into the right and left subcostal areas. Via the trocar in the right upper quadrant, the left lobe of the liver is retracted to allow dissection of the hiatus. The left lateral trocar is used to pull the stomach and especially the gastroesophageal junction caudally to achieve good exposure of that area. Then via another two trocars for the passage of scissors and grasping forceps the gastroesophageal junction and especially if present the hiatal hernia is dissected. The preparation begins to the left from the angle of His cranially to the right. Care is taken not to damage the branches of the vagal nerve. The dissection of the lower esophageal sphincter and the pillars of the hiatal crus are brought over to the right. These structures must be clearly identified. The proximal fundus is also mobilized toward the spleen, but without extensive dissection of the small gastric vessels along the spleen. Then it must be possible for the fundic flap (hemifundoplication) to be pulled with ease across the lower esophageal sphincter toward the right crus of the hiatus. If that cannot be accomplished easily, mobilization of the fundus must be expanded, but usually this is not necessary. The posterior area of the esophagus is then dissected by pulling the gastroesophageal junction up with a Babcock clamp placed through the middle trocar using the left lateral trocar for dissection of the hiatal crus. If necessary, and in most cases it is, posterior hiatal approximation and suturing are performed with two U-stitches by an extracorporeal technique (Fig. 1). Then the fundic flap is fixed with two or three nonresorbable endosutures at the middle portion of the lower esophageal sphincter. The right lateral portion of the flap is fixed on the right crus with another two or three sutures. Again these sutures are closed with an extracorporeal tying technique. The antireflux 180-degree anterior hemifundoplication procedure is then complete (Fig. 2).

In case of a defective lower esophageal sphincter, mobilization of the fundus is carried out farther down for a complete Nissen wrap, dissecting the short gastric vessels between clips. When the fundus is completely mobilized, a floppy wrap is possible. If necessary a closure of the hiatus posterior to the abdominal esophagus is also performed. Then the posterior portion of the fundus is brought around the posterior wall of the esophagus with a Babcock clamp and taken over at the level of the right crus with another Babcock (Fig. 3). Then 360-degree fundoplication is completed by tying one U-stitch with a nonresorbable-0 suture in a sandwich technique over two stents (Fig. 4). This also involves the anterior right lateral wall of the lower esophageal sphincter. To make the wrap as loose as possible, a 45 Fr bougie is placed into the cardia through the mouth and esophagus during that suturing procedure.

DISCUSSION

Early functional results show an improvement in lower esophageal sphincter pressure with less effect on sphincter length. Symptomatic improvement of the patients has been compared with that achieved with laparotomy. The recovery time during the initial postoperative period after the laparoscopic procedure has been shortened, as has been shown for other laparoscopic operations,[26] so patients can be discharged sooner. However, long-term results must be studied objectively before deciding whether the laparoscopic techniques, especially 180-degree hemifundoplication, have a better long-term outcome than long-term drug treatment. Until then, laparoscopic antireflux procedures should be performed in centers under controlled conditions to gather as much objective data as possible.

Widespread application of laparoscopic techniques in antireflux surgery, especially without objective as-

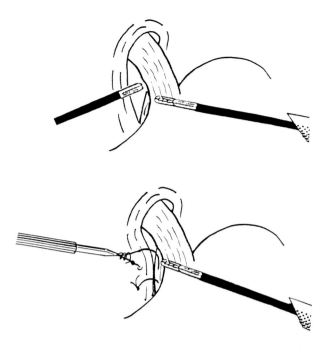

Fig. 1. Approximation of pillars of hiatal crus and posterior hiatoplasty with two endosutures.

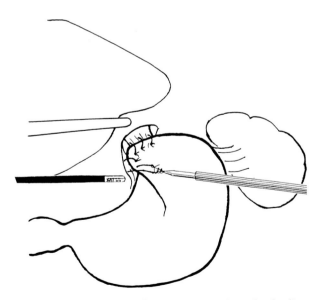

Fig. 2. Diagram of 180-degree anterior hemifundoplication with fixation of fundic flap to lower esophageal sphincter and right crus.

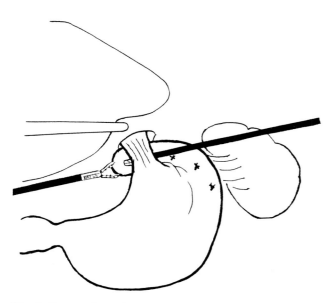

Fig. 3. Preparation of gastroesophageal junction for 360-degree Nissen fundoplication.

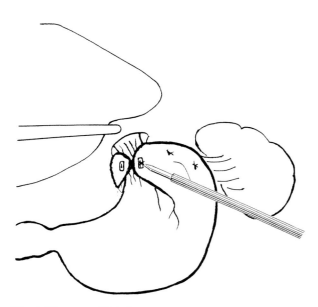

Fig. 4. Diagram of 360-degree wrap according to DeMeester-Nissen fundoplication sandwich technique.

sessment of the functional defects of those patients with no clear indications, can result in a poor postoperative outcome. This can have disastrous consequences, since it generates a negative opinion of laparoscopic techniques. The latter, however, can only be prevented if these operations are performed after extensive training and with the proper indications. Patients must not be compromised in order to perform minimally invasive techniques.

REFERENCES

1. Jamieson GG, Duranceau AC. In Jamieson GG, ed. The Development of Surgery for Gastroesophageal Reflux Disease in Surgery of the Oesophagus. London: Churchill-Livingstone, 1988, pp 233-245.
2. Allison PR. Reflux esophagitis, sliding hiatus hernia and the anatomy of repair. Surg Gynecol Obstet 92:419-431, 1951.
3. Richter JE, Castell DO. Gastroesophageal reflux: Pathogenesis, diagnosis and therapy. Ann Intern Med 97:93-103, 1982.
4. DeMeester TR. Gastroesophageal reflux disease. In Moody FG, Carey LC, Jones RS, et al., eds. Surgical Treatment of Digestive Disease. Chicago: Year Book Medical Publishers, 1985, pp 132-158.
5. Lortat-Jacob JL. Le traitement chirurgical des maladies du reflux gastro-oesophagien: Malpositions cardiotubérositaires, hernies hiatales, brachyoesophages. Presse Med 65:455-456, 1957.
6. Hill LD, Tobias JA. An effective operation for hiatal hernia: An eight year appraisal. Ann Surg 166:681-692, 1967.
7. Hill LD. Intraoperative measurement of lower esophageal sphincter pressure. J Thorac Cardiovasc Surg 75:378-382, 1978.
8. Bonavina L, Evander A, DeMeester TR, et al. Length of the distal esophageal sphincter and competency of the cardia. Am J Surg 151:25-34, 1986.
9. Zaninotto G, DeMeester RR, Schwizer W, et al. The lower esophageal sphincter in health and disease. Am J Surg 155:104-111, 1988.
10. Joelsson BE, DeMeester RR, Skinner DB, et al. The role of the esophageal body in the antireflux mechanism. Surgery 92:417-424, 1982.
11. Kahrilas PJ, Dodds WJ, Hogan WG, et al. Esophageal peristaltic dysfunction in peptic esophagitis. Gastroenterology 91:897, 1986.
12. Schwizer W, Hinder RA, DeMeester TR. Does delayed gastric emptying contribute to gastroesophageal reflux disease? Am J Surg 157:74-81, 1989.
13. Boesby S. Relationship between gastroesophageal acid reflux, basal gastroesophageal sphincter pressure and gastric acid secretion. Scand J Gastroenterol 12:547-551, 1977.

14. Barlow AP, DeMeester TR, Boll CS, et al. The significance of the gastric secretory state in gastroesophageal reflux disease. Arch Surg 124:937-940, 1989.

15. Cuschieri A. Endoskopische Mikrochirurgie. Chirurgie 62:248-252, 1991.

16. Fuchs KH. Die chirurgische Therapie der gastroösophagealen Refluxkrankheit. In Fuchs KH, Hamelmann H, eds. Gastrointestinale Funktionsdiagnostik in der Chirurgie. Berlin: Blackwell, 1991, pp S 86-98.

17. Stein HJ, DeMeester TR, Naspetti R, et al. Three-dimensional imaging of the lower esophageal sphincter in gastroesophageal reflux disease. Ann Surg 209:374-384, 1991.

18. Nissen R. Gastropexy and fundoplication in surgical treatment of hiatal hernia. Am J Dig Dis 6:954-961, 1961.

19. DeMeester TR, Bonavina L, Albertucci M. Nissen fundoplication for gastroesophageal reflux disease. Evaluation of primary repair in 100 consecutive patients. Ann Surg 204:19, 1986.

20. Skinner DB, Belsey RHR. Surgical management of esophageal reflux with hiatus hernia: Long-term results with 1,030 cases. J Thorac Cardiovasc Surg 53:33-54, 1967.

21. DeMeester TR, Fuchs KH. Comparison of operations for uncomplicated reflux disease. In Jamieson GG, ed. Surgery of the Oesophagus. London: Churchill-Livingstone, 1988, pp 299-308.

22. Toupet A. Technique d'oesophago-gastroplastie avec phrénogastropexie appliquée dans la cure radicale des hernies hiatales et comme complément de l'opération d'Heller dans les cardiospasmes. Mem Acad Chir 89:394, 1963.

23. Angelchik JP, Cohen R. A new surgical procedure for the treatment of gastroesophageal reflux and hiatal hernia. Surg Gynecol Obstet 148:246-248, 1979.

24. Watson A, Jenkinson LR, Ball CS, et al. A more physiological alternative to total fundoplication for the surgical correction of resistant gastro-oesophageal reflux. Br J Surg 78:1088-1094, 1991.

25. Fuchs KH, Freys SM, Thiede A. Laparoskopische Antirefluxoperation an der Cardia. In Fuchs KH, Hamelmann H, Manegold BC, eds. Chirurgische Endoskopie im Abdomen. Berlin: Blackwell, 1992, pp 415-420.

26. Fuchs KH, Freys SM, Heimbucher J, et al. Laparoskopische Cholecystektomie—Lohnt sich die laparoskopische Technik in "schwierigen" Fällen? Chirurgie 63:296-304, 1992.

104 *Laparoscopic Nissen Fundoplication*

Alberto Del Genio, Vincenzo Landolfi, Andreina Martella, Natale Di Martino, Antonio Nuzzo, and Giuseppe Angiluetta

Laparoscopic surgery, which has become the main procedure for many gastrointestinal diseases, is gradually becoming the preferred approach to the correction of functional esophageal disorders, which until recently were treated exclusively by means of an open operation. In our department in the last 15 months, we have used a "calibrated Nissen" procedure performed through a laparoscopic approach. The surgical steps are identical to those followed for open operation.

MATERIALS AND METHODS

After obtaining informed consent, we performed calibrated Nissen fundoplication by laparoscopy on 25 patients (18 female, 7 male). Of these, 13 had symptomatic second-degree esophagitis, and 24-hour pH monitoring revealed supine or bipositional gastroesophageal reflux. After 6 months of well-conducted nonoperative therapy, these patients had not experienced any clinical improvement of the reflux disease. Twelve patients showed achalasia and therefore underwent Heller cardiomyotomy and Nissen fundoplication.

The patient is placed in the lithotomy position, and anesthesia is administered through endotracheal intubation. A gastroscope is positioned so that the stomach can be decompressed and, by means of transillumination, the esophagogastric junction can immediately be visualized. The surgeon stands between the patient's legs; the first assistant stands on the surgeon's right and the second assistant to the left of the surgeon.

A 15 mm Hg pneumoperitoneum is obtained and a 10 mm trocar is positioned in the midline halfway between the xiphoid appendix and the umbilicus. The laparoscope is introduced through the trocar, and the abdominal cavity is examined to rule out the presence of other conditions. We use a stationary device, but in the near future it will probably be replaced by instruments with a rotating end. The operating table is put in a 40-degree anti-Trendelenburg position, and four additional 10 mm trocars are placed with the aid of transillumination to avoid vascular injuries of the abdominal wall. One trocar is positioned into the left hypochondrium and another one into the right 3 cm from the costal margin; the third one is placed in the midline just below the xiphoid appendix and the fourth is placed in the left upper quadrant at the joining point between a transverse line from the umbilicus and the anterior axillary line. The use of the 10 mm trocars is necessary because we use instruments of different diameters and must change the visual angle during the different stages of the operation, which we model, as much as possible, on the stages of the classic open procedure.

After lifting the left hepatic lobe with a retractor inserted through the right trocar, we can easily identify the esophageal hiatus, thanks to the endoscope that previously was positioned. The stomach is pulled down with a Babcock forceps, and the peritoneal reflection plica is sectioned with a hook or scissors. Once the anterior wall of the esophagus is exposed, the right diaphragmatic crus, which is shifted away from the right lateral esophageal wall, can be identified. With the esophagus free from the left diagphragmatic crus, the posterior esophageal wall is prepared and attention paid to identifying the right vagus nerve and the left pleura.

When gastroesophageal reflux is associated with hiatal hernia, the stomach is reduced into the abdomen, and a posterior hiatal repair with one or two stitches is performed.

Once the esophagus has been completely mobilized, a Babcock clamp is passed behind it from right to left while another clamp picks up the anterior wall of the gastric fundus and moves it into the jaws of the posterior forceps. The latter grasps the gastric fundus, rotating it for 360 degrees around the esophagus. After verifying that there is no excessive traction, the surgeon performs the plication using a monofilament suture, which must not pierce the esophageal wall. The operation is concluded with a manometric control measurement to verify the calibration of the plication. The peritoneal cavity is irrigated with antibiotic solution, the trocars are removed under direct vision to verify the absence of bleeding, and the CO_2 is released. The skin is sutured with disposable clips.

In patients with achalasia after the preparation of the esophagus, the anterior longitudinal and circular muscular fibers are sectioned. The myotomy is prolonged downward on the stomach to include Helvethius fibers. For this procedure, intraoperative endoscopy is useful, since it allows identification of all muscular fibers and verification of mucosal integrity. Intraoperative manometry ensures total sphincteric pressure annulment so that a Nissen fundoplication can be performed.

RESULTS

Only in two cases were we compelled to convert to an open procedure, one because of pleural perforation (a patient with severe adhesions from previous surgical procedure) and another for esophageal perforation during the Heller myotomy. An intraoperative complication that did not require conversion to an open procedure was a microperforation during a Heller procedure. It was treated with a mucosal suture.

Operating time varied from 45 minutes to 4 hours. Postoperative pain was moderate, and there was no need to administer drugs. Patients were able to walk by the end of the operative day when intravenous liquids were discontinued. Oral feeding was allowed on the third postoperative day. We have noticed a reduction in recovery time and an early return to normal activities with this procedure.

All patients reported the disappearance of reflux-related symptoms, and patients with achalasia noted the absence of dysphagia. The use of intraoperative manometry in the cases that we have just described documented a satisfactory calibration of the antireflux procedure, which therefore has never been modified.

DISCUSSION

Abnormal acid gastroesophageal reflux can be treated with several different surgical procedures, even if the most effective one for the cure or prevention of reflux is the Nissen fundoplication. Several modifications have been applied to the original procedure. Among the most significant are those of Nissen's disciple Rossetti, who suggests the following: not to treat the esophageal hiatus, not to section the vasa brevia, not to open the gastrohepatic ligament, to use only the anterior wall of the gastric fundus for plication, not to include the esophageal wall in the suture, and to suture the inferior margin of the plication to the lesser curvature.

The impression—which many surgeons share—that the Nissen procedure causes obstruction to esophagogastric transit has prompted several others to suggest a "floppy Nissen." Our experience with the traditional operation favors a Nissen fundoplication using only the anterior wall of the gastric fundus (Nissen-Rossetti). We do not usually mobilize either the gastric fundus or the lesser curvature. The fundoplication is calibrated to the desired values by routine use of intraoperative manometry, a method we have advocated and followed since 1972. On the basis of intraoperative manometric pressure values, we define *normocalibrated Nissen* as the procedure with pressure values between 10 and 20 mm Hg and *hypercalibrated Nissen* as the one with pressure values between 21 and 40 mm Hg. Having documented a certain percentage (28.6%) of reflux relapse after the normocalibrated Nissen procedure, we now perform only hypercalibrated procedures. The hypercalibration can always avoid reflux, although the incidence of dysphagia was 4.2%; however, this dysphagia disappeared within 6 to 12 months.

Guided by intraoperative manometry during a traditional approach, we have performed 166 hypercalibrated Nissen fundoplications: 80 after Heller myotomy; 64 for reflux esophagitis; 17 in patients with diverticulum (10 after cardiomyotomy and seven for associated gastroesophageal reflux); one in a patient with diffuse esophageal spasm after a Heller myotomy; and four reoperations (one was our only case of reflux relapse caused by a disrupted Nissen fundoplication and three had been operated on elsewhere for achalasia).

On the basis of this long experience in traditional surgery, we decided to follow the laparoscopic route, not to compare two different techniques that are basically similar but to prove that after adequate experience it is possible to obtain through laparoscopy the same effectiveness and the same results as with the traditional technique but with additional advantages comparable to those of laparoscopic cholecystectomy. Even if our experience is brief, the preliminary results prove that these patients do not complain of postoperative pain. They show better respiratory activity; they are dismissed on the third postoperative day; and after 7 days they can do any type of normal physical activity. They had better cosmetic results and none of the complications associated with laparotomy. As for manometry, its results are not influenced in a statistically significant manner by the presence of pneumoperitoneum, as we observed in a series of patients who had laparoscopic cholecystectomy. In these patients preoperative and postoperative manometric values did not show significant variations. In the cases in this study the manometric parameters were always satisfactory, and it was never necessary to modify the fundoplication.

CONCLUSION

Laparoscopic surgery has in the last few years become a routine approach, particularly in the gastroenteric field, even for operations that had always been performed in the traditional way. Based on an extensive "traditional" experience, we started 1 year ago to perform laparoscopic Nissen fundoplication to cure or prevent gastroesophageal reflux. Twenty-five patients (13 for the cure of gastroesophageal reflux and 12 for the prevention of reflux after Heller myotomy) underwent laparoscopic operations. The surgical technique, which is similar to the traditional one, has been described and the advantages and validity of the laparoscopic approach emphasized.

REFERENCES

1. Del Genio A. L'elettromanometria esofagea intraoperatoria. Atti Soc Ital Chir 6:252-266, 1990.
2. Landolfi V, Di Martino N, Izzo G, et al. Nissen ed Heller calibrate per via laparoscopica. Atti Congr Naz S:IP:I:G:C: Ischia, 1992.
3. Dallemagne B, Weerts JM, Jehaes C, et al. Laparoscopic Nissen fundoplication: Preliminary report. Surg Laparosc Endosc 3:138-143, 1991.
4. Del Genio A, Landolfi V, Martella A, et al. La fundoplicatio sec. Nissen per via laparoscopica nel paziente anziano. Atti VI Congr Naz Soc It Chir Ger Napoli, Sept. 23-26, 1992.
5. Zucker KA. Laparoscopic Surgery. St. Louis: Quality Medical Publishing, 1991.
6. Cuschieri A, Buess G, Perissat J. Operative Manual of Endoscopic Surgery. New York: Springer-Verlag, 1992.

105 *Laparoscopic Management of Gastroesophageal Reflux Disease*

Mario Morino, Maurizio De Giuli, Valentino Festa, Corrado Garrone, and Claudio Miglietta

Minimally invasive surgery has rapidly developed as a feasible and safe method of managing a number of different functional diseases of the upper gastrointestinal tract.

In particular, a posterior truncal vagotomy with lesser curvature anterior gastric myotomy by videocoelioscopy has been performed by Katkhouda for the treatment of chronic duodenal ulcer.[1] Dubois has described a technique of bilateral truncal vagotomy by videothoracoscopy for the same disease.[2]

Cuschieri reported a technique of laparoscopic cardiopexy for the cure of gastroesophageal reflux disease. Furthermore, Nouaille has described an antireflux procedure laparoscopically performed by realizing an anterior hemifundoplication,[3,4] while Dallemagne reported 12 cases of symptomatic reflux disease treated by laparoscopic Nissen fundoplication.[5]

In our institute a laparoscopic Nissen-Rossetti fundoplication has been performed in 11 patients with gastroesophageal reflux disease.

We present a consecutive series of eight patients with a postoperative follow-up of 3 months.

MATERIALS AND METHODS

Between December 1991 and December 1992, eight Nissen-Rossetti fundoplication procedures were performed laparoscopically in our department.

Indications for surgery were established on the basis of symptoms, endoscopy, and 24-hour pH-manometric evaluation, demonstrating an abnormal pattern of esophageal acid exposure in all patients (Table 1). None of the patients evidenced esophageal stricture on endoscopy or an esophageal motility disorder on manometry.

Table 1. Presenting symptoms in eight patients with gastroesophageal reflux disease requiring operation*

Symptom	No. of Patients
Persistent heartburn	8/8
Dysphagia	3/8
Grade 1 esophagitis	1/8
Grade 2 esophagitis	6/8
Grade 3 esophagitis	1/8
Hiatal hernia	3/8
Reflux on barium enema	5/8
Positive 24-hour pH monitoring test results	8/8

*Mortality, 0; morbidity, 0.

Table 2. Side effects of the operation

Side Effect	No. of Patients
Inability to belch	2/8
Inability to vomit	0/8
Temporary swallowing discomfort	3/8
Symptomatic gas bloat	0/8
Persistent dysphagia	0/8

TECHNIQUE

As is done for laparoscopic cholecystectomy, patients are placed in the supine position with their legs in low stirrups. The pneumoperitoneum is established with a Veress needle inserted just beside the umbilicus.

Five trocars are placed into the upper abdominal cavity to allow the insertion of a 10 mm video camera and the operative instruments (Fig. 1).

The surgeon stands between the patient's legs, with the two assistants on each side. The procedure exactly reproduces the well-tested laparotomy operation.

The left liver ligament is not divided. The operation is begun by dividing the reflection of the parietal peritoneum from the diaphragm onto the esophagus (phrenoesophageal ligament). The distal esophagus is then dissected free from its vascular and fibrous connections within the posterior mediastinum. Particular care must be taken to avoid any injuries to vagal nerves. The dissection is carried on until both right and left diaphragmatic crura are identified and exposed. The gastrophrenic ligament is then divided and the fundus of the stomach is mobilized, without dividing the short gastric vessels.

A soft string is passed around the esophagus to facilitate retraction.

The esophageal hiatus is closed with a nonabsorbable monofilament interrupted suture to approximate the left and the right limbs of the crura, behind the esophagus.

The anterior wall of the fundus is passed behind the esophagus in a 360-degree fundoplication (Fig. 2). A nonabsorbable monofilament interrupted suture is placed to secure the plication after a 60 Fr bougie is passed down the esophagus into the stomach to size the diameter of the gastric wrap. The height of the gastric wrap should not be more than 2 cm to reduce the risk of postoperative dysphagia.

Two gastrogastric sutures are placed from the gastric wrap fold to to maintain the plication in place.

A nasogastric tube is placed into the stomach and left in place for 24 to 48 hours. The patient is discharged on the third or fourth postoperative day when an x-ray evaluation has demonstrated adequate esophagogastric emptying.

RESULTS

There was no mortality or early postoperative morbidity in our series.

Patients were discharged between the third and fifth postoperative days. One patient experienced a postoperative transient dysphagia, which spontaneously regressed a month later (Table 2).

All patients returned to work within 15 to 20 days.

Postoperative clinical, endoscopic, and pH-manometric evaluation performed 3 months after the operation documented a complete recovery of the esophageal mucosa and a normal pattern of esophageal acid exposure with a normal distal sphincter activity. In particular, the first postoperative DeMeester score was less than 18 in every patient; the mean distal esophageal sphincter pressure was 24.1 ± 6 mm Hg, compared with a preoperative mean pressure of 9.4 ± 4.7 mm Hg.

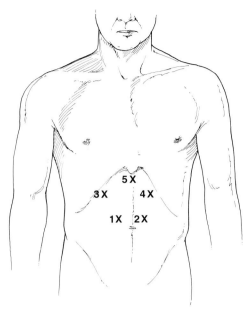

Fig. 1. Sites for trocar insertion. The instruments used through each trocar are (1) 10-11 mm trocar, 30-degree forward oblique laparoscope; (2) 10-11 mm trocar, scissors, hook, pledget swab, needle holder; (3) 5 mm trocar, atraumatic grasping forceps; (4) 5 mm trocar, atraumatic grasping forceps; and (5) 5 mm trocar, suction-aspiration cannula.

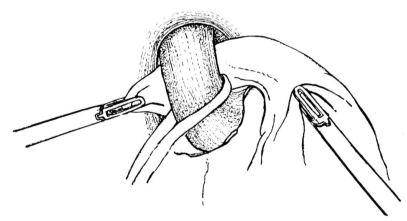

Fig. 2. The upper and anterior portion of the gastric fundus is grasped with an atraumatic forceps and passed through the window created behind the esophagus during the previous dissection of the intra-abdominal esophagus. This tongue of fundus in then grasped on the right side and the plication is completed anteriorly with one nonabsorbable suture placed from the plicated (right) edge of the anterior fundus to the (left) anterior fundic fold created by the plication maneuver. The suture is tied over a 60 Fr intraluminal esophageal bougie and Teflon pledgets (DeMeester's sandwich technique).

DISCUSSION

Following the success of laparoscopic cholecystectomy as the elective treatment of gallbladder stones, various minimally invasive procedures have been suggested for treating upper gastrointestinal disorders.

The feasibility and efficacy of the laparoscopic approach has been proved for the treatment of peptic ulcer, hiatal hernia, and gastroesophageal reflux disease. The procedures seem to maintain the same advantages as in celioscopic cholecystectomy: reduced operative trauma, shortened hospital stay, and early return to normal activities, as well as cosmetic advantages.

Our preliminary results confirm that the use of laparoscopic Nissen-Rossetti fundoplication for the treatment of gastroesophageal reflux disease can be feasible, safe, and efficient when performed by teams well experienced in minimally invasive surgery.

Three months' follow-up data seem to suggest that functional results will be superior to those obtained through traditional procedures.[6]

REFERENCES

1. Katkhouda N, Mouiel J. A New Technique of Surgical Treatment of Chronic Duodenal Ulcer Without Laparotomy by Videocoelioscopy. Am J Surg 161:361-364, 1991.
2. Dubois F. La chirurgie de l'ulcere duodenal non compliquè. In Testas P, Delaitre B. Chirurgie Digestive par voie Coelioscopique. Paris: Maloine, 1991.
3. Cuschieri A, Nathanson LK. Laparoscopic ligamentum teres cardiopexy for intractable gastrooesophageal reflux disease. Br J Surg (in press).
4. Nouaille JM. La chirurgie du hiatus oesophagien. In Testas P, Delaitre B. Chirurgie Digestive par voie Coelioscopique. Paris: Maloine, 1991.
5. Dallemagne B, Weerts JM, Jehees S. Laparoscopic Nissen fundoplication: Preliminary report. Surg Laparosc Endosc 1:138, 1991.
6. DeMeester TR, Bonavina L, Albertucci M. Nissen fundoplication for gastroesophageal reflux disease: Evaluation of primary repair in 100 consecutive patients. Ann Surg 204:10-20, 1986.

106 *A Prospective Randomized Study Comparing Teres Cardiopexy With Nissen Fundoplication as Surgical Therapy for Gastroesophageal Reflux Disease*

I.M.C. Janssen, D.J. Gouma, P. Klementschitsch,† M.N. van der Heyde, and H. Obertop

Most patients with gastroesophageal reflux disease can be treated successfully by lifestyle modification and medical therapy.[1] Maintenance therapy is essential, since relapse occurs as a rule after treatment is discontinued.[1,2] Since omeprazole is a very potent drug with an excellent success rate, some patients face lifelong omeprazole treatment.[3] On the other hand, antireflux surgery can restore distal esophageal sphincter competence, and after a successful procedure no further therapy is required.[4,5] Thirty-five years after its introduction, the Nissen fundoplication is still the gold standard for surgical treatment with which newer techniques should be compared. Results of the Nissen procedure vary with the authors' experience; postoperative sequelae include dysphagia and gas bloating, while even such complications as gastric fistula have been reported.[6,7] Other techniques are constantly being developed or modified, but none of them has proved superior.[2,8] Narbona has developed an antireflux procedure by using the ligamentum teres hepatis as a sling around the esophagus, anchoring the lower esophagus into the intra-abdominal position—the teres cardiopexy.[9-13] It is hypothesized that using this technique improves the gastroesophageal valve mechanism; remarkable results were reported in a retrospective study, with only 3% to 4% reflux recurrence rate.[12,13] The procedure was reported to be associated with minimal morbidity, with no long-term side effects such as dysphagia and gas bloat syndrome.

---

†Deceased.

The technique has never been validated by others or compared with other techniques. After a pilot study (30 patients), we found the teres cardiopexy a technically feasible procedure with minimal postoperative morbidity and promising short-term results. Therefore a prospective randomized clinical trial was initiated to assess the effect of teres cardiopexy (Narbona) as compared with fundoplication (Nissen) for the treatment of esophageal reflux disease in patients whose conditions were resistant to medical treatment. The trial was discontinued when interim analysis showed significantly more recurrence in the cardiopexy group after 1 year.

MATERIALS AND METHODS

Twenty patients (14 men, 6 women, with a mean age of 48 years [range, 24 to 64 years]) were referred for surgical treatment of gastroesophageal reflux disease that was resistant to medical therapy and entered the trial during the period February 1986 to February 1988. These patients all fulfilled the preoperative criteria (see below). They were randomized, and 10 patients underwent Narbona cardiopexy while the other 10 underwent Nissen fundoplication.

Patient Selection

All patients had persistent symptoms of esophageal reflux disease, even after intensive medical treatment for more than 6 months including at least 3 months' treatment with an H_2-receptor antagonist. No patients had previously undergone upper abdominal or esophageal surgery. Patients with ulcer disease and other gastric abnormalities were excluded after endoscopic examination. Patients with gallstone disease were also excluded, as were patients with abnormal esophageal motility diagnosed by manometry and abnormal gastric emptying diagnosed by radionuclide scintigraphy.

Preoperative and Postoperative Evaluation

Evaluation was carried out by a system of symptom scoring (at 0, 3, and 12 months), 24-hour pH recording (at 0 and 12 months), and endoscopic score of esophagitis (at 0 and 12 months).

Symptom score. The symptom score was calculated by adding the scores of these four symptoms: (A) retrosternal pain, (B) regurgitation, (C) dysphagia, and (D) heartburn (see box at right). The maximum score (A + B + C + D) was 13; the minimum score 0.

Endoscopy score. Through endoscopy of the esophagus the severity of esophagitis was scored using the following criteria: (0) no esophagitis, (1) erythema,

(2) linear erosions, maximum three, (3) more than three erosions, and (4) stricture. Endoscopy was performed by an independent endoscopist. However, at endoscopy the endoscopic aspects of cardiopexy and fundoplication were different and easily recognized.

Twenty-four-hour esophageal pH recording. A continuous 24-hour pH recording was performed with a glass electrode, connected in most patients to a portable recorder. The pH electrode was inserted through the nose, with the tip positioned 5 cm above the lower esophageal sphincter (LES). The LES was localized by manometry. The ambulatory 24-hour pH recording was performed without treatment and with no further restrictions on an outpatient basis. In view of the results of a recent study by Masclee et al.[14] who used the percentage of the total time with pH below 4 as the single determinant for gastroesophageal reflux, this criteri-

---

PREOPERATIVE AND POSTOPERATIVE EVALUATION CRITERIA

Symptom score = A + B + C + D (total score: 0-13)

A. Restrosternal pain	0	Absent
	1	Once a day or less
	2	Necessitating medical treatment
	3	Disabling patient in daily living
B. Regurgitation	0	Absent
	1	Once a day or less
	2	Predictable at certain posture or action
	3	Periods of aspiration or chronic cough
	4	Recurrent periods of pneumonia
C. Dysphagia	0	Absent
	1	Once a day or less
	2	Requiring liquids for swallowing
	3	Periods of esophageal obstruction
D. Heartburn	0	Absent
	1	Once a day or less
	2	Necessitating medical treatment
	3	Disabling patient in daily living

on was used as a parameter for comparison of the pH monitoring results in the present study.[16]

Surgical Procedures

Nissen fundoplication was performed as a "floppy" fundoplication, described by Donahue et al.[15] A midline upper abdominal incision was used. The esophagus was mobilized, and if indicated, a crural repair was performed. A complete fundic wrap was brought around the esophagogastric junction and fixed to a corresponding fold of the fundus. A fundic wrap 4 cm long was loosely constructed to allow the passage of at least an index finger within the fundoplication alongside the esophagus.

Teres cardiopexy was performed according to the technique that had been described by Narbona-Arnau,[12,13] who visited the Netherlands before the start of this study to explain and show this new technique.[12,13] The surgical procedure was standardized according to his videotape. The esophagus was mobilized in the same way as for the Nissen procedure, and crural repair was performed when indicated. The teres ligament was mobilized, starting in the falciform ligament up to the umbilical insertion, where it was divided. The ligament was passed dorsal to the esophagogastric junction, around the esophagus from right to left, and fixed to the cardia on both sides. Then the ligament was fixed to the anterior gastric wall, parallel to the lesser curvature. Care was taken to preserve the vascular supply of the ligament.

Randomization

Randomization was performed by the principal investigator (IMCJ) 1 day before surgery by drawing envelopes for either the Nissen or the Narbona procedure. Stratification was achieved for the participating hospitals. Informed consent was obtained from all patients who entered the trial. It was originally suspected that the morbidity and side effects and probably also the recurrence rate after the Narbona procedure would be lower than after the Nissen procedure, but the trial could be discontinued on the basis of results from an interim analysis.

Statistics

Values of the various scoring systems are presented as mean (SEM). Statistical comparison was performed with Student's t-test, and values less than $p < 0.05$ were taken to be statistically significant.

RESULTS
Preoperative Findings

The preoperative findings for both groups are summarized in Table 1. There were no differences in age, weight, length, and average period of nonoperative treatment between the two groups. The endoscopy score showed no significant differences either. The symptom score was slightly higher in the Narbona group, but the difference was not significant ($p = 0.06$). The percentage of total time with pH <4 was significantly higher in the Narbona group.

Table 1. Comparison of preoperative findings for patients undergoing a cardiopexy or fundoplication procedure

Preoperative Findings	Cardiopexy (n = 10)	Fundoplication (n = 10)
Male/female	6/4	8/2
Age (yr)	51 (range, 30-64)	45.2 (range, 24-64)
Height (cm)	169	176
Weight (kg)	73	84.3
Cons. treatment (mo)	25.4	32.6
Symptom score	7.8 (0.87)	5.7 (0.59)*
Endoscopy score	1.9 (0.18)	1.5 (0.27)
Percent of total time pH <4	34.34 (7.1)	16.4 (2.4)†

Values are means, with SEM in parentheses.
*$p = 0.06$.
†$p <0.01$.

Surgical Procedure

We encountered no technical problems during the operations. Blood loss was the same in both groups: 150 ml and 120 ml after cardiopexy and fundoplication, respectively. Crural repair was performed in two patients in the cardiopexy group and five patients in the fundoplication group. Mortality was zero; three patients (all after cardiopexy) suffered from minor complications (wound infection). The hospital stay was not significantly different for the two groups, 12.3 days and 9.5 days, respectively, after cardiopexy and fundoplication.

Symptom Score

The symptom score decreased significantly after 3 months in both groups (Fig. 1) and was not different in the two groups (1.1 versus 0.2). After 1 year only two patients in the cardiopexy group had no symptoms, while the mean symptom score was significantly higher than in the fundoplication group (3.9 versus 0.33; $p <0.01$) in which all patients were without symptoms. When the two groups were studied separately at the various time intervals, significantly lower symptom score as compared with preoperative values were found in both groups after 3 months, suggesting a good short-term clinical result. However, at one year after operation there was a significant increase in the symptom score in the cardiopexy group, whereas results in the

fundoplication group were persistently good (Table 2; Fig. 1).

Endoscopy

After 1 year 16 patients (nine cardiopexy, seven fundoplication) consented to evaluation by endoluminal endoscopy. After cardiopexy only one patient had a normal esophagus, whereas no signs of esophagitis were found in all except one patient after fundoplication (Fig. 2). Reduction of the mean endoscopy score was only found in the fundoplication group, but not in the cardiopexy group (see Table 2).

Twenty-Four-Hour pH Monitoring

After 1 year 16 patients (9 cardiopexy, 7 fundoplication) consented to 24-hour pH recording. The percentage total time with pH <4 was significantly higher in the cardiopexy group than in the fundoplication group (23.97 versus 3.77; $p <0.05$). When the two groups were studied separately, no reduction in the mean percentage of total time with pH <4 was found in the cardiopexy group, while a significant decrease was found in the fundoplication group (Table 2; Fig. 3).

Follow-up

After 1 year's follow-up, six patients in the cardiopexy group underwent reoperation because of recurrent re-

Table 2. Comparison of symptom score, percentage of total time with pH <4, and endoscopy postoperatively and at 3 and 12 months' follow-up for patients undergoing a cardiopexy or fundoplication procedure

Follow-up	No.	Postoperative	No.	3 Months	No.	12 Months
Symptom score						
Cardiopexy	10	7.8 (0.87)†	10	1.1 (0.62)‡	10	3.9 (0.81)*
Fundoplication	10	5.7 (0.59)†	10	0.2 (0.13)	9	0.33 (0.17)*
Endoscopy						
Cardiopexy	10	1.9 (0.18)			9	1.88 (0.31)
Fundoplication	10	1.5 (0.27)			7	0.29 (0.29)§
Percent of total time with pH <4						
Cardiopexy	10	34.34 (7.1)			9	23.97 (6.89)
Fundoplication	10	16.4 (2.4)			7	3.77 (3.06)‡

Values are means with SEM in parentheses.
*$p < 0.01$ 0 versus 12 months.
†$p < 0.01$ 0 versus 3 months.
‡$p < 0.05$ 3 versus 12 months.
§$p = 0.01$ 0 versus 12 months.

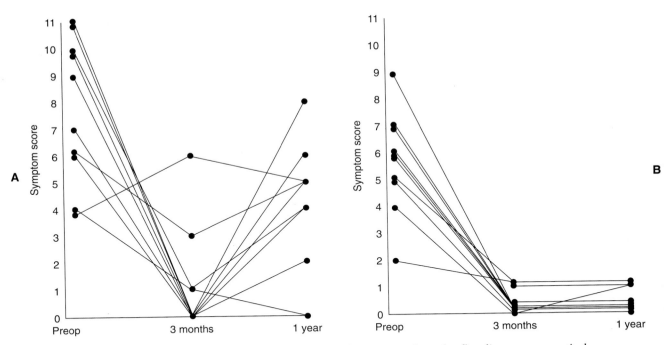

Fig. 1. Symptom scores of patients with complicated gastrooesophageal reflux disease preoperatively and after 3 and 12 months postoperatively. **A,** Cardiopexy. **B,** Fundoplication.

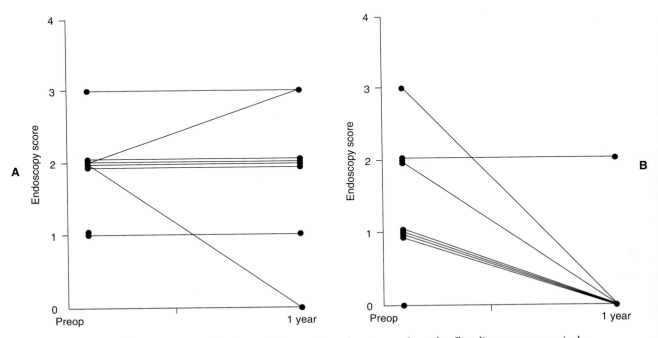

Fig. 2. Endoscopy scores of patients with complicated gastroesophageal reflux disease preoperatively and after 1 year. **A,** Cardiopexy. **B,** Fundoplication.

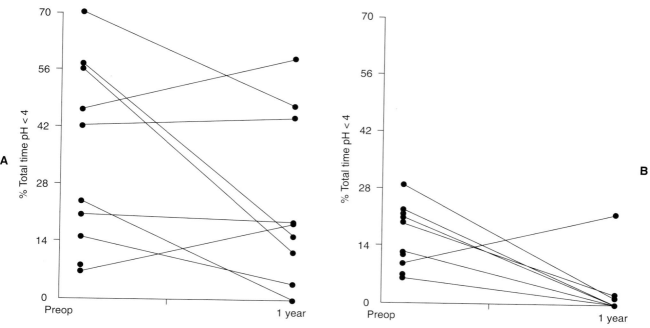

Fig. 3. Percentage of total time with pH <4 for patients with complicated gastroesophageal reflux disease preoperatively and after 1 year. **A,** Cardiopexy. **B,** Fundoplication.

flux disease with severe complaints despite conservative treatment. In these patients a fundoplication was performed without postoperative complications. One patient in the fundoplication group had an abnormal endoscopy (esophagitis plus Barrett's) and pH monitoring but a low symptom score; after 1 year a refundoplication was performed.

In three patients in the Nissen group and one patient in the Narbona group pH monitoring and endoscopy could not be performed, but these patients were free of symptoms one year after surgery.

DISCUSSION

In this study, the results 3 months after cardiopexy and fundoplication, evaluated by using the symptom score, were good for both groups. These good results were comparable with those from a pilot study in 30 patients (data not shown here) that had been performed before the prospective randomized study was initiated. These satisfactory "early" results are very much in accordance with the literature and show the potential value of teres cardiopexy as well as of fundoplication.[12,13,16,17] However, after one year, 6 of the 10 patients with cardiopexy re-

quired a second antireflux procedure (fundoplication). The mean symptom score 1 year after cardiopexy (3.9) was significantly higher than after fundoplication (0.33) and also significantly higher than the results after 3 months. Objective criteria such as esophagitis scored during endoscopy and percentage of total time with pH <4 showed a significant difference between the two groups of patients, which favored fundoplication markedly. Findings relating to the endoscopy score and during 24-hour pH monitoring had not improved 1 year after cardiopexy when compared with the preoperative findings. The disappointing results of cardiopexy after 1 year led to discontinuation of the trial after an interim analysis. The results of this analysis show that cardiopexy was, in our hands, significantly less effective for the treatment of gastroesophageal reflux disease.

These results are in sharp contrast with the excellent results reported by Narbona.[12,13] In his extensive experience with this technique, a low 3% to 4% recurrence after 10 to 15 years' follow-up was reported. Ten percent of his patients had symptoms possibly related to reflux, but no recurrence by objective criteria. Endoscopy and pH-metry were performed postoperatively in, respectively, 47% and 29% of the patients, but results of these investigations are unfortunately not available.

The differences between Narbona's results and those of the present study are remarkable and difficult to understand. They may result from technical aspects, despite the fact that experience was obtained in a pilot study. Three frequent technical errors are mentioned by Narbona[13]: (1) postoperative necrosis of the teres ligament because of damage to the blood supply, (2) poor fixation of the ligament, and (3) poor positioning of the sling in the angle of His. These technical aspects, however, were extensively discussed before starting this trial, and one of the principal investigators attended in nearly all procedures during the pilot study and the trial. The acceptable results after 3 months suggest that the initial procedure was performed correctly. Persistent traction on the ligament, in combination with the constant movement in the area where the sling is located, could result in damage (fibrosis) to the ligament after a longer period of time. A possible role of ischemia or progressive laxating of the teres ligament has also been suggested.[13]

Despite the negative results of this trial the sling principle is an interesting "new" method. The procedure would be of more interest if the excellent results reported by Narbona could be obtained by others, especially since postoperative morbidity in his study was minimal.[15-18] The results of this trial are also of special importance in view of recent developments in laparoscopic surgery, which have led to adaptation of these two techniques for surgical laparoscopic treatment of gastroesophageal reflux disease.[19,20] Both techniques have recently been described, and the cardiopexy procedure in particular can probably be performed laparoscopically without too many difficulties, although the authors did not draw any conclusions regarding long-term benefits of the procedure.[19,20] Because of the excellent results reported by Narbona, cardiopexy will deserve much attention in the development of a laparoscopic approach for surgical treatment of reflux disease. The results of the present trial, however, suggest that more objective prospective data should be obtained before teres cardiopexy can be advised for the surgical treatment of gastroesophageal reflux disease, regardless of whether it should be performed by laparoscopic or open surgery.

REFERENCES

1. Tytgat GNJ, Nicolai JJ, Reman FC. Efficacy of different doses of cimetidine in the treatment of reflux oesophagitis. Gastroenterology 99:629-634, 1990.

2. Richter JE. Surgery for reflux disease—reflections of a gastroenterologist. N Engl J Med 326:825-827, 1992.

3. Maton PN. Omeprazole. N Engl J Med 324:965-975, 1991.

4. Shirazi SS, Schulze K, Soper RT. Long-term follow-up for treatment of complications of chronic reflux oesophagitis. Arch Surg 122:548-552, 1987.

5. DeMeester TR, Bonavinia L, Albertucci M. Nissen fundoplication for gastroesophageal reflux disease. Ann Surg 204:9-19, 1986.

6. Skinner DB. Complications of surgery for gastroesophageal reflux. World J Surg 1:485-491, 1977.

7. Negre JB. Postfundoplication symptoms. Ann Surg 146: 635-637, 1983.

8. Maddern GJ, Myers JC, McIntosh N, Bridgewater FHG, Jamieson GG. The effect of the Angelchik prosthesis on esophageal and gastric function. Arch Surg 126:1418-1422, 1991.

9. Pedinelli L. Triatment chirurgicale de la hernie hiatal par la "technique de collet." Ann Chir 18:1461, 1964.

10. Rampall M, Perillat P, Rouzaud R. Notes preliminiare sur une nouvelle technique de cure chirurgicale des hernies hiatales. La cardiopexie par le ligament rond. Marsielle Chirurgical 16:488, 1964.

11. Helsdingen GCF. Hiatal herniorrhaphy with posterior gastropexy utilizing the ligamentum teres hepatis. Intern Surg 50:128, 1968.

12. Narbona-Arnau B, Olavarietta L, Lloris JM. Reflujo gastro esofagioco hernia hiatal. Rehabilitacion quirurgica del musculo esofagico mediante pexia con el ligamento redondo. Resultados (1143 operados en 15 anos). Bol Soc Val Digest 1:21-28, 1980.

13. Narbona-Arnau B. The sling approach to the treatment of reflux peptic oesophagitis. In Nyhus LIM, Condon RE, eds. Hernia, 3rd ed. Philadelphia: JB Lippincott, 1989, pp 668-682.

14. Masclee AAM, De Best ACAM, De Graaf R, Cluysenaer OJJ, Jansen JBMJ. Ambulatory 24-hour pH-metry in the diagnosis of gastroesophageal reflux disease. Scand J Gastroenterol 25:225-230, 1990.

15. Donahue PE, Samelson S, Nyhus LM, Bombeck CT. The floppy Nissen fundoplication. Arch Surg 120:663-668, 1985.

16. Spechler SJ. Comparison of medical and surgical therapy for complicated gastroesophageal reflux disease in veterans. N Engl J Med 326:786-793, 1992.

17. Breumelhof R, Smout AJPM, Schyns MWRJ, Bronzwaer PWA, Akkermans LMA, Jansen A. Prospective evaluation of the effects of Nissen fundoplication on gastro-esophageal reflux. Surg Gyn Obstet 171:115-120, 1990.
18. Hill LD, Aye RW, Ramel S. Antireflux surgery: A surgeon's look. Gastroenterol Clin North Am 19:745-773, 1990.
19. Nathanson LK, Shimi S, Cuschieri A. Laparoscopic ligamentum teres (round ligament) cardiopexy. Br J Surg 78:947-951, 1991.
20. Cuschieri A, Shimi S, Nathanson LK. Laparoscopic reduction, crural repair, and fundoplication of large hiatal hernia. Am J Surg 163:425-430, 1992.

107   *Current Procedures in Bariatric Surgery*

John G. Kral

Surgical treatment of severe obesity *(bariatric surgery)* is justified by the greatly increased morbidity, mortality, and impaired quality of life associated with excess weight (45 kg or more above standard, established in life insurance tables) or with manifest serious complications of obesity. Unfortunately, with nonsurgical methods most patients cannot maintain a clinically significant weight loss over the long term, thus further justifying surgical treatment.

Since the causes of obesity are not known, surgical treatment is only symptomatic and cannot be curative unless it could permanently affect neuroregulation of appetite. Gastrointestinal procedures for severe obesity have different regulatory effects limiting ingestion of calories either by gastric restriction or, in malabsorptive procedures that stimulate neurohumoral mechanisms influencing appetite regulation, by limiting uptake of calories.

The approach most commonly used is *gastric restriction*, although gastric bypass, which relies on a combination of restriction, maldigestion, and poor absorption, is more effective in achieving and maintaining weight loss by causing food aversion secondary to dumping and intestinal distention.

GASTRIC BYPASS

Since its introduction in 1966, gastric bypass has undergone numerous modifications.[1] Initially a proximal gastric pouch was created by transecting the stomach horizontally and creating a loop gastrojejunostomy. With the introduction of stapling instruments, the pouch was created by in-continuity stapling without transection. The loop gastrojejunostomy was abandoned in favor of a Roux-Y construction to avoid bile reflux into the pouch and also into the distal esophagus in those patients with weak lower esophageal sphincter (LES) tone secondary to obesity. Further modifications mainly have shrunk the size of the proximal pouch (currently with a measured volume of 15 to 25 ml) and the diameter of the gastroenterostomy (presently approximately 10 mm).[2]

Developments

Extremely obese patients—the *superobese*—and some other severely obese patients typically lose only a moderate amount of weight or regain significant weight during a follow-up period of 5 years or more after gastric bypass. For this reason more aggressive operations have been attempted. Biliopancreatic bypass or diversion, invented by Scopinaro of Genoa, consists of gastrectomy with a long-limb Roux-en-Y gastroileostomy plus ileoileostomy anastomosing the blind, biliopancreatic limb end to side 50 cm from the ileocecal valve.[3] This operation creates more maldigestion and malabsorption than conventional gastric bypass.

The principle of biliopancreatic diversion, which has its foundation in intestinal bypass operations, was incorporated into variants of conventional Roux-en-Y gastric bypass without performance of an irreversible gastrectomy. This *distal gastric bypass*[4] or *long-limb gastric bypass*[5] operation is still being evaluated for use in selected obese patients. Because of the potential for se-

583

vere malnutrition within the first 2 to 3 years, patients require vigilant monitoring and occasionally need intravenous supplementation.

Another strategy for increasing the efficacy of gastric bypass is to reinforce the gastroenterostomy by external banding to increase the gastric restrictive component of the operation.[6] This same effect can be achieved by combining banded gastroplasty with gastric bypass.[7] Recognition of breakdown of staple lines as a cause of failure of gastric bypass has prompted several surgeons to revert to dividing the stomach and oversewing the cut edges.[8] Some use this as their preferred method for reoperation, whereas others divide primarily.[9]

In summary, the standard gastric bypass operation currently is Roux-en-Y gastric bypass with a 20 ml stapled proximal gastric pouch anastomosed to a 50 cm efferent limb of jejunum. Modifications involve lengthening the efferent limb significantly, increasing the malabsorptive component of the operation and stomal reinforcement, and increasing the restrictive mechanism. It is probable that stomal reinforcement and transection of the stomach will become standard in gastric bypass surgeries.

GASTRIC RESTRICTION
Gastroplasty

In 1971 Mason introduced gastroplasty as a gastric restrictive operation created by transecting the fundus, leaving a gastrogastric opening or a channel along the greater curvature.[10] Significant failure among the 59 patients was already evident within 6 months, and the operation was abandoned. Gastroplasty was reintroduced in 1977, using stapling techniques to create a smaller pouch and reinforcing the greater curvature gastrogastrostomy channel with a suture. Once again it became apparent that weight loss maintenance was unsatisfactory.

The next modification of gastroplasty was the vertical banded gastroplasty (VBG), since 1981 the most widely performed bariatric procedure.[11] As the name implies, it consists of a vertically oriented stapled gastric pouch with a volume of 10 to 15 ml created by two double-stapled lines oriented distally from the angle of His, with an externally banded stoma with approximately a 9 to 10 mm inner diameter (Fig. 1). Variants of this operation include Silastic ring vertical gastroplasty,[12] the Long gastroplasty using Mersilene sutures instead of banding,[13] and one version using a divided vertical staple line.

Banding

In an attempt to simplify gastric restriction further, Wilkinson[14] applied an external circumferential band sutured to itself, thus avoiding violating the integrity of the gastric mucosa, in a dog study reported in 1978. Significant dilation of the proximal stomach pouch prompted him to abandon this method in favor of wrapping the entire stomach with Silastic mesh or a prosthetic cast after imbrication ("Nissenizing") from the lesser curvature.[15] This complex operation is difficult to reverse and has raised concerns about erosions in the long term.

In spite of Wilkinson's failure, numerous surgeons have performed gastric banding in large numbers of patients. In one of the rare studies comparing banding with gastroplasty, the latter was found superior with respect to weight loss maintenance. An animal study revealed a propensity of external bands to erode,[16] which also has been reported anecdotally in humans.

The most meticulous and methodically sound approach to banding has been developed by Kuzmak,[17] who has patented devices to calibrate precisely the size of the stoma and the pressure of Silastic band. His clin-

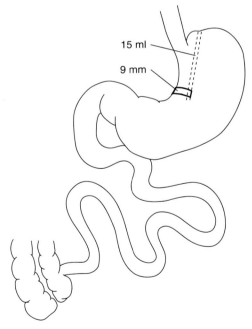

Fig. 1. Vertical gastroplasty demonstrating volume of stapled gastric pouch and inner diameter of externally banded outlet.

ical results with 10 years' follow-up are superior to other studies of banding and need replication by other investigators.

Developments

Recognizing the importance of stomal diameter for determining rate and magnitude of ingestion and noticing postoperative expansion of the inner diameter of the banded stoma, Kuzmak developed his band further,[18] making it inflatable. This adjustable gastric band is attached by tubing to an implanted saline solution–filled port, which can be injected or aspirated during fluoroscopy to modify stoma size. This procedure has been used by Kuzmak in more than 150 patients with a maximum follow-up time of 5 years with promising results. His technique is currently being evaluated at several centers in Europe and the United States.

Rarely, gastric restrictive operations must be reversed; however, the fact that a patient can "out-eat" the restriction of the procedure does not mandate surgical reversal. However, if patients develop intercurrent diseases with which gastric restriction is incompatible, if they have complications, or if they simply do not tolerate gastric restriction, it may become necessary to reverse the operation. To avoid the increased risk of reoperative surgery Dr. Kuzmak has modified the adjustable band so that it can be removed entirely by exposing the subcutaneous port with the use of a local anesthetic; a formal laparotomy is not required. This reversible stoma-adjustable gastric band has been tested recently in dogs[19] and is being prepared for clinical use.

MINIMALLY INVASIVE SURGERY

With the advent of laparoscopic techniques, there is a great interest in developing bariatric procedures because of the complication rates associated with laparotomy of severely obese patients. Although such patients have varying degrees of respiratory compromise that might pose problems during hyperinflation of the abdomen and although hepatomegaly and enlarged intra-abdominal fat deposits might encumber access through a laparoscopic approach, it seems feasible to perform some type of circumgastric banding. Such a technique should allow calibration of stomal size and band tension, drawing on the experience of Kuzmak with conventional banding. Perfection of such minimally invasive techniques potentially would expand the indications for surgical intervention.

LIMITATIONS OF GASTRIC RESTRICTION—METHODS FOR PREVENTION

The main limitation of gastric restriction is failure of the patient to lose adequate weight and maintain the weight loss although results of gastric restriction are far superior to those of nonoperative treatment. The main reasons for weight loss failure are behavioral: (1) ingestion of calorically dense liquid or soft or melting food (the "soft calorie syndrome") that readily empties through the stoma without causing pouch distention and (2) eating to the "limit," which over time causes expansion of the pouch. Pouch expansion can be substantial so that a large total amount of food can be eaten, even though emptying through the banded stoma is delayed. Some attempts have been made to prevent excessive stretching by wrapping the gastroplasty pouch. This did not improve results sufficiently to justify this more complex operation. Consequently it can be reasoned that pouch expansion is not a major factor in failure and that the soft calorie syndrome is a more important cause of failure.

There is no technical method for overcoming the soft calorie syndrome, unless the stoma were made tight enough to limit ingestion of liquids. However, this method cannot be tolerated indefinitely. With stoma-adjustable banding, it would be possible to periodically tighten the band sufficiently to cause weight loss despite consumption of calorically dense liquids.

Animal experiments have shown that drinking behavior[20] and nutrient selection[21] are strongly influenced by a truncal vagotomy. In a small study of obese patients, truncal vagotomy was similarly demonstrated to affect liquid consumption.[22] The total weight loss experience with vagotomy alone was poor. However, adding vagotomy to gastroplasty has significantly potentiated weight loss over the long term.[23] It is likely that vagotomy causes a change in neuroregulation of fluid intake sufficient to improve the results of gastric restriction.

STAGED SURGERY

The heaviest patients (superobese) have a higher failure rate after conventional gastric restriction and gastric bypass procedures. It is not possible from available data to determine the risk/benefit ratio of more aggressive primary operations in these patients. The immediate risks of performing more complex operations on the superobese and the long-term risks of more "malnutritive" operations have not been evaluated.

Apart from the degree of overweight, there are no criteria for predicting long-term outcome. Sugerman et al.[24] have noted that patients with high consumption of sweets lose more weight after gastric bypass surgery than after gastroplasty. Their data do not allow preoperative identification of patients who will have inadequate weight loss after gastric bypass, although sweet consumption and ethnicity are predictors of poorer outcome.

In the absence of outcome predictors and risk/benefit analyses, a *staged* approach to surgical treatment of obesity has been proposed.[25] With this approach, all patients primarily are given the simplest procedure and the one with least long-term sequelae. Patients who have recurrence of comorbidity and/or significant weight regain are then considered for more aggressive procedures. The ultimate goal is to maintain sufficient weight loss to ameliorate comorbidity and to increase the duration and quality of life.

CONCLUSION

Gastric restriction, either by gastroplasty or circumgastric banding, and gastric bypass provide better weight control than any nonsurgical treatment of clinically significant obesity. Gastric restriction, because of its relative simplicity and low morbidity, is used most often. Because of long-term failure of weight loss maintenance, techniques have been developed to improve the efficacy of gastric restrictive operations. Perfection of laparoscopic techniques may expand the use of gastric restriction in obese patients. However, subgroups of severely obese patients probably require a staged approach for long-term management of their disease, justifying increasingly malnutritional operations. In the absence of preventive measures, there is a great need for long, controlled studies of surgical treatment for this prevalent, crippling, and killing disease to assess the risk/benefit ratio and to identify outcome predictors. Because of the multifactional etiology of obesity, there is no procedure of choice, and it will always be necessary to individualize treatment.

REFERENCES

1. Mason EE, Ito C. Gastric bypass. Ann Surg 170:329-339, 1969.
2. Linner JH. Gastric operations: Specific techniques. In Linner JH. Surgery for Morbid Obesity. New York: Springer-Verlag, 1984, pp 65-85.
3. Scopinaro N, Gianetta E, Civalleri D, et al. Partial and total biliopancreatic bypass in the surgical treatment of obesity. Int J Obes 5:421-429, 1981.
4. Sugerman HJ, Starkey JV, Birkenhauer R. A randomized prospective trial of gastric bypass versus vertical banded gastroplasty for morbid obesity and their effects on sweets versus non-sweets eaters. Ann Surg 205:613-624, 1987.
5. Brolin RE, Kenler HA, Gorman JH, et al. Long-limb gastric bypass in the superobese. Ann Surg 215:387-395, 1992.
6. Linner JH. Overview of surgical techniques for the treatment of morbid obesity. Gastroenterol Clin North Am 16:253-272, 1987.
7. Salmon PA. Gastroplasty with distal gastric bypass: A new and more successful weight loss operation for the morbidly obese. Can J Surg 31:111-113, 1988.
8. MacLean LD, Rhode BM, Forse RA. Late results of vertical banded gastroplasty for morbid and super obesity. Surgery 107:20-27, 1990.
9. Pories WJ, MacDonald KG, Flickinger EG, et al. Is type II diabetes mellitus (NIDDM) a surgical disease? Ann Surg 215:633-643, 1992.
10. Printen KJ, Mason EE. Gastric surgery for relief of morbid obesity. Arch Surg 106:428, 1973.
11. Mason EE. Morbid obesity: Use of vertical banded gastroplasty. Surg Clin North Am 67:521-537, 1987.
12. Willbanks OL. Long-term results of silicone elastomer ring vertical gastroplasty for the treatment of morbid obesity. Surgery 101:606-610, 1987.
13. Long M, Collins JP. The technique and early results of high gastric reduction for obesity. Aust N Z J Surg 50:146, 1980.
14. Wilkinson LH. Reduction of gastric reservoir capacity. Am J Clin Nutr 33:515-517, 1980.
15. Wilkinson LH, Peloso OA. Gastric (reservoir) reduction for morbid obesity. Arch Surg 116:602-605, 1981.
16. Coelho JCU, Solhaug JH, Moody FG, et al. Experimental evaluation of gastric banding for treatment of morbid obesity in pigs. Am J Surg 149:228-231, 1985.
17. Kuzmak LI. Gastric banding. In Dietel M, ed. Surgery for the Morbidly Obese Patient. Philadelphia: Lea & Febiger, 1989, pp 225-259.
18. Kuzmak LI. Stoma adjustable silicone gastric banding. Probl Gen Surg 9:298-317, 1992.
19. Abramson DL, Thelmo W, Kuzmak LI, et al. Subcutaneously removable stoma-adjustable silicone gastric banding (in preparation).
20. Kraly FS, Gibbs J, Smith GP. Disordered drinking after abdominal vagotomy in rats. Nature 258:226-228, 1975.
21. Sclafani A, Kramer TH. Aversive effects of vagotomy: A conditioned taste aversion analysis. Physiol Behav 34:721-725, 1985.

22. Gortz L, Bjorkman A-C, Andersson H, et al. Truncal vagotomy reduces food and liquid intake in man. Physiol Behav 48:779-781, 1990.
23. Gortz L, Kral JG. Vagotomy improves weight reduction after gastroplasty. Int J Obes 14(Suppl 2):160, 1990.
24. Sugerman HR, Londrey GL, Kellum JM, et al. Weight loss with vertical banded gastroplasty and Roux-Y gastric bypass for morbid obesity with selective versus random assignment. Am J Surg 157:93, 1989.
25. Kral JG. Overview of surgical techniques for treating obesity. Am J Clin Nutr 55:552S-555S, 1992.

108 Current Therapeutic Strategies in the Treatment of Bleeding Esophageal Varices in Infants and Children and Twenty Years' Results of Endoscopic Paravariceal Sclerotherapy

Karl-Joseph Paquet and Aristotel Lazar

The treatment of portal hypertension in children presents challenges such as small vessel size, which renders creation of surgical portosystemic shunts difficult, unknown long-term tolerance of portosystemic shunts, and possible spontaneous regression of varices as the patient matures.

Portal hypertension is one of the most important causes of bleeding from esophagogastric varices. Most reports on this problem address the choice, timing, and complications of surgery and have led to increasing dissatisfaction with portosystemic shunt procedures. In the area of the terminal esophagus, where more than 90% of esophageal bleeding occurs, paravariceal endoscopic sclerotherapy (PES) represents an acceptable alternative therapeutic approach.[1-3]

ANATOMICAL CONSIDERATIONS FOR PARAVARICEAL ENDOSCOPIC SCLEROTHERAPY

Causes of bleeding from varices in the distal 5 cm of the esophagus have been identified through anatomical studies.[4-7] In normal patients four distinct venous zones have been established in the distal esophagus and proximal stomach (Fig. 1). Of these, the palisade zone and the perforating zone are most important in the development and rupture of esophageal varices. The palisade zone begins at the gastroesophageal junction and extends 2 to 3 cm cephalad. The veins within this zone

are longitudinally arranged in the lamina propria. Blood flow within the palisade zone is bidirectional and accommodates the variable pressures of the gastroesophageal junction associated with the respiratory cycle, coughing, and Valsalva maneuver. Thus blood from the palisade zone alternately drains into the gastric zone (into the portal system) or into the perforating zone, which extends 3 to 5 cm proximal to the gastroesophageal junction. In the perforating zone four distinct layers of veins have been identified (Fig. 2). Fine, superficial, arborized intraepithelial veins drain capillary beds in the epithelium into a superficial venous plexus. Blood subsequently flows into three to five large-caliber, deep intrinsic veins. Blood from these intraesophageal veins is directed into periesophageal veins through perforating veins, which have valves that direct flow.

These normal vascular relationships are altered significantly in a patient with portal hypertension. Dilation and high pressure in the periesophageal veins cause the valves in the perforating veins to become incompetent; this allows retrograde flow into the deep intrinsic veins and their tributaries. These conditions result in increased blood flow and turbulence in the intrinsic venous trunks. The dilated deep intrinsic veins displace the superficial venous plexus and assume a subepithelial position, a condition that results in the tortuous, large variceal trunks often seen at endoscopy.[5-8] Dilation of the intraepithelial veins results in endo-

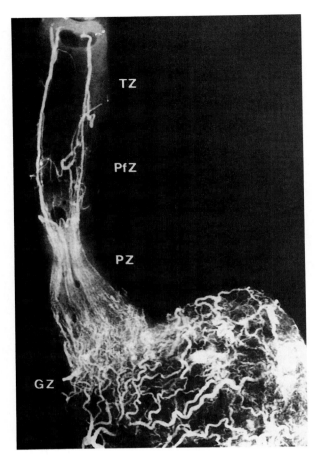

Fig. 1. Radiograph of venous circulation in human gastroesophageal junction after barium injection. No perforating veins are seen in palisade zone. (*GZ*, Gastric zone; *PZ*, palisade zone; *PFZ*, perforating zone; *TZ*, truncal zone.) (From Vianna A, Hayes PC, Moscoso G, et al. Normal venous circulation of the gastroesophageal junction. Gastroenterology 93:876, 1987.)

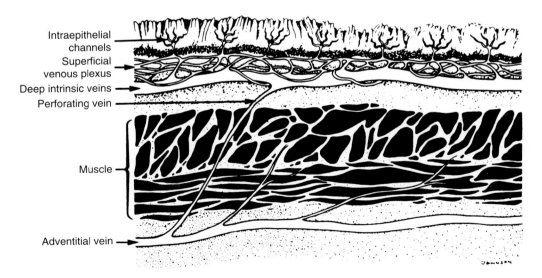

Fig. 2. Diagram of layers of veins at human distal esophagus. (From Kitano S, Terblanche J, Kahn J, et al. Venous anatomy of lower esophagus in portal hypertension: Practical implications. Br J Surg 73:525, 1986.)

scopically recognizable telangiectases or minivarices,[8] "cherry-red spots," "red wales," or "varices upon varices."[9] Dilation and increased pressure in the perforating zone cause blood to flow caudally into the palisade zone. The palisade zone, however, must also accommodate the increased gastrosplenic blood flow associated with portal hypertension. Consequently blood flow in the palisade zone is more turbulent in patients with portal hypertension. High pressures and turbulent flow in superficially located dilated vessels in the distal 5 cm of the esophagus (the palisade and perforating zones) contribute to the likelihood of variceal rupture.

PATHOPHYSIOLOGICAL FACTORS IN BLEEDING VARICES

Sclerotherapy is used to obliterate the varices of the distal esophagus and gastroesophageal junction that are most likely to bleed. This is accomplished by injection of a sclerosant in and/or around the varices to cause thrombosis and mucosal fibrosis. However, the incompetent perforating veins that connect the intrinsic venous trunks to the periesophageal veins are not effectively obliterated, and new collateral channels may form in the distal esophagus.

Our group[1-3,10] has introduced the concept of paravariceal endoscopic sclerotherapy, in which the lower part of the esophagus and the esophagocardiac junction are endoscopically injected with sclerosant. This technique rarely causes thrombosis of the vascular channels and induces the formation of fibrous subepithelial layers that cover the non-occluded necessary portal systemic collaterals (Fig. 3). Varices in the esophageal subepithelium and submucosa can be protected by these fibrous layers. Effects on gastric varices are unlikely to occur.[11]

We present our study of 71 infants and children with portal hypertension who were referred to the Department of Surgery of the University of Bonn from January 1, 1972 to January 1, 1982 and to the Heinz-Kalk Hospital, Bad Kissingen, from January 1, 1982 to January 1, 1992.

MATERIALS AND METHODS

In 1972, at the initial resurgence of sclerotherapy by our group, flexible pediatric endoscopes were not available. We constructed and used rigid endoscopic instruments of two different sizes, one for use in infants and the other for older children. A general anesthetic was administered to the patient. These rigid instruments were used to suction large amounts of blood during emergency sclerotherapy and to compress the bleeding varix after

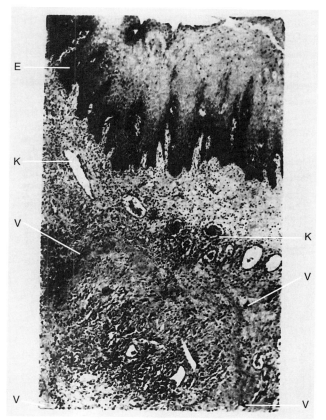

Fig. 3. Histological specimen from 3 cm of resected terminal esophagus 1 to 4 cm above the esophagocardiac junction. Note preservation of subepitheal and submucosal varices and vascular channels. Intraepithelial channels are completely obliterated or substituted by fibrous tissue. (*V,* Varices; *K,* collateral; *E,* epithelium.) (From Paquet KJ, Lindecken KD, Göcke H. Massive Ulkusblutung aus der Speiseröhre nach Dislokation einer Doppelballonsonde—Diagnostik und Therapie. Kinderchir 27:303, 1979.)

paravariceal injection.[12] Because training for rigid esophagoscopy is no longer widely available, endoscopists who are inexperienced with the rigid instrument may experience higher complication rates than with the flexible endoscope, which became more widely used in the late 1970s.

Today the flexible pediatric endoscope is the instrument of choice for emergency and elective sclerotherapy. General anesthesia is required for infants and children younger than 6 years of age; in older children, intravenous sedation is sufficient. In elective cases the procedure can be performed on an outpatient basis during long-term maintenance sessions.

The choice of the sclerosant and its concentration (0.5% to 1.0% polidocanol), the number of injections per session, the frequency of sessions per phase, and the follow-up sclerotherapy schedule have been described.[10,11,13] Endoscopic sclerotherapy was performed under fluoroscopic control in the first 20 children to confirm the injection site of the sclerosant beside the varix (Fig. 4). Injections of sclerosant (the first of which was administered at the esophagocardiac junction) were repeated 30 to 50 times, and a helical arrangement of weals developed as the endoscope was withdrawn. The injections should be limited to the distal esophagus and the cardia unless a more proximal bleeding site is identified.

From January 1, 1972, to January 1, 1992, 72 consecutively examined infants and children with bleeding esophagogastric varices were referred to our hospital. The youngest infant was 10 months of age, and the oldest child was 15 years of age (median age, 8.6 years). The causes of portal hypertension and the number of previous episodes of gastrointestinal hemorrhage before referral for endoscopic sclerotherapy are listed in Table 1. All cases are based on the results of liver biopsy. More than 70% of these patients had portal obstruction (group Ia) as a result of injury to the portal vein (from neonatal venous catheterization, omphalitis, blunt trauma, or abdominal infection). There were two cases of congenital hepatic fibrosis (group Ib), five cases of cholestatic cirrhosis, 11 of postnecrotic cirrhosis, and one case of Wilson's disease (group II). Emergency surgical interventions had been performed to stop variceal bleeding in 30 children from groups Ia and Ib and in six children from group II. Elective procedures to stop bleeding were performed in 43 children from group I and in 10 from group II.

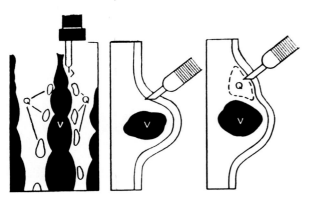

Fig. 4. Technique of paravariceal injection sclerotherapy in esophageal wall. Injection is made beside varices.

RESULTS

Emergency or elective endoscopy was performed when the general condition of the child was adequate and be-

Table 1. Causes of portal hypertension and number of episodes of hemorrhage in 71 children before referral for endoscopic sclerotherapy

Group	Cause	Number*	Percent	Previous Episodes of Hemorrhage
Ia	Portal obstruction	50	70.0	1-4
Ib	Congenital hepatic fibrosis	2	3.0	1-2
II	Cholestatic cirrhoses	—	—	—
	Extrahepatic biliary atresia	5	7.0	1-8
	Alpha-1 antitrypsin deficiency	1	1.5	1-2
	Cystic fibrosis	1	1.5	1-2
	Postnecrotic cirrhoses	11	15.5	1-3
	Chronic hepatitis	—	—	—
	Autoimmune cirrhosis	7		
	HBsAG-positive cirrhosis	3		
	Serum-negative cirrhosis	1		
	Wilson's disease	1	1.5	1

*Some cases had multiple causes.

cause flexible endoscopes were available (Table 2). Our supplementary therapeutic strategy is summarized in the box below. Of 29 children (41% of pediatric patients studied) with spurting varices, control of hemorrhage was achieved in 28 cases (96.5%) after emergency paravariceal sclerotherapy. In a 7-year-old boy with portal thrombosis that resulted from neonatal umbilical catheterization, bleeding stopped after emergency sclerotherapy and the introduction and inflation of the Sengstaken-Blakemore tube for 12 hours. Care was taken not to induce overtransfusion, because a hemoglobin level >9.5 g/dl may be a factor in recurrent bleeding. In children with cirrhosis, neomycin and lactulose were administered by gastric tube, and/or magnesium sulfate or lactulose enemas were given. Posthemorrhagic ascites and the subsequent risk of bacterial peritonitis were prevented by alternate infusions of human albumin and packed red blood cells.

Complications of paravariceal endoscopic sclerotherapy (Table 3) were analyzed with respect to time (1 day to 1 month and 1 month to 1 year) and were separated according to the causes of portal hypertension. The primary early complications in both groups were from pleural effusion (22.5%), substernal pain (12.5%), and ulcerations >5 mm (12.5%). Ulcerations with bleeding and stricture occurred in 3%, and no case of mediastinitis (and thus no fatal complication) occurred.

Primary complications that developed within one month to one year of treatment included recurrent bleeding despite continued sclerotherapy in three patients (4%) and dysmotility in two patients (3%). Bougienage of a stricture was necessary for two patients (3%)

THERAPEUTIC STRATEGY FOR TREATMENT OF ESOPHAGOGASTRIC VARICEAL HEMORRHAGE

1. Hospital admission to intensive care unit
2. Shock prophylaxis and/or therapy
3. Gastric tube and suction
4. Emergency endoscopy or sclerotherapy
5. Balloon tamponade (and/or intravenous glypressin therapy)
6. No transfusion over the level of 9.5 g/dl
7. Neomycin and lactulose through gastric tube*
8. Magnesium sulfate or lactulose enema*
9. Alternate infusions of human albumin and packed red blood cells*

*In infants and children, used only with intrahepatic block.

Table 2. Number and type of emergency operations performed in 36 children before referral for sclerotherapy

Type of Operation	Group I: Prehepatic Block (n = 52)		Group II: Intrahepatic Block (n = 19)	
	Number	Percent	Number	Percent
Shunts (different types)	15	35	5	50
Variceal ligation and/or devascularization	18	42	2	20
Splenectomy	9	21	2	20
Splenic arterial ligation	1	2	1	10
TOTALS	43 (in 30 children)		10 (in 6 children)	

Table 3. Complications of paravariceal endoscopic sclerotherapy

Time of Occurrence	Type of Complication	Group I		Group II		Total	
		Number	Percent	Number	Percent	Number	Percent
1 day to 1 month after sclero-therapy	Substernal pain	6	11.5	3	16.0	9	12.5
	Pleural effusion	11	21.0	5	26.5	16	22.5
	Mediastinitis	0	0	0	0	0	0
	Ulceration (<5 mm)	6	11.5	3	16.0	9	12.5
	Ulceration with bleeding	1	2.0	1	5.25	2	3.0
	Stricture	1	2.0	1	5.25	2	3.0
	TOTALS	25	48.0	13	69	38	53.5
1 month to 1 year after sclero-therapy	Recurrent bleeding	1	2.0	2	10.5	3	4.0
	Stricture	0	0	1	5.25	1	1.5
	Dysmotility	1	2.0	1	5.25	2	3.0
	TOTALS	2	4.0	4	21.0	6	8.5

Table 4. Causes of early and late mortality after paravariceal endoscopic sclerotherapy in infants and children (n = 71/66)*

	Group I (n = 52)		Group II (n = 19)	
	Number	Percent	Number	Percent
Early (iatrogenic) mortality	0	0	0	0

	Group I (n = 50)			Group II (n = 16)		
	Number	Percent	Cause of Death	Number	Percent	Cause of Death
Late mortality	1	2	Renal failure	3	18.75	Liver failure
				1	6.25	Sepsis
TOTAL	1	2		4	25.0	

*66 of 71 patients were followed.

within 1 day to 1 month of sclerotherapy and in one patient (1.5%) within 1 month to 1 year of sclerotherapy.

There was no hospital mortality in the series (Table 4). Of the original 71 children studied, 66 infants and children could be followed for 20 years. Nine foreign children were included in the study: seven from Italy, one from Belgium, and one from Switzerland. Three children from Italy were lost to follow-up. One girl with congenital hepatic fibrosis died 8 years after the first endoscopic sclerotherapy; the cause of death was renal failure and its sequelae. This patient had been treated with hemodialysis for 3 years and was not a candidate for kidney transplantation.

Late mortality for group I was 2% for the entire period studied. The mortality for group II patients was 25%; causes of death were liver failure 3, 5, and 7 years after initiation of continuing endoscopic sclerotherapy in three children with postnecrotic cirrhosis. No do-

Table 5. Procedures necessary during follow-up of children primarily managed by paravariceal endoscopic sclerotherapy in group I (n = 52/50)

Number	Time of Follow-up Procedure After PES	Indication	Procedure
1	8 mo	Recurrent hemorrhage from esophageal ulcer localized in a varix	Transthoracic resection of 3 cm esophageal segment, end-to-end anastomosis, and fundoplication
1	6 yr	Recurrent hemorrhage despite continued PES	Warren shunt
1	8 yr		Mesocaval interp
1	10 yr		Warren shunt
1	11 yr		Splenomesenter

Table 6. Surgical procedures necessary during follow-up of infants and children managed primarily by paravariceal endoscopic sclerotherapy in group II (n = 19/16)

Number	Time of Follow-up (yr)	Indication for Procedure	Procedure
1	3	Recurrent hemorrhage in spite of continued sclerotherapy	Warren shunt
1	5	Recurrent hemorrhage in spite of continued sclerotherapy	Warren shunt
1	3	Liver insufficiency	Liver transplantation (no donor)
1	5	Liver insufficiency	Liver transplantation (no donor)
1	7	Liver insufficiency	Liver transplantation (no donor)
1	8	Liver insufficiency	Successful liver transplantation

nor for liver transplantation was available for any of these three patients. One 6-year-old girl with extrahepatic biliary atresia died 5 years after operation; the cause of death was enterocolitis with sepsis.

We have analyzed the surgical procedures performed during the follow-up of the infants and children who underwent long-term PES in group I and group II by number of procedures, the time between interventions, the indications, and the surgical procedure required. In group I a 10-year-old boy underwent a transthoracic resection of a 3 cm esophageal segment, end-to-end anastomosis, as well as fundoplication 8 months after the first sclerotherapeutic intervention. These procedures were performed because of recurrent hemorrhage from an esophageal ulcer in a varix (Table 5). In four children 12, 13, 15, and 16 years of age, shunt operations were performed because of recurrent variceal hemorrhage despite continued endoscopic sclerotherapy. In these procedures, two Warren shunts, one mesocaval interposition shunt and one splenomesentericorenal shunt were used. Thus a 10% frequency was noted for early or late surgical intervention during repeat endoscopic sclerotherapy; this was determined by a 20-year follow-up of 50 children with portal obstruction. In group II (19 infants and children) two Warren shunt placements were performed 3 and 5 years after the initiation of repeated endoscopic sclerotherapy because of recurrent variceal hemorrhage (Table 6). In this

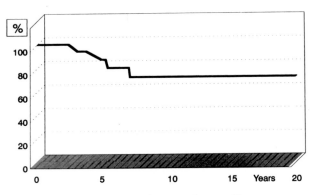

Fig. 5. Survival curve of group II.

group shunt placement was necessary in 10% of patients. Liver insufficiency occurred 3, 5, 7, or 8 years after initiation of endoscopic sclerotherapy group, and liver grafts failed because organ donors were not available in three cases (1975, 1976, and 1985). In one 1982 case liver transplantation was successful. Life expectancy according to Kaplan-Meier in group I patients was 95%, and in group II it was 70% for 10 and 20 years (Fig. 5).

DISCUSSION

This is the first report describing the application of continuing PES in infants and children in a 20-year follow-up of 93% of cases studied. Analysis of this series also provides data on the long-term follow-up and prognosis of children with portal obstruction and chronic liver disease who have undergone operations such as elective shunt operation (when PES fails) or liver grafts (in the end-stage of chronic liver disease). In both groups, variceal bleeding was successfully stopped in 96.5% of cases for 4 weeks through emergency and repeat PES at weekly intervals. The early and long-term results of PES show that varices in the esophageal subepithelium and submucosa are protected by fibrous layers.

The number of complications that occurred within 1 month of PES was high—48% in group I and 53.5% in group II. However, in the majority of cases, no therapy was necessary, and no complication caused a fatality. Late complications that occurred from 1 month to 1 year after PES also required no therapy and caused no fatalities. In one such case, an urgent transthoracic resection of 3 cm of the terminal esophagus, a reanastomosis and fundoplication were performed because of

recurrent esophageal bleeding from an ulcer in a varix despite repeat and emergency PES and application of a Sengstaken-Blakemore tube.

During the follow-up of group I cases, elective shunt operations were performed in four children (10% who ranged in age from 12 to 16 years) because of recurrent hemorrhage despite repeat PES. In group II, shunt procedures were performed in two children (11% who ranged in age from 1 to 14 years) because of the same indication. Four children of this group (25%) required liver transplantation, but because of organ shortage, only one child underwent successful surgery; the other three died as a result of hepatic failure.

Thus the risk of recurrent hemorrhage is reduced to a high extent. With the combined use of repeat PES and very urgent devascularization (and with elective shunt if repeat PES fails), life expectancy for 10 to 20 years is >95% in children with portal obstruction. If liver grafts are also available to correct liver failure, life expectancy is approximately 70% in children with chronic liver disease.

Despite these results, the choice of treatment for esophageal varices remains controversial. Primary surgery and sclerotherapy are considered competing modalities. However, more than two thirds of the children treated with surgery on varices or variceal vessels will experience recurrent bleeding.[14,15] Splenectomy alone is a worthless and dangerous procedure.[14,16] Attention has focused on the relative merits of portosystemic shunting and injection sclerotherapy.

Portosystemic surgical shunts stop bleeding, but they are associated with significant morbidity and mortality.[17-21] Mortality varied from 0% to 22%, and rates of recurrent bleeding varied from 2% to 47% in six recent series[22,23] conducted from 1980 to 1986. Shunt thrombosis, which occurred in 6% to 47% of these cases was often observed in children <10 years of age.

Dissatisfaction with portosystemic shunting is not confined solely to shunt thrombosis and recurrent bleeding; in children with cirrhosis, deterioration in liver function and hepatic encephalopathy are additional hazards. In a series of 37 children originally diagnosed with portal obstruction or congenital hepatic fibrosis, one died in the early postoperative period with hepatic encephalopathy, and in nine of 31 children with a patent shunt, encephalopathy developed during a mean follow-up period of 5 years; three of these nine patients died.[20] Hazards also occur from splenectomy performed

Table 7. Results of endoscopic sclerotherapy in children in studies published 1984-1990

Author	Number	Previous Operations for Portal Hypertension	Mortality Rate From Bleeding and ES (%)	Rate of Recurrent Bleeding (%)	Time of Follow-up (yr)
Spence et al.[27]	18	7	11	5.5	0.6-3.0
Stellen and Lilly[28]	25	9	4	0	0.8-6.0
Stray and Fausa[29]	9	3	0	22.0	0.5-4.8
Vane et al.[30]	13	7	0	8.0	2.0-4.5
Donovan et al.[31]	16	3	6	25.0	1.1-6.2
Howard et al.[32]	108	19	4	5.0 (after obliteration)	0.2-7.8

during a Linton splenorenal shunt construction during the Sugiura procedure.[23,24] Studies of adult patients[25,26] have shown that side effects, may not result from a more selective portosystemic anastomosis like that used with the Warren shunt or the narrow lumen mesocaval interposition shunt. However, too few of these series have been evaluated and the patients studied are too select (children >10 years of age in whom sclerotherapy had failed).

The results of portosystemic shunt operations can be contrasted with those of endoscopic sclerotherapy (Table 7), which indicate mortality rates of 0 to 11% (median 4.1%) and recurrent bleeding rates of 0 to 25% (median 10.9%).[27-32] A greater proportion of children with extrahepatic portal hypertension who have a better prognosis are presented in the surgical series cited.[17-21] In addition, surgical researchers have often been more selective in their reports. For example, Bismuth et al.,[17] who have published the best results with portosystemic anastomosis, excluded the outcome in 10 of 90 children studied in whom shunting was impossible. A further important aspect that supports PES is spontaneous development of fibrous subepithelial layers that cover portosystemic collaterals.[32,33] In PES, the need for a shunting procedure is eliminated as children with portal obstruction become adults.

Additional merits of endoscopic sclerotherapy include reduction of the risk of early recurrent bleeding to 5% to 10% if the endoscopically confirmed varices are obliterated or are completely covered by fibrous tissue after repeat intraendoscopic sclerotherapy or paravariceal endoscopic sclerotherapy. Mortality from variceal bleeding in this series was 0%, it was 1% in a recently published report[32] with an 8-year follow-up of 97 children. The number of complications in this report are high, and although one complication resulted in emergency surgery, no fatalities occurred. PES may cause temporary or permanent motility disorders in rare cases, but these sequelae are asymptomatic and H_2-antagonist therapy is rarely required.

If PES is combined with elective and selective shunt surgery,[25,34] recurrent variceal hemorrhage can be avoided, as we demonstrate in this study. Liver transplantation can be performed more easily and with lower morbidity and mortality if primary portosystemic shunt surgery is avoided.

CONCLUSION

Endoscopic sclerotherapy—in which an associated mortality of 0 to 1% results from bleeding and in which a recurrent bleeding rate of 5% to 10% is noted—is the current treatment of choice for primary management of bleeding esophageal varices from both portal vein obstruction and chronic liver disease in infants and children. Underlying liver disease and bleeding determine the prognosis; however, if liver transplantation is available, the prognosis can be improved. Results with endoscopic sclerotherapy are better than those of primary surgical management, which should be reserved for sclerotherapy failures.

REFERENCES

1. Paquet KJ, Raschke E. Experiences in the management of the acute or impending hemorrhage from esophageal varices using the esophagoscopic sclerosing method. In Urgent Endoscopy of Digestive and Abdominal Diseases. International Symposia, Prague/Carlsbad, 1971. Basel: Karger, 1972, p 184.

2. Paquet KJ, Raschki E. Management of hemorrhage from esophageal varices using the endoscopic sclerosing method. Ann Surg 117:99, 1973.

3. Paquet KJ, Harler B. Die Therapie der akuten und drohenden Ösophagusvarizenblutung durch Wandsklerosierung der Speiseröhre im Kindesalter. Monatsschr Kinderheilkd 125:298, 1977.

4. Butler H. Gastro-esophageal haemorrhage in hepatic cirrhosis. Thorax 7:159, 1952.

5. Kitano S, Terblanche J, Kahn J, et al. Venous anatomy of the lower esophagus in portal hypertension. Practical implications. Br J Surg 73:525, 1986.

6. Sarin SK, Sachdev G, Nauda R, et al. Endoscopic sclerotherapy in the treatment of gastric varices. Br J Surg 75:747, 1988.

7. Vianna A, Hayes PC, Moscoso G, et al. Normal venous circulation of the gastroesophageal junction. Gastroenterology 93:876, 1987.

8. Paquet KJ. Prophylactic endoscopic sclerosing treatment of the esophageal wall in varices: A prospective controlled randomized trial. Endoscopy 14:4, 1982.

9. Beppu K, Inochuki K, Goyna G, et al. Prediction of variceal hemorrhage by esophageal endoscopy. Gastrointest Endosc 27:213, 1981.

10. Paquet KJ, Lindecken KD. Wandsklerosierung der Speilseröhre bei Ösophagusvarizenblutung im Kindesalter. Z Kinderchir 23:269, 1978.

11. Paquet KJ, Oberhammer E. Sclerotherapy of bleeding esophageal varices by means of endoscopy. Endoscopy 10:7, 1978.

12. Paquet KJ. Ein neues Instrument zur Wandsklerosierung von Ösophagusvarizen im Kindesalter und erste Ergebnisse. In Henning, H, ed. Fortschritte der Gastroenterologischen Endoskopie. Baden-Baden: Witzstrock, 1978, p 95.

13. Paquet KJ, Koussouris P. Ten years' experience with paravariceal injection sclerotherapy of esophageal varices in children. J. Pediatr Surg 20:109-112, 1985.

14. Fonkalsrud EW. Surgical management of portal hypertension in childhood. Arch Surg 115:1042, 1980.

15. Aoyama K, Myers NA. Extrahepatic portal hypertension: The significance of variceal hemorrhage. Aust Paediatr J 18:17, 1982.

16. Webb LJ, Sherlock S. The etiology, presentation and natural history of extrahepatic portal venous obstruction. Q J Med 48:627, 1979.

17. Bismuth H, Franco D, Alagille D. Portal diversion for portal hypertension in children. Ann Surg 192:18, 1980.

18. Tocornal J, Cruz F. Portosystemic shunts for extrahepatic portal hypertension in children. Surg Gynecol Obstet 153:52, 1982.

19. Alvarez F, Bernard O, Brunelle F, et al. Portal obstruction in children. II. Results of surgical portosystemic shunts. J Pediatr 103:703, 1983.

20. Bernard O, Alvarez F, Alagille D. Resultats des anastomoses portosystemiques dans les cirrhoses de l'enfant. Arch Fr Pediatr 42:249, 1985.

21. Heloury Y, Valayer J, Hax JM, et al. Hypertension portale chez l'enfant. Chir Paediatr 27:143, 1986.

22. Fonkalsrud EW, Myers NA, Robinson MJ. Management of extraheptic portal hypertension in children. Ann Surg 180:487, 1974.

23. Ulshen MH. To shunt or not to shunt? Gastroenterology 87:446, 1984.

24. Ohi R, Mochizuki I, Komatsu K, et al. Portal hypertension after successful hepatic portoenterostomy in biliary atresia. J Pediatr Surg 21:271-274, 1986.

25. Paquet KJ, Mercado MA, Koussouris P, et al. Improved results with selective distal splenorenal shunt in a highly selected patient population: A prospective study. Ann Surg 210:184, 1989.

26. Paquet KJ, Lazar A, Hotzel B. Rebirth of the mesocaval interposition shunt using narrow-lumen-PTFE-prosthesis in cirrhotics with recurrent variceal hemorrhage in spite of long-term injection sclerotherapy: A prospective study. Gastroenterology 100:A783, 1991.

27. Spence RAJ, Johnston GW, Odling-Smee GW, et al. Bleeding oesophageal varices with long-term follow-up. Arch Dis Child 59:336, 1984.

28. Stellen GP, Lilly JR. Esophageal endosclerosis in children. Surgery 98:970, 1985.

29. Stray N, Fausa O. Injection sclerotherapy of bleeding oesophageal and gastric varices in children. Scand J Gastroenterol 20 (Suppl 107):36, 1985.

30. Vane DW, Boles T, Clatworthy HW. Esophageal sclerotherapy: An effective modality in children. J Pediatr Surg 20:703, 1985.

31. Donovan TJ, Ward M, Sheperd RW. Evaluation of endoscopic sclerotherapy of esophageal varices in children. J Pediatr Gastroenterol Nutr 5:696, 1986.

32. Howard ER, Springer MD, Mowat AP. Assessment of injection sclerotherapy in the management of 152 children with oesophageal varices. Br J Surg 75:404, 1988.

33. Henderson JM, Kutner MH, Millikan U, et al. Endoscopic variceal sclerosis compared with distal splenorenal shunt to prevent recurrent variceal bleeding in cirrhosis: A prospective randomized trial. Ann Intern Med 112:262, 1990.

34. Paquet KJ, Mercado MA, Gad HA, et al. Surgical procedures for bleeding esophagogastric varices when sclerotherapy fails: A prospective study. Ann J Surg 160:43, 1990.

109   *Stoma-Adjustable Silicone Gastric Banding: A New and Less Invasive Operation for Severe Obesity*

F. Favretti, Giuliano Enzi, Gianni Segato, Claudio Belluco, Luca Busetto, and Mario Lise

Gastric partition procedures produce good results in the treatment of severe obesity.[1,2] Stoma-adjustable silicone gastric banding (SASGB) is a recently introduced gastric restrictive procedure.[3,4] The band* is applied around the subcardial area, creating a small measured upper pouch and a calibrated stoma. The operation is fully reversible, and the diameter of the outlet can be adjusted to the patient's needs.

Meticulous measurement of the upper gastric pouch and stoma sizes during the operation is extremely important, as it is in any gastric restriction surgical procedure.[5]

This is a report on the results achieved in our series of 123 SASGB patients. We also stress some important technical aspects to minimize the morbidity rate. Regular supervision is essential in maintaining the efficacy of the technique.

MATERIALS AND METHODS
Patient Selection and Follow-up

The operation and the risks involved were fully described to prospective SASGB patients. Detailed instructions were given on what patients should expect during the postoperative period and what kinds of adjustments would be needed in their eating habits.

All patients were at least 160% of their ideal weight as defined by their height (Ideal Height and Weight Tables from Metropolitan Life Insurance Co.).[6]

Between April 1990 and March 1993 at the Department of Surgery, Padua University, SASGB was performed as a primary operation for weight loss on 123 severely obese patients (89 females, 34 males; mean age, 38 years, range, 16 to 60) who were refractory to dietary and medical regimens and group therapy. Patient demographics are summarized in Tables 1 and 2.

The follow-up consisted of clinical control and body weight measurement 2 and 4 weeks postoperatively and then every 2 months. Body weight was expressed in kilograms and as a percentage of the ideal body weight (IBW). The body mass index (BMI) was also calculated. Because the aim of any treatment for obesity is loss of excess body weight, we used the percentage of excess weight lost (% EWL) to show postoperative weight loss. Means and standard deviations were calculated for all the parameters considered.

The Stoma-Adjustable Silicone Gastric Band

The SASGB (Fig. 1) consists of a Dacron-reinforced silicone band that is 22.5 cm long, 1 cm wide, and 0.3 cm thick. The Dacron mesh incorporated into the SASGB

Table 1. Patient demographics for April 1990–March 1993 series

No. of patients	123 (F, 89; M, 34)
Age (yr)	38 (16-60)
Body weight (kg)	129.5 ±25
% Ideal body weight	207.8 ±31
Body mass index	46.7 ±8.7
Mean follow-up (days)	483

Table 2. Obesity demographics

Morbidly Obese

No. of patients	91
Body weight (kg)	121.2 ±15
% Ideal body weight	196.2 ±17

Superobese

No. patients	32
Body weight (kg)	154.7 ±21
% Ideal body weight	247.7 ±19

---

* The SASGB is manufactured by Bioenterics Corporation, 1035A Cindy Lane, Carpinteria, CA 93013.

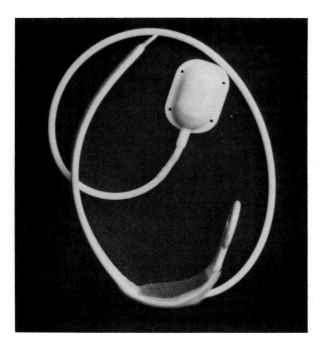

Fig. 1. Stoma-adjustable silicone gastric band. (Courtesy L. Kuzmak, M.D., and Bioenterics Corporation.)

provides strength and limits distention. The exterior surface of the entire band is made of soft silicone elastomer, chosen for its biocompatibility and inertness. The SASGB is radiopaque. An inflatable silicone section 4 cm long is outlined on the band by heavy contrast blue markers. A radiopaque nonkinking 60 cm tube is attached to connect the inflatable section to the subcutaneous reservoir. The self-sealing injection reservoir is for percutaneous band volume adjustment.

Calibrating Tube and Electronic Sensor

The upper gastric pouch and stoma are calibrated with the calibrating tube and electronic sensor (see Fig. 6). The calibrating tube has two separate parts, one of which has a balloon that can be inflated to measure the pouch size (25 cc). Below the balloon is an air chamber that is connected to the electronic sensor during the stoma calibration. The diameter of the air chamber is 13 mm. When the band is tightened over the stomach, the air chamber is compressed. Compression of the air chamber activates different lights on the electronic sensor (gastrostenometer), with each particular light cor-

responding to a specific stoma-diameter size. A fourth light indicates that the stoma diameter is 12.5 mm, which is the stoma size currently used.

Surgical Procedure

SASGB was performed using Kuzmak's technique[7] in all patients (Fig. 2).

An upper midline incision is made, extending from the xyphoid process to the umbilicus and through the subcutaneous tissue to the linea alba. A pocket (for later placement of the self-sealing reservoir) is made on the right rectus sheath by dissecting the subcutaneous tissue approximately 10 cm from the anterior rectus sheath, using cutting cautery. After the dissection of the subcutaneous tissue is completed, a small part of the rectus sheath is opened transversely, and a small part of the rectus muscle is incised with cutting cautery to form a pocket for later placement of the reservoir. The midline fascia is next incised from the xyphoid process to the umbilicus. The peritoneum is opened and the abdomen inspected.

The abdominal retractors are inserted to obtain good exposure of the subdiaphragmatic area and gastroesophageal junction.

Before mobilization of the stomach, the adhesions to the spleen should be secured and transected to avoid splenic injury during dissection. The stomach is inspected, and a small opening is made in the avascular portion of the hepatogastric ligament. The thumb is inserted through an opening below the pedicle of the gastric vessels underneath the stomach. By blunt dissection with the thumb, a tunnel is made toward the gastrophrenic ligament proximal to the short gastric vessels. With the index finger, an opening is made in the gastrophrenic ligament proximal to the short gastric vessels (Fig. 3).

A Penrose drain is placed through these openings and around the stomach (Fig. 4). Further mobilization of the pouch is carried out. In a few cases it may be necessary to secure and transect the short gastric vessel to obtain the proper-sized pouch.

After sufficiently mobilizing the fundus, a small opening is made at the edge of the lesser curvature, 2 cm below the gastroesophageal junction and medial to the gastric vessels and vagus nerve. The index finger is inserted behind the stomach and lesser curvature for traction. A kidney pedicle is used to puncture the tissue next to the stomach. No attempt should be made

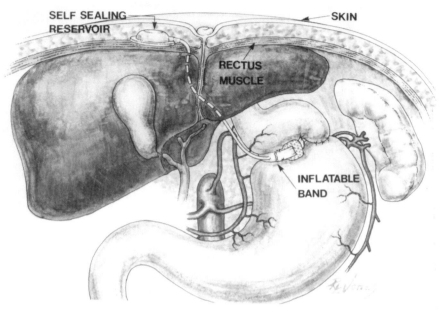

Fig. 2. Placement of stoma-adjustable silicone gastric banding. (Courtesy L. Kuzmak, M.D., and Bioenterics Corporation.)

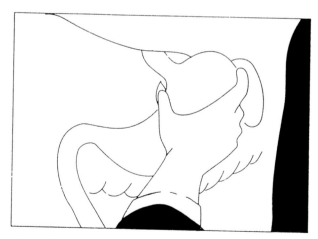

Fig. 3. Blunt dissection of the gastrophrenic ligament. (Courtesy L. Kuzmak, M.D., and Bioenterics Corporation.)

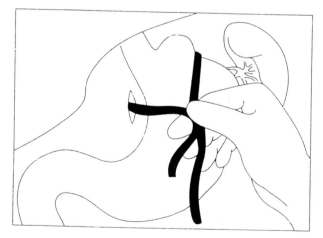

Fig. 4. Placement of Penrose drain. (Courtesy L. Kuzmak, M.D., and Bioenterics Corporation.)

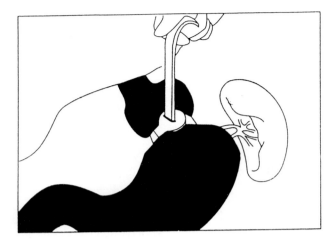

Fig. 5. Manually pulling gastric band strap. (Courtesy L. Kuzmak, M.D., and Bioenterics Corporation.)

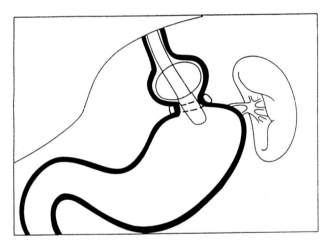

Fig. 6. Cross section of the stomach with calibration tube and gastric band in place. (Courtesy L. Kuzmak, M.D., and Bioenterics Corporation.)

Fig. 7. Band tightening tool and band holder. (Courtesy L. Kuzmak, M.D., and Bioenterics Corporation.)

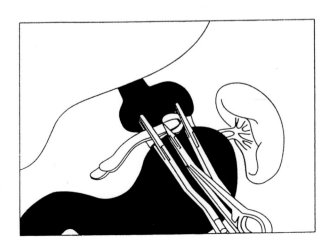

to puncture the tissue blindly, because to do so may perforate the lesser curvature. The edge of the lesser curvature must be seen during the procedure. The opening produced should be only large enough barely to allow introduction of the gastric band, because overdissection may result in movement of the band and require reoperation.

The Penrose drain is relocated through the opening around the stomach. At that point, the silicone band is prepared for implantation by irrigating the inflatable part and the silicone tube with saline solution to purge the air. The band is then preinflated with 0.8 to 1 ml of saline solution and the silicone tube clamped with a rubber-shod clamp. The prepared band is threaded through the opening next to the lesser curvature and around the stomach (Fig. 5).

At this point, the anesthesiologist inserts the calibrating tube. The pouch volume is measured by inflating the balloon, which is retracted against the gastroesophageal junction. The stomach is pulled down, and the band is tightened by hand just below the balloon (Fig. 6). The mobilized greater curvature is sutured initially with one 3-0 silk suture to the pouch to stabilize the position of the band. On the pouch the suture must be placed superficially to avoid accidental puncturing of the inflated balloon (see Fig. 2).

Stoma calibration is done by tightening the band around the stomach and the air chamber on the calibrating tube. When the calibrating tube is connected to the electronic sensor, the band is tightened, using the band-tightening tool (see Fig. 6).

At activation of the fourth light on the sensor, the banding instrument is secured with a screw, and the band holder is placed to hold the band together (Fig. 7). The banding instrument and the calibrating tube are removed, and the band is easily sutured together. Four 2-0 Ethibond sutures (Ethicon) are used. The excess of the band and the buckle are excised, at which point two or three seromuscular, 3-0 silk sutures are used to suture the mobilized greater curvature to the pouch to prevent migration of the band (see Fig. 2). The silicone tube is then placed over the pouch and under the diaphragm, where it is secured with 3-0 chromic sutures. With a long clamp, the posterior rectus sheath is then punctured proximal to the space previously prepared for the injection port implantation. The silicone tube is threaded to that space, trimmed to the proper length, and connected to the injection port, which has been filled and irrigated with saline solution. The injection port is then implanted within the prepared space, and its position is secured with one or two sutures to the posterior rectus sheath. The area of banding is irrigated with antibiotic solution, and the incisions are closed in the usual fashion.

RESULTS

The mortality rate with SASGB was zero. Early and late complications are summarized in Tables 3 and 4. A surgical revision without removal of the band was made in the two patients with band slipping and in the six patients with stoma stenosis and pouch dilation. The SASGB was removed in one patient with band erosion and in one with proximal gastric herniation. One patient with an ulcer on the neostoma and one with an ulcer in the upper pouch were treated medically. The injection part was removed from a patient who experienced an injection port infection. A leakage in the reservoir appeared in two patients who had a replacement of the injection port.

Weight loss for all the patients (Table 5) and for the morbidly obese (Table 6) and superobese (Table 7)

Table 3. Early complications

Condition	Number
Outlet stenosis	1
Reservoir-related leak	2
Bronchopneumonia	7
Superficial venous thrombosis	6

Table 4. Late complications

Condition	Number
Slipping of band	2
Outlet stenosis and pouch dilation	6
Band erosion	1
Proximal gastric herniation	1
Infected injection port site	1
Upper pouch ulcer	1
Neostoma ulcer	1

groups is shown as a variation of body weight, %EWL, and BMI.

DISCUSSION

The creation of a small proximal gastric pouch is an effective method to achieve weight reduction.[1,2] Among gastric restrictive procedures, SASGB appears promising because it allows the surgeon to create a small upper pouch with a well-calibrated stoma. The procedure does not involve the use of staples, nor is the stomach wall cut or crushed. Moreover, the neostoma can be adjusted to each patient's needs, and the operation is fully reversible.[7]

In our series of 123 consecutive patients the mortal-

Table 5. Weight loss (123 patients)

Time	0	1 yr	2 yr	3 yr
No. of patients	123	94	46	15
BW (kg)	129.5 ±25	101.0 ±21	90.6 ±20	89.3 ±14
EWL (%)	—	41.1 ±19	54.6 ±23	59.0 ±21
IBW (%)	207.8 ±30	163.6 ±31	147.5 ±30	145.9 ±26
BMI	46.7 ±9	36.4 ±7	32.8 ±7	32.3 ±6

BW = body weight; EWL = excess weight lost; IBW = ideal body weight; BMI = body mass index.

Table 6. Weight loss in morbidly obese group

Time	0	1 yr	2 yr	3 yr
No. of patients	91	64	34	11
BW (kg)	121.2 ±15	93.4 ±15	85.6 ±15	89.7 ±13
EWL (%)	—	45.7 ±18	57.7 ±22	60.6 ±21
IBW (%)	196.2 ±17	152.6 ±21	141.5 ±22	140.5 ±22
BMI	43.8 ±4	34.0 ±5	31.4 ±5	31.1 ±5

BW = body weight; EWL = excess weight lost; IBW = ideal body weight; BMI = body mass index.

Table 7. Weight loss in superobese group

Time	0	1 yr	2 yr	3 yr
No. of patients	32	25	10	4
BW (kg)	154.7 ±21	121.2 ±23	110.7 ±21	99.2 ±14
EWL (%)	—	35.3 ±18	48.9 ±23	54.5 ±24
IBW (%)	247.7 ±19	195.6 ±30	176.6 ±34	161.0 ±33
BMI	55.0 ±4	43.4 ±6	39.2 ±8	35.7 ±8

BW = body weight; EWL = excess weight lost; IBW = ideal body weight; BMI = body mass index.

ity rate was zero, and early morbidity was negligible. Two patients were reoperated because the original band slipped upward around the cardia, thus requiring replacement. Because this complication apparently is caused by early postoperative vomiting, an attempt should be made to control the patients' eating habits in the immediate postoperative period.

Six patients underwent further surgical revision without removal of the band because of stoma stenosis with pouch dilation and one patient because of stoma stenosis only. These complications were caused by overtight banding and incorrect neostoma calibration at the initial operation. All these patients underwent SASGB during our initial experience.

The calibration instructions specified by the suppliers must be followed with care.

There are no standard criteria for assessing the success of surgery in terms of weight loss, but it is generally accepted that if the patient's weight decreases to within 140% of IBW, most of the obesity-related health hazards will be circumvented and the operation can be considered successful, provided the weight loss can be maintained. More than 80% of our patients with a follow-up of at least 12 months moved from the high-risk to the low-risk group. The average of our patients reaches a body weight 147 ±29% of IBW 2 years after the operation.

The band eroded in one patient; we have not been able to find an explanation for this complication, which required the removal of the SASGB.

Another patient, with a body weight of 70 kg, who experienced proximal gastric herniation, requested removal of the SASGB. Overdissection on the lesser curve caused this complication.

The two patients with an ulcer in the upper pouch and at neostoma level were taking FANS despite different medical advice. They were treated with anti-H_2-blockers.

The patients' body weight decreased from a mean of 121.2 kg (morbidly obese group) and 154.7 kg (superobese group) to 85.7 and 99.2 kg, respectively, at 3 years (see Tables 6 and 7). The percent of EWL reached 60.6% and 54.5% in the morbidly obese and superobese groups at 3 years, with a corresponding change in BMI.

Although the results reported here are preliminary, our findings show that weight loss after SASGB is comparable to that produced by more extensive operations.[5]

Our patients were monitored closely every 2 months, and their eating habits were investigated carefully. If no weight loss occurred for 2 to 3 months, the band was readjusted nonsurgically. We believe that regular supervision is important in maximizing the efficacy of this technique.

CONCLUSION

The surgical treatment of morbid obesity by SASGB is a safe and effective means of producing successful weight reduction and social rehabilitation. The long-term aim is dietary modification, and the operation is the initial treatment. Since there is no long-term information available on the outcome of SASGB, longer clinical trials are required.

REFERENCES

1. Mason EE. Vertical banded gastroplasty. In Proceedings of the American Society for Bariatric Surgery, annual meeting. San Francisco: 1985, The Society, pp 181-188.
2. Deitel M, Jones BA, Petrov I, et al. Vertical banded gastroplasty: Results in 233 patients. Can J Surg 29:322-324, 1986.
3. Kuzmak L. Silicone gastric banding: A simple and effective operation for morbid obesity. Contemp Surg 28:13-18, 1986.
4. Kuzmak L. Gastric banding. In Deitel M, ed. Surgery for the Morbidly Obese Patient. Philadelphia: Lea & Febiger, 1989, pp 225-259.
5. Mason EE, Maher JW, Scott DH, et al. Ten years of vertical banded gastroplasty for severe obesity. In Mason EE, ed. Surgical Treatment of Morbid Obesity, vol 9. Philadelphia: JB Lippincott, 1992, pp 280-289.
6. 1983 Metropolitan Height and Weight Tables. Stat Bull Metropolitan Ins Co 64:2, 1983.
7. Kuzmak L. Stoma adjustable silicone gastric banding. In Mason EE, ed. Surgical Treatment of Morbid Obesity, vol 9. Philadelphia: JB Lippincott, 1992, pp 298-317.

XVI

Videoendoscopic
Gastroduodenal Surgery

110 *Preliminary Results of Laparoscopic Repair of Perforated Duodenal Ulcers*

Ara Darzi, P. Declan Carey, N. Menzies-Gow, and John R.T. Monson

The widespread success of laparoscopic cholecystectomy has led to the development of a wide range of laparoscopic surgical procedures such as hernia repair,[1,2] colectomy,[3] Nissen fundoplication,[4] and vagotomy.[5]

In peptic ulcer disease complicated by anterior duodenal perforation, laparoscopic repair could offer a number of advantages. First, laparoscopy would confirm the diagnosis. Second, a better view of the anterior peritoneal cavity with the video laparoscope would allow a more thorough washout of the peritoneal cavity. Finally, the lack of an upper abdominal incision, especially in elderly patients who are often frail, should allow early mobilization and reduction of postoperative complications.

This report documents our initial experience with an attempt to perform laparoscopic repair of a perforated duodenal ulcer in six consecutive patients with peritonitis admitted through the emergency department. The evolution of the different techniques used, the difficulties encountered, and patient outcome are described.

MATERIALS AND METHODS

Six patients underwent laparoscopically assisted repair of a perforated duodenal ulcer. The mean age was 62 years. All were admitted with acute abdominal pain with no previous history of peptic ulcers. Clinical and radiological findings were suggestive of duodenal perforation. After an initial period of resuscitation and correction of fluid and electrolyte disturbances, patients were prepared for emergency laparoscopy. All patients received prophylactic antibiotics at the time of anesthesia induction.

All procedures were carried out under general anesthesia, with endotracheal intubation and full muscle relaxation. All patients had a urinary catheter inserted to empty the bladder and monitor urinary output. A large-bore nasogastric tube was inserted into the stomach, and gastric contents were aspirated to ensure that the stomach was empty.

Patients were placed in the supine position with legs spread apart. This is similar to the technique we have adopted for laparoscopic cholecystectomy. The operating surgeon stood between the legs of the patient, and an assistant was stationed on the left side of the patient. A second assistant was positioned on the patient's right. The operating room was set up so that the light source, insufflator, and video monitors were in direct view of the entire surgical team. Patients were prepared and draped as for open laparotomy.

A pneumoperitoneum was established with CO_2; the intraperitoneal pressure was maintained at or below 15 mm Hg. The insufflation needle was introduced through the umbilicus or just below.

The first port (10 mm) was located at the umbilicus and was used to introduce the forward-viewing laparoscope. Then, under direct vision, the remaining trocars were inserted through the abdominal wall. A 5 mm port was placed just below and to the right of the xiphoid process and was used for introducing blunt-nosed retractors or an aspiration-lavage probe. A 10 mm port was located in the left upper quadrant at the anterior axillary line, which allowed for insertion of an atraumatic Babcock clamp. This was used to retract the gastric antrum downward and to the left to expose the first part of the duodenum. Two more 10 mm ports were located to the right and left of the umbilical port at the midclavicular line, for the insertion of grasping forceps and needle holders. On occasion the laparoscope was interchanged between the umbilical port and the port to the left of the umbilicus.

The operative procedure was similar in many ways to the traditional open operation. The abdominal cavity was first explored with the video laparoscope to determine the degree of peritoneal soiling and the site of perforation, since acute duodenal perforations are usually anterior and easily identified through the laparoscope. Abdominal fluid was obtained for bacterial culture and sensitivity testing. After the peritoneal cavity was irrigated copiously with warm saline solution, the perforation was closed. Simple closure can be achieved by using a laparoscopic needle holder with a 2-0 synthetic braided suture either on a ski needle or a curved needle. One or two additional sutures are placed, with knots tied intracorporeally or extracorporeally, approximating the omentum over the site of perforation with each suture, in the traditional manner. The pneumoperitoneum was desufflated and the abdominal punctures were closed.

The nasogastric tube was left in place for a minimum of 48 hours following closure of an acute duodenal perforation. All patients received a conventional regimen of H_2 antagonist.

RESULTS

As of September 1991, we have performed six operations for perforated duodenal ulcer with no mortality and minimal morbidity. Two patients were given a Gastrografin meal 48 hours after the repair to ensure that there was no leakage. The mean hospital stay was 6 days. Repeat upper GI endoscopy was performed in all patients 6 to 8 weeks after operation, which confirmed that the ulcer had healed. Two patients had postoperative respiratory tract infections. No other septic complications were recorded.

DISCUSSION

Laparoscopic surgery has already revolutionized the practice of biliary procedures and is likely to have an ever-increasing impact on many gastrointestinal operations.[6] Although laparoscopic cholecystectomy has been undeniably successful, it would seem reasonable to suggest that even greater benefits might be achieved in the treatment of patients who were septic with peritonitis. Following laparoscopic cholecystectomy the considerable reduction in postoperative pain has led to rapid recovery with an attendant decrease in complications such as chest infections and particularly wound sepsis.[7,8] If this was also to be reflected in patients undergoing repair of perforated duodenal ulcers it would certainly represent a therapeutic and possibly economic advance. In addition, a significant number of patients with perforated duodenal ulcers are frail and elderly, which makes a laparoscopic procedure even more attractive. Our initial experience would tend to confirm this supposition in those patients in whom the operation could be successfully performed laparoscopically. The complete absence of wound sepsis in our patients has been most gratifying, as indeed has been the low incidence of other septic complications. Early mobilization was a marked feature in this series with nearly all patients being fully mobile within 72 hours of the operation. Our efforts have also allowed us to identify some defects in the instrumental technology of laparoscopic surgery that require further refinement. In the first four patients we adopted a technique of intracorporeal knot tying, which seemed to be tedious and time consuming. In the last two patients we adopted a technique of extracorporeal knot tying, and the knot was then pushed into position with a special knot pusher. Both techniques were equally effective.

Some investigators have suggested that if the perforation is less than 12 hours old an acid-reducing procedure should be contemplated, either a truncal or selective vagotomy, depending on the operative findings and the experience of the surgeon. However, we believe that simple closure is adequate in the emergency setting except in patients with associated duodenal stricture and gastric outlet obstruction.

CONCLUSION

It is clear from this series that the operation is technically feasible in the majority of patients. In addition, it is associated with greatly reduced postoperative discomfort and a rapid return to mobility. Morbidity appears to be reduced, particularly with regard to septic complications. Our preliminary experience leads us to suggest that as laparoscopic technology improves and surgical expertise is gained, this minimally invasive approach will become the operation of choice for perforated duodenal ulcers.

REFERENCES

1. Nyhus LM. Laparoscopic hernia repair: A point of view. Arch Surg 127:137, 1992.
2. Paget GW. Laparoscopic repair of inguinal hernia. Med J Aust 156:508-510, 1992.
3. Monson JRT, Drazi A, Carey PD, et al. Prospective evaluation of laparoscopic assisted colectomy in an unselected group of patients. Lancet 1:831-833, 1992.
4. Cuschieri A, Shimi S, Nathanson LK. Laparoscopic reduction, crural repair and fundoplication of large hiatal hernia. Am J Surg 163:425-430, 1992.
5. Katkhouda N, Mouiel J. A new technique of surgical treatment of chronic duodenal ulcer without laparotomy by videocoelioscopy. Am J Surg 161:361-364, 1991.
6. Tompkins RK. Laparoscopic cholecystectomy: Threat or opportunity? Arch Surg 125:1245, 1990.
7. Myers WC, Branaum GD, Farouk M, et al. A prospective analysis of 1518 laparoscopic cholecystectomies. N Engl J Med 324:1073-1078, 1991.
8. Peters JH, Ellison EC, Innes JT, et al. Safety and efficacy of laparoscopic cholecystectomy. A prospective analysis of 100 consecutive patients. Ann Surg 213:3-12, 1990.

111 *Posterior Truncal Vagotomy and Denervating Anterior Vertical Linear Strip Gastrectomy: A New Laparoscopic Technique for Treating Chronic Duodenal Ulcers*

Fernando Gomez-Ferrer

FIRST EXPERIMENTAL STUDY

It is currently accepted that surgery constitutes a valid alternative to continuous antisecretory treatment in young patients with ulcers who are otherwise healthy. Admittedly, medical treatment is rarely unsuccessful when full doses of antisecretory medication are administered over prolonged periods; however, these medications occasionally cause side effects such as diarrhea, steatorrhea, or diminished libido, and as a result many patients discontinue treatment.

Just as gastroenterologists comment on the cost of surgery, its complications, and recurrences, surgeons may speak of identical problems with the use of antisecretory drugs. Often complications develop as a result of duodenal ulcers and recurrence of ulcers, and the mortality rate in such instances is quite high. Gastroenterologists admit that surgery provides a better means to prevent and treat the complications of duodenal ulcers; in effect, surgeons are better equipped to alter the natural course of the disease and reduce mortality while securing a positive cost-benefit relationship.

The expected outcome of surgery includes zero mortality (after all, the disease is regarded as benign), low morbidity, a very low recurrence rate, and a technically acceptable result. These requirements are not always satisfied, even when the most complete procedure available to date is performed—that is, vagotomy and antrectomy. In any event, such surgery is advisable for recurrences in patients undergoing medical treatment, when cicatrization cannot be achieved, even with correct medical protocol, and in the case of prepyloric ulcers. Young patients with ulcers who are otherwise healthy and who respond favorably to medication in the event of a recurrence are ideal candidates for vagotomy. But the question remains: Why a vagotomy?

Proximal gastric vagotomy (PGV) is the most highly regarded option presently available. However, it should be stressed that the success achieved with this technique depends largely on the experience of the surgeon who performs it; that is, it continues to pose inconveniences, and as a result only 17% of surgeons in Great Britain choose this option. However, it has been accepted that the results achieved with a combination of vagotomy and pyloroplasty are superior to those achieved with supraselective denervation. With the aim of avoiding pyloroplasty, in the early 1970s other techniques were adopted, including Griffith's technique[1] (posterior truncal vagotomy [PTV] and selective anterior denervation), the Hill-Barker technique[2] (PTV with supraselective anterior denervation), and Taylor's second technique[3] (PTV with anterior seromyotomy). As a result, nerve regeneration has been reported following parietal cell vagotomy.[4,5]

In 1985 I realized that there were no reports in the literature on possible nerve regeneration of the anterior gastric surface following seromyotomy of the lesser curvature. The following year I suggested that PTV be performed with continuous and vertical anterior seromyotomy of the lesser curvature to the upper part of the greater tuberosity. I likewise proposed a modification of this approach, in which the seromyotomy was replaced by gastrotomy along the same trajectory as described earlier. In this technique we sectioned all layers of the gastric wall with eversion suturing after appropriate hemostasis. This method achieved maximum sectioning of the vagal fibers, interrupting the nerve branches descending from the mediastinal esophagus toward the gastric plexuses, thus preventing any possible regeneration through either these fibers or the serosa.[6,7] The purpose of the first experimental study was to evaluate denervation and possible nerve regeneration of the anterior gastric wall following PTV with either seromyotomy or anterior gastrotomy.

Methods

Twenty-eight preadult male Wistar rats (220 ± 10 g) were randomly divided as follows: group I (control: laparotomy and reference suture on the anterior gastric wall; n = 4), group II (seromyotomy of the lesser gastric curvature, with PTV; n = 12), and group III (gastrotomy of the lesser gastric curvature with the use of eversion sutures, with posterior truncal vagotomy; n = 12). The animals were fasted for 24 hours before operation. Anesthesia was achieved with sodium pentobarbital (40 mg/kg intraperitoneally). All operations were performed at approximately the same time of day, that is, at the same point in the circadian rhythm of the rats (12-hour light-darkness cycles; 22° C).

Seromyotomy. Following a vertical midline laparotomy, the stomach wall was exposed after displacing the liver upward. The serosa and oblique and circular muscle layers were sectioned parallel to the lesser gastric curvature from the antrum to the upper fundus region. A scalpel was used in all cases for the serosal incision, whereas the muscle layers were cut with a scalpel or blunt scissors. Following full-thickness sectioning of the gastric wall, hemostasis was achieved with catgut 4/0 sutures. In one rat a small mucosal orifice required suturing. Electrocoagulation was not performed; slight pressure applied with hydrophilic cotton was found to be useful. To provide a good separation between nerve fibers (3 to 4 mm), the serosa was not sutured as described by Taylor et al.[3]

Gastrotomy. In group III all stomach layers were sectioned from the crow's foot to the upper part of the greater gastric tuberosity. Following hemostasis the wall was closed with slowly reabsorbing eversion sutures (4/0). Postoperatively the rats were housed individually and given chow ad libitum (83.1% carbohydrates, 6.1% vegetable proteins, 6% animal proteins, 4% vitamin and mineral supplement). Body weight was monitored every 5 days. All animals gained approximately 30 g during the first 2 postoperative months; at this point the surgical specimens were harvested under anesthesia as described previously. Following removal, the pieces were fixed in neutral 1% formaldehyde and embedded in paraffin.

Immunohistochemistry. Sections of fixed tissue, 5 μm thick, were deparaffined and hydrated for peroxidase/antiperoxidase (PAP) immunostaining. Endogenous peroxidase was inhibited by treating the sections with 1% methanol-hydrogen peroxide for 30 minutes at room temperature. The sections were then washed successively in Tris-saline buffer, 0.05 mol/L (pH 7.6), and covered with nonimmune 20% horse serum (Oxoid) for 20 minutes to inhibit nonspecific collagen staining. The specimens were then covered in sequence with the following diluted antisera: rabbit serum against bovine

S-100 protein (1/200), swine serum against rabbit immunoglobulins (1/50), and rabbit PAP complex (1/100). Specimens were incubated for 3 to 5 minutes at room temperature.

After several washings in buffer, peroxidase activity was assayed by the benzidine method (3,3-diaminobenzidine, DAB) (50 mg DAB dissolved in 0.2 mol/L Tris buffer, pH 7.4, and adding 30 μl of hydrogen peroxide). The sections were incubated in the recently prepared medium for 3 to 5 minutes, followed by washing in tap water, and contrasting the nuclei with hematoxylin-eosin stain. Finally the pieces were dehydrated, rinsed in saline, and embedded in synthetic resin. Positive and negative control sections (from malignant melanomas) were included and processed along with the rest of the study material.

Results

Postoperative mortality and morbidity were zero. There were no wound infections or dehiscences. At sacrifice, all rats subjected to either seromyotomy or gastrotomy with PTV had marked gastric dilation. Sternberg's method showed anterior wall innervation to be normal among the control animals (group I) (Figs. 1 and 2). Total denervation was achieved after surgery in groups II and III (Fig. 3). The denervation achieved was similarly complete in both the seromyotomy and gastrotomy groups (Fig. 4); amputation neuromas were observed, but no nerve regeneration was seen (Fig. 5). Finally, partial or total sectioning of the lesser curvature again failed to influence the possible passage of nerve fibers from healthy areas to the denervated region (Figs. 6 and 7).

Discussion

The results of our study reflect good denervation of the gastric corpus and fundus after both seromyotomy and gastrotomy with eversion suturing. At sacrifice, 2 months after operation, no nerve regeneration was noted. The 2-month period is equivalent to 3 years in humans.[8] With the aim of promoting possible nerve regeneration, the animals were operated on during their period of maximum vitality. Nerve reparation phenomena were seen occasionally, and a number of amputation neuromas and Schwann cells were noted. However, in no case were nerve fibers observed to pass from healthy zones to the denervated region. Moreover, in the event of morphological evidence of reinnervation, long-term functional tests would be required to certify possible functional regeneration.

To secure maximum sectioning of the nerve plexus

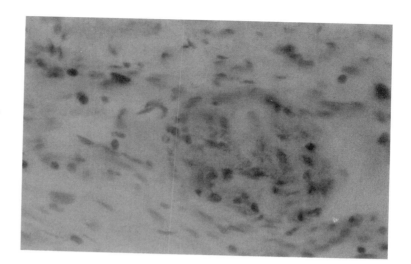

Fig. 1. Normal nerve section showing transversely sectioned Schwann cells and nerve filaments. (Sternberg stain [peroxidase/antiperoxidase] for protein S-100 antigen.)

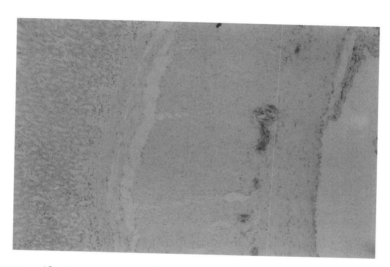

Fig. 2. Higher magnification of the normal gastric wall, with mucosa on the right and intramuscular plexus on the left.

Fig. 3. Gastric wall of a rat subjected to seromyotomy. Innervation has completely disappeared. Only nuclei are observed, with no antigen activity.

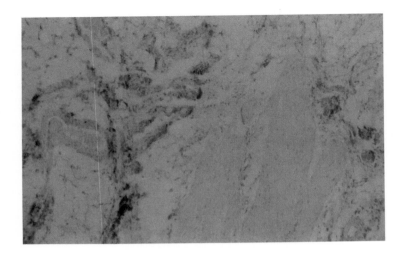

Fig. 4. Large mass of disoriented filaments with occasional sectioned nerves. Note filaments exhibiting focal regeneration to produce amputation neuromas.

Fig. 5. Section zone with oblique scar. Musculature lacking nerves.

Fig. 6. Scar tissue with suture points. Completely denervated zone appears on the left; right side is healthy.

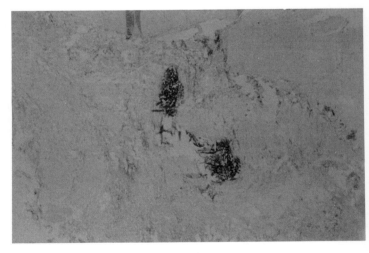

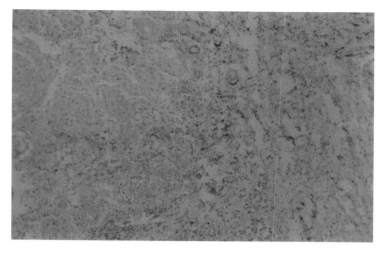

Fig. 7. Detail showing isolated cells, granulation tissue with total lack of organization. Occasional disoriented Schwann cells are seen.

of the gastric wall and to completely avoid any possible nerve regeneration, we used a technique derived from gastrotomy with eversion suturing. This approach involves removal of a full-thickness strip of anterior wall of the lesser curve with a mechanical stapler. The technique is easy to perform, and we think it offers the same advantages as highly selective vagotomy and seromyotomy: it is nonaggressive and has no profound functional consequences. However, its efficacy in diminishing the risk of recurrences is perhaps more relevant, since the denervation achieved is more extensive in length and depth than that of seromyotomy. We have used this procedure under laparoscopic guidance, further simplifying the postoperative course.

SECOND EXPERIMENTAL STUDY

Since functional tests may be more useful in the long run than morphological evaluation of surgical outcome, we decided to complement operation with an experimental study of gastric secretion. The second technical variant, called *anterior linear-strip gastrectomy* (ALG) (i.e., sectioning of all gastric layers and suturing), is easier to perform by removing a full-thickness strip of gastric wall with staplers. Hemostasis is achieved at stapling, thus sealing the stomach and preventing any possible peritoneal contamination. The risk of dehiscence is minimal. We used this experimental model to study the influence of ALG with PTV on gastric secretion, transit, body weight, and nerve regeneration.

Methods

Thirty-one male Wistar rats (184 g average birth weight), housed under identical conditions, were subjected to gastric intubation with neonatal 8/10 catheters to determine gastric pH. The animals were divided into four groups according to the surgical technique performed following sodium pentobarbital anesthesia (40 mg/kg). Surgery in group I (control, n = 7) was limited to PTV. In group II (n = 8) surgery involved PTV with continuous anterior seromyotomy of the lesser curvature and fundus and use of a low-voltage electric scalpel. Group III (n = 8) underwent PTV with ALG according to the following protocol: A reference-traction silk stitch was placed at the vertex of the fundus and another at the origin of the crow's foot; this delineated a fold parallel to the lesser curvature reaching the fundus. Traction was exerted on the stitches (an additional central stitch was applied as required) and the fold was carefully raised. The TA-30 stapler arms were placed in the open position so that a small "pinched" gastric wall fold stood out. The stapler was then closed and the trigger pulled, followed by resection of the raised fold with a manual scalpel, thus leaving a 4 to 5 mm linear gastrectomy. Finally, hemostasis was completed with U-sutures. In group IV (n = 8) surgery involved PTV with ALG, as in the preceding group, but a GIA-50 stapler was used. Gastric pH was evaluated weekly for 3 months in all rats. Esophagogastroduodenal transit was studied in one rat from each group to evaluate gastric emptying, transit rate, and possible leakage. Under superficial anesthesia, 5 ml of barium sulfate was injected with a sonde catheter, followed by x-ray evaluation after 5, 15, 30, and 45 minutes. Each animal was weighed after surgery, and weight changes were recorded over the next 3 months. The rats were sacrificed 3 months after surgery, and the stomachs were prepared for light-microscopic histological study of the anterior gastric region with hematoxylin-eosin, periodic acid–Schiff, and Masson trichrome stains. Denervation was evaluated immunohistochemically with S-100 protein and gastrin markers.

Results

There were no deaths between the time of surgery and when the rats were sacrificed 3 months later. The postoperative course was optimal in all cases. There were two laparotomy wound infections in group II. In all cases the transit rate was normal, and no differences in fecal color or consistency were noted after surgery. No diarrhea was observed.

Gastric pH. Mean gastric pH for all four groups was 2.86. Table 1 shows the mean pH corresponding to weekly recordings over a 3-month period (i.e., the mean of 12 postoperative determinations) in group I. Fig. 1 shows the mean for each rat. The net mean pH value in group I was 3.73 ± 0.64. Corresponding information is provided for group II in Table 2 and Fig. 2, where the mean pH for all animals was 4.71 ± 0.69, and for group III in Table 3 and Fig. 3, where the mean pH for all animals was 5.02 ± 0.65. Finally, Table 4 shows the mean pH for the eight rats in group IV, whereas Fig. 4 reflects the mean pH for each individual animal. Mean pH in this group was 5.33 ± 0.60. Table 5 shows the compar-

Table 1. Comparative pH results before and after surgery (pH 0) in group I (control)

	pH 0	R1	R2	R3	R4	R5	R6	R7
$\bar{x}$	2.86	3.34	3.52	4.34	4.21	3.82	3.99	2.94
	±0.10	±0.41	±0.45	±0.60	±0.46	±0.38	±0.47	±0.34
Maximum	4.85	5.33	5.41	6.59	5.32	5.50	5.98	4.05
Minimum	2.18	2.59	2.22	3.18	2.80	2.72	3.04	2.18
SD	0.60	0.77	0.84	1.11	0.86	0.70	0.87	0.63
%VC	0.20	0.23	0.23	0.25	0.20	0.18	0.21	0.21

$p < 0.05.$

Table 2. Comparative pH results before and after surgery (pH 0) in group II (electric scalpel)

	pH 0	R8	R9	R10	R11	R12	R13	R14	R15
$\bar{x}$	2.86	3.76	5.29	4.54	4.09	5.60	5.02	4.46	4.97
	±0.10	±0.58	±0.38	±0.47	±0.62	±0.27	±0.65	±0.79	±0.57
Maximum	4.85	5.98	6.56	5.76	5.83	6.28	6.32	7.10	6.12
Minimum	2.18	2.29	4.21	2.79	2.50	4.90	2.53	2.50	2.88
SD	0.60	1.07	0.71	0.88	1.15	0.50	1.20	1.46	1.06
%VC	0.20	0.28	0.13	0.19	0.28	0.80	0.23	0.32	0.21

$p < 0.05.$

Table 3. Comparative pH results before and after surgery (pH 0) in group III (TA-30 stapler)

	pH 0	R16	R17	R18	R19	R20	R21	R22	R23
$\bar{x}$	2.86	5.13	3.85	5.26	4.15	5.34	5.33	5.48	5.65
	±0.10	±0.75	±0.50	±0.66	±0.54	±0.45	±0.34	±0.45	±0.36
Maximum	4.85	7.25	5.09	6.71	5.82	6.66	6.09	6.57	6.32
Minimum	2.18	3.10	2.27	3.19	2.56	3.74	4.00	3.45	4.10
SD	0.60	1.39	0.92	1.22	1.01	0.84	0.64	0.83	0.67
%VC	0.20	0.27	0.23	0.23	0.24	0.15	0.12	0.15	0.11

$p < 0.05$.

Table 4. Comparative pH results before and after surgery (pH 0) in group IV (GIA-50 stapler)

	pH 0	R24	R25	R26	R27	R28	R29	R30	R31
$\bar{x}$	2.86	5.09	5.11	6.21	5.25	5.69	4.95	5.33	5.08
	±0.10	±0.38	±0.72	±0.34	±0.47	±0.53	±0.51	±0.32	±0.51
Maximum	4.85	6.04	7.04	6.87	6.25	6.82	6.12	6.04	6.37
Minimum	2.18	4.03	2.35	5.18	3.75	3.87	3.37	4.43	3.28
SD	0.60	0.71	1.33	0.64	0.87	0.99	0.95	0.60	0.94
%VC	0.20	0.13	0.26	0.10	0.16	0.17	0.19	0.11	0.18

$p < 0.05$.

Table 5. Final comparative results for all groups*

	pH 0 (n = 31)	pH Group I (n = 7)	pH Group II (n = 8)	pH Group III (n = 8)	pH Group IV (n = 8)
$\bar{x}$	2.86	3.73	4.71	5.02	5.33
	±0.10	±0.64	±0.69	±0.65	±0.60
Maximum	4.85	4.34	5.60	5.65	6.21
Minimum	2.18	2.94	3.76	3.85	4.95
SD	0.60	0.82	1.00	0.94	0.87
%VC	0.20	0.21	0.21	0.18	0.16

$p < 0.05$.
t (group I) = 1.94.
t (groups II, III, and IV) = 1.83.
*pH increase was significantly greater following anterior linear gastrectomy, where TA-30 and GIA-50 mechanical staplers were used.

ative results for all four groups, and Fig. 5 shows the mean group pH.

Body weight. All animals gained weight normally during the postoperative period, and there were no statistically significant differences in comparison with control values.

Gastroduodenal transit. Postoperative gastrointestinal transit showed no marked differences with respect to normal values. In all cases x-ray films showed a normal-sized stomach and normal duodenal transit times.

Nerve regeneration. All animals in groups II to IV showed gastric lesions of the anterior wall consisting of clear linear atrophy of the gastric mucosa and parietal fibrosis. The nerve fibers and plexus were absent with no signs of nerve regeneration. Thus, although the anterior gastric wall was denervated in all rats in groups II to IV, mucosal atrophy was greater (with a diminished parietal cellularity) when ALG was performed. Immunohistochemistry showed no signs of vagal reinnervation of the anterior gastric wall in rats subjected to linear gastrectomy. No regeneration zones were observed within the postoperative scar, and there was no apparent increase in nerve fibers in the vicinity of the surgical wound.

Discussion

Our results show a significant decrease in gastric acid output following PTV and ALG (pH 5.17). This decrease in acidity was greater than that after PTV and anterior seromyotomy with a low-voltage electric scalpel (pH 4.71). Mean control pH was 2.86. The pH obtained for each animal was the average of 12 determinations (weekly evaluations over 3 months). Why results were more consistent when ALG was performed with the GIA-50 stapler than with the TA-30 instrument is not clear. The study was concluded 3 months after surgery; in the rat this is the equivalent of 4 human years. With the aim of promoting nerve regeneration, all rats were in the maximum-vitality preadult stage at surgery. Minimum ALG performed with mechanical staplers is an important technical advance with respect to gastrotomy and eversion suturing, since it avoids bleeding and opening of the gastric cavity. All rats showed a normal weight gain during the postoperative period. X-ray examination of the stomach and duodenum with barium contrast medium showed normal gastric emptying; no diarrhea was observed. Our results indicate that total denervation of the anterior gastric body and fundus was achieved; in no case were nerve fibers noted to leave healthy gastric wall and penetrate denervated areas. This approach offers the following advantages: it is faster and simpler to perform than highly selective vagotomy or seromyotomy and does not require careful dissection of the abdominal esophagus. The technique poses no risk of either lesser curvature necrosis (as occurs in highly selective vagotomy) or damage to Latarjet's nerve. It is easily reproduced and requires no significant prior experience. The anatomical variations of the anterior vagus need not be taken into account in ALG; the technique sections each and every anterior vagal branch with greater ease than seromyotomy. The use of stapling devices and laparoscopic sectioning may also facilitate a laparoscopic approach. For these reasons we have been using this laparoscopic approach in humans since January 1992.

SURGICAL TECHNIQUES
Open Technique

With this technique a standard laparotomy is performed, the abdominal cavity is explored, and the duodenum is freed. Duodenal amplitude is evaluated following its extensive liberation. We consider it very important to preserve the pars condensa of the lesser omentum to leave the vagal branches intact. The posterior vagal trunk is isolated and ligated, and a segment is removed for histopathological study. The absence of the "criminal" nerve of Grassi is always checked. The crow's foot and Latarjet's nerve are located, the latter always being carefully preserved. The antrum is identified, and a series of Allis forceps are positioned 1 to 1.5 cm from the lesser curvature; a fold on the anterior aspect of the stomach is raised, extending the dissection toward the vertex of the fundus. A TA-90 stapler is positioned and fired to remove the elevated strip of anterior gastric wall. We prefer to excise the strip with a scalpel, applying hemostatic sutures where required. We then position a TA-50 stapler and work it up to the vertex of the fundus. A rectangle is thus removed, the length of which must equal that of both staplers combined. This guarantees sectioning of both nerve plexuses of the anterior stomach wall.

After this technique was used for open surgery in 20 patients, we applied the occlusive (EndoGIA) stapler to the distended stomach of the pig. The technique was determined to be safe for use in humans with this instrument.

Laparoscopic Technique

This technique is performed with the patient under general anesthesia and with antibiotic prophylaxis. Urethral and nasogastric catheters are positioned, and the monitor is placed at the left at the head of the patient. After exploring the abdominal cavity, the assistant holds the liver with an atraumatic instrument so that the surgeon with both hands can section the lesser omentum and gain access to the epiploon cavity, either preserving or sectioning the pars nervosa of the lesser omentum. The right diaphragmatic crus is visualized and the phreno-esophageal membrane is sectioned. The posterior esophagus is bluntly separated—the pneumoperitoneum aiding in the dissection process. The posterior vagus nerve and if necessary the "criminal" nerve of Grassi are identified. The latter is sectioned, whereas the former is coagulated and sectioned.

To perform denervating minimal linear gastrectomy, the surgeon is positioned on the right, and with a pair of forceps through the right subcostal access a point is grasped on the anterior wall of the stomach at the crow's foot, some 6 or 7 cm from the pylorus and 1 to 1.5 cm from the lesser curvature. The first assistant grasps another point that is then raised to form a fold. The surgeon introduces the EndoGIA stapler, opens it, and then closes the instrument so as to place the tissue transection 1 cm from the anterior vertex of the linear vertical fold. The EndoGIA stapler is fired and a first strip of folded anterior gastric wall is separated from the remaining stomach along the distal gastric curvature. With the action of the GIA, both the strip of folded gastric wall and the remaining body of the stomach are stapled closed on both sides of the transection (Fig. 8). Through the angle remaining between this first strip and the remainder of the stomach, the endoGIA stapler is again introduced and the fold sectioned parallel to the lesser curvature, toward the fundus. This maneuver is repeated until the fundus is reached (Figs. 9 to 11).

It is important to not work too close to the cardia.

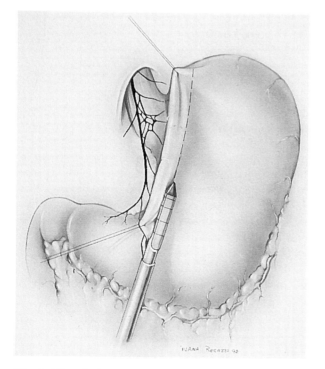

Fig. 8. The EndoGIA stapler is placed and fired and an anterior strip of the fold is separated as a result.

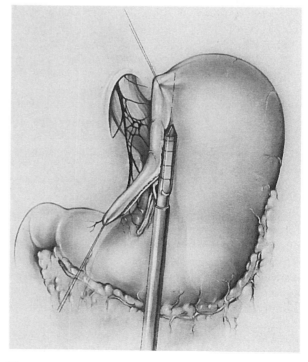

Fig. 9. Working of the EndoGIA stapler toward the fundus.

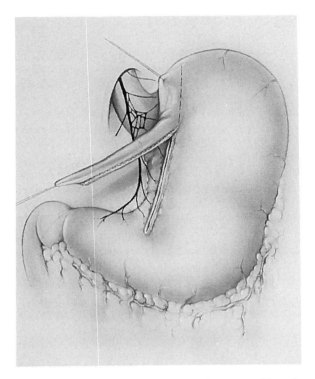

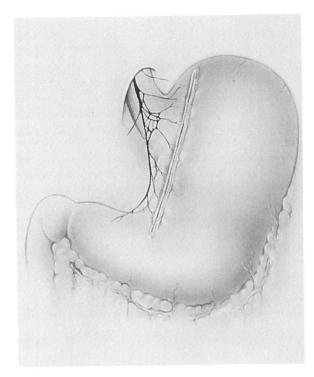

Fig. 10. Separation of the gastric strip on reaching the vertex of the fundus.

Fig. 11. Final presentation after excision of the strip of gastric wall.

Removal of the rectangle of gastric wall should reach the fundus and even extend beyond it, to section all branches that may descend from the esophagus. In this way a strip of anterior gastric wall is obtained in the form of a long, stapled, folded strip.

DISCUSSION

Minimal linear gastrectomy represents an important technical advance with respect to gastrotomy and eversion suturing, since it avoids both bleeding and contamination. Minimal linear gastrectomy offers a number of advantages over supraselective vagotomy and seromyotomy in both open and laparoscopic procedures. It is very simple to perform and is quick. It requires no careful esophageal dissection and involves no necrosis of the lesser curvature or damage to Latarjet's nerve. The technique is easily reproduced and requires no extensive prior experience with either open or laparoscopic technique. Finally, there is no risk of perforation or necrosis of the mucosa as a result of electrocoagulation. Serosal suturing is not required. Minimal linear

gastrectomy secures adequate hemostasis and sutures the gastric wall layers prior to removal of the rectangular strip of stomach. The technique is therefore easy to perform, safe, and reproducible in the treatment of chronic duodenal ulcers and constitutes a valid option for both the gastroenterologist and the patient. The only apparent disadvantage is the cost, which is counterbalanced by the safety features and amount of time saved. This method should be further evaluated in a larger series.

REFERENCES

1. Griffith CA, Harkins HN. Partial gastric vagotomy: An experimental study. Gastroenterology 32:96-102, 1957.
2. Hill GL, Barker MCJ. Anterior highly selective vagotomy with posterior truncal vagotomy: A simple technique for denervating the parietal cell mass. Br J Surg 65:702-708, 1978.
3. Taylor TV, Macleod DAD, Maclennan L. Anterior lesser curve seromyotomy and posterior truncal vagotomy in the

treatment of chronic duodenal ulcer. Lancet 1:844-848, 1982.

4. Cuesta MA, Doblas M, Rodriguez M, et al. Vagal regeneration after parietal cell vagotomy. An experimental study in dogs. World J Surg 11:94-100, 1987.

5. Joffe SN, Crocket A, Dyle D. Morphologic and functional evidence of reinnervation of the gastric mucosa parietal cell mass after parietal cell vagotomy. Am J Surg 143: 80, 1982.

6. Gómez-Ferrer F. Estudio de la denervación de la cara anterior del estómago producida por la seromiotomía o la gastrotomía de curvadura menor solas o combinadas con vagotomía. Surgical Department Study. Valencia University, 1986.

7. Gómez-Ferrer F, Anton V, Llombart A. Estudio de la denervación de la cara anterior del estómago producida por seromiotomía o gastrotomía. II. Presented at the Spanish-Portuguese Meeting of the Collegium Internationale Chirurgiae Digestivae. Alicant: November 20, 1987.

8. Baker J, Lindsey J, Weishoth S. The Laboratory Rat, vol. I. New York: Academic Press, 1980, pp 78-79.

112 *Laparoscopic Gastrectomy and Gastrojejunostomy (Billroth II Procedure)*

Patrice H. Lointier

We will describe a technique of total intra-abdominal laparoscopic gastrectomy. The continuity of the upper gastrointestinal tract was reestablished by gastrojejunostomy (Billroth II procedure) using the EndoGIA stapler. This procedure warrants inclusion in the surgeon's armamentarium for treating recurrent gastric ulcers.

MATERIALS AND METHODS

A subtotal gastrectomy was performed in a 53-year-old white male who had no prior abdominal surgery. He was referred because of a refractory gastric ulcer for which he was receiving drug treatment (omeprazole). Multiple biopsies showed no dysplasia.

In addition to the standard laparoscopic equipment, we used a 12 mm EndoGIA stapler (Autosuture) and a dissector, forceps, and retractor (Storz and Autosuture). The operation was performed through four ports (one 5 mm, one 10 mm, and two 12 mm).

TECHNIQUE

Laparoscopy was performed with the patient under general anesthesia. An endotracheal tube and nasogastric suction tube were placed. The patient was positioned supine, with legs spread apart and in low stirrups (Fig. 1, *A*). He was prepared and draped for both laparoscopic and open gastric resection. An insufflation needle was inserted through a small skin incision 3 cm below the umbilicus. The abdomen was insufflated with CO_2 to a maximal pressure of 14 mm Hg. After establishing the pneumoperitoneum, a 10 mm laparoscopic cannula was inserted through the same puncture site, which was enlarged after the needle was removed. A 0-degree (10 mm) rigid laparoscope with an attached video camera was introduced into the peritoneal cavity. The operator stood between the patient's legs with the camera assistant on the patient's right and the nurse on the left. A video monitor was placed to the right of the head of the table. Trocars were inserted under visual guidance and positioned as shown in Fig. 1.

The assistant used the right subcostal port to retract the liver and control the video endoscope, which was passed through the infraumbilical port. The surgeon used the two 12 mm operating paraumbilical ports in a two-handed approach to the stomach. At the beginning of the procedure the patient was placed in a reverse Trendelenburg position with the table at a 30-degree tilt. This position allowed the transverse colon and the greater omentum to be kept out of the operative field.

After completing a laparoscopic survey of the abdomen, we located the gastric ulcer. The greater curvature of the stomach was mobilized by means of electrocautery for dissection of the vessels from the omentum, which were secured with a clip applier before being

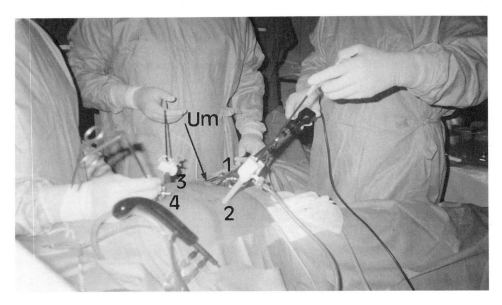

Fig. 1. Trocar placement. (*Um* = umbilicus.)

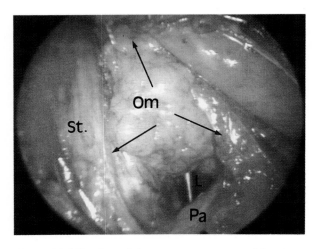

Fig. 2. Mobilization of the greater curvature of the stomach. (*OM* = greater omentum; *L* = lesser sac entered; *St* = stomach; *Pa* = pancreas.)

divided. In this way the distal two thirds of the greater curvature was mobilized. The posterior wall of the stomach was exposed by entering the lesser sac through the gastrocolic ligament (Fig. 2). The proximal 2 cm of the duodenum were freed from connective tissue and vessels by sharp dissection and cauterization. To visualize the pyloric vessels the laparoscope was introduced through the right 12 mm port (Fig. 3). The vessels were

secured with a 30 V EndoGIA vascular stapler. When the posterior wall of the duodenum was mobilized it was transected with two applications of the EndoGIA 30 stapler (Fig. 4). The gallbladder was grasped with forceps and the duodenum was then pulled securely into the jaws of the stapler. For this the laparoscope was removed and placed in the medial 10 mm port, and the EndoGIA stapler was introduced via the right 12 mm port. The lesser curvature was then easily mobilized from the distal to the proximal aspect using traction of the stomach to the left and up to the abdominal wall.

The transverse colon was displaced superiorly and the duodenojejunal junction was located. A proximal loop of jejunum was chosen, brought up through a "window" created in the colonic mesentery and held adjacent to the posterior wall of the stomach before its transection (Fig. 5). The intestinal loop was first approximated to the stomach by means of a superior external slipknot suture of 2-0 polypropylene. Two stab wounds were then created—one in the stomach and one in the jejunum—at one end of the projected anastomotic line. This was done by use of monopolar electrocauterization applied with laparoscopic scissors, followed by sharp incision of the protruding mucosa. The EndoGIA stapler was positioned with one jaw in each stab wound, first in the jejunum using the narrow portion of the stapler jaws (Fig. 6). The stapler was closed and fired after anterior and posterior positions were symmetrical-

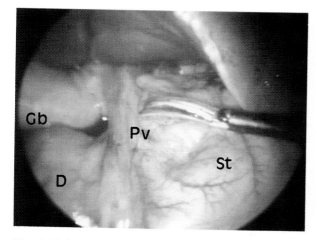

Fig. 3. Pyloric vessels seen through 12 mm port. (*PV* = pyloric vessels; *Gb* = gallbladder.)

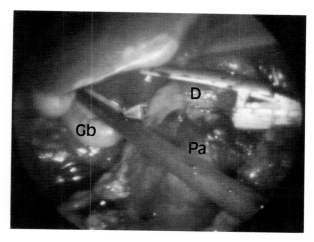

Fig. 4. Division of the duodenum with a linear stapler.

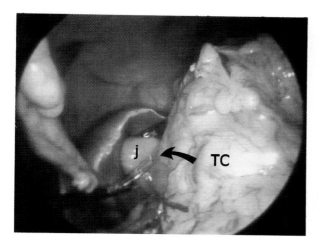

Fig. 5. Proximal jejunum *(j)* brought up posterior to the colon *(TC)*.

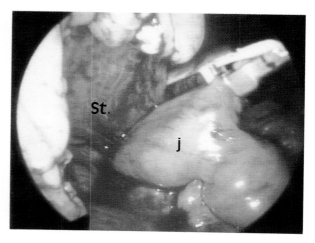

Fig. 6. Billroth II gastrojejunostomy. Introduction of the linear stapler.

Fig. 7. Laparoscopic inspection of the anastomosis and enterotomies.

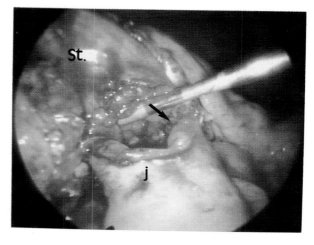

ly aligned and examined. The anastomosis was inspected after irrigation (Fig. 7). The lips of the now single stab wound were joined together by means of extracorporeally tied sutures and were closed with three applications of the EndoGIA 30 stapler along the edges of the intestinal wound. The sutures were used to hold the edges together for positioning of the stapler (Fig. 8). Then the stomach was transected distal to the anastomosis (Fig. 9). Thick areas of lesser omentum and the descending branch of the left gastric vessels required division with the EndoGIA stapler after gastric tran-

section from the greater curvature. The resected stomach specimen was temporarily placed above the right lobe of the liver (Fig. 10).

The level of gastric resection was determined by the ulcer location and the end of the left gastroepiploic vessels and was accomplished with four applications of the 30 mm EndoGIA stapler. The nasogastric tube was carefully withdrawn proximal to the line of resection before the stapler was fired. The anastomotic line and gastric stump were examined for leaks by inflating the stomach with air and methylene blue (Fig. 11). The en-

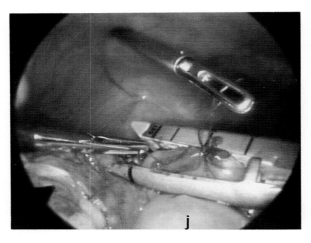

Fig. 8. Stay sutures are used to hold the lateral margins of the enterotomies. An EndoGIA stapler is then placed and fired.

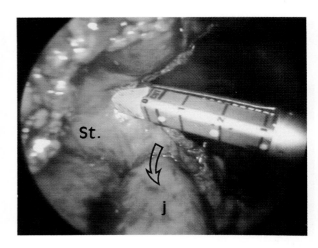

Fig. 9. Division of the stomach.

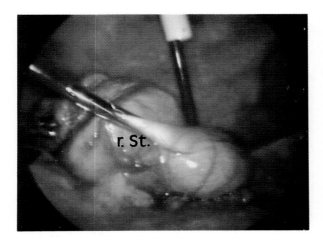

Fig. 10. Resected stomach (*r. St.*) specimen was placed above the right lobe of the liver.

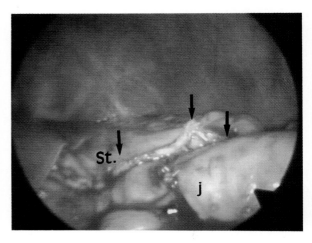

Fig. 11. Completed anastomosis is checked for leaks using intragastric filling with methylene blue.

tire abdomen was inspected for bleeding, then washed, and aspirated. The patient lost approximately 200 to 300 ml of blood. A drain was placed through the right 12 mm port. The resected stomach specimen was extracted through a small incision in the 12 mm laparoscope trocar wound, which was extended to 3 cm near the umbilicus. The intraoperative course was uneventful. The duration of the procedure was 4 hours. The patient had no abdominal pain, but did complain of headache and ached all over for 48 hours.

The nasogastric tube was removed on day 2. The patient passed gas on day 3, at which time he was fed clear liquids. A swallow test using hydrosoluble contrast material was done on day 6, and the anastomosis was examined for patency. The patient was then begun on a normal diet. The drain was removed on day 8 and the patient was discharged.

Based on findings in the present case and our experience with laparoscopic esophagogastrointestinal operations,[1-5] we agree with Goh et al.[6,7] that laparoscopic gastric resection can offer a safe and reasonable alternative to long-term medical management of gastric ulcers. New instruments such as the EndoGIA stapler allow safe intestinal and vascular transection and closure.[8-10] Nonetheless, more patients and additional follow-up will be necessary before this procedure can be accepted as standard treatment.

REFERENCES

1. Lointier P, Bail JP, Bourlier P, et al. Thoracoscopic dissection of the esophagus in human cadavers. J Laparoendosc Surg (in press).
2. Lointier P. Oesophagectomie sous thoracoscopie droite (film). Presented at the Ninety-fourth Congres Francais de Chirurgie. Paris: Sept. 1992.
3. Lointier P, Fatton B, Ferrier C, et al. Laparoscopic subtotal colectomy. Presented at the Second European Congress of Viscerosynthesis. Minimally Invasive Surgery and New Technology. Luxembourg: Sept. 1992.
4. Lointier P, Ferrier C, Dapoigny M, et al. Colectomie subtotale sous laparoscopie. J Chir (in press).
5. Lointier P, Lechner C, Ferrier C, et al. Recto-colectomie gauche périnéale assistée par laparoscopie. Chirurg Endosc 7:10-14, 1992.
6. Goh P, Tekant Y, Isaac J, et al. The technique of Billroth II gastrectomy. Surg Laparosc Endosc 2:16-23, 1992.
7. Goh P, Tekant Y, Kum CK, et al. Totally intra-abdominal laparoscopic Billroth II gastrectomy [Letter]. Surg Endosc 6:160, 1992.
8. Lathrop JC, Felix EJ, Lauber D. Laparoscopic Janeway gastrotomy utilizing an endoscopic stapling device. J Laparoendosc Surg 6:355-359, 1991.
9. Mouiel J, Katkhouda N, White S, et al. Endolaparoscopic palliation of pancreatic cancer. Surg Laparosc Endosc 2:241-243, 1992.
10. Leahy PF, Furman RH, Pennino RP. Laparoscopically assisted gastrectomy [Abstract]. Surg Endosc 6:102, 1992.

113 *Laparoscopic Gastroenterostomy for Malignant Duodenal Obstruction*

Robert Graeme Wilson and J.S. Varma

Simple gastrojejunal bypass is an established surgical procedure for palliative treatment of patients with unresectable malignant duodenal obstruction. Although surgical bypass is the only effective therapeutic option for such patients, the need for laparotomy has hitherto been an unwelcome event.

We will describe a laparoscopic technique of anterior gastroenterostomy for palliation of patients with inoperable malignant gastric outlet obstruction. This

operation has been performed in three patients, with complete resolution of the symptoms of gastric outlet obstruction and minimal postoperative discomfort. Each operation took nearly 2 hours to perform, with a postoperative hospital stay ranging from 4 to 10 days. This minimally invasive technique provides ideal palliation for patients with advanced pancreatic or duodenal malignancy without the need for laparotomy.

MATERIALS AND METHODS

The first patient was an 82-year-old woman with a 3-month history of weight loss and vomiting. Investiga-

Based on Wilson RG, Varma JS. Br J Surg 79:1348, 1992.

tions revealed an occluding adenocarcinoma in the third portion of the duodenum. CT scan confirmed the presence of a duodenal lesion with local infiltration into the pancreas. The second patient was a 78-year-old man with mature onset diabetes and severe ischemic heart disease. He had vomiting and weight loss. A barium meal demonstrated extrinsic compression at the junction of the third and fourth portions of the duodenum with evidence of reverse peristalsis and gastric stasis. He was initially managed nonoperatively, but after admission for profound vomiting, precipitating an episode of hyperglycemic coma, he was referred for laparoscopic gastroenterostomy. The third patient, a 79-year-old woman, had a duodenal obstruction 2 months after placement of a biliary stent for carcinoma of the head of the pancreas.

In the first patient, laparoscopy confirmed the presence of a tumor mass arising from the duodenum with infiltration into the pancreas. In the second patient, small tumor metastases were present in the liver and underneath the right diaphragm. These had not been detected previously by ultrasonography. Paraffin section biopsy confirmed the presence of metastatic carcinoma.

SURGICAL TECHNIQUE

The operations were performed under general anesthesia with endotracheal intubation and a nasogastric tube in situ. Preoperative antibiotic prophylaxis (cefotaxime, 1 g and metronidazole, 400 mg) was given intravenously. Patients were placed in the Lloyd-Davies position with a minor degree of reverse Trendelenburg tilt. The principle operator stood between the patient's legs and the assistant on the right side.

Three laparoscopic cannulae were used for access. A 10 mm cannula was placed below the umbilicus for a 10 mm laparoscope and attached endocamera to perform general laparoscopy. A 5 mm cannula was inserted in the left subcostal area in the anterior axillary line. A 12 mm disposable cannula was similarly situated in the right subcostal area.

Using atraumatic graspers introduced via the working cannulae, the transverse colon was elevated and the duodenojejunal flexure identified. After "walking" the forceps down the jejunum for approximately 30 cm, a suitable length was elevated over the transverse colon and apposed to the inferior margin of the greater curvature of the stomach with two transabdominal stay sutures mounted on a straight cutting needle (2-0 prolene, Ethicon). Each stay suture was passed through the abdominal wall lateral to one of the accessory cannulas. Once the abdominal wall was penetrated, the needle was grasped intracorporeally with an endoscopic needle holder and placed through the seromuscular layers of the adjacent stomach and jejunum. By reversing the suture back through the abdominal wall, it was possible to maintain the selected segment of jejunum in close apposition to the stomach while leaving the accessory cannulas free for the introduction of instruments (Fig. 1).

The antecolic gastroenterostomy was created by cut-

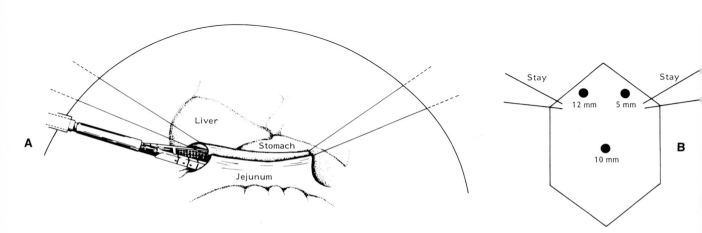

Fig. 1. A, Transabdominal stay sutures and laparoscopic stapling technique. **B,** Relative positions of the ports and stay sutures.

ting a small enterotomy through the adjacent stomach and jejunum with scissors or hook diathermy introduced through the right subcostal port. While maintaining traction on the right-hand stay suture, an EndoGIA stapler (U.S. Surgical Corp.) was inserted via the 12 mm port into the adjacent stomach and small bowel, closed, and fired. In the first patient a single firing of the 30 mm cartridge was used; in subsequent patients two firings were used to create a longer anastomosis. The EndoGIA stapler was then withdrawn and the laparoscope inserted through the right upper quadrant port to inspect the gastroenterostomy and check hemostasis.

The resulting small defect in the stomach and jejunum was closed using a continuous, full-thickness 2-0 nurolon suture mounted on a 30 mm round-bodied needle (Ethicon). The suture was first prepared by trimming it to a short length and tying a jamming loop slipknot on the end.[1] Suturing was performed with a 5 mm endoscopic needle holder and atraumatic grasping forceps via the right and left subcostal cannulas. Taking an equal bite of stomach and jejunum, the needle was passed through the loop of the slipknot, which was then tightened by traction on the tail of the suture. A continuous suturing technique was used, and the suture line was completed with an Aberdeen knot.[2]

RESULTS

All operations were completed in less than 2 hours. The nasogastric tubes were removed the next day and fluids were introduced by mouth after 48 hours. A full diet was begun within 4 days for the first patient and within 3 days for subsequent patients. In all patients postoperative pain was controlled with simple oral analgesia. The first patient was discharged on the fifth postoperative day and the second on the fourth, whereas the third patient remained in the hospital for a total of 10 days because of adverse home circumstances.

Patients underwent gastroscopy 4 weeks after the operation at which time they reported no vomiting since surgery. All stomas appeared to be patent. However, in the first patient the stoma was considered to be small and balloon dilation was performed.

The first patient remains alive with a functioning stoma 8½ months postoperatively; the second and third patients died of metastatic disease at 4 and 5 months, respectively, with no further vomiting.

DISCUSSION

Laparotomy with antecolic anterior gastroenterostomy is an accepted surgical procedure for obstruction of the duodenum. The laparoscopic approach reported here uses the same principles for formation of the anastomosis with stapling devices as open surgery.[3] The significant difference with the laparoscopic procedure is that it avoids an abdominal incision. In the first patient, a good functional result was achieved with a single firing of the EndoGIA stapler. However, the relatively small size of the stoma at gastroscopy prompted us to create a 60 mm anastomosis in the second and third patients, since this more closely duplicates the size of a linear stapled gastroenterostomy at open operation. Although it would be technically feasible to perform the procedure solely by suturing, the introduction of the endoscopic stapling and anastomosing device greatly facilitates the procedure. Endoscopic suturing of the defect used to introduce the stapling device remains the most technically demanding part of the procedure. However, with practice and the use of a continuous suture, this can be performed quickly and safely. Although the operations took nearly 2 hours to perform, this is likely to decrease with experience.

The palliative nature of this surgery makes the laparoscopic approach particularly desirable, inasmuch as it eliminates the discomfort and debilitation of a laparotomy. Our patients recovered quickly from the procedure, and their gastroenterostomies functioned rapidly without postoperative vomiting or obstruction.

This report demonstrates that currently available laparoscopic techniques and instrumentation allow duplication of the surgical techniques used at laparotomy to perform a stapled gastroenterostomy. Furthermore patients who require palliative bypass, by the very nature of their disease, stand to gain the most from the reduced hospitalization and minimal convalescence period achieved with our technique.

REFERENCES

1. Shimi S, Banting S, Cuschieri A. Laparoscopy in the management of pancreatic cancer: Endoscopic cholecystojejunostomy for advanced disease. Br J Surg 79:317-319, 1992.
2. Paterson-Brown S, Dudley HF. Knotting in continuous mass closure of the abdomen. Br J Surg 73:679-680, 1986.
3. Steichen FM, Ravitch MM. Contemporary stapling instruments and basic mechanical suture techniques. Surg Clin North Am 64:425-440, 1984.

XVII

Reconstructive and Corrective Procedures in the Upper Gastrointestinal Tract

114 *Reconstruction After Esophagectomy*

Jean-Marie Collard, J.B. Otte, and P.J. Kestens

Various digestive organs such as the stomach, colon, and jejunum can be used to restore continuity after esophagectomy. Any possible substitute has to fulfill two conditions: (1) to be of sufficient length to reach the remaining part of the esophagus or the pharynx without excessive tension, and (2) to receive excellent blood supply from its supporting vascular pedicle.

MATERIALS AND METHODS

Over an 8-year period, 245 patients underwent esophageal resection at the University of Louvain Hospital. Indications for surgery included cancers of the laryngopharynx (n = 17), cancers of the esophagus (n = 150), cancers of the esophagogastric junction (n = 64), caustic esophagites (n = 9), peptic esophagitis (n = 2), instrumental perforation (n = 1), benign esophagotracheal fistula (n = 1), and restoration of the digestive continuity after total gastrectomy complicated by leakage of the esophagojejunal anastomosis (n = 1).

Two hundred forty-six esophageal resections were performed on 245 patients, one patient having been reoperated for proximal cancer extension after distal esophagectomy. One caustic esophagitis patient who had previously undergone a colon bypass operation was admitted for complementary esophagectomy. One patient with a benign esophagotracheal fistula underwent segmental esophagectomy with end-to-end esophago-esophageal anastomosis. This made a total of 246 esophagectomies, 245 esophageal anastomoses, and 244 esophageal substitutes on 245 patients.

Esophagectomy was total (n = 17), subtotal (n = 162), distal (n = 66), or segmental (n = 1). It was carried out by right thoracotomy (n = 124), left thoracophrenolaparotomy (n = 72), combined transhiatal and transcervical approach (n = 38), median sternotomy (n = 5), and right thoracoscopy (n = 6).

Digestive continuity was restored using nine different types of transplants: long gastric tube (n = 102), short gastric tube (n = 18), entire stomach with denudation of the lesser curvature (n = 57), separated gastric tube (n = 2) isoperistaltic colon segment (n = 13), reverse colon transplant (n = 3), Roux-en-Y jejunal loop (n = 23), interposed jejunal loop (n = 25), and nontypical gastric transplant (n = 1).

The esophageal substitute was placed either in the substernal space (n = 49) or in the posterior mediastinum (n = 195). One hundred seventy-six esophageal anastomoses were performed in the neck and 69 in the chest. They were hand-sewn in all patients but three, in whom the EEA stapler was employed. Manual anastomoses were performed using a single-layer interrupted or running suture technique, taking the full thickness of the esophageal wall and the extramucosal layers of the esophageal substitute.

Long Gastric Tube With Resection of the Lesser Curvature[4,5]

The greater omentum is dissected off the gastrocolic ligament. All vascular pedicles but the right gastroepiploic vessels are severed at their root. The lesser curvature is denuded 3 to 4 cm proximal to the pylorus for application of a GIA 50 stapler or a PLC 50 stapler on the gastric wall (Fig. 1). The stomach is then simultaneously incised and stapled along the free edge of the lesser curvature up to the left side of the cardia (Fig. 2). The staple line is oversewn using seroserosal permanent interrupted sutures; a running suture could shorten the gastric transplant. Pyloroplasty or pyloromyotomy is performed as a drainage procedure. The portion of the greater omentum located left of the vascular arcade of the greater curvature is removed. However, upper fringes are usually maintained to wrap the cervical anastomosis and to create a barrier that protects pleural cavities and the proximal mediastinum or the substernal space from any septic contamination from the neck in the event of leakage of the cervical anastomosis.

Short Gastric Tube With Proximal Gastric Resection

The short gastric tube is used to reestablish continuity after a limited esophagogastrectomy for advanced cancer of the cardia. It is based on the right gastroepiploic vessels. The proximal part of the lesser curvature and the subcardial area of the stomach are resected us-

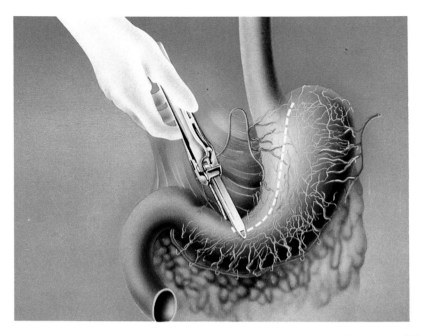

Fig. 1. Following separation of the greater omentum from the gastrocolic ligament and ligation of all vessels, except for the right gastroepiploic vessels and the entire gastroepiploic arcade, the GIA stapler is applied and activated at a right angle to the lesser curvature, some 3 to 4 cm proximal to the pylorus. This maneuver starts the resection of the lesser curvature.

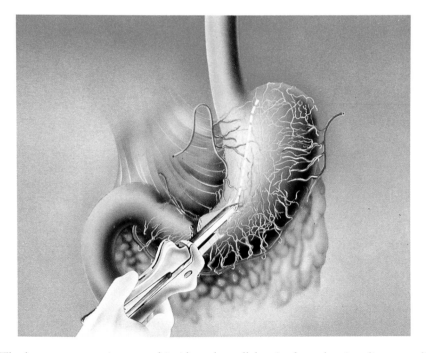

Fig. 2. The lesser curvature is resected inside and parallel to its free edge, in a line extending from below upward to the left of the cardia, by repeated applications of the GIA or PLC stapler.

ing a stapling technique similar to that described for long gastric tubes. The staple line is oversewn using a seroserosal running suture, since the distance to the remaining part of the thoracic esophagus is short. Pyloroplasty or pyloromyotomy is the rule. Gastroesophageal acid reflux may sometimes be prevented by wrapping the distal segment of the remaining esophagus with redundant stomach.

Entire Stomach With Denudation of the Lesser Curvature[6]

This is a gastroplasty technique we have experimented with for more than 3 years. The terminal rami of both the right and left gastric vessels are severed flush with the gastric wall from the pylorus up to the cardia to radically remove lymph nodes in the lesser omentum and to unfold the right side of the stomach (Fig. 3). The thoracic esophagus is separated from the stomach by application of a single-cartridge GIA-50 or PLC-50 stapler on the cardia (Fig. 4). The short staple line is oversewn using interrupted sutures. The top of the entire stomach is vascularized by the right gastroepiploic vessels through the whole submucosal vascular network that has been maintained. Pyloroplasty or pyloromyotomy is routinely done.

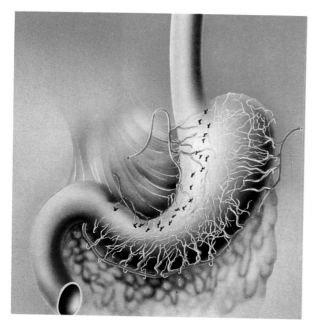

Fig. 3. The terminal rami of the right and left gastric vessels are ligated and transsected flush with the lesser curvature wall from the pylorus to the cardia. The lesser omentum and all lymph nodes along the lesser curvature are removed with the specimen.

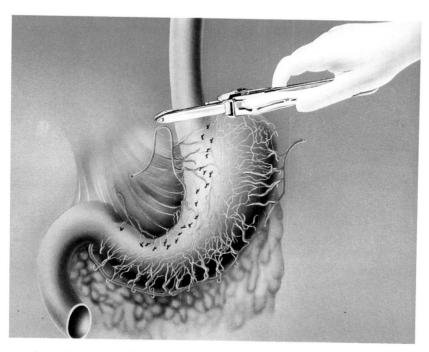

Fig. 4. The esophagus is separated from the stomach of the cardia with the GIA or PLC instrument.

Separated Gastric Tube

This technique, as described by Ioshida and Iwatsuka,[7] was used on some patients with a caustic stenosis of both the esophagus and antrum and in whom the proximal two thirds of the stomach were intact. The antrum is removed by stapling division of the duodenum distal to the pylorus and of the stomach 2 cm proximal to the burned antral area. The proximal stomach is tubulized by stapling resection of the proximal part of the lesser curvature, and a Roux-en-Y loop is anastomosed to the distal edge of the gastric pouch. The latter remains vascularized by the upper rami of the right gastroepiploic vessels and the arcade of the greater curvature.

Colon Substitute[8-11]

Different segments of the colon can be used for substitution. In most cases we use the transverse part and the right angle of the colon based on the left ascending colic vessels. Variations in the vascularity of the mesocolon may lead to elevate the right colon based on the midcolic vessels. In such an instance, appendectomy is mandatory. When the left colic vessels are small in diameter, the transverse colon and the left angle based on the midcolic vessels can be transposed in an anisoperistaltic fashion. In patients with a history of right hemicolectomy, the descending colon based on the left colic vessels may be used. The lower anastomosis is performed to the posterior wall of the intact stomach. The distal end of the colon segment is connected with the duodenum or a Roux-en-Y loop in previously gastrectomized patients.

Temporary occlusion of the vascular pedicle to be divided and, palpation of the vascular arcade are critical steps to follow before making the final choice of the segment that will be pulled up to the neck. Colonic continuity is reestablished by end-to-end anastomosis between the two portions of the remaining colon.

Jejunal Loop

A jejunal loop was used to reestablish continuity after distal esophagectomy and total gastrectomy for cancers of the cardia. The mesenteric vessels of the proximal few jejunal loops are inspected using transillumination. Depending on individual local anatomy, one or two vascular pedicles are divided as far from the jejunum as possible after a trial occlusion to ensure that there is an adequate blood supply to the area corresponding to the future proximal end of the loop. The jejunum is transsected at this level using a GIA-50 or PLC-50 stapler after division of the local marginal vessels. The staple line is oversewn with a continuous inverting suture. The jejunal loop is elevated through an incision in the mesocolon.

The proximal anastomosis is performed end to side between the remaining part of the distal esophagus and a short lateral opening in the loop just distal to its proximal stapled end. In Roux-en-Y loops, the proximal duodenum is closed by application of a single cartridge of the TA stapler or the RL stapler, and the jejunum distal to the ligament of Treitz is anastomosed end to side to the efferent jejunum leaving 60 cm of jejunal loop between esophagus and the Y anastomosis.

In other instances a 60 cm jejunal loop is interposed between the esophagus and the duodenum. The esophagojejunal anastomosis is made end to side, and the jejunoduodenal anastomosis is done end to end in a single layer running suture. Jejunal continuity is then restored by end-to-end jejunojejunal anastomosis.

RESULTS

Postoperative Mortality (Table 1)

Seven patients (2.8%) died from a postoperative complication during the hospital stay—two within the first 30 postoperative days (0.8%), three during the second month (1.2%), and two afterward (0.8%). Four of the seven patients were 70 years or more in age. In addition, a 73-year-old patient died from an unexplained cause the day before he had planned to leave the hospital for social reasons after a long postoperative course. The results of the postmortem examination were unremarkable. The remaining 237 patients were discharged from the hospital.

Technical Complications (Table 2)

Technical complications included esophageal anastomosis fistulas (5.4%) and strictures (12.5%), various types of fistulas (2.1%), and necrosis of the transplant (0.8%) or perforation of the transplant (0.4%).

Esophageal anastomosis strictures occurred more frequently in the neck than in the chest (15.9% versus 2.8%; $p < 0.01$); most of these developed in long gastric tubes. All but two subsided after a few (two or more) sessions of endoscopic dilations. The two others, one cervical and one intrathoracic, required surgical revision.

Cervical esophageal anastomosis fistulas presented as weeping of saliva through the cervical drain. Only one was complicated by cervical sepsis. These were treated by total parenteral nutrition and prolonged fasting.

Table 1. Causes of death from postoperative complications

Period	No. of Patients	Cause of Death
<30 days	2 (0.8%)	Respiratory failure (1)
		Accidental chest tube disconnection (1)
>30 days/<60 days	3 (1.2%)	Hepatic failure (2)
		Respiratory failure (1)
>60 days	2 (0.8%)	Aspiration pneumonia (1)
		Respiratory failure (1)

Table 2. Technical complications according to type of esophageal substitute

Esophageal Substitute	Necrosis of the Transplant	Esophageal Anastomosis Fistula	Esophageal Anastomosis Stenosis	Other Fistulas	Perforation of the Transplant
Long gastric tube (102)	1	8	20	2	0
Entire stomach (57)	1	0	5	0	1
Ioshida gastric tube (2)	0	0	1	0	0
Nontypical gastric transplant (1)	0	0	1	0	0
Colon transplant (16)	0	1	1	1	0
Short gastric tube (18)	0	2	1	0	0
Interposed jejunal loop (25)	0	1	1	2	0
Roux-en-Y jejunal loop (23)	0	1	0	0	0
TOTAL (244)	2	13	30	5	1

Three of the four intrathoracic anastomotic fistulas were seen only as radiological findings in postoperative contrast medium swallow examinations. They were treated medically. The fourth one required emergency rethoracotomy: the absence of local sepsis allowed a new anastomosis to be performed after excision of the two margins.

There were five fistulas other than esophageal ones: partial leakage of the pyloroplasty suture line of a gastric transplant (n = 2), of the colocolic anastomosis after colon interposition (n = 1), and of the jejunoduodenal anastomosis after jejunal interposition (n = 2). All five fistulas were treated appropriately by surgical revision.

Necrosis of the upper part of a gastric transplant occurred in two patients. Surgical treatment consisted of a Thorek operation in one patient. In the patient who had been operated on by esophagolaryngopharyngectomy, the cervical part of the gastric transplant was resected, and digestive continuity was finally restored using a musculocutaneous tube after necrosis of a free jejunal loop. Both patients had concomitant severe arteritis and a past history of myocardial infarction. In addition, mucosal ischemia in a nontypical gastric transplant resolved spontaneously.

Perforation of a gastric transplant was Boerhaave-like: it occurred in the course of a severe epilepsy crisis, and there was no evidence of wall ischemia at rethoracotomy. Simple suture of the perforation site was successful.

DISCUSSION

Critical to selection of the appropriate esophageal substitute after esophagectomy are the underlying disease, the upward extent of the esophageal tumor, the need for a concomitant gastrectomy, the individual vascularity of the segments, the patient's surgical history (i.e., previous gastrectomy or colectomy), and the surgeon's level of experience.

Gastric Transplant

The stomach is probably the most commonly used substitute following total or subtotal esophagectomy. Major arguments for using the stomach include its extraordinary plasticity and stretchability and the richness of its submucosal vascular network made of numerous anastomotic pathways. Nevertheless, anatomical variations in patients' gastric anatomy due to ethnic factors were documented by Goldsmith and Akiyama in 1979.[12] They may explain the need in white patients, for using various lengthening techniques to elevate the stomach up to the neck, and especially to reach the base of the tongue after esophagopharyngolaryngectomy.[1]

Three kinds of procedures may be used for pulling the stomach up to the neck: (1) those which lengthen the cardiopyloric distance, (2) those which facilitate upward mobilization of the stomach toward the unmovable anatomical structures, and (3) those which facilitate transthoracic elevation of the tailored stomach.

1. Four major techniques may be employed for gastric lengthening. Gastric tubulization by resection of the lesser curvature using stapling devices permits the remaining part of the stomach to be unfolded. The staple line has to be placed close to the free edge of the lesser curvature to maximize the tube diameter and to maintain as much submucosal vascular network as possible, since the main anastomotic pathways between the antrum and the fundus have been shown to be located in the right part of the stomach.[13]

The three other lengthening techniques are stapling division of the right side of the stomach by application of a GIA stapler at right angles to the lesser curvature,[14] transverse and longitudinal seromyotomies,[15] and denudation of the lesser curvature, with which we have experimented.[6] The latter method unfolds the right side of the stomach and lengthens the cardiopyloric distance by 23% on average. Maintenance of the entire capacity of the gastric reservoir significantly reduces the incidence of the sensation of early fullness during or after a meal, a symptom which is frequently reported by patients who have a gastric tube.[16,17] In the same way maintenance of the whole submucosal vascular network affords optimal blood supply to the gastric fundus; as a consequence, the incidence of anastomotic stenosis resulting from chronic ischemia has been lowered in our own experience. The only contraindication to this technique is resection of a lower-third tumor, which is liable to spread microscopically into the cardial area. In such an instance, stapling resection of the lesser curvature and the subcardial area of the stomach is recommended.

2. Upward mobilization of the stomach may be facilitated by division of the right gastric vessels, the contribution of which to the blood supply to the fundus has been shown to be negligible.[18] The Kocher maneuver, section of the mesenteric root, and division of the adhesions between the inferior vena cava and the portal vein allow elevation of the duodenopancreatic bloc up to the subdiaphragmatic area of the abdomen and an upward shift of the hepatic pedicle. Downward mobilization of the right angle of the colon may also be helpful.[19] Finally, division of the antrum with drainage of the isolated proximal stomach by a Roux-en-Y loop, as described by Ioshida and Iwatsuka,[7] may elevate the fundus to the desired level when the other procedures have proved ineffective.

3. The tailored stomach has to be pulled up to the neck. In this regard, the posterior mediastinal route has been shown to be the shortest.[20,21] A residual indication of the substernal route is restoration of digestive continuity after incomplete resection of an esophageal tumor. Insertion of the stomach into a plastic bag prevents the epiploic fringes along the vascular arcade of the greater curvature to be caught in mediastinal structures such as the aortic arch or the carina.

Colon Transplant

Fifteen years ago, colon transplant was the esophageal substitute of choice after subtotal or total esophagectomy.[8-10] Even more recently, critical steps for accurate performance of the procedure have been reported and outstandingly illustrated by T. DeMeester.[11] However, it has been abandoned by many surgical teams in favor of gastric transplant because of the need for three anastomoses instead of one with the stomach, the potential for contamination of the operative field by the colon contents, the individual variations in the vascularity of the mesocolon, and the possibility of kinking of the colon segment above the diaphragm in the long run. The most common vascular abnormality consists of an early branching midcolic vein on the superior mesenteric vein. Excising a button of superior mesenteric vein and suturing the branches together to maintain the patency between them has been described.[11] In some instances of poor venous return, neck microanastomosis of a mesocolic vein to the internal jugular vein may be helpful.

In our opinion, a residual indication of a colon transplant is restoration of the digestive continuity after combined total gastrectomy and subtotal esophagectomy in previously gastrectomized patients or after necrosis of a gastric transplant, and in the exceptional situation of a short stomach that could not be pulled up to the base of the tongue after esophagopharyngolaryngectomy.

Although the role of residual motor activity remains controversial, most colon transplants are constructed in an isoperistaltic fashion and are based on the left colic or midcolic vessels. Reverse transplant should be only used as a salvage procedure after necrosis of an isoperistaltic colon transplant, or in patients with a past history of segmental colectomy for another disease.

Jejunum Transplant

Although in Oriental patients jejunal loops can be pulled up to the neck,[20] the carina is the uppermost level that can be reached by a pedicled jejunal loop in most white people. Mesenteric vascularity may exceptionally be segmental. This abnormality was present in only one patient in our series. Therefore we limited gastric resection to the proximal part of the stomach and restored digestive continuity using the remaining distal part instead of a jejunal loop.

PREVENTION AND MANAGEMENT OF TECHNICAL COMPLICATIONS

Esophageal anastomosis strictures and fistulas are the most common complications after esophageal replacement. They occur more frequently in the neck than in the chest.[23] The repercussions of intrathoracic fistulas on vital functions is much more severe than that of cervical fistulas, which usually result in local sepsis or weeping of saliva only.

Predisposing factors include (1) catabolic status, which may compromise the healing phase; (2) poor intrinsic vascularity of the esophageal substitute and its external compression, both conditions resulting in inadequate blood supply to the anastomotic site; (3) narrowness of the cervical esophagus lumen in nonobstructive diseases; and (4) inflammatory changes in the pharyngeal wall secondary to caustic burn, resulting in progressive narrowing of an initially large-diameter cervical anastomosis.

The role of the mode of suturing (manual versus mechanical) remains controversial.[24,25]

Preventive measures include (1) preoperative restoration of a positive nitrogen balance to any patient with severe dysphagia and poor general condition (total parenteral nutrition); (2) absence of any tension on the suture line (see the description of elevating and lengthening procedures); (3) excellence of the blood supply to the anastomotic site (not crushing the wall of the transplant with forceps not to damage the submucosal vascular network,[18] trial occlusion of the vascular pedicle before division, maintenance of a good fluid balance to ensure adequate blood flow to the esophageal substitute while protecting the lungs against any fluid overload); (4) prevention of any external compression of the transplant (resection of the sternal notch or head of the clavicle,[10] large mediastinal tunnel; (5) wrapping of the anastomosis using the greater omentum whenever possible; (6) intraoperative testing of the intrathoracic anastomoses by methylene blue–stained water instillation through a nasoesophageal catheter; and (7) intraoperative enlargement of a small-diameter esophageal lumen (finger intralumenal dilation, muscular wall relaxation by intravenous administration of glucagon).

Both cervical and radiological intrathoracic fistulas are usually healed within a few days or weeks when the patient is kept in a fasting state and given total parenteral nutrition. A gross defect at an intrathoracic anastomosis level requires emergency rethoracotomy, a new anastomosis can be performed when local sepsis is minimal. In other instances, a Thorek operation has to be performed as a salvage procedure.

Most anastomotic strictures are simple narrowings of a suture line that subside after a few endoscopic dilations; surgical revision is seldom necessary.

Necrosis of the transplant is an exceptional situation. It may be related either to poor arterial blood flow in patients with severe arteritis or to poor venous return. The latter has to be suspected when digestive juice in the nasogastric or nasocolic catheter becomes bloody in the early postoperative period. Such a critical situation theoretically leads to the necessity for removing the necrotic area, replacing the lower part of the transplant into the abdomen, and performing a cervical esophagostomy and a feeding jejunostomy. However, as documented in one of our own patients, necrosis of the cervical part of the transplant after esophagopharyngolaryngectomy may be treated by segmental resection and reestablishment of digestive continuity using either a free digestive transplant or a musculocutaneous tube.

CONCLUSION

More than one digestive segment is available for restoring continuity after esophagectomy. The development of stapling devices has played an important role in the evolution of techniques through the past decade. We have discussed only guidelines for constructing the different esophageal substitutes. Long-standing experience with esophageal surgery is required to adapt the various techniques to each individual case. Meticulousness in the performance of the multiple steps of such a complex operation is critical to minimize the risk of postoperative life-threatening complications or death.[26]

REFERENCES

1. Collard JM, Lerut T, Otte JB, et al. Traitement des tumeurs du carrefour oesopharyngolaryngé par oesopharyngolaryngectomie: Expérience commune de l'UCL et de la KUL. Lyon Chir 85:285-288, 1989.
2. Collard JM, Otte JB, Reynaert M, et al. Feasibility and effectiveness of en bloc resection of the esophagus for esophageal cancer: Results of a prospective study. Int Surg 76:209-213, 1991.
3. Michel L, Collard JM. Oesophagus: Perforation, Boerhaave's syndrome, and Mallory-Weiss syndrome. Oxford Textbook of Surgery. Oxford: Oxford University Press, 1992.
4. Akiyama H, Miyazono H, Tsurumaru M, et al. Use of the stomach as an esophageal substitute. Ann Surg 188:606-610, 1978.
5. Collard JM, Otte JB, Reynaert M, et al. Long gastroplasties with the GIA stapler in esophageal surgery. In Ravitch M, Steichen F, Welter R, eds. Current Practice in Surgical Stapling. Philadelphia: Lea & Febiger, 1991, pp 183-187.
6. Collard JM, Otte JB, Kestens PJ. From the tubulized gastroplasty to the denuded entire stomach. In Inouye T, Fukuda H, Sato T, et al., eds. Recent Advances in Bronchoesophagology. Amsterdam: Elsevier, 1990, pp 577-581.
7. Ioshida M, Iwatsuka M. Separated and pedicled wide gastric tube as an esophageal substitute. In Siewert J, Hölsher A, eds. Diseases of the Esophagus. Berlin: Springer-Verlag, 1988, pp 451-454.
8. Belsey R. Reconstruction of the esophagus with left colon. J Thorac Cardiovasc Surg 49:33-53, 1965.
9. Postlethwait RW. Colonic interposition for esophageal substitution. Surg Gynecol Obstet 156:377-383, 1983.
10. Otte JB, Lerut T, Collard JM, et al. Les plasties coliques de l'oesophage. Acta Chir Belg 82:389-396, 1982.
11. DeMeester TR, Johansson KE, Franze I, et al. Indications, surgical techniques, and long-term functional results of colon interposition or by-pass. Ann Surg 208:460-474, 1988.
12. Goldsmith HJ, Akiyama H. A comparative study of Japanese and American gastric dimensions. Ann Surg 190:690-693, 1979.
13. Koskas F, Gayet B. Etude anatomo-technique avec injection vasculaire des oesophagoplasties gastriques rétrosternales chez le cadavre. Actualités Digestives 2:67-68, 1985.
14. Giraud RMA, Berzin S. The reversed gastric esophagoplasty in palliation of carcinoma of the esophagus. Surg Gynecol Obstet 165:111-115, 1987.
15. Ancona E, Rossi M, Finco C, et al. Lengthening of gastric tube for esogastroplasty by extramucosal myotomy. Second International Symposium on Stapling [Abstract], p 59.
16. Collard JM, Otte JB, Reynaert M, et al. Quality of life three or more years following esophagectomy for cancer. J Thorac Cardiovasc Surg (in press).
17. Collard JM, Otte JB, Kestens PJ. Gastric pull-up to the neck after total or subtotal esophagectomy. A comparison of two methods of reconstruction (in preparation).
18. Liebermann-Meffert D, Rashcke M, Siewert JR. How well vascularized is a gastric tube from the greater curvature? Fourth World Congress of the ISDE, Chicago, 1989 [Abstract], p 1.
19. Hay JM, Maillard JN. Etude anatomique des gastroplasties. J Chirurgi Colombes (communication), 1983.
20. Ngan SYK, Wong J. Lengths of different routes for esophageal replacement. J Thorac Cardiovasc Surg 91:790-792, 1986.
21. Maillard JN, Hay JM. Surgical anatomy of available routes for oesophageal by-pass. In Jamieson GG, ed. Surgery of the Oesophagus. Edinburgh: Churchill Livingstone, 1988, pp 723-726.
22. Wong J. The use of small bowel for oesophageal replacement following oesophageal resection. In Jamieson GG, ed. Surgery of the Oesophagus, Edinburgh: Churchill Livingstone, 1988, pp 749-760.
23. Segol P, Gignoux M, Marchand P, et al. Oesophagectomie pour cancer de l'oesophage. Etude comparative de l'oesophagectomie subtotale et de l'oesophagectomie partielle. The Belsey Seventy-fifth Celebration Meeting, Louvain (communication), 1985.
24. Giuli R. Enquête du groupe O.E.S.O. In Giuli R, ed. Les Cancers de l'Oesophage en 1984: 135 Questions. Paris: Maloine, 1984, pp 401-424.
25. Peracchia A, Tremolada C. Anastomose intrathoracique, fistules et sténoses, anastomose manuelle versus anastomose mécanique. Actualités Chirurgicales, 86ème Congress Français de Chirurgie, Paris, 1985, p 41.
26. Collard JM, Otte JB, Reynaert M, et al. Esophageal resection and by-pass: A 6 year experience with a low postoperative mortality. World J Surg 15:635-641, 1991.

115 Reconstruction After Total Gastrectomy With Mechanical Sutures

Aldo Leggeri, Mauro Roseano, and Marina Bortul

Reconstruction after total gastrectomy presents various problems—both of digestive physiopathology and of surgical technique.

As far as physiopathological problems are concerned, several techniques have been proposed to avoid the *postgastrectomy syndrome*. Reconstruction modalities can be divided into two groups, depending on whether duodenal transit is maintained. Studies have demonstrated that the maintenance or exclusion of duodenal transit influences neither functional results nor nutritional effects.[1-3]

However, sophisticated investigations into postgastrectomy biliopancreatic physiology have demonstrated that maintenance of the duodenal transit may be the most physiological modality of reconstruction because it affects the hormonal mechanism regulating biliopancreatic secretion.[4,5] Therefore the choice of reconstruction must take into account both the best quality of life for the patient and the higher incidence of potential complications resulting from increasing complexity of various reconstruction modalities and the correspondingly rising number of anastomoses required.

As far as the surgical technique is concerned, the introduction of stapling devices has helped with the performance of complex operations. In total gastrectomy the surgical problem concerns esophagojejunal anastomosis, since the anastomosis must be performed at the level of the esophageal hiatus, which is a narrow and deep surgical field. The structure of the muscular esophageal wall and the terminal modality of vascularization make it difficult for surgical sutures to hold. Many technical solutions for these problems have been achieved by using manually placed sutures (e.g., transverse rather than vertical execution of the suture on the esophageal wall and the execution of a second esophagojejunal suture so that the first suture line can be protected). However, the stapler is both easier to handle and more reliable than manual suturing.

MATERIALS AND METHODS

Our personal experience with staplers dates from October 1979. We have performed 105 total gastrectomies for gastric neoplasms with stapling devices. In the first years of our experience (1979 to 1983), we used the Russian SPTU device in 12 cases; then (1984 to 1989) we used the American end-to-end anastomosis (EEA) device with disposable cartridges, and then wholly disposable devices (76 cases). More recently curved end-to-end anastomosis (CEEA) devices have been used routinely (17 cases). For reconstruction we prefer the interposed jejunal loop as described by Mouchet-Camey in younger patients and in patients at an early tumor stage with a long life expectancy. The jejunal loop must be at least 50 cm long. In the other patients we used a Roux-en-Y reconstruction with a jejunal loop at least 60 cm long. The Hoffmann technique was used in only two cases: both were elderly patients in poor health (Table 1).

The esophagojejunal anastomosis was performed with an end-to-side technique. After preparation of the distal esophagus, the lumen was calibrated using Hegar dilators of increasing size so that the anvil of the stapler could be inserted without causing mucosal lesions, which can lead to stenosis. Purse-string suturing was carried out (easy to perform using the disposable purse-string instrument). Anvil No. 25 of the disposable stapler was introduced into the esophagus and the purse-string suture tied. The jejunal loop was then passed through an avascular area of the mesocolon. Particular attention was paid to avoid any twisting of the jejunal loop on its vascular pedicle. Without its anvil and

Table 1. Reconstruction after total gastrectomy

Technique	Cases
Roux-en-Y	79
Mouchet-Camey	24
Hoffmann	2
TOTAL	105

fitted with a trocar, the stapler was inserted into the open lumen of the jejunum to perforate the wall at least 6 to 7 cm from the upper jejunal margin. After the trocar was removed, the anastomosis was completed. The open end of the jejunal loop was closed with a TA stapler, avoiding a large cul de sac and obtaining an end-to-side esophagojejunal anastomosis.

Care must be taken when the CEEA stapler is closed to avoid any intraoperative complication such as catching the lateral wall of the jejunal loop, which would lead to stenosis of the anastomosis. In addition, during the purse-string preparation and the esophageal lumen calibration, it is important to avoid causing mucosal tears that might result when traumatic forceps are used. This part of the operation now is less traumatic because of the disposable purse-string device.

We also used stapling devices in the jejunoduodenal anastomosis and in only 30 cases of jejunojejunal anastomosis; we now prefer to use manual sutures. In all the cases of the Roux-en-Y reconstruction the duodenum was closed using a TA stapler.

RESULTS

During the 105 total gastrectomies performed, we had no problems associated with poor working of the stapling devices (e.g., staples failing to advance, defective closure of staples, or annular blades failing to cut the inverted visceral surfaces).

Table 2 illustrates postoperative complications. They were more serious during the first phase of our experience when we used the SPTU device (three cases out of 12 [25%]). Serious complications fell sharply when American staplers were used (for EEA and ILS, five cases out of 76 [6.5%], and for CEEA, one case out of 17

[5.8%], giving a total of nine anastomotic leaks [8.5%]). With the reconstruction type of total gastrectomy there were six leaks out of 79 cases (8.7%) using the Roux-en-Y technique and three out of 24 (12%) using the Mouchet-Camey technique.

Treatment of fistulas was conservative, using suctioned drainage placed near the anastomosis during the operation and total parenteral nutrition. Dehiscence of the anastomosis led to the patient's death in only one case (11%).

Stricture occurred in one patient with an esophagojejunal anastomosis with a Hoffmann loop and was secondary to severe alkaline reflux. The problem was resolved by medical therapy and endoscopic dilations.

In other anastomoses requiring total gastrectomy, two leaks were found at the level of the jejunoduodenal anastomosis (8.3%) and one at the level of the jejunojejunal anastomosis (3.3%). No patient died.

DISCUSSION

Widespread use of stapling devices in gastric surgery necessitates critical evaluation of their use, especially in terms of cost/benefit ratio. In the case of reconstruction after total gastrectomy it also is important to evaluate data from the literature regarding the incidence of complications and mortality after manual and mechanical methods of anastomosis. Authors have been especially concerned with esophagojejunal anastomosis because it is with this procedure that the manual technique has resulted in a high incidence of fistulas, ranging from 6% to 23%,[6-8] even if a reduction of incidence has been demonstrated recently.[9,10] Experiences with stapling devices have shown that the rate of occurrence of these incidents has fallen to much lower levels (0% to 10%).[11-13] Moreover, examination of numerous case studies shows that dehiscence mainly occurs during the initial phase of various authors' experience and then falls to much lower levels once greater experience in using the instrument has been acquired and when disposable instruments, which are highly reliable, are available. Complications connected to poor functioning of the stapler are now very rare with the use of new disposable devices. Mortality as a consequence of leakage of the anastomosis has fallen significantly in the changeover from manual to mechanical suturing.[14,15] This decrease has resulted because the rupture of manual sutures usually occurs widely, if not totally, whereas it is more limited with mechanical suturing. In addition, parenteral nutrition can be used for long periods of time,

Table 2. Postoperative complications after total gastrectomy

Complication	Cases	Operative Mortality
Anastomotic dehiscence		
Radiological	2	—
Clinical	7	1
Stricture	1	—
Hemorrhage	—	—

something that was not possible earlier, during the time of manual suturing only.

Our experience further demonstrates that the use of highly improved instruments has greatly reduced the incidence of complications.

Authors have been less concerned with manual versus mechanical suturing in cases of other anastomoses performed during total gastrectomies since in these cases the use of staplers does not lead to a real benefit in terms of incidence of fistulas in comparison with manual suturing. In our experience the incidence was reduced in jejunojejunal anastomoses, whereas we found a higher number of leaks in cases of jejunoduodenal anastomosis. However, complications were again higher in the first phase of our experience when we used SPTU staplers.

CONCLUSION

We favor the use of staplers in total gastrectomies. As far as esophagojejunal anastomosis is concerned in particular, there is no doubt that technological features of the disposable devices, especially the curve of the CEEA stapler, facilitate the operation. At the level of the esophageal hiatus where the surgical field is narrow and deep, mechanical suturing renders execution of the anastomosis simple, rapid, and, above all, safe, whereas manual techniques require greater attention and do not guarantee the same hold. Although defective performance of more recent staplers can now be ruled out, the result of the suturing depends on correct technique of execution, which includes careful preparation of the viscera that will be anastomosed, precise execution of the purse-string suturing, choosing the correct-caliber instrument, respecting the vascularization of the loop, and maintaining complete absence of tension along the suture line.

For the prevention of strictures, it is essential to remember the importance of using medium-caliber staplers except in an esophagus with a greatly reduced diameter in which a lower caliber is required. Moreover, the use of long jejunal loops that impede alkaline reflux prevents stricture caused by esophagitis.

As far as the use of stapling devices in other anastomoses is concerned, we support their use in the elderly or in patients in poor health because their only advantage is that of more rapid execution.

REFERENCES

1. Troidl H, Kusche J, Westweber K, et al. Pouch versus esophagojejunostomy after total gastrectomy: A randomized clinical trial. World J Surg 11:699, 1987.
2. Miholic J, Meyer HJ, Kotzerke J, et al. Emptying of gastric substitute after total gastrectomy. Am Surg 210:165, 1989.
3. Stael von Holstein C, Walther B, Ibrahimbegovic E, et al. Nutritional status after total and partial gastrectomy with Roux-en-Y reconstruction. Br J Surg 78:1084, 1991.
4. Nishiwaki H, Satake K, Kitamura T, et al. Postprandial plasma secretion response in patients following gastrectomy. Surg Gynecol Obstet 156:69, 1983.
5. Itani KMF, Akwari DE, Burch W, et al. Gastric emptying, glucose tolerance and insulin response after duodenojejunostomy. J Surg Res 42:521, 1987.
6. Ekbom GA, Gleysteen JJ. Gastric malignancy: Resection for palliation. Surgery 88:476, 1980.
7. Papachristou DN, Forner JG. Anastomotic failure complicating total gastrectomy and esophagogastrectomy for cancer of the stomach. Am J Surg 151:244, 1986.
8. Saario I, Shroeder T, Tolppanen E, et al. Total gastrectomy with esophagojejunostomy. Analysis of 100 consecutive patients. Am J Surg 151:244, 1986.
9. Seufert RM, Schmidt-Matthiesen A, Beyer A. Total gastrectomy and esophago-jejunostomy—A prospective randomized trial of hand sutured versus mechanically stapled anastomoses. Br J Surg 77:50, 1990.
10. Fujimoto S, Takahashi M, Endoh F, et al. Stapled or manual suturing in esophagojejunostomy after total gastrectomy: A comparison of outcome in 379 patients. Am J Surg 162:256, 1991.
11. Campion JO, Grossetti D, Launois B. Circular anastomosis stapler: An alternative to purse-string suture. Arch Surg 119:232, 1984.
12. Ulrich B, Kochel N. Maschinelle oesophagusanastomosen. Clin Gastroenterol 2:47, 1986.
13. Leggeri A, Roseano M, Bortul M. Le anastomosi esofagodigiunali meccaniche. Chirurgie 1:251, 1988.
14. Junginger T, Walgenbach S, Pichlmaier H. Die zirkulare Klammernahtanastomose (EEA) nach Gastrektomie. Chirurg 54:161, 1983.
15. Partenski C, Champetier P, Faure JL. L'anastomose esojéjunale termino-terminale mécenique a l'EEA. Aspects techniques et complications spécifiques. Lyon Chir 84:169, 1988.

116 *Reconstruction After Pancreatectomy*

Christian Partensky and Aly el Arini

Pancreatectomies are currently divided into three categories: distal pancreatectomy, pancreaticoduodenectomy (Whipple procedure), and total pancreatectomy. However, two new operations have been developed during the last few years and now belong to the spectrum of pancreatic resections: isthmic pancreatectomy, which consists of segmental resection of the pancreatic isthmus, and regional pancreatectomies, which are resections that extend to the surrounding vascular structure.

Once these various resection procedures have been performed, continuity must be restored wherever pancreatic, biliary, and digestive flow has been interrupted. Moreover, vascular reconstruction is needed after regional pancreatectomies, particularly in patients with severe stenosis or thrombosis of the celiac axis who are referred for pancreaticoduodenectomy.

Regardless of the complexity of the reconstruction, the very specific technical point remains restoration (or interruption) of pancreatic flow, since the consequences of a pancreatic fistula may be dramatic and life threatening. Treatment of the pancreatic remnant is the critical step in the operation. Consequently it is not surprising that most controversies regarding reconstruction after pancreatic resections concern the reconstruction after pancreaticoduodenectomy.

DISTAL PANCREATECTOMY

Distal pancreatectomy is usually considered to be the simplest type of resection with the lowest morbidity. However, the extent of the resection may vary considerably from 30% to 90% and the dissection, which is usually simple when the operation is performed for small lesions of the tail of the pancreas, may become extremely difficult when segmental portal hypertension as a result of splenic vein occlusion is present.

In most cases, Wirsung's duct drains freely into the duodenum and the procedure can be performed without any reconstruction. After transection of the pancreatic parenchyma, the pancreatic duct is identified and ligated, and the pancreatic surface is closed with running or interrupted sutures. The use of staplers for transection and closure of the pancreas must be considered

with caution because of the risk of fragmentation of pancreatic tissue unless the pancreatic parenchyma is atrophic and thin. We favor closure with running, slowly resorbing sutures.

On the other hand, pancreatic drainage into the digestive tract must be restored after left pancreatectomy when Wirsung's duct is obstructed either at the papilla or in the cephalic remnant by chronic calcifying pancreatitis. This obstruction can be demonstrated by catheterization of the dilated Wirsung's duct and injection of dye under fluoroscopy. In this case the Du Val procedure, which consists of a pancreaticojejunal anastomosis with a Roux-en-Y loop, is the procedure of choice. As a consequence of the chronic inflammatory process, the pancreatic parenchyma is easy to suture and the risk of fistula is very low. Consequently this mode of reconstruction does not usually generate any technical problems. The anastomosis can be performed end to end, at the level of the pancreatic transection, or side to side, after opening of Wirsung's duct in the direction of the papilla, a maneuver that may facilitate the extraction of juxtapapillary pancreatic calculi.

PANCREATICODUODENECTOMY

Since Whipple's original description of a two-stage operation in 1935, pancreaticoduodenectomy remained a formidable procedure until the last decade when technical refinements led to a considerable decline in the operative mortality, as reported throughout the world literature.[1] Although extension of the resection toward the tail may vary, it usually preserves enough islets to prevent diabetes, which is the main intent, and is superior to the total pancreatectomy procedure.

Pylorus-preserving pancreaticoduodenectomy (PPPD) has become an increasingly accepted alternative, since its original description by Traverso and Longmire.[2] It has become the procedure of choice for benign conditions because of its technical simplicity compared with partial gastrectomy, and the improvement in postoperative comfort it provides. Moreover, it can be used for malignant tumors that do not invade the first portion of the duodenum and the perigastric lymph nodes, such as periampullary tumors and stage I and II pancreatic carcinomas.[3,4] Our personal experience with PPPD currently includes 75 patients (Table 1).

There are a number of acceptable methods for restoring continuity following pancreaticoduodenal resection. Reconstruction has always been considered a key point after the Whipple procedure, since most causes of operative mortality and morbidity are closely related to failure of the anastomosis, especially the pancreaticodigestive anastomosis. Occlusion of the distal Wirsung's duct with neoprene or fibrin glue has been advocated by some investigators. We and others have limited experience with this procedure and believe it is technically more demanding than a drainage procedure.

A considerable number of technical reconstructive procedures have been described in the literature. One of the most popular is the Child procedure. The jejunum is brought to the region of the pancreas in a retro-colic manner or in an antecolic position. We favor the antecolic position because it does not require opening and subsequent closing of the mesocolon. We routinely transect the pancreas with an ultrasonic dissector for the following two reasons: (1) elective dissection and hemostasis of small pancreatic vessels with bipolar coagulation or ligature, and (2) isolation and dissection of Wirsung's duct at 1.5 to 2 cm above the pancreatic surface (Fig. 1). Reconstruction begins with an end-to-end anastomosis between the pancreas and the jejunum. We use one layer of running 0000 monofilament absorbable sutures, although interrupted and nonabsorbable sutures have been advocated by many.[5] We routinely insert a catheter into Wirsung's duct before suturing and remove it at the end of the anastomosis procedure. The second anastomosis is the end-to-side hepaticojejunostomy, which is usually performed at a distance of 15 to 25 cm from the pancreatic anastomosis, according to the anatomic relationship. We use 4-0 or 5-0 absorba-

Table 1. Personal experience with pancreaticoduodenectomy (October 1981 to August 1992)

Pathological Condition	PPPD No. of Cases	Whipple Procedure No. of Cases	Total
Malignant			
Pancreatic exocrine carcinoma	23 (1)	7 (0)	30 (1)
Ampullary carcinoma	15 (1)	3 (0)	18 (1)
Pancreatic endocrine carcinoma	4 (1)	1 (0)	5 (1)
Cystic benign pancreatic tumor	5 (0)	1 (0)	6 (0)
Duodenal carcinoma	3 (1)	0	3 (1)
Metastatic pancreatic carcinoma	2 (0)	0	2 (0)
Biliary carcinoma	2 (0)	2 (0)	4 (0)
Endocrine ampullary carcinoma	2 (0)	1 (0)	3 (0)
Gastric carcinoma	0	1 (0)	1 (0)
Benign			
Chronic pancreatitis	13 (0)	3 (0)	16 (0)
Endocrine pancreatic tumor	4 (0)	0	4 (0)
Benign ampulloma	1 (0)	0	1 (0)
Pancreatic trauma	1 (0)	0	1 (0)
Radioinduced pancreatitis	0	1 (0)	1 (0)
TOTAL	75 (4)	20 (0)	95 (4)

PPPD = pylorus-preserving pancreaticoduodenectomy.
Operative mortality figures in parentheses.

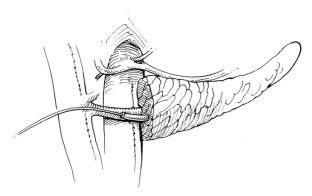

Fig. 1. Transection of the pancreas during pancreatico-duodenectomy with isolation of Wirsung's duct (using ultrasonic dissection), leaving a 1.5 to 2 cm stump above the cut surface of the pancreas.

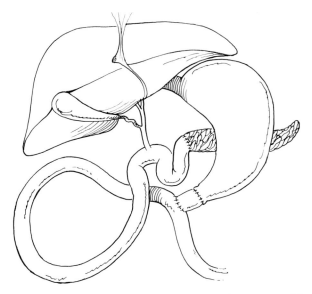

Fig. 3. Pylorus-preserving pancreaticoduodenectomy with pancreaticojejunal anastomosis.

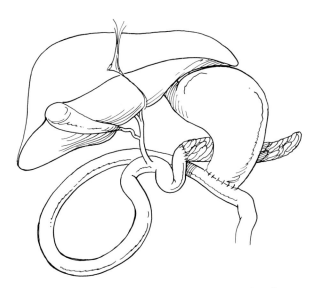

Fig. 2. Whipple operation with pancreaticojejunal anastomosis according to Child.

biliary tree. The gastro- or duodenojejunostomy is performed in an ordinary fashion, that is, with a single layer of 4-0 sunning absorbable sutures (Figs. 2 and 3). A nasogastric tube is left in place, and two small suction drains are inserted to allow drainage of tissue fluids and lymph.

A large number of alternative methods of reconstruction have been reported. Some of them concern the methodology of pancreaticojejunostomy, end to side rather than end to end, with mucosa-to-mucosa approximation, with a stent or a tube that is brought through the skin. Other procedures concern the order of the anastomosis, the length of the intestinal loop between the pancreatic and biliary anastomoses, and the placement of pancreatic and biliary anastomoses into separate jejunal limbs.

The most interesting of these proposed modifications is the creation of a pancreaticogastrostomy rather than a pancreaticojejunostomy.[6-9] Such encouraging results have been reported that we and others have recently switched our standard technique from pancreaticojejunostomy to pancreaticogastrostomy.[10-12] The procedure is easy to perform and in fact seems to be more accurate from a technical standpoint than pancreaticojejunostomy (Figs. 4 and 5). A number of theoretical and technical advantages supporting the use of

ble running sutures and do not place any tubes in the bile duct. In the case of a small bile duct, we use interrupted sutures and temporarily intubate the anastomosis with a catheter, which is removed at the end of the procedure. The last type of reconstruction concerns end-to-side duodenojejunal (or gastrojejunal) anastomosis, which is located 50 to 60 cm from the biliary anastomosis to prevent reflux of gastric contents into the

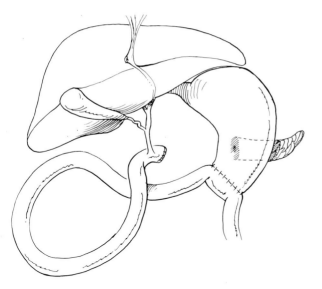

Fig. 4. Whipple operation with pancreaticogastric anastomosis.

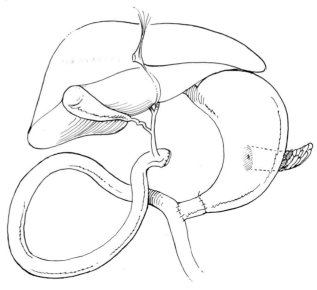

Fig. 5. Pylorus-preserving pancreaticoduodenectomy with pancreaticogastric anastomosis.

Table 2. Results of pancreaticogastrostomy after pancreaticoduodenectomy

Investigator	Year	No. of Cases	Pancreatic Fistula	Bleeding at the Anastomosis Site	Operative Deaths
Waugh	1946	1	0	0	0
Milbourn	1959	7	0	0	0
Mackie	1975	2	1	0	2
Flautner	1985	27	0	1	0
Kapur	1986	31	0	2	2
Icard	1988	17	0	1	0
Delcore	1990	45	0	1	1
Sauvanet	1991	27	1	1	1
Arnaud	1992	26	0	0	2
Partensky	1992	10	0	0	0

pancreaticogastrostomy include the anatomical proximity of the posterior gastric wall to the pancreatic remnant, the security of suturing the pancreas into the stomach, and the postoperative decompression of the stomach, which prevents build-up of pancreatic secretions. Our preliminary results have been satisfactory, and pancreaticogastrostomy has become standard procedure in our current practice (Table 2).

TOTAL PANCREATECTOMY

Total pancreatectomy is usually considered with great reluctance because of the metabolic consequences, which can be disastrous. However, it can be attempted as a mode of technical resolution when softness and friability of the pancreatic parenchyma make pancreaticodigestive anastomosis hazardous and as a second-step procedure when the postoperative course is complicated by pancreatitis or pancreaticodigestive fistula. The pylorus can be preserved occasionally, that is, when the same criteria as those for the Whipple procedure are met. This was the case in five of our patients.

Autotransplantation of the tail has been advocated to decrease the risk of severe diabetes, but this time-consuming, complicated, and hazardous procedure has not achieved widespread acceptance in our surgical community.

SEGMENTAL ISTHMIC PANCREATECTOMY

This modality of limited conservative therapy, that is, segmental isthmic resection of the pancreas, has the advantage of avoiding a major resection in the treatment of benign tumors of the pancreatic isthmus.[13] The original description was of a limited pancreatic resection centered on the neck, with restitution of exocrine function by an end-to-end anastomosis between the tail of the pancreas and a Roux-en-Y loop. The cephalad pancreas is closed by a single layer of running delayed-absorption sutures. Our personal experience with this operation includes 12 patients, six with pancreatic cystadenoma, five with focalised chronic pancreatitis, and one with insulinoma.[14] The first 11 patients underwent reconstruction with a Roux-en-Y loop; the remaining patient underwent pancreaticogastrostomy for a non-enucleable isthmic insulinoma (Figs. 6 and 7). This latter procedure appeared to be very simple and secure. Our impression is that it may be considered the procedure of choice for reconstruction after segmental isthmic pancreatectomy, as has become the case after pancreaticoduodenectomy.

REGIONAL PANCREATECTOMY

Regional pancreatectomies have been described by Fortner et al.[15] These operations include various modalities of more or less complex vascular resection(s) and subsequent reconstruction(s), which have been classified into the following four types: *type I*, resection of the portal vein; *type IIa*, resection of both the portal vein and the superior mesenteric artery; *type IIb*, resection of both the portal vein and the hepatic artery; and *type IIc*, resection of the portal vein plus the superior mesenteric artery plus the hepatic artery. The least unusual of these major procedures is type I, which consists of an en bloc pancreatic portal vein and lymph node resection. Reconstruction of the portal vein can be achieved by various means including direct end-to-end anastomosis, venous graft, or prosthetic graft. The use of arterial grafts

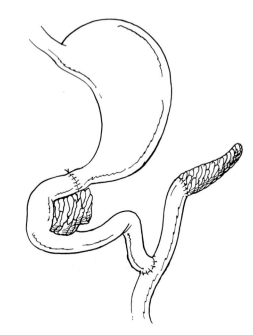

Fig. 6. Segmental isthmic pancreatectomy with pancreaticojejunal Roux-en-Y anastomosis.

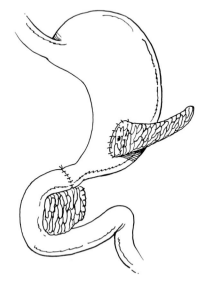

Fig. 7. Segmental isthmic pancreatectomy with pancreaticogastric anastomosis.

collected from a cadaver donor has been advocated for arterial reconstruction.

PANCREATICODUODENECTOMY AND CELIAC OCCLUSIVE DISEASE

As far as exceptional procedures are concerned, vascular reconstruction may also be needed in the particular association of pancreaticoduodenectomy and celiac occlusive disease. Sectioning of the gastroduodenal artery interrupts the collateral pathways that develop in response to chronic celiac insufficiency, with the subsequent risk of hepatic failure and breakdown of the anastomosis. As a consequence of this hemodynamic disturbance, restoration of blood flow to the upper abdominal viscera becomes necessary. Stenosis of the celiac axis as a result of median arcuate ligament obstruction may be treated by simple resection of the median arcuate ligament, which immediately restores pulsations and thrill in the hepatic left gastric and splenic arteries.[16] In contrast, strong consideration should be given at the time of pancreaticoduodenal resection to simultaneous celiac revascularization in the case of complete obstruction of the celiac axis. A splenic-to-mesenteric artery reimplantation technique has been advocated in this case by Thompson et al.[17]

REFERENCES

1. Trede M, Schwall G, Saeger HD. Survival after pancreatoduodenectomy. 118 consecutive resections without an operative mortality. Ann Surg 211:447-458, 1990.
2. Traverso LW, Longmire WP. Preservation of the pylorus in pancreaticoduodenectomy. Surg Gynecol Obstet 146:959-962, 1978.
3. Partensky C, Champetier P, Faure JL. Peut-on élargir les indications de la conservation pylorique? Ann Chir 42:313-317, 1988.
4. Roder JD, Stein HJ, Hüttl W, et al. Pylorus-preserving versus standard pancreaticoduodenectomy: An analysis of 110 pancreatic and periampullary carcinomas. Br J Surg 79:152-155, 1992.
5. Jordan GL. Pancreatic resection for pancreatic cancer. Surg Clin North Am 69:569-597, 1989.
6. Flautner L, Tihanyl T, Szecseny A. Pancreaticogastrostomy: An ideal complement to pancreatic head resection with preservation of the pylorus in the treatment of chronic pancreatitis. Am J Surg 150:608-611, 1985.
7. Kapur BM. Pancreaticogastrostomy in pancreaticoduodenal resection for ampullary carcinoma: Experience in thirty-one cases. Surgery 100:489-492, 1986.
8. Mackie JA, Rhoads JE, Park CD. Pancreaticogastrostomy: A further evaluation. Ann Surg 181:541-545, 1975.
9. Dubois F, Icard P. Un méthode sûre de traitement du moignon pancréatique après duodénopancréatectomie céphalique: l'anastomose pancréaticogastrique. Ann Chir 42:319-321, 1988.
10. Delcore R, Thomas JH, Pierce GE, et al. Pancreaticogastrostomy: A safe drainage procedure after pancreaticoduodenectomy. Surgery 108:641-647, 1990.
11. Sauvanet A, Belghiti J, Gayet B, Fekété F. L'anastomose pancreatico-gastrique après duodénopancréatectomie céphalique. Ann Chir 45:889-893, 1991.
12. Arnaud JP, Casa C, Pousset JP, et al. Pancreaticogastrostomy: A safe drainage procedure after pancreaticoduodenectomy. Br J Surg (Suppl) 79:S116, 1992.
13. Fagniez PL, Kracht M, Rotman N. Limited conservative pancreatectomy for benign tumours: A new technical approach. Br J Surg 75:719, 1968.
14. El Arini A, Velecela E, Frering V, et al. Pancréatectomie segmentaire pour tumeur de l'isthme du pancréas [Abstract]. Ann Chir 46:535-536, 1992.
15. Fortner JG, Kim DK, Cubilla A, et al. Regional pancreatectomy. En bloc pancreatic, portal vein and lymph node resection. Ann Surg 186:42-50, 1977.
16. Fortner JG, Watson RC. Median arcuate ligament obstruction of celiac axis and pancreatic cancer. Ann Surg 194:698-700, 1981.
17. Thompson NW, Eckhauser FE, Talpos G, et al. Pancreaticoduodenectomy and celiac occlusive disease. Ann Surg 193:399-406, 1981.

117 *Endoluminal Endoscopic Electrosurgical Management of Postoperative Anastomotic Strictures of the Upper Gastrointestinal Tract*

Karl-Joseph Paquet and Aristotel Lazar

The causes of postoperative strictures in the upper GI tract include marginal ulcerations or anastomotic edema and fibrosis in patients who have undergone esophageal or gastric resection and esophagogastrostomy, or gastroenterostomy for acid induced peptic disease, premalignant, or malignant conditions. Most patients are seen with a variable increase in postprandial pain, reflux symptoms, nausea and vomiting, or weight loss. Traditionally surgery has been the primary therapeutic option for benign esophageal or esophagogastric outlet obstruction, but operative treatment cannot be performed without mortality and morbidity. More recently, however, balloon dilation of benign stenoses has been used in an attempt to correct such obstructions with less morbidity and mortality.[1,2] As an alternative to balloon dilation, we have developed two different procedures in which a polypectomy snare is used. In this chapter we describe the techniques and report our results in the first 15 patients over a 5-year period.

MATERIALS AND METHODS

Any solid-state electrosurgical unit suitable for polypectomy is acceptable. We used a small snare, 3.2 cm long and widening to 1 cm. For resection of anastomotic scar tissue (technique 1) by polypectomy technique (Fig. 1), a larger snare, 6.2 cm long and widening to 3 cm, is sometimes required. For resection of anastomotic scar tissue, two forces must act simultaneously: one is the heat supplied by the electrosurgical unit, and the other is the shearing action produced when the wire loop is closed by squeezing the snare handle assembly. Either of these two forces acting alone will not result in satisfactory resection of anastomotic scar tissue. Heat without the mechanical force of a wire transection will not result in resection, and the shearing force alone may result in resection but will not achieve the desired hemostatic effect provided by heat.

Anastomotic strictures occurring after an operative procedure present difficulties that cannot in every case be successfully managed by technique 1. Therefore technique 2 was developed (Fig. 2), which uses the same instrumentarium. After the gastroscope is introduced, the poloypectomy snare is partially opened or subtotally closed and localized with its center in the stenosis. Thereafter, under endoscopical view, longitudinal electrocautery incisions are made at the 3-, 7-, and 11-o'clock positions to a depth of 3 to 5 mm (see Fig. 2, B). There is little danger of perforation or deep secondary necrosis, because the anastomosis is usually surrounded by fibrotic tissue. Methods for handling the electrosurgical unit and the polypectomy snare have been described previously. The primary results of the enlarged lumen immediately after the three incisions is shown in Fig. 2, C. One week later, during an outpatient endoscopic control study, the lumen, which was originally 5 mm,

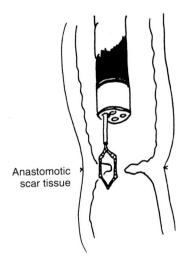

Anastomotic scar tissue

Fig. 1. Resection of anastomotic scar tissue by polypectomy snare (intrathoracic esophageogastric anastomotic stricture after resection for carcinoma of the cardia or terminal esophagus).

has been enlarged dramatically to 20 to 30 mm, and the three incisions were partially or totally covered by epithelium or mucosa.

The indications for primary operations that may result in the early or late postoperative development of anastomotic strictures are listed in Table 1. In detail, nine men (median age, 63.5 years) and six women (median age, 66.4 years) underwent some type of gastrectomy for the following reasons: cancer in four, resection of the cardia in four, cancer of the terminal esophagus in three and the middle third of the esophagus in

two, achalasia with dysplasia in one, and therapy-resistant peptic stenosis of the terminal esophagus in one. The types of anastomoses performed are shown in Table 2: nine intrathoracic anastomoses between the stomach and esophagus, four partially intrathoracic anastomoses between the esophagus and jejunum, and two gastroesophageal anastomoses in the neck without thoracotomy.

RESULTS

Minor bleeding was an early complication observed in three patients (Table 3), but it stopped spontaneously during the endoscopic procedure. No perforations were observed. All patients were followed for at least 1 year

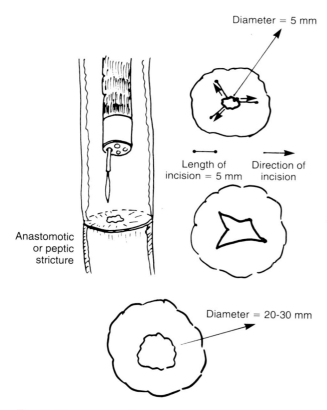

Fig. 2. Management of postoperative anastomotic or peptic stricture. Incisions with a subtotally closed or partially opened polypectomy snare longitudinally at the 3-, 7-, and 11-o'clock positions. **A,** The endoscope is introduced and the polypectomy snare is partially opened or subtotally closed. **B,** Longitudinal incision of the stricture (into the anastomotic tissue) at the 3-, 7-, and 11-o'clock positions. The stick (incision) should not be deeper than 5 mm! **C,** Primary results. **D,** Result after 1 week. The diameter of the lumen is enlarged from 5 mm to 20 to 30 mm. The incisions are subtotally or completely covered by epithelium or mucosa.

Table 1. Indications for primary operation

Indication	Number	Percent
Carcinoma of the cardia	4	26.50
Carcinoma of the stomach	4	26.50
Carcinoma of the terminal esophagus	3	20.00
Carcinoma of the middle third of the esophagus	2	13.50
Achalasia with dysplasia	1	6.75
Therapy-resistant peptic stenosis of the terminal esophagus	1	6.75
TOTAL	15	

Table 2. Type of anastomosis performed after gastrectomy, cardia, or esophagus resection because of cancer (n = 13), achalasia (n = 1), and peptic stenosis (n = 1)

Type of Anastomosis	Number	Percent
Gastroesophageal		
At the neck	2	13.5
Intrathoracic	9	60.0
Esophagojejunal, partially intrathoracic	4	26.5
TOTAL	15	

Table 3. Complications after endoluminal endoscopic electrosurgical management of postoperative anastomotic strictures

Complication	Number	Percent
Minor bleeding	3	20.0
Perforation	0	0

Table 4. Long-term results (over at least 1 year) of endoscopic endoluminal electrocautery dilation of postoperative anastomotic strictures in the upper gastrointestinal tract

Result	Number	Percent
Recurrence	2	13.5

(Table 4). After 1 and 3 months, respectively, two strictures redeveloped. The restenosis after 1 month was suspected to be the result of an inadequate longitudinal incision during the first electrocautery dilation procedure. Both restenoses were successfully managed with the same methodology.

DISCUSSION

Anastomotic strictures after surgery, particularly if they are localized in the neck after an esophagogastric anastomosis or intrathoracically following a gastroesophageal anastomosis are difficult to treat. Guidewire techniques that use metal dilators (olives, Eder-Puestow) or firm polyvinyl chloride tapered dilators with a hollow core (American or Savary-Gillard system) or hydrostatic balloons are dangerous and often unsuccessful. Sometimes, particularly if the stenosis is located in the neck, general anesthesia is necessary. Occasionally it is not possible to pass a guidewire or balloon catheter through the stricture. The disadvantage of metal dilators is their rigidity, which provokes multiple fissures and lesions in the stricture, which heal with the production of fibrotic scar tissue and result in restenosis. The rigidity of such stenoses prevents their successful dilation with hydrostatic balloons. Under all these circumstances, di-

lation must sometimes be performed at weekly intervals.

Our group has therefore developed two new techniques. In the first technique, anastomotic scar tissue can be safely resected with a polypectomy snare. In the second technique, three longitudinal incisions with a partially opened polypectomy snare are made at the 3-, 7-, and 11-o'clock positions to a depth of 3 to 5 mm. With this technique, strictures with a diameter of 5 mm can be enlarged to a diameter of 20 to 30 mm in one session. Our experience in 15 consecutive patients (nine men and six women) demonstrates that this technique is safe, quickly learned, and easy to perform. It can be applied in any endoscopical department where there is an electrosurgical unit for polypectomy. It is preferable to use this technique in postoperative strictures, since it often challenges traditional dilation methods such as the guidewire technique or more recently the application of hydrostatic balloons. These two new techniques can be combined for the definitive management of difficult strictures. Thus surgery, which is often associated with high morbidity and mortality, can be avoided.

CONCLUSION

A new technique of endoluminal endoscopic electrosurgical management of postoperative anastomotic strictures in the upper gastrointestinal tract is presented. Over a period of 5 years, 15 consecutive patients (nine men and six women) were observed weeks or months after gastrectomy for the following reasons: resection of the cardia because of cancer, resection of the terminal or middle third of the esophagus because of cancer, resection because of achalasia with dysplasia, or therapy-resistant peptic stenosis of the terminal esophagus. The locations of the anastomoses were as follows: in the neck in two patients, intrathoracic in nine, and partially intrathoracic or at the level of the diaphragm in four. In technique 1 resection of anastomotic scar tissue by a completely extended and thereafter subtotally extended polypectomy snare—comparable to a polypectomy procedure—is performed and can be repeated. In technique 2 a partially open or subtotally closed polypectomy snare is introduced with its middle part in the stenosis; thereafter a longitudinal incision is made at the 3-, 7-, and 11-o'clock positions to a depth of 3 to 5 mm. Three instances of minor bleedings (20%) were observed, which stopped spontaneously during the endoscopic procedure. During a follow-up period of at least 1 year, there were two recurrences: one after 1 month and one after 3 months; both were managed successfully with the same technique. These techniques are safe, easy to learn, and simple to perform. It is preferable to apply them in postoperative strictures, thus avoiding the need for reoperation. In the majority of cases treatment is definitive.

REFERENCES

1. Barkin J, O'Phelan CA. Advanced Therapeutic Endoscopy. New York: Raven Press, 1990, pp 1-105.
2. Mion F, Lambert R. Therapeutic Endoscopy in the oesophagus. Curr Opin Gastroenterol 8:606, 1992.

XVIII

Videoendoscopic Techniques in Operations on the Pleura, Lungs, and Mediastinum

118 Videoendoscopic Thoracic Operations and Endostapling for Diagnostic and Therapeutic Lung Resection

Hendrik Dienemann, Hans Hoffmann, Christian Mueller, Guenther Meyer, and Volker Lange

Recent improvements in video camera technology and endoscopic instruments, including the development of endoscopic stapling devices, have expanded the diagnostic and therapeutic applications of thoracoscopy. Although videothoracoscopic surgery (VTS) is an exciting new adjunct in the management of intrathoracic disease, adequate treatment with VTS may be achieved only in a specific group of patients. Most important, patients with malignant or metastatic pulmonary disease must be very carefully selected. VTS technique should not compromise the long-term benefits that can be achieved with standard thoracotomy procedures. We have reviewed our recent experience with wedge excisions of the lung by means of VTS to define appropriate indications.

MATERIALS AND METHODS

From October 1991 to January 1993, a total of 107 patients underwent 110 videothoracoscopic operations. Indications for pulmonary wedge resections were diagnosis and/or treatment of indeterminate peripheral solitary or multiple pulmonary nodules, diffuse interstitial lung disease including patients with lung transplants, and spontaneous and iatrogenic pneumothorax. Other procedures included excision of the pericardium, biopsy of pleural or mediastinal masses, drainage of hemothorax, and dorsal thoracic sympathectomy (Table 1). Peripheral pulmonary nodules were located by high-resolution spiral computed tomography (CT). In other patients preoperative CT was not mandatory.

All procedures were performed under general anesthesia with a double-lumen endotracheal tube. Patients were placed in the usual lateral decubitus position for standard thoracotomy and prepared to allow maximum flexibility for access. A 1 cm incision was made in the fourth or fifth intercostal space at the midaxillary line. After ipsilateral collapse of the lung was achieved by discontinuation of mechanical ventilation and insufflation of CO_2 through a Veress needle, a 10 mm trocar (Surgiport, United States Surgical Corporation) was

introduced through the incision to create access for the thoracoscope. A 10 mm 30-degree rigid endoscope and a CCD video camera (UTV-S2, Olympus Corporation) attached to a video monitor were used. After thoracoscopic examination, suitable sites for placement of additional trocars were selected. Usually a 5 mm trocar and a 12 mm trocar were inserted under direct vision between the posterior margin of the pectoralis muscle and the anterior margin of the latissimus muscle. Wedge excision was achieved by means of an endoscopic stapling device (EndoGIA) with 3.5 mm staples. The staple lines were inspected for air leakage during reinflation of the lung. In selected patients with pneumothorax, pleurodesis was performed with cauterization.

A constant positive pressure of 4 to 6 mm Hg was maintained by intermittent CO_2 insufflation through one of the trocars (OP-Pneu, Heraeus). On completion of the operation, a chest tube (size 20 to 28 Charrière) was inserted through the 10 mm trocar site, and the lung

Table 1. Indications for thoracoscopy

Disorder	No. of Patients
Solitary lesion/infiltrate	28
Multiple lesions/infiltrates	11
Diffuse interstitial disease (including posttransplant infiltrates)	14
Pneumothorax	32
Biopsies from pleura and mediastinum	17
Pericarditis (fenestration)	1
Hemothorax	1
Hyperhidrosis (upper extremities)	2
Occlusive disease (upper extremities)	1

Table 2. Tissue diagnosis by videothoracoscopic wedge resections

| | Pulmonary Nodules | | | |
	Solitary		Multiple	
History of malignancy	Yes	No	Yes	No
Diagnosis	(12)	(13)	(4)	(7)
Benign	7	12	1	3
Metastasis	4	None	2	1
Lung cancer	1	1	1	3
Thoracotomy	1	1	None	1

In three patients, histological studies revealed primary lung cancer; these patients then underwent thoracotomy and lung resection.

was reexpanded under full visualization. Trocar incisions were closed with nonabsorbable sutures.

RESULTS
Wedge Resection for Pulmonary Nodules

All solitary pulmonary nodules excised were less than 3 cm in diameter and were located in the periphery of the lung. Using tissue obtained at VTS a diagnosis was made or definitive operative therapy was achieved in 25 patients. Tissue diagnoses were as follows: benign in 19 patients, metastatic cancer in four, and bronchial carcinoma in two. The two patients with peripheral bronchial carcinoma underwent thoracotomy and open formal lung resection with lymph node dissection. It is noteworthy that of 12 patients with solitary pulmonary nodules and a history of malignancy, seven were found to have benign coin lesions after resection (Table 2).

In four patients with multiple pulmonary nodules, the lesions were benign. Three patients had metastatic cancer and four had primary lung cancer with pulmonary metastasis (Table 2).

Diffuse Pulmonary Disease

In 14 patients thoracoscopic wedge resection was performed for the diagnosis of diffuse parenchymal disease including acute rejection or infection following lung transplantation. Diagnosis by means of VTS was achieved in all patients, despite the fact that two of them had end-stage adult respiratory distress syndrome with densely consolidated lungs. In these patients one of the

trocar sites was enlarged, and a wedge resection of the lingula was performed with a conventional stapler.

Pneumothorax

Eleven patients underwent thoracoscopy for spontaneous pneumothorax type I according to Vanderschüren (no visible bullae).[1] In these patients apical wedge resection and partial pleurodesis with cauterization were performed. Patients with type III disease according to Vanderschüren (bullae <2 cm in diameter) had apical wedge resection only. Accompanying pleurodesis was performed in selected patients when additional nonresectable bullae were found. All three patients with type IV bullous disease according to Vanderschüren (bullae >2 cm in diameter) diagnosed thoracoscopically underwent an open procedure because of inadequate control of air leaks from the ruptured bullae. Moreover, two of these patients had multiple type IV bullae with a need to reduce parenchymal resection to a minimum. One patient required a more extensive procedure in terms of segmental resection (segments 4 and 5, left side). In four patients with iatrogenic pneumothorax, including two patients following heart-lung transplantation, the parenchymal air leak was sealed successfully with staples. Follow-up was complete in all patients and ranged from 2 to 62 weeks. None of the patients has had a recurrence.

Conversion to Thoracotomy

In 15 patients conversion to open thoracotomy (Table 3) became necessary for the following reasons: dense

Table 3. Indications for conversion to open thoracotomy

Cause	No. of Patients
Dense pleural adhesions	6
No atelectasis achieved	2
Lesion not identified	2
Pneumothorax with multiple bullae	3
Lung cancer identified on frozen section	2

pleural adhesions (n = 6), stiff lung syndrome (n = 2), small nodules that could not be located thoracoscopically (n = 2), multiple bullae that were deemed unsafe for thoracoscopic wedge resection (n = 3), or diagnosis of primary lung cancer (n = 2).

COMPLICATIONS

There was one significant intraoperative complication that required immediate thoracotomy for bleeding when the aortic arch was injured with a cauterization instrument. Three patients had prolonged air leaks (more than 3 days). Two of these patients required reoperation Postoperative morbidity and pain were reduced in comparison with open thoracotomy. The mean period of chest tube drainage was 1.5 days. The mean postoperative hospital stay after elective procedures performed in well patients was 2.5 days. There were no deaths. None of the patients had postoperative infections.

DISCUSSION

Based on successful experiences with video-assisted laparoscopic surgery, VTS has already become an accepted new modality in the diagnosis and treatment of thoracic disease. Controversy currently exists regarding the indications for VTS in patients with initial spontaneous pneumothorax or patients with pulmonary nodules that are found to be metastatic cancer or primary lung cancer.

Generally accepted indications for VTS include recurrent spontaneous pneumothorax, persistent air leak, and incomplete reexpansion of the lung with chest tube treatment. However, because of the high rate of recurrence (30%) with chest tube treatment only, some investigators advocate videothoracoscopic examination in all cases of initial spontaneous pneumothorax to ensure identification of all blebs.[2,3] Alternatively, standard thoracotomy causes postoperative pain and compromises lung function over a long period.[4] With the esthetically favorable small incision in the axillary region, evaluation of the caudal lung surface is not possible. Therefore, because of the minimally invasive nature of VTS and the reduced morbidity compared with open thoracotomy procedures, this technique should be offered as standard approach to patients with recurrent pneumothorax as a result of apical blebs. However, we currently believe that thoracoscopic wedge resection is unsafe for multiple bullae, and they require an open procedure.

Thoracoscopic wedge resection of pulmonary metastases may be performed as a diagnostic or curative procedure. The diagnostic value of thoracoscopic wedge excision in the management of undiagnosed lesions has received widespread acceptance. Controversy exists as to whether a peripheral nodule may be diagnosed as a solitary pulmonary nodule by preoperative CT, and videothoracoscopic wedge resection may be accepted as a curative procedure. It has been demonstrated that there is a 10% incidence of malignant nodules found at thoracotomy by careful palpation that are not detected by preoperative CT.[8] This is due to the low resolution of conventional CT. New improved spiral CT technology promises detection limits comparable to those of palpation.[9] All of our patients with peripheral pulmonary lesions underwent preoperative spiral CT. We believe that with this prerequisite thoracoscopic wedge resection for solitary pulmonary nodules may prove to be adequate. If more than one nodule is detected and resection is required, we currently prefer open procedures (Fig. 1).

We believe that VTS is not currently an option for treatment of primary lung cancer. A higher recurrence rate has been demonstrated in patients with lung cancer treated with wedge excision only as compared with those treated with formal lung resection.[7] Therefore when primary lung cancer is diagnosed from the wedge resection of a peripheral nodule, we proceed to thoracotomy and open formal lung resection with lymph node dissection. Thoracoscopic wedge resection may

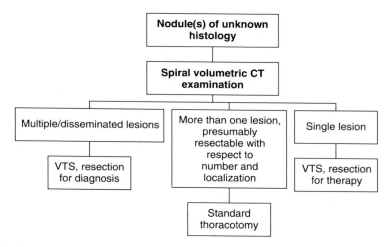

Fig. 1. VTS for diagnostic or therapeutic purposes and indications for standard thoracotomy depending on number and resectability of lesions based on nodules detected by spiral volumetric CT examination.

be an acceptable form of treatment in a highly select group of patients with impaired lung function or at high operative risk.

CONCLUSION

Videothoracoscopic wedge resection of peripheral pulmonary nodules can be performed with low morbidity and high diagnostic accuracy. In addition, thoracoscopic wedge resection may be adequate treatment for benign pulmonary lesions and in selected patients with metastatic pulmonary nodules.

REFERENCES

1. Vanderschueren RG. Le talcage pleural dans le pneumothorax spontané. Poumon-Coeur 37:273, 1981.
2. Merkle NM, Vogt-Moykopf I, Baumeister RGH, et al. Pneumothorax. In Heberer G, Schildberg FW, Sunder-Plassmann L, et al., eds. Lunge und Mediastinum. Berlin: Springer-Verlag, 1991, p 500.
3. Swierenga J, Wagenaar JPM, Bergstein PGM. The value of thoracoscopy in the diagnosis and treatment of diseases affecting the pleura and lung. Pneumology 151:11, 1974.
4. Singh VS. The surgical treatment of spontaneous pneumothorax by parietal pleurectomy. Scand J Thorac Cardiovasc Surg 16:75, 1982.
5. Meyer G, Dienemann H, Sunder-Plassmann L. Der Spontanpneumothorax. Focus MHL 6:9, 1990.
6. Landreneau RJ, Hazelrigg SR, Ferson PF, et al. Thoracoscopic resection of 85 pulmonary lesions. Ann Thorac Surg 54:415, 1992.
7. Miller DL, Allen SM, Trastek VF, et al. Videothoracoscopic wedge excision of the lung. Ann Thorac Surg 54:410, 1992.
8. McAfee MK, Allen MS, Trastek VF, et al. Colorectal lung metastases: Results of surgical excision. Ann Thorac Surg 53:780, 1992.
9. Costello P, Anderson W, Blume D. Pulmonary nodule: Evaluation with spiral volumetric CT. Radiology 179:875, 1991.

119 *The Current Role of Video-Assisted Thoracoscopy in the Diagnosis and Treatment of Chest Disease*

Douglas R. Norman and Jose M. Velasco

Since its initial use in 1910 by Jacobaeus, thoracoscopy had been used primarily for the diagnosis and treatment of pleural diseases.[1] Its most common indication was pleurolysis to enhance therapeutic pneumothorax in tuberculous lung collapse therapy.[2] Thoracoscopy was largely neglected until the early 1980s, when the development of modern video optics and microchip cameras, coupled to high-resolution video monitors, allowed a major expansion of the indications for video-assisted thoracoscopy or video-assisted thoracic surgery (VATS). We present our experience with this procedure at Rush North Shore Medical Center.

MATERIALS AND METHODS

Between September 1991 and August 1992, a total of 49 patients underwent VATS at our center. Patient ages ranged from 33 to 82 years; there were 28 men and 21 women in this group.

All patients underwent general anesthesia for the procedure. Unless a flexible fiberoptic bronchoscopy had been previously performed, we did this routinely at this point to assess for an intraluminal pathological condition. A double-lumen endotracheal tube was inserted in all cases to permit collapse of the lung. Monitoring was done in all patients by radial artery catheter, digital oximeter, and capnograph. In most patients a thoracic epidural catheter was inserted for control of pain. A pediatric bronchoscope was available for intraoperative use through the endotracheal tube as needed. Most patients were positioned in the lateral decubitus position unless otherwise indicated. Patients signed an informed consent for standard thoracotomy.

An initial 10 mm trocar was inserted in the midaxillary line at the seventh or eighth intercostal space for initial exploratory thoracoscopy. CO_2 insufflation was not used.

The equipment used included a 0-degree thoracoscopic lens attached to a microchip camera with a xenon light source, two video monitors placed on either side of the operating table, and a video-recorder and photoprinter. An assortment of trocars, scissors, graspers, and retractors was used. The EndoGIA stapling instrument was particularly useful.

The indication for video-assisted thoracoscopy was primarily for pulmonary masses (Table 1). Altogether, 53 procedures were performed (Table 2).

Table 1. Indications for video-assisted thoracoscopy

Lesion	No. of Patients
Pulmonary masses	26
Pleural effusion	6
Empyema/loculated effusion	5
Diffuse pulmonary infiltrates	4
Mediastinal tumor	3
Enlarged aortopulmonary lymph nodes	2
Massive pericardial effusion	1
Vertebral body lesion (combined)	1
Pleural mass	1

Table 2. Procedures performed

Procedure	No. of Procedures
Wedge resection	18
Lobectomy	1
Mediastinal tumor biopsy (malignant)	3
Aortopulmonary lymph node biopsy	2
Pleural biopsy ± pleurodesis	7
Debridement of empyema/loculation	5
Pericardial window drainage	1
Exploratory VATS	4
Exploratory VATS immediately before thoracotomy	12

RESULTS
Pulmonary Masses

There were 26 patients with pulmonary masses: primary lung cancer (16), metastases (4), histoplasmosis (3), Wegener's granuloma (1), inflammatory mass (1), and hamartoma (1). Fifteen patients underwent VATS resections (14 patients had a total of 18 wedge resections; one patient underwent right lower lobectomy).

Primary Lung Cancer

The 16 patients with primary lung cancer underwent initial screening with bronchoscopy, with or without mediastinoscopy, and chest and brain CT and bone scans. Video-assisted thoracoscopy was performed at the time of the bronchoscopy and mediastinoscopy for initial staging in 6 of 16 patients and used to evaluate chest wall invasion (2), and enlarged aortopulmonary lymph nodes (2). Two additional patients scheduled for resection were found to have unexpected pleural seeding, thus rendering their lesions unresectable; unnecessary open thoracotomy was therefore prevented in these cases. VATS was used at the time of definitive resection in 10 of 16 patients. Three patients underwent definitive resection (one lobectomy and two peripheral wedge resections) with the remaining 7 of 10, proceeding to open thoracotomy because a VATS resection was not felt appropriate. Two of these patients had their diagnosis of peripheral adenocarcinoma made by VATS wedge resection immediately before open thoracotomy. Reasons for conversion to open resection included the need for more radical resection, a large or deeper seated tumor, adhesions, or poorly developed fissures.

Metastasis to the Lungs

Four patients presented with multiple pulmonary metastases. The primary site was colon (2), retroperitoneal sarcoma (1), and breast (1). Wedge resection was diagnostic in three patients and allowed adequate tissue for oncological sensitivity and chemoreceptor studies. These three patients were not deemed candidates for complete resection of their lesions because of distant disease elsewhere. The one patient with metastatic sarcoma had undergone previous resection of her primary tumor 2 years earlier. Thoracoscopy allowed evaluation of a potentially unresectable lesion, which, however, proved resectable. Complete resection of five bilateral lesions was then accomplished through a midline sternotomy approach.

Diffuse Pulmonary Infiltrates

Four patients underwent wedge resection for diffuse pulmonary infiltrates. The pathological examination revealed interstitial fibrosis (3), and bronchiectasis with fibrosis (1). One patient in this group with progressive diffuse interstitial fibrosis died 3 weeks after the diagnosis was made despite intensive medical therapy.

Mediastinal Masses

Of three patients with mediastinal tumors, two had a diagnosis of Hodgkin's disease, and one had metastatic lung cancer with superior vena cava syndrome. All three had large pleural effusions and, after initial biopsy, tube thoracostomy was instituted for an average of 2 days. One patient with a large mediastinal metastatic cancer associated with superior vena cava syndrome died 6 days later after a progressively and rapidly downhill course.

Pleural Effusion

Six patients underwent definitive diagnostic and therapeutic thoracoscopy for effusions associated with primary lung carcinoma (2), metastasis from carcinoma of the breast (2), persistent post coronary bypass effusion (1), and nonspecific inflammatory effusion (1). Definitive biopsies were obtained followed by reexpansion of the lung under direct vision. In malignant cases, talc pleurodesis was accomplished using a slurry of 2 g of sterile purified talc in 100 ml saline. No recurrence was seen in follow-up.

Debridement of Empyema/Loculation

Five patients were treated definitively for empyema (3) and bloody loculated fluid (2). Evacuation and debridement of the typical gelatinous and fibrinous material was obtained, with reexpansion confirmed on the monitor. Tube drainage was maintained an average of 6.5 days. Follow-up chest x-ray evaluation and/or CT scans confirmed reexpansion without recurrence.

Aortopulmonary Window Lymph Node Enlargement

Two patients underwent aortopulmonary lymph node biopsies for enlarged lymph nodes noted on CT scans during workup for primary lung cancer. Thoracoscopy was done after mediastinoscopy biopsy proved negative. In both patients, biopsies of the AP window nodes were also negative for metastatic tumor. The chest tube was removed the following day.

Pleural Mass

One patient underwent direct biopsy of a pleura-based mass (benign hyaline plaque). Tube drainage was used overnight.

Massive Pericardial Effusion

One patient with known metastatic carcinoma of the breast developed a large pericardial effusion with tamponade. She underwent anterior and posterior pericardial windows by the video-assisted technique. No malignant cells were found on pathological examination. Tube drainage of the left pleural space was instituted for 5 days.

DISCUSSION

Video-assisted thoracic surgery is a natural development of the modern technology that has fostered minimally invasive surgery. With VATS, patient discomfort appears diminished and postoperative morbidity is significantly reduced when compared with open thoracotomy.[3,4] Many patients had VATS during the course of a prolonged hospitalization, but if they were admitted solely for thoracoscopy, their hospital stay was decreased. The procedure appears ideally suited for poor-risk patients, particularly those with compromised pulmonary function.[5] We have found the use of the thoracic epidural catheter to be of significant benefit in minimizing the postoperative pain and atelectasis, which is associated more commonly with a standard thoracotomy. The economic impact of VATS procedures is not clear, since the cost of additional equipment may offset the shorter hospital stay.

The role of VATS procedures in the treatment of primary lung cancer is of particular interest. It was particularly useful in two elderly patients with severely compromised pulmonary function: one had a small peripheral adenocarcinoma and the other a small typical carcinoid tumor. Both were considered prohibitive risks for standard thoracotomy elsewhere. A simple wedge resection was easily and safely performed in both. In another patient, a formal lobectomy was undertaken through a minimal non-rib-spreading incision for a right lower lobe adenocarcinoma. The usual staging was performed. Of interest were two patients who underwent exploratory thoracoscopy at the time of planned resection, only to find unexpected pleural seeding. An open thoracotomy was avoided in these patients.

Thoracoscopy is a valuable adjunct in the staging of primary lung cancer but should not be used in place of mediastinoscopy where indicated. In addition, thoracoscopy might allow curative resection provided the basic oncologic surgical techniques are respected.[6,7,13] This role will undoubtedly be expanded as more experience is gained. The use of exploratory thoracoscopy immediately before planned resection provides useful information and aids in the decision making process concerning open versus VATS resections.

VATS appears to be the procedure of choice for metastatic lesions to the lung where a simple diagnosis is all that is needed.[5] If complete resection of multiple or bilateral metastasis is planned, surgical palpation may be necessary, thus mandating an open thoracotomy.[7]

Increasing experience with the complete excision of localized mediastinal tumor masses, via thoracoscopy, is being reported.[12] Invasive mediastinal tumors can be easily biopsied using this technique since visibility is considerably improved to allow appropriate tissue sampling. The use of the classic limited access Chamberlain procedure is becoming increasingly rare.[8]

VATS is ideally suited for wedge biopsy of the lung in cases of diffuse pulmonary infiltrates and other unknown lesions.[9] Adequate tissue can readily be obtained for appropriate laboratory examination. In cases of biopsy-proven benign lesions (i.e., granuloma, hamartoma), the procedure is definitive. If a peripheral malignancy is detected, more formal resection can then be performed either using the VATS technique or by opening the chest in the conventional manner.

Pleural effusions and lesions can be readily evaluated and an accurate diagnosis made. In patients with a known distant primary carcinoma, we prefer thoracoscopy to rule out metastatic disease. The diagnostic yield of VATS is much higher than that of simple thoracentesis or percutaneous pleural biopsy. Tube drainage with talc pleurodesis can be instituted immediately to lessen morbidity.[10,11] An additional benefit is the ability to procure sufficient tissue for chemoreceptor and sensitivity studies.

REFERENCES

1. Jacobaeus HC. Ueber die Moeglichkiet der Zystoskopischen Untersuchung seroeser Hoehlunger anzuwenden. Munch Med Wochenschr 40:2090,1910.
2. Jacobaeus HC. The cauterization of adhesions in artificial pneumothorax therapy of tuberculosis. Am Rev Tuberculosis 6:871, 1922.

3. Hazelrigg SR, LoCicero J, Nunchuck S, et al. The Video Assisted Thoracic Surgery Study Group data. Presented at the 29th Annual Meeting of the Society of Thoracic Surgeons, San Antonio, January 1993.

4. Landreneau RJ, Hazelrigg SR, Mack MJ, et al. Differences in postoperative pain, shoulder function, and morbidity between video-assisted thoracic surgery and muscle-sparing open thoracotomies. Presented at the 29th Annual Meeting of the Society of Thoracic Surgeons, San Antonio, January 1993.

5. Mack MJ, Aronoff RJ, Acuff TE, et al. Present role of thoracoscopy in the diagnosis and treatment of diseases of the chest. Ann Thorac Surg 54:403-409, 1992.

6. Lewis RJ, Caccavale RJ, Sisler GE, et al. Video-assisted thoracic surgical resection of malignant lung tumors. J Thorac Cardiovasc Surg 104:1679-1687, 1992.

7. Rice TW. Thoracoscopy and pulmonary surgery. Presented at the 29th Annual Meeting of the Society of Thoracic Surgeons, San Antonio, January 1993.

8. McNeill TM, Chamberlain JM. Diagnostic anterior mediastinotomy. Ann Thorac Surg 2:532-539, 1966.

9. Newhouse MT. Thoracoscopy: Diagnostic and therapeutic considerations. Pneumologie 43:48-52, 1989.

10. Page RD, Jeffrey RR, Donnelly RJ. Thoracoscopy: A review of 121 consecutive surgical procedures. Ann Thorac Surg 48:66-68, 1989.

11. Webb WR. Thoracoscopy. Chest Surg Clin North Am 2:679-689, 1992.

12. Landreneau RJ, Dowling RD, Castillo WM, et al. Thoracoscopic resection of an anterior mediastinal tumor. Ann Thorac Surg 54:142-144, 1992.

13. Roviaro GC, Varoli F, Rebuffat C. Videoendoscopic major pulmonary resections pneumonectomy-lobectomy: The Italian experience. Presented at the First International Symposium of Thoracoscopic Surgery, San Antonio, January 1993.

120 Diagnostic Thoracoscopy: Advantages in the Community Hospital

Raymond A. Dieter, Jr.

Frequently we see patients with thoracic problems that are not readily diagnosed from chest x-ray films; CT scans, bronchoscopy, and other procedures often fail to yield a diagnosis for the patient who has an abnormal chest x-ray film or progressive symptomatology. Invasive procedures, including bronchoscopic biopsy, needle aspiration biopsy, and thoracotomy, are used in these patients. Thoracoscopy was introduced in the early 1900s as an alternative diagnostic procedure, but it has rarely been used since then. Over the years open thoracotomy and lung or pleural biopsy have become the standard procedures (see box). However, more recently less invasive or minimally invasive procedures have progressed in their diagnostic and therapeutic capabilities (see box), and thoracoscopy is now being reconsidered as an option for some patients. In well-selected individuals this may be the procedure of choice to reduce the risk, the potential for complications, and the expense, yet diagnose the problem and determine the appropriate treatment.

We report our findings over the past 20 years in a series of patients in whom thoracoscopy was performed in a community hospital setting.

MATERIALS AND METHODS

Seventy-nine patients were seen in five community hospitals for pulmonary or pleural problems; in these patients it was thought best to proceed with diagnostic and possibly therapeutic thoracoscopy. There were 43 men and 36 women, ranging in age from 16 to 80 years of age, with the majority between 50 and 79 years of age.

During the past 20 years the technique has been refined, and therefore the number of procedures has slowly increased. A large number of patients were cared for at one hospital and were referred by more than 25 different attending physicians.

INVASIVE PROCEDURES

Bronchoscopy with biopsy, brushing, and washing
Thoracentesis—Cope's needle biopsy
Scalene/mediastinal biopsy
Percutaneous biopsy
Bone marrow
Open thoracotomy or chest tube

SUITABLE FOR MULTIPLE DISEASES

Diagnostic	Therapeutic
Pleura	Effusion
Lung	Foreign body
Mediastinum	Lung tumors
Therapeutic	Cysts
	Neurectomy
	Blebs

Preoperative chest x-ray films, CT scans, thoracentesis, and other diagnostic evaluations were performed as indicated. Patients were operated after adequate preoperative evaluation and consideration of the anesthetic to be used. Most patients were given a general anesthetic—occasionally with the use of a Carlens double-lumen endotracheal tube. The side to be operated was elevated on a sandbag or an IV bag. If a pleural effusion was present, thoracentesis was carried out to determine its exact location. An incision was made and the chest was entered through the appropriate interspace.

During the first few years this procedure was accomplished with a chest trocar or a laparoscopic setup and trocar. Initially a rigid or flexible bronchoscope was used for the procedure, but as laparoscopes and thoracoscopes became available, the appropriate equipment was utilized. With the recent availability of the video screen, video-assisted procedures are now performed. When the pleural cavity was entered, fluid, if present, was suctioned from the chest. If no fluid was present, the lung was collapsed with either Carlen's tube single-lung ventilation or CO_2 compression of the affected lung. Under direct vision, second or third chest ports

were created at appropriate distances for additional manipulation of the lung, for insertion of additional instruments, and for performance of the procedure. On insertion of the instruments, appropriate visualization of the pleural cavity and lung was achieved. Where present and potentially a hindrance to the procedure, adhesions were lyzed with a cauterization technique or with scissors. Afterward the appropriate procedure (pleural biopsy, diaphragmatic biopsy, lung or mediastinal biopsy, or removal of a foreign body) was carried out. Occasionally C-arm guidance was used for thoracoscopic needle biopsy of the lung. Tissue cultures, pleural abrasion, or tetracycline instillation was carried out where appropriate. Bleeders were coagulated and on completion of the procedure, one or two chest tubes were placed through either the port used for the thoracoscopic procedure or through new posteroinferior ports. If the appropriate result could not be achieved, other diagnostic or therapeutic procedures were carried out including open thoracotomy. Routine postoperative chest x-ray films were obtained. Patients were monitored, and Heimlich flutter valves were attached to chest tubes that could not be removed but the patient was otherwise able to be discharged.

PATIENT CHARACTERISTICS AND RESULTS

The most prominent symptoms were shortness of breath in 44 patients, chest pain in 26, cough in 16, weakness in 18, weight loss in nine, a chest mass in four, and fever in four (Table 1). Other symptoms included postural hypotension, anemia, jaundice, loss of appetite, coma, dizziness, hyperglycemia, abdominal pain and distention (in three patients), hemoptysis (two patients), respiratory infection, wheezing (two patients), diarrhea (three patients), congestive heart failure (two patients), respiratory distress (two patients), bronchitis, dysphagia (two patients), pneumonia, night sweats, tingling in the mouth, rib fractures, shaking, chills, nausea and vomiting, headache, back pain, and chronic pleurisy (two patients). In addition, these patients had other concomitant medical problems, including diabetes mellitus, a history of tuberculosis, seizure disorders, smoking, gastric resection, *Blastocystis hominis*, a history of asbestos exposure, nephropathy, or a positive skin test for tuberculosis.

Chest x-ray films showed effusion in 71 patients, which was increasing in volume in most of them (Table 2). Some had a small amount, whereas others had a

Table 1. Major symptomatology

Symptom	Number
Shortness of breath	44
Cough	16
Chest pain	26
Weakness	18
Weight loss	9
Chest mass	4
Fever	4

Table 2. Major radiological findings

Finding	Number
Effusion	
Bilateral	5
Right	37
Left	29
Pericardial	2
Consolidation/atelectasis	3
Densities: pulmonary/pleural	6
Pneumothorax	6
Infiltrate (unilateral/bilateral)	7
Chronic lung disease/emphysema	4
Other	8

massive amount of effusion with opacification of the chest. Many of these effusions were bloody. Five were bilateral and three were pericardial. Thirty-seven effusions were on the right side and 29 were on the left. A few patients had no effusion at all. Consolidation or atelectasis of the lung was noted in three patients. One or more pulmonary densities or nodules were noted in six patients. Pneumothorax with blebs or emphysema was noted in six patients and was associated with catamenia in one. Pulmonary infiltrates were noted in six patients. Other findings included the absence of a lung in one patient with a bronchopleural fistula and the presence of a pleural mass or process in two. Congestive heart failure, a chronic lung problem, a foreign body in a woman with a catamenial pneumothorax, and a chronic tubercular process with fistula were also seen. An elevated diaphragm, a destroyed lung, a mass in front of the trachea, and a ventricular aneurysm were all noted on x-ray films.

Preoperative diagnoses included undiagnosed effusion in 39 patients, spontaneous pneumothorax in five, congestive heart failure in three, metastatic carcinoma in 11, fistula in three, and neoplasm in six. Additional diagnoses included a pacemaker, diabetes mellitus, benign prostatic hypertrophy, a foreign body, bronchopleurocutaneous fistula, a history of tuberculosis, pneumonia, cardiomyopathy, probable lymphoma, a history of carcinoma of the lung, and Hodgkin's disease. When metastatic carcinoma was considered, the most likely sources were the breast, ovary, thyroid gland, or endometrium.

The preoperative diagnostic procedures performed in these patients were numerous and varied (Table 3). A large number (50) had bronchoscopy with brushing, biopsy, or washing. Thoracentesis was performed in at least 29 patients, with the majority of the results being nondiagnostic, negative, or class I, II, or III cytology. Many of the patients with carcinoma had negative thoracentesis, normal cytologic findings, and were found to have gross tumor on thoracoscopy. Patients with blastomycosis, lymphomatosis, and metastatic pancreatic carcinoma had negative thoracentesis. Occasionally a patient would have class III or IV (suspected carcinoma) cytological findings, and endoscopic examination was required for further definition. At least 12 patients had had prior nondiagnostic Cope's needle biopsies. Other procedures included esophagoscopy with biopsy for carcinoma, cardiac catheterization, sternal bone marrow biopsy, scalene node biopsy, axillary biopsy, cervical node biopsy, partial mastectomy or modified radical mastectomy, excision of a lesion in the forearm or the chest wall, pericardial tap, oophorectomy, chest tube insertion on the opposite side, unroofing of the abscess, right nephrectomy, and renal angiography.

The most common procedure performed in addition to thoracoscopy was biopsy of the pleura or chest wall in 70 patients (Table 4). Pleural sclerosing techniques were used in 30 patients—usually 1 or 2 g of tetracycline diluted to 100 cc. In three patients pleural abrasion and Atabrine were used. A lung biopsy was performed in 23 patients and lysis of adhesions in six. Biopsy of the diaphragm was done in five patients and tis-

Table 3. Other invasive procedures

Procedure	Number
Bronchoscopy (biopsy/brush/wash)	50
Thoracentesis	29
Cope pleural biopsy	13
Open thoracotomy/biopsy/lobectomy	11
Scalene node biopsy	5
Sternal biopsy	3
Portacath	Many

Table 4. Thoracoscopic procedure

Procedure	Number
Pleural/chest wall biopsy	70
Tetracycline	27
Biopsy cultures	4
Lung biopsy	23
Lysis of adhesions	6
Diaphragm biopsy	5
Chest tubes	95%
Cytology/cell block	Most
Scope–open thoracotomy	5(?)
Remove foreign body	1

sue cultures in four. In most patients cytologic or cell block examinations were performed. One patient underwent bilateral simultaneous thoracoscopies, and one had the procedures performed on two different days. Two patients demonstrated large blebs, but we were unable to delineate the air leak and therefore open thoracotomy was performed at the same sitting. Subsequent to biopsy, one patient had a therapeutic open thoracotomy. One patient had a biopsy of a retrosternal mass and another had a mediastinal biopsy. An attempt to enter the pleural space with the thoracoscope was unsuccessful in two patients, and therefore open thoracotomy with biopsy was performed. One patient had a foreign body removed by means of the C-arm fluoroscopic technique. Two patients had a percutaneous thora-

coscopic guided needle biopsy. One patient had a segmental resection. Forty-eight patients had a right-sided approach, 31 had a left-sided approach, and two had a bilateral approach. All patients had chest tubes placed and positioned under direct view. Seven patients underwent open thoracotomy for either diagnostic or therapeutic purposes—particularly for blebs or large diagnostic samples. One patient had an azygous lobectomy, and in another patient with radiation fibrosis diagnosis was difficult.

The postoperative diagnosis was pleuritis in 28 patients: acute, subacute, or chronic in 13, empyema in four, fungus or tuberculosis in three, and chronic mesothelial hyperplasia in five; radiation effects were noted in three. Neoplasm was diagnosed in 60 patients: adenocarcinoma in 39, mesothelioma in eight, metastatic carcinoma in eight, retrosternal carcinoma in two, and possible/suspected carcinoma of the lung in three. One patient with a thoracoscopic diagnosis of acute pleuritis was found at open biopsy to have carcinoma of the lung. The group with adenocarcinoma included patients with metastasis from the breast, lung, ovary, or thyroid gland. Metastatic tumors were also found to be from cystosarcoma phyloidis, the larynx (squamous cell), or the pancreas. Other diagnoses included pneumonia in three patients, adhesions in three, fistula in two, and emphysematous bullae or blebs in five. As noted, it was possible for a patient to have more than one diagnosis. Types of fungi included Candida and Penicillium in one patient and pleural Blastomyces infection in another (probably the first reported case to be diagnosed by thoracoscopy). Other findings included lymphomatosis, granulomatosis, pulmonary abscess, chronic pulmonary/pleural inflammation, and amyloidosis. Patients were also found to have aspiration pneumonia, lung fibrosis, a carcinoma fistula, a tubercular fistula, and emphysema. Care must be taken in patients with emphysematous bullae to avoid inadvertent puncture of the lung. Pleural adhesions (three patients), congestive heart failure in hyperthyroidism (two patients), pleural Hodgkin's disease, recurrent postcobalt effusion, and cirrhotic esophageal varices were also seen.

DISCUSSION

Complications in these patients were minimal and the vast majority had none. Inability to make a diagnosis on the basis of the specimens submitted was a concern with closed procedures such as thoracentesis and Cope's

RESULTS OF DIAGNOSTIC THORACOSCOPY IN 79 PATIENTS

Accuracy good
Large samples
62 of 79 had malignancy
2+ diagnoses in some
Few false negative findings (the surgeon must be alert)
Much greater accuracy than with previously established
  procedures

POSTOPERATIVE COURSE

In this series, following diagnostic thoracoscopy
patients were:
  Ambulatory after the procedure/same day
  Eating on postoperative day 1
  Requiring fewer narcotics and medications because
    of less discomfort
  Breathing easier—less use of oxygen/respirators was
    required
  Quickly self-sufficient

EXPENSES REDUCED

Shorter time in the operating room with a surgeon who
  has experience in thoracoscopy
No intensive care unit stay
Less medication/fewer dressings
Fewer days in the hospital
Fewer major side effects
Less nursing care required

INCISIONS

Small—thus small scar
Less painful
Aesthetically pleasing
Multiple incisions are required
Less conspicuous

needle biopsy. This was not the case with the thoracoscopic tissue samples, since they were generally large workable specimens—sometimes 1 cm or more of tissue (see box). One patient with effusion had false negative findings and 9 months later was proved to have carcinoma of the extreme apex of the lung. Multiple negative preoperative diagnostic findings were noted in several patients. Therefore one wonders whether a single direct approach such as thoracoscopy might be more appropriate in many of these patients.

One patient with severe lung disease and marked respiratory insufficiency had postoperative ECG changes characteristic of an acute myocardial infarction. One severely ill patient with previously undiagnosed terminal carcinoma underwent diagnostic biopsy before her death. We were unable to locate the persistent air leak in one patient; therefore an open procedure was performed at the same time. One patient had postoperative pneumonia and responded to treatment. Patients were usually ambulatory, eating, and self-sufficient the night of surgery. In essence, the equivalent of a chest tube procedure was performed under anesthesia (usually general) with the additional benefit of a biopsy or therapeutic modality. A positive biopsy-proven diagnosis was established in most patients before they left the operating room (frozen section).

Only respirator-dependent or open-thoracotomy patients were placed in the intensive care unit (see box). This reduced the potential morbidity and expense to the patient by avoiding a major open surgical procedure (see box). Such an approach therefore reduces the size of the incision (and thus the scar) (see box), reduces the period of hospitalization, and reduces the incidence of postoperative complications. With the patient diagnosed and eating, appropriate therapy could be initiated the same day or the next day. Patients were able to return to the home and community environment rapidly and safely—occasionally with intrapleural tubes still in place. This minimally invasive diagnostic procedure proved to be highly reliable, safe, quick, and simple and was readily accepted by the patient.

121 *Videothoracoscopic Treatment of Recurrent Pneumothorax*

Piero Borasio, Francesco Ardissone, Bruno G. Audino, Giorgio Chiampo, Claudio Ferraro, Roberto Giardino, Elena Manzone, Claudio Mossetti, and Corrado Novello

Spontaneous pneumothorax is a commonly observed condition affecting 9 of every 1000 persons per year,[1] primarily males, at a rate of 5 to 1 compared with females. The diversity in pathological conditions and symptoms has led to a great variety of treatment approaches for both first episodes and recurrences. These range from simple observation in asymptomatic cases with modest parenchyma collapse, to thoracotomy with pleural abrasion or pleurectomy in cases of multiple relapses or persistent air leak. The essentially benign nature of the disease has prompted an ongoing search for the most effective and least traumatic treatment. Surgical thoracoscopy, which allows visualization of the complete lung and pleura, as well as treatment of bullae and pleurodesis, is an alternative to conventional surgery in treating recurrent spontaneous pneumothorax. Endoscopic treatment combines the advantages of a low rate of recurrence with reduced anatomical and functional impairment and shortened postoperative hospitalization.

MATERIALS AND METHODS

From March 1990 to January 1992 at the San Luigi Gonzaga Hospital in Turin, we treated 10 patients who had recurrent spontaneous pneumothorax. The condition was right sided in seven cases and left sided in three. There were nine men and one woman in this series; they ranged in age from 14 to 37 years. Five had suffered multiple recurrences, with a maximum of five episodes, while in four this was a first occurrence.

Two patients, who had already undergone thoracic drainage with persistent air leak, underwent operations 5 and 8 days after admission. The remaining patients were treated 24 to 72 hours after onset of symptoms. All underwent videoendoscopic pleural abrasion; in three this treatment was combined with evaporization of apical bullae by endoscopic Nd:YAG laser.

The mean postoperative stay was 5 days, with a minimum of 3 and maximum of 8 days. Four cases showed a slight postoperative air leak, which resolved spontaneously. The operations took an average of 90 minutes.

Postoperative antalgic treatment was limited to the use of antispasmodic medications. No other special drugs were used. A follow-up control conducted 1 to 10 months later did not reveal any recurrence or sequelae associated with the surgery.

TECHNIQUE

General anesthesia is required, with double-lumen endotracheal intubation and selective pulmonary ventilation. The patient is placed on the operating table in the lateral decubitus position. Two monitors are used, one at the side of the patient's head and one at the feet.

With the patient in the appropriate lateral decubitus position, the surgeon stands in back of the patient with the assistant placed opposite. After positioning a 10 mm non-gas-tight trocar at the fourth intercostal space of the medial axillary line, a 0-degree optical lens connected to the video camera is introduced. A 12 mm trocar is placed at the fifth space of the posterior axillary line to permit use of grasping forceps and eventual endoscopic Nd:YAG therapy. If a parenchyma resection is necessary, a trocar is placed at the fourth to fifth intercostal space of the anterior axillary line for the introduction and use of the EndoGIA (Figs. 1 and 2).

The lung is inspected carefully, especially at the apex. Any adhesions are lyzed and air leak sources are carefully examined by irrigating the constantly ventilated lung with a physiological saline solution. Small subpleural blebs are not treated. If there are bullae, atypical resection by endoscopic Nd:YAG therapy is undertaken. Then superficial abrasion of the entire accessible pleura is performed using an abrasion brush mounted on grasping forceps, using all available pleurotomies in sequence.

An unabraded area remains around the pleurotomies that is inaccessible with the instruments currently used but that can be treated using a broad, curved dissection forceps with a mounted brush; this is introduced

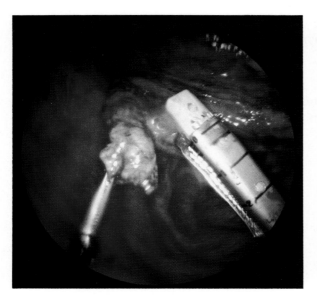

Fig. 1. A group of apical blebs in the process of resection through their parenchymal base with the help of an EndoGIA stapler.

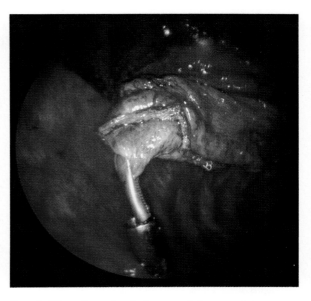

Fig. 2. The triangulated closure of the remaining parenchymal apex is aerostatic and hemostatic.

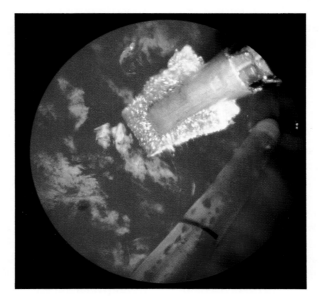

Fig. 3. Pleural abrasion is performed with an appropriately tailored brush-sponge carried by a grasping forceps. The chest tube is placed through the most oblique chest opening into an optimal drainage site under direct vision.

through the pleurotomies and rotated in a circular motion. The abrasion will produce slight bleeding while preserving the integrity of vascular and nervous structures. Finally, a multiple-windowed drain tube is positioned under visual control through the most oblique chest opening. The remaining chest incisions are sutured.

Thoracic drainage is maintained continuously with suction of $-20\,cm/H_2O$; the drain is removed on the fourth postoperative day or whenever the air leak has stopped. The thorax is evaluated radiographically each day to ensure full expansion of the lung.

DISCUSSION

In about 30% of the cases of spontaneous pneumothorax, parenchyma collapse is less than 20%; if the patient does not show signs of respiratory insufficiency, simple observation is indicated. However, more than 70% of patients have a collapsed lung of greater significance, and suction drainage is the most commonly used treatment.[2] This method, while adequate for immediately resolving the problem, may result in persistent air leak in 2% to 3% of cases and in 10% to 50% of recurrences.[3,4] To circumvent this drawback, we considered thoracoscopic examination of all patients with pneumothorax. We also considered using talc[5] or tetracycline[6] for pleurodesis in those without bullae. The recurrence rate for the first group was less than 6.6% and for the second 16%. We do not consider this method suitable, because it causes irreversible pleurodesis in young patients who are potential candidates for thoracic surgery later in life.

Surgery is indicated in cases of failed reexpansion of the lung because of persistent air leak (4% to 14%); unilateral recurrence, increasing from 16% following the first episode to 80% after the third; and simultaneous contralateral pneumothorax.[7] We also believe that this therapy should be extended to patients in high-risk activities or who live in distant areas.

Through a videothoracoscopic procedure, the surgeon can identify the causes of the air leak; determine using methods that allow maximal preservation of the parenchyma; and implement measures to induce stable adhesion of visceral and parietal pleura (pleurodesis). Surgery ensures a stable cure in almost all patients and has a recurrence rate of less than 1%.[8] Nevertheless, the procedure has a mortality rate of 1% and results in significant functional damage (reduction of volume estimated at about 10%), notwithstanding the use of low-impact methods, such as axillary thoracotomy.[9]

We believe that a minimally invasive approach could eliminate these drawbacks while ensuring similar therapeutic potential. Surgical thoracoscopy in fact allows complete visualization of the lung and pleura, treatment of blebs and bullae that are causing air leaks, performance of mechanical pleurodesis or pleurectomy that will guarantee a stable result with a low recurrence rate, and results in minimal discomfort for the patient.[10] For treating bullae, we opted for linear suturing (Figs. 1 and 2) because it is more secure than simple coagulation and less risky than ligature. This also makes it possible to remove a sample of pulmonary parenchyma to send to the anatomical pathologist. Small diffuse blebs were not treated; it is our experience that their coagulation does not guarantee adequate aerotaxis. Apical pleurectomy, as proposed by other authors,[7] was not deemed useful, since these were young patients whose need for an ulterior thoracotomy could not be excluded. The lack of a means for treating the pleura near pleurotomies imposes the need for technical devices similar to the one we have proposed.

The results obtained confirm the applicability of the method.

FURTHER EXPERIENCE

From February 1992 to this writing, we have treated 28 more cases of recurrent pneumothorax using the method previously described. The patient group comprised 25 men and 3 women. Their ages ranged from 16 to 45 years; 10 had right-sided pneumothorax and 18 had left-sided pneumothorax; in 8 patients this episode was the first occurrence; the remaining 20 had had multiple recurrences, with a maximum of six episodes. Exceptional among these was a 24-year-old quadriplegic man who had been on assisted-respiration therapy for more than a year; this was his fourth relapse. Twenty of these patients underwent simple pleural abrasion and eight underwent abrasion combined with treatment of bullae.

There were complications in three patients from this last group; in one patient, bleeding from the 12 mm trocar site with hemothorax required an axillary thoracotomy 48 hours after the endoscopic procedure. In a second patient, a persistent air leak caused by failure to identify bullae at the paramediastinal superior left lobe required an axillary thoracotomy on postoperative day 5. The third patient had a unilateral recurrence 90 days after the endoscopic intervention, with subtotal parenchyma collapse, and was treated by axillary thoracotomy.

The additional experience reinforced our conviction that the videothoracoscopic approach represents the treatment of choice in recurrent spontaneous pneumothorax in young patients. However, we feel it is useful to point out several technical innovations that could improve and facilitate the procedure:

1. Use of 30-degree optical telescope to visualize and treat all the parietal pleura
2. Meticulous identification of the bullae hidden from direct vision because of adhesions that require transsection
3. Use of short valveless trocars, previously unavailable
4. Careful initial maintenance of hemostasis of the ports to avoid bothersome and persistent fogging of the telescope; complete hemostasis of the termination of the procedure, especially of the chest openings.

REFERENCES

1. Sabiston DC, Spencer FC. Surgery of the Chest, 5th ed. Philadelphia: WB Saunders Co, 1990, p 445.
2. Brooks JW. Open thoracotomy in the management of spontaneous pneumothorax. Chest 57:65, 1970.
3. Seremetis MG. The management of spontaneous pneumothorax. Chest 57:65, 1970.
4. Swierenga J, Wagenaar JPM, Bergstein PGM. The value of thoracoscopy in the diagnosis and treatment of diseases affecting the pleura and lung. Pneumologie 151:11, 1974.
5. Vanderschueren RG. Le talcage pleural dans le pneumothorax spontan. Poumon-Coeur 37:273, 1981.
6. Olsen PS, Andersen HO. Long-term results after tetracycline pleurodesis in spontaneous pneumothorax. Ann Thorac Surg 53:1015, 1992.
7. Nathanson LK, Shimi SM, Wood RB, Cuschieri A. Videothoracoscopic ligation of bulla and pleurectomy for spontaneous pneumothorax. Ann Thorac Surg 52:316, 1991.
8. Deslauries J, Beaulieu M, Despres JP, Lemieux M, Lablanc J, Desmeules M. Transaxillary pleurectomy for treatment of spontaneous pneumothorax. Ann Thorac Surg 30:569, 1980.
9. Cass F, Cham B, Van den Brande P, Welch W. Transaxillary thoracotomy for treatment of spontaneous pneumothorax. Acta Chir Belg 87:137, 1987.
10. Melvin WS, Krasna MJ, McLaughlin JS. Thoracoscopic management of spontaneous pneumothorax. Chest 102:1875, 1992.

122 *Pleurodesis for Recurrent Pneumothorax*

Thomas M. Daniel

The type of pleurodesis used in the thoracoscopic surgical approach to recurrent pneumothorax is determined by its pathological characteristics: primary or secondary. Primary pneumothorax is defined as resulting from a rupture of localized bleb disease of the lung, with normal remaining lung parenchyma. Secondary pneumothorax is defined as an air leak from a bleb or bullous lesion associated with extensive underlying pulmonary emphysema or fibrosis.

A patient's first episode of *primary pneumothorax* at our institution is generally treated with tube thoracostomy. No specific attempt at pleurodesis is undertaken in that the chest tube itself creates a pleural reaction. Indications for thoracoscopic surgical treatment of primary pneumothorax include (1) persistence of air leak following chest tube treatment of an initial episode, (2) recurrent ipsilateral pneumothorax, or (3) primary pneumothorax occurring for the first time in a patient whose contralateral lung has already been treated for primary pneumothorax. Under these circumstances general anesthesia, double-lumen endotracheal intubation, and lateral decubitus positioning of the patient are performed. Thoracoscopic surgical identification and endostaple excision of the offending localized blebs are undertaken. Pleurodesis in this clinical setting is performed most commonly by mechanical abrasion of the parietal pleura. This is achieved by removing the thoracoscopic trocar and inserting a tightly folded 2 × 2 compress, secured on a curved clamp, instead and mechanically abrading the pleura overlying the first five ribs under thoracoscopic visualization. Occasionally electrocauterization is used to supplement the pleurodesis. The parietal pleura overlying the ribs is cauterized. Care is taken to avoid cauterizing the intercostal muscle to avoid thermal injury to the adjacent intercostal vessels and nerves. Experiments are currently being performed in the laboratory with the argon beam coagulator, and its clinical use has been described by Quinlan et al.[1] Initial results suggest that this method of pleurodesis is rapid and avoids injury to the underlying intercostal vessels; can therefore be applied diffusely over the parietal pleura. The method has no untoward complications when used under the conditions of thoracoscopic surgery.

Nd:YAG laser production of pleurodesis has been reported by Toree et al.[2] Nd:YAG laser pleural treatment for recurrent pneumothorax is not used at our institution because its depth of penetration has been associated with intercostal vessel and nerve injury, and we have achieved similar effects with electrocauterization when pleurodesis is limited to the intercostal rib surfaces. Talc pleurodesis has not been chosen routinely for cases of recurrent primary pneumothorax with normal underlying lung tissue because its very effectiveness creates a pleural seal that would make elective lung surgery later in the patient's life a significant challenge. However, there is no evidence that talc applied in amounts of 4 g or less to the pleural space produces chronic fibrothorax with secondary restrictive lung disease.

When *secondary pneumothorax* occurs, pleurodesis is created thoracoscopically by talc poudrage. Initial treatment of pneumothorax in this setting is generally with tube thoracostomy. When the air leak is persistent there is in essence a chronic bronchopleural fistula, and talc has been found to be an effective agent if no significant large air space is present within the pleural cavity.[3,5] Tschopp et al.[4] have also reported on the effectiveness of talc poudrage in a setting of chronic postoperative bronchopleural fistula.

Thoracoscopic surgical technique for the application of talc pleurodesis in patients with secondary pneumothorax involves general anesthesia, double-lumen endotracheal intubation, and lateral decubitus positioning of the patient. These patients are difficult to anesthetize because of their pulmonary insufficiency, and single-lung ventilation is resorted to only intermittently and minimally during the surgical procedure. A significant hazard in a thoracoscopic approach to

this problem is the creation of additional bronchopleural fistulas by inadvertent laceration of the underlying lung parenchyma during trocar insertion or subsequent lung manipulation. By using extreme caution and intermittent single-lung ventilation these complications are generally avoided. It is often impossible to recognize the site of persistent air leak. If the leak is located, attempts at staple excision of the tissue surrounding the air leak in a setting of underlying diseased parenchyma often produces additional parenchymal injuries. Therefore the primary focus of thoracoscopic surgery in the setting of recurrent pneumothorax for persistent air leak is to create a pleurodesis and not to close the air leak. Occasionally fibrin glue is sprayed over the lung surface before talc pleurodesis in hopes of decreasing or stopping the air leak without resorting to stapling or endoscopic suturing. Talc for pleurodesis is obtained from a pharmaceutical company in an asbestos-free state. It is sterilized by one of two methods. Heat sterilization is achieved with a dry-oven technique, since steam sterilization will cause the talc to become putty-like in consistency. A second method of sterilization involves gamma irradiation, which is performed at a specialized institution and delivered to our medical center. Talc is applied through an atomizer with care being taken to deliver no more than 6 g; often 2 to 4 g will suffice for limited pleural surfaces. Talc applied as a powder is very effective in diffusely coating the visceral and parietal pleural surfaces, but care must be taken to avoid allowing the sprayer tip to come in contact with fluid, since this will create a pastelike mixture of fluid and talc that will limit further application of powder through the atomizer tubing.

A very significant change in the philosophy of selection for talc pleurodesis of patients with secondary recurrent pneumothorax has occurred at the University of Virginia Health Sciences Center since the advent of clinical lung transplantation. None of the patients in the pediatric or adult populations who are potential candidates for single- or double-lung transplantation are treated with talc pleurodesis. The very effectiveness of this modality makes subsequent lung resection in the setting of transplantation a prohibitively tedious surgical procedure, with the potential for significant blood loss. The likelihood of phrenic nerve injury secondary to the extensive pleurodesis is also increased. These patients are now treated with a combination of mechanical pleural abrasion and thoracoscopic application of fibrin glue.

RESULTS

From 1981 to 1992, thoracoscopic surgical procedures were performed in 133 patients at the University of Virginia: 22 of these patients (17%) underwent pleurodesis for recurrent pneumothorax, 20 underwent talc pleurodesis, one underwent fibrin glue application for bronchopleural fistula, and one underwent apical blebectomy and mechanical pleurodesis. Therapeutic success—defined as cessation of air leakage within 4 days of surgery—was achieved in 19 of the 22 patients (86%). The three patients in whom treatment was unsuccessful required open thoracotomy for resolution of chronic air leaks. There were no deaths or empyemas.

REFERENCES

1. Quinlan DM, Naslund MH, Brendler CB. Application of argon beam coagulation in urological surgery. J Urol 147:410-412, 1992.
2. Torre M, Belloni P. Nd:YAG laser pleurodesis through thoracoscopy: New curative therapy in spontaneous pneumothorax. Ann Thorac Surg 47:887-889, 1989.
3. Daniel TM, Tribble CG, Rodgers BM. Thoracoscopy and talc poudrage for pneumothoraces and effusions. Ann Thorac Surg 50:186-189, 1990.
4. Tschopp JM, Ev'Equoz D, Karrer W, et al. Successful closure of chronic BPF by thoracoscopy after failure of endoscopic fibrin glue application and thoracoplasty. Chest 97:745-746, 1990.
5. Weissberg S. Handbook of Practical Pleuroscopy. Mt. Kisco, NY: Futura Publishing, 1991.

123 Minimally Invasive Resection of Lung Parenchyma in the Treatment of Spontaneous Pneumothorax

Detlev-Wilhelm Schröder and Ronald-Joachim Elfeldt

The rate of relapse after treatment of spontaneous pneumothorax by chest tube drainage alone has compelled thoracic surgeons to look beyond the obvious cause and search for effective therapy. However, confusion concerning optimal methods of treatment is almost unparalleled. According to some investigators,[1] approximately six different procedures are currently being used to treat a first occurrence or a relapse of spontaneous pneumothorax. This wide range of treatment options is in part the result of individual variable morphological changes that occur as a result of pathological conditions in the bronchial tree, the lungs, or the chest wall. Kjaergaard[2] characterized juvenile pneumothorax as idiopathic, since the diagnostic methods available at that time did not provide a clear explanation of the cause. Both the unknown etiological factors and the extent of the changes in the lungs caused Gänger[3] to consider pleurectomy as a therapeutic option.

This wide variety of treatments can also be explained by the lack of long-term studies and the low incidence of the condition (5 to 45/100,000) in Europe,[4] which limits evaluation of various therapeutic options in controlled studies. Our assessment of the validity of therapeutic options, specifically a comparison of staples versus manual sutures in resection procedures, is based on clinical observations over a 10-year period. Although parenchymal resection is the most effective procedure, it is only one element in a total concept, in which pleurectomy also has some value. The criteria for our diversified mode of treatment and the early indications for operative intervention will be presented along with our therapeutic results.

RESULTS

Between 1979 and 1989, we performed a total of 192 procedures, with follow-up investigation in 90% of all patients (n = 172) for a minimum of 2 years. Of these 172 patients, 75 were admitted from other hospitals after unsuccessful tube thoracostomy drainage (Table 1). The 30-day mortality rate from primary complications of pneumothorax was 3% (n = 6). These patients, who were over the age of 65 years, had a high degree of morbidity. In only two patients were the complications lead-

Table 1. Therapeutic procedures in first episode and recurrent pneumothorax in 172 cases investigated during follow-up

Therapy	First Episode	Previously Treated	Recurrence Rate
Intercostal tube drainage	63	2	27 (42%)
Thoracoscopy (without cyst resection)	14	10	12 (50%)
Primary thoracotomy	20	48	2 (3%)
Thoracoscopy with cyst resection (EndoGIA)	13	2	2 (13%)
TOTAL EPISODES	110	62	43 (25%)

Table 2. Recurrence rate after treatment of first pneumothorax

Therapy	No. of Patients	Relapse	Percent
Intercostal tube drainage	63	25	40
Thoracoscopy (without cyst resection)	14	7	50
Thoracotomy	20		
TOTAL	97		

ing to death directly attributed to the operative treatment (1%; 2/172). Four patients died of cardiorespiratory failure after an atypical pulmonary resection, which was performed following unsuccessful chest tube drainage for old age emphysema with pneumothorax.

Results of Chest Tube Drainage

Among 97 patients admitted with a first episode of pneumothorax during a period of 10 to 2 years, prior to this review, 34 patients had already been treated unsuccessfully with chest tube suction drainage, which was applied continuously for 7 days. In principle, a macrocalibrated underwater sealed drainage system was used with continuous suction through a 20 cm-or-higher water column. Drainage therapy was successful in 63 patients at the time; however, 25 of them had a subsequent relapse (Table 2). Ten of these patients were eventually treated with another chest tube drainage procedure, and the remaining 15 underwent a longer operation, thus indicating an unsatisfactory success rate for drainage therapy in these patients. The combined results of 25 late relapses and 34 primary unsuccessful therapy attempts yields a failure rate of 61% for tube thoracostomy and drainage therapy. This rate might be higher

Table 3. Interval between initially successful drainage therapy and recurrent episodes (n = 63) (1978 to 1988)

Interval (Years)	No. of Patients	Percent
0-1	15	60
1-2	3	12
2-3	5	20
>3	2	8
TOTAL	25	100

Date of follow-up January 1, 1990.

in view of the fact that follow-up was carried out in only 90% of patients (Table 3).

Results of Thoracoscopy and Thoracotomy

Until 1991 thoracoscopy was performed mainly as a diagnostic procedure. Endocoagulation or isolated ligation of cysts, partial abrasion of the pleura, and chemical pleurodesis were possible in only a few select cases. Thoracoscopic treatment was suitable for small isolated pathological changes in the lung tissue. Attempts at definitive elimination of the leak or total pleurodesis were unsuccessful with this method. Major pathological transformations of the lung parenchyma, in both size and number, could not be satisfactorily controlled through thoracoscopy. In four cases it was determined during subsequent thoracotomy that the cause of the pneumothorax had been missed. This is reflected in the 50% relapse rate after thoracoscopy.

THORACOTOMY

The open operation rate for all patients with a first occurrence of pneumothorax was 42%. Ablation of cysts proved to be the most effective procedure with a recurrence rate of 3%. Tissue-sparing resection of affected lung parenchyma is sufficient in cases of uncomplicated pneumothorax, which are mostly the result of solitary cysts in the lung apices and upper lobes. These cysts evolved from localized changes that develop with no substantial structural loss of parenchyma. Therefore tissue-sparing resection and manual suturing of the base can be performed with few technical problems. It is remarkable that in young patients with subpleural cysts, underlying fibrosis is frequently found rather than classic emphysema. In these cases at least the marginal areas of the cysts are more resistant and can be managed more easily with regard to suture techniques. A stapling device can simplify the suturing process, as has previously been reported for resections through fissures.[5]

The technical problems encountered in the surgical treatment of pneumothorax are related mainly to the extent of the elastic fibrous webs within lung tissue and the functional pulmonary impairment due to parenchymal loss and compression from blebs and bullae; that is, they are predominantly associated with degenerative emphysema of the elderly patient. This functional impairment entails increased operative morbidity. Care must be taken to ensure that parenchyma is not lost in the resection of emphysematous lung tissue. However, this is difficult to accomplish, since the thin-walled cystic network and the underlying marginal lung parenchyma are susceptible to rupture. Therefore the resection must be extended into an area of grossly healthy lung tissue to attain safe suture or staple lines. The problem of minimal lung parenchyma resection in emphysema-induced pneumothorax is mainly determined by the physical properties of the transition zone of ab-

normal to grossly normal tissue. This poses a specific problem with regard to suture technique. The therapeutic objective is therefore defined by a compromise between the air-sealed transsegmental and intersegmental ablation of atrophic cystic tissue and the thrifty resection of healthier parenchyma.

When emphysematous and cystic areas extend over a major portion of the lungs, the mechanical suture technique is clearly superior to manual sutures. Because of the fragility of the transition zone lung tissue, the needle puncture and the leverage of driving it through tissue adds to tissue injury with manual suturing, which can result in additional parenchymal lacerations and leaks during expansion of the lung. Furthermore, the thread placement is irregular and it punctures minute thin-walled, underlying cystic areas. Thus further opening of acinous areas is unavoidable. An airtight seal and the stability of the parenchymal closure lines can be ensured by using a double row of equally spaced staples. Parenchymal leaks cannot be adequately sealed with running manual sutures or single interrupted sutures. This problem can be significantly reduced or even avoided by the use of a tangential mechanical suture technique with GIA and TA staplers. The transition zone and absolute minimum amount of parenchyma that must be resected is easily determined by the anesthesiologist's withholding of active ventilation for a short time. With this so-called one-stage procedure, an airtight and hemostatic suture can be achieved, compared with manual sutures because of the uniform parenchymal compression preceding staple placement. Remaining air leaks along puncture channels in the stapled lines can be easily sealed with fibrin glue.

THORACOSCOPIC LUNG RESECTION

The EndoGIA stapler complies with requirements for the successful use of mechanical sutures via the thoracoscope. We consider the minimally invasive thoracoscopic technique to be a safe alternative to open resection, and we have used this method in 15 patients since 1991. Thus open surgical intervention, which would otherwise have been necessary, was avoided in 95% of all cases.

Ventilation with the double-lumen endotracheal tube and technique is an important requirement to make thoracoscopy possible without time and space constraints. Furthermore, often a bronchopleural fistula can be located only by specific ventilation of the affected collapsed lung.

DISCUSSION

Morphological findings in pneumothorax can range from small subpleural defects to major bullous emphysematous loss of parenchyma. Thus the difference between the so-called idiopathic and the symptomatic, emphysematous pneumothorax is a clinically established phenomenon. A single, nosologically strictly defined entity has not yet been substantiated and may well never be proven.

Our findings indicate that an acceptable standard of care cannot be expected or achieved with thoracostomy tube drainage (see Table 1). An important reason for this is that for almost all cases of pneumothorax there is a perceptible cause. In so-called idiopathic conditions this cause can be observed only by means of thoracoscopy.

Structural defects including pleural changes, have been found in virtually all patients, and could be spatially related to parenchymal or bronchial fistulas. The fact that these defects frequently are isolated within healthy lung tissue questions the necessity for pleurectomy in principle. Ferguson et al.[6] in 1981 reported excellent long-term results after ablation of cysts in cases of complicated spontaneous pneumothorax. Similar results were reported in 1987 by Krumhaar et al.,[7] who found that only a partial pleurectomy was necessary for recurrences of pneumothorax after unsuccessful operations.

In our patients we only resected the cysts and planned to perform a pleurectomy later on, except in cases of diffuse small cystic emphysema. The advantage of a low rate of recurrence after this intervention is offset by the risk of considerable postoperative bleeding; however, this occurred in only 4% of our patients. Furthermore, a problem of operative technique can be present after pleurodesis, when patients must undergo additional chest surgery at a later time in life.

Long-term results were satisfactory for both parietal pleurectomy and cyst resection, whether they were performed individually or in combination. Thus resection of areas transformed by cysts has been proved to be sufficient in the treatment of spontaneous pneumothorax. Exceptions may involve patients with mucoviscidosis and histiocytosis X. A lung parenchymal resection should be avoided in these patients because of related complications resulting from the underlying disease. In addition, the structural changes caused by cysts are frequently so diffuse and small that resection is contraindicated. These minor defects can be coagulated focally or resected sparingly at the margins. Also, in some patients filling of small cysts with fibrin glue has proved to be effective.

The obstructive ventilation disorder in mucoviscidosis induces subpleural changes and also results in bronchiectasis. Because of the loss of elasticity and the inflammatory peribronchial changes, the lung is found to be rigid and does not collapse completely. Parenchymal resection should be performed sparingly and is indicated only for localized, major cysts, which develop at the surface of the lung.

Focal cysts located subpleurally are difficult to control. Each of them can be the starting point for a recurrence of pneumothorax. Therefore, pleurectomy is considered to be the only option to avoid a recurrence of pneumothorax in these cases. Since lung transplantation may have to be considered later, indications for pleurectomy must be carefully evaluated in these patients. Often the cysts are confined to the apical area of the lungs. This is typical of young patients. The majority of patients with spontaneous pneumothorax still belong to this group.

The literature over the past year contains only sporadic references to a possible link between so-called spontaneous pneumothorax and smoking.[8-10] We confirmed this hypothesis in a case-control study of our own.[11] The proportion of smokers among our male patients with spontaneous pneumothorax was significantly increased compared with a random population in a comparable age distribution. The association between smoking and pneumothorax has led us to question whether localized areas of cystic transformation in the lungs could also be associated with cigarette smoking (Table 4).

Table 4. Relative percentages of smokers among men, aged 15 to 45 years

Status	Control	No. of Patients	Total
Nonsmokers	33 (41%)	6 (12%)	39
Ex-smokers	10 (12%)	2 (4%)	12
Smokers	38 (47%)	43 (84%)	81
TOTAL	81 (100%)	51 (100%)	132

$p < 0.01$.

Table 5. Localization of cysts in men, aged 15 to 45 years

Location	Smoker	Nonsmoker	Total
Upper lobe	33	6	39
Total lung	6	10	16
TOTAL	39	16	55

$p < 0.01$.

Our study involved patients whose lungs could be examined macroscopically by thoracoscopy or thoracotomy. The smoking history was known for all of them. As shown in Table 5, the cysts in smokers and ex-smokers were located significantly more frequently in the upper lobe or the apical area of the upper lobe as compared with nonsmokers.

This phenomenon had been demonstrated previously in smokers with emphysema. We know from this disease that the bullous changes begin primarily in the upper lobe and spread caudally over time.[12] The discovery that cystic changes in young patients who smoke occur predominantly in the apical areas of the lung was particularly significant with regard to the success of minimally invasive procedures in thoracic surgery. The procedure to resect lung cysts thoracoscopically with an EndoGIA stapler has become routine. Based on 15 patients who were operated on thoracoscopically, we established that even apical cysts are suitable for endoscopic resection, since this area can be reached and resected easily with the EndoGIA stapler. The advantage of this method over thoracotomy, with regard to the patient's postoperative state, is obvious.

Based on the preceding results, we believe a differentiated concept is indicated concerning operative methods in spontaneous pneumothorax. The combination of a young male who is a cigarette smoker and who presents with spontaneous pneumothorax represents an indication for early thoracoscopic intervention, particularly in a first occurrence. Almost all patients can be adequately treated endoscopically and derive the most from minimally invasive thoracoscopic resection.

REFERENCES

1. Elfeldt RJ, Schröder D, Meinicke O. Spontanpneumothorax-Überlegungen zur Ätiologie und Therapie. Chirurgie 62:540-546, 1991.
2. Kjaergaard H. Spontaneous pneumothorax in the apparently healthy. Acta Scand Med (Suppl 53), 1932.
3. Gänger KH. Der Spontanpneumothorax. Schweiz Rundschau Med (Praxis) 68:782-785, 1979.
4. Mattila S, Kostianen S. Spontaneous pneumothorax. Scand J Thorac Cardiovasc Surg 11:259-263, 1977.
5. Schröder DW. Technische Hilfen durch Nahtmaschinen in der Lungenchirurgie. Langenbecks Arch Chir (Suppl II):389-391, 1989.
6. Ferguson LJ, Imrie CW, Hutchinson J. Excision of bullae without pleurectomy in patients with spontaneous pneumothorax. Br J Surg 68:214-216, 1981.
7. Krumhaar D, Mollinedo J, Gau A. Primäre thorakotomie beim spontanpneumothorax. Z Herz Thorax Gefässchir 1:53-55, 1987.
8. Bense L, Eklund G, Wiman LG. Smoking and the increased risk of contracting spontaneous pneumothorax. Chest 92:1009-1012, 1987.
9. Jansveld CAF, Dijkman HJ. Primary spontaneous pneumothorax and smoking. Br Med J 42:559-560, 1975.
10. Nakamura H, Izuchi R, Hagiwara T, et al. Physical constitution and smoking habits of patients with idiopathic spontaneous pneumothorax. Jpn J Med 22:2-8, 1983.
11. Elfeldt RJ, Schröder. Relation between smoking and idiopathic pneumothorax: A case-control study. Theor Surg (in press).
12. Cockcroft DW, Horne SL. Localization of emphysema within the lung. Chest 82:483-487, 1982.

124 *Thoracoscopic Treatment of Spontaneous Pneumothorax and Bullous Emphysema*

W. Coosemans, D. Van Raemdonck, and T. Lerut

Spontaneous pneumothorax results from the rupture of a subpleural bleb or bulla without a known cause such as trauma, infection, or malignancy.[1-3] The aims of treatment are to alleviate symptoms, obtain full reexpansion of the lung, and prevent recurrence. Modes of treatment have been under discussion since the beginning of the nineteenth century when Itard and Laennec first described the clinical picture. Conservative measures, including observation, needle aspiration, and intercostal drainage alone, have yielded a substantial failure rate and are associated with recurrence in 30% to 50% of cases.[4] Chemical pleurodesis is more effective, but visualization, which is necessary to achieve optimal results, is limited. Moreover, the cause of the problem, the air leak, is not addressed, and the long-term effects of some of the agents used are uncertain.[5] Thoracotomy provides the opportunity to deal with the cause that means closing the air leak. Recurrence is rare after parietal pleurectomy, but complications in both the short and long term are not uncommon.[6,7] Pleural abrasion produces a milder inflammatory response and may minimize the chance of complications and allow earlier ambulation and discharge.[8] Recently a new technique was proposed—treatment by videoendoscopy. Modern videoendoscopic technology and percutaneous techniques of exposure and dissection have been applied in abdominal surgery with favorable results. Application of this technology and corresponding instrumentation has opened new horizons in the field of thoracic surgery as well.

MATERIALS AND METHODS

During general anesthesia with full relaxation, a double-lumen endobronchial Carlens tube is introduced. The patient is positioned in the lateral decubitus position as for a formal lateral thoracotomy. A 2 cm incision is made, usually in the fifth or sixth intercostal space in the midaxillary line. Digital palpation is used to enter the thoracic cavity so as to avoid any laceration of adherent lung tissue. A 10 mm 0- or 30-degree telescope is advanced through an 11 mm cannula after ipsilater-

al lung collapse has been achieved. A xenon light source provides illumination so that the image captured by the low-light capability CCD-chip video camera is transferred to two high-resolution television monitors, allowing both the surgeon and the assistant to have simultaneous unobstructed views of the intrathoracic exposure. There is no need for CO_2 insufflation, inasmuch as the rib cage is not collapsed and work space is ample. Additional cannulas are preferentially placed in "poor muscle" regions. Usually two and sometimes three grasping forceps and scissors with an electrocautery adapter, clip appliers, and endoloop applicators are variably introduced and if necessary the CO_2 laser (Sharplan 1060). The pleura is treated by evaporization with the defocused CO_2 laser at 10 watts or by pleurectomy. Hydrodissection—that is, injection of a water solution between the parietal pleura and the chest wall—may facilitate the pleurectomy. However, abrasion of the entire parietal pleura with a sponge is currently the method of choice.

Emphysematous bullae or blebs are treated by laser coagulation, ligation with a catgut Roeder endoloop, or more recently by resection with an endolinear stapler and cutting device. After completion of the procedure, one or two chest tubes (28 Fr) are inserted and a control x-ray film of the chest is always obtained before extubation to ensure complete lung expansion.

RESULTS

From August 1989 to August 1992, we treated 32 patients by a thoracoscopy for pneumothorax. During the same period, thoracotomy was performed in three additional patients with generalized bullous emphysema; in these patients a thoracoscopic approach was judged to be inadequate. In two patients the thoracoscopy was converted to an open procedure during the same operation. Respectively, a major persistent air leak and incomplete lung reexpansion at the end of the thoracoscopy procedure were considered too high a risk, and therefore a thoracotomy with wedge resection and pleurectomy of the apical dome of the pleura were per-

Table 1. Methods of treating pneumothorax

Condition	CO₂ Laser (n = 16)	Hydrodissection and Pleurectomy (n = 7)	Abrasion (n = 7)
Bulla			
Ligation	3	2	0
Laser coagulation	4	0	0
EndoGIA stapler	0	0	7
No treatment	1	1	0
No bulla	8	4	0

formed in both of them. The thoracoscopic procedure was completed in 30 patients.

There were eight women and 22 men ranging in age from 17 to 80 years, with a mean of 35 years. The pneumothorax was left sided in 12 and right sided in 18. Indications for intervention were as follows:

- First spontaneous pneumothorax with a persistent air leak with incomplete lung reexpansion in 10 patients and recurrence of lung collapse immediately after removal of the chest drain in three patients, one of whom had an enormous bulla of 10 cm of the inferior lobe (this patient had an inoperable carcinoma of the head of the pancreas).
- First recurrence of homolateral pneumothorax in eight patients, one of whom had a recurrence after surgical abrasion.
- Two or more recurrences in eight patients, one of whom had a catamenial pneumothorax.
- One elective procedure on specific request of the patient, who feared a recurrence while working in third world countries.

Four patients were considered high risk: One had severe coronary artery disease necessitating continuous intravenous administration of medication. A second patient (77 years of age) had a large intrathoracic goiter with tracheal compression and deviation with an arterial PO_2 of 50 mm Hg and a PCO_2 of 60 mm Hg at the time of admission. The third and fourth patients were already known to have significant chronic obstructive lung disease secondary to emphysema.

In 16 patients evaporization of the parietal pleura by CO_2 laser was performed, hydrodissection and pleurectomy were used in seven patients, and abrasion of the pleura in seven (Table 1). Twelve patients had as-

sociated pulmonary ligation and/or resections of blebs and bullae at the time of the operation: three patients had laser evaporisation and ligation of the bulla by Roeder endoloop, two underwent pleurectomy and ligation by endoloop, and seven had abrasion and resection of the bleb with an endostapler.

The results of thoracoscopic treatment for spontaneous pneumothorax are shown in the box. Mean follow-up for these 30 patients was 16 months, mean hospital stay after treatment was 9 days, and mean time for removal of chest drains was the sixth postoperative day. In one patient a partial recurrence was noted at the lower portion of the hemithorax; this was treated with tube drainage, and the problem was resolved within 4 days with no further complications.

Five major persistent problems were seen. Two persistent and significant air leaks required a thoracotomy. In one patient the leak persisted after thoracoscopic CO_2 laser treatment of the pleura and ligation of two bullae with the endoloop technique. After 3 days a thoracotomy was performed because of the magnitude of the residual air leak. Only one catgut ligature was found in place; it was thought that the other ligature had probably slipped off by the time the lung was reexpanded. Another patient had a thoracotomy 30 days postoperatively because of a small but persistent air leak. A wedge resection was performed to resect a leaking bulla that was missed at the time of thoracoscopy. In three patients pneumothorax recurred after hospital discharge. One patient had a recurrence after 18 days and was treated with thoracotomy and pleurectomy. Two other patients had a recurrence after 60 and 120 days, respectively. Both were treated with talc pleurodesis. There was no mortality or major morbidity. The overall success rate for

---

RESULTS OF TREATMENT FOR PNEUMOTHORAX (n = 32)

Air Leak/Recurrent Pneumothorax

D3   Major persistent air leak
D30 Persistent air leak   ⎫
D18 Early recurrence after discharge ⎬ Thoracotomy
D60 Recurrence   ⎭
D120 Recurrence   ⎫ Talc pleurodesis
                                  ⎭

COMPLICATIONS IN RELATION TO SURGICAL TECHNIQUE

Laser evaporization of pleura
  Without bulla laser   1 early recurrence (D18)   ⎫
    treatment   ⎬
  With bulla laser   1 late recurrence (D60)   ⎬ 3/16 = 18.7%
    treatment   ⎬
  With bulla ligation   1 major air leak (D3)   ⎭
Hydrodissection and pleurectomy without bullectomy
                             1 partial recurrence (D23)   ⎫
                             1 major recurrence (D120)   ⎬ 3/7 = 42.8%
                             1 small persistent leak (D30) ⎭
  Abrasion and application of endostapler   0/12 = 0%

---

completed procedures was 83%. Correlating complications and surgical technique (see the box) showed a failure rate of 18.7% for CO_2 laser evaporation with or without ligation or laser coagulation of the bulla. There were major problems in 42.8% of the patients treated with hydrodissection and pleurectomy, but no recurrences were seen with pleural abrasion and bullectomy with the endostapler. Therefore this technique has now become the treatment of choice.

DISCUSSION

Recurrent spontaneous pneumothorax occurs in 4.3/10,000 patients a year, with a male:female ratio of 5:1. A pneumothorax of less than 20% of the ipsilateral hemithorax volume "in an otherwise healthy" adult who is not short of breath is best managed by observation. However, more than 70% of patients have a lung collapse greater than 25% and require active management mostly with intercostal tube drainage.[6]

Surgical intervention is indicated if the lung fails to reexpand mostly because of persistent air leak in 4% to 14%.[9] Ipsilateral recurrence, with likely increases from 16% after the first episode to 80% after the third episode, heterolateral pneumothorax, bilateral spontaneous pneumothorax, which is a life-threatening condition, and pneumothorax in special risk groups, for example, flight crews and truck drivers, are other indications for surgical treatment.

Thoracotomy with parietal pleurectomy (first described by Gaemsler[10] in 1956) or pleural abrasion (first performed by Tyson and Crandall[11] in 1941), if necessary combined with excision, oversewing, ligature, or stapling of any visible blebs, is an effective well-validated procedure. The advantage of pleural abrasion over standard pleurectomy relates to the incidence of complications and the dubious logic of treating an abnormality of the lung by removing a large area of normal pleura.[8] Long-term studies with follow-up of up to 8 years showed no recurrences and no serious impairment of the mechanics of respiration.[12] However, there is a distinct decrease up to 16% in vital capacity in the early postoperative period, which returns to preoperative values only at 5 months. This is attributed to the trauma of the thoracotomy, which impairs lung function. With the video-assisted thoracoscopic approach the same operative technique as in open surgery can be used, presumably without the negative aspects of the thoracotomy itself.[13]

We have been using three different techniques with varying results. Initially CO_2 laser evaporization was used with laser coagulation or ligation by an endoloop of the bullae if necessary. The failure rate of 18.7% correlates very well with data from Wakabayashi et al.,[14] who treated 24 patients with an overall success rate of 83.0%.

Some investigators, however, prefer to use the Nd:YAG laser.[11,15,16] This laser may be more advantageous for more extensive lesions because it is more readily absorbed by the hemoglobin pigment, leading to a superior potential for coagulation especially in hemorrhaghic surgical fields. Because of the good results achieved with pleurectomy in open surgery[16] and because of the development of better instruments for thoracoscopic purposes, we switched to thoracoscopic pleurectomy with or without ligation with an endoloop as advocated by Cushieri (personal communication). Inderbitsi et al.[17] treated 49 patients with a recurrence rate of only 6.1%. Our own results, however, were not so favorable with up to 42.8% having major problems. The reason for this high failure rate was twofold: some minor bullae or blebs were overlooked and the Roeder knot slipped off, although it has been demonstrated that chromic catgut tied with the Roeder slipknot can withstand a tension of approximately 1000 g before slipping occurs.

In light of the development of the linear endostapler device and because of the favorable results achieved with pleural abrasion in open surgery for pneumothorax (Maggi et al.[16] described no recurrences in 80 patients), we have switched our technique to this latter method. Abrasion is a quick and safe procedure, normally lasting no longer than 30 minutes. It also has the distinct advantage of minimally affecting the pleural space.[18] This will render subsequent reintervention in the thoracic cavity much easier to perform, which is indeed very important since some of these patients will eventually become candidates for traditional lung surgery and transplantation. Seven of our patients were treated with this method with no subsequent problems. A recurrence rate of 3.2% to 6.7% was noted by Wieser.[19]

Inasmuch as the mechanism of the so-called spontaneous pneumothorax is usually attributed to the rupture of an apical subpleural bleb or bulla,[3] treatment of the bleb or bulla itself is of paramount importance. In this respect it is essential to obtain as much information as possible preoperatively. A standard chest x-ray film will show major bullous deformities. Much more precise information will be obtained from a CT scan of the thorax.[2,15] When a CT scan confirms diffuse bullous emphysema, we do not choose a thoracoscopic approach. In this series, blebs larger than 4 cm in diameter were also considered contraindications for thoracoscopy. For this reason in three patients we decided to immediately perform an open procedure instead. However, it is clear that currently, with the introduction of the new generation of 60 mm endostaplers, the scope of thoracoscopic surgery, especially in the treatment of more significant bullae, will be enlarged.

CONCLUSION

Many operative procedures that are traditionally performed through open thoracotomy can now be done by videothoracoscopic surgery with equally good results; this is especially the case in the treatment of spontaneous pneumothorax. Although video-assisted thoracoscopy is more difficult and tedious to perform, its main benefits seem to be an apparent shortened recovery time and a decreased frequency of the side effects commonly seen in conventional open surgery, for example, post-thoracotomy pain, impaired postoperative pulmonary function, and/or shoulder girdle impairment.

REFERENCES

1. Laurenzi GA, Turino GM, Fishman AP. Bullous disease of the lung. Am J Med 32:361-377, 1962.
2. Lesur O, Delarue N, Formaget JM, et al. Computed Tomography in the etiologic assessment of idiopathic spontaneous pneumothorax. Chest 98:341-347, 1990.
3. Torre M, Pierangelo Belloni P. Nd:Yag laser pleurodesis through thoracoscopy: New curative therapy in spontaneous pneumothorax. Ann Thorac Surg 47:887-889, 1989.
4. Getz SB Jr, Beasly WE III. Spontaneous pneumothorax. Am J Surg 145:823-827, 1983.
5. Atassi K, Pilorget A, Lemarie F, et al. Thoracostomy tube pleurodesis by collagen instillation. Intensive Care Med 12:335-336, 1986.
6. DeMeester TR, LaFontaine E. The pleura. In Sabiston DC, Spencer FC, eds. Surgery of the Chest. Philadelphia: WB Saunders, 1990.
7. Deslauries J, Leblanc P, McClish A. Bullous and bleb diseases of the lung. In Shields TW, ed. General Thoracic Surgery. Philadelphia: Lea & Febiger, 1989.

8. Seaton A, Seaton D, Leitch AG. Pneumothorax. In Seaton A, ed. Crafton & Douglas' Respiratory Diseases, 4th ed. Oxford: Blackwell Scientific, 1989, p 776.
9. Singh VS. The surgical treatment of spontaneous pneumothorax by parietal pleurectomy. Scand J Thorac Cardiovasc Surg 16:75-80, 1982.
10. Gaemsler EA. Parietal pleurectomy for recurrent pneumothorax. Surg Gynecol Obstet 102:293, 1956.
11. Tyson MD, Crandall WB. The surgical treatment of recurrent idiopathic spontaneous pneumothorax. J Thorac Surg 10:566, 1941.
12. Terminology, definitions, and classification of chronic pulmonary emphysema and related conditions: A report of the conclusions of a CIBA guest symposium. Thorax 14:286-299, 1959.
13. Nathanson LK, Shini SM, Wood RAB, et al. Videothoracoscopic ligation of bulla and pleurectomy for spontaneous pneumothorax. Ann Thorac Surg 52:316-319, 1991.
14. Wakabayashi A, Brenner M, Wilson F, et al. Thoracoscopic treatment of spontaneous pneumothorax using carbon dioxide laser. Ann Thorac Surg 50:786-790, 1990.
15. Locicero J III, Hartz R, Frederiksen J, et al. New applications of the laser in pulmonary surgery: Hemostasis and sealing of air leaks. Ann Thorac Surg 40:546-550, 1985.
16. Maggi G, Ardissone F, Oliaro A, et al. Pleural abrasion in the treatment of recurrent or persistent spontaneous pneumothorax. Int Surg 77:99-101, 1992.
17. Inderbitsi R, Furrer M, Striffelen H. Die Operative Thoracoskopie. Indikationen and Technik. Chirurgie 63: 334-341, 1992.
18. Nkere U, Griffin SC, Fountain SW. Pleural abrasion: A new method of pleurodesis. Thorax 46:596-598, 1991.
19. Wieser O, Wieser CO. Indikationen zur Thoraskopic bein sekundären spontaneous Pneumothorax. Pneumologie 43:92-95, 1989.

125   *Thoracoscopic Treatment of Pneumothorax*

Martin Hürtgen, Andreas Schäfer, Christian J. Lukosch, and Konrad Schwemmle

Indications for and the principles of a surgical procedure should be the same for endoscopic and conventional surgery. Surgeons performing endoscopic operations should be familiar with the corresponding open procedure and thus be capable of managing complications. An unbiased decision for endoscopic or open procedure might be compromised by lack of experience in either one of these two approaches. With this in mind, the trauma of surgical access for treatment of pneumothorax may be reduced by use of the thoracoscopic approach. Since January 1990 we have tested whether thoracoscopy really combines less trauma with a lower rate of recurrence and complications as compared with known data for conventional operative treatment of pneumothorax.[1]

INDICATIONS

In accordance with the principles mentioned previously, we selected patients with recurrent spontaneous pneumothorax or persisting air leak during tube thoracostomy drainage, thus including only those patients who would otherwise have undergone thoracotomy. Excessive risk by thoracotomy, mostly due to reduced lung function in secondary pneumothorax, is also a contraindication for thoracoscopic treatment.

MATERIALS AND METHODS
Preoperative Management

Thoracoscopy immediately on admission in suitable patients is feasible in only a few centers. Furthermore, a thorough inspection of the whole lung under local anesthesia is not very pleasant for the patient. Therefore we primarily insert a chest drain to reexpand the collapsed lung. In marginal pneumothorax this may be omitted. The entry point of the drain should be in the third intercostal space in the midclavicular line to avoid infection of incisions in the potential operative area on the lateral thoracic wall. After reexpansion of the lung a CT scan of the thorax is added to the standard preoperative workup to determine the extent of the bullous changes (Fig. 1) and to complement the information obtained by thoracoscopic exploration of the lung.

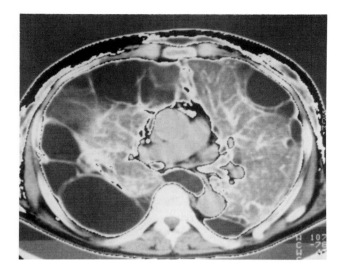

Fig. 1. Preoperative CT scan of bullous emphysema.

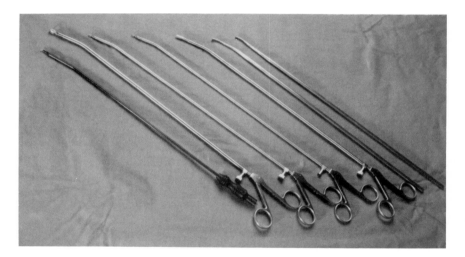

Fig. 2. Angled instruments.

Anesthesia

Double-lumen intubation with single-lung ventilation is mandatory. Intraoperative monitoring is the same as in major open surgery; this makes the job for the anesthesiologist more demanding than in standard surgery for pneumothorax. The anesthesiologist should be experienced in thoracic surgery; without these premises thoracoscopic surgery is not advisable.

Instrumentation

A video camera must be connected to the thoracoscope to allow coordinated action of surgeon and assistant, similar to laparoscopic surgery. Special angled instruments are now available (Fig. 2), which allow the surgeon to reach almost anywhere in the thorax. The previously used straight instruments derived from laparoscopy made the lateral thoracic wall a no man's land. The diameter of the instruments varies from 5 to 12 mm. Thinner instruments are preferable, because they offer greater mobility in the sometimes narrow intercostal space. Instruments may be introduced directly through the incisions, but we prefer the use of trocars. Multiple changes of instrument cause tissue damage on the unprotected incision sites. Without a trocar, the lens

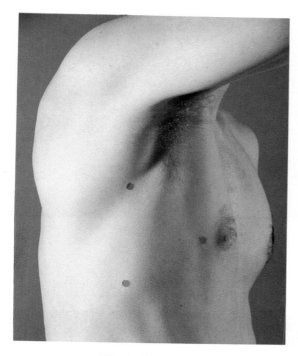

Fig. 3. Trocar sites.

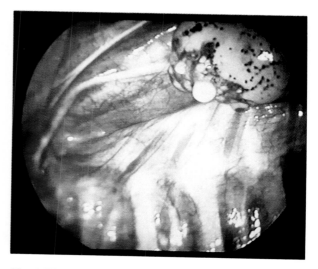

Fig. 4. Typical apical bullae in spontaneous pneumothorax.

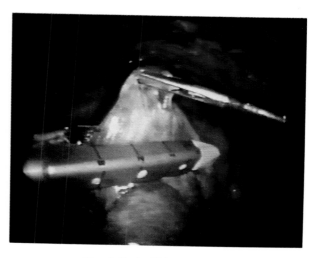

Fig. 5. EndoGIA application.

is frequently smeared with blood. Low-pressure insufflation, not exceeding 5 mm Hg, requires air-tightness and in selected cases facilitates the procedure. With higher pressure the tension pneumothorax might induce dramatic hemodynamic changes, resulting in low cardiac output or even arrest.

Operative Technique

Position. The patient is placed in a lateral position, as for standard thoracotomy, with the surgeon and assistant at the front and the monitor at the back of the patient. A second monitor on the opposite side is helpful if the surgeon wants to change sides during the operation. This may be appropriate for manipulation of the ventral inner thoracic wall.

The patient's upper arms should be elevated as much as possible to the front. Abduction to the side, as is usually done, would hinder passage of instruments through the axillary trocar sheath.

Trocar sites. The first incision is made most cranial at the ventral border of the latissimus dorsi muscle in the fourth or fifth intercostal space. Opening the parietal pleura bluntly almost precludes injuring the lung. Additional trocars are inserted under direct vision in the fifth to eighth intercostal space in the ventral and dorsal axillary line (Fig. 3). The precise site depends on the location of the pulmonary changes. In general, the area on the lateral thoracic wall, which is almost free of muscles, should be used.

Resection. An identified air leak or bullae should be resected as in open surgery. Small bullae (Fig. 4) may be ligated; larger areas require several applications of an EndoGIA instrument (Fig. 5). Applying fibrin glue or coagulating the bullae has shown a high rate of relapse.[2]

Pleurodesis. The second principle in operative treatment of pneumothorax is this: only if the changes of the lung are well defined and circumscribed, resection alone may preclude recurrent pneumothorax. Idiopathic pneumothorax without visible bullae and unidentified air leak or vast bullous changes as usually encountered in secondary pneumothorax requires pleurodesis.[3] This may be achieved by several means.

Fibrin glue or chemical pleurodesis is not very effective; only talcum pleurodesis is effective, but this method is reserved for patients with a limited life expectation[4] because of the sometimes extensive fibrous reaction.[5]

Surgical pleurodesis is done mostly by pleurabrasion with a swab or by pleurocoagulation by electrocautery or laser (Fig. 6). Pleurabrasion by thoracoscopy is quite boresome. Pleurocoagulation offers greater comfort for the patient, but the depth of tissue damage is difficult to define. Too much would interfere with subpleural structures; too little could mean insufficient pleurodesis. Thus the result of the procedure is very much dependent on the experience of the surgeon. Pleurectomy offers a standardized and firm pleurodesis. It can be done thoracoscopically even better than by open operation, because the dissection in the right plane and bleeding on the lateral thoracic wall are better controlled. If later lung transplantation is ruled out for the patient, pleurectomy has become our first choice for pleurodesis after performing principally pleurocoagulation during the first 2 years of our experience.

Pleurocoagulation is done with an isolated suction probe, with the coagulation current set to low levels to avoid adherence of the probe to the pleura and facilitate continuous, smooth movements. Carbonization with higher voltages should be avoided. The argon beam coagulator or Nd:YAG laser did not show any advantages in our hands and are more expensive.

The pleurectomy is carried out with dissectors and graspers after the margins of the pleurectomy are marked with the coagulation hook (Fig. 7). The extent of pleurodesis corresponds with the extent of the changes of the lung.

Saline is injected in the subpleural space or hydrodissection with low pressure is done to open the right plane of dissection; this usually prevents severe bleeding. At the end of the procedure a chest drain (at least 24 Fr) is inserted and the lung is reexpanded under direct vision. Partial atelectasis would require bronchoscopy. An imprisoned lung needs decortication.

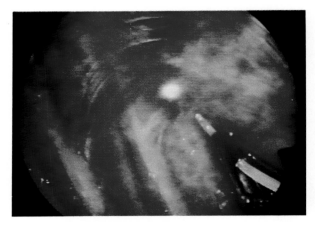

Fig. 6. Laser coagulation for pleurodesis.

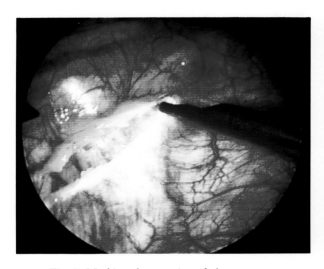

Fig. 7. Marking the margins of pleurectomy.

POSTOPERATIVE CARE

An x-ray evaluation is obligatory immediately after operation. No antibiotic agents are administered. The intravenous catheter is removed on the afternoon of the operation. The chest drain is necessary for 1 to 4 days, depending on the kind of pleurodesis and the resulting amount of drained fluid. After the chest drain is removed, patients only rarely require analgesics. The

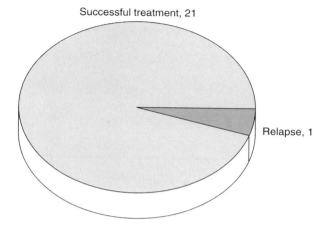

Fig. 8. Results of thoracoscopic treatment for idiopathic pneumothorax in 22 patients.

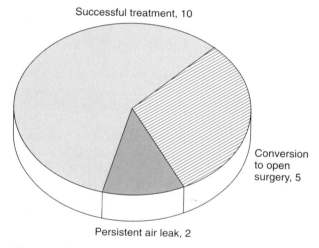

Fig. 9. Results of thoracoscopic treatment for secondary pneumothorax in 17 patients.

patient is discharged after the chest drain has been removed and an x-ray evaluation has yielded normal results. Repeat x-ray evaluation is advisable 1 week later.

RESULTS

Since January 1990 we have performed 39 operations on 37 patients. In 22 cases with idiopathic pneumothorax (Fig. 8), only one relapse has occurred. This man had bullae in the apex of the upper lobe but refused any procedure other than fibrin glue application. Originally he was sent for removal of an interpleural lost catheter. The relapse was treated by thoracotomy. Seventeen patients with secondary pneumothorax (Fig. 9) demonstrated the limitations of thoracoscopy: in five cases conversion to an open procedure was necessary as a result of vast adhesions or disseminated bullous changes with an unidentifiable air leak. Two more patients had a persistent air leak after thoracoscopy and required prolonged suction therapy. Nevertheless, about two thirds of the patients with secondary pneumothorax had the benefit of less trauma and no relapse. The other third had no disadvantage compared with primary open operation. Complications have been very rare to date. One patient with secondary pneumothorax had an intraoperative reversible cardiac arrest caused by excessive insufflation. In another case, local infection of one incision healed after removal of the suture without further treatment.

CONCLUSION

In secondary pneumothorax, thoracoscopic treatment is an alternative to open surgery. Since in one third of our patients thoracoscopy fails, a restrictive indication is proposed. CT scanning provides important information. For patients in very poor condition who have extensive bullous changes and persisting air leak, thoracoscopic talcum pleurodesis under local anesthesia is one consideration.

In all patients with primary pneumothorax, thoracoscopy is our treatment of choice. Bullae are resected and lung biopsy sometimes reveals prior unknown underlying lung disease, such as silicosis or malignancy. We now offer thoracoscopic treatment to our patients even after the primary manifestation of idiopathic pneumothorax. This avoids unsuccessful suction treatment or relapse and may be performed bilaterally. The risk of conversion to open procedure or development of complications is minimal in these patients.

REFERENCES

1. Krumhaar D, Mollinedo J, Gau A. Therapie des Spontanpneumothorax—Chirurgische Therapie. Langenbecks Arch Chir (Suppl) 2:501-503, 1988.
2. Elfeldt RJ, Schröder D, Meinicke O. Spontanpneumothorax—Überlegungen zur Ätiologie und Therapie. Chirurgie 62:540-546, 1991.

3. Inderbitzi R, Furrer M, Striffeler H. Die operative Thora-coskopie—Indikation und Technik. Chirurgie 63:334-341, 1992.
4. Daniel TM, Tribble CG, Rodgers BM. Thoracoscopy and talc poudrage for pneumothoraces and effusions. Ann Thorac Surg 50:186-189, 1990.
5. Lange P, Mortensen J, Groth S. Lung function 22-35 years after treatment of idiopathic spontaneous pneumothorax with talc poudrage or simple drainage. Thorax 43:559-561, 1988.

126 *Videoendoscopic Techniques in the Diagnosis and Treatment of Spontaneous Pneumothorax*

Andrea Sortini, Mirco Santini, Giuseppe Navarra, Savino Occhionorelli, and Ippolito Donini

The introduction of new videoendoscopic technology and minimally invasive surgery have enabled the use of thoracoscopy as both a diagnostic and a therapeutic procedure.[3,4] Today, thoracoscopic technique is the gold standard in the diagnosis and therapy of spontaneous pneumothorax.

Videoendoscopic-supported thoracic surgery is based on the following principles:

1. Careful preoperative evaluation of the patient who has possible contraindications for open thoracic surgery must be done because the operation may have to be converted to classic thoracotomy.
2. The patient must be able to undergo general anesthesia with an endotracheal Carlens tube that excludes the lung on the surgically treated side.

OPERATIVE TECHNIQUE FOR VIDEOENDOSCOPIC THORACIC SURGERY

With the patient placed as for a classic anterolateral thoracotomy, a telescope–camera port is placed into the fifth intercostal space and the anterior axillary line; a second 5 mm working port is placed into the third or fourth intercostal space and midclavicular line. A third 12 mm trocar sleeve is usually introduced into the sixth or seventh intercostal space in the midaxillary line when the lesion is at the apical level or in another site according to the position of the lesion (Fig. 1). A grasping for-

ceps is used through the 5 mm trocar sleeve to grasp the parenchyma easily.

When the lesion is found, a forceps is used to lift and stretch the zone.

With an endogauge forceps introduced through the operative 12 mm trocar, we measure the portion of the parenchyma that must be removed, and then we crush it to facilitate the surgical resection.

The EndoGIA 30 multifire stapler is introduced through the 12 mm trocar and is positioned on the resection rim to be effected; the trace left by the endogauge is followed. We then close the stapler and fire. A section and a suture with a double or triple line of 3.5 mm staples result. Margins are clear-cut and hemostatic (Fig. 2).

When the resection must be enlarged, the stapler is extracted and is reloaded with a new charge unit, and the parenchymal suture is redone.

The resected parenchyma is removed by an extracting forceps introduced through the operative trocar sleeve. Abrasion with a coagulator is performed to induce adherence between the two pleural sheets as prophylaxis for complete lung collapse if a relapse of pneumothorax occurs. The anesthesiologist then reexpands the lung. We control the resection margins, suction the blood from the pleural cavity, and place a chest tube that passes through the lowest wound. The drain, which contains many holes, is pulled up to the apex.

Closure of the parietal incisions completes the operation. The pleural drain is kept in place for a mean time

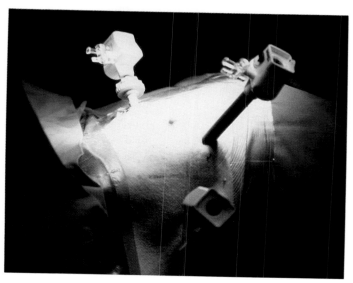

Fig. 1. Complete insertion of trocars to treat spontaneous pneumothorax caused by a bleb on the superior lobe of right lung.

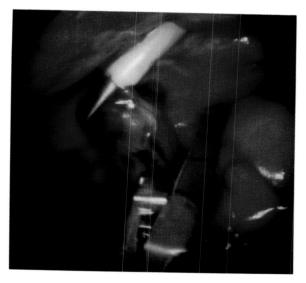

Fig. 2. EndoGIA stapling device *(below)* used in bleb resection with double lines of staples.

Table 1. Ferrara University case series
(January-December 1992)

	Number
Patient profile	26
Male	19
Female	7
Mean age (yr)	51
Hospital stay (days)	6
Diagnosis	
Spontaneous pneumothorax	9
Peripheral pulmonary neoplasms	10
Pleural effusion of unknown cause	7
Procedure	
Minimally invasive thoracoscopic resection	12
Biopsy and drainage	7
Thoracotomy after minimally invasive approach	7
Complication	
Delayed lung reexpansion (sixth postoperative day)	2

of 5 days. Even thoracoscopy can result in complications. For example, during trocar introduction, parenchymal rupture or perforation can occur. (Care should be taken not to injure the liver during the introduction of the lowest trocar in a patient with concurrent hepatomegaly.) Acute cardiac or respiratory failure may occur during the operation or in the early postoperative period. We feel that local metastatic dissemination is impossible because of the small dimension of the lesions. Infection of the pleural cavity may also occur.

We have had only two cases of delayed reexpansion of the lung on the sixth postoperative day (Table 1). All patients were completely recovered when they were discharged from the hospital (mean length of hospital stay, 6 days).

We believe in the value of video-supported thoracoscopic surgery, which we consider to be the gold standard for the therapy of pneumothorax that results from bleb rupture. This method has much promise.

REFERENCES

1. Jacobeus HC. Uber die Moglichkeit, die Zystoskopie bei untersuchung seroser Hohlungen anzuwenden. Munch Med Wschr 57:2090, 1910.
2. Jacobeus HC. The practical importance of thoracoscopy in surgery of the chest. Surg Gynecol Obstet 34:280-296, 1912.
3. Lewis RJ, Caccavale RJ, Sisler GE. Special report: Video-endoscopic thoracic surgery. N J Med 88:473-475, 1991.
4. Wakabayashi A. Expanded applications of diagnostic and therapeutic thoracoscopy. J Thorac Cardiovasc Surg 102:721-723, 1991.
5. Coltharp WH, Arnold JH, Alford WC Jr, et al. Video-thoracoscopy: Improved technique and expanded indications. Ann Thorac Surg 53:776-778, 1992.
6. Sampietro R. La Videotoracoscopia Interventistica. Il Polso 4:24-26, 1992.
7. Sortini A, Santini M, Occhionorelli S, et al. Atypical pulmonary resection performed with video-supported thoracoscopic surgery. Eurosurgery '92, Brussels, June 5-6, 1992.
8. Sortini A, Santini M, Donini A, et al. Resezione polmonare atipica eseguita con chirurgia toracoscopica videoguidata. Primi risultati. In Proceedings of the National Congress of the Italian Society of Surgery. Rome: Oct. 1992, The Congress.
9. Sortini A, Donini A, Santini M, et al. Resezione polmonare atipica in videotoracochirurgia. Atti Convegno "Le nuove tecniche miniinvasive. Diagnostica e Terapia." Milano: Nov. 5-6, 1992, pp 361-364.
10. Sortini A, Donini A, Navarra G, et al. Pulmonary Videosurgery. Initial Results. New Delhi: World Congress of the International College of Surgeons, 1992.

127 Comparative Study of Manual and Mechanical Sutures in Traditional Surgery for Spontaneous Pneumothorax: Analysis of 594 Procedures

Jesús Loscertales, Francisco J. Ayarra, Rafael Jimenez-Merchan,
Fernando Jose Garcia-Diaz, Carlos J. Arenas-Linares, Jose M. Cuaresma-Ferrete,
Antonio Rico-Alvarez, and Juan Carlos Giron-Arjona

Use of staple sutures in lung surgery began after World War II, with studies carried out in Moscow under the guidance of the Scientific Research Institute for Experimental Apparatus and Instruments.[1,2] However, it was not until the studies of Smith et al.[3] that staplers were sufficiently evaluated to achieve the high standards currently demanded. One of the main reasons that use of the mechanical suture has become common is that it significantly decreases dehiscence of the bronchial stump, one of the most frequent and serious complications of thoracic surgery. However, the most notable results effected by the staplers in the field of surgery are a significant shortening of the duration of operative procedures and a decrease in postoperative complications, particularly with regard to sectioning and suturing of lung parenchyma. Also relevant is the ease of application, since it is not necessary to take into account segmental planes, and the technical difficulties that often accompany dissection.[4]

The aim of our study was to compare results achieved with mechanical sutures in the treatment of bullae or apical blebs, which are the cause of spontaneous pneumothorax, with our previously used procedures of capitonnage or exeresis and manual sutures.

MATERIALS AND METHODS

Between January 1976 and December 1991, 594 cases of spontaneous pneumothorax were treated at the University Hospital of Seville. There was a predominance of male patients: 538 (90.6%) men and 56 (9.4%) women, a male/female ratio of 9.6/1 (Fig. 1).

The age distribution is shown in Fig. 2; there is a clear predominance of patients in their teens and twenties. The youngest patient was 14 years of age and the oldest was 89, with a median age of 31 years.

The sites of pneumothorax were as follows (Fig. 3): 307 cases on the right side, 248 on the left, 10 simulta-

neous bilateral, and 29 alternate bilateral, which refers to the presence of a spontaneous pneumothorax in one hemithorax followed some time later by a new one occurring on the opposite side.

Clinical symptoms were present in practically all of our patients, with an intensity that was generally in proportion to the size of the chamber of the pneumothorax. Pain and dyspnea, sometimes accompanied by cough in an intermittent crisis, was the usual clinical mode of presentation.

It should be noted that 163 of our patients had had previous episodes of pneumothorax that were studied radiographically: one episode in 88 patients, two episodes in 38, three episodes in 21, and more than three episodes in 16 (Fig. 4).

The diagnosis of pneumothorax was based on clinical history and physical examination (triad of Galliard). In addition, it was confirmed by radiographic examination. Based on results of x-ray examination four cate-

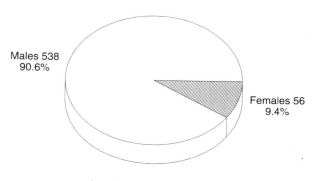

Males 538
90.6%

Females 56
9.4%

Ages 14-89 (mean 31 years)

Fig. 1. Patient demographic data; note predominance of males.

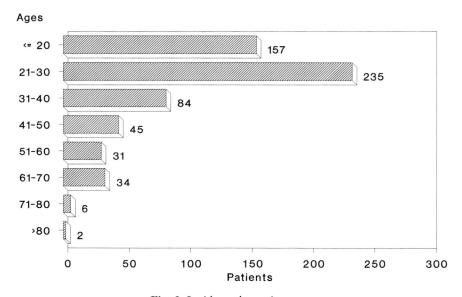

Fig. 2. Incidence by patient age.

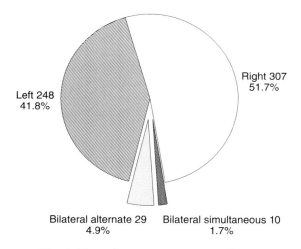

Fig. 3. Sites of spontaneous pneumothorax.

Table 1. Surgical approaches

Approach	No. of Patients
Axillary thoracotomy	14
Lateral thoracotomy	571
Posterolateral thoracotomy	2
Middle sternotomy	7
TOTAL	594

gories of pneumothorax were established, depending on the size of the pleural air chamber within the hemithorax: (1) smaller than one third, 150 patients; (2) between one third and two thirds, 326 patients; (3) larger than two thirds, 118 patients, and (4) tension pneumothorax, which was observed in 96 patients (Fig 5).

For our patients with pneumothorax, the thoracotomy procedure chosen most frequently was the lateral thoracotomy of Noirclerc in the fifth and sixth intercostal spaces; it was used in 571 patients. Axillary thoracotomy was performed in 14 patients, posterolateral thoracotomy in two patients, and median sternotomy for the treatment of bilateral pneumothorax in seven patients (Table 1).

For treatment of causal lesions in pneumothorax (Fig. 6), we initially used bleb exeresis and manual sutures; we also performed exeresis and capitonnage of large bullae in 78 patients (exeresis and sutures in 58 and capitonnage in 20). Mechanical sutures were used in 493 patients. Over the past 12 years, sutures were used in 579 patients. Since the beginning we have used the TA (thoracoabdominal) device (U.S. Surgical Corp.), available in 30, 55, and 90 mm lengths and which uses 3.5 mm staples. Recently we have added the RL stapler (Ethicon), available in 30, 60, and 90 mm. The RL presents several options for height of the staples, depend-

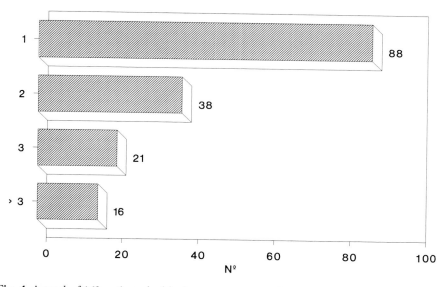

Fig. 4. A total of 163 patients had had one or more previous incidences of pneumothorax.

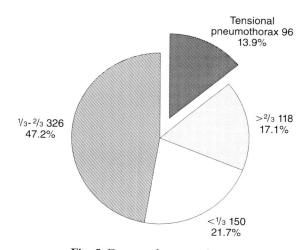

Fig. 5. Degree of pneumothorax.

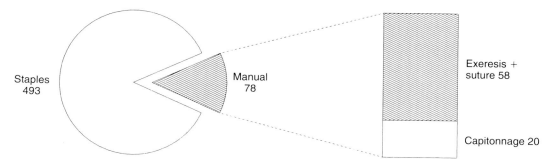

Fig. 6. Suture types in 493 patients over 12 years.

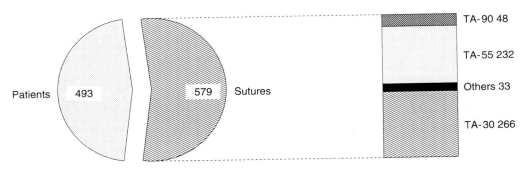

Fig. 7. Various staplers used.

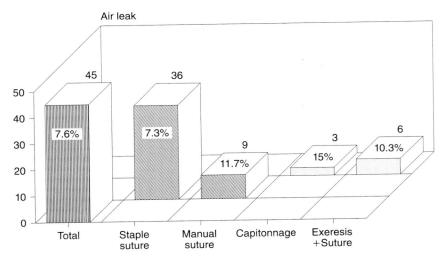

Fig. 8. Incidence of air leaks by type of suture used.

ing on the tension of the screw of the machine. The frequency with which each is used is shown in Fig. 7.

Pleurodesis was always performed by means of pleural abrasion with a plastic sponge; occasionally the visceral pleura was brushed with iodine in patients with remaining parenchymal disease to speed symphysis.

RESULTS

The parameters evaluated in this study are those inherent in this type of procedure: the presence of persistent air leaks is directly related to the presence of residual blebs or bullae and determines the length of the postoperative hospital stay.

There were a total of 45 extended air leaks in our study

(7.6%). They always occurred in patients with underlying parenchymal disease, and all diminished with prolonged drainage.

The distribution of air leaks according to the type of suture used was as follows (Fig. 8): 36 patients (7.3%) with staples, nine patients (11.5%) with manual sutures, six patients (10.3%) with exeresis and sutures, and three patients (15%) with capitonnage of large bullae.

Although these differences between groups were not significant, it is evident that the number of air leaks was lower in the group with mechanical sutures. If manual sutures were used more often, these differences would probably be greater. However, because of the availability of staples and their high degree of safety, they are used

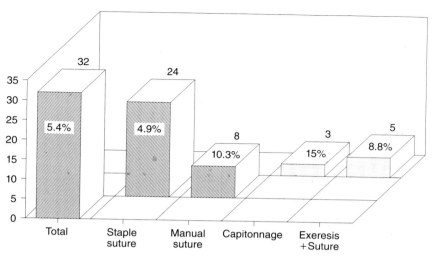

Fig. 9. Incidence of apical residual air spaces by type of suture used.

routinely, and we have essentially abandoned the use of manual sutures, except for capitonnage of large bullae.

The presence of residual pleural air chambers should also be mentioned. They can be directly linked to air leakage, inasmuch as all of the chambers appeared in patients with prolonged air leakage after removal of the superior drainage tube.

When stapling was performed for extirpation of a lesion, 24 chambers appeared (4.9% of the group). However, when manual sutures were used eight residual chambers appeared (10.3% of the group). In the groups with capitonnage or exeresis, three (15%) and five (8.8%) residual chambers appeared, respectively, with manual sutures (Fig. 9).

Of the 32 (5.4%) residual chambers observed in our study, all were small, and 28 resolved with respiratory physiotherapy. They disappeared between 15 and 30 days after patients were discharged from the hospital. The other four small chambers were not diminished, and a minimal apical pleural enlargement remained that did not cause any functional sequelae.

The usual duration of stapling procedures was 49 minutes, whereas for manual sutures the time increased up to 73 minutes. This is another advantage of mechanical sutures.

The hospital stay was also shorter when staple sutures were used, with a ratio of 8 days versus 11 days in those with manual sutures.

Concerning relapse after resolution, we found only one small apical chamber (<2 cm) 3 months after manual sutures were used, which resolved with physiotherapy. We do not believe that the type of suture has as much influence on the recurrence of air chambers as the quality of the pleural abrasion.

The type of suture used had no influence on the mortality rate; no patients died in either group.

DISCUSSION

The treatment of spontaneous pneumothorax has ranged from very conservative to overly aggressive; for example, in 1954 Myers[5] recommended a year of bed rest for one patient following treatment of pneumothorax, with no resolution of the episode. By contrast, Baronofsky et al.[6] and Kalnins et al.[7] proposed systematic bilateral thoracotomy for patients with unilateral pneumothorax.

The aim of operative treatment of spontaneous pneumothorax is twofold[8]: (1) to suppress the air leak, that is, to treat the lesion through which air escapes from the lung into the pleural cavity, and (2) to achieve the most perfect symphysis possible between the two sides of the pleura (parietal and visceral) in such a way that the pleural cavity disappears, and to eliminate any possibility of recurrence of the pneumothorax.

The first of these goals can be achieved by extirpation of the lesion causing the pneumothorax. Until we began using staplers, we employed a technique based on extirpation of the emergent cupulae of the blebs that were found during suturing of the parenchymal base with loose stitches of polyglycolic acid 000. For large bullae, lung suturing is performed after opening and exeresis of the emergent cupula. When treating these lesions, one must preserve the parenchyma during resectioning. The reason for this is that in young patients with pneumothorax, extirpation of small apical blebs is sufficient, and in older patients pneumothorax occurs in dystrophic lungs. These patients have poor functional respiratory reserve, which is why preservation of the parenchyma during exeresis is critical. Thus exeresis in these cases may be suitable only when a lesion has destroyed the parenchyma of an entire segment or lobe, making recovery impossible.

Since 1980 we have treated these lesions with staple sutures. Concerning the presence of air leaks and residual chambers—complications inherent in this kind of surgery—we have found important differences compared with the anterior technique, as well as a considerable decrease in the duration of the leaks and persistence of the chambers. They probably would have been larger if we had continued to use exeresis and manual sutures. The stapler is simple to operate, which shortens the duration of the operation and implies a shorter hospital stay.

CONCLUSION

Before concluding this report, we must mention thoracoscopic surgery. With the advent of new developments in the treatment of spontaneous pneumothorax, conventional surgery is no longer used. The reason for this lies in the development of proper instrumentation with endoscopic clips and staplers, as well as the possibility of electrocoagulation and photocoagulation with the Nd:YAG laser,[9] which offers guarantees similar to those of open surgery. This type of surgery has been performed on our service for 1 year, and we no longer use thoracotomy as a means of access to the pleural cavity.

REFERENCES

1. Amosov NM, Berezosky KK. Pulmonary resection with mechanical suture. J Thorac Cardiovasc Surg 41:325-328, 1961.
2. Andronov PI. New instruments for thoracic surgery. Dis Chest 44:550, 1963.
3. Smith RN, Faraci RP, Aubrey H. Bronchial stump closure techniques following pneumectomy. A serial comparative study. Ann Surg 116:206-211, 1976.
4. Steichen FM, Ravitch MM. Stapling in Surgery. Chicago: Year Book Medical Publishers, 1984.
5. Myers JA. Simple spontaneous pneumothorax. Dis Chest 26:420, 1954.
6. Baronofsky ID, Warden HG, Kaufman JL, et al. Bilateral therapy of unilateral spontaneous pneumothorax. J Thorac Cardiovasc Surg 34:310-315, 1957.
7. Kalnins I, Torda TA, Wright JS. Bilateral simultaneous pleurodesis by median sternotomy for spontaneous pneumothorax. Ann Thorac Surg 15:202-208, 1973.
8. Loscertales AJ. Neumotórax espontáneo. Monografía Ed. Elba S.A. Madrid, 1988.
9. Torre M, Belloni P. Nd:YAG laser pleurodesis through thoracoscopy: New curative therapy in spontaneous pneumothorax. Ann Thorac Surg 47:887-889, 1989.

Endoscopic Treatment of Empyema

Paul Damien Ridley

Pus in the chest, like murder, will out. Sometimes it outs out-wards (empyema necessitatis) and sometimes it outs inwards (bronchopleural fistula). Never let the sun go down on pus in the chest.

Russell Brock, c. 1950

Improved antibiotic treatment has resulted in a reduction in the incidence of empyema thoracis[1] and an alteration in the responsible pathogens.[2-4] However empyema thoracis remains a condition with a significant morbidity and mortality.[5] Although antibiotics are effective in treating pneumonia and have therefore reduced the incidence of empyema, their value in established nontuberculous empyema with frank pus in the pleural cavity is unproven.[3] In complex empyemas such as those associated with esophageal rupture and mediastinitis antibiotics are required. Early, adequate, dependent drainage with subsequent sterilization of the pleural cavity remains the essential principle in successful management. Reexpansion of the lung reduces the size of the empyema space, improves chances of resolution and is desirable.[6]

It is advisable for all cases of empyema to be referred to a thoracic surgeon at an early stage.[4] Patients with pleural effusions are usually referred to chest physicians. Therefore empyema is usually treated initially by multiple transthoracic aspirations or closed (underwater seal) drainage. In some cases this management results in successful resolution; however, these measures often prove inadequate and delays definitive treatment.

The wide variety of surgical approaches that have been advocated testifies to the persistent challenge presented by this condition. These approaches include rib resection and open drainage,[5,7] open window thoracostomy,[8,9] decortication,[10] thoracoplasty,[11,12] intrathoracic muscle transposition,[13] and cyclical irrigation.[14] Thoracoscopy with[15] or without[16] cyclical irrigation of the thoracic cavity has also been described in the management of empyema thoracis. All these techniques aim to drain pus, sterilize the thoracic cavity, or reduce the size of the empyema cavity by filling the cavity (with muscle or expanded underlying lung) or collapsing it by resection of ribs.

THORACOSCOPY: A MINIMALLY INVASIVE TECHNIQUE

The thoracoscope provides an opportunity to perform minimally invasive surgery. It is increasing in popularity and being employed in an expanding role.[17] The thoracoscope was originally described by Jacobaeus more than 80 years ago[17,18] but was little used until the early 1970s,[20] when it was generally limited to a diagnostic role. In recent years there has been renewed interest in therapeutic thoracoscopy in the management of other pathological conditions of the pleura[21,22] and the lung parenchyma.[23]

Thoracoscopy is usually performed with the patient under general anesthesia. The patient is placed into the appropriate lateral decubitus position. A double-lumen endotracheal tube allows the lung on the affected side to be collapsed, improving visualization of the empyema cavity. It is not necessary to insufflate gas into the pleural cavity; tension in the pleural cavity impairs cardiac function. For the same reason sealed ports used in laparoscopy are not necessary when performing thoracoscopy. Inflating the cuff around the endobronchial tube to the good lung is important to avoid spillage from the empyema cavity in the event of a bronchopleural fistula. It is useful to insert a Saugmann's needle (GU Instruments) into the empyema cavity to determine its extent and locate the most dependent site where the lung is displaced from the chest wall and unlikely to be damaged by instrumentation; typically the fifth or sixth intercostal space in the posterior axillary line represents this point. A number of excellent thoracoscopes are available. It has been our practice to employ a standard laparoscope/thoracoscope (Jacobs-Palmer Fibre Light Operating Laparoscope FW4937-V; Wolf).[24] The large bore of this instrument allows better debridement. Its superior lighting and field of view and its offset parallel eyepiece allows easier manipulation of the biopsy forceps and aspiration handles.

Advantages of Thoracoscopy

Thoracoscopy allows removal of foreign bodies, biopsy, assessment of lung expansibility, debridement, accurate drain placement, and postoperative irrigation.

Thoracoscopy may reveal previously unsuspected underlying etiologies for empyema. In an early description of the merits of thoracoscopy in the management of empyema, Weissberg[16] described a patient in whom thoracoscopy revealed a surgical sponge (35 × 35 cm) that had been left in the pleural cavity during a coronary artery bypass operation (performed at another institution) 2 years earlier. It was possible to remove the foreign body with the thoracoscope, resulting in complete resolution of the empyema. In a second patient, Weissberg describes thoracoscopic identification of pus and undigested food particles in the right pleural cavity and the diagnosis of a previously unrecognized perforation of a malignant tumor of the lower esophagus.

Thoracoscopic biopsy has been shown to be an effective method of diagnosing malignancy, which reduces the need for formal diagnostic thoracotomy.[25] The etiology of empyema is frequently in doubt, particularly in patients who are debilitated and unable to give a clear history. Thoracoscopy allows routine multiple pleural biopsies under direct vision to be taken in all patients with empyema. Such biopsy specimens are larger and more accurate than those obtained by blind percutaneous pleural biopsy; thus the chances of overlooking an underlying malignancy such as mesothelioma or advanced lung malignancy are reduced.

The chronicity of the empyema is reflected in the expansibility of the underlying lung. Empyema classically commences as infection of a low viscosity pleural effusion with an underlying lung that is fully expansile. Subsequently the fluid becomes more turbid, and a thin layer of fibrin starts to cover the lung and pleural surface. Further organization occurs as fibroblasts and capillaries invade the fibrin peel covering the lung and pleural surfaces. Eventually a thick, fibrous-walled cavity containing viscous pus is produced, and expansion of the underlying lung is extremely limited. This process typically takes place over a period of 6 weeks. The transition from a thin-walled, fibrin-covered cavity containing thin, infected pleural effusion to a thick, fibrous-walled cavity containing viscous pus represents a spectrum of pathological conditions. The patient may be seen at any stage of this evolution.

The expansibility of the underlying lung may be assessed at thoracoscopy. Thus some indication of further management requirements may be obtained. These findings may alter treatment, distinguishing patients with early empyema that is likely to resolve with thoracoscopic debridement and tube drainage[15,17] from those with late empyema and a nonexpansile lung that might benefit from decortication.

Thoracoscopy allows full debridement (and thus adequate drainage), because with the tip of the instrument and long-handled forceps, loculi of pus and adhesions can be broken down under direct vision. The empyema cavity can be repeatedly washed out with warm saline during the procedure. Full debridement is possible because of the wide bore of the thoracoscope cannula, any debris becoming lodged in the cannula being readily removed with long-handled forceps.

Accurate drain placement, impossible to determine by x-ray evaluation alone, can be ensured as drains are positioned under direct vision. Thus dependent drainage can be ensured. If postoperative pleural irrigation[15] is employed, an apical 12 Fr Argyle drain can be placed under direct vision to infuse irrigation fluid; then the thoracoscope is replaced with a 32 Fr Argyle drain, at or near the base of the empyema cavity, that fits the hole made by the thoracoscope trocar without fluid or pus leaking around it. Sideholes cut in this basal chest tube allow drainage over a 15 cm length of tube, with the lowest hole 2.5 cm inside the parietal pleura. The advantage of the Argyle drain is that at 37° C it is supple and is tolerated intercostally for weeks if necessary. Early rib resection, mandatory with stiffer tubing, becomes unnecessary. If open drainage subsequently becomes necessary, this can sometimes be achieved simply by shortening the basal drain without rib resection.

The technique of repeated irrigation ensures that the basal drain is effectively dependent. Thoracoscopy combined with cyclical irrigation should be considered a success only if complete resolution is obtained by this technique alone. Rapid symptomatic improvement is obtained by removal of pus and infected material so that the patient is better able to withstand subsequent surgical interventions. This is particularly obvious when a bronchopleural fistula is present. A bronchopleural fistula would make complete resolution with thoracoscopic debridement and pleural irrigation very unlikely. However, the patient is rapidly rendered less toxic and better able to withstand subsequent surgical intervention.

Early thoracoscopy should be considered in patients

presenting with empyema thoracis. Thorough debridement with rapid removal of pus results in rapid resolution of the patient's toxicity and accurate dependent drainage is possible under direct vision. It is a relatively atraumatic procedure that, with modern anesthesia, is well tolerated even in severely debilitated patients. It allows easy determination of lung expansibility and a search for factors underlying the condition. Subsequent surgical procedures are not precluded by this relatively atraumatic technique, and it is hoped that the relatively noninvasive nature of the surgery involved will encourage physicians to refer cases of empyema thoracis directly to a thoracic surgeon.

REFERENCES

1. Elving G. A comparison of the frequency of lung abscess, pneumonia, acute bronchitis and acute pleural empyema. Acta Chir Scand 107:454-455, 1954.
2. Bartlett J, Gorgach S, Thadepalli H, Finegold S. Bacteriology of empyema. Lancet 1:338-340, 1974.
3. Neild J, Eykyn S, Phillips I. Lung abscess and empyema. Q J Med 57(224):875-882, 1985.
4. Smith J, Mullerworth M, Westlake G, Tatoulis J. Empyema thoracis: 14-year experience in a teaching center. Ann Thorac Surg 51:34-38, 1991.
5. Lemmer J, Botham M, Orringer M. Modern management of adult thoracic empyema. J Thorac Cardiovasc Surg 90:849-855, 1985.
6. Clagett OT GJ. A procedure for the management of adult thoracic empyema. J Thorac Cardiovasc Surg 90:849-855, 1985.
7. Ridley P, Myers C. Braimbridge M. Empyema thoracis. Prof Nurs Nov:73-76, 1989.
8. Bayes A, Wilson J, Chiu R, Errett L, Hedderich G, Munro D. Clagett open-window thoracostomy in patients with empyema who had and had not undergone pneumonectomy. Can J Surg 30:329-331, 1987.
9. Cicer R, del Velcchio C, Porter J, Carreno J. Open window thoracostomy and plastic surgery with muscle flaps in the treatment of empyema thoracis. Chest 89:374-377, 1986.
10. Hoover E, Hsu H, Ross M, Gross A, Webb H, Ketosugbo A, Finch P. Reappraisal of empyema thoracis surgical intervention when the duration of illness is unknown. Chest 90:511-515, 1986.
11. Gregoire R, Deslauriers J, Beaulieu M, Piaux M. Thoracoplasty: Its forgotten role in the management of non-tuberculous postpneumonectomy empyema. Can J Surg 30:343-345, 1987.
12. Sarkar S, Sharma T, Singh H, Singh A, Purohit S, Sharma V. Thoracoplasty with intercostal myoplasty for closure of an empyema cavity and bronchopleural fistula. Int Surg 70:219-221, 1985.
13. Pairolero P, Arnold P, Trastek V, Meland N, Kay P. Postpneumonectomy empyema: The role of intrathoracic muscle transposition. J Thorac Cardiovasc Surg 99:958-968, 1990.
14. Rosenfeldt F, McGibney D, Braimbridge M, Watson D. Comparison between irrigation and conventional treatment for empyema and pneumonectomy space infection. Thorax 36:272-277, 1981.
15. Ridley P, Braimbridge M. Thoracoscopic debridement and pleural irrigation in the management of empyema thoracis. Ann Thorac Surg 51:461-464, 1991.
16. Weissberg D. Pleuroscopy in empyema: Is it ever necessary? Poumon-Coeur 37:269-272, 1981.
17. Jacobaeus H. Ueber die Möglichkeit die Zystoskopie bei Untersuchung seroser Hohlungen anzuwenden. Munchen Med Wochenscher 57:2090-2092, 1910.
18. Jacobaeus H. Endopleurale Operationen unter der Leitung des Thorakoskops. Beitr Klin Tuberk 35:1-35, 1915.
19. Miller J, Hatcher CJ. Thoracoscopy: A useful tool in the diagnosis of thoracic disease. Ann Thorac Surg 26:68-72, 1978.
20. Daniel T, Tribble C, Rodgers B. Thoracoscopy and talc poudrage for pneumothoraces and effusions. Ann Thorac Surg 50:186-189, 1990.
21. Wakabayashi A, Brenner M, Wilson A, Tadir Y, Berns M. Thoracoscopic treatment of spontaneous pneumothorax using carbon dioxide laser. Ann Thorac Surg 50:786-790, 1990.
22. Landreneau R, Herlan D, Johnson J, Boley T, Nawarawong W, Ferson P. Thoracoscopic neodynium-aluminum garnet laser–assisted pulmonary resection. Ann Thorac Surg 52:1176-1178, 1991.
23. Wakabayashi A. Expanded application of diagnostic and therapeutic thoracoscopy. J Thorac Cardiovasc Surg 102:721-723, 1991.
24. Sang C, Braimbridge M. Thoracoscopy simplified using the laparoscope. Thorac Cardiovasc Surg 29:129-130, 1981.
25. Hucker J, Bhatnagar N, Al-Jilaihawi A, Forrester-Wood C. Thoracoscopy in the diagnosis and management of recurrent pleural effusions. Ann Thorac Surg 52:1145-1147, 1991.

129 Challenges in Thoracoscopic Diagnosis and Treatment of Lung Nodules

Renato De Angelis, Paolo Tabbi, Paolo Aurello, Francesco D'Angelo, Stefano Valabrega, Giuseppe Pozzi, and Gianfranco Fegiz

The renewed interest in minimally invasive surgery through modern videoendoscopic techniques has expanded the field of long-established thorascopy or pleuroscopy methods in thoracic operations. The aim of this new technique is to reduce operative trauma and the cost of health care.[1] The advantages are evident in the field of thoracic surgery, especially in patients with poor pulmonary function or severe cardiovascular disease. The new instrumentation and the increased experience of surgeons make this approach to many thoracic diseases possible. Among these diseases, the treatment of lung nodules represents one of the main challenges. Resecting a pulmonary nodule by operative thoracoscopy makes possible a definitive diagnosis and perhaps even treatment of the disease.[2]

MATERIALS AND METHODS

We present a consecutive series of seven patients with nine nodules observed and treated in the First Department of Surgery of the University ("La Sapienza") of Rome from October 1991 to July 1992. Table 1 lists the patients' age, sex, definitive pathology reports, modality of identification, and operative procedure undertaken.

RESULTS

All patients except case No. 1 were scheduled for operation with no definite preoperative diagnosis and were classified as having a coin lesion. Patient No. 1, previously operated on for tibial osteogenic sarcoma, presented with multiple (three) bilateral metastases and was scheduled for operative thoracoscopy to avoid having to undertake a median sternotomy approach or a staged bilateral thoracotomy.

Resection of the nodules was carried out in all patients. In two cases (Nos. 6 and 7), a minimal thoracotomy was necessary for nodule identification and removal.

Definitive pathological diagnosis confirmed three metastatic lesions in patient No. 1 and one in patient No. 7. Benign lung lesions were found in all the other cases.

The lung nodules were identified by running instruments over the surface of the lung to feel the nodule indirectly beneath the pleural surface or by placing a finger through the trocar site to palpate the lung directly. In the final two patients we started a protocol of nodule identification consisting of preoperative comput-

Table 1. Patient demographic data

Patient No.	Age	Sex	Pathology	Identification	Procedure
1	16	M	Bilateral metastases (3)	Visual	Closed exeresis and stapling
2	22	M	Fibrosis	Visual	Closed exeresis and stapling
3	40	M	Chondroma	Visual	Closed exeresis and stapling
4	41	F	Mesothelioma	Wire guide	Closed exeresis and stapling
5	68	M	Chondroma	Wire guide	Closed exeresis and stapling
6	64	M	Fibrosis	Visual	Thoracotomy
7	66	F	Metastases	Wire guide	Thoracotomy

ed tomography (CT) scan–assisted positioning of a percutaneous hook wire into the lesion.

No morbidity was associated with the various procedures.

The median postoperative inpatient stay was 4 days (range, 3 to 6 days) for patients who underwent operative thoracoscopy.

DISCUSSION

The diagnosis and treatment of pulmonary nodules by operative thoracoscopy is a valid concept. The degree of success still depends on two factors: nodule identification and use of appropriate instruments.

Nodule identification. Nodule identification is always difficult except when the lesion is visible on the pleural surface. The search for deeper seated lesions can lead to unacceptably prolonged operative times and the need for conversion to open operations. In our series, patients Nos. 6 and 7 were converted to thoracotomy because it was impossible to identify the nodule by videoendoscopy.

In July 1992 we began a protocol of preoperative nodule localization with CT scan–assisted percutaneous positioning of a hook wire into the lesion.[2,3] Patients 4 and 5 were operated on after the hook-wire positioning, resulting in easy nodule identification and a quicker procedure. Furthermore, the wire guide allows the surgeon to choose the best place for trocar insertion and can be used as a supplementary tool for traction.

Instrumentation. In our experience, thoracoscopic instrumentation still must be perfected. Major problems are related to the absence of instruments specifically adapted to thoracoscopy. Stapling instruments must be adapted to and refined for intrathoracic use. The EndoGIA stapler is not always easy to place at the required angle or onto thick lung tissue and a rotating stapling device could be of great help.

Although our experience is limited to a small number of cases to date, we think that the treatment of lung nodules by operative thoracoscopy could compete with the open thoracotomy procedure in terms of reduced surgical trauma, shorter postoperative in-hospital stay, accelerated recovery, and reduction of health care cost.

Videoendoscopic intrathoracic techniques in association with adjuvant techniques such as wire-guided CT scan localization could permit thoracoscopy to become the approach of choice in diagnosis and treatment of benign and metastatic lung nodules.

REFERENCES

1. De Angelis R, D'Angelo F, Aurello P, et al. La toracoscopia operativa in oncologia toracica. Inc Oncol Chir 4:3-6, 1991.
2. De Angelis R, Tabbi P, Aurello P, et al. La video-toracoscopia attualita' e prospettive. Presented at the 94th Congresso della Societa' Italiana di Chirurgia, Oct. 25-29, 1992.
3. Mack MJ, Gordon MJ, Postma TW, et al. Percutaneous localization of pulmonary nodules for thoracoscopic lung resection. Ann Thorac Surg 53:1123-1124, 1992.

130 *Limited Resection in the Surgical Treatment of Lung Cancer*

J. Borelly, F. Martin, G. Grosdidier, and T. Routiot

Surgery remains the most basic of all therapies for lung cancer and at present offers almost the only chance of extending survival time for the patient. In opposition to the concept of removing a maximal amount of tissue is the minimalist attitude represented by limited resections. These procedures reduce the functional cardiorespiratory limitations that follow anatomically regulated operations such as pneumonectomy, lobectomy, or bilobectomy, and often preclude such operations if severe cardiopulmonary conditions exist before operation. Limited or tissue-sparing pulmonary resections offer a chance of survival to such patients if the TNM staging is favorable to a more localized excision (T1 N0 M0).

The study, from 1969 to 1991, of 70 patients on whom a limited pulmonary resection was performed, allows judgment of the value of this approach.

MATERIALS AND METHODS

Seventy limited pulmonary resections were performed in our series. The average age of the patients, 66 men and 4 women, was 56.3 years (range, 24 to 76). These procedures were distributed as follows: 65 typical or anatomically regulated resections (32 segmentectomies, 15 bisegmentectomies, and 6 lingulectomies with 16 associated radical hilar node dissections) and 17 atypical or tissue-sparing resections in which we removed the tumor with a healthy parenchymal tissue margin, without taking into consideration any lymphatic node dissection.

Data from the preoperative functional respiratory examinations in 40 patients contraindicated a large pulmonary resection for seven of these patients. Each patient was given the benefit of a complete clinical preoperative examination; data from the imaging investigations allowed us to eliminate any patients with preoperative metastatic dissemination.

The procedure frequently was performed using selective tracheal intubation through a posterolateral or lateral thoracostomy, with or without rib resection. The decision to do an anatomical resection or an atypical resection was made based on the site of the tumor, ganglionic invasion macroscopically suspected, and the extent of intrathoracic involvement of the lesion.

The atypical resections were done in a cuneiform mode with two applications of TA30, TA55, or TA90 staplers or sometimes with a single application of forceps for a tangential wedge. The typical resections followed the conventional thoracic surgery rules.

RESULTS

The pathological study of the 70 tumors revealed that 41 were epidermoid cancers, 20 were adenocarcinomas, three were unclassified carcinomas, two were anaplastic cancers with small cells, two were bronchioalveolar cancers, and two were malignant carcinoids. For five patients with epidermoid cancer, the presence of a previous epidermoid (ENT) cancer (four cases), and of a previous keratinizing urothelial cancer of the bladder (one case) did not allow us to confirm with complete certainty the primary character of the pulmonary lesion.

According to the topography of the tumor/node/metastasis (TNM) classification system, our 70 observations included 39 T1, 25 T2, and six T3 classifications. Fifty-eight patients had no ganglionic invasion (N0), with the remaining 12 patients classified as follows: nine N1, two N2, and one N3. Hepatic metastasis discovered during the autopsy of a patient operated on in 1969 allows classification of only 87 of 88 patients as M0.

The early postoperative mortality was 4.3% (three cases, two caused by pneumopathies with severe hypoxia and one by myocardial infarction). These three deaths happened among the group of patients who had undergone the 53 anatomical segmentations (6%). No death was reported in our patient group of 17 atypical resections.

The postoperative morbidity was 20% (14 cases). The

postoperative complications (without counting mortality) are given in the list below:

Postoperative Mortality

Tracheobronchial congestion	5
Pneumopathies, infectious syndrome	3
Hematoma, postoperative hemorrhage	2
Pneumothorax	1
Cardiac problems	1
Infected hematoma	1
Phlebitis	1

In reality, we accept as specific morbidity of these limited resections only the two postoperative hemorrhagic complications and the pulmonary abscess complicating a hematoma on the edge of resection.

We observed incomplete tumor margins in 4 of the 53 anatomically regulated resections (7.6%). The bronchial line of section on the specimen was positive in 3 cases of the 53 (5.6%). A local recurrence was reported in eight cases of 67 (12%), happening after an average delay of 20.1 months (range, 1 month for an unclassified carcinoma, histologically T3 N0, to 66 months for an adenocarcinoma, T1 N0).

The global survival rate to 2 years was 64.8% (35/54); to 5 years, 44.2% (19/43); and to 10 years, 25% (8/32), with three patients surviving in excess of 15 years (two at 17 years, including one N+, and one at 16 years N0). For the 35 patients classified T1 N0, the survival rate to 2 years is 78.5% and to 5 years is 51%.

DISCUSSION

The advantages of anatomically reduced and of atypical limited resections are to offer the possibility of a curative attempt for patients with limited operability levels by reason of age, tumor location, and cardiopulmonary function. This technique provides a chance of survival in the best condition to a greater number of patients.

The problem of the limited resections has been pondered for more than 10 years. In 1992 the North American Lung Cancer Study Group was not able to reach any conclusion despite a random study including more than 400 patients. No formal argument was presented in terms of survival in favor of the limited resections compared with lobectomies for the treatment of peripheral bronchiogenic cancers, T1 N0.

The type of observed lesions, the opposed therapies for tumors, and our own diversified statistics do not pretend to allow formal conclusions but give rise to a certain number of speculations. The analysis of these series shows a difference in mortality and morbidity between the atypical resections for which the numbers are fewer and the anatomically regulated resections, which are more difficult and delicate, especially if they are associated with a ganglionic dissection. In our own study we did not have any deaths resulting from atypical resection. The three deaths in our study followed regulated segmentectomies, but we cannot arrive at a formal statistical conclusion.

Many criteria are important in deciding whether to perform a limited tissue-sparing resection. In contrast to other series we did not allow the high age of patients (>70 years old) or the limited preoperative functional explorations to determine whether we would use this procedure. For these patients, our results were comparable with those of the large resections in terms of mortality, morbidity, and survival.

Because of the heterogeneity of the patients and the long period of study, the decision for a regulated or atypical resection was often taken only on perioperative verification. For the same reason, the indication for secondary treatment is difficult to systematize. We used radiotherapy as a therapeutic complement in only nine cases. Theoretically, the use of secondary radiation was justifiable for all the patients with parietal or ganglionic extension (N2, N3, and some distal N1) or with a positive bronchial margin.

One of the major arguments against limited resections is that they are carcinologically incomplete and therefore they favor local recurrence (10% to 27% of the local recurrence results from insufficient resection of peritumoral lymphatic tissue and from the persistent presence of neoplastic vascular microemboli). We reported 8 local recurrences in 67 patients (12%). We analyzed the following factors to determine how they affected local recurrence, and they do not seem to have influenced recurrence significantly:

- Histology: 18.1% of the epidermoid epitheliomas, 19.4% of the adenocarcinomas, and 23.1% of the unclassified anaplastic cancers (which represented no more than two cases in nine) recurred locally.
- Ganglionic invasion: Of eight recurrences, we count seven N0 and one N1.
- Incomplete tumor margins were observed in four patients. Only two patients of these had a local recurrence (25%). These patients were not systematically the object of adjuvant treatment.

We cannot connect in a statistically significant way the positive bronchial margins and the local recurrence.

Only one patient in three with a positive margin presented a local recurrence, but it was a T3 lesion (with parietal extension).

The most important factor in the incidence of a local recurrence, apparently, is the size of the tumor. Indeed, one T1 in 39 (only 2.5%) compared to five T2 in 25 (20%) and two T3 in six (33%) locally recurred.

These local recurrences were particularly serious. For patients having a local recurrence, the global survival time is 21.4 months. When the local recurrence is diagnosed, the average survival time is only 4.1 months (range, 1 to 11 months). Finally, these local recurrences led to resection in four patients (50%). Two of them died following a pneumonectomy.

CONCLUSION

When can we proceed with a limited resection? Mainly, the tumor must be peripherally located beyond the bronchial division on the bronchial tree. The local area must be conducive to tumor removal.

Classically, these procedures do not apply to the anaplastic forms of cancer, but the histological diagnosis of such a form is not always done preoperatively. One of our three patients who were anaplastic, operated on by "mistake," is still alive 80 months after posterior segmentectomy of the right superior lobe!

These limited procedures must be proposed to the patients for whom the respiratory functional state contraindicates larger resections. Review of the literature shows that in these "insufficient respiratory patients" the risk and consequences of such procedures do not jeopardize the quality of a good survival.

Finally, and this is perhaps the essential point, the surgeon who practices these procedures must be ready to offer to his or her patient a real chance of survival. These small lesions require, of necessity, close and regular long-term supervision.

131 *Videothoracoscopic Pulmonary Lobectomies for Cancer*

Giancarlo Roviaro, Carlo Rebuffat, Federico Varoli, Contardo Vergani,
Marco Maciocco, Fabrizio Grignani, Silvio Marco Scalambra, and
Claudio Mariani

Major pulmonary resections are usually carried out through ample thoracotomies. However, extensive section of muscles and even the removal of a rib usually result in significant postoperative pain that is sometimes protracted for a few months, with functional impairment and poor cosmetic results. The recent development of miniature cameras has allowed perfection and greater use of surgical videoendoscopic techniques. Widely employed in abdominal surgery,[1,2] such sophisticated technology has been applied in thoracic surgery only for atypical pulmonary exeresis or for treatment of pneumothorax.[3] Careful training in endoscopic surgery and a vast experience with over 2500 cases in open chest operations led us to apply operative videothoracoscopy to performing classic lobectomies in selected cases.[4,5] In this paper we report our preliminary results. (Our paper here is after the series reported in references 4 and 5.)

MATERIALS AND METHODS

We decided to try videoendoscopic pulmonary lobectomies in patients with benign pulmonary disease, lung metastasis requiring pulmonary lobectomies, and primary lung neoplasm at the T1, N0, M0 stage. In the Department of General Surgery, University of Milan–S. Giuseppe Hospital, from September 1991 through July 1992, we performed nine pulmonary lobectomies and one anatomically regulated segmentectomy. Four patients had benign disease, five patients were suffering from primary lung malignancies, and one from lung metastasis. Their average age was 53 years (range, 20 to 74 years). All patients underwent preoperative chest x-ray evaluation and CT scanning to assess the exact location and anatomical relationship of the lesion. They also underwent routine bronchoscopy. A patient with recurrent hemoptysis also had a selective transfemoral arteriography, which demonstrated the presence and location of an arteriovenous fistula. Patients with lung malignancies followed routine staging evaluation.

TECHNIQUE

Once intubated with a double-lumen Carlens tube, all patients are positioned in the lateral decubitus position, as for a classic posterolateral thoracotomy. The table is set to provide adequate lateral flexion of the truncus. Thoracoscopic maneuvers are facilitated by the presence of a double video system, which allows optimal visualization for all members of the surgical team.

The video camera is always inserted through a 10 mm trocar positioned in the midaxillary line and the seventh intercostal space to permit suitable exploration of the pleural cavity. The introduction of the first trocar produces a pneumothorax, thus permitting lung collapse, which is further facilitated by ventilatory exclusion of the selected lung by means of the Carlens tube. Two or three other 10 mm trocars are then inserted into the fifth intercostal space on the anterior and posterior axillary line. Pleural adhesions may be lysed with endoscopic scissors.

At the very beginning of the intervention in all patients, a 3 to 4 cm inframammary incision, which we call a "utility thoracotomy," is carried out (Fig. 1). This is necessary for extraction of the specimen and allows insertion of battle-proven surgical chest instruments not available in endoscopic version and perhaps not needed in a new version, because the utility incision is wide enough to permit comfortable intrathoracic placement. Videothoracoscopic lobectomy follows the same steps as an open operation (Figs. 2 through 4). After careful

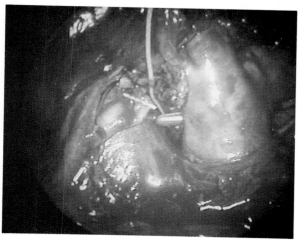

Fig. 2. Isolation of the major pulmonary artery. Once isolated, the artery is encircled with a thread using a roticulator forceps as a ligature carrier. Gentle traction on the thread greatly facilitates the positioning of the endoscopic stapler.

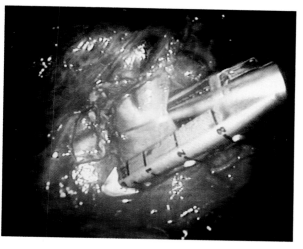

Fig. 3. The artery, isolated and encircled, is secured with an EndoGIA. Positioning of the stapler may be difficult, and sometimes it is necessary to change to another trocar site to find the best direction for controlling the procedure.

Utility
thoracotomy
site

Fig. 1. Position of the trocars and the site of the utility thoracotomy along the inframammary fold.

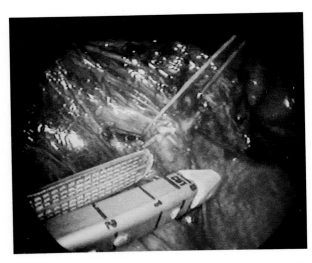

Fig. 4. With a technique similar to that for the vessels, the bronchus is isolated, encircled, and stapled.

exploration of the pleural cavity and mediastinum, all lobar and/or segmental vessels are isolated and divided with the vascular EndoGIA. The bronchus corresponding to the lobe or segment is similarly closed and divided with an EndoGIA stapler.

The specimen is inserted in a plastic bag to facilitate its extraction, thus preventing tumor spoiling. The cavity is washed and a chest drain is positioned to conclude the operation.

RESULTS

Of 14 patients with lobar lesions who underwent videothoracoscopy, a pulmonary lobectomy was carried out in 10 patients by this method. They consisted of three right lower lobectomies (two squamous cell cancers and one adenocarcinoma of the lung), two left lower lobectomies (one for arteriovenous fistula, one for renal clear cell carcinoma metastasis, and two for bronchiectasis) and one superior segmentectomy of the right lower lobe for squamous cell cancer.

In four cases conversion to an open procedure was necessary (28.5%): in one patient, during a right upper lobectomy, after having isolated the superior division of the right pulmonary artery and the pulmonary vein from the upper lobe, displacement of the Carlens tube and irreversible reinflation of the lung prevented isolation of the segmental branches and securing of the

posterior ascending artery. In another case of left upper lobectomy, an incomplete fissure precluded isolation of the pulmonary artery even though the superior pulmonary vein had already been secured with an EndoGIA. In the third case (left upper lobectomy), the left pulmonary artery was accidentally injured during dissection in the fissure. In the fourth case (right upper lobectomy), dissection of the posterior ascending artery was impossible because of an incomplete fissure.

The average time of endoscopic operations was 205 minutes (range, 150 to 240 minutes). In these cases the average postoperative hospital stay was 11 days (range, 4 to 18 days). All the thoracoscopically treated patients had uneventful postoperative courses with little pain and rapid functional recovery. Furthermore, the minimal incision always healed with excellent cosmetic results. No operative or postoperative death occurred in the 10 patients who underwent pulmonary lobectomy.

DISCUSSION

Traditional thoracotomy offers excellent exposure of the thoracic cavity and guarantees good control of hilar structures; nevertheless, it necessitates long incisions as well as large division of muscle and spreading of the ribs, which is often complicated by fractures. Postoperative pain added to pulmonary parenchymal resection limits respiratory function, which is often already severely compromised in elderly patients, who therefore cannot tolerate thoracotomy and resection. However, even in the absence of functional problems, wide thoracotomies imply severe and protracted pain and greatly reduced respiratory movements and leave unsightly scars.

The application of minimally invasive technology in thoracic surgery has recently brought about new perspectives in the treatment of pulmonary lesions. Notwithstanding the lack of stereoscopic vision and a global view of the entire field in close-up shots, the highly sophisticated cameras and monitors provide excellent quality of definition and magnification. The recent development of endoscopic devices such as endoclips and the EndoGIA allow the surgeon to safely secure large vessels, pulmonary parenchyma, and bronchi.

To date, videoendoscopic pulmonary surgery has been limited to removal of bullae or to wedge resection of peripheral lesions. To our knowledge, no major pulmonary resections (segmentectomies, pneumonectomies, or lobectomies) have been reported in the literature as of this writing. Our first 10 videoendoscopic lobectomies allow evaluation of the various problems related to this innovative technique.

Major problems include (1) diffuse pleural adhesions, (2) incomplete fissure, (3) the possibility of emergency conversion to thoracotomy in case of vascular accident, and (4) lymphadenectomy in case of malignancy. Usually, limited pleural adhesions are easily sectioned and cauterized; diffuse pleural adhesions can prevent lung collapse and prevent introduction of the camera and instruments. An incomplete or thick fissure also constitutes a major problem, since it hinders the identification of lobar arteries, thus making their isolation and safe control difficult. In addition, rigidity of the ribs and restricted intercostal spaces highly limit movements of the long, rectilinear, nonflexible endoscopic instrumentation specifically designed for laparoscopic surgery.

In our resections we have also used conventional instruments, usually inserted through the utility thoracotomy, which is necessary anyway for extraction of the specimen. New endoscopic dissectors, nontraumatic clamps, various mounted swabs, and, above all, endoscopic staplers slender enough to slip under the intrafissural arteries and long enough to ensure easy completion of the fissures are now indispensable. Probably, the development of endoscopic dissecting clamps and endostaplers with different sizes and adjustable curvatures would render dissection of the arteries of the anterior segment of the upper left lobe technically possible. These are in fact too short to be isolated for a sufficient length and divided with present instruments. In case of vascular accident this is not controllable endoscopically,

a clamp may be inserted through the utility thoracotomy, which also allows rapid extension into an emergency thoracotomy if the need arises.

In the present series, all patients with malignancies had T1, N0, M0 neoplasms; nevertheless, lymphadenectomy may be performed in cases of malignant hilar lymphadenopathy by a videoendoscopic thoracic approach.

The development of specialized thoracoscopy devices would permit surgeons to overcome most current problems. This will probably make way for further progress in this technique, which still remains an avant garde procedure. Nevertheless, marked reduction of functional impairment, minimal surgical trauma, and consequently little postoperative pain, with ready resumption of normal activity, make it a concrete opportunity for treatment.

REFERENCES

1. Olsen DO. Laparoscopic cholecystectomy. Am J Surg 161:399-444, 1991.
2. Zucker KA. Surgical Laparoscopy. St. Louis: Quality Medical Publishing, Inc, 1991.
3. Nathanson LK, Shimi SM, Wood AB, Cuschieri A. Videothoracoscopic ligation of bullae and pleurectomy for spontaneous pneumothorax. Ann Thorac Surg 52:316-319, 1991.
4. Roviaro GC, Rebuffat C, Varoli F, Vergani C, Mariani C, Maciocco M. Videoendoscopic pulmonary lobectomy for cancer. Surg Laparosc Endosc (in press).
5. Roviaro GC, Rebuffat C, Varoli F, Vergani C, Maciocco M, Grignani F, Scalambra SM, Mariani C, Pezzuoli G. Videoendoscopic thoracic surgery. Int Coll Surg (in press).

132   Results of Mechanical Suture in Thoracic Surgery: Thirteen Years' Experience

Jesús Loscertales, Francisco J. Ayarra, Rafael Jimenez-Merchan,
Fernando Jose Garcia-Diaz, Carlos J. Arenas-Linares, Jose M. Cuaresma-Ferrete,
Antonio Rico-Alvarez, and Juan Carlos Giron-Arjona

Because one of the gravest and most frequent complications in thoracic surgery is leakage from the bronchial stump, with the development of a bronchopleural fistula, staples have become a very desirable substitute to manual sutures for bronchial stump closure.

In 1942 Rienhoff, Cannon, and Sherman,[1] studying the results of bronchial closure in dogs on which a pneumonectomy had been performed, concluded that, independent of the technique used, the failure of the bronchial closure was caused by gradual erosion of the sutures through the bronchial cartilages caused by the springlike action that makes the forcefully collapsed semicircular cartilages return to their natural shape. Later Sweet[2] completed these studies, emphasizing the importance of closing the stump's ends flush with the parent bronchus, to avoid complications through stasis and poor drainage in a long, blind stump.

However, it was not until after World War II that the first studies appeared in which sutures with staples were used. They were carried out in Moscow under the leadership of the Scientific Research Institute for Experimental Apparatus and Instruments.[3,4] The original instrument, called *UKB-25*, applied a single row of clips perpendicular to the cut edge of the bronchus; later it was shown that better results were achieved with the UKL-40, with two rows of staples placed parallel to the cut section of the stump. But it was with Smith's study[5] that American suture machines began to develop sufficient credibility and to achieve the perfection of the currently used devices (TA, GIA, RI).

Later publications confirmed experimentally the suitability of staple closures, because manually placed sutures were spaced and tied unevenly and resulted in an irregular edge to the bronchial section, which makes the appearance of fistulas more common.[6,7] Since lobectomies have been performed with staplers, the frequency of bronchial fistulas has decreased notably.[8]

Staplers have been of great efficacy in surgery, notably shortening operative time and as a consequence reducing the postoperative complications. The stapler can be used in sectioning the lung parenchyma, since it is not necessary to take into account the segmental planes and the technical difficulty that sometimes accompanies the blunt dissection of lung parenchyma.[9] Vascular staples have also proved completely hemostatic and perform quickly when applied on vascular structures.[10]

MATERIALS AND METHODS

We have used surgical staplers during the last 13 years on 1463 of our patients, 1211 men and 252 women, aged 14 to 84 years (average, 47). From the beginning we have used devices of American origin: TA and GIA (U.S. Surgical Corp.).

In our early experience we used the TA and after that the TA Premium device, without any remarkable difference in results between the two. With the RL or TAII-55, the results were the same in spite of the theoretical advantage of being able to graduate the pressure with the RL.

The diagnoses of the patients operated on using staplers can be seen in Fig. 1, with lung cancer and spontaneous pneumothorax the most frequent.

The surgical techniques performed are listed in Fig. 2, and mechanical sutures were employed in almost all of them, usually for several structures, resulting in a total of 3286 staple lines (Fig. 3). When they were used for bronchial closures, as noted in Fig. 4, the bronchial section was performed at different levels, as required by the intervention, resulting in staple placements in 740 bronchi.

Fig. 5 shows the operative field for a left pneumonectomy in which bronchial, arterial, and venous stapled closures can be seen.

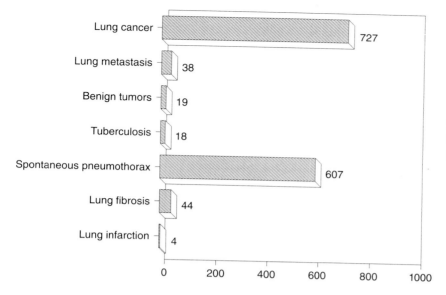

Fig. 1. Diagnoses in patients on whom stapling closure techniques were employed.

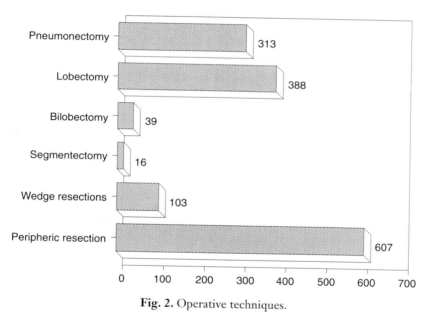

Fig. 2. Operative techniques.

Fig. 3. Applications of staple sutures.

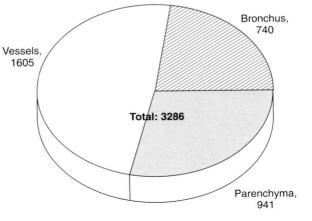

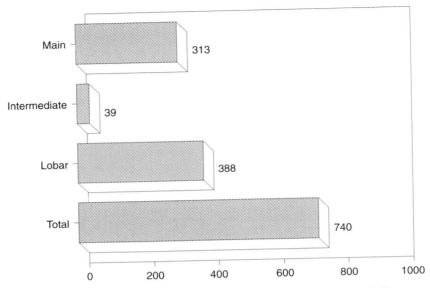

Fig. 4. Bronchial levels in which sutures were mechanically applied.

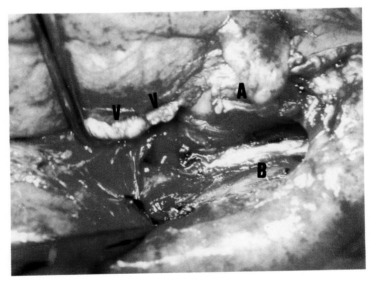

Fig. 5. Intraoperative view showing stapling of main left bronchus *(B)*, pulmonary artery *(A)*, and veins *(V)*.

RESULTS

Before we had surgical staplers in our department, we closed bronchial stumps manually, following Sweet's technique (i.e., interrupted reabsorbable sutures with 3 to 4 mm between each one). Later we substituted the mechanical suture for that kind of closure, and in the last 98 pneumectomies we have applied mixed sutures (i.e., we added a manual suture to the mechanical closure by leaving, when possible, a minimally longer stump to make this double closure line possible).

When we used manual sutures in 90 pneumonectomies, we had nine bronchial leaks, which represent 10% of the cases. Since our pneumonectomies have been performed using staplers, out of 313 bronchial closures, 33 patients (10.5%) have experienced dehiscence. However, 14 of these developed bronchial leaks 3 months to 1 year after the operation. Thus it may be that other factors (e.g., local cancer recurrence, infection of the stump, hypoproteinemia, tuberculosis) have some kind of influence on the appearance of these fistulas over such a long period of time. Therefore data cannot be interpreted to mean that leakage is an absolute consequence of the type of suture used: we relate the aforementioned complication to the method used only when it appears within 1 month or less after the procedure. Thus considered, a total of 19 (6.07%) leaks could be defined as a complication of the stapled closure. This complication thus decreases to almost half the rate with the manual suture. We have not found differences in the results depending on the stapler used—TA, TA Premium, RL, or TAII-55.

Recently, whenever possible (with almost all patients), we have used a combination of both methods of suture, because, as we explained previously, leaving a stump a few millimeters longer obtains better results than when only metal sutures are applied flush with the cut section of the bronchus. Out of 98 patients receiving pneumectomies, five have had bronchopleural fistulas; the rate of fistulous occurrence was 5.1%, an even greater decrease of this dangerous complication. We used this combined technique to diminish the force of tension that tended to open the bronchus, believing that tension is perhaps one of the factors contributing to produce dehiscence in the suture. In fact, after placement of the mechanical sutures, the stump left distal to the staples splits along its sides. This is repaired with additional manual sutures. On the other hand, postpneumonectomy bronchopleural fistulas have appeared more often on the right side than on the left side (21 right, 12 left), just as Kaplan[11] stated. The closures

on inferior lobar and intermediate bronchi, in a total of 427 operations, have not presented dehiscence problems, either partial nor total, in any case.

From the beginning we have applied staplers to important vascular structures that we previously occluded with a double ligature of silk, and in case of doubt we completed the process with a continuous vascular suture. We have used staplers both intrapericardially and extrapericardially (Fig. 6) for suturing arteries and veins or the atrial wall (28 occasions), using excision when necessary up to one third of its volume (Fig. 7).

Three of our patients (0.2%) had postoperative hemorrhage that was controlled in two cases (one originating in an artery and the other in a vein) with a manual vascular suture applied urgently. The other patient died because there was no time for reoperation. The autopsy revealed that the origin of the hemorrhage was a torn vein at the proximal line of staples.

One of the most important fields of application of these devices is the transsection and suture of lung parenchyma, which when performed manually inevitably produces hemorrhage and air leaks that in some cases are difficult to control. However, mechanical sutures applied with a stapler, since they are performed before or at the same time as the transsection, avoids much of the potential for hemorrhage and air leaks.

Thus we use the TA and RL instruments for the exeresis of bullae and small peripheral lesions. The GIA instruments, which apply two rows of staples and section in between simultaneously, are used for wedge resections and to open fissures to guarantee hemostasis and pneumostasis proximal and distal to the section of both edges. With their use in wedge resections, the resected area does not bleed peripherally on the specimen while the second or third row of staples is placed. We have also used the TA stapler in segmentectomies.

We have applied the stapler in 941 cases for parenchymal transsection. The majority of these procedures was for bullectomy (607 occasions) (Fig. 8). The other applications were performed on 109 occasions for opening fissures and always were carried out with a 90 mm or 60 mm GIA stapler, which was also used on 103 occasions for wedge resections of lung lesions and in 11 cases to perform lung resection and suturing during segmentectomy.

The rest of the parenchymatous sutures (see Fig. 8) were performed with linear suture instruments (TA or RL) of adequate length. Five segmentectomies were done with a TA-90.

Complications inherent to these techniques are de-

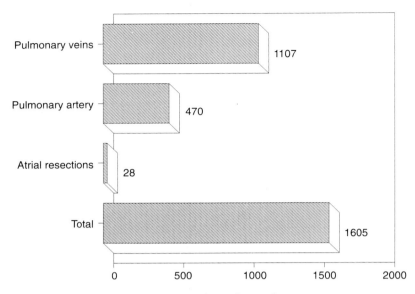

Fig. 6. Uses of vascular staples.

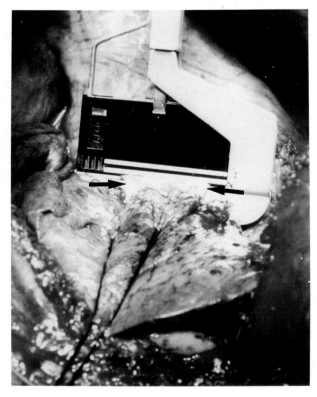

Fig. 7. Stapling both pulmonary veins at the atrial level *(arrows).*

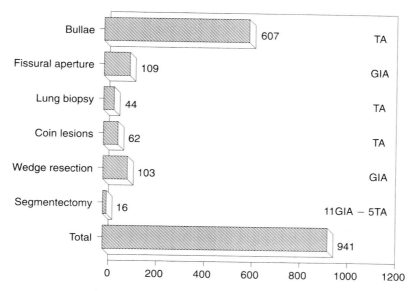

Fig. 8. Distribution of parenchymal resections.

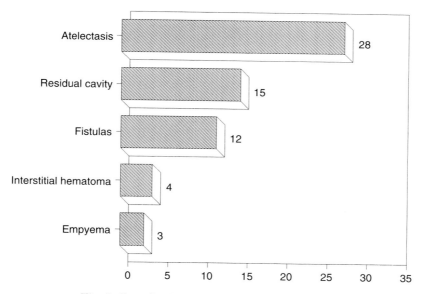

Fig. 9. Complications with stapling of parenchyma.

tailed in Fig. 9, although we know that in most of the cases the stapler is not responsible for the complication. Nevertheless, when we compared the number of complications that can be direct consequences of such sutures (e.g., residual cavities and extended leaks), the number was one third of that when we performed the operations manually in emphysematous patients, in big superficial bullae resections, and in peeling for lobar or segmental resections.

DISCUSSION

Surgical staplers constitute great technological progress in lung surgery. They are reliable, easily applied, efficient, and time saving and safe during their use for either closure of hilar structures or parenchymatous sutures.

The results achieved in the stapling of lobar bronchi have been totally satisfactory, with no inherent complications associated with the staples. At this point we concur with other studies published.[8-12]

At present we close the main bronchus with stapling devices in all cases when a pneumonectomy is needed, leaving manual sutures for use in those limited cases in which application of a suture machine is not advisable (i.e., mainly when there is limited space and the suture would stay very close to the neoplasic lesion without an oncological security margin). In any case the frozen section biopsy of the edge of the bronchial section will reveal whether or not there is an invasion, in which case a bronchial recut using manual suturing of the stump is necessary. This happened 16 times in our cases.

We also use manual sutures when we estimate that it is necessary to inspect the bronchial lumen before closure and in cases in which there is an excessive rigidity of the bronchus, because the strength of the jaws of the stapler risks devitalizing the bronchial stump. In the majority of comparative studies of both methods of bronchial closure, results favor the staples because of the uniformity in the surface of the suture.[6,13,14] The stapler maintains a constant compression without anatomical deformations. In addition, the closure of the staples does not cause tissue ischemia. In our experience the incidence of bronchopleural fistulas decreased remarkably when staples are compared with manually placed sutures.

From the beginning we were inclined to use staples in vascular structures, thus achieving hemostasis, saving time, and clearing the surgical field.[10] When the in-

trapericardiac section must be performed, the pulmonary veins can be sutured together as a trunk, with only one application of the device (see Fig. 7).

If the surgical time and complications have been remarkably reduced in any one field of lung surgery, it is in techniques on the lung parenchyma, achieving better aerostasis and hemostasis because of the double or triple row of staples. The easy application of these techniques can save from 25 minutes to 1 hour in certain operations,[15] diminishing at the same time the complications inherent with the use of extended anesthesia, thus allowing comfort and safety in superficial resections (apical bullae, superficial nodules, wedge resections in biopsies, transsections of incomplete fissures, segmentectomies, and transegmentectomies).[16]

REFERENCES

1. Rienhoff WF Jr, Cannon J Jr, Sherman I. Closure of the bronchus following pneumectomy. Ann Surg 116:481-531, 1942.
2. Sweet RH. Closure of the bronchial stump following lobectomy or pneumectomy. Surgery 18:82-86, 1945.
3. Amosov NM, Berezosky KK. Pulmonary resection with mechanical suture. J Thorac Cardiovasc Surg 41:325-328, 1961.
4. Andronov PI. New instruments for thoracic surgery. Dis Chest 44:550, 1963.
5. Smith RN, Faraci RP, Aubrey H. Bronchial stump closure techniques following pneumectomy. A serial comparative study. Ann Surg 116:206-211, 1976.
6. Peterffy A, Calabrese E. Mechanical and conventional manual sutures of the bronchial stump. A comparative study of 298 patients. Scand J Thorac Cardiovasc Surg 13:87-91, 1979.
7. Scott RN, Faray RP, Aubrey H. Bronchial stump closure techniques following pneumectomy. A serial comparative study. Ann Surg 116:206-211, 1976.
8. Takaro T. Use of staplers in bronchial closure. In Grillo HC, Eschapasse M, eds. International Trends in General Thoracic Surgery, vol 2. Major Challenges. Philadelphia: WB Saunders, 1987, pp 452-457.
9. Steichen FM, Ravitch MM. Stapling in Surgery. Chicago: Year Book, 1984.
10. Ricci C, Rendina EA, Venuta F, et al. La suturatrici meccaniche nella chirugía di exeresis del cancer del polmone. G Chir 11:138-140, 1990.
11. Kaplan K. Pulmonary resection using automatic stapler. Eur J Cardio-Thorac Surg 1:152-157, 1987.
12. Paolini A, Lefore M, Riccardelli F, et al. 100 casi di suture meccaniche bronchiali. G Chir 11:135-137, 1990.

13. Takaro T. Use of staples in pulmonary surgery. Surg Clin North Am 64:461-466, 1984.
14. Bazelly B, Donceau-Gouge GP, Dausdy M, et al. Suture mechanique et manuelle des moignons bronchiques dans la peneumectomie. Etude comparative. Noveau Presser Med 10:3.647-648, 1981.
15. Dehnel RNW. Staple suturing vs conventional suturing. AORN 18:296-299, 1973.
16. Hood RM. Techniques in general thoracic surgery. Philadelphia: WB Saunders, 1985, pp 97-99.

133 *Videothoracoscopic Exeresis of Mediastinal Masses*

Giancarlo Roviaro, Carlo Rebuffat, Federico Varoli, Contardo Vergani,
Marco Maciocco, Fabrizio Grignani, Silvio Marco Scalambra,
and Claudio Mariani

Advances in optics, endoscopic television monitoring, and instrumentation has led to the development of minimally invasive videoendoscopic surgery. While the laparoscopic approach is revolutionizing surgery,[1,2] at present thoracic videoendoscopic techniques are generally limited to resection of pleural bullae, to pleurectomies, or to small pulmonary wedge resections.[3] Mediastinal masses are usually removed through wide thoracotomies; the postoperative course is painful, there is functional impairment, and cosmetic results are poor. Therefore a minimally invasive approach seems advisable.[4,5]

MATERIALS AND METHODS (Figs. 1-3)

From September 1991 to July 1992 we performed 62 videoendoscopic operations in the chest. Of these we removed seven mediastinal masses: three thymomas, one thymic cyst, one pleuropericardial cyst, one thoracic disembryoma, and one thoracic lipoma. Average age of the patients was 53 years of age, with a range of 27 to 76 years of age.

The patient is placed in the lateral decubitus position as for a conventional posterolateral thoracotomy and is intubated with a double-lumen Carlens tube for the separate one-lung ventilation, which avoids the necessity of a CO_2-induced pneumothorax. Two wide-screen monitors are usually employed to ensure the best view for all members of the team. The position of the surgeons changes according to the kind of operation and the phase of the procedure. A microcamera connected to the thoracoscope provides excellent exposure of the pleural cavity and mediastinum and magnifies the operative field. Two or three additional cannulas permit insertion of instruments. The number and position of the trocars vary according to the case or to the size of the mass. The trocar for the telescope is usually positioned in the seventh intercostal space on the midaxillary line. The low position of the camera gives the best operative vision both for the surgeon and for the assistants. Electrocoagulating scissors, endoscopic mul-

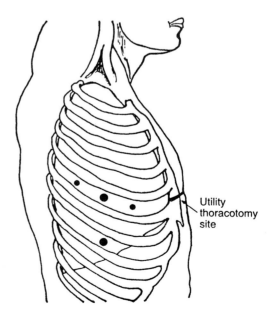

Fig. 1. Position of the trocars and of the utility thoracotomy along the inframammary fold.

Utility thoracotomy site

tifire clip appliers, and endoscopic staplers are frequently used in the course of the operation.

An additional incision is essential for the removal of large specimens. In these cases, at the very beginning of the operation we usually perform a minimal (3 to 4 cm) inframammary incision that we call a "utility thor-

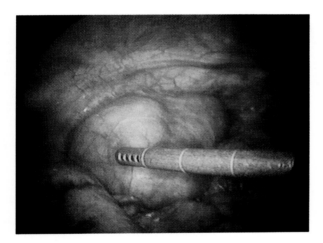

Fig. 2. The camera is introduced through the trocar in the seventh intercostal space; this offers a superb view of the mediastinum, which is occupied by a large thymic neoplasm. The latter is carefully explored and palpated with endoscopic instruments.

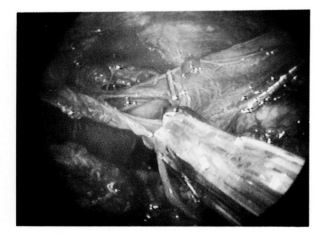

Fig. 3. Isolation of the neoplasm proceeds until exposure of the superior thymic veins of Keynes is achieved; these can then be safely clipped and severed.

acotomy," since it permits the insertion of nonendoscopic instruments (Fig. 1). This small incision greatly simplifies all maneuvers.

In case of neoplasms, the specimen must be inserted in a plastic bag before extraction to avoid the possibility of spreading the tumor. Excision of masses is always performed with gentle blunt dissection and with electrocoagulating scissors.

Apart from the approach, a videoendoscopic technique of removal does not differ from open chest surgery. Mediastinal cysts are excised after positioning occlusive clips to secure vascular pedicles, when necessary. In thymectomy, the thymic pedicle was isolated and divided after positioning occlusive clips to ensure hemostasis. In all cases of thymoma and that of disembryoma we performed the utility thoracotomy directly at the beginning of the procedure. Washing the cavity and positioning a chest drain concludes the operation.

RESULTS

No operative or postoperative deaths occurred in our series. The average operative time was 125 minutes (range, 75 to 200 minutes). We observed no postoperative complications.

The average postoperative hospital stay was 5.1 days (range, 4 to 9 days). All patients had little postoperative pain and very good cosmetic results.

DISCUSSION

Even though videothoracoscopic surgery has only recently been introduced, it has already had a wide diffusion for the treatment of many thoracic diseases. At present some videothoracoscopic operations such as treatment of pulmonary bullae, recurrent pneumothorax and metastatic lesions are commonly accepted and performed throughout the world. Surgical removal of well-encapsulated mediastinal tumors usually gives few technical problems, since no great vessels have to be divided and the mass may easily be enucleated from the fatty mediastinal tissue because of the constant presence of a cleavage plane.

Use of the double-lumen Carlens tube, which we usually employ in open chest surgery, greatly simplifies all procedures. It allows for separate lung ventilation and easy collapse of either lung when required, thus sparing an artificial CO_2-induced pneumothorax. It is therefore possible to work without interference from the collapsed lung and without the difficulties of a positive-pressure closed system. Nevertheless, knowledge of anatomy and utmost care are mandatory to dissect the vascular thymic pedicle, to identify and secure the veins of Keynes, and to preserve the phrenic nerves.

Similarly, excision of pleuropericardial or mediastinal cysts is usually easily performed. Videothoracoscopy provides an excellent transpleural approach to the mediastinum, thus allowing careful removal of the mass by combined blunt and sharp dissection. Safe performance of the procedure is possible only after training in open chest surgery, because the paramount importance of mediastinal organs requires a perfect command of anatomy and a wide experience of mediastinal pathology.

The utility thoracotomy is sometimes necessary to extract the specimen. In this case we advocate its performance at the very beginning of the procedure. Pleuropericardial and serous cysts usually do not require a utility thoracotomy.

In our experience the excision never gave any great difficulty, and complete removal of the lesion was always performed without any great problems. Neoplasms were extracted within a plastic bag. The videoendoscopic approach undoubtedly offers functional and cosmetic advantages and avoids the sequelae of wide thoracotomies: pain is much reduced and respiratory function is far better. Furthermore, a utility thoracotomy, if performed along the inframammary sulcus, does not compromise cosmetic results, which are very satisfactory.

Considering that mediastinal masses are often be-

nign and asymptomatic and their discovery usually incidental, videothoracoscopic approach seems particularly advisable.

CONCLUSION

Videothoracoscopic excision seems particularly indicated for benign mediastinal growths, since the operative technique does not imply any difficulty and the exposure of the field through wide screen monitors is superb. Functional and cosmetic advantages for the patients are unquestionable.

REFERENCES

1. Zucker KA. Surgical laparoscopy. St. Louis: Quality Medical Publishing, Inc, 1991.
2. Olsen DO. Laparoscopic cholecystectomy. Am J Surg 161:399-444, 1991.
3. Nathanson LK, Shimi SM, Wood AB, Cuschieri A. Videothoracoscopic ligation of bulla and pleurectomy for spontaneous pneumothorax. Ann Thorac Surg 52:316-319, 1991.
4. Roviaro GC, Rebuffat C, Varoli F, Vergani C, Mariani C, Grignani F. Videothoracoscopic excision of a mediastinal thymoma. Surg Laparosc Endosc (in press).
5. Roviaro GC, Rebuffat C, Varoli F, Vergani C, Maciocco M, Grignani F, Scalambra SM, Mariani C, Pezzuoli G. Videoendoscopic thoracic surgery. Int Surg (in press).

XIX

Thoracoscopic Sympathectomy and Vagotomy

134 *Thoracoscopic Sympathectomy: An Established Minimally Invasive Technique*

William John Byrne

Thoracoscopic sympathectomy is the treatment of choice for palmar and axillary hyperhidrosis. It produces excellent long- and short-term results, and patients experience the benefits of minimally invasive surgery. The development of surgical sympathectomy mirrors that of minimally invasive surgery as a whole. It has evolved from the recognition of the efficacy of sympathectomy through an open technique, to a thoracoscopic approach as the best treatment for palmar and axillary hyperhidrosis.

Traditional approaches to surgical sympathectomy have involved the supraclavicular or cervical approach, the transaxillary approach, and the dorsal approach, with the cervical approach previously being the procedure of choice in the United Kingdom and Ireland. The cervical approach, however, is associated with an incidence of permanent Horner's syndrome ranging from 1% to 57%.[1,2] Brachial plexus contusion, phrenic nerve palsy, and major vessel damage have also been reported[3] as a result of the cervical approach, which is rapidly being replaced by the thoracoscopic technique.

The main indication for surgical sympathectomy today is palmar or axillary hyperhidrosis. Sympathectomy in the treatment of Raynaud's phenomenon has fallen into disrepute. It is occasionally required in the treatment of intractable causalgia and arterial occlusive disease of the upper limb. Since 1980 the approach of choice in our unit has been thoracoscopic sympathectomy. Although we have used the alternative terms *transthoracic electrocautery* and *endoscopic transthoracic sympathectomy*, the term *thoracoscopic sympathectomy* accurately reflects the instruments used and the technique.

THORACOSCOPIC TECHNIQUE

Careful attention to preoperative workup is essential in patients undergoing thoracoscopic sympathectomy. In all cases of patients with primary palmar and axillary hyperhidrosis, it is essential to rule out an underlying pathologic cause for the condition. All patients routinely undergo a whole blood count and evaluations for urea and electrolytes, blood glucose, and thyroid function as well as outpatient chest x-ray evaluation. The patient must be informed of the potential complications of the operation, such as postoperative pain, possible pneumothorax or hemithorax requiring insertion of a chest drain, and some degree of compensatory hyperhidrosis. Patients with evidence of pleural adhesions revealed by chest x-ray films should not undergo operation, although in our experience of thoracoscopic sympathectomy, especially when the ages and patient profiles are considered, this has not been a problem.

As demonstrated by Jdeikin et al.,[4] anesthesia is essential for successful completion of this procedure, which is performed with the patient under general anesthetic and with a double-lumen endotracheal tube inserted. The patient is placed in the supine position with both arms abducted to a 90-degree angle. Blood pressure, heart rate, electrocardiography, pulse oximetry, end-tidal CO_2 concentration, and peak inspired airway pressure are monitored throughout the operation. An artificial pneumothorax is established by insufflating 500 ml of CO_2 through a Veress needle in the fourth intercostal space after the ipsilateral portion of the endotracheal tube is disconnected from the ventilator. A small incision is made in the fourth intercostal space in the anterior axillary line, and a thoracoscope is introduced through a cannula. More CO_2 is introduced, and the upper lobe of the lung is observed as it collapses. Flimsy adhesions are often encountered at this stage; they can safely be cut with a diathermy scissors. Major apical adhesions may be difficult to cut and may even render the operation impossible.

The sympathetic chain is usually seen under the parietal pleura as it runs down over the necks of the second to the sixth ribs. A unipolar diathermy probe is inserted (usually in the midclavicular line) through a separate stab incision. If the chain is not easily seen as a result of subpleural fat, it can be located by stroking the diathermy along the neck of the rib. The chain is then felt as it slips out from under the tip of the probe. The pleura over the chain can be incised with diathermy, and the second, third, and fourth thoracic ganglia and intervening chain are electrocoagulated until they present a charred appearance. This differs from the approach of Kux and co-workers,[5] who at this stage of the operation attempt to remove the chain with a grasping forceps and dissecting scissors. Kao[6] has also described the use of the fiberoptic CO_2 laser at this stage of the operation to destroy the sympathetic chain. Phenol injections have been used, less successfully, for the same purpose. If axillary hyperhidrosis is also a problem, the fifth ganglion should also be removed for adequate denervation of the axilla. Stellate ganglion injury is not a problem when the thoracoscopic technique is used; the ganglion is covered by a characteristic yellow fat pad and is not seen at the time of operation.

When operation on the first side is complete, the endotracheal tube is reconnected and the lung is reinflated so that CO_2 escapes through the cannula. Reinflation of the lung is then checked through the thoracoscope, and when the lung is fully inflated, the incision is closed with a single nylon suture. The procedure is repeated on the opposite side under the same anesthetic.

This technique has not resulted in problems in our experience. The patient must be monitored closely throughout the procedure to prevent inadvertent pneumothorax, and the CO_2 line pressure must not exceed 10 cm H_2O. In experienced hands, the procedure can be performed in 30 to 35 minutes.

A chest radiograph, which is performed on all patients in the recovery area after the operation, must be viewed by the operating surgeon before the patient is returned to the ward. Chest drains are not routinely placed unless there has been a specific indication, such as significant pneumothorax or troublesome oozing during the operation that could not be contained by direct pressure. In our experience this has occurred rarely. Another chest radiograph is performed 24 hours after surgery, and the patient is usually discharged on the second postoperative day.

RESULTS

The results of successful sympathectomy are dramatic. The hyperhidrotic patient awakens to dry, warm hands. Usually the success of this operation is apparent by the first postoperative day. However, we also examined the long-term efficacy of the procedure.

In our series in Dublin[7] we reviewed 112 patients who had undergone thoracoscopic sympathectomy for palmar and axillary hyperhidrosis refractory to treatment.

All patients completed a questionnaire inquiring into all aspects of their condition and how they had fared after surgery. In all but one patient, the hands were recorded as being dry on return from the operating room. In one early case the procedure was unsuccessful and had to be repeated. Seventy-eight of the 85 patients on whom follow-up was completed reported immediate satisfaction with the procedure. No mortality and no serious morbidity occurred in our series. Horner's syndrome occurred in three patients; it resolved in two patients within 6 weeks after surgery and by 6 months after surgery in one patient. Surgical emphysema was noted in three patients, and a significant pneumothorax requiring a chest drain occurred in one patient. Other transient postoperative phenomena included chest pains (eight patients), back pains (four patients), and transient well-described Raynaud's phenomenon (four patients). The mean length of hospital stay was 3.1 days (range, 1 to 7 days), although when the procedure is performed by surgeons experienced in the technique almost all patients return home on the first postoperative day. Long-term results for the procedure are equally gratifying. Our mean follow-up period was 43 months (range, 3 to 95 months). Subjective patient assessment of the effectiveness of surgery was impressive (Table 1).

Patient satisfaction with the cosmetic results of the procedure was impressive; 80% of patients graded their result as "good," and no patient expressed dissatisfaction with the cosmetic result. However, 64% of patients described some degree of compensatory hyperhidrosis; all patients who consider undergoing the procedure must be made aware of this possibility before surgery. Twelve patients in our group described gustatory sweating.

Table 1. Patient assessment of surgical result

Categories of Assessment of Patient's Condition	Assessment Immediately After Operation	Assessment at Follow-up
Much improved	67	65
Moderately improved	11	7
Slightly improved	3	7
Unchanged	2	2
Worse	2	3

CORROBORATION WITH OTHER SERIES

Our experience with thoracoscopic sympathectomy has been repeated in other centers. Kux[5] reported that 55 of 59 patients in his review group were satisfied with their result but that there was a 48% incidence of compensatory sweating. He reported no cases of Horner's syndrome, wound infection, or pneumothorax requiring a chest drain. Claes and Gothberg[8] reported similar results in their series, in which they used a slight modification of the previously described technique. They reported that of the 100 cases in their series, all were dry after the operation, and that at follow-up, 80% reported "good" results, 15% reported "improved" results, and no patient regretted having undergone the operation. Two patients required insertion of a chest tube, but no other complications occurred. In a preliminary communication, Bannerjee et al.[9] reported a similarly satisfactory experience: 95% of patients reported their postsurgical condition as being "improved" if only their hands were affected as opposed to 77% of those who indicated an "improved" result if both hands and axillae were affected. Thirty-eight of their 50 patients reported some degree of compensatory hyperhidrosis, and 24 mentioned gustatory sweating. One patient developed transient Horner's syndrome. Masters and Rennie[10] have also published data on 50 patients; they indicated that 92% of patients with palmar hyperhidrosis gained symptomatic relief but that when axillae were also involved, ≤20% reported residual sweating. Compensatory sweating occurred in 75% of their treated group, and gustatory sweating in 48% of patients; one transient Horner's syndrome occurred. Adams et al.[11] reported similar results in 26 patients; only one transient Horner's syndrome occurred in their series.

CONCLUSION

All surgeons performing routine surgical sympathectomy should be familiar with thoracoscopic sympathectomy. The technique can be performed as a single-stage bilateral procedure with minimum morbidity and can avoid the cosmetically deforming complications of the cervical approach, such as permanent Horner's syndrome,[1] as well as more life-threatening complications, such as subclavian vessel damage.[3] It also avoids the need for the costotransversectomy that is inherent in the dorsal approach.[12] Thoracoscopic sympathectomy is a relatively easy operation to perform, results in few complications, and can be performed rapidly (usually in 30 to 35 minutes by an experienced surgeon). The procedure requires a short hospital stay and produces a cosmetically acceptable long-lasting result. Thoracoscopic sympathectomy should be regarded as the approach of choice for surgical sympathectomy.

REFERENCES

1. Adar R, Kurchin A, Zweig A, Mozes M. Palmar hyperhidrosis and its surgical treatment. Ann Surg 186:34-41, 1977.
2. Conlon KC, Keaveny TV. Upper dorsal sympathectomy for palmar hyperhidrosis. Br J Surg 74:651, 1987.
3. Hashmonai M, Kopelman D, Kein O, Schein M. Upper thoracic sympathectomy for primary palmar and axillary hyperhidrosis: Long-term follow-up. Br J Surg 79:268-271, 1992.
4. Jdeikin R, Olsfanger D, Shachor D, Mansoor K. Anaesthesia for transthoracic endoscopic sympathectomy in the treatment of upper limb hyperhidrosis. Br J Anaesth 69:349-351, 1992.
5. Kux M. Thoracic endoscopic sympathectomy in palmar and axillary hyperhidrosis. Arch Surg 113:264-266, 1978.
6. Kao MC. Laser endoscopic sympathectomy for palmar hyperhidrosis. Lasers Surg Med 12:308-312, 1992.
7. Byrne J, Walsh TN, Hederman WP. Endoscopic transthoracic electrocautery of the sympathetic chain for palmar and axillary hyperhidrosis. Br J Surg 77:1046-1049, 1990.
8. Claes G, Gothberg C. Endoscopic transthoracic electrocautery of the sympathetic chain for palmar and axillary hyperhidrosis [letter]. Br J Surg 78:760, 1991.
9. Bannerjee AK, Edmondson R, Rennie JA. Endoscopic transthoracic electrocautery of the sympathetic chain for palmar and axillary hyperhidrosis [letter]. Br J Surg 77:1435, 1990.
10. Masters A, Rennie JA. Endoscopic transthoracic sympathectomy for idiopathic upper limb hyperhidrosis. Clin Autonomic Res 2:349-352, 1992.
11. Adams DC, Wood SJ, Tulloh BR, Baird RN, Poskitt KR. Endoscopic transthoracic sympathectomy: An experience in the southwest of England. Br J Surg 6:558-562, 1992.
12. Shih C, Wang Y. Thoracic sympathectomy for hyperhidrosis: A report of 457 cases. Surg Neurol 10:291-296, 1978.

135 *Thoracoscopic Surgery of the Neurovegetative System*

R. Wittmoser†

Almost all the peripheral autonomic nervous system—sympathetic and vagus—lies on the inner walls of the large body cavities and is covered only by the thin transparent pleura parietalis in the thoracic cavity.

Thoracoscopic adhesiolysis was first carried out in 1913 by Jacobaeus; in the 1930s Kremer also performed the procedure in cases such as pulmonary tuberculosis. Thoracoscopic sympathectomy was first performed in 1941 by Goetze and after 1949 by Kux. From 1951 we developed various methods of endoscopic selective sympathectomies and selective ramisections of the vagus system and coined the term *endoscopic surgery* for these techniques.

METHOD

With the patient lying prone, the thoracic cavity is entered by means of a parascapular incision, and the sympathetic trunk under the pleura parietalis on the heads of the ribs is thoracoscopically exposed. At the dorsal edge of the ganglia the rami communicantes grisei and albi between T1 and T2 can be dissected under the magnifying glass of the endoscope and electrosurgically eliminated, as can the trunci interganglionares and the splanchnic nerve roots between T5/6 and T11 or the splanchnic nerve trunks.

Endoscopic surgery of the autonomic nervous system can be used for a great many indications for which major surgical access to the deep-lying structures would scarcely be adequate. Furthermore, operative trauma is minimized because of the precision of dissection that can be achieved with the endoscopic lens, which can approach to within millimeters of the surgical site. The surgical site is also magnified by the optical system, so microsurgery can be performed. The relatively fine nerve structures of the sympathetic and vagus systems can be dissected much more precisely and selectively by endoscopy than with macrosurgical techniques, where the eye is 30 to 40 cm from the surgical site.

In circulatory disturbances, especially Raynaud-type functional disturbances, the stellate ganglia are in no danger because the vasomotor fibers ascend from the third to the fifth thoracic neural segment, as was demonstrated by Foerster in the 1920s. They can be thoracoscopically eliminated here, preganglionically in the rami communicantes. According to our knowledge of physiology, this promises better long-term results, and this is confirmed by electrothermograms and rheograms. The early results are positive in almost 100% of cases, so that a negative early result can almost certainly be attributed to an operative-technical deficiency.

For hyperhydrosis, the affected sweat zones can be selectively eliminated for the most part. The second thoracic neural segment carries the fibers for head and neck. The third neural segment innervates the armpit by means of short segmental fibers that can only be accessed in the rami communicantes.

The hand and arm are supplied by the third to the fifth thoracic sympathetic neural segments; long fibers ascend to the stellate ganglia and connect to the brachial plexus.

Innervation of the trunk is, by contrast, segmental, through short sympathetic nerve fibers. Depending on the indications, it is possible to perform thoracoscopic eliminations as far as the horizontal line through the mamillae (T5) or the navel (T10) or even under certain circumstances as far as T12 (i.e., suprapubically).

In pain syndromes at various locations the sympathetic innervation is a determining factor. In Sudeck-type posttraumatic sympathicogenic reflex dystrophies, endoscopic sympathectomy in the area of the rami communicantes encompasses not only the nocitropic but also the vasoconstrictive and the sudomotor fibers (i.e., the most commonly occurring triads associated with pain, circulatory disturbances, and hyperhidrosis).

The pain path for the organs of the epigastrium is through the nervi splanchnici. For various therapy-resistant epigastric pain syndromes, endoscopic splanchnicotomy can be a very effective, low-stress operation.

Certain forms of chronic pancreatitis in which pain syndromes with phagodolophobic cachexia is prominent are a rewarding but still too rarely heeded indication for splanchnicotomy.

†Deceased.

720

In technical terms, thoracoscopic access to the splanchnic nerve, well away from the epigastric adhesion region, represents such a minimization of this operation that it can also be tolerated well by very weak patients and has so far proved nonlethal. The elimination should be extended sufficiently caudally, as far as T11, because our experience has shown that the autonomic pain path from the pancreas also runs through the lowest thoracic neural segments. Left-sided elimination usually suffices in the case of pancreatitis.

The vagus, with its various branches, has also been made ever more selectively accessible to thoracoscopic surgery. For ulcus pepticum jejuni, thoracoscopic splanchnicotomy-vagotomy can already be described as the procedure of choice.

Because we are now able to differentiate between dorsal and ventral abdominal vagus trunks, it has become possible to perform a semiselective thoracoscopic vagotomy for the stomach region, avoiding the liver and antrum branches. In combination with splanchnicotomy, this has also resulted in a new, especially mild therapy concept for duodenal ulcers.

In the case of bronchial asthma the rami bronchiales can be selectively dissected and cut without any danger of harming the rami abdominales.

VIDEOENDOSCOPY

We demonstrated the first color videoendoscopy in 1969 at the Erlanger Endoscopy Congress, with three-tube camera, specially developed articulated optic lens system and 1-inch tape recorder. From 1987 we used second- and third-generation minicameras with 300,000 to 400,000 pixels and ¾-inch U-matic cassette recorders. Since 1990 we have used a fourth-generation chip camera with 1.4 million pixels and Betacam SP recording equipment as a highly superior standard method.

---

136 *Thoracoendoscopic Truncal Vagotomy*

F. Dubois

Thoracic vagotomy is not a new procedure: Wittmoser[1] began performing many truncal vagotomies by this method in 1950, but did not publish his experience at the time. The development of laparoscopic surgery, specifically laparoscopic vagotomy, encourages a rediscovery of the thoracic approach.

MATERIALS AND METHODS

For thoracoendoscopic truncal vagotomy the patient is placed under general anesthesia. Selective endotracheal intubation is done with the patient placed in a lateral decubitus position, as for posterolateral thoracotomy. The left-sided approach is more commonly employed.

After pneumothorax is initiated, a 10 mm trocar is inserted in the seventh intercostal space at the posterior axillary line for the endoscope; two 5 mm trocars are placed under direct vision at the midaxillary line (MAL) as far as possible from each other to allow for passage of a forceps and a hook or scissors. A fourth (5 mm) trocar is placed at the anterior axillary line for a retractor. All are introduced through the seventh (or sixth) intercostal space.

The mediastinal pleura is opened between the aorta and the pericardium, down to the diaphragm. The esophagus is easily identified and dissected all around by blunt dissection. The vagus nerves are clearly recognized; usually there are two main trunks and two smaller ones in a plexiform aspect. A short segment of each is obtained for histological examination. These are dissected, electrocoagulated, and cut. There is little bleeding in this avascular area, so no drains are necessary. The operation ends with the evacuation of the pneumothorax. The procedure is very quickly and easily performed. If the pulmonary parenchyma remains intact during the procedure, chest tube drainage is not required.

Postoperatively, a nasogastric tube is left in place for 24 hours to avoid eventual acute gastric dilation and to allow measurement of gastric acidity. Oral fluids are permitted as soon as the tube is removed, and alimentation is progressively restored. The patient leaves the hospital on the fourth day.

DISCUSSION

After Dragstedt, truncal vagotomy alone acquired a bad reputation because of its side effects and the risk of gastric stasis.

Because of the risk of diarrhea, this procedure is contraindicated for patients with a history of diarrhea. There is undoubtedly a risk of postoperative gastric stasis resulting from atony of the antrum more than from a pylorospasm, which was evaluated by Dragstedt at 40%, and which necessitates a drainage procedure. In fact, the risk of major complications is less than 10% and can be palliated by endoscopic balloon dilation of the pylorus.

In 1991 and 1992 we performed 21 thoracoscopic vagotomies (19 for recurrent duodenal ulcers and three for postoperative anastomotic ulceration). All ulcers healed. In our series, one phrenic paralysis occurred in a patient who had strong pleural adhesions. Two patients required pyloric dilation. In the first case the procedure was done preventively; in the second it was done out of necessity for persistent gastric atony. We now prefer to wait and to perform selective dilation only if necessary.

It is too early to assess long-term results, but our purpose is to emphasize the ease and benignity of thoracic truncal vagotomy.

REFERENCES

1. Wittmoser R. Thoracoscopic sympathectomy and vagotomy. In Cuschieri A, ed. Operative Manual of Endoscopic Surgery, Vol 1. Berlin: Springer-Verlag, 1992, pp 110-133.
2. Dubois F. Chirurgie de l'ulcère duodénal non compliqué. In Testas P, Delaitre B, ed. Chirurgie Digestive par Voie Coelioscopique, Vol 1. Paris: Maloine, pp 127-136, 1991.

XX

New Technology in Vascular Surgery

137 *Endoluminal Arterial Prosthesis: An Experimental Study*

György Weber

It is well known that every second patient with arterial insufficiency of the legs suffers from vascular occlusive disease in the femoropopliteal segment. Arterial occlusions in this location warrant particular attention, not merely because of their frequency but also because of the special problems associated with their surgical correction.[1,2]

Balloon angioplasty or surgical thromboendarterectomy is accepted as a safe and effective treatment for carefully selected patients, but in patients with diffuse, multiple stenoses or occlusion of long segments of the superficial femoral artery, a successful endarterectomy or balloon dilation is unlikely and long-term results are poor.[3-7]

Currently, the autogenous saphenous vein graft offers the best long-term results in this condition, but it is likely to be unavailable or unsuitable for approximately one third of the patients who need it.[8,9] When a vein is not available, the problem arises of what to use. Grafting in the femoropopliteal region with a synthetic prosthesis is often unsuccessful because of insufficient elasticity of the graft and late progressive fibrosis at the site of the distal anastomosis.[10,11] However, inasmuch as extensive superficial femoral artery occlusions in general represent a more advanced stage of systemic arterial disease, these patients also have involvement of the coronary and cerebral vessels.[1,12] These factors demonstrate the need for an alternative method of femoropopliteal reconstruction.

The basic concept of this method is that after endarterectomy or balloon angioplasty of the occluded femoral artery, an ultra–thin-walled prosthesis is inserted intraluminally.[13-15] The endoluminal prosthesis with its smooth, nonthrombogenic flow surface is thought to improve long-term patency because it covers the remaining thrombogenic arterial layers and provides favorable hemodynamic conditions, allowing the blood flow to follow a natural course with no diversions.

This procedure requires a shorter operating time than other types of femoropopliteal reconstruction. It can be especially useful in patients with contraindications to bypass surgery, because only an inguinal incision is required and in certain instances a local anesthetic may be used. The distal end of the inserted prosthesis does not have to be exposed, because it is glued to the arterial wall and held by intraluminal pressure. The endarterectomized or dilated segment and the position of the inserted prosthesis are controlled by angioscopy or angiography.

Advantages of this technique include the following:

1. The operative trauma is reduced and the operating time is shorter than with other types of reconstruction.
2. Because extensive dissection can be avoided, damage to the lymphatic vessels is minimal.
3. The vasa vasorum are preserved, reducing ischemic injury to the vessel wall. We can then hope to reduce the ultimate neointimal hyperplasia that directly affects the long-term graft patency rate.

MATERIALS AND METHODS

This report summarizes the results of short-term preclinical studies in animals with this method. We have investigated the healing characteristics of the following intraluminal prostheses: a polytetrafluoroethylene (PTFE) thin-walled vascular graft with a 3 mm inner diameter (ID) and a 0.39 mm wall thickness (Gore-Tex) and two types of expanded PTFE grafts with a 4 mm ID—one standard vascular graft with a 0.64 mm wall thickness and one thin-walled vascular graft with a 0.39 mm wall thickness (Gore-Tex and Impra). Ten adult mongrel dogs and 10 young pigs, with an average weight of 20 to 30 kg, were used for these experiments. The 20 animals were divided into four groups to evaluate PTFE prostheses with different wall thicknesses and inner diameters.

Five dogs and five pigs each received a 4 cm length of standard graft, 4 mm ID, which was inserted into one carotid artery; an equal length of thin-walled graft, 3 mm ID, was inserted into the contralateral artery. Another five dogs and five pigs each received a 4 cm length of thin-walled Impra graft, 4 mm ID, which was inserted into one carotid artery, and a thin-walled Gore-Tex graft of equal length and inner diameter, which was in-

Table 1. Experimental data

No. of Dogs	No. of Pigs	Type of Prosthesis	Inner Diameter (mm)	Wall Thickness (mm)
5	5	Standard Gore-Tex	4 (carotid artery)	0.64
		Thin-walled Gore-Tex	3 (contralateral artery)	0.39
5	5	Thin-walled Impra	4 (carotid artery)	0.45
		Thin-walled Gore-Tex	4 (contralateral artery)	0.39
10	10			

serted into the contralateral artery (Table 1). The carotid arteries of these animals, which have internal diameters of 4 to 5 mm, were exposed through a midline cervical incision. After arteriotomy and intima scratching, the graft was inserted intraluminally in a distal direction (Fig. 1). When the prosthesis was in position the carotid artery was transected at the level of the arteriotomy, and an end-to-end anastomosis was created between the proximal end of the vessel and the proximal end of the inserted graft (Fig. 2).

No anticoagulants or antiplatelet agents were used. One graft in each group was removed at 7 days, two at 14 days, two at 21 days, two at 42 days, two at 84 days, and one at 300 days after implantation.

RESULTS

The gross descriptions revealed more similarities than differences between the standard and thin-walled vascular prostheses. The specimens were found to be embedded into normally formed connective tissue, with no noticeable periarterial reaction. In general the thin-walled prothesis appeared to be better incorporated by the host tissues. The poorer adherence of the vascular wall to the standard graft was probably due to the wall thickness. For this reason, the best choice to cover the injured remaining vessel wall would be a filmlike, electron-negative material with sufficient strength to withstand intraluminal pressure. Unfortunately, at this time this type of material with this wall thickness is not available commercially.

The process of endothelialization of the luminal surface seen by light microscopy appeared similar for both Gore-Tex and Impra prostheses. There was no sign of endothelium covering the grafts at 1 week (Fig. 3). At 14 days (Fig. 4) a single layer of immature endothelial cells extended from the host carotid artery onto the sur-

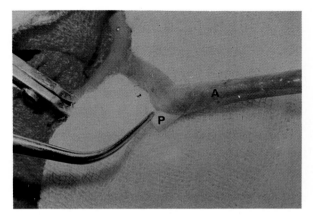

Fig. 1. Insertion of prosthesis *(P)* into carotid artery *(A)*.

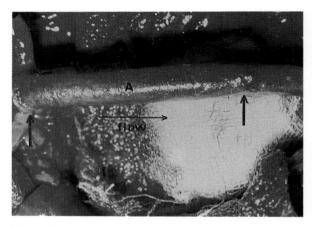

Fig. 2. Inserted prosthesis in intraluminal position. *Arrows* show the two ends of the implanted graft.

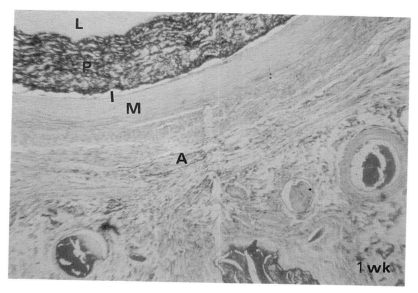

Fig. 3. Harvested graft after 1 week. (L = lumen; P = prosthesis; I = intima; M = media; A = adventitia.)

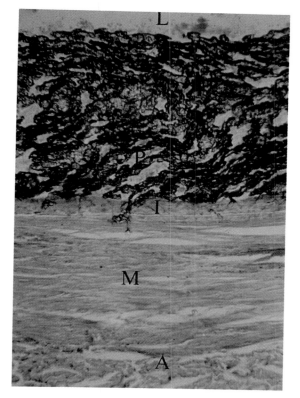

Fig. 4. Section of intraluminal graft at 2 weeks. Inner surface of the graft is covered by a fibrin-platelet layer and interstices of the graft wall are filled with acellular fibrin matrix. (L = lumen; P = prosthesis; I = intima; M = media; A = adventitia.)

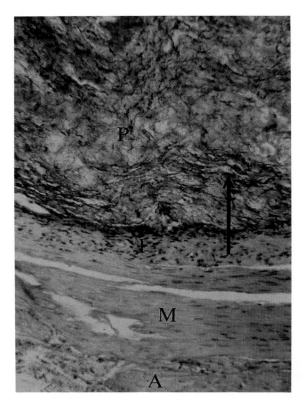

Fig. 5. Prosthesis implanted for 3 weeks. Section shows extension of different cells into the prosthesis wall. (*P* = prosthesis; *I* = intima; *M* = media; *A* = adventitia.)

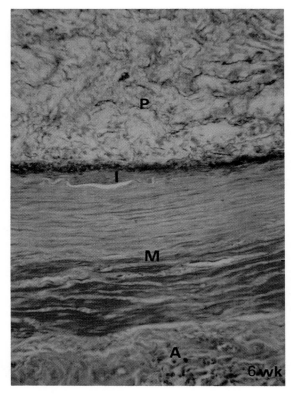

Fig. 6. At 6 weeks the endoluminal graft is characterized by firmly adherent tissue along its outer surface, with complete interstitial ingrowth. (*N* = neointima; *P* = prosthesis; *I* = intima; *M* = media; *A* = adventitia.)

faces of the prosthesis, whereas the remaining surface at the midportion of the graft was covered by a fibrin-platelet matrix. At 21 days (Fig. 5) a new endothelium was seen extending over the surface of the graft. This process was slower in the dogs. At 42 days (Fig. 6) the inner surface of the graft was covered by a nonthrombogenic, smooth, glistening coating and endothelia-like cells. Most of the neointimal tissue adhered well to the surface of the graft. The same general pattern was observed at 84 (Fig. 7) and 300 days (Fig. 8) as after 42 days, in both the dogs and the pigs. The average patency of thin-walled grafts compared with standard grafts was somewhat higher but not significantly so.

DISCUSSION

Despite exciting new developments in technology, a restenosis rate of 45.4% remains the major limitation to long-term success with various endovascular procedures.[16] Methods used to solve this problem include

longer balloon inflation times, oversizing of balloons, atherectomy devices, laser-assisted angioplasty, use of angioscopy, and pharmacological manipulation including use of steroids and prostaglandin inhibitors.[3-5,16] Although complete data are not available, initial results indicate that these approaches are only marginally successful in altering the natural history of arterial injury following endovascular reconstruction.[16,17] This lack of success can be easily understood if we analyze the process induced by endothelial injury.

Although platelets do not normally adhere to intact endothelium, damage to this surface results in platelet adhesion to the exposed and highly thrombogenic subendothelium.[18] Platelet adhesion is followed by platelet aggregation and degranulation with release of several factors including platelet-derived growth factor. This factor is a very potent mitogen, and its release results in prompt migration and proliferation of subendothelial fibroblasts and smooth muscle cells. Elegant

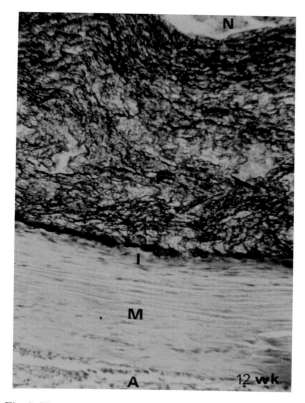

Fig. 7. Harvested graft after 12 weeks. (N = neointima; P = prosthesis; I = intima; M = media; A = adventitia.)

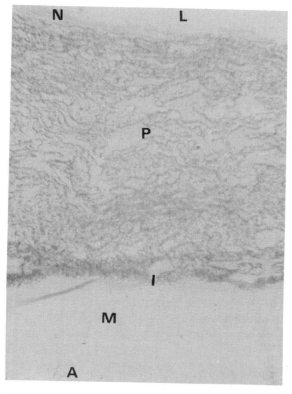

Fig. 8. Section of intraluminal graft at 300 days. (N = neointima; L = lumen; P = prosthesis; I = intima; M = media; A = adventitia.)

microscopic studies by Imparato[19] demonstrated that within 24 hours of the endothelial injury, smooth muscle cells within the media begin to proliferate. Between 2 and 4 days after injury, proliferating smooth muscle cells begin to migrate through clefts in the internal elastic lamina into the lumen, which results in narrowing of the lumen.

On the basis of the above-mentioned process, it is clear that prompt covering of the damaged surface with an electronegative material might prevent the platelet adhesion and hinder the local response to endothelial injury. This simple overlaying function of this so-called endoluminal graft means that it can be only a few microns in size. Theoretically the vessel wall could be painted with this material under angioscopic guidance.

The nutritional requirements of the arterial walls are also of considerable importance in relation to the endoluminal graft. It is well known that the vasa vasorum usually arise from branches of the artery as they pass through the adventitia. They subdivide and connect with one another in the adventitia and send out arteriolar twigs that penetrate the media and provide a capillary network through the external two thirds of the arterial wall. In the healthy young artery the intima and the central portion (approximately one third) of the media are avascular tissues deriving their oxygen and nutrients by diffusion from the blood in the lumen, but in atherosclerotic vessels, because of impaired oxygen transport by the circulating blood, the entire media and intima may be vascularized.[1] This explains why the dilated vessel wall can be covered without any consequences. After thromboendarterectomy, when the inner third of the vessel wall is removed, the endoluminal graft is probably better incorporated. If a truly passive and nonthrombogenic synthetic material could be devised, there would be no need to promote healing (pore diameter) of vascular implants. There have been many efforts to produce a material that would be totally resistant to blood clotting, but no satisfactory solution has yet been found. Some of the suggested methods have been very imaginative, for example, the use of heparin-impregnated plastics or the coating of grafts with hydrophilic gels, but none of these has been successful. Although principally from a totally different standpoint, intraluminal grafting of vessels is not a new idea. It was first used experimentally by Dotter[20] in 1969. His graft, which was made of coiled stainless-steel wire, was introduced into the femoral artery of dogs, mounted coaxially over a guidewire, and positioned with a pusher catheter. This early device and the ones that followed[21-29] also consisted of tubes formed by coiled wire. All of these stents were designed to be placed in a location remote from the site of insertion and positioned with the aid of fluoroscopy. The intent of this purely mechanical approach with these stents was to support and prevent recoil of the dilated arterial wall.

A serious problem exists, however, in that the more electronegative the material, the more thromboresistant it becomes. Unfortunately, most negatively charged metals are very corrosive. Conversely, most noncorrosive metals are positively charged and therefore have a propensity for thrombosis.[26,27] For these reasons metal stents are not suitable for our purpose.

Biomaterials are routinely used for research in animal models to evaluate the clinical efficacy of prosthetic devices. The selection of an appropriate animal model is critical to such research. Sauvage et al.[30] implanted arterial prostheses in humans and in experimental animals. They found that humans have the slowest rate of healing, whereas pigs, calves, and baboons heal very rapidly. The rate of healing in dogs more closely approximates the rate in humans compared with the other three species. For our experiments we chose the dog and the pig because we wanted to investigate and follow both slow and rapid incorporation of intraluminal prostheses. We found no significant differences in healing characteristics between the two species.

The potential applications of this method are largely speculative at the present stage of vascular graft development, but we believe that the concept of endoluminal prosthesis implantation is promising, since it could be a valuable alternative to classical surgical treatment of both obstructive and aneurysmal arterial lesions. Results of our experiments demonstrated good tissue incorporation and endothelialization with intraluminal PTFE prostheses and indicated that this method could be an effective alternative in arterial reconstruction; however, further investigations with thinner material and long-term follow-up are needed.

REFERENCES

1. Vollmar J. Reconstructive Surgery of the Arteries, 3rd ed. Stuttgart: Thieme-Stratton, 1980.
2. Morin JF, Johnston KW, Wasserman L, et al. Factors that determine the long-term results of percutaneous transluminal dilatation for peripheral arterial occlusive disease. J Vasc Surg 4:68, 1986.
3. Cumberland DC. Percutaneous transluminal angioplasty: A review. Clin Radiol 34:25, 1983.
4. Roth FJ, Heimig TH, Berliner P, et al. Perkutane Rekanalisation peripherer Arterien. In Günther RW, Thelen M, eds. Interventionelle Radiologie Stuttgart: Thieme, 1988, pp 20-44.
5. Rutherford RB, Patt A, Kumpe DA. The current role of percutaneous transluminal angioplasty. In Greenhalgh RM, Jamieson CW, Nicolaides AN, eds. Vascular Surgery: Issues in Current Practice. London: Grune & Stratton, 1986, p 229.
6. Spence RK, Freiman DB, Gatenby R, et al. Long-term results of transluminal angioplasty of the iliac and femoral arteries. Arch Surg 116:1377, 1981.
7. Zeitler E, Richter EI, Roth F, et al. Results of percutaneous transluminal angioplasty. Radiology 146:57, 1983.
8. Taylor LM, Edwards JM, Porter JM. Present status of reversed vein bypass grafting: Five-year results of a modern series. J Vasc Surg 11:193, 1990.
9. Veith FJ, Gupta SK, Ascer E, et al. Six-year prospective multicenter randomized comparison of autologous saphenous vein and expanded PTFE grafts in infrainguinal arterial reconstructions. J Vasc Surg 3:104, 1986.
10. Charlesworth PM, Brewster RC, Darling JG, et al. The fate of PTFE grafts in lower limb bypass surgery: A six year follow-up. Br J Surg 72:896, 1985.
11. Quinones-Baldrich WJ, Busuttil RW, Baker JD, et al. Is the preferential use of PTFE grafts for femoro-popliteal bypass justified? J Vasc Surg 8:219, 1988.
12. Weber G, Kiss T. Intraoperative balloon angioplasty. Eur J Vasc Surg 3:153, 1989.
13. Weber G. New type of dilation balloon catheter and its application: New possibility in femoro-popliteal reconstruction. Proceedings of the International Congress of Angiology. Athens: 1985, p 145.
14. Weber G, Rozsos I. Intraluminal prosthesis: New conception in arterial reconstruction. In Maurer PC, Becker HM, Hoffman G, et al., eds. What is New in Angiology. Mnchen-Bern-Wien-Mnchen: W. Zuckschwerdt Verlag, 1986, p 138.
15. Weber G, Rozsos I. Intraluminal prosthesis: New conception in arterial reconstruction—experiments in animals. Proceedings of the Second International Vascular Symposium. London: 1986, p 26.

16. Miller BV, Sharp WJ, Shamma AR, et al. Surveillance for recurrent stenosis after endovascular procedures. Arch Surg 26:867, 1991.
17. Palmaz JC, Sibbitt RR, Reuter SR, et al. Expandable intraluminal graft: A preliminary study. Radiology 156:73, 1985.
18. Castaneda-Zuniga WR, Fromanek A. Tadawarthy M. The mechanism of angioplasty: A new concept. Radiology 135:565, 1980.
19. Imparato TJ. Electron microscopic studies of experimentally produced fibromuscular arterial lesions. Surg Gynecol Obstet 139:497, 1974.
20. Dotter CT. Transluminally placed coilspring endarterial grafts: Long term patency in canine popliteal artery. Invest Radiol 4:329, 1969.
21. Dotter CT, Buschmann RW, McKinney MK, et al. Transluminal expandable Nitinol coil stent grafting: Preliminary report. Radiology 147:259, 1983.
22. Cragg A, Lund C, Rysavy J, et al. Non-surgical placement of arterial endoprosthesis. A new technique using Nitinol wire. Radiology 147:261, 1983.
23. Maass D, Zolikoffer CL, Largiader F, et al. Radiological follow-up of transluminally inserted vascular endoprostheses: An experimental study using expanding spirals. Radiology 152:659, 1984.
24. Charnsangaved C, Wallace S, Wright KC, et al. Endovascular stent for use in aortic dissection: An in vitro experiment. Radiology 157:323, 1985.
25. Wright KC, Wallace S, Charnsangaved C, et al. Percutaneous endovascular stents: An experimental evaluation. Radiology 156:69, 1985.
26. Palmaz JC, Sibbitt RR, Reuter SR, et al. Expandable intraluminal grafting: A feasibility study. Surgery 99:199, 1986.
27. Palmaz JC, Windeler SA, Garcia F, et al. Arteriosclerotic rabbit aortas: Expandable intraluminal grafting. Radiology 160:723, 1986.
28. Rousseau H, Joffre J, Puel J, et al. Percutaneous vascular stent: Experimental studies and preliminary clinical results in peripheral arterial diseases. Intr Angiol 6:153, 1987.
29. Sigwart U, Puel J, Mirkovitch V, et al. Intravascular stents to prevent occlusion and restenosis after transluminal angioplasty. N Engl J Med 316:701, 1987.
30. Sauvage LR, Berger K, et al. Interspecies healing of porous arterial prostheses: Observations. Arch Surg 109:698, 1974.

138 *Banding of Aortoiliac Aneurysms in High-Risk Patients: A Minimally Invasive Alternative?*

Albert Verhulst, Hugh A. Crispin, and Alex Hubens

Prosthetic materials used as cardiovascular conduits are not as ideal as the natural alternatives for the following reasons: (1) They are all more or less recognized as foreign material, evoking in the host an inflammatory response reaction with fibrous tissue formation and encapsulation, and (2) even more important, since they are in direct contact with blood and its constituents, their surfaces must be nonthrombogenic, and with regard to hemodynamics they must mimic arterial compliance as closely as possible. The slightest mismatch in viscoelastic properties may cause significant alteration of blood flow resulting in formation of thrombus. For replacement of aortic segments, however, no natural alternative is available, and before the era of resec-

tion and prosthetic grafting a number of banding, wrapping, and wiring techniques were described in an effort to prevent aneurysmal rupture. These procedures consisted of placing foreign material in close proximity to the anterior and lateral walls of the aneurysm to promote irritation and fibrosis; cellophane film, diethylphosphate, polyvinyl sponge, cutis graft, and fascia lata were all tried with very little success because of uncertainty regarding formation of scar tissue. For the most part, these operations fell into disuse with the introduction of resection and graft replacement techniques.

Since the introduction of synthetic prostheses in clinical vascular surgery in the mid-1950s, aneurysms of the thoracic and abdominal aorta—when diagnosed in time—were radically extirpated and replaced with grafts of various materials and dimensions. However, it was gradually realized that it was not necessary to remove the aneurysm entirely, and in the never-ending sinusoidal curve of discovery, decline, and rediscovery, a more conservative approach seemed appropriate; that is, a grafting procedure that could be carried out safely by leaving part or even all of the aneurysmatic wall in place, and *endoaneurysmorraphy*, the procedure that has become the gold standard in the management of aneurysmal disease.

External grafting (wrapping) is one step closer to a more conservative approach without aortic resection; it consists of surrounding the diseased arterial segment with a well-fitting tube of synthetic material to provide a stable support and prevent further dilation from cyclical pulsatile wall stresses. The segment is not resected and is left in continuity with the remainder of the cardiovascular conduit.

These techniques were originally used by Blalock and Taussig as adjunctive treatment in certain congenital heart deformities. Afterward they were reintroduced by Vargas and Deterling, who placed a nylon net around large aneurysms of the thoracic aorta in two patients with poor results. Bahnson and Nelson also used this technique in the ascending aorta. In 1968 Krippaehne reintroduced the concept of circumferential wrapping with various materials under certain conditions such as high operative risks, involvement of the renal arteries, and/or poor arterial run-off. Robicsek has been the leading advocate over the past two decades; he has applied the same technique to small and medium-sized fusiform aneurysms of the thoracic and abdominal aorta, and even to the entire aortic arch, and he has published some interesting long-range observations.

This procedure remains controversial; although foreign material does not have to come into direct contact with blood, the aneurysm remains in place with the laminated thrombus inside, and even with no rupture or significant distal embolization during long-term follow-up studies, the idea of leaving a *curable* abdominal tumor in situ does not satisfy our pursuit of optimal treatment. Also, most aneurysms are suitable for external wrapping, but some are so densely adherent to the vena cava or to the anterior vertebral column that safe dissection in those areas is precluded because of the risk of turning a safe limited procedure into a major catastrophe. We therefore wanted to determine whether ex-

---

AMERICAN SOCIETY OF ANESTHESIOLOGISTS CLASSIFICATION

Class I	Normal patient with surgical pathology without systemic repercussions or any important antecedents
Class II	Age over 75 or under 1 year or medical history without actual systemic repercussion or surgical pathology with systemic repercussion
Class III	Chronic illness, nontreated medical pathology, or beginning of organic failure
Class IV	Life threatening
Class V	Patient dies without treatment within 24 hours

---

ternal reinforcement or banding of nonruptured abdominal aortoiliac aneurysms is a feasible alternative to conventional prosthetic replacement procedures in selected high-risk patients, as advocated by Robicsek in the early 1970s.

In a prospective study we selected five high-risk patients with an ASA score of III or more (see the box) who had aneurysmal disease; we included nonruptured aneurysms of the abdominal aorta and/or iliac arteries that were at least 4 and 3 cm in diameter respectively. In an elective procedure, the aneurysm was carefully mobilized circumferentially through a midline laparotomy incision and banded with a continuous sheet of prosthetic material; initially a longitudinally opened Dacron prosthesis and later a commercially available Teflon or Marlex mesh (Bard, U.S. Surgical) material was fitted around the aneurysm, just tightly enough to contain the pulsatile wall expansion (Figs. 1 and 2). When necessary this on-site tailored design was modified with a segment above the renal arteries. Care was taken to secure the proper banding position. No aortic cross-clamping was used and no anastomosis was required. All procedures except one were completed within 2 hours. There was no substantial blood loss and no transfusion of blood products was necessary, except in one case because of technical difficulties in dissecting an adherent inferior vena cava.

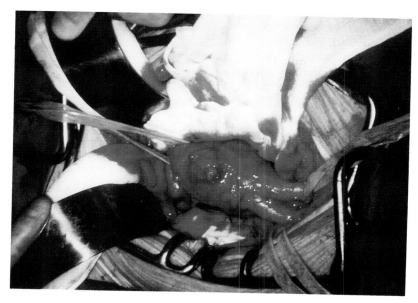

Fig. 1. Isolated aneurysm before banding.

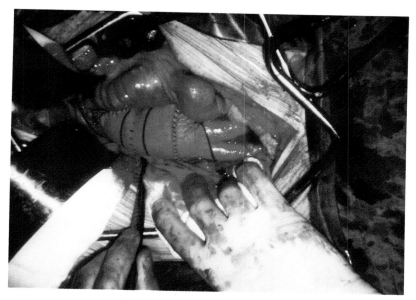

Fig. 2. Banding completed. Foreign material is placed around the circumferentially mobilized aneurysm just tightly enough to contain pulsatile wall expansion.

Six aneurysms in five patients (mean age 74.4 years, male:female ratio 4:1; Tables 1 through 3) were operated on from January 1988 to December 1991 using this technique; there were five aortic aneurysms and one iliac aneurysm. One patient died 9 months postoperatively of severe bronchopneumonia unrelated to the procedure; the others are still alive and were seen every 3 months for ultrasonography during the first year. Later they were seen every 6 months and underwent routine intravenous aortography once a year (mean follow-up 24.4 months, Kaplan-Meier statistic). Feared late complications were not encountered, and no late ruptures or aortoduodenal fistulas were seen. One distal embolization was observed in a patient with severe distal arterial insufficiency; this was treated with a minor toe amputation and classic femoropopliteal reconstructive surgery. All patients are free of symptoms at the present time.

Table 1. Patient profile and history

Patient	Sex	Age (yr)	Medical History
G.F.	Male	74	COPD, cardiac decompensation with inferolateral ischemia on ECG, pulmonary embolism, DVT
V.F.	Male	64	Severe COPD, duodenal ulcers with gastrointestinal bleeding, DVT, arterial hypertension, ethyl abuse
T.F.	Male	79	Severe COPD (corticosteriod dependent), pneumonia, angina pectoris, liver steatosis, severe obesity, severe arterial insufficiency of lower extremities
K.M.	Female	75	COPD, arterial hypertension, pancreatitis, severe arterial insufficiency of lower extremities
J.D.	Male	81	Myocardial infarction, curative lobectomy for lung cancer (unknown anatomicopathological specification)

COPD = chronic obstructive pulmonary disease; *DVT* = deep venous thrombosis.

Table 2. Patient intraoperative data

Patient	Aneurysm	Dimension	Graft Material	Duration of Operation (min)	Transfusion
G.F.	Infrarenal aorta	4 cm diameter	Longitudinally cut ABP	110	None
V.F.	Infrarenal aorta Heavily calcified	5.5 cm diameter	Teflon mesh	140	None
T.F.	Infrarenal aorta Right iliac artery	7 × 3 cm 3.5 cm diameter	Marlex mesh Dacron DV	130 60	None None
K.M.	Abdominal aorta Heavily calcified	5 cm diameter	Marlex mesh	180	4 units PC
J.D.	Abdominal aorta	8 × 10 cm	Marlex mesh	130	None

PC = packed cells.

In comparing our limited results with data published in the literature (Tables 4 and 5), one immediately observes significant postoperative morbidity and mortality in all series, especially from complications not involving the aorta itself but reflecting the precarious condition of these selected high-risk patients. Feared late complications, however, such as aortoduodenal fistula and rupture, or arterial insufficiency of the lower extremities and distal embolization, appear to be minimal or nonexistent, despite the alarming notion that the aneurysm remains in situ and more important in continuity with the blood flow; the inside of this *tumor* is still filled with an amorphous mass of thrombotic material, as seen on the postoperative control angiograms.

Table 3. Patient data on complications

Patient	Postoperative Complications	Late Complications	Mortality
G.F.	None	None	Alive
V.F.	None	Arterial insufficiency in lower limbs	Alive
T.F.	None	None	Alive
K.M.	Bleeding	Arterial insufficiency in lower limbs Distal emboli	Alive
J.D.		Unrelated to operation	Died (pneumonia)

Table 4. Comparison of patient data with that of other published series

Author	Number of Patients	Localized Thoracic Aorta	Localized Abdominal Aorta	Localized Iliac Artery	Mean Age (yr)
Krippaehne	9		9		Unknown
Smith	33	4	28	8	66
Robicsek	69	2	67		63
Our series	6	0	5	1	74

Table 5. Comparison of results with that of other published series

Author	No Blood Transfusions	Postoperative Morbidity	Postoperative Mortality	Follow-up (mo)	Late Morbidity	Late Mortality Related/Unrelated
Krippaehne	Unknown	Unknown	11%	30	None	None
Smith	58%	45%	6.1%	48	9%	9/27%
Robicsek	Unknown	"Severe"	7.8%	120	None	1.5/18%
Our series	83%	17%	None	25	17%	0/17%

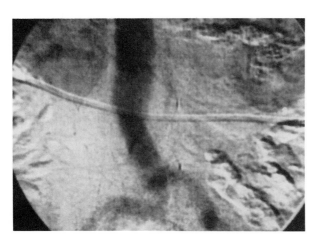

Fig. 3. Routine postoperative control subtraction angiography after 6 months. Stabilized situation. Note outline of the aneurysm wall and near-perfect *reorganization* of the amorphous thrombus into a *neobifurcation*.

After banding, however, this plastic mass seems to remodel itself into a quasiperfect neobifurcation inside the existing dilation (Fig. 3). Bluth et al.[1] analyzed the flow pattern inside a fusiform dilated aorta by means of color Doppler flow imaging and in an in vitro model. They found two distinct patterns—a smooth laminar type and a turbulent circuitous form—depending on the type and rate of inflow. Turbulent flow, initially observed at the distal aspect of the aneurysm, propagated proximally as the flow rate increased, but when pulsatile wall movement was restricted, laminar flow predominated. This may be an explanation for the near-perfect *reorganization* of the amorphous thrombus into a *neobifurcation* inside the immobilized aneurysm.

The precise scope of the indications for this procedure remains unclear; although Robicsek advocates the use of this technique, either in conjunction with a resection, for external reinforcement or as an independent procedure for small fusiform aneurysms ("too small to remove and too big to leave without treatment") and for small to medium-sized aneurysms in high-risk patients, especially with poor run-off. Smith and et al. re-

strict banding to aneurysms with involvement of the renal (or visceral) arteries in elderly and high-risk patients. According to the latter, external grafting has no place in the management of a *conventional* infrarenal aortic aneurysm, even in a high-risk population. In our limited experience, we feel encouraged to use this technique in older patients, in poor health, with calcified aneurysms and/or poor run-off; dimensions and location of the aneurysm(s) are not major determining factors.

Perhaps in the future, with a better understanding of the physiopathological and hemodynamic problems involving aneurysmal formation and further dilation and with new developments in anesthesiology, blood recuperation techniques, and prosthetic materials science, this procedure will become obsolete, but at the present time, and based on our experience, we conclude that external grafting should not be regarded as a quick, simple alternative to standard endoaneurysmorraphy; however, in selected high-risk patients with a nonruptured abdominal aneurysm, banding can provide a reliable, safe, and simple means of preventing catastrophic rupture.

REFERENCES

1. Bluth EI, Murphey SM, Hollier LH, et al. Color flow Doppler in the evaluation of aortic aneurysm. Int Angiol 9:8, 1990.
2. Robicsek F. Wall reinforcement (external grafting) in the management of aneurysms of the great vessels. In Nyhus LM, Baker RJ, eds. Mastery of Surgery, chap 169. Boston: Little, Brown & Company, 1987, p 1372.
3. Robicsek F. Fusiform aneurysm of the entire aortic arch. A new surgical approach. J Thorac Cardiovasc Surg 43:756, 1972.
4. Robicsek F. Long-range observations with external aortic grafts. J Cardiovasc Surg 17:195, 1976.
5. Robicsek F. Is there a place for wall reinforcement in modern aortic surgery? Arch Surg 105:824, 1972.
6. Wylie EJ, Kerr E, Davies O. Experimental and clinical experiences with the use of fascia lata applied as a graft about major arteries after thrombo-endarterectomy and aneurysmorrhaphy. Surg Gynecol Obstet 93:257, 1951.
7. Robicsek F, Tam W, Daugherty HK, et al. The applicability of Bernoulli's law in the process of enlargement and rupture of aortic aneurysms. J Thorac Cardiovasc Surg 61:472, 1971.

J. Marzelle

Angioscopy has been used in the superficial femoral artery for many years, as well as in the control of vascular surgery procedures. Inasmuch as fluid irrigation allows visualization of the iliac arteries, and as smaller atraumatic optic fibers allow safe visualization of the tibial arteries, new areas have opened for the use of angioscopy in peripheral vascular disease. This technique has been proved to be useful as a diagnostic tool, as a control device in new endovascular procedures, and as a therapeutic instrument.

TECHNIQUE
Catheters

Modern angioscopes are made of flexible optical fibers. Sizes range from 0.5 to 3 mm (Fig. 1). The main problem is enabling visualization in a bloodless field. Fluid irrigation with heparinized saline is delivered through a channel in fibers larger than 1.8 mm or through a coaxial catheter in smaller fibers. A balloon catheter can temporarily stop blood flow. The irrigation channel can be used to pass guidewire or small instruments. Some fibers have a deflectable tip. An angle of 10 degrees can help visualize tortuous vessels, but straight fibers passed over a wire provide an adequate view in most cases.

Complications

Direct trauma from the stiff tip of the fiber or from the pressure of irrigation can create intimal tears. Spasm can occur when the size of the fiber is too similar to the size of the vessel, but the thinnest scope may not be the best for the task because of its limited optical properties.

Fluid overload can be dangerous in patients with cardiac or renal failure. After several procedures, the surgeon learns how to limit the amount of fluid infused to less than 500 ml in most instances. Certain techniques are very helpful, such as retrograde angioscopy, compression of inflow and backflow, and scope positioning at the level of the lesion under fluoroscopic guidance. In the iliac arteries fluid irrigation only is sufficient below a tight stricture. After treatment the inflow can make it more difficult to obtain a bloodless field; in such instances temporary occlusion by a balloon may be necessary. Control angioscopy after endovascular therapy is safer if the scope is passed over a wire left in place across the lesion because of the risk of dissection that can be worsened by fluid irrigation. A "foggy" image, small streaks like those seen after surgical endarterectomy, and blood suffusions from the wall of the

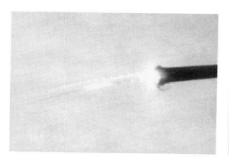
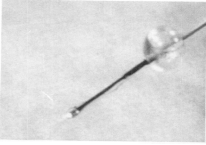

Fig. 1. Angioscopy catheters (Baxter Edwards). *Left,* Fluid irrigation is delivered through a channel inside the catheter. This channel also allows over-the-wire control angioscopy after endovascular procedures. *Right,* Fluid irrigation is delivered though a coaxial catheter. A balloon at the distal portion of this catheter allows temporary occlusion of arterial flow. The atraumatic tip of the fiber has a hole through which a guidewire can be passed.

media must be noted early so that the angioscopy can be stopped before an extensive dissection occurs.

ANGIOSCOPY IN CONVENTIONAL VASCULAR SURGERY

White et al.[1] found angioscopy more reliable than angiography in as many as 21% of patients undergoing vascular surgery. Grundfest et al.[2] showed that intraoperative angiography often misses intimal flaps at the level of the anastomosis (14%), residual valves in "in situ" vein bypasses (48%), or residual thrombus after embolectomy (85%). Nothing justifies correction of all abnormalities seen, but angioscopy has simplified femorodistal bypass and thromboembolectomy.

Thromboembolectomy

White et al.[3] have shown that angioscopic monitoring of thromboembolectomies is quicker and more reliable than intraoperative repeat angiography. It allows better diagnosis of thrombi. It avoids overinflation of Fogarty balloon catheters and provides clear evidence of residual thrombi. Proper placement of the embolectomy catheter from a short femoral approach avoids the additional procedure involving the popliteal artery and its branches. In some cases it shows failure of the Fogarty balloon catheter, when the balloon slips on an adherent thrombus. In those instances angioscopy helps guide more efficient instruments such as Vollmar rings

(Fig. 2) or Fogarty adherent to clot catheters. In bypass occlusions, thrombolysis is a time consuming and often results in hemorrhagic complications, necessitating a complementary procedure (percutaneous transluminal angioplasty [PTA] or surgery), in most cases to correct the cause of the occlusion. Angioscopy through a limited approach allows rapid graft thrombectomy with the use of Vollmar rings. Through the same incision the surgeon can simultaneously perform PTA, patch angioplasty of the anastomosis, or a complementary bypass procedure to provide good outflow to the bypass.

Femorodistal Bypass

Angioscopy has proved to be useful in quantifying the flow after venous graft valvulotomy. Chin et al.[4] have shown that the quality of the valvulotomy is important, especially when the vein is small. In elderly patients, we perform angioscopy of the saphenous vein at the beginning of the intervention, through a short incision. It often helps to detect abnormalities (wall thickening, old adherent thrombi, fibrous diaphragms, and webs) that preclude the use of the vein (see Fig. 2) as a bypass conduit. We use prosthetic bypass grafts with better results than if we had used a diseased vein. When an "in situ" bypass is performed, angioscopy helps localize the tributaries. They can be ligated through short incisions, thus avoiding problems with wound healing and edema related to the extent of the incisions.

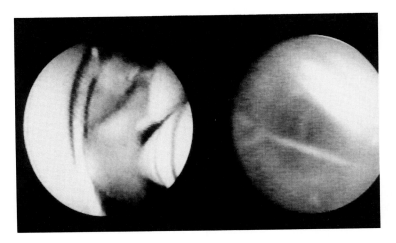

Fig. 2. Angioscopy and conventional vascular surgery. *Left,* Angioscopic monitoring of a prosthetic graft thrombectomy. Vollmar rings are used to retrieve adherent clots. *Right,* Angioscopy of a saphenous vein prior to in situ bypass. Fibrous webs can be seen and the use of a prosthetic graft will be preferred for this severely diseased vein.

ANGIOSCOPY AND ENDOVASCULAR PROCEDURES

Angioscopy is a very valuable imaging tool in endovascular procedures. It allows evaluation of the results and failures with these new techniques. Rees et al.[5] compared angioscopy and angiography in the monitoring of laser angioplasty and atherectomy procedures. Angioscopy is more reliable than angiography in identifying the nature of an arterial occlusion, that is, whether it is thrombotic or atheromatous, before a procedure. Angioscopy helps identify thrombi, flaps, and dissection after completion of the procedure, yet angiography is more precise in quantifying the degree of stenosis. In more than 150 infrainguinal endovascular procedures, we performed angioscopy in 40% of patients. In the iliac arteries angioscopy was attempted in 30% of patients. The lesion could be visualized in all patients before the procedure but in only 30% after restoration of normal blood flow.

Guidance

Abela et al.[6] have suggested that combining a scope with a laser fiber could be useful. White et al.[7] have shown that angioscopic guidance of a hot-tip laser is difficult once the catheter has crossed the first centimeter of the occlusion. Even if angioscopy aids in understanding the action of endoluminal techniques, it cannot replace angiographic monitoring of the procedures. Hydrophilic wires (Glidewire) have reduced the failure rate of recanalization of total occlusions (Fig. 3); nevertheless, they carry a risk of dissection. Angioscopy can monitor the positioning of the wire, since it often shows a small hole at the origin of the occlusion. It also helps to identify side branches when misleading of the guide occurs.

Choice of Type of Procedure

In coronary arteries[8] angioscopy is useful for comparing the results of thrombolysis with those of percutaneous transluminal angioplasty in lesions where the precise nature of the occlusion cannot be identified on the angiogram. In peripheral arteries thrombolysis[9] carries a 1% to 3% risk of fatal cerebral hemorrhage and should be avoided whenever another type of treatment is possible. A distinction between atheromatous occlusions and fresh thrombi is thus mandatory (see Fig. 3). Thrombolysis is used in too many lesions that could be treated with catheter thrombosuction or simple PTA. Angiography and preoperative duplex scanning are better than angioscopy in determining the degree of stenosis. Angioscopy is more useful in choosing the best therapy—directional atherectomy[10] of an eccentric fibrous plaque or high-speed rotational atherectomy[11] of an atheromatous occlusion of a tibial artery.

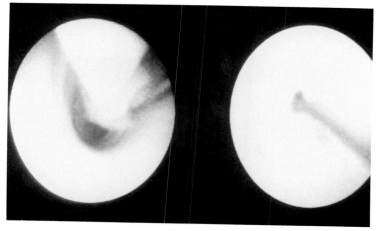

Fig. 3. Angioscopy before endovascular procedures. *Left,* Thrombotic occlusion of the superficial femoral artery. PTA or atherectomy carries a risk of distal embolization; primary thrombosuction through an 8 Fr catheter will be followed by complementary PTA of the short stenosis below the thrombotic occlusion. *Right,* Angioscopic guidance of the recanalization of an atheromatous occlusion by means of a hydrophilic guidewire.

Control After Procedure

The fair results of conventional PTA prove that many lesions created by this technique (flaps, plaque rupture) heal, but this "healing" can nevertheless lead to a stricture. The cause of this stricture can be blood disturbances, when the residual lesion is hemodynamically significant, or myointimal hyperplasia induced by modifications of the arterial wall at the site of PTA. Angiography misses some of the residual lesions that could explain early "mysterious" technical failure such as occlusions or emboli originating at the treatment site. No comparative study exists between PTA with and without angioscopic monitoring, with and without correction of abnormalities. For this reason experience helps to determine which lesions need further correction and which ones can be left as is without risk.

Ablation of adherent thrombi without significant stenosis is very likely useless. In contrast, identification of fresh thrombi (Fig. 4) is important. These thrombi can be due to a circulating dissection, sometimes seen on angiograms obtained at various angles, and repeated prolonged PTA or placement of a stent (Fig. 5) is necessary in such dissections. Fresh thrombi also carry a risk of migration, and careful removal by thrombosuction through a catheter may be prudent.

Flaps can be fibrin deposits or intimal tears. In most cases they are not occlusive and are very likely to disappear during the ensuing weeks, as shown on repeat duplex scanning. Overcorrection of such abnormalities can be hazardous since it carries a risk of dissection.

In most cases, plaque rupture does not require a complementary procedure as long as it is deemed part of the "normal" process of PTA. It allows contact of the media layers with circulating blood, which can lead to further development of intimal hyperplasia. Repeated PTA or stent placement will not prevent restenosis as long as these procedures do not prevent contact between the media layers and circulating blood. When a plaque rupture occurs, patients are carefully monitored with serial color-flow duplex scans at 1, 3, and 6 months. They are kept on a proper antithrombotic therapeutic regimen (low-molecular-weight heparin and aspirin) for at least 1 month. When the control duplex scan shows no evidence of thrombus or progression of restenosis, they are given aspirin therapy alone. In some instances a plaque rupture give the appearance of arterial lamination on the angiogram. It often leads to a residual stricture (see Fig. 4) and thus requires further treatment.

When a circulating dissection is suspected, flushing through the irrigation port of the angioscope should be done with caution because of the risk of extensive dissection. The optic fiber should be passed over a wire crossing the lesion in all control angioscopies after endoluminal procedures to avoid this risk. Circulating dissections are at high risk of abrupt closure or significant residual stenosis. Repeat PTA sometimes leads to immediate recoil because of the persistence of thrombus in the false lumen. Placement of a stent is sometimes necessary.[12] Proper positioning of the stent over the en-

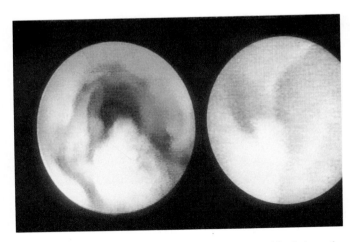

Fig. 4. Control angioscopy after endovascular procedures. *Left,* Residual thrombus after PTA. The underlying cause may be iatrogenic dissection. This type of thrombus carries a risk of distal embolization. *Right,* Plaque fracture causing residual stenosis.

tire length of the dissection is essential. Angioscopy allows better identification of the entry site of the dissection than angiography. However, in the iliac arteries, where angioscopy is not always feasible, intravascular ultrasound imaging (Fig. 6) is quite reliable.

Sometimes control angiography shows a narrowed lumen after the procedure. Angiography alone is not reliable in determining whether the image is related to recoil, thrombus, dissection, or spasm. Angioscopy allows determination of the true cause and the choice of an adequate therapy. We have previously noted that recoil or dissection is amenable to repeated PTA or stent

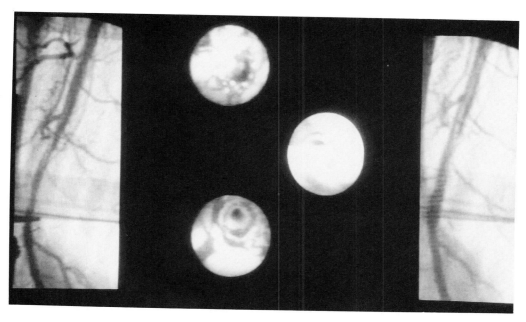

Fig. 5. Control angioscopy after placement of a Palmaz stent.

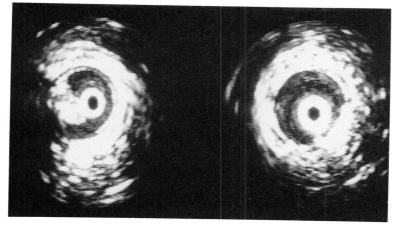

Fig. 6. Intravascular ultrasound imaging after iliac artery PTA. *Left,* Iatrogenic dissection with intraluminal atheroma at 9 o'clock. *Right,* Control after stent placement. Ultrasound is better than angioscopy for evaluation of the arterial wall and assessment of stenoses.

placement. Thrombi can either be left in place or retrieved by thrombosuction. A spasm is a contraindication to repeat PTA because of the risk of worsening the degree or extent of the spasm. Vasodilating drugs are usually very effective within minutes, and a control angiogram will then verify the absence of residual stricture.

THERAPEUTIC ANGIOSCOPY

The following instruments have been used in gastrointestinal or bronchial endoscopy, as well as in urology: biopsy forceps, prehensile forceps, scissors, Dormia baskets, and brushes. They should be evaluated in peripheral arteries as long as miniaturization allows their use through the irrigation port of the scope or alongside the fiber. A sheath avoids open arteriotomy and prevents arterial damage at the site of entry of the instruments. It can be placed percutaneously, but a short cutdown incision under local anesthesia is preferred when the size of the sheath (over 9 Fr) carries a risk of postoperative hematoma. Significant hematomas after percutaneous placement of a sheath can require blood transfusion or surgical closure of the arterial defect and are less cosmetically pleasing than a short incision. Af-

ter endovascular procedures the frequency of hemorrhagic complications is related to the perioperative use of an antithrombotic regimen such as heparin associated with aspirin or in some cases thrombolytic agents.

Among the instruments, biopsy forceps[7] can help retrieve intimal flaps. Care must be taken when removing those flaps, because removal of a small flap can provoke extensive wall damage with a risk of dissection. Because of its optical properties, angioscopy has a tendency to overestimate the size of the abnormalities seen, as shown in 12 cases where results were compared with those of intravascular ultrasonographic imaging. Whenever an arterial wall biopsy is indicated,[13] a directional atherectomy catheter allows a safer procedure than biopsy forceps. Specimens are kept in a small chamber, at the distal portion of the catheter, and their size is usually sufficient for pathological examination. Prehensile forceps (Fig. 7) are very useful for retrieving small adherent thrombi. They are also valuable in iatrogenic situations such as breakage of the distal portion of a guidewire or an atherectomy device. Improper stent placement may sometimes be corrected as long as the stent has not been totally expanded against the wall. Vascular brushes can be useful[14] during graft thrombecto-

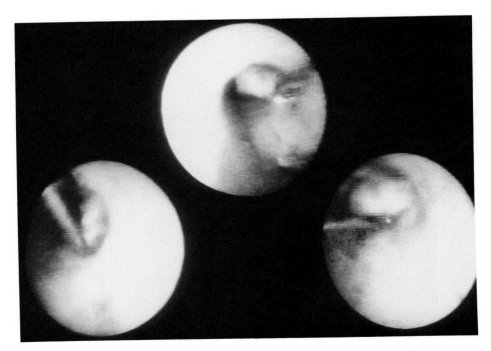

Fig. 7. Angioscopic monitoring of thrombus retrieval with prehensile forceps.

my to retrieve adherent fibrous material; however, we would be reluctant to use such brushes in a native artery.

The Dormia basket catheter is usually too small to retrieve thrombi. The Fogarty adherent clot catheter uses a metallic structure similar to the shape of the Dormia catheter. Its rubber coating allows atraumatic expansion along the wall and appears to be a good alternative when the conventional Fogarty balloon catheter fails to retrieve adherent thrombi. It is also useful in graft thrombectomies with the same efficacy as Vollmar rings. Vollmar rings have been used for years in blind endarterectomies. Vollmar and Storz[15] described iliac endarterectomy through a femoral approach, and in some cases they checked the efficacy of the endarterectomy by means of a rigid scope. Angioscopy is now the safest adjunct to the technique of closed or semiclosed endarterectomy. Retained plaque or thrombus after endarterectomy can cause early occlusion or distal embolization. If necessary, repeated use of Vollmar rings or biopsy forceps can help achieve a neat endarterectomy.

Scissors can be used for valvulotomy during in situ venous bypasses. We pass them alongside the angioscope. Other valvulotomy devices exist. Many surgeons are reluctant to use the Mills valvulotome blindly. This hook-shaped valvulotome (Fig. 8) can easily become trapped in a tributary and create extensive intimal lacerations with a high risk of thrombus formation. Modified Mills valvulotomes, mounted on a flexible metallic wire, have been developed. During valvulotomy we insert the valvulotome through a short venotomy, at the distal portion of the saphenous vein, at the ankle level. We insert the angioscope in the proximal portion of the vein at the groin (Fig. 9). Fluid irrigation helps to identify the valves, inasmuch as the irrigation is delivered retrograde. Angioscopic monitoring of the valvulotomy is then simple, inasmuch as the hook of the valvulotome can cut the entire valve leaflet. The tributaries are identified during the progression of the angioscope by stopping the irrigation, which allows backbleeding. A small incision is made as the light of the scope becomes visible through the skin (Fig. 10). Chin and Fogarty[16] reported on a device (Fig. 11) integrating the valvulotome inside the angioscope; small prongs, emerging from the catheter whenever the scope identified a valve, cut the leaflets.

Thrombosuction can be performed through an 8 Fr catheter under fluoroscopic guidance. Angioscopic

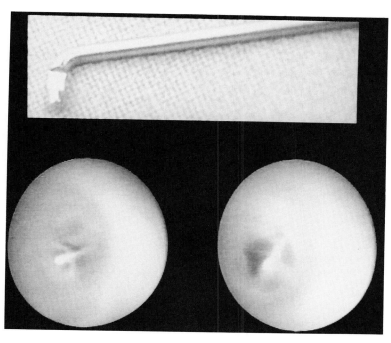

Fig. 8. Angioscopic monitoring of vein valvulotomy by means of a Mills valvulotome.

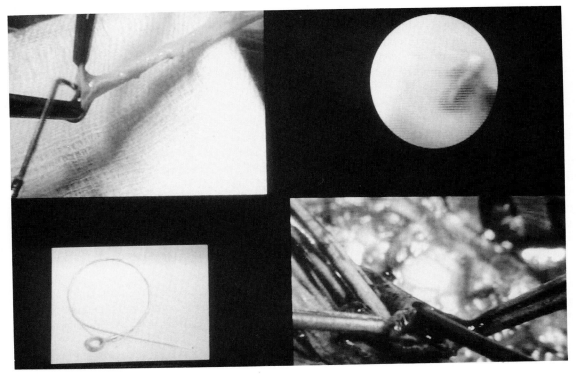

Fig. 9. A simplified technique of vein preparation before in situ bypass to the tibial arteries. Valvulotomy by means of a modified Mills valvulotome.

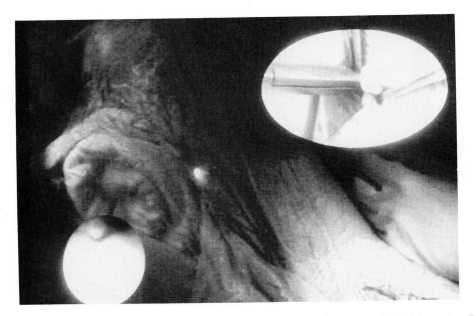

Fig. 10. A simplified technique of vein preparation before in situ bypass to the tibial arteries. Ligation of tributaries after localization under angioscopy.

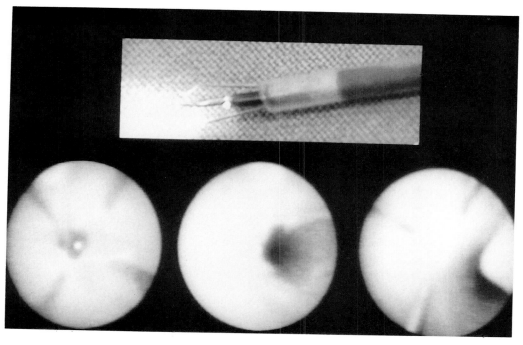

Fig. 11. Valvulotomy by means of the Fogarty-Chin angioscope (Baxter Edwards).

monitoring of this procedure has several advantages. Irrigation is useful since it loosens adherent clots. The risk of distal embolization is small, inasmuch as the thrombus is larger than the artery below. Among eight patients with cardiac arrhythmias undergoing this type of treatment for femoropopliteal and tibial emboli, there was no evidence of distal embolization to the foot arteries on control angiograms. Angioscopy avoids the need for repeat angiography during this procedure and is quite reliable in diagnosing residual thrombus.

CONCLUSION

Angioscopy allows better understanding of a variety of endoluminal lesions seen in atheromatous peripheral disease, as well as in vascular surgery and endovascular procedures. It enhances a certain number of vascular interventions such as thromboembolectomy and femorodistal bypass. In a modern operating room angioscopy does not replace angiography, but these two imaging techniques are complementary. They help the vascular surgeon who performs simpler procedures. They provide patients with a less invasive type of surgery.

The results of endovascular techniques are good in selected lesions, but much research remains to be done in this field. Angioscopy guides the choice of a technique well suited to the lesion. It detects cases in which complementary procedures are needed to obtain optimal short- and long-term results. The indications and results of angioscopic therapy may be less dramatic than those of other surgical specialties, inasmuch as instruments adapted to peripheral vascular disease have yet to be developed. Nevertheless, the angioscope can no longer be considered merely an intriguing bit of technological hardware in the vascular surgeon's armamentarium.

REFERENCES

1. White GH, White RA, Kopchok G, et al. Intraoperative video angioscopy compared with arteriography during peripheral vascular operations. J Vasc Surg 6:488-495, 1987.
2. Grundfest WS, Litvack F, Glick D, et al. Intraoperative decisions based on angioscopy in pheripheral vascular surgery. Circulation 78(Suppl):1-13, 1988.
3. White GH, Kopchok GE, Wilson SE. Angioscopic thromboembolectomy: Preliminary observations with a recent technique. J Vasc Surg 7:318-325, 1988.
4. Chin AK, Mayer DN, Goldman RK, et al. The effect of valvulotomy on the flow rate through the saphenous vein graft: Clinical implications. J Vasc Surg 8:316-320, 1988.
5. Rees MR, Gehani A, Ashley S, et al. Percutaneous angioscopy of peripheral arteries. Lancet 1:695, 1988.

6. Abela GS, Seeger JM, Barbieri E, et al. Laser angioplasty with angioscopic guidance in humans. J Am Coll Cardiol 8:184-192, 1986.

7. White GH, White RA, Kopchok GE, et al. Endoscopic intravascular surgery removes intraluminal flaps, dissections, and thrombus. J Vasc Surg 11:280-288, 1990.

8. Tomaru T, Uchida Y, Sugimoto T. Fiberoptic study on the effects of transluminal angioplasty in experimental occlusive arterial thrombosis. Am Heart J 115:312-317, 1988.

9. Marzelle J, Combe S, Gigou F, et al. Results of thrombolysis in the treatment of arterial ischemia of the limbs according to mode of administration. Int Angiol 8:179-187, 1989.

10. Schwarten DE KB, Simpson JB, Cutcliff WB. Simpson catheter for percutaneous transluminal removal of atheroma. Am J Roentgenol 150:799-801, 1988.

11. Ahn SS, Auth D, Marcus DR, et al. Removal of focal atheromatous lesions by angioscopically guided high-speed rotary atherectomy: Preliminary experimental observations. J Vasc Surg 7:292-300, 1988.

12. Becker GJ, Palmaz JC, Rees CR, et al. Angioplasty-induced dissections in human iliac arteries: Management with Palmaz balloon-expandable intraluminal stents. Radiology 176:31-38, 1990.

13. Garratt KN EW, Kaufmann UP, Vliestra RE, et al. Differential histopathology of primary atherosclerotic and restenotic lesions in coronary arteries and saphenous vein bypass grafts: Analysis of tissue obtained from 73 patients by directional atherectomy. J Am Coll Cardiol 17:422-448, 1991.

14. Crispin HA. Experience with the vascular brush. J Cardiovasc Surg 28:45-49, 1987.

15. Vollmar JF, Storz LW. Vascular endoscopy: Possibilities and limits of its clinical application. Surg Clin North Am 54:111-122, 1974.

16. Chin AK, Fogarty TJ. Specialized techniques of angioscopic valvulotomy for in situ vein bypass. In White GH WR, ed. Angioscopy: Vascular and Coronary Applications. Chicago: Year Book Medical Publishers, 1988, pp 76-83.

XXI

Ethics

140 *The Foundation and Principles of Ethics in Medical Practice and Technological Progress*

Hans-Wilhelm Schreiber, Roger Welter, and Felicien M. Steichen

The health sciences have the mission to prevent disease or to treat—and ideally heal—sick human beings. If this optimal result is beyond the reach of available means, the mission extends to the compassionate treatment of the patient's pain, suffering, and functional and mental restrictions. This concept is governed by criteria of quality and allows value judgments as soon as the patient or legal guardian, of his or her own free will, accepts the recommendations and actions made by the physician. The care of an individual's health, elevated to a human right by modern society, becomes a partnership between the physician and the patient, with well-delineated reciprocal duties and responsibilities that exist only after free consent by both parties involved. This has a corollary legal implication, as defined by the legislature. Patients (and society as a whole) have become increasingly and beneficially aware of the sovereign character of the human being, sick or healthy.

During the nineteenth and twentieth centuries the empirical, clinical art or craft of medicine and surgery has experienced a radical yet essential change, with scientific exploration and basic research into pathological states such as infection, trauma, genetic malfunction, neoplasia, and harm resulting from physical and chemical agents. With these advances medicine and surgery have become a biological science concerned with the anatomical, physiological, and pathological basis of disease.

The humanistic side of the individual—his or her psyche, social condition, environmental well-being, behavior, hopes, and ambitions—forms another important part of what constitutes each complex human being. This anthropological understanding of health and illness creates a new dimension: biology and humanism encompass all human activities and increase the demands and elevate the mission of the healer—an awesome call, made but poorly understood and appreciated by the public and our political leaders.

The doctor-patient relationship or partnership, the use of scientific biological principles in diagnosis and treatment, and the need to include all relevant humanistic considerations leads to the necessity for a code of ethics. In this age of burgeoning technological developments, it is not only appropriate but also essential that we reiterate that an immutable code of ethics is fundamental to the practice of medicine and surgery. This code has to respond to the currently weakening one-on-one doctor-patient relationship, which has been increasingly replaced by anonymous care given by physicians who have been gathered into a practice group primarily because of economic considerations. The code has to govern the conduct and interpretation of experimental and clinical studies, the transfer to clinical practice of new, valid findings, and the use of sometimes helpful (and at other times domineering) technology and techniques.

FOUNDATION AND PRINCIPLES OF ETHICS

Despite their many admirable attributes, humans seemingly have a sense of incompetence regarding themselves and their relationship to their environment. Humans' instinctive behaviors do nothing to assist societies in determining and delineating the roles and responsibilities of the individual to society and of society to the individual. Humans require guidance by a code that assists in the shaping of their lives. Four facts are worthy of consideration in this respect:

1. Within the world that surrounds them, people have created a living space, commonly called civilization or culture.
2. People can change nature and control it in many but not all areas. Natural disasters, accidents, and illness are testimony to our vulnerability.
3. The human is supposedly the only being who is aware of his or her mortality.
4. The human is a social creature who fulfills his existence as a *Homo sapiens* with the help of other humans, not in isolation.

Therefore codes of ethics have been established to define *or* establish the mores and principles for governing increasingly complex societies and to make each individual's life a morally and materially recognizable success. Such a code should ensure these optimal results prospectively and should not serve as a guide for retrospective critiques after an action—good or bad—has been taken. To define and implement its principles, the code of ethics can call on two powerful human resources: *reason*, the most beautiful flower in the garden of virtues (Thomas of Aquinas), and *moral-philosophical conviction*.

Historically the twin concept of ethics and law in medicine existed in 2000 BC in ancient Mesopotamia and was promulgated in Babylonia as the Code of Hammurabi. Socrates (469-399 BC) was said by Aristotle (384-322 BC) to have carried philosophy and the science of life from the heavens into the cities and homes of mankind. He taught the love of truth, justice, and virtue, recognizing that the motivation for these qualities does not exist naturally but has to be reasoned. However, a code of ethics can be for the common good only if it is respected by all and is equally beneficial to all.

The rules of ethics are fundamental to the safe development and growth of life within a society, the natural environment, and a humane civilization. Each human being has a unique dignity to be respected and recognized; his or her life cannot be arbitrarily terminated, shortened, or changed. All of these principles correspond to the content of the Hippocratic oath and have direct consequences:

1. Whoever does not accept the code of ethics lives dangerously for himself or herself and others, has to live in fear of others, and can anticipate only a haphazard destiny.
2. For the sick, the will and right of self-determination are preeminent.
3. A dying person is a patient who possesses human dignity to the highest degree, deserving compassion and mercy, emotional support, and personal comfort in passing from life to death. He or she requires protection from all pressures that would not respect the right to individual dignity.

Without ethical conviction, trust among mankind is impossible. Our conscience is the safe harbor of this conviction. At times the problems encountered by physicians can stress the individual's conscience beyond its resources. This is a time for consultation with theologians, philosophers, lawyers, and members of an ethics commission. The code of ethics is *timeless* and *absolute*; it cannot be adapted to political dictates or economic contingencies or be subject to the vagaries of the philosophical-religious beliefs of each era. Historically, as new needs and values arise, we do not bend the rules of ethics to accommodate changing events; rather, we *modify events* so as to respect the immutable laws of ethics.

ETHICS OF SURGICAL TECHNOLOGY IN DIAGNOSTIC AND THERAPEUTIC METHODS

Advances in technology and ever more sophisticated diagnostic and therapeutic methods create new values and may cause potential conflicts in the decision-making process. However, *new technology and new methods do not require adjustments in the code of ethics*. Bertold Brecht, in his play, had Galileo state: "New science, new ethics"; this is an opinion frequently repeated by colleagues or incompletely informed people, including those who shape opinions and have the power to make decisions. Nothing is more dangerous than to bend the rules of ethics and morality to accommodate the use of dangerous new technology and in its wake, the implementation of unproven surgical methods, regardless of how brilliant, ingenious, and creative the advances may be. Such conduct has always led to moral and philosophical dilemmas and to human disaster.

It is also often stated that the technical aspects create an ethical and practical fence between the physician and the patient. New techniques and the means to implement them should enrich human civilization; medicine and surgery are an integral part of this. Technical advances serve human needs just as much (perhaps surprisingly so in this context) as does the memory of tradition. New methods and instruments are created by humans for the well-being of humans. Such advances have significantly raised the quality of life in mankind's endeavors, including the health sciences, where patient and physician alike have become equally dependent on technical progress.

However, when the charge of excessive use of critical and radical care—based on lifeless technology (symbolized for many by the computer)—is made, the real face of conflict is hidden. The true conflict is the tension that exists:

- Between an anguished patient and a methodical physician
- Between apprehensive individuals and an impersonal hospital
- Between available technology and limited means or actual needs

- Between an information only–oriented media and those concerned with real public education

All of these conflicts have the potential to explode into an ethical crisis unless in each situation the physician understands the often competing forces and masters and coordinates them to serve the patient for the best possible outcome. Medical technology does not of itself function in opposition to ethics. On the contrary, the same reasons that impose rules of ethical behavior on the physician recommend that he or she be interested in technical advances. The danger is not in developing new techniques and instruments but in the injudicious use we may make of them, a use that can be misguided by lack of knowledge, a low sense of responsibility, carelessness, poor intellectual discipline, misplaced pride, or refusal to provide objective and understandable information to the individual and the public.

For the surgeon the solution is professional realism and individual concern: authoritative mastery of the art or craft and science of surgery as they relate to and govern indications, strategies, and techniques of diagnosis and treatment, to heal or give comfort to an individual patient, and to reassure his or her family.

PRACTICAL CONCLUSIONS

In daily practice a surgeon is guided as an individual and as a member of a larger community, usually a clinic or hospital, by a code of ethics. This relationship becomes more sensitive when the personal involvement is elevated to a collective level in consultations, interdisciplinary therapeutic trials, cost-reducing strategies, emergency coverage, lists of available medications and surgical treatment modalities, organizational changes, and a host of problems related to labor policies, hospital governance, and the economy and political will of society. In all of these dilemmas and apparent conflicts, one must ask, "Who is helped and who is hurt?"

If a satisfactory conclusion seems impossible for an individual or extends well beyond the level of responsibility the individual can or should assume, then an ethics committee, created along the principles of the Helsinki declaration of the World Medical Association, should stand ready to debate, advise, and recommend standards of ethical behavior, especially in the areas of transfer from science to practice, clinical research, and extraordinary prolongation of life. Many of these latter problems have been solved by the use of living wills and advance directives and by the participation of the patient's family members, an all-important factor in ethical decision making. The ethics committee can be hospital or university based or be composed of members of a regional medical society. Often all three types, individually or in various compositions, are active and have different areas of competence. While they do make recommendations, they never relieve the individual physician of personal responsibility. They are living testimony to the absolute principle that research on the human will only take place with the most rigid observation of an eternally and immutably valid code of ethics.

Since ethics has become such an integral part of modern medicine and contemporary life, ethics courses should be integrated in medical school curricula and offered regularly in continued medical education symposia with the participation of physicians, theologians, philosophers, social workers, lay representatives or ombudsmen, and perhaps even politicians and lawyers.

In its modern practical application, the code of ethics governs the physician-patient relationship as well as their place within an overall health care system. The patient and his or her family, better informed than ever, are offered a wide choice of means to care for their health. They have a real personal and collective responsibility to make wise decisions that respect their individual right to health as well as that of society. They should demonstrate personal discipline in accepting established and recognized preventive measures for themselves as well as in their daily contacts with others, and they should never, as individuals or as a group, knowingly contaminate or harm the natural and animal environment of the world.

Just as society at large, doctors, nurses, and other health care personnel have an obligation to protect the individual, each individual human being has a sacred obligation to use advantages provided by health care plans honestly and to follow prescriptions and recommendations by doctors and nurses unless there is a good—and clearly stated—reason to question such prescriptions.

In the final analysis, the code of ethics is guided by the simple yet difficult biblical commandment, "Love thy neighbor as thyself," and the Apostle Paul's recommendation to "examine everything and keep what is good" (1 Thess. 5:21).

Index